extra-helical terminal peptide

b_1 a_4 a_3

Collagen in Health and Disease

Collagen in Health and Disease

EDITED BY

Jacqueline B. Weiss
MSc, DSc, DCC
Reader in Medical Biochemistry to the Departments of Rheumatology and Medical Biochemistry, University of Manchester.

Malcolm I. V. Jayson
MD, FRCP
Professor of Rheumatology, Rheumatic Diseases Centre, University of Manchester.

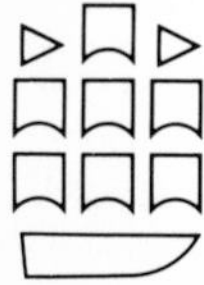

CHURCHILL LIVINGSTONE
EDINBURGH LONDON MELBOURNE AND NEW YORK 1982

CHURCHILL LIVINGSTONE
Medical Division of Longman Group Limited

Distributed in the United States of America by Churchill Livingstone Inc., 1560 Broadway, New York, N.Y. 10036, and by associated companies, branches and representatives throughout the world.

First published 1982

ISBN 0 443 02142 2

British Library Cataloguing in Publication Data
Collagen in health and disease.
1. Genetics 2. Collagen
I. Weiss, Jacqueline B.
II. Jayson, Malcolm I.V.
591.1'852 QH430

Library of Congress Cataloging in Publication Data
Main entry under title:
Collagen in health and disease.
Includes index.
1. Collagen diseases. 2. Collagen.
I. Weiss, Jacqueline B. II. Jayson, Malcolm I. V.
[DNLM: 1. Collagen — Metabolism. 2. Collagen diseases. WD 375 C697]
RC924.C53 1983 616.7'7 82-9628

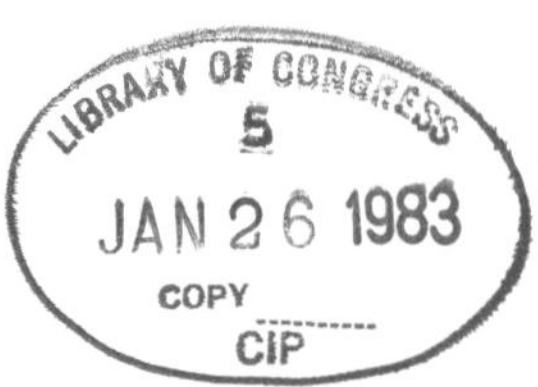

Printed in Singapore by Kyodo Shing Loong Printing Industries Pte Ltd

Preface

Collagen is the most abundant protein in the animal world. It is part of the structural connective tissue in every organ in the body. However, interest in collagen, in the world outside the specialist workers in the field, has been cautious. Only very recently has collagen been given adequate coverage in textbooks of biochemistry and physiology and in many of the cases where coverage has been given it is regrettable that it has been given incorrectly. The purpose of this book is to present collagen *toute entière* as it were, to medical and scientific workers in a form which brings into focus current knowledge of the many aspects of collagen biochemistry. It is hoped to relate this knowledge to specific tissues and systems in the body where abnormalities of collagen metabolism occur.

In the last decade it has been realised that there are a variety of genetically distinct collagen types and that different organs and systems either have tissue specific collagen within them or contain the same collagens as are present in other tissues but in unique ratios. The specific arrangements of the various collagens in individual tissues has lead to research in alterations of matrix in diseased tissues which may arise through suppression of one collagen phenotype and expression of another in the same cell. This facet of collagen research has also been valuable to developmental biologists. Much more exact information has recently become available as to the physiological mechanisms of the degradation of collagen, and the type of cells which are involved in this process. Again, such knowledge has been rapidly applied to disease states. In the biosynthesis of collagen, a variety of enzymes have been isolated and studied which are involved in the numerous post-translational modifications of collagen and this has led quite rapidly to a new appreciation of the many possibilities for inherited defects in the synthesis of this protein. Again, new information has become available as to the mechanism of binding of collagen to the cell associated proteins such as fibronectin. It is interesting that some proteins have been found to contain collagenous sequences within them although they do not function themselves as collagens and it is quite possible that as more knowledge of structure of proteins becomes available more proteins of this type will be discovered. Understanding of the biomechanical properties of collagen, which probably contribute to its adoption as the universal structural protein in vertebrates and invertebrates, has resulted from the increased precision of X-ray diffraction methodology. More information as to the sequences of amino acids in the various types of collagen from different animal species becomes available at fairly regular intervals either from peptide, mRNA or gene sequencing. For this reason the lay out of the appendix, which gives all the sequences known at the time of publication, has been designed so that new sequences can be filled in by the reader as and when they are published.

We hope this book will be of value as a reference work for people involved in the medical sciences as well as for connective tissue biochemists, cell biologists and biophysicists.

We would like to express our gratitude to Sarah Godfrey for her invaluable secretarial assistance in the preparation of this book.

Manchester, 1982

J.B.W.
M.I.V.J.

Contributors

Eileen Adamson PhD
La Jolla Cancer Research Foundation
La Jolla
California
USA

Shirley Ayad PhD
Research Fellow
Department of Rheumatology
Medical School
University of Manchester
Manchester
UK

Michael Barnes PhD
Stangeways Research Laboratory
Cambridge
UK

Eugene Bauer MD
Associate Professor of Medicine
Division of Dermatology (EAB, AZE)
Washington University School of Medicine
St Louis
Missouri
USA

Henning Birkedhal-Hansen DDS PhD
Associate Professor of Dentistry
School of Dentistry
Department of Oral Biology
University of Alabama in Birmingham
Birmingham
Alabama
USA

Robert A. Brown PhD
Blood Products Laboratory
National Blood Transfusion Service
Elstree
Borehamwood
Herts
UK

Robert Burgeson PhD
Assistant Professor of Pediatrics
Department of Pediatrics
UCLA Medical Center
Los Angeles County Harbor
Torrance
California
USA

Kathryn S. E. Cheah PhD
Research Fellow
Imperial Cancer Research Fund
Lincoln's Inn Fields
London
UK

Milos Chvapil MD PhD
Professor and Head of Section of
Surgical Biology
Department of Surgery
University of Arizona
College of Medicine
Tucson
Arizona
USA

Ronald Crystal MD
Chief
Section of Pulmonary Biochemistry
National Heart and Lung Institute
Bethesda
Maryland
USA

Peter F. Davison PhD
Director
Department of Fine Structure
Boston Biomedical Research Institute
Boston
Massachusetts
USA

Ian L. Freeman PhD
Assistant Professor of Ophthalmology
Pittsberg
Pennsylvania
USA

Diane Galloway MA
54 Windmill Drive
Croxley Green
Hertfordshire
UK

Steffen Gay MD
Associate Professor of Medicine
Thomas Kresina Institute of Dental Research
Department of Medicine
University of Alabama in Birmingham
Birmingham
Alabama
USA

Michael E. Grant PhD
Professor of Medical Biochemistry
Department of Medical Biochemistry
University of Manchester
Manchester
UK

Godfrey Heathcote PhD
Development Biology Laboratory
Harvard University Medical School
Massachusetts General Hospital
Boston
Massachusetts
USA

David W. L. Hukins PhD
Senior Lecturer in Medical Biophysics
Department of Medical Biophysics
Medical School
University of Manchester
Manchester
UK

David Jackson PhD
Professor of Medical Biochemistry
Department of Medical Biochemistry
Medical School
University of Manchester
Manchester
UK

Malcolm I. V. Jayson MD
Professor of Rheumatology
Department of Rheumatology
Rheumatic Diseases Centre
University of Manchester
Salford
UK

Nicholas A. Kefalides MD PhD
Professor
Department of Medicine and Biochemistry
University of Pennsylvania
University City Science Centre
Philadelphia
USA

Karik Kivirikko MD PhD
Professor of Medical Biochemistry
Department of Biochemistry
University of Oulu
Oulu
Finland

Hynda K. Kleinman PhD
Department of Health Education and Welfare
Public Health Services
National Institute of Health
Bethesda
Maryland
USA

Thomas F. Linsenmayer PhD
Associate Professor
Developmental Biology Laboratory
Harvard University Medical School
Massachusetts General Hospital
Boston
Massachusetts
USA

John O'D. McGee PhD MD
Professor of Morbid Anatomy
Department of Pathology
University of Oxford
John Radcliffe Hospital
Headington
Oxford
UK

Richard Mayne PhD
Assistant Professor of Anatomy and Biochemistry
Institute of Dental Research
Department of Anatomy
University of Alabama in Birmingham
Birmingham
Alabama
USA

Raili Myllylä PhD
Docent in Medical Biochemistry
Department of Biochemistry
University of Oulu
Oulu
Finland

Ruy Pérez-Tamayo MD
Head of Department of Pathology
Instituto de la Nutricion
Hospital de Enfer Medades de la Nutricion
Av San Fernando you Viaducto Italpan
Mexico

Kenneth B. M. Reid PhD
MRC Immunochemistry Unit
Department of Biochemistry
University of Oxford
Oxford
UK

Stephen I. Rennard MD
Senior Staff Fellow
Section of Pulmonary Biochemistry
National Heart and Lung Institute
Bethesda
Maryland
USA

R. Kent Rhodes PhD
Institute of Dental Research
Department of Biochemistry
University of Alabama in Birmingham
Birmingham
Alabama
USA

Simon P. Robins PhD
Rowett Research Institute
Bucksburn
Aberdeen
UK

Seizaburo Sakamoto DDS PhD
Principal Research Assistant in Oral Biology
Harvard School of Dental Medicine
Boston
Massachusetts
USA

Jouni Uitto MD PhD
Associate Professor of Medicine
Department of Medicine
University of California at Los Angeles
UCLA School of Medicine
Torrance
California
USA

Jacqueline B. Weiss DSc
Reader in Medical Biochemistry
Departments of Rheumatology & Medical Biochemistry
Rheumatic Diseases Centre
University of Manchester
Salford
UK

Zena Werb PhD
Associate Professor
Laboratory of Radiobiology
University of California
San Francisco
California
USA

Charlotte Wilkes PhD
Department of Health Education and Welfare
Public Health Services
National Institute of Health
Bethesda
Maryland
USA

John Woodhead-Galloway PhD
The Medical Research Council
Park Crescent
London
UK

J. Fred Woessner PhD
Professor of Biochemistry and Medicine
Department of Biochemistry
University of Miami
School of Medicine
Miami
Florida
USA

Contents

1

An introduction to collagen

J. B. WEISS and S. AYAD

INTRODUCTION

How does one introduce collagen? It is possible to say that the Greeks had a word for it and in a sense they did. The word collagen derives from the Greek, Kolla meaning glue and the term 'glue former' or 'collagen' was originally used in the 19th Century for the component in skin and bone, cartilage and tendon, which when the tissues were boiled in water and the extracts evaporated produced glue. The Romans too knew all about collagen as a source of glue, for in AD 50 Pliny wrote, 'Glue is cooked from the hides of bulls' (Bogue, 1922). Modern day photographic dry mounting paper still makes use of gelatin as a glue source, though synthetic polymers have mainly replaced it for other uses.

Collagen is a protein present throughout the animal kingdom. Most of the body scaffolding in mammals is composed of collagen and in this sense it can be thought of as analogous to chitin in orthoptera and to cellulose in plants. However, collagen should not be considered in isolation since it is only one of the constituents of connective tissue and the function of the different connective tissues depends on the number, nature and microanatomical arrangements of the constituent macromolecules collagen, proteoglycan and noncollagenous glycoproteins. Cogently involved in this interaction are a number of small molecules in particular water.

Collagen itself is a glycoprotein, somewhat unique in this classification since it contains no amino sugars and in fact has only two types of carbohydrate residues — glucose and galactose — in its structure. Until fairly recently it was supposed that collagen was a single protein type but in the last decade it has become clear that it is polymorphic and that there are four major genetically distinct forms of the protein and at least 4 other minor genetic variants Type V, 1α 2α 3α, CPS, 7-S etc., and this latter number is likely to increase. It is a common cliché to talk of collagen as a fibrillar protein but this is not true of basement membrane collagen which does not form fibrils in vitro and which does not exist in a fibrillar form in the body. However, it is certainly true that the fibrillar nature of the other major collagen types makes them uniquely suitable for their structural roles. True for all collagens — basement membrane and interstitial alike — is the helical structure of the molecule itself in which each of its three constituent α chains coils in a left handed minor helix each minor helix then coiling with two others to form a right handed super helix.

Perhaps because of its primary structural function in the body, collagen is peculiarly resistant to attack by neutral proteinases and other enzymes. Only one mammalian enzyme is known which is capable of cleaving the helical body of the major interstitial collagen molecules and this enzyme, collagenase, cleaves solely at one site along the whole length of the molecule. On the other hand a bacterial enzyme, bacterial collagenase, *is* able to degrade native collagen into small fragments, although it has virtually no action at all on other proteins. This incidentally provides a useful test in establishing the possibly collagenous nature of an isolated protein since if it is bacterial collagenase sensitive it is almost certainly collagen — though there may be exceptions in the case of collagens which are highly disulphide bonded (Risteli et al, 1980; Furuto & Miller, 1981).

The nomenclature of collagen is complex and it has therefore seemed worthwhile to include a glossary of terms, both in date and out, which may help the reader who is unfamiliar with the field.

GLOSSARY OF COLLAGEN TERMS

Acid soluble collagen. Collagen extracted from tissues by dilute acid. It is released from the insoluble polymer by rupture of acid-labile bonds. This collagen contains inter-molecular cross-links.

Alpha chains. The constituent chains of the collagen molecules.

Amianthoid. Very large diameter collagen fibrils seen in ageing hyaline cartilage.

Collagenase. There are two distinct classes of collagenases — those of vertebrate origin and bacterial enzymes. Vertebrate collagenases are endopeptidases and make a single cleavage at a point approximately three quarters of the length of the molecule from the amino terminal end, thus dividing the molecule into two fragments. Bacterial collagenases, on the other hand, attack the collagen molecule from both ends cleaving at multiple foci and reducing the molecule to small fragments. 'Classical' mammalian collagenase of the type found in skin and synovia cannot degrade types IV and V collagen which presumably lack the specific cleavage sequence. However, enzymes capable of degrading type IV collagen have been found in tumours. (See Ch. 7).

Collagentsia. A term applied to those persons interested in or involved with collagen research (Professor J. Ball personal communication).

Crimp. The waveforms seen in certain fibres. (For its relevance to collagen, particularly tendon collagen see Ch. 4).

Cross-links. Cross-links occur between individual collagen molecules. The ϵ-amino groups of specific lysine, hydroxylysine or glycosylated hydroxylysine residues in the non-helical extension peptides are initially oxidised to an aldehyde form by the action of the extracellular enzyme lysyl oxidase. These aldehyde groups can subsequently react with the ϵ-amino group of a lysine or hydroxylysine residue in the helix of an adjacent molecule to form intermolecular crosslinks. Some of these crosslinks have been well characterised (see Ch. 9). However other crosslinks (for example between the helices of adjacent molecules) are possible, particularly in mature tissues, but these have not been isolated. Chains of type III and type IV collagen are also crosslinked by disulphide bonds.

Cyanogen bromide peptides. Each collagen α chain contains relatively few methionine residues. Cyanogen bromide selectively cleaves the peptide bond immediately following a methionine residue to yield homoserine at the carboxy terminal end. The peptides produced have lengths equal to the distances between the methionine residues. The number and size of these peptides are characteristic for each α-chain and act as a 'fingerprint' for the collagen type.

Dentine. The collagen of teeth.

Elastoidin. A collagen which forms the fin rays of the elasmobranchs. This collagen consists of three identical α-chains.

FLS-fibrous long spacing collagen. An artificial fibrillar precipitate of collagen molecules with a periodicity greater than 67nm and in which all the molecules are not pointing in the same direction. There are several forms of FLS all having different periodicities. It is worth pointing out that abnormal fibrillar structures, generally with perodicity greater than 67nm, seen in situ in diseased tissue are frequently referred to as FLS, though there is no evidence that this is collagen. It is equally probable that these structures are fibrin or some other fibrillar protein.

Gelatin. The denatured or random coil form of collagen. Treatment of soluble collagen by exposure to a temperature of 40°C for a few minutes will convert it to gelatin.

Lathyrogen. A substance which when administered systemically to animals inhibits the formation of cross-links in collagen. β-aminopropionitrile is the usual lathyrogen and has been used in order to obtain easily extracted soluble collagen. Lathyrogens inhibit the enzyme lysyl oxidase which is essential for the formation of crosslinks.

Microfibril. The smallest fibrillar collagen structure formed which can be visualised in the electron microscope. Models for the microfibril include a tetramer model and a pentafibril model.

Native collagen. Natural, non-denatured collagen molecules.

Neutral salt soluble collagen. Collagen extracted from tissues by neutral sodium chloride solutions (0.1 to 1M). This collagen represents the most newly synthesised form and contains very few intermolecular cross-links.

Nonhelical terminal peptides. Short nonhelical regions at each end of the tropocollagen molecules. These are an integral part of the molecule and should not be confused with the extension peptides in the procollagen molecule.

Osteoid. The collagen of bone.

Pepsin extracted collagen. Collagen extracted from pepsin digested tissue. This collagen lacks all or part of the nonhelical terminal peptides.

Polymeric collagen. Insoluble collagen which has been extracted from the tissue after breaking the calcium mediated electrostatic linkages between the collagen fibres and the interfibrillar proteoglycan matrix. The collagen is extracted intact into acetic acid where it exists as a polymer suspension. Collagen fibrils can be 'spooled out' if the suspension is neutralised. The collagen molecules retain their nonhelical terminal peptides.

Preprocollagen. Precursor form of procollagen containing an additional hydrophobic amino terminal sequence which probably binds to the rough endoplasmic reticulum. The preprotein sequence is removed intracellularly.

Procollagen. The secreted precursor form of collagen which has bulky extension peptides at either end of a tropocollagen molecule. Procollagen is 'processed' in the extracellular matrix by specific proteases which remove the extensions.

P_N collagen. Procollagen from which the carboxy terminal extension peptide has been removed but in which the amino terminal peptide remains.

P_C collagen. Procollagen from which the amino terminal peptide has been cleaved but in which the carboxy terminal peptide remains intact.

Procollagen peptidases. Two endopeptidases amino and carboxy peptidases which exist in the extracellular matrix and which convert procollagen to tropocollagen.

Propeptides. The extension peptides at each end of the procollagen molecule.

Protocollagen. Newly synthesised collagen in which the proline residues have not yet been hydroxylated and which therefore cannot be secreted from the cell.

Reconstituted collagen. Under the correct conditions of temperature, pH and ionic strength, collagen forms 'gels' in which the collagen fibrils appear identical to native fibrils in the electron microscope.

Reticulin. Thin, fine branched, argyrophilic fibres observed in developing tissues. It has been suggested that reticulin is type III collagen.

SLS-segment long spacing collagen. An artificial precipitate of collagen in which the molecules are assembled into a crystallite in such a manner that like features of each molecule are in accurate transverse register. Positive staining of these crystallites enables the collagen molecule to be visualised in a laterally extended form in the electron microscope.

Symmetric fibrils. Fibrils in which some of the molecules are pointing in opposite directions. Such fibrils have been shown to arise, in vitro, from molecules which have been assembled after the amino terminal nonhelical peptide has been specifically removed by aminopeptidases. They are also seen in preparations of reconstituted fibrils from pepsin treated collagen.

Tactoids. Cigar shaped collagen aggregates formed, in vitro, from collagen molecules from which the carboxy terminal peptide has been specifically cleaved by carboxypeptidases. Such aggregates can be polarised or symmetric or a mixture of both in the same tactoid. If the carboxy terminal residues only are removed and the nonhelical amino terminal peptides are intact they will be polarised. If both nonhelical terminal peptides are removed they will be a mixture. Tactoids can also occur as a result of interaction of intact collagen molecules with proteoglycans.

Telopeptides. (Greek — telos = end). A rather old fashioned though not necessarily obsolete term for the nonhelical terminal peptides.

Tropocollagen. (Greek — tropos = form). The intact triple helical collagen molecule. It contains the short nonhelical terminal peptide regions at each end which are an integral part of the collagen molecule. Unfortunately it is also used loosely to refer to pepsin solubilised collagen molecules from which these extrahelical regions have been lost.

HISTORICAL BACKGROUND

Early work on the chemistry of collagen was mainly confined to the glue and gelatin industries and to the leather tanning trade (Eastoe, 1967). As collagen was then solubilised by boiling, only gelatin, which is the denatured form of the protein, was known. It was accepted that connective tissues, in particular tendon, swelled when immersed in acid solution (Zaccharides, 1900) but Nageotte (1927) was the first to isolate a native soluble collagen by extracting rat tail tendon with cold dilute acetic acid. In a sense it could be said that Nageotte was fortunate in his choice of animal since immature rat tail tendon is peculiarly soluble in acetic acid, whereas bovine and human tendon are much more resistant to solubilisation. Nageotte was able to demonstrate that the solubilised collagen, when dialysed against tap water or neutral salt solutions precipitated as fibres apparently indistinguishable from those seen in the original tendon by light microscopy. This reconstituted collagen was the first evidence of the inherent ability of the collagen molecule to assemble into fibrils in vitro. At the start of the 1940's several workers using electron microscopy observed that collagen fibrils displayed a constant periodicity of approximately 67nm (Schmitt et al, 1942). This periodicity had also been inferred from early X-ray diffraction studies. (Wyckoff & Corey, 1936; Bear, 1942).

Studies on the solubilisation of collagen showed that it could be solubilised to some extent by neutral salt solutions as well as by citric acid or acetic acid extraction. These solubilised collagens represented only a fraction of the total collagen and the amount which could be extracted varied with the age of the animal and with the type of tissue extracted. The amount of neutral salt soluble material was always smaller than that obtained from acid extraction. Jackson (1957) in studies on carrageenin induced granulomas showed that the neutral salt soluble fraction had a turnover rate higher than that for the acid extracted collagens. This work was later extended by Jackson & Bentley (1960) who proposed that the neutral salt soluble collagen represented the most newly synthesised form of the protein. Previously it had been shown that neutral salt extraction of collagen fibres did not in any way alter their structural organisation whereas extraction with acetic acid led to swelligg and disruption (Gross, Highberger & Schmitt, 1954). Thus it seemed reasonable to suppose, as Jackson and Bentley did, that the salt soluble collagen had not yet become incorporated into the fibril. Elegant physicochemical studies carried out at approximately the same time deduced that the native collagens in solution were all composed of molecules containing three α-chains arranged in a triple helical configuration and behaving in solution as rigid rods (Boedtker & Doty, 1956). Sedimentation velocity studies from other laboratories on denatured collagen (gelatin) showed that there were at least three disparate fragments in the solution with molecular weights approximately 100 000, 200 000 and 300 000. These fragments were termed α, β and γ components respectively (Mathews et al, 1954; Orekhovich & Shpikiter, 1955, 1958; Altgelt et al, 1961; Grassman et al, 1961; Veis et al, 1962). Chromatographic analysis of gelatin on ion exchange resins confirmed the presence of α chains (100 000 MW) and β components which consisted of either two identical α chains cross-linked together (β_{11}) or two dissimilar α chains also as cross-linked dimers ($\beta_{1,2}$). The concept of a trimer of two similar and one dissimilar α chains being the fundamental collagen molecule was thus established.

Early amino acid analysis of collagen showed that it contained glycine in very high proportions, approximately one third of all residues being glycine. This led, naturally, to the idea that every third residue in the molecule would be glycine. Very little tyrosine was detected and initially it was thought that no cystine or half cystine residues were present, though this latter point is now known to be true for only some of the collagens present in the animal kingdom (see Appendix). Two rather unusual amino acids, hydroxyproline and hydroxylysine were shown to account for a considerable percentage of all the amino acids in the molecules, 10 to 12 per cent and 0.3 to 0.5 per cent respectively (Eastoe, 1967).

Earlier work on an artificial precipitate of native collagen — segment long spacing collagen (SLS) — had given evidence for the concept that collagen existed in solution as a monomer (tropocollagen). SLS is a highly ordered crystallite of collagen (see glossary) which can be precipitated from an acidic collagen solution either with ATP or with triphosphoric acid. These artificial assemblies of collagen molecules in which like features are in accurate transverse register enable the charge profile along the length of the molecule to be determined in the electron microscope (Hodge & Schmitt, 1960). Direct optical synthesis of the collagen fibrillar band pattern with that of SLS gave rise to the concept that molecules were 'staggered' in relation to one another within the length of the molecule. (Hodge & Schmitt, 1960; Hodge & Petrushka, 1963). Subsequently the 'stagger' or periodicity of the collagen fibril was established as being the length of 234 residues and this period is now referred to as D. (See Ch. 3.)

In 1956 Boedtker and Doty had suggested that collagen molecules had 'dangling chain peptide appendages' at one or both ends which were not in a triple helical conformation. Treatment with proteolytic enzymes caused the viscosity of collagen solutions to decrease and this led Hodge and his colleagues (Hodge et al, 1960; Hodge & Schmitt, 1960) to propose that a depolymerisation of the fibrils had occurred. They suggested that this was a limited attack, confined to nonhelical regions of the molecule and that the main body of the molecule remained intact. Rubin

(Rubin et al, 1963) observed that pepsin treatment of a collagen solution led to almost total loss of the β components. They proposed that at each end of the collagen molecule there were nonhelical terminal regions (telopeptides — see glossary) which contained intramolecular interchain bonds and that these regions were destroyed by pepsin.

So much then for the soluble forms of collagen. By far the largest bulk of the collagen fibre had resisted solubilisation and had not been studied. However, several workers now showed that treatment of the residual collagen, after neutral salt and acid extraction, with proteolytic enzymes such as pepsin or pronase enabled considerably more solubilisation to take place (Kühn et al, 1966; Drake et al, 1966; Steven, 1966).

At a time when it seemed that knowledge of collagen chemistry was nearing completion came the surprising observation that cartilage collagen was different from the collagen previously known and was therefore probably a genetically different type (type II), (Miller & Matukas, 1969). Collagen cannot be solubilised from cartilage by neutral salt or dilute acid extraction but Miller and Matukas had used young lathyritic chicks; chicks treated with lathyrogen, β-aminopropionitrile, which inhibits biological cross-linking (Tanzer, 1965) as their tissue source. A substantial portion of the collagen from these young chicks could be solubilised in neutral salt solutions. This soluble collagen did not appear to contain the expected ratio of two $\alpha 1$ chains to one $\alpha 2$ chain. On the contrary the proportion of the $\alpha 1$ chain appeared to be considerably higher. Furthermore, examination of the cyanogen bromide peptides (see glossary) from the $\alpha 1$ chains of cartilage collagen showed them to contain peptides which were not present in the previously characterised $\alpha 1$ chain and $\alpha 2$ chains. Thus the concept of genetically distinct collagens was born. Cartilage collagen was therefore described as type II collagen and the previously characterised collagen as type I. Type II collagen contained approximately three times the content of hydroxylysine than type I collagen and was comparatively highly glycosylated. In addition it appeared to consist of three identical α chains (Trelstad et al, 1970; Miller, 1971). The behaviour of these new chains on carboxymethyl cellulose chromatography was similar to that of the $\alpha 1$ chains and this led to the classification of the new α chains as $\alpha 1$(II). (Miller, 1976a).

In 1971 Miller and his colleagues reported that repeated pepsin extraction of skin collagen had revealed yet another polymorph —type III collagen. This collagen was again a triplet containing three $\alpha 1$ type chains but their amino acid content and cyanogen bromide peptide pattern were different from those in either type I or type II collagen. A particularly striking difference was the presence of cysteine residues. Today there are no less than 6 genetically distinct collagens and more are expected.

In the late 60's and in the 70's research has concentrated upon discovering the nature, number and position of the cross-links of collagen (Tanzer, 1976). Also biosynthetic studies have revealed a precursor form of collagen, procollagen (Prockop et al, 1976) in which extension peptides are present at each end of the molecule giving rise to a much more soluble form of the protein. A function of procollagen is to act as a soluble 'transport' form of the molecule and to ensure that fibril formation does not occur prematurely during biosynthesis. Specific extracellular peptidases remove the extensions when required.

Collagen is particularly noteworthy in that it requires considerable post-translational modification both at the intracellular and extracellular levels and studies of the enzymes involved in these various modifications represent some of the more important recent aspects of collagen research (Kivirikko & Myllylä, 1979; Siegel, 1979).

PRIMARY STRUCTURE OF COLLAGEN

Determination of the primary sequences of the many collagen types has been a tedious and lengthy process. Collagen is such a large molecule and the presence of glycine as every third residue has not helped. Approximately 10 per cent of other residues in collagen are proline and a further 10 to 12 per cent hydroxyproline. If the repeating sequence of glycine is written as a triplet $(X–Y–Gly)_{333}$ then it is interesting that with very few exceptions proline is always present in the X position and hydroxyproline in the Y position. These cyclic imino acids limit the rotation of the peptide backbone of the molecule and determine the left handed helix structure for the separate α chains. In addition the hydroxyproline residues stabilise the structure of the triple helix itself as well as contributing a stabilising hydrogen bond cross-link between neighbouring triple helical chains (Bansal et al, 1975; Ramachandran et al, 1975; Ramachandran & Ramakrishnan, 1976). The remaining residues in the primary sequence of collagen tend to cluster in groups of charged and hydrophobic residues and these influence the assembly of the molecule into its quaternary fibrillar structure. The amino acid sequences of the type I collagen α chains represented in the form of a positively stained fibril, as seen in the electron microscope where charged residues would pick up the electron dense stains, are shown in the diagram on the end papers. (Chapman et al, 1981).

Mathews (1980) has pointed out that the triple helical regions of collagen α chains are generally conserved in evolution. Charged residues are strongly conserved throughout the entire range of animal species and this is reflected in the banding patterns of positively stained SLS crystallites as seen in the electron microscope. It can be seen (Fig. 1.1) that the similarities of SLS crystallites from collagens of a variety of vertebrates and invertebrates is far

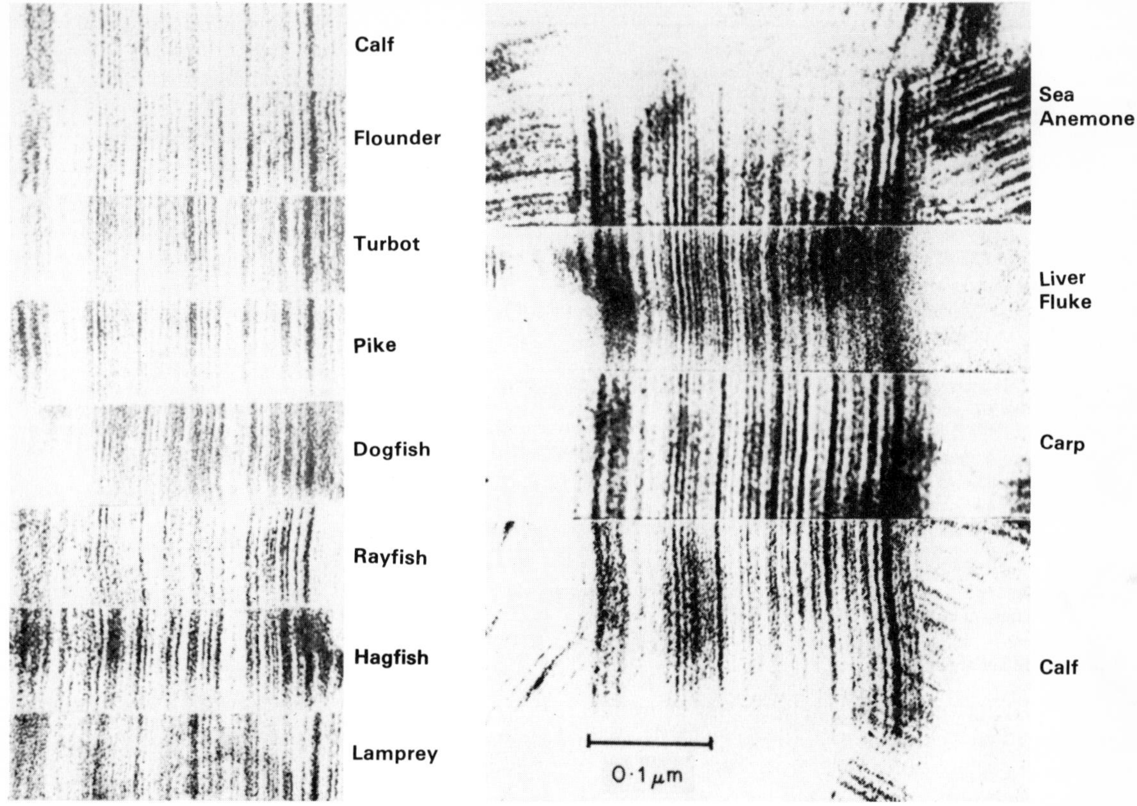

Fig. 1.1 Comparison of segment long spacing crystallites of collagen showing general similarity of distribution of charged and apolar groups along the alpha chains of the collagen molecule from both vertebrates and invertebrates (Mathews, 1980).

greater than the differences which are, in most cases, not immediately apparent (Mathews, 1975).

Glycosylation of collagen is through the hydroxylysine residues some of which exist as the single sugar glycoside — galactosylhydroxylysine and some as the disaccharide glycoside — glucosylgalactosylhydroxylysine. The extent of glycosylation of the hydroxylysine residues varies with the different collagen types.

COLLAGEN TYPES

At least six genetically distinct collagen types co-exist in the body. These collagens exist either singly or together in different proportions in the various connective tissues. Individual fibroblasts, in culture, have been shown to be capable of synthesising two different collagen types (Church et al, 1973). Fibroblasts from adult skin and human fetal lung synthesise types I and III collagens in the same proportion as found in the tissue (Penttinen et al, 1975; Hance et al, 1976; Lichtenstein, et al, 1975). It has been pointed out that the ability of fibroblasts to synthesise these different types of collagen in rigidly controlled proportions over many passages indicates that the coding genes are simultaneously controlled (Penttinen et al, 1980).

The tissue sources of the known collagen types are given in Table 1.1.

Interstitial collagens

Early work on collagen was performed on neutral salt soluble and acid soluble collagens derived from tissues which were either wholly made up of type I collagen (tendon) or in which type I collagen was the predominant *soluble* species. Collagen was thus originally thought to be a single genetic species.

However, characterisation of the peptides obtained after cyanogen bromide digestion of collagen (see glossary) from chick cartilage (Miller & Matukas, 1969) and subsequently from human cartilage and skin (Miller et al, 1971) revealed the presence of additional α-chains: α1(II) in cartilage and α1(III) in skin. Cartilage collagen is therefore called type II and consists of 3 identical α1(II) chains: $(\alpha1(II))_3$ and skin contains (in addition to type I) a collagen consisting of 3 identical α1(III) chains — type III or $(\alpha1(III))_3$.

Fractionation by precipitation at different salt concentrations enabled the various collagen types, solubilised from the same tissue, to be identified (Chung &

Table 1.1 Distribution and molecular configuration of collagen types

Collagen type	*Molecular configuration*	*Tissue or organ source**
Interstitial		
I	$(\alpha 1(I))_2\alpha 2(I)$	Skin, bone, tendon, cornea, annulus fibrosus, placental tissue, lung, liver, muscle
I trimer	$(\alpha 1(I))_3$	Skin, tumour, tendon, liver
II	$(\alpha 1(II))_3$	Cartilage, annulus fibrosus, nucleus pulposus, vitreous body
III	$(\alpha 1(III))_3$	Fetal skin, aorta, uterus, placental tissues, synovia, heart, liver, lung, nerve
V	$(\alpha 1(V))_2\alpha 2(V)$	Placental tissues, skin, bone, tendon, synovia, cornea, aorta, nerve, lung, liver, muscle
	$(\alpha 1(V)\alpha 2(V)\alpha 3(V))$	Placental villi and uterus
Basement membrane		
IV	$\alpha 1(IV)$ and $\alpha 2(IV)$	Lens capsule, glomerulus, placenta, tumour, aorta
	or possibly $(\alpha 1(IV))_3$	Descemet's membrane
Other collagens		
1α, 2α, 3α	unknown	Cartilage, annulus fibrosus, nucleus pulposus
High molecular weight aggregate	unknown	Placental tissues, skin, liver, uterus
7-S	unknown	Lens capsule, tumour, placenta
CPS-1	$(33K)_3$-part of larger molecule?	Cartilage, annulus fibrosus, nucleus pulposus, vitreous

*References for tissue or organ source include: Interstitial collagens — Burgeson et al (1976); Brown et al (1978); Epstein and Munderloh (1975); Eyre and Muir (1977); Freeman (1978); Bornstein and Sage (1980); Uitto (1979).
Basement membrane collagen — Heathcote et al (1978); Kefalides et al (1979); Bornstein and Sage (1980).
Other collagens — Ayad et al (1981); Burgeson and Hollister (1979); Furuto and Miller (1980); Laurain et al (1980); Risteli et al (1980); Rojkind et al (1979).

Miller, 1974; Epstein, 1974). The distribution of the three main interstitial collagen types (I, II and III) could therefore be established for each tissue. Type I collagen is the main constituent of tendon and bone, whilst type II collagen predominates in cartilage, the nucleus of the intervertebral disc and in the vitreous of the eye. Type III collagen occurs together with type I in skin, blood vessels, synovia, and placental tissues (Miller, 1976a). All 3 types have been well characterised (see Appendix) and form characteristic fibrils with a 67 nm periodic banding pattern. These three collagens make up the bulk of the interstitial collagens.

Type V (AB) collagen is a relatively minor component accounting for less than 10 per cent of the total collagen in any tissue in which it has been found and although almost certainly of interstitial origin, it has not yet been so well characterised. Rigorous fractionation of pepsin solubilised collagen resulted in the isolation of two genetically distinct α-chains; αA and αB (Burgeson et al, 1976; Chung et al, 1976). These chains were subsequently found to occur in most tissues to the extent of 1 to 8 per cent of the total tissue collagen. In placental villi a third chain αC copurifies with the collagen containing the A and B chains (Ayad et al, 1980; Sage & Bornstein, 1979). However, recent work in our own laboratory indicates that type C collagen probably derives from the uterus and is a contamimant of the placental villi (Abedin et al, 1981). AB collagen is now known as type V collagen and the B and A chains as $\alpha 1(V)$ and $\alpha 2(V)$ respectively (Bornstein & Sage, 1980). Whether the $\alpha 1(V)$ and $\alpha 2(V)$ occur within the same molecule as suggested by Burgeson et al (1976) and Bentz et al (1978) or in different molecules (Rhodes & Miller, 1978) is not yet certain. Recent evidence from biosynthetic studies however, strongly favours the idea of a single molecule $(\alpha A(\alpha B)_2)$ or in new terminology $(\alpha 1(V))_2\alpha 2(V)$, as the major form of type V collagen (Kumamoto & Fessler, 1980). The αC chain is now called $\alpha 3(V)$.

However, these synthetic studies also provide evidence for a separate molecule consisting of three αB chains $(\alpha 1(V))_3$. Such a conformation of α chains is reminiscent of a rare form of type I collagen in which three $\alpha 1(I)$ chains have been shown to constitute the molecule. This collagen has been called type I trimer.

Type I trimer was first observed in a polyoma induced mouse tumour (Moro & Smith, 1977) and subsequently in cirrhotic but not normal liver (Rojkind et al, 1979) and in human skin (Uitto, 1979). The relevance of this form of type I collagen is not yet clear.

The association of $\alpha 1(V)$ with either itself or with $\alpha 2(V)$ and of $\alpha 1(I)$ as a trimer or a molecule associated in a 2:1 ratio with $\alpha 2(I)$ has been studied by Kuhn and coworkers. These workers showed that when type I collagen was denatured and the separated α chains allowed to renature over a period of time, then $\alpha 1(I)$ could renature into a stable molecule $(\alpha 1(I))_3$ whereas $\alpha 2(I)$ could not (Tkocz & Kühn, 1969). Using very similar experimental methodology recent work from the same laboratory has shown that the $\alpha 1(V)$ chain can also renature into an independent molecular form $(\alpha 1(V))_3$ whereas $\alpha 2(V)$ can not (Bentz et al, 1978).

Basement membrane collagen(s) (type IV collagen)

The collagen of basement membranes has a distinct amino acid composition, is highly glycosylated and lacks the distinctive 67nm fibrillar structure of interstitial collagens (Kefalides et al, 1979). Moreover, until recently, it was believed to consist of three identical α chains and was designated type IV collagen (or $(\alpha 1(IV))_3$). However, in the last 2 years the number of papers on the nature of type IV collagen has escalated and the majority of them suggest that there are two genetically distinct α(IV) chains ie: α1(IV) and α2(IV).

Difficulties in determining the structure of basement membrane type IV collagen arise because basement membrane contains weak nonhelical regions within the triple helix (Schuppan et al, 1980). (This is in contrast to the interstitial collagens where the nonhelical regions are limited to the terminal extensions of the molecule.) These regions are susceptible to pepsin and as a result of digestion with this enzyme a number of discrete fragments can be obtained. The major fragments are of the same order of size as the interstitial alpha chains (Dixit, 1979; Kresina & Miller, 1979; Sage et al, 1979). Studies on the amino acid analysis of the separated denatured forms of these fragments suggest that the high molecular weight forms represent two dissimilar collagenous chains and that lower molecular weight fragments derive from one or the other of these distinct chains. Similarly the cyanogen bromide patterns confirm the probability that two genetically distinct α(IV) chains exist — α1(IV) and α2(IV).

Biosynthetic studies have shown that basement membrane collagen is incorporated directly into the matrix as a procollagen (Heathcote et al, 1978) and that there are two distinct procollagen chains (Heathcote et al, 1980). It is not certain whether the two genetically distinct type IV α chains occur within the same giant molecule or exist as separate molecular entities.

Recently electron microscopic examination of polymeric type IV collagen by rotary shadowing, suggests that four triple helical molecules are joined by disulphide and other covalent linkages (Kuhn et al, 1981).

Other workers have suggested that one of the isolated chains (α2(IV)) may be an artefact (Kefalides, Ch. 17). However, the body of evidence which supports the contention that there are two genetically distinct basement membrane collagen chains far outweights that put forward to support an artifactual theory.

Compositional similarities between types IV and V collagens

There are certain similarities in amino acid composition between types IV and V collagens. They both have low alanine and high hydroxylysine content and both are highly glycosylated. This led to the initial belief that type V collagen was of basement membrane origin (Chung et al, 1976). However, type V collagen possesses many properties characteristic of interstitial collagens (Bentz et al, 1978; Ayad et al, 1980) and can be isolated from synovia which has no basement membrane (Brown et al, 1978). Furthermore, no type V collagen has ever been isolated from a pure basement membrane such as lens capsule. Differences and similarities between the two collagen types are detailed in Table 1.2.

Immunofluorescent studies with type V collagen on

Table 1.2 Similarities and differences between type IV and V collagens

Method of characterisation	*Type IV collagen*		*Type V collagen*		
1. Amino acid analysis [1, 2]					
	α1(IV) (C-chain)	α2(IV) (D-chain)	α2(V) (αA)	α1(V) (αB)	α3(V) (αC)
% proline hydroxylation	59	60	51	44	48
% lysine hydroxylation	89	89	64	75	74
% hydroxylysine glycosylation	92	86	62	65	55
2. Susceptibility of helix to enzymic degradation					
i) pepsin	Susceptible		Resistant		
ii) human skin collagenase [2, 3]	Resistant		Resistant		
3. Presence of disulphide bonds	Present		Absent		
4. Solubility at acid pH(2.8) [4]	Insoluble at 1.2M NaCl		Insoluble at 1.2M NaCl		
5. Solubility at neutral pH(7.4) [2]	Insoluble at 1.7–2.0M NaCl		Insoluble at 4.5M NaCl		
6. Solubility in phosphate buffer [5]	Soluble		Insoluble		
7. Solubility in low ionic strength buffers [4, 6]	Soluble		Insoluble		

1. Human placenta (Kresina and Miller, 1979)
2. Human placenta (Sage and Bornstein, 1979)
3. Sage et al (1979)
4. Rhodes and Miller (1978)
5. Abedin et al (1981, 1982)
6. Hong et al (1979)

cartilage indicated an association of this collagen with the chondrocytes and for this reason it has been classified by some workers as a pericellular collagen (Gay et al, 1980 see also Ch. 15).

In our own laboratory immunofluorescent studies with type V collagen on placenta (Abedin, in preparation) and other studies on human skin (Black, personal communication) are at variance with this observation. It may be that this is a feature unique to cartilage. It is perhaps relevant to point out that type V collagen has only been isolated from immature cartilage (Rhodes & Miller, 1978) and has not been found in adult specimens (Ayad et al, 1981).

Other collagens

Cartilage contains in addition to type II collagen several minor collagens. The first of these to be described were three α chains, two of which appeared to be similar at first sight to type V collagen. These alpha chains — 1α and 2α have however distinct characteristics which differentiate them from type V collagen (see Ch. 18) (Burgeson & Hollister, 1979). The third chain, 3α, is similar to $\alpha1(II)$ chain and may represent a form of this collagen which is differently glycosylated. It is interesting that a more heavily glycosylated form of type I collagen has been observed in corneal tissue and it is possible that the extent of glycosylation may have important physiological connotations (Freeman, 1978; Ch. 21).

1α, 2α and 3α collagen chains have also been observed in the annulus and nucleus of the intervertebral disc (Ayad et al, 1981). It is possible that the 1α, 2α and 3α collagens have a structural or functional relationship with type II collagen, whereas type V collagen is related only to collagen types I or III.

With the exception of type IV collagen which appears to exist in the procollagen form, all the collagen types described so far have the basic tropocollagen structure and have molecular weights of the order of ± 300 000. Other collagens have however been described which are highly glycosylated high molecular weight aggregates of much smaller subunits linked by disulphide bonds. Chung et al (1976) first isolated this type of collagen from human placenta and the aortic intima. The subunits have since been shown to consist of both acidic and basic chains (Furuto & Miller, 1980). Similar collagens have also been found in liver (Rojkind et al, 1979) and calf skin (Laurain et al, 1980; Ayad et al, unpublished data). Reports as to the number and size of the subunits of these high molecular weight aggregates vary in different laboratories, but in general two to three subunits are observed in the molecular weight range 30–50 000. Since these collagens appear to be intimately associated with non collagenous proteins and are isolated from pepsin digests of tissues, it is possible that reported differences in molecular weights reflect different amounts of non collagenous glycoprotein-bound material. The proportion of these high molecular weight aggregates varies with tissue source, comprising only 0.3 per cent of the total collagen in calf skin (Ayad et al, unpublished data) but 2 to 3 per cent in placental tissues (Furuto & Miller, 1980; see also Ch. 26). The molecular configuration and function are not yet known. SLS of the high molecular weight aggregate isolated from placental tissue is fibrous and appears to consist of ordered collagenous regions linked together by disordered, probably nonhelical portions which may or may not be collagenous (Weiss, J. B. personal communication).

It should be noted that these high molecular weight aggregates are distinct from another recently described collagen designated 7–S (Risteli et al, 1980).

7–S collagen is also a highly glycosylated and disulphide bonded macromolecule but is a constituent of basement membranes only and has an amino acid composition very similar to type IV collagen. Unlike the high molecular weight aggregates previously described, it is reduced to a range of subunits varying from 27 000 to more than 153 000 molecular weight each differing in size by a regular increment of 25–27 000.

Recently Kuhn et al (1981) have suggested that the 7–S collagen is a central domain linking the end regions of four type IV collagen molecules (see p. 7).

The placenta is a highly complex tissue and contains basement membrane structures as well as interstitial collagen (Ch. 26). Hence both the high molecular weight aggregate and 7–S collagen are found in this tissue. They can however, be separated: 7–S collagen possesses similar solubility properties to type IV collagen whereas the high molecular weight aggregate tends to co-purify with type V collagen.

A highly soluble glycosylated and disulphide bonded collagen, called CPS–1 collagen, has recently been isolated from cartilage and the intervertebral disc (Ayad et al, 1981). It has a molecular weight of approximately 100 000, but on reduction gives rise to fragments of ± 33 000 MW. Chromatographic analyses and electron microscope observation of its SLS crystallites indicate that it is a short triple helical molecule, approximately one-third the length of the conventional tropocollagen molecule and consists of 3 identical chains of 33 000 MW linked by interchain disulphide bonds (Fig. 1.2).

CPS–1 collagen is almost certainly identical to another reported by Shimokomaki et al, (1980) and wrongly described as a collagen of three identical α chains each of ± 110 000 MW.

More recently a second cartilage collagen has been identified (Ayad et al, 1982). This latecomer CPS–2 consists of three chains of 16K, 10K and 8K linked together by disulphide bonds. Whether CPS–1 and CPS–2 are constituents of a larger molecule has not yet been determined.

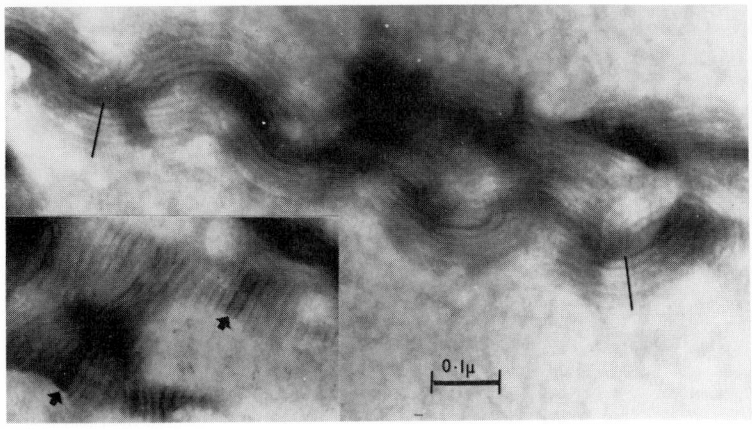

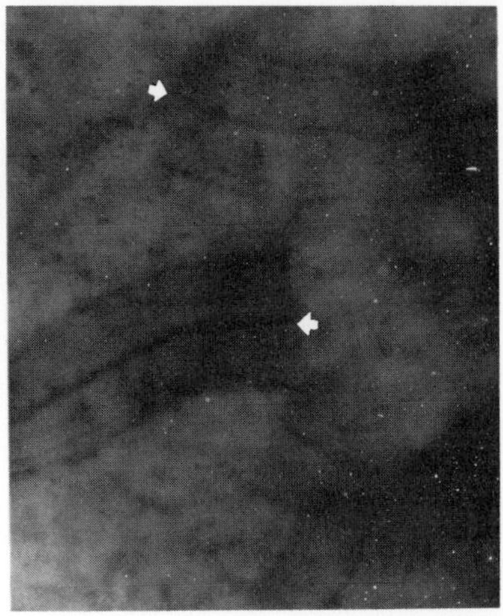

Fig. 1.2 Segment long spacing (SLS) crystallites of C–PS1 collagen from (A) cartilage and (B) vitreous. Lines indicate the approximate length of the molecule. Inset shows dimerisation of these short segments in cartilage. The vitreous molecule only occurred in a dimerised form. (Arrows indicate point of dimerisation.)

Chemical characterisation of collagen types

Old tissues, particularly old human tissues, are singularly difficult to solubilise. For this reason the majority of work on the isolation of collagen types has been done on younger animals. Generally a limited pepsin digest is used to solubilise the collagen fibres (Epstein, 1974). The product of such a digestion is a mixture of different collagens which can then be separated by a combination of various methods. These include:

1. Differential salt precipitation at acid pH (Rhodes & Miller, 1978; Sage & Bornstein, 1979) or at neutral pH (Epstein, 1974).
2. Dialysis against 0.02 M disodium hydrogen phosphate pH 9.2 (Abedin et al, 1981, 1982) or against phosphate buffered saline at 4° (Chiang et al, 1979).
3. Ion exchange chromatography in the native state using either CM cellulose or DEAE cellulose (Bentz et al, 1978; Kresina & Miller, 1979).

The characterisation of the different collagen types in these separation procedures is listed in Table 1.3.

Amino acid analysis and quantitation of the extent of glycosylation of the various collagens is obviously the ideal way of characterising them. Details of amino acid sequences known for the different types are given in Appendix. The extent of post translational modifications of the α chains can vary for the same collagen type, that is for collagen of identical primary structure, in different tissues. This is mainly reflected in the extent of lysine hydroxylation and glycosylation (Appendix).

Gel electrophoresis in sodium dodecyl sulphate (SDS) gives characteristic patterns for most of the denatured α, β and γ components of the various collagens. Collagen, like all glycoproteins, behaves in a somewhat anomalous fashion on SDS gels such that the position of the separated chains and components need not reflect their molecular weight accurately (Furthmayr & Timpl, 1971; Rhodes & Miller, 1979). Ion exchange chromatography has also proved useful in separating the denatured α chains in sufficient quantity for preparative work involving chemical characterisation (Bentz et al, 1978; Kresina & Miller, 1979; Miller, 1976(b); Sage & Bornstein, 1979). Cyanogen bromide digestion of the denatured or native collagens gives rise to a number of peptides, the size of which, ideally, represents the length of the sequences between methionine residues. The patterns of peptides, separated by molecular sieve electrophoresis or ion exchange chromatography, are characteristic for the denatured dissociated chains but are more difficult to interpret on native collagens where cross-linking between chains influences the molecular size of the peptides (Piez, 1976; Bornstein & Traub, 1979). Recently an enzymatic method has been described for characterising the collagen types using digestion with a specific mast cell protease to obtain similarly defined fragments of differing molecular weight. (Sage & Bornstein, 1979; Bornstein & Sage, 1980).

The banding patterns of SLS segments of the various collagens seen in the electron microscope show considerable similarity, nevertheless there are sufficient differences, often in intensity of staining of some of the bands, to provide a characteristic 'finger print'.

With the possible exception of 7–S collagen, all the collagens isolated can be completely degraded by digestion with bacterial collagenase.

PROCOLLAGEN

Collagen is initially secreted into the extracellular matrix in the form of procollagen (Ch. 6). Procollagen has extension peptides at both carboxy and amino terminal ends. These

Table 1.3 Solubility and ion exchange characteristics of native collagen types

Collagen type	*Molar NaCl concentration for precipitation at:* acid pH (2.8) (a), (b)	neutral pH (7.4) (c)	*Solubility by dialysis against:* 0.02M Na_2HPO_4 (pH9.2) (a) (c)	phosphate buffered saline (d)	*Molar NaCl concentration for elution in the native state on:* carboxymethyl cellulose 0.04M sodium acetate, 2M urea pH4.8 (e) (f)	diethylamino ethyl cellulose 0.05M tris-HCl, 2M urea pH8.6 (g)
Interstitial						
I	0.7–0.9	2.4–2.6	insoluble	soluble	0.09–0.1	0
I Trimer[(h)]	0.7–0.9	4.0	insoluble	soluble	—	—
II[(i)]	0.7–0.9	3.5–4.4	insoluble	soluble	0.09–0.1	0
III	0.7–0.9	1.5–1.7	insoluble	soluble	0.09–0.1	0
V	1.2	4.0–4.5[(j)]	insoluble[(j)]	insoluble	0.09–0.1	0.08–0.1
Basement membrane						
IV	1.2	1.7–2.0[(k)]	soluble[(l)]	soluble[(l)]	0.04	0
Other collagens						
$1\alpha2\alpha3\alpha$[(m)]	1.2	4.0–4.5[(f)]	insoluble[(f)]	insoluble[(n)]	0.15–0.17	—
High molecular weight aggregate[(o)]	1.8–2.0	4.5–5.0	insoluble	—	—	0.08–0.1[(n)]
7–S[(p)]	—	1.7–2.0	—	—	—	—
CPS-1[(f)]	2.0	4.5–5.0	soluble	soluble	0.11–0.15	—
CPS-2[(q)]	2.0	3.7–4.0	soluble	soluble	0.11–0.15	—

[(a)] Chung et al (1976) [(b)] Rhodes and Miller (1978) [(c)] Epstein (1974) [(d)] Chiang et al (1980) [(e)] Kresina and Miller (1979) [(f)] Ayad et al (1981) [(g)] Bentz et al (1978) [(h)] Uitto (1979) [(i)] Miller and Lunde (1973) [(j)] Burgeson et al (1976) [(k)] Glanville et al (1979) [(l)] Abedin et al (1981) [(m)] Burgeson and Hollister (1979) [(n)] Ayad et al — unpublished data [(o)] Furuto and Miller (1980) [(p)] Risteli et al (1980) [(q)] Ayad et al (1982)

peptides are moderately large and their amino acid sequences are now known (see Appendix). The procollagen molecules are exported from the cell in the form of a non-fibrillar but structured aggregate (Trelstad & Hayashi; 1979). It seems likely that the bulky extension peptides actually inhibit fibril formation such that the fibril assembly process does not take place until the peptides have been excised. Two very specific endopeptidases, amino and carboxy terminal proteases, remove these extensions in the extracellular space (Ch. 6).

Procollagens which have only been partially processed in the extracellular matrix have been termed P_N and P_C collagens respectively, the former having the amino terminal extension only and the latter the carboxy terminal peptide.

Procollagens of types I, II, III and V collagen have been identified in the medium of tissue cultured cells (Olsen et al, 1977; Merry et al, 1976; Burke et al, 1977; Kumamoto & Fessler, 1980). However, although there is evidence for high molecular weight forms of type IV collagen (180 000 MW) in the media from cultured intact rat lenses (Heathcote et al, 1978; 1980) and in cultured amniotic fluid cells (Crouch & Bornstein, 1979), these procollagen forms appear to incorporate intact into the permanent basement membrane structure (Heathcote et al, 1980). It would seem therefore that endopeptidases are not present which are capable of converting type IV procollagen to a form similar to that found for the interstitial collagens.

Neutral salt solutions of collagens extracted from young tissues which represent newly synthesised protein, often contain some unprocessed procollagen α chains. Type III procollagen has been isolated from neutral salt solutions of rat skin (Byers et al, 1974; Timpl et al, 1975) and procollagens have been identified in several tissues by immunofluorescence (Nowack et al, 1976). Recently type V procollagen has been observed in neutral salt preparations of foetal calf skin (Elstow et al, 1982).

FIBRILLAR COLLAGEN

Native tropocollagen solutions of types I, II and III collagens can precipitate under suitable conditions of temperature and ionic strength into fibrils. These fibrils when examined in the electron microscope appear to have identical fine banding patterns. The only apparent difference is that type III collagen generally precipitates as somewhat smaller diameter fibrils than those from type I collagen. However this fact may have no physiological significance since the diameter of fibrils in vitro and in vivo may not be strictly comparable. For example, although type II collagen usually appears in vivo as much finer fibrils than those of type I collagen it can be precipitated in vitro as fibrils of the same width as type I collagen (Eyre 1979).

The collagen gels prepared in vitro show changes with age which may be similar to processes occurring in the tissue collagens. Thus reconstituted collagen fibrils become increasingly insoluble with age, indicating that formation of crosslinks is occurring, as a function of time, between contiguous molecules (Sopata et al, 1974).

Removal of the nonhelical terminal peptides by pepsin digestion has a profound effect on the ability of the collagen to form fibrils and fibrils formed from some pepsin solubilised collagen are atypical. Type I collagen from which the nonhelical terminal peptides have been removed forms either symmetric fibrils or a mixture of polarised and symmetric tactoids (Leibovich & Weiss, 1970). For a definition of symmetric fibrils and tactoids see glosstary. Type III collagen, on the other hand, which is prepared after pepsin digestion of the tissue forms what appear to be perfectly polarised fibrils, though of narrow diameter. However fibrils prepared from type V collagen, also extracted after pepsin digestion, are symmetric (Weiss, Abedin & Ayad, personal observation). This raises some interesting questions. Is in vitro fibril formation from type III collagen unaffected by removal of its nonhelical terminal ends, because of the presence of cross-links between the amino terminal *helical* region of the molecule and an intramolecular disulphide bonded carboxy terminal nonhelical region of another molecule? Such a cross-link has been identified (Nicholls & Bailey, 1980) from type III collagen extracted from pepsin digested fetal calf skin. This cross-link may stabilise the molecule in some manner which maintains its polar integrity.

Ever since the observations that the fibrils formed from soluble collagen solutions had the same characteristic 67nm periodicity of the fibres seen in intact tissues, research has centred on the mechanism of fibril formation in vitro in the hope of explaining fibrillogenesis in vivo. The limitations to this type of study are that the collagen used has often been an acid soluble extract which consists of only type I collagen and has ignored the presence of more than one type of collagen in nearly every tissue.

Ironically, the X-ray diffraction studies of natural collagen fibres have nearly all been on tendon, which with the exception of bone, is the only tissue in the body to contain only one major type of collagen — type I collagen.

In tissues in which more than one collagen type is present, as for example skin in which there are both types I and III collagens, each may affect the rate and extent of fibril formation of the other. It is not yet clear whether the different collagen types form independent fibre bundles or whether they precipitate together as mixed fibrils.

There is some evidence that reticulin, thin silver staining branched fibrils seen in young developing tissues, may consist of type III collagen (Fietzek & Kühn, 1976). If so it would lend credence to the idea that the collagen types form independent and not mixed fibrils, though it has been suggested that reticulin is the template for the organisation and maintenance of fibre orientation (Eastoe, 1967).

The fact that acid soluble collagen from fetal and adult skin contains only type I collagen suggests either, that type I and III collagens are in singular fibres having dissimilar cross-links with differing acid lability, or that type I collagen molecules are on the outside of a mixed type I/type III fibre. The latter suggestion seems the most feasible particularly, as in embryonic skin at least, types I and III collagen have been shown to possess the same cross-link, hydroxylysino-5-keto-norleucine (Bailey and Sims, 1976), though, of course, there may be additional stable cross-links in type III collagen which have not yet been identified.

It may be relevant that two types of SLS crystallites are formed from mixed solutions of types I and III collagen, each having the typical appearance of SLS from one or other of the collagen types (Weiss, personal observations).

An important question yet to be answered, concerns the minor collagens whose main function in fibrillogenesis could be to form the infrastructure for fibres from types I and III collagen. So far no information on this point is available.

Fibril morphology in vivo

It certainly seems likely that the different characteristics of the various tissues are conferred by, among other things, the proportion of the different types of collagen present. Kuhn & Glanville (1980) have pointed out that the collagen fibrils in calf skin are of relatively large diameter and are packed parallel to one another into fibres whereas the collagen in bone tissue is in the form of thin fibrils, irregularly arranged. They conclude that as type I collagen is present in both tissues, the macromolecular organisation of the fibres cannot be regulated by the primary sequence of the molecule. However this still leaves a number of other possibilities. The presence in skin of type III collagen may be important for the arrangement of type I collagen molecules into large diameter parallel fibres. Alternatively the other components of the extracellular matrix different in bone and skin, may be the mediators.

It has already been mentioned that collagen should not be considered in isolation since it is only one of different connective tissue macromolecules. Scott (1975) pointed out the importance to tissue function of the relationship between collagen and the soluble polymers, proteoglycans, which are dissolved in the interfibrillar fluids. Recently Scott and his associates (Scott et al, 1981) have demonstrated an inverse relationship between tendon fibre diameter and the dermatan sulphate content in the tissue. This aspect of collagen morphology may be of great importance in inherited diseases such as Ehlers-Danlos type 1 syndrome in which very wide diameter fibrils are observed although no collagen abnormality has so far been detected.

COLLAGEN CROSS-LINKS

Two categories of collagen cross-links have been described. These are the 'reducible' cross-links, and the 'stable' cross-links. The former have been identified after treatment of the collagen with tritiated borohydride which conveniently labels the cross-links and enables them to be identified in digests of the protein. Much less is known about the stable cross-links and there is controversy as to whether these arise through stabilisation of reducible cross-links or are new entities arising at different sites in the molecule.

The two amino acids concerned in reducible cross-link formation in collagen are lysine and hydroxylysine. Cross-links are generally between the aldehydes derived from these two residues and another lysine or hydroxylysine residue. The aldehydes are formed by the action of the enzyme lysyl oxidase. Siegel (1974) found that lysyl oxidase was only active on insoluble native collagen and could not form aldehydes from lysine or hydroxylysine residues in soluble collagen. This observation led to the suggestion that lysyl oxidase binds to the molecule next to the one which it is using as substrate and that for this reason a fibrillar collagen is required (Light & Bailey, 1980).

Cross-links occur between residues which are in areas of sequence homology along the molecule. The lysine aldehyde precursors occur in the amino and carboxy terminal nonhelical regions of the molecules. The molecules are probably aligned during the formation of the cross-links by nearby hydrophobic interactions between residues on either molecule (Light & Bailey, 1980).

The two major reducible cross-links are dehydro-hydroxylysinonorleucine (dehydro-HLNL) which is an aldimine derived from the condensation of one lysine and one hydroxylysine residue and hydroxylysino-5-keto-norleucine (HLONL) a keto imine derived from two hydroxylysine residues. The structure of these and other minor reducible cross-links is dealt with in detail in Chapter 9.

Each tissue in the body contains different proportions of reducible cross-links and it has been suggested that the extent of hydroxylation of the lysine residues in the nonhelical terminal peptide may be the key factor in determining the ratio of the two cross-links. Skin contains mainly dehydro-hydroxylysinonorleucine and in this tissue the extent of hydroxylation of the relevant lysine residue is low (Barnes et al, 1971). However, in bone and cartilage, where the hydroxylation is substantial, the major cross-link is hydroxylysino-5-keto-norleucine (Mechanic et al, 1971; Barnes, 1973; Light & Bailey, 1980).

It has been shown that both the relative amounts of the two major cross-links and their total number change with age of the animal (Bailey & Robins, 1972; Robins et al, 1973).

Embryonic skin contains HLONL as the predominant cross-link but this is replaced after birth by dehydro-HLNL which increases in early post natal life. However the quantity of both cross-links decreases during maturation. This decrease in reducible cross-links with age has been established for many tissues (Light & Bailey, 1980).

With the decrease in reducible cross-links new stable bonds appear to form and these lead to the almost complete insolubility of aged tissue collagens. Human synovial collagen has been shown to become progressively resistant to pepsin digestion with increasing age, reaching a maximum resistance at 35 yrs. (Table 1.4) (Weiss et al, 1980).

Table 1.4 Relationship of tissue age with the amount of collagen which can be solubilised by pepsin digestion (Human synovial collagen, Weiss et al, 1980)

Age	*Collagen solubilised* (%)
7 months	98
1 yr	96
4 yr	76
8 yr	36
18 yr	15
29 yr	6.5
36 yr	3.2
47 yr	0.8
53 yr	0
60 yr	0
64 yr	0
66 yr	0
67 yr	0
70 yr	0

The pepsin resistance suggests that the stable cross-links, unlike the reducible ones are not between residues in the amino terminal nonhelical regions and helical regions of the collagen molecule. If they were pepsin would cleave the terminal nonhelical peptides and effectively solubilise the collagen. However, no confirmed report of a helix to helix cross-link has so far surfaced.

There have been reports on the isolation of helical-helical cross-linked peptides from digests of insoluble collagen (Becker et al, 1975; Scott et al, 1976) but no further evidence for these is yet available. It is hard not to believe that such cross-links do occur, if only because of the resistance of older collagens to solubilisation with enzymes which cleave the nonhelical terminal peptides. An important consideration is the relative instability of the reducible cross-links in collagen as compared with other types of covalent bonds. It is feasible that they could form, break and reform under applied stress.

Reports of changes in the nature of the cross-links with maturation of the tissue suggest that adult animal collagen contains different cross-links from embryonic and immature forms (Robins et al, 1973; Fujii & Tanzer, 1974; Mechanic et al, 1971). Also, the total number of reducible cross-links decreases with increasing age, suggesting either that they are replaced by more stable bonds, although these have not yet been characterised, or that the reducible cross-links themselves are modified to a stable form (Light & Bailey, 1980).

COLLAGEN DEGRADATION IN VIVO

Mammalian collagenase is the only mammalian enzyme known to cleave the helical portion of types I, II and III collagen. However, it is not capable of attacking either type IV or type V collagen. Recently, evidence for other animal collagenases specific for these latter collagens has been obtained (Liotta et al, 1979; Mainardi et al, 1980).

In the tissues, collagenase exists as one of a group of neutral proteinases which, acting in concert, are capable of degrading the insoluble fibres. Collagenase together with its associated neutral proteinases probably exists in the extracellular matrix in an inhibited form as an enzyme inhibitor complex or procollagenase bound to the collagen fibres themselves (See Ch. 7). There is some evidence for a dynamic interchange between the enzymes and their inhibitors (Steven & Podrazky, 1978) and this may have some relevance in inflammatory diseases. An inhibitor, which is specific for collagenase and which has no effect on other neutral proteinases has been demonstrated in normal human serum (Woolley et al, 1976). The role of this circulating inhibitor, a β_1 globulin is not yet clear.

DISORDERS OF COLLAGEN METABOLISM: INHERITED OR ACQUIRED DISEASES

As more knowledge has been acquired of the mechanisms of collagen bisoynthesis and of its polymorphism, a number of genetic disorders of collagen metabolism have been characterised. Sometimes however it has worked the other way round. For example the first indication for a procollagen molecule was from studies of collagens extracted from the skin of dermatosparactic cattle (Lenaers et al, 1971).

Nowadays inherited diseases of collagen metabolism (synthesis or degradation) can be seen to fall into four main categories; genetic abnormalities in the procollagen DNA, defects at the level of translation or transcription of procollagen mRNA, failure or partial failure of the intracellular and extracellular post translational modifications of procollagen and genetically determined variations of collagenase activity. Examples of diseases within each of the above categories can be seen in Table 1.5 and these diseases will be dealt with at length elsewhere in this book.

Acquired diseases may result from abnormalities in the cellular immune response to collagen but at present less is known about this very important group of diseases although antibodies to type II collagen have been demonstrated in patients with rheumatoid arthritis. Mechanisms for the regulation of synthesis and secretion of procollagens are also not yet well understood. It is possible that a failure in this control may be involved in the lesion of progressive systemic sclerosis (scleroderma) (Jayson & Weiss, 1979) and possibly in pulmonary fibrosis.

In addition there are the inflammatory diseases such as rheumatoid arthritis and gout in which normal cells have been shown to synthesise an excess of collagenase in response to stimulation by monoctyes.

CONCLUSIONS

Collagen, as may be seen, is a complex protein. As more information becomes available relating to its polymorphism and mechanisms and control of its biosynthesis and degradation so we may expect to more fully understand its complex functions, which are surely not simply structural. Such an understanding may help to elucidate the causes of many inherited or acquired diseases.

Table 1.5 Examples of inherited diseases of collagen biosynthesis, processing and degradation

Level of defect	*Example*
DNA abnormality	Ehlers–Danlos syndrome type VII. Substitution at the amino terminal cleavage site of the procollagen $\alpha 2$ chain[1]
Transcription and translation	Ehlers–Danlos syndrome type IV. Decreased synthesis of type III collagen[2, 3]
Intracellular post translational modification	Ehlers–Danlos syndrome type VI. Lysyl hydroxylase deficiency[4]
Extracellular post translational modification	Cutis laxa. Defect in lysyl oxidase[5]
Genetic variations of collagenase	Epidermolysis bullosa dystrophica[6]

1. Tuderman et al (1979)
2. Byers et al (1979)
3. Pope et al (1975)
4. Quinn and Krane (1976)
5. Byers et al (1976)
6. Bauer (1977)

REFERENCES

Abedin M Z, Ayad S, Weiss J B 1981 Type V collagen: The presence of appreciable amounts of α3(V) chain in uterus. Biochemical and Biophysical Reasearch Communications 102: 1237-45

Abedin M Z, Ayad S, Weiss J B 1982 Isolation and native characterisation of cystein-rich collagens from bovine placental tissues and uterus and their relationship to types IV an V collagens. In press.

Altgelt K, Hodge A V, Schmitt F O 1961 Gamma tropocollagen: A reversibly denaturable collagen molecule. Proceedings of the National Academy of Science, USA 47: 1914-19

Ayad S, Abedin M Z, Grundy S, Weiss J B 1981 Isolation and characterisation of an unusual collagen from hyaline cartilage and intervertebral disc. FEBS Letters 123: 195-9

Ayad S, Abedin M Z, Weiss J B 1980 Non-basement-membrane collagen A, B and C α-chains: types V and VI collagen? Biochemical Society Transactions 8: 324-5

Ayad S, Abedin M Z, Weiss J B, Grundy S M 1982 Characterisation of another short-chain disulphide bonded collagen from cartilage, vitreous and intervertebral disc. FEBS Letters in press.

Bailey A J, Lapiere C M 1973 Effect of additional peptide extension of the N-terminus of collagen from dermatosparactic calves on the crosslinking of the collagen fibres. European Journal of Biochemistry 34: 91-100

Bailey A J, Robins S P 1972 Embryonic skin collagen. Replacement of the type of aldimine crosslinks during the early growth period. FEBS Letters 21: 330-2

Bailey A J, Sims T J 1976 Chemistry of the collagen crosslinks. Nature of the crosslinks. Biochemical Journal 153: 211-5

Bansal M, Ramakrishnan C, Ramachandran G N 1975 Stabilisation of the collagen structure by hydroxyproline residues. Proceedings of the Indian Academy of Sciences Section A82: 152-64

Barnes M J 1973 In: Hard Tissue Growth, Repair and Remineralisation. Elsevier, Amsterdam, p 247-61

Barnes M J, Constable B J, Morton L F, Kodicek E 1971 Hydroxylysine in the N-terminal telopeptides of skin collagen from chick embryo and new born rat. Biochemical Journal 125: 925-8

Bauer E A 1977 Recessive dystrophic epidermolysis bullosa: Evidence for an altered collagenase in fibroblast cultures. Proceedings of the National Academy of Science, USA 74: 4646-50

Bear R S 1942 Long X-ray diffraction spacing of collagen. Journal of the American Chemical Society 64: 727

Becker U, Furthmayr H, Timpl R 1975 Tryptic peptides from the cross-linking regions of insoluble calf skin collagen. Hoppe-Seyler's Zeitschrift für Physiologische Chemie 356: 21-32

Bentz H, Bächinger H P, Glanville R, Kühn K 1978 Physical evidence for the assembly of A and B chains in human placental collagen in a single triple helix. European Journal of Biochemistry 92: 563-9

Boedtker H, Doty P 1956 The native and denatured states of soluble collagen. Journal of the American Chemical Society 78: 4267-80

Bogue R H 1922 The chemistry and technology of gelatin and glue. McGraw-Hill, New York

Bornstein P, Sage H 1980 Structurally distinct collagen types. Annual Review of Biochemistry 49: 957-1003

Bornstein P, Traub W 1979 The chemistry and biology of collagen. In: Neurath H, Hill R L (eds) The Proteins 3rd edn, Vol IV. Academic Press, New York and London, p 411-632

Brown R A, Shuttleworth C A, Weiss J B 1978 Three new alpha chains of collagen from a non-basement membrane source. Biochemical and Biophysical Research Communications 80: 866-72

Burgeson R E, El Adli F A, Kaitila I I, Hollister D W 1976 Foetal membrane collagens: identification of two new collagen alpha chains. Proceedings of the National Academy of Science, USA 73: 2579-83

Burgeson R E, Hollister D W 1979 Collagen heterogeneity in human cartilage: identification of several new collagen chains. Biochemical and Biophysical Research Communications 87: 1124-31

Burke J M, Balian G, Ross R, Bornstein P 1977 Synthesis of types I and III procollagen and collagen by monkey aortic smooth muscle cells in vitro. Biochemistry 16: 3243-9

Byers P H, Holbrook K A, McGillvray B, MacLeod P M, Lowry R B 1979 Clinical and ultrastructural heterogeneity of type IV Ehlers-Danlos syndrome. Human Genetics 47: 141-50

Byers P H, McKenney K H, Lichtenstein J R, Martin G R 1974 Preparation of type III procollagen and collagen from rat skin. Biochemistry 13: 5243-8

Byers P H, Narayanan A S, Bornstein P, Hall J G 1976 An X-linked form of cutis laxa due to deficiency of lysyl oxidase. Birth Defects 12: 293-8

Chapman J A, Holmes D F, Meek K M, Rattew C J 1981 Electron-optical studies of collagen fibril assembly. In: structural aspects of recognition and assembly in biological macromolecules. Proceedings of the Seventh Annual Katzir — Katchalsky conference. The Weizmann Institute of Science, Rehovot and Nof Ginossar — Israel February 24th-29th 1980

Chiang T M, Mainardi C L, Seyer J M, Kang A H 1980 Collagen platelet interaction. Type V (AB) collagen induces platelet aggregation. Journal of Laboratory and Clinical Medicine 95: 99-107

Chung E, Miller E J 1974 Collagen polymophism: characterisation of molecules with the chain composition $(\alpha 1(III))_3$ in human tissues. Science 183: 1200-1

Chung E, Rhodes R K, Miller E J 1976 Isolation of three collagenous components of probable basement membrane origin from several tissues. Biochemical and Biophysical Research Communications 71: 1167-74

Church R L, Tanzer M L, Lapière C M 1973 Identification of two distinct species of procollagen synthesised by a clonal line of calf dermatosparactic cells. Nature New Biology 244: 188-90

Crouch E, Bornstein P 1979 Characterisation of type IV procollagen synthesised by human amniotic fluid cells in culture. The Journal of Biological Chemistry 254: 4197-204

Dixit S N 1979 Isolation and characterisation of two alpha-chain size collagenous polypeptide chains C and D from glomerular basement membrane. FEBS Letters 106: 378-84

Drake M P, Davison P F, Bump S, Schmitt F O 1966 Action of proteolytic enzymes on tropocollagen and insoluble collagen. Biochemistry 5: 301-12

Eastoe J E 1967 Composition of collagen and allied proteins. In: Ramachandran G N (ed) Treatise on Collagen, Vol 1. Chemistry of collagen. Academic Press, New York, p 1-72

Elstow S F, Ayad S, Abedin M Z, Weiss J B 1982 Isolation and chemical characterisation of neutral salt soluble type V collagen from foetal calf skin — in preparation

Epstein E H 1974 $(\alpha 1(III))_3$ Human skin collagen. Release by pepsin digestion and preponderance in foetal life. The Journal of Biological Chemistry 249: 3225-31

Epstein E H, Munderloh N H 1975 Isolation and characterisation of CNBr peptides of human $(\alpha 1(III))_3$ collagen and tissue distribution of $(\alpha 1(I))_2\alpha 2$ and $(\alpha 1(III))_3$ collagens. The Journal of Biological Chemistry 250: 9304-12

Eyre D R 1979 Biochemistry of the intervertebral disc. In: Hall D A, Jackson D S (eds) International Review of Connective Tissue Research, Vol 8. Academic Press, New York and London, p 227-91

Eyre D R, Muir H 1977 Quantitative analysis of types I and II collagens in human intervertebral discs at various ages. Biochimica et Biophysica Acta 491: 29-42

Fessler J H, Doege K J, Siegel R C, Fessler L I 1977 Procollagen associations into supramolecular structures. Federation Proceedings 36: 680

Fietzek P P, Kuhn K 1976 The primary structure of collagen. In Hall D A, Jackson D S (eds) International Review of Connective Tissue Research, Vol 7.Academic Press, New York and London, p 1-60

Freeman I L 1978 Collagen polymorphism in mature rabbit cornea. Investigative Ophthalmology and Visual Science. St Louis 17: 171-7

Fujii K, Tanzer M L 1974 Age-related changes in the reducible crosslinks of human tendon collagen. FEBS Letters. 43: 300-2

Fuller F, Boedtker H 1981 Sequence determination and analysis of the 3′ region of chicken proα_1 type I and proα_2 Type I. Biochemistry, 20: 996-1006

Furuto D K, Miller E J 1980 Isolation of a unique collagenous fraction from limited pepsin digests of human placental tissue. The Journal of Biological Chemistry 255: 290-5

Furuto D K, Miller E J 1981 Characterisation of a unique collagenous fraction from limited pepsin digests of human placental tissue: molecular organisation of the native aggregate. Biochemistry 20: 1635-40

Furthmayr H, Timpl R 1971 Characterisation of collagen peptides by sodium dodecylsulphate-polyacrylamide electrophoresis. Analytical Biochemistry 41: 510-6

Gay S, Gay R, Miller E J 1980 The collagens of the joint. Arthritis and Rheumatism 23: 937-41

Glanville R W, Rauter A, Fietzek P P 1979 Isolation and characterisation of a native placental basement-membrane collagen and its component α chains. European Journal of Biochemistry 95: 383-9

Grassman W, Hannig K, Engel J 1961 Quantitative behaviour between α and β components of denatured soluble collagen in ultracentrifugation as well as a description of a more rapidly sedimentable component. Hoppe-Seyler's Zeitschrift fur Physiologische Chemie 324: 284-8

Gross J, Highberger J H, Schmitt F O 1954 Collagen structures considered as states of aggregation of a kinetic unit. The tropocollagen particle. Proceedings of the National Academy of Science, USA 40: 679-87

Hance A J, Bradley K, Crystal R G 1976 Lung Collagen heterogeneity. Synthesis of Type I and Type III collagen by rabbit and human lung cells in culture. Journal of Clinical Investigation 57: 102-11

Heathcote J G, Bailey A J, Grant M E 1980 Studies on the assembly of rat lens capsule. Biosynthesis of a cross-linked collagenous component of high molecular weight. Biochemical Journal 190: 220-37

Heathcote J G, Sear C H, Grant M E 1978 Studies on the assembly of rat lens capsule. Biosynthesis and partial characterisation of the collagenous components. Biochemical Journal 176: 283-94

Hodge A J, Highberger J H, Deffner G G J, Schmitt F O 1960 The effects of proteases on the tropocollagen macromolecule and its aggregation properties. Proceedings of the National Academy of Science, USA 46: 197-205

Hodge A J, Petrushka J A 1963 Recent studies with the electron microscope on ordered aggregates of the tropocollagen macromolecule. In: Ramachandran G N (ed) Aspects of Protein Structure. Academic Press, London and New York, p 289-300

Hodge A J, Schmitt F O 1960 The charge profile of the tropocollagen macromolecule and the packing arrangement in native type collagen fibrils. Proceedings of the National Academy of Science, USA 46: 186-97

Hong B S, Davison P F, Cannon D J 1979 Isolation and characterisation of a distinct type of collagen from bovine foetal membranes and other tissues. Biochemistry 18: 4278-82

Jackson D S 1957 Connective tissue stimulated by carrageenin 1. The formation and removal of collagen. Biochemical Journal 65: 277-84

Jackson D S, Bentley J P 1960 On the significance of the extractable collagens. The Journal of Biophysical and Biochemical Cytology 7: 37-42

Jayson M I V, Weiss J B 1979 Progressive systemic sclerosis: Metabolism of connective tissue. In: Clinics in Rheumatic Diseases. W B Saunders Company Ltd, London, p 185-200

Kefalides N A, Alper R, Clark C C 1979 Biochemistry and metabolism of basement membranes. International Review of Cytology 61: 167-228

Kivirikko K I, Myllyla R 1979 Collagen Glycosyl transferases. In: Hall D A, Jackson D S (eds) International Review of Connective Tissue Research, Vol 8.Academic Press, New York and London, p 23-72

Kresina T F, Miller E J 1979 Isolation and characterisation of basement membrane collagen from human placental tissue. Evidence for the presence of 2 genetically distinct collagen chains. Biochemistry 18: 3089-97

Kuhn K, Fietzek P, Kuhn J 1966 The action of proteolytic enzymes on collagen. Biochemische Zeitschrift 344: 418-22

Kuhn K, Glanville R W 1980 Molecular structure and higher organization of different collagen types. In: Viidik A, Vuust J (eds) Biology of Collagen Academic Press, New York and London, p 1-14

Kuhn K, Wiedermann H, Timpl R, Risteli J, Dieringer H, Voss T and Glanville R W 1981 Macromolecular structure of basement membrane collagens. Identification of 7S collagen as a cross-linking domain of type IV collagen. FEBS Letters 125: 123-8

Kumamoto C A, Fessler J H 1980 Biosynthesis of A, B procollagen. Proceedings of the National Academy of Science, USA 77: 6434-38

Laurain G, Delvincourt T, Szymanowicz A G 1980 Isolation of a macromolecular collagenous fraction and AB_2 collagen from calf skin. FEBS Letters 120: 44-8

Leibovich S J, Weiss J B 1970 Electron microscope studies of the effects of endo- and exopeptidase digestion on tropocollagen. A novel concept of the role of terminal regions in fibrillogenesis. Biochimica et Biophysica Acta 214: 445-54

Lenaers A, Ansay M, Nusgens B V, Lapière C M 1971 Collagen made of extended α-chains, procollagen, in genetically-defective dermatosparaxic calves. European Journal of Biochemistry 23: 533-43

Lichtenstein J R, Byers P H, Smith B D, Martin G R 1975 Identification of the collagenous proteins synthesised by cultured cells from human skin. Biochemistry 14: 1589-94

Light N D, Bailey A J 1980 Molecular structure and stabilization of the collagen fibre. In: Viidik A, Vuust J (eds) Biology of Collagen. Academic Press, London and New York, p 15-38

Liotta L A, Abe S, Robey P G, Martin G R 1979 Preferential digestion of basement membrane collagen by an enzyme derived from a metastatic murine tumour. Proceedings of the National Academy of Science, USA 76: 2268-72

Mainardi C L, Seyer J M, Kang A H 1980 Type-specific collagenolysis: A type V collagen degrading enzyme from macrophages. Biochemical and Biophysical Research Communications 97: 1108-115

Mathews M B 1975 Connective Tissue. Macromolecular Structure and Evolution. Springer-Verlag, New York, Heidelberg and Berlin

Mathews M B 1980 Coevolution of collagen. In: Viidik A, Vuust J (eds) Biology of collagen. Academic Press, London and New York, p 193-209

Mathews M B, Kulonen E, Dorfman A 1954 Studies on procollagen. II Viscosity and molecular weight. Archives of Biochemistry and Biophysics 52: 247-53

Mechanic G L, Gallop P M, Tanzer M L 1971 The nature of cross-linking in collagen from mineralized tissues. Biochemical and Biophysical Research Communications 45: 644-53

Merry A H, Harwood R, Woolley D E, Grant M E, Jackson D S 1976 Identification and partial characterisation of the non-collagenous amino- and carboxy-terminal extension peptides of cartilage procollagen. Biochemical and Biophysical Research Communications 71: 83-90

Miller E J 1971 Isolation and characterisation of collagen from chick cartilage containing three identical chains. Biochemistry 10: 1652-9

Miller E J 1976a Biochemical characteristics and biological significance of the genetically distinct collagens. Molecular and Cell Biochemistry 13: 165-92

Miller E J 1976b Separation of collagen fractions on carboxymethyl cellulose. In: Hall D A (ed) The Methodology of Connective Tissue Research. Joynson-Bruvvers Ltd, Oxford, p 197-203

Miller E J, Epstein E H, Peiz K A 1971 Identification of three genetically distinct collagens by cyanogen bromide cleavage of insoluble human skin and cartilage collagen. Biochemical and Biophysical Research Communications 42: 1024-9

Miller E J, Lunde L 1973 Isolation and characterization of the cyanogen bromide peptides from the $\alpha 1$(II) chain of bovine and human cartilage collagen. Biochemistry 12: 3153-9

Miller E J, Matukas V J 1969 Chick cartilage collagen: A new type of $\alpha 1$ chain not present in bone or skin of the species. Proceedings of the National Academy of Science, USA 65: 1264-8

Moro J, Smith B S 1977 Identification of collagen $\alpha 1$(I) trimer and normal type I collagen in a polyoma virus — induced mouse tumour. Archives of Biochemistry and Biophysics 182: 33-41

Nageotte J 1927 Coagulation fibrillaire in vitro due collagène dissous dans un acide dilué. Comptes Rendus Academie des Sciences 184: 115

Nicholls A C, Bailey A J 1980 Identification of cyanogen bromide peptides involved in intermolecular crosslinking of bovine type III collagen. Biochemical Journal 185: 195-201

Nowack H, Gay S, Wick G, Becker U, Timpl R 1976 Preparation and use in immunohistology of antibodies specific for type I and type III collagen and procollagen. Journal of Immunological Methods 12: 117-24

Olsen B R, Guzman N A, Engel J, Condit C, Aase S 1977 Purification and characterization of a peptide from the carboxyterminal region of chick tendon procollagen type I. Biochemistry 16: 3030-6

Orekhovich V N, Shpikiter V O 1955 Study of some properties of denatured procollagen with the ultracentrifuge. Doklady Akademii Nauklady SSSR 101: 529-32

Orekhovich V N, Shpikiter V O 1958 Sedimentation and diffusion of the α and β components of procollagen and their quantitative ratio in procollagen. Biokhimiya 23: 266-71

Peltonen L, Palotie A, Prockop D J 1980 A defect in the structure of type I procollagen in a patient who had osteogenesis imperfecta: Excess mannose in the COOH-terminal propeptide. Proceedings of the National Academy of Science, USA 77: 6179-83

Pentinnen R P, Frey H, Aalto M, Vuorio E, Marttala T 1980 Collagen synthesis in cultured cells. In: Viidik A, Vuust J (eds) Biology of Collagen Academic Press, London and New York, p 87-103

Piez K A 1976 Primary structure. In: Ramachandran G N, Reddi A H (eds) Biochemistry of Collagen Plenum Press, New York and London, p 1-44

Pope F M, Martin G R, Lichtenstein J R, Penttinen R P, Gerson B, Rowe D W, McKusik V A 1975 Patients with Ehlers-Danlos syndrome type IV lack type III collagen. Proceedings of the National Academy of Science, USA 72: 1314-6

Prockop D J, Berg R A, Kivirikko K I, Uitto J 1976 Intracellular steps in the biosynthesis of collagen. In: Ramachandran G N, Reddi A H (eds) Biochemistry of collagen. Plenum Press, New York and London, p 163-273

Quinn R A, Krane S M 1976 Abnormal properties of collagen lysyl hydroxylase from skin fibroblasts of siblings with hydroxylysine-deficient collagen. Journal of Clinical Investigation 57: 83-93

Ramachandran G N, Bansal M, Ramakrishnan C 1975 Hydroxyproline stabilises both intra-fibrillar structure as well as inter-protofibrillar linkages in collagen. Current Science 44: 1-3

Ramachandran G N, Ramakrishnan C 1976 Molecular structure: In Ramachandran G N, Reddi A H (eds) Biochemistry of Collagen. Plenum Press, New York and London, p 45-84

Rhodes R K, Miller E J 1978 Physical characterisation and molecular organisation of collagen A and B chains. Biochemistry 17: 3442-8

Rhodes R K, Miller E J 1979 The isolation and characterisation of the cyanogen bromide peptides from the B chain of human collagen. The Journal of Biological Chemistry 254: 12084-7

Robins S P, Shimokomaki M, Bailey A J 1973 The chemistry of the collagen cross-links. Age-related changes in the reducible components of intact bovine collagen fibres. Biochemical Journal 131: 771-80

Rojkind M, Giambrone M-A, Biempica L 1979 Collagen types in normal and cirrhotic liver. Gastroenterology 76: 710-19

Risteli J, Bächinger H P, Engel J, Furthmayr H, Timpl R 1980 7-S collagen: characterisation of an unusual basement membrane structure. European Journal of Biochemistry 108: 239-50

Rubin A L. Pfahl D, Speakman P T, Davison P F, Schmitt F O 1963 Tropocollagen. Significance of protease-induced alterations. Science 139: 37-9

Sage H, Bornstein P 1979 Characterisation of a novel collagen chain in human placenta and its relation to AB collagen. Biochemistry 18: 3815-22

Sage H, Woodbury R G, Bornstein P 1979 Structural studies on human type IV collagen. The Journal of Biological Chemistry 254: 9893-900

Schmitt F O, Hall C E, Jakus M A 1942 Electron microscope investigations of the structure of collagen. Journal of Cellular and Comparative Physiology 20: 11

Schuppan D, Timpl R, Glanville R W 1980 Discontinuities in the triple helical sequence Gly-X-Y of basement membrane (type IV) collagen. FEBS Letters 115: 297-301

Scott J E 1975 Composition and structure of the pericellular environment. Physiological function and chemical composition of pericellular proteoglycan (an evolutionary view). Philosophical Transactions of the Royal Society London B 271: 235-42

Scott J E, Orford C R, Hughes E W 1981 Proteoglycan-collagen arrangements in developing rat tail tendon. Biochemical Journal 195: 578-81

Scott P G, Veis A, Mechanic G L 1976 The identity of a cyanogen bromide fragment. A bovine dentine collagen containing the site of an intermolecular crosslink. Biochemistry 15: 3191-8

Shimokomaki M, Duance V C, Bailey A J 1980 Identification of a new disulphide bonded collagen from cartilage. FEBS Letters 121: 51-4

Siegel R C 1974 Biosynthesis of collagen cross-links. Increased activity of purified lysyl oxidase with reconstituted collagen fibrils. Proceedings of the National Academy of Science, USA 71: 4826-31

Siegel R C 1979 Lysyl oxidase. In: Hall D A, Jackson D S (eds) International Review of Connective Tissue Research, Vol 8. Academic Press, New York and London, p 73-118

Sopata I, Wojtecka-lukasik E, Dancewicz A M 1974 Solubilisation of collagen fibrils by human leocoyte collagenase activated by rheumatoid synovial fluid. Acta Biochemica Polonica 21: 283-9

Steven F S 1966 The depolymerising action of pepsin on collagen. Molecular weights of the component polypeptide chains. Biochimica et Biophysica Acta 130: 190-5

Steven F S, Podrazky V 1978 Evidence for the inhibition of trypsin by thiols: The mechanism of enzyme inhibitor complex formation. European Journal of Biochemistry 83: 155-61

Tanzer M L 1965 Experimental Lathyrism. In Hall D A, Jackson D S (eds) International Review of Connective Tissue Research, Vol 3.Academic Press, New York and London, p 91-112

Tanzer M L 1976 Cross-linking. In: Ramachandran G N, Reddi A H (eds) Biochemistry of Collagen. Plenum Press, New York and London, p 137-62

Timpl R, Glanville R W, Nowack H, Wiedemann H, Fietzek P P, Kühn K 1975 Isolation, chemical and electron microscopical characterisation of neutral-salt-soluble type III collagen and procollagen from foetal skin. Hoppe-Seyler's Zeitschrift für Physiologische Chemie 356: 1783-92

Tkocz C, Kühn K 1969 The formation of triple helical collagen molecules from $\alpha 1$ and $\alpha 2$ polypeptide chains. European Journal of Biochemistry 7: 454-62

Trelstad R L, Hayashi K 1979 Tendon collagen fibrillogenesis: Intracellular subassemblies and cell surface changes associated with fibril growth. Developmental Biology 71: 228-42

Trelstad R L, Kang A H, Igarashi S, Gross J 1970 Isolation of two distinct collagens from chick cartilage. Biochemistry 9: 4993-8

Tuderman L, Steinmann B, Peltonen L, Martin G, Prockop D J 1979 Evidence for a structural mutation in the procollagen synthesised by a patient with Ehlers Danlos syndrome type VII. Federation Proceedings 38: 1407

Uitto J 1979 Collagen polymorphism. Isolation and partial characterisation of $\alpha 1(I)$ trimer molecules in normal human skin. Archives of Biochemistry and Biophysics 192: 371-9

Veis A, Anesey J, Cohen J 1962 The characterisation of the γ component of gelatin. Archives of Biochemistry and Biophysics 98: 104-10

Veis A, Anesey J, Yuan L, Levy S J 1973 Evidence for an amino-terminal extension in high molecular-weight collagens from mature bovine skin. Proceedings of the National Academy of Science, USA 70: 1464-7

Weiss J B 1976 Enzymic degradation of collagen In: Hall D A, Jackson D S (eds) International Review of Connective Tissue Research, vol 7. Academic Press, New York and London, p 102-49

Weiss J B, Sedowofia K, Jones C 1980 Collagen degradation: a defended multi-enzyme system. In: Viidik A, Vuust J (eds) Biology of Collagen Academic Press, London and New York, p 113-34

Woolley D E, Roberts D R, Evanson J M 1976 Small molecular weight β_1 serum protein which specifically inhibits human collagenases. Nature 261: 325-7

Wycoff R W G, Corey R B 1936 X-ray diffraction pattern from reprecipitated connective tissue. Proceedings of the Society for Experimental Biology and Medicine 34: 285

Zaccharides M P A 1900 Des actions diverses des acides sur la substance conjonctive. Comptes Rendus Societe Biologie 52: 1127

2

Proteins containing collagen sequences

K. B. M. REID

INTRODUCTION

With the exception of the well defined collagen molecules, only two proteins have been extensively characterized which are considered to contain collagen-like amino acid sequences, in the form of a triple helix, as part of their structure. These two proteins, C1q and acetylcholinesterase, appear to be quite unrelated in terms of the functions that they perform. They also differ significantly in terms of structure, since in C1q the collagen-like sequences and globular type sequences are found, in approximately the same proportion, within the same polypeptide chain whereas for acetylcholinesterase this does not appear to be the case. The precise reasons for the presence of triple helical regions in either protein is not clear but studies, such as those involving collagenase digestion, indicate that these regions are of considerable importance for the expression of full biological activity.

A third protein which clearly has collagen-like amino acid sequences (two short sections of approximately 60–70 residues) alternating with non-collagenous sequences is the 62 000 molecular weight glycoprotein isolated from lung lavage material of patients with alveolar proteinosis (Bhattacharyya, 1980). However, it is not known if these short sections of collagen-like sequences are involved in triple helix formation and the biological role of this glycoprotein, which is also found in the lung lavage and lameller bodies of normal animals, is unknown.

C1q: LOCATION, PRIMARY FUNCTION AND INITIAL OBSERVATIONS WHICH INDICATED SOME SIMILARITY TO COLLAGEN

C1q, a glycoprotein of 410 000 molecular weight, is a subcomponent of the classical pathway of complement (Porter & Reid, 1979) and is present in serum at a concentration of approximately 80 mg/l. C1q has an unusual amino acid composition, for a serum protein, since it contains 17 per cent glycine, 5 per cent 4-hydroxyproline and 2.1 per cent hydroxylysine (Yonemasu et al, 1971; Calcott & Müller-Eberhard, 1972; Reid et al, 1972), the hydroxylated amino acids not having been found, so far, in other well characterized serum proteins. The finding that approximately 80 per cent of the hydoxylysine residues in C1q are glycosylated by glucosylgalactosyl disaccharides or galactose monosaccharides (Shinkai & Yonemasu, 1979) is another indication of the similarity between a portion of C1q and some of the basement membrane collagens. Further similarity between C1q and the collagens can be seen in electron microscopy studies since a single molecule of C1q has the appearance of a bunch of flowers in which the lower half is composed of collagen-like 'stems' bunched together which then branch out, in the upper half, to give six separate collagen-like 'stems' each of which is joined to a globular 'head' (Shelton et al, 1972; Knobel et al, 1975; see Fig. 2.2 for a diagram giving the electron microscopy measurements). Another indication that there might be triple helical structure in C1q was obtained when it was found that bacterial collagenase fragmented the 'stems' of the molecule causing loss of activity (Reid et al, 1972; Brodsky-Doyle et al, 1976).

Probably the most important role that C1q plays in the blood is to recognize, and bind to, activators of the classical pathway of complement and thus bring about the activation of subcomponent C1r. The C1r and C1s subcomponents, which are both proenzymes of molecular weight 83 000, form a calcium dependent tetrameric complex-$C1r_2$-$C1s_2$which, in association with C1q yields C1, the first component of complement. C1q has not been shown to have any enzymic activity. C1q is able to bind, probably via its six globular 'heads', suitable activators such as immune aggregates containing immunoglobulin G, and bring about the activation of proenzyme C1r which in turn activates proenzyme C1s, thus allowing the sequential utilization of the later components in the pathway to take place (for review, see Porter & Reid, 1980). Therefore C1q acts as a link between the immune system and the complement system.

Human C1q has been used for most of the structural and

functional studies, however C1q has also been purified from the ox, dog, rat, guinea pig and frog. Even the frog C1q, which is interchangeable with human C1q in the in vitro haemolytic assays, possesses the unusual collagen-like features and has a similar shape to human C1q when viewed in the electron-microscope (Alexander & Steiner, 1980).

STRUCTURAL STUDIES AND MOLECULAR MODEL OF HUMAN C1q

Human C1q has a molecular weight of 410 000 in non-dissociating conditions and is composed of 18 polypeptide chains, each having a molecular weight of approximately 23 000 (Reid et al, 1972; Reid & Porter, 1976). There are three types of chain present in equimolar amounts thus yielding six A, six B and six C chains per molecule. Each C1q molecule contains nine disulphide-linked dimers of these chains, i.e. six A-B dimers and three C-C dimers, since there is a disulphide bond joining the A and B chains via the half-cystine residues at positions A4 and B4 and another between the half-cystine residues at two C4 positions and there are no other interchain disulphide bonds in the molecule (Figs. 2.1 and 2.2; Reid & Thompson, 1978). In each of the three types of chain, after a short N-terminal section of non-collagen-like amino acid sequence of two to eight residues, there is a region of approximately 80 residues of typical collagen-like sequence (which is broken at one point in each chain) followed by approximately 110 residues of globular type sequence which extends to the C-terminal (Figs. 2.1 and 2.2). All the hydroxyproline and hydroxylysine present in C1q is located in the collagen-like regions (Reid, 1979) and approximately 80 per cent of the hydroxylysine residues are glycosylated.

The imino acid contents of the A, B and C collagen-like regions are 14, 23 and 26 per cent respectively which is of the same order as that found in vertebrate collagens. Thus two of the most important requirements for the formation of a stable collagen-like triple helix, i.e. glycine as every third residue (with the exceptions noted below) and a high imino acid content, are present in C1q. The helical regions of the collagen molecules have been found to be formed from three polypeptide chains each containing strictly continuous stretches of the -Gly-X-Y-, repeating triplet, type of amino acid sequence. In contrast, the B and C chains of C1q show the presence of alanine at positions where glycine might be expected in their collagen — like sequences (at positions B9 and C36, Fig. 2.1). The A chain also has the continuity of it's collagen-like sequence broken, in this case by the insertion of a threonine residue between positions 38 and 39 (Fig. 2.1). Any model proposed for the structure of C1q would have to account for these 'breaks' in the A, B and C chain collagen-like regions.

Strong evidence for the view that these collagen-like sequences, found in C1q, do form triple helical structure comes from a variety of studies: limited proteolysis of the molecule with pepsin and bacterial collagenase; circular dichroism studies; electron microscopy studies.

1 10 20 30
A-chain Glu-Asp-Leu-Cys-Arg-Ala-Pro-Asp-Gly-Lys-Hyl- Gly- Glu-Ala- Gly-Arg-Hyp-Gly-Arg-Arg-Gly-Arg-Hyp-Gly-Leu-Hyl-Gly-Glu-Gln-Gly-Glu-Hyp-
B-chain Glu-Leu-Ser-Cys-Thr-Gly-Pro-Hyp-Ala-Ile- Hyp- Gly- Ile- Hyp- Gly- Ile- Pro- Gly- Thr- Pro-Gly-Pro-Asp-Gly-Gln-Hyp-Gly-Thr-Hyp-Gly-Ile-Hyl-
C-chain Asn-Thr-Gly-Cys-Thr-Gly-Ile-Hyp-Gly-Met-Hyp-Gly-Leu-Hyp-Gly-Ala-Hyp-Gly-Lys-Asp-Gly-Tyr-Asp-Gly-Leu-Hyp-Gly-Pro-Hyp-Gly-Glu-Pro-

40 50 60
A-chain -Gly- Ala- Hyp- Gly- Ile- Arg- Thr- Gly-Ile-Gln————————Gly-Leu-Hyl-Gly-Asp-Gln-Gly-Glu-Hyp-Gly-Pro-Ser-Gly-Asn-Hyp-Gly-Lys-Val-Gly-Tyr-
B-chain -Gly-Glu-Hyl-Gly- Leu- Hyp————Gly-Leu-Ala-Gly-Asp-His-Gly-Glu-Phe-Gly-Glu-Hyl- Gly-Asp- Pro-Gly-Ile-Hyp-Gly-Asp-Hyp-Gly-Lys-Val-Gly-Pro-
C-chain -Gly-Ile-Hyp-Ala-Ile-Hyl———————Gly-Ile-Arg————————Gly-Pro-Hyp-Gly-Gln-Hyl-Gly-Glu-Pro-Gly-Leu-Hyp-Gly-His-Hyl-Gly-Lys-Asp-Gly-Pro-

70 80 90
A-chain -Hyp-Gly-Pro-Ser-Gly-Pro- Leu- Gly- Ala- Arg- Gly- Ile- Hyl- Gly- Ile- Hyl- Gly-Thr- Hyp- Gly- Ser- Pro-Gly-Asn-Ile-Lys-Asp-Gln-Pro-Arg-Pro-Ala-Phe-
B-chain -Hyl-Gly-Pro-Met-Gly-Pro-Hyl-Gly-Pro-Hyp-Gly-Ala-Hyp-Gly-Ala-Hyp-Gly- Pro-Hyl-Gly- Glu-Ser-Gly-Asp-Tyr-Lys-Ala-Thr-Gln-Lys-Ile-Ala-Phe-
C-chain -Asn-Gly-Pro-Hyp-Gly- Met-Hyp-Gly-Val-Hyp-Gly-Pro-Met-Gly-Ile-Hyp-Gly-Glu-Pro-Gly-Glu-Glu-Gly-Arg-Tyr-Lys-Gln-Lys-Phe-Gln-Ser-Val-Phe-

After the phenylalanine residue, equivalent to position 97, there are approximately 100 residues of non-collagen-like amino acid sequence to the C-terminus of each of the chains.

Fig. 2.1 The N-terminal amino acid sequences of the A-, B-, and C- chains of human C1q.
The numbering of amino acid residues in all three chains is based on the B-chain sequence. The optimal alignment for showing the maximum homology between the three chains is obtained if a gap is left between positions 38 and 39 in the B- and C- chain sequences to allow for the extra threonine in the A- chain sequence; a triplet gap is left between residues 41–45 in the A- and C- chain sequences to allow for an 'extra' triplet in the B-chain sequence. The sequences shown are from Reid (1979). All, except three (at positions B-50, B-65 and C-38) of the 14 hydroxylysine residues found in the collagen — like sequences appear to be glycosylated.

FRAGMENTS PRODUCED BY LIMITED DIGESTION OF C1q WITH PEPSIN OR BACTERIAL COLLAGENASE

The non-triple-helical regions of collagen or procollagen are readily fragmented to yield small peptides on incubation with pepsin, at low temperatures, in dilute acid, while the triple helical-regions are, in general, left intact. Digestion of human C1q with pepsin at pH 4.4, at 37°C, was found to fragment most of the C-terminal globular 'head' regions of the molecule to small peptides while leaving the collagen regions intact (Reid, 1976). This large peptic fragment of approximately 176 000 molecular weight was shown by amino acid sequence studies (Reid, 1976), circular dichroism and electron microscopy studies (Brodsky — Doyle et al, 1976) to be composed of the six connecting strands plus the fibril like end-piece of the C1q molecule (Fig. 2.2).

When C1q is digested with bacterial collagenase at pH 7.4, at 37°C, for 6–20 hours, then most of the collagen-like regions of the molecule are reduced to small peptides while the six peripheral globular 'heads' are left intact (Fig. 2.2; Reid et al 1972; Knobel et al, 1974; Hughes — Jones & Gardner, 1979; Pâques et al, 1979). Each peripheral globular 'head', of molecular weight 37 000–45 000 is considered to be composed of three non-covalently linked fragments i.e. the C-terminal region from each of the three types of chain found in C1q (Fig. 2.2).

These large fragments of C1q produced by limited proteolysis have proved useful in functional studies as well as in the chemical and physical studies. The collagen-like peptic fragment has been shown to inhibit the reconstitution of whole C1 activity from its C1q, C1r and C1s subcomponents which indicates that some portion of the collagen-like regions of the molecule may be employed in the binding of the tetrameric $C1r_2$-$C1s_2$ complex and in the activation of proenzyme C1r (Reid et al, 1977). Studies on preparations of the isolated globular 'head regions show that these regions contain the binding sites, present in C1q, for the Fc region of aggregated immunoglobulin G (Hughes — Jones & Gardner, 1979; Pâques et al, 1979).

Circular dichroism and electron microscopy studies

The circular dischroism spectra and extrema obtained, for intact C1q and the collagen-like peptic fragment of C1q, are consistent with the presence of triple helical structure since they are similar to those obtained for lathyritic rat skin collagen (Brodsky — Doyle et al, 1976). This was most clearly demonstrated with the peptic fragment which gave a positive band at 223 nm and a negative band at 200 nm (with magnitudes of mean residue ellipticity of + 2200 and − 16450 respectively) compared with lathyritic rat skin collagen which gave a positive band at 220 nm and a negative band at 198 nm (with magnitudes of +6000 and − 50 000 respectively). From the amino acid sequence data (Fig. 2.1) it can be calculated that approximately 84 per cent of the residues in the peptic fragment are in the form of -Gly-X-Y- repeating triplet sequences, yet the magnitudes of both extrema are considerably less (one-quarter at 200 nm, one-half at 223 nm) than that expected for a sample of unaggregated collagen molecules containing 80 per cent triple helical structure. However, if the 16 per cent of the residues in the peptic fragment that do not have collagen-like sequences are in an α-helical or β-conformation, this could in part explain the low ellipticity observed at 223 nm since typical α-helical structures and β-structures show a high mean residue ellipticity at 223 nm. Aggregation of the triple helices, thought to be present in C1q, could also have some effect on the magnitude of the mean residue ellipticity since it has been found that aggregated α-helices give a considerably lower value than that found for unaggregated α-helices.

The band at 230 nm in the circular dichroism spectrum of the peptic fragment of C1q can be readily abolished by bacterial collagenase or heat treatment (Brodsky — Doyle et al, 1976), however both the intact C1q and the peptic fragment of C1q show a higher melting temperature (by approximately 10°C) than that observed for lathyritic rat skin collagen. Therefore it is possible that aggregation of the six triple helices, postulated to be present in a single C1q molecule, (Fig. 2.2) stabilizes the molecule against heat denaturation.

Electron micrographs of C1q (Shelton et al, 1972; Knobel et al, 1975) indicate quite clearly that the molecule is divided into two distinct types of structure i.e. six globular 'heads', each connected by strands to a central fibril-like region (Fig. 2.2). Electron micrographs of the peptic fragment shows that all the collagen-like region of C1q is located in the connecting strands and fibril-like region (Brodsky — Doyle et al, 1976). It is of interest that even after the six globular heads have been removed that the postulated triple — helical regions still appear to bend approximately half-way along their length (Brodsky — Doyle et al, 1976).

Molecular model proposed for human C1q

From the studies described above it is probable that approximately 40 per cent of the C1q molecule is composed of collagen-like triple helical structure which is formed from the 81-residue-long stretches of collagen-like sequence found in the six A, six B and six C chains. Three regions of collagen-like sequence, one from each chain, could yield a triple helix of dimensions 81×0.29 nm = 23.4 nm long and 1.5 mn in diameter (0.29 nm and 1.5 nm being taken as the length and diameter respectively of the cross-section of a one residue long stretch of collagen triple helix — Traub & Piez, 1971). Two triple helices, formed in this manner,

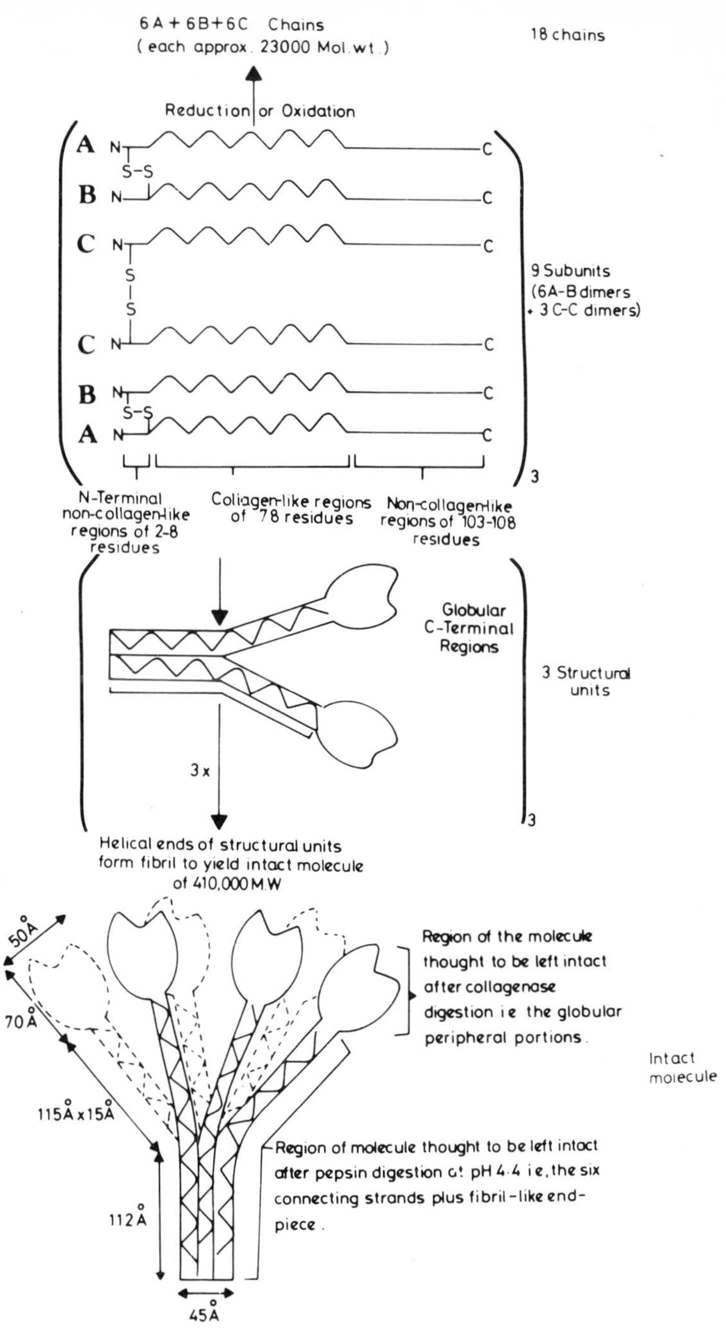

Fig. 2.2 Structure of human C1q.

The dimensions given are averages of those estimated from electron miscroscopy studies (Shelton et al, 1972; Knobel et al, 1975). It is proposed that the three different types of collagen — like sequence present in C1q will form triple helical regions as are found in collagen. ∼ , indicates the collagen-like regions of the molecule proposed to be in a triple helix.

Length of collagen-like connecting strand + length of fibril-like end-portion = 11.5 nm + 11.2 nm = 22.7 nm.

Length of triple helix proposed from the sequence studies = 81 × 0.29 nm = 23.4 nm.

This figure is taken from Reid and Porter (1976), note that 10 Å = 1 nm.

would have to be disulphide-linked via the bond located between the two C chains at position four in each of the C chains (Figs. 2.1 & 2.2). Then, six triple helices, lined in parallel along their N-terminal halves, could give a region of approximately 11.2 nm long and 4.5 nm in diameter which could correspond to the fibril-like end piece (Fig. 2.2). The remaining halves of each of the six individual triple helices, which were not involved in fibril formation, could represent the six connecting strands (11.5 × 1.5 nm each) seen in the electron microscopy studies (Fig. 2.2). The reason why each of the connecting strands appears to be set at an angle to the fibril — like central portion can be predicted from the sequence data which shows the presence of an alanine at position C36 and a threonine at position A39 (Fig. 2.1). These residues break the continuity of -Gly-X-Y- repeating triplet sequences in the C and A chains at a predicted position of 11.2 nm from the N-terminal end of the helix, if it is assummed that the initial glycine in each chain is involved in triple helix formation. This break in the continuity is likely to cause a distortion in each triple helix and thus cause the 'bends' seen in the collagen-like regions (Fig. 2.2). Each connecting strand is joined to one of the six peripheral globular 'heads'. Each 'head' is probably composed of the C-terminal 110 residues of one A, one B and one C chain (Fig. 2.2).

ACETYLCHOLINESTERASE: LOCATION, PRIMARY FUNCTION AND INITIAL OBSERVATIONS WHICH INDICATED SOME SIMILARITY TO COLLAGEN

Acetylcholinesterase (acetylcholine hydrolyase EC3. 1.1.7) catalyses the hydrolysis of choline esters and is primarily associated with the cells of nerve and muscle tissue. It can however be found in many other tissues and in whole blood there is a particulate form of the enzyme associated with red blood cell membranes (for review, see Rosenberry, 1975). Acetylcholinesterase's most important role is in controlling ionic currents in excitable membranes, and it has been shown by histochemical techniques that the enzyme is associated with both classes of excitable membrane i.e. conducting membrane and postsynaptic membrane. However it appears to be most concentrated in the endplates of the neuromuscular junction where it functions by terminating impulse transmission by hydrolysing the neurotransmitter acetylcholine. The enzyme appears to be associated with the acetylcholine receptor, in about equal concentrations, in the synaptic regions of excitable membrane. The enzyme and receptor, although they show some similarity in ligand binding properties, are distinct glycoproteins which can be extracted and isolated separately. However, while the receptor behaves as an integral membrane protein, in that it requires denaturing agents for its extraction and continued solubility during subsequent fractionation, the enzyme could be considered to be an extrinsic, or peripheral, membrane protein in that much of it is relatively easily removed by high ionic strength, or limited proteolysis, and it does not require denaturants to keep it in solution after removal from the membrane. The observation that acetylcholinesterase activity was at least three to six times higher in the end plate regions of postsynaptic plasma membranes led to the examination of the electric organs of electric fish. These organs are phylogenetically derived from muscle and very high concentrations of acetylcholinesterase were detected in them. Thus it has proved convenient to use the electric organs of the electric rays (Torpedo marmorata and Torpedo californica) or the electric eels (Electrophorus electricus) in the isolation of large amounts of acetylcholinesterase by affinity chromatography, on acridinium resin columns, of partially purified salt extracts (Daudi & Silman, 1974; Rosenberry & Richardson, 1977).

Initially, acetylcholinesterase, as isolated from electric organ tissue, was considered to be a globular protein with a sedimentation coefficient of 11S. However the use of very fresh tissue, and the development of affinity chromatography procedures, allowed the isolation of forms of the enzyme with sedimentation coefficients of 18S, 14S and 8S, all of which could be converted by mild proteolysis with trypsin to the globular 11S form (Massoulié & Reiger 1969; Massoulié et al, 1970). The 18S, 14S and 8S forms all differed from the globular 11S form in that they appeared as elongated structures in the electron microscope in which a multisubunit head was attached to a 'tail' which was approximately 50 nm long. The 18S form of the enzyme thus resembles a bunch of flowers in which 12 globular heads appear to be connected via three strands to a long 'tail' (Cartand et al, 1975; Rieger et al, 1973; Daudi et al, 1973; see Fig. 2.3 for a diagram giving the electron microscopy measurements). The appearance of the strands and 'tail', in these electron microscopy studies, was therefore suggestive that there might be triple-helical structures in the acetylcholinesterase molecule. The finding of approximately 1 per cent hydroxyproline and 0.7 per cent hydroxylysine in the 18S and 14S forms and no hydroxylated amino acids in the globular 11S form was further indirect evidence that the 'tail' might be composed of collagen-like amino acid sequences (Anglister & Silman, 1978; Rosenberry & Richardson, 1977; Lwebuga — Mukasa et al, 1976). The 'tail' region appears to contain sites which are susceptible to bacterial collagenase (Anglister & Silman, 1978) and a further similarity between collagen and the 'tail' region is indicated by the finding that the 18S + 14S forms of the enzyme, but not the 11S form, have antigenic sites in common with collagen isolated from rat tendon (Anglister et al, 1979).

STRUCTURAL STUDIES AND MOLECULAR MODEL OF ACETYLCHOLINESTERASE FROM THE ELECTRIC EEL

The 18S form of acetylcholinesterase has a molecular weight of approximately 1 100 000 and is composed of about 12 globular catalytic subunits, each of approximately 75 000 molecular weight, and a fibrous 'tail' (30–50 nm long) which is considered to be around 100 000 molecular weight. The 'tail', which may contain collagen-like triple helical structure, has not been isolated as a distinct structure free of all the catalytic subunits. Limited proteolysis of the 18S form of the enzyme can give rise to a number of different forms i.e. 14S, 8S and 11S which are all enzymically active. The 18S, 14S and 8S forms of the enzyme which all contain the 'tail' structure and are considered to contain 12, 8 and 4 globular catalytic subunits respectively (Bon et al, 1976; Daudi et al, 1973; Bon et al, 1973). The 11S form is considered to be composed of only four globular catalytic subunits and the rise in sedimentation coefficient from 8S to 11S on the loss of the 'tail' from the 8S form is attributed to the marked change in shape from an elongated structure to a completely globular type of structure.

Six of the twelve catalytic subunits in the 18S form of the enzyme are present as disulphide linked dimers which appear to be non-covalently bound to the rest of the molecule (Rosenberry & Rosenberry, 1977; Anglister & Silman, 1978) while the remaining six catalytic subunits are covalently attached to the 'tail' of the molecule via disulphide bonds. It is not absolutely clear if the six catalytic subunits, which are covalently attached to the 'tail', are also disulphide linked to each other in the same manner as the catalytic subunits which are not covalently attached to the 'tail'. In one model proposed for acetylcholinesterase it is suggested that each catalytic subunit has only one of its half-cystine groups involved in the formation of an interchain disulphide bond and that this half-cystine group would therefore be utilized in either linking one catalytic unit to another catalytic unit or to the 'tail' structure (Rosenberry, 1975; Rosenberry & Rosenberry 1977; Fig. 2.3).

The catalytic subunits, on their own, contain no hydroxylated amino acids and have a significantly lower

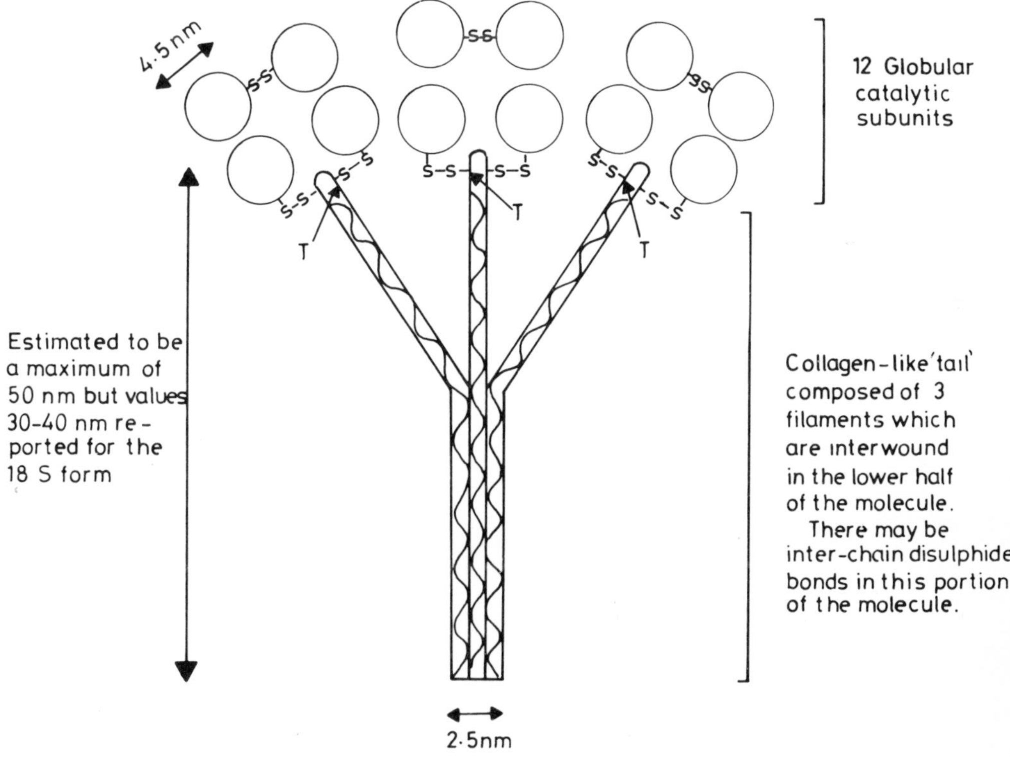

Fig. 2.3 Structure of acetylcholinesterase from the electric eel.
The dimensions given are averages of those estimated from electron microscopy studies (Cartaud et al, 1975; Rieger et al, 1973; Daudi et al, 1973). The model shown for the 18S form of acetylcholinesterase is taken from the models proposed by Rosenberry & Rosenberry (1977) and Anglister & Silman (1978). ∼ , indicates the collagen-like regions of the molecule proposed to be in a triple helix. T: represents the posssible sites of limited proteolysis by trypsin.

glycine content compared to the 18S and 14S forms of the enzyme (Rosenberry & Rosenberry, 1977; Anglister & Silman, 1978). The amino acid composition of the 'tail' structure can be estimated indirectly by calculating the difference in amino acid composition between a sample of 'tail' structure plus covalently bound catalytic subunits and a sample composed of only catalytic subunits (Rosenberry & Rosenberry, 1977). This procedure indicated that the 'tail' structure contained 7.2 per cent 4-hydroxyproline, 6.8 per cent hydroxylysine and 30.6 per cent glycine which would be consistent with a structure composed of at least 90 per cent collagen-like sequence. By examination of reduced and alkylated samples of the 18S molecule, before and after bacterial collagenase digestion, it was concluded that two polypeptide fractions, of apparent molecular weights 40 000 and 44 000, may contain these collagen-like sequences. The molecular weight estimations were made by SDS-polyacrylamide gel electrophoresis so that, in view of the anomalous behaviour of collagen-like polypeptides on SDS-gels, the true molecular weight of these polypeptides could be as low as 25 000 (Furthmayer & Timpl, 1971). If of the order of 90 per cent of these chains is in the form of -Gly-X-Yrepeating triplet sequence then it is possible that acetylcholinesterase contains collagen-like regions each of which is approximately 200 residues long, and which, if in the form of a triple helix, could give a collagen-like structure of 200 × 0.29 nm = 58 nm. (This value would more than accommodate the maximum length of 50 nm calculated for the 'tail' structure seen in the electron microscope studies.) As regards the number of triple helices whigh might be present in the 'tail', some of the electron microscopy studies (Cartaud et al, 1975) give the impression that there could be three since it was observed that the 'tail' structure of the 18S molecule appears to split into three individual filaments each of which was associated with one tetramer of globular catalytic subunits (Fig. 2.3). The filaments appeared to be interwound in the lower half of the molecule and thus a diameter of 2.5 nm would be consistent with the presence of three triple helices aligned in parallel (in a similar manner to that suggested for C1q). A molecular model of the type shown in Figure 2.3 (taken from: Rosenberry & Rosenberry, 1977; Anglister & Silman, 1978; Cartand et al, 1975) would predict that the 'tail' may be composed of three triple helices having a total molecular weight of 220 000 (which is about double the estimates that have been made). However, much further work is required before it can be seen if this type of model is correct since it has not been directly established that there is -Gly-X-Y-repeating triplet sequence in acetylcholinesterase, although studies such as those showing digestion of the 'tail', or part of the 'tail', with bacterial collagenase have provided strong indirect evidence.

It has been shown that acetylcholinesterase activity is associated with filamentous components of the basement membrane matrix, and that bacterial collagenase digestion will release the enzyme therefore it has been suggested that the role of the tail is to anchor the enzyme, possibly via the basement membrane, onto the cell surface (Silman, 1976).

HUMAN C1q IN HEALTH AND DISEASE

C1q has been shown to be synthesized by a wide variety of cells in culture, such as fibroblast, macrophages, monocytes and columner epithelial cells (see Porter & Reid, 1980 for a review). The finding that 2, 2′-dipyridyl markedly reduced C1q secretion by macrophages (Muller et al, 1978) is consistent with C1q and collagen being synthesized and secreted in a similar manner. A single major site of synthesis of the C1q found in the blood has not been identified but in view of its concentration (150 mg/l) and relatively high rate of catabolism (Kohler & Müller-Eberhard, 1972) an abundant cell type, like the fibroblast could be considered as a possible source. However fibroblast cell lines appear to synthesize and secrete a C1q molecule which is larger than that normally found in serum (Reid & Solomon, 1977) which may indicate that there is a 'pro' form of C1q.

In normal individuals the C1q serum levels full within quite a narrow range and in a study on the effect of age on C1q levels it was found that cord sera had approximately 60 per cent of the total normal mean level and that soon after birth the level rose to normal and stayed there up to the age of 40 years, after which it gradually increased (Yonemasu et al, 1978).

Deficiencies of C1q

Defects of the early acting components of the complement system, such as the genetic deficiencies of C1r, C4 or C2, are usually associated with immune complex diseases with vasculitis and lupus — like syndromes (for review, see Lachmann & Rosen 1978). Defects of other complement components, such as C3 or C3b inactivator, may cause recurrent bacterial infections or, in the case of defects involving the components C5, C6, C7 or C8, recurrent infections due to Neisserian organisms. Low plasma C1q levels have been reported in diseases such as systemic lupus erthematosus, chronic urticaria and a few well-characterized genetic immunodeficiency states. In these conditions, displaying low C1q levels, signs of utilization of the other early acting complement components, besides C1q, are present. However in two reports of a complete deficiency of C1q activity the lack of the functionally active C1q cannot be explained by the normal activation of the classical complement pathway since the components acting after C1q were found to lie within the normal range. In one case, a complete functional and immunological absence of C1q was found in a child who suffered from skin disease and recurrent sepsis (Berkel et al, 1977) but the genetic basis of this abnormality was not established (Berkel et al, 1979; Loos et al, 1980) since nine members of his family, including the parents and two healthy siblings, had close to normal C1q and total complement levels. In the other report, a brother and sister were found to completely lack functionally active C1q and immunochemical evidence was obtained which indicated the presence of a non-functional form of C1q in the patients' sera (Thompson et al, 1980). The brother (age 4) suffered from a lupus like syndrome and developed glomerulonephritis and has been successfully treated with oral prednisolone. His younger sister (age 2), who also lacked C1q and thus classical complement pathway activity, has only recently developed similar symptoms. The non-functional form of C1q was detected in both parents and another brother, who had close to normal and half-normal levels of C1 respectively, but was not detected in one other sister who had a normal C1 level. Therefore these functional and immunochemical studies on the complement levels of the members of this family, although not completely unambiguous, suggest that the defect described is the con an antigenically deficient, nonfunctional, molecule and which is expressed as a co-dominant allele. The parents, who would be obligate heterozygotes for the abnormal gene, have normal total complement levels and are clinically well. The total lack of functional C1q in two of the children followed by the development of an immune-complex renal disease, illustrates the importance of the classical complement pathway in clearing such complexes.

Although there are many similarities between C1q and collagen, in terms of their structure and biosynthesis, no clinical abnormalities in the collagen metabolism of any of the C1q deficient patients has been reported. Also, observations made of C1q levels, under conditions where there was a defect or impairment of collagen biosynthesis, suggests an apparent disassociation between C1q and collagen biosynthesis. For example in a family affected by Ehlers-Danlos syndrome type VI, the structure and function of the collagenous portion of C1q appears to be unimpaired (Hanauske-Abel & Rohm, 1980). As there is a reduction in the hydroxylysine content, but not the hydroxyproline content, of the collagen (types I and III) produced by fibroblast cultures obtained from patients suffering from this disease (Krieg et al, 1979; Quinn & Krane, 1979) (See Ch. 16), it might have been expected that the patients' C1q would also be affected in a similar manner.

Another example of the apparent disassociation between C1q biosynthesis and collagen biosynthesis is the retention of normal C1q levels in guinea pigs suffering from an acute vitamin C deficiency (Bates et al, 1978). Therefore under conditions where the synthesis of interstitial collagen was markedly impaired, due to the reduction in ascorbate-dependent prolylhydroxylase activity, the C1q and C1 apparently remained structurally and functionally unaffected. Possible reasons for this apparent disassociation between C1q and collagen biosynthesis have been discussed by Hananuske-Abel and Rohm (1980).

Possible functions of the collagen-like portion of C1q

In addition to being involved in the binding, and possibly activation, of the proenzymes C1r and C1s during activation of the classical complement pathway, the collagen-like portion of C1q may have other functions in the blood-stream. After the C1 complex, containing C1q and the proenzyme forms of C1r and C1s, has been activated then the activated forms of C1r and C1s are readily dissociated from C1q by the action of the C1-inhibitor present in the blood (Sim et al, 1979). The C1q remains bound to the activating agent, probably via its globular 'heads', and its collagen-like portion should now be free of any possible association with the $C1r_2$-$C1s_2$ complex. It is possible that the collagen-like portion may then interact with suitable receptors, such as those found on platelets or lymphoid cells.

Effects of C1q on platelet — collagen interaction

Platelets adhere readily to collagen and this binding causes the release of the contents of the platelet amine storage granules, the released ADP then contributes to platelet aggregation (see Barnes, Ch. 10, for a review). Intact native C1q, and the collagen — like peptic fragment of C1q, inhibit collagen-induced platelet aggregation (Cazenave et al, 1976; Wautier et al, 1977). The concentrations of C1q used to give good inhibition in those experiments were less than those which occur in plasma which suggests that it may be of some physiological significance that C1q can compete with collagen for specific sites on the platelet surface. It has been found that the region in C1q responsible for the interaction with platelets is located principally in the A chain section of the collagen-like portion of the molecule (Wautier et al, 1980).

Receptors for C1q on lymphoid cells

It has been reported that there are receptors for C1q on B-derived lymphoblastoid cells and peripheral lymphocytes (mainly non-T cells) (Ghebrehiwet & Müller-Eberhard, 1978; Gabay et al, 1979). Surface immunoglobulins do not appear to be involved in the C1q binding and the binding takes place via the collagen — like portion of C1q (Gabay et al, 1979).

Cross-reactivity of C1q with human collagen

Humoral and cellular reactivity to collagen has been demonstrated in several diseases such as scleroderma and rheumatoid arthritis. The finding of cross-reactivity of human type I collagen with the collagen-like portion of C1q suggests a possible involvement of C1q in these diseases (Menzel et al, 1980).

CONCLUSION

Although, so far, it has only been shown directly, by amino acid sequence studies, that C1q has -Gly-X-Y- repeating triplet sequences contained within the same polypeptide chain as non-collagen-like sequences, it is possible that the polypeptide chains in the 'tail' of the acetylcholinesterase molecule will show a similar mixture of sequences. However the studies in the case of acetylcholinesterase suggest that the 'tail' is composed almost entirely of collagenous material and that it is disulphide linked to the rest of the molecule. The finding of a mixture of the two types of amino acid sequence in one molecule is not very unexpected in view of the presence in procollagen chains of N-terminal extensions composed of both helical and non-helical regions and C-terminal extensions composed of entirely non-helical regions. Also discontinuities, of from one to eight amino acid residues, have been located within the triple helical regions of basement membrane (type 1V) collagen (Schuppan et al, 1980). It is probable that other proteins, such as the glycoprotein isolated from lung lavage material (Bhattacharyya, 1980), will be found to contain certain collagen-like features although they are not true collagens. Indeed, there is evidence that C1q may be responsible for only 45 per cent of the protein bound hydroxyproline present in human serum and that the remaining 55 per cent is associated with protein, or polypeptides, which differ from C1q in solubility at low ionic strength, electrophoretic mobility, size and reactivity to anti-C1q (Rosano & Hurwitz, 1977; Rosano et al, 1979). This protein, or polypeptide, serum fraction, if it is not derived from the breakdown products produced by the relatively high rate of catabolism of C1q (Kohler & Müller-Eberhard, 1972) could contain another, as yet uncharacterized, molecule with collagen-like features. Similarly, acetylcholinesterase may prove not to be unique among enzumes by its possession of a disulphide-linked, collagen-like, 'tail' and that perhaps this structure will turn out to be a common feature among other membrane associated enzymes.

REFERENCES

Alexander R J, Steiner L A 1980 The first component of complement from the bullfrog, Rana Catesbeiana: functional properties of C1 and isolation of subcomponent C1q. Journal of Immunol. 124: 1418

Anglister L, Silman I 1978 Molecular structure of elongated forms of electric eel acetylcholinesterase. Journal of Molecular Biology 125: 293

Anglister L, Tarrab-Hazdai R, Fuchs S, Silman I 1979 Immunological cross-reactivity between electric-eel acetylcholinesterase and rat-tail-tendon collagen. European Journal of Biochemistry 94: 25

Bates C J, Levene C I, Oldroyd R G, Lachmann P J 1978 Complement component C1q is insensitive to acute vitamin C deficiency in guinea pigs. Biochimica et Biophysica Acta 540: 423

Berkel A I, Sanol Ö, Thesen R, Loos M 1977 A case of selective C1q deficiency. Turkish Journal of Pediatrics 19: 101

Berkel A I, Loos M, Sanol Ö, Mauff G, Gungen Y, Örs U, Ersoy F, Yegin O 1979 Clinical and immunological studies in a case of selective complete C1q deficiency. Clinical and Experimental Immunology 38: 52

Bhattacharyya S N 1980 Characterization of collagenous and non-collagenous peptides of a glycopeptide isolated from alveoli of patients with alveolar proteinosis. Biochem. J. 193: 447

Bon S, Rieger F, Massoulié J 1973 Proprietes des formes allongée de l'acétylcholinestérase en solution. Rayon de Stokes, densite et masse. European Journal of Biochemistry 35: 372

Bon S, Huet M, Lemonnier M, Rieger F, Massoulié J 1976 Molecular forms of Electrophorous Acetylcholinesterase-Molecular weight and composition. European Journal of Biochemistry 68: 523

Brodsky-Doyle B, Leonard K R, Reid K B M 1976 Circular-dichroism and electronmicroscopy studies of human subcomponent C1q before and after limited proteolysis by pepsin. Biochemical urnal 159: 279

Calcott M A, Müller-Eberhard H J 1972 C1q protein of human complement. Biochemistry 11: 3443

Cartaud J, Rieger F, Bon S, Massoulie J 1975 Fine structure of electric eel acetylcholinesterase. Brain Research 88: 127

Cazenave J-P, Assimeh S N, Painter R H, Packham M A, Mustard J F 1976 C1q inhibition of the interaction of collagen with human platelets. Journal of Immunology 116: 162

Daudi Y, Silman I 1974 Acetylcholinesterase. Methods in Enzymology 34: 571

Daudi Y, Herzberg M, Silman I 1973 Molecular structures of acetylcholinesterase from electric organ tissue of the electric eel. Proceedings of the National Academy of Science, USA 70: 2473

Furthmayr H, Timpl R 1971 Characterization of collagen peptides by sodium dodecylsulphate-polyacrylamide electrophoresis. Analytical Biochemistry 41: 510

Gabay Y, Perlmann H, Perlmann P, Sobel A 1979 A rosette assay for the determination of C1q receptor-bearing cells. European Journal of Immunology 9: 787

Ghebrehiwet B, Müller-Eberhard H J 1978 Lysis of C1q-coated erythrocytes by human lymphoblastoid cell lines. Journal of Immunology 120: 27

Hanauske-Abel H M, Rohm K H 1980 The collagenous part of C1q is unaffected in the hydroxylysine deficient collagen disease. Federation of European Biochemical Societies Letters 110: 73

Hughes-Jones N C, Gardner B 1979 Reaction between the isolated globular subunits of the complement component C1q and IgG complexes. Immunochemistry 16: 697

Knobel H R, Heusser C, Rodrick M I, Isliker H 1974 Enzymatic digestion of the first component of human complement (C1q). Journal of Immunology 112: 2094

Knobel H R, Villiger W, Isliker H 1975 Chemical analysis and electron microscopy studies of human C1q prepared by different methods. European Journal of Immunology 5: 78

Kohler P F, Müller-Eberhard H J 1972 Human C1q-Studies in hypogammaglobulinemia, myeloma and systemic lupus erthyematosus. Journal of Clinical Investigation 51: 868

Krieg T, Feidmann U, Kessler W, Müller P K 1979 Biochemical characteristics of Ehlers-Danlos syndrome type VI in a family with one affeced infant. Human Genetics 46: 41

Lachmann P J, Rosen F S 1978 Genetic defects of complement in man. Springer Seminars in Immunopathology 1: 339

Loos M, Laurell A-B, Sjöholm A G, Mp8rtensson U, Berkel A I 1980 Immunochemical and functional analyses of a complete C1q deficiency in man. Journal of Immunology 124: 59

Lwebuga-Mukasa J S, Lappi S, Taylor P 1976 Molecular forms of acetylcholinesterase from Torpedo californica: their relationship to synaptic membranes. Biochemistry 15: 1425

Massoulié J, Rieger F 1969 L'acétylcholinestérase des organes électrique de poissons (torpille et gymnote), complexes membranaires. European Journal of Biochemistry 11: 441

Massoulie J, Rieger F, Tsuji S 1970 Solubilisation de l'acétylcholinestérase des organes électriques de gymnote-Action de la trypsine. European Journal of Biochemistry 14: 430

Menzel E J, Smolen J S, Reid K B M 1980 Immunological cross-reactivity between the collagen-like peptic fragment of human C1q and human type I collagen. Submitted for publication

Müller W, Hanauske-Abel H, Loos M 1978 Biosynthesis of the first component of complement by human and guinea pig peritoneal macrophages: evidence for an independent production of the C1 subunits. Journal of Immunology 121: 1578

Pâques E P, Huber R, Priess A, Wright J K 1979 Isolation of the globular region of subcomponent C1q of the first component of complement. Hoppe-Seyler's Zeitshrift fur Physiologie Chemie 360: 177

Porter R R, Reid K B M 1979 Activation of the complement system by antibody-antigen complexes: the classical pathway. Advances in Protein Chemistry 33: 1

Quinn S R, Krane S M 1979 Collagen synthesis by cultured skin fibroblasts from siblings with hydroxylysine deficient collagen. Biochimica et Biophysica Acta 585: 589

Reid K B M 1976 Isolation, by partial pepsin digestion, of the three collagen-like regions present in subcomponent C1q of the first component of complement. Biochemical Journal 155: 5

Reid K B M 1979 Complete Amino acid sequences of the three collagen-like regions present in subcomponent C1q of the first component of complement. Biochemical Journal 179: 367

Reid K B M, Porter R R 1976 Subunit composition and structure of subcomponent C1q of the first component of human complement. Biochemical Journal 155: 19

Reid K B M, Solomon E 1977 Biosynthesis of the first component of complement by human fibroblasts. Biochemical Journal 167: 647

Reid K B M, Thompson E O P 1978 Amino acid sequence of the N-terminal 108 amino acid residues of the B chain of subcomponent C1q of the first component of human complement. Biochemical Journal 173: 863

Reid K B M, Lowe D M, Porter R R 1972 Isolation and characterization of C1q, a subcomponent of the first component of complement, from human and rabbit sera. Biochemical Journal 130: 749

Reid K B M, Sim R B, Faiers A P 1977 Inhibition of the reconstitution of the haemolytic activity of the first component of human complement by a pepsin-derived fragment of subcomponent C1q. Biochemical Journal 161: 239

Rieger F, Bon S, Massoulié J 1973 Observation par microscopie électronique des formen allongées et globulaires de l'acétylcholinesterase de gymote (Electrophorus electricus) European Journal of Biochemistry 34: 539

Rosano C L, Hurwitz C 1977 Separation of hydroxyproline-containing protein from C1q (a subcomponent of complement) in serum. Clinical Chemistry 23: 1335

Rosano C L, Parhami N, Hurwitz 1979 Determination of C1q in human sera. Journal of Laboratory and Clinical Medicine 94: 593

Rosenberry T L 1975 Acetylcholinesterase. Advances in Enzymology 43: 103

Rosenberry T L, Richardson J M 1977 Collagen-like subunits in acetylcholinesterase. Structure of 18S and 14S acetylcholinesterase. Identification of collagen-like subunits that are linked by disulphide bonds to catalytic subunits. Biochemistry 16: 3550

Rotundo R L, Fambrough D M 1979 Molecular forms of chicken embryo acetylcholinesterase in vitro and in vivo. Journal of Biological Chemistry 254: 4790

Schuppan D, Timpl R, Glanville R W 1980 Discontinuities in the triple helical sequence Gly-X-Y of basement membrane (type 1V) collagen. FEBS Letters 115: 297

Shelton E, Yonemasu K, Stroud R M 1972 Ultrastructure of the human complement component, C1q. Proceedings of the National Academy of Science, USA 69: 65

Shinkai H, Yonemasu K 1979 Hydroxylysine-linked glycosides of human complement subcomponent C1q and of various collagens. Biochemical Journal 177: 847.

Silman I 1976 Molecular structure of acetylcholinesterase. Trends in Biochemical Sciences 1: 225

Sim R B, Arlaud G J, Colomb M G 1979 C1 Inhibitor-dependent dissociation of human complement component C1 bound to immune complexes. Biochemical Journal 179: 445

Thompson R A, Haeney M, Reid K B M, Davies J G, White R H R, Cameron A H 1980 A genetic defect of the C1q complement subcomponent associated with childhood (immune complex) nephritis. New England Journal of Medicine, 303: 22

Traub W, Piez K A 1971 The chemistry and structure of collagen. Advances in Protein Chemistry 25: 243

Wautier J-L, Souchon H, Reid K B M, Peltier A P, Caen J P 1977 Studies on the mode of reaction of the first component of complement with platelets: interaction between the collagen-like portion of C1q and platelets. Immunochemistry 14: 763

Wautier J-L, Reid K B M, Legrand Y, Caen J P 1980 Region of the C1q molecule involved in the interaction between platelets and subcomponent C1q of the first component of complement. Molecular Immunology, 17: 1399

Yonemasu K, Kitagina H, Tanabe S, Ochi T, Shinkai H 1978 Effect of age on C1q and C3 levels in human serum and their presence in colestrum. Immunology 35: 523

Yonemasu K, Stroud R M, Niedermeier W, Butler W T 1971 Chemical studies on C1q: A modulator of immunoglobulin biology. Biochemical and Biophysical Research Communications 43: 1388

3

Structure of the collagen fibril: an interpretation

J. WOODHEAD-GALLOWAY

> How odd it is that anyone should not see that all observation must be for or against some view if it is to be of any service.
>
> Charles Darwin (1861): letter to Henry Fawcett

> See the value of imagination said Holmes . . . we imagined what might have happened, acted upon the supposition and find ourselves justified. Let us proceed.
>
> Sir Arthur Conan Doyle: Silver Blaze

INTRODUCTION

My aim in this chapter is to give an idea of how collagen molecules interact with one another and how some of these interactions result in the formation of the collagen fibril by self assembly. I shall do this by showing how simple theoretical ideas may illuminate observations made under the electron microscope or using X-ray diffraction.

ELECTRON MICROSCOPY AND X-RAY DIFFRACTION

Both electron microscopy and X-ray diffraction are means of observing structure on a small scale. To some extent the methods are complementary in the degree of detail each can reveal (Fig. 3.1). Roughly speaking X-ray diffraction covers the range 1Å (0.1 nm) to about 1000 Å (100 nm) and the electron microscope that from about 30 Å (3 nm) in tissues to 10 000 Å (1000 nm = 1 μm) where the optical microscope has taken over. Since both techniques present some problems of interpretation, the overlap of applicability in the mid-range is valuable — it allows comparisons of what each of the techniques purports to be revealing, and many important features of collagen fall within this range. Both methods rely on the scattering power of the electrons within the atoms of the specimen. In X-ray diffraction a beam of X-rays is scattered by the object and falls on a photographic film to form a diffraction pattern. For the microscope, a beam of electrons is used which are focused before and after scattering by electromagnetic lenses. A book such as Lipson and Lipson's *Optical Physics* explains the relationship between the principles on which the two methods are based. Interpretation of electron micrographs is relatively direct. It is customarily presumed that the micrograph is a snapshot of the object. Interpretation of an X-ray diffraction pattern is rarely accomplished so immediately (see below).

A beam of electrons is not scattered strongly by the atoms usually found in biological structures — much of the energy is absorbed by the specimen. Thus the specimen at once is vulnerable to the destructive power of the beam and has little contrast. To obviate both these drawbacks the material is usually fixed and stained with heavy-metal salts (or shadowed with heavy-metal atoms). We shall be concerned only with the former method.

Positive staining involves a fairly long immersion of the specimen in the salt solution followed by removal of excess stain — some remains stuck to the specimen. As will be seen later, the stain often adheres rather specifically, for example in proteins it binds to those amino acids with charged side chains. *Negative* staining merely uses the stain to *outline or fill* topological features of the specimen. Figure 3.2 illustrates and contrasts the appearance of the collagen fibril using the two methods.

X-rays are not particularly destructive to tissues, which is fortunate since patterns may take hours or even days to produce (whereas electron micrographs take only a few seconds). The chief practical problem in obtaining a pattern is to keep the specimen in the state in which it existed in the animal until a picture is produced. Specimens are, for that reason, always encased in 'wet cells'. For many purposes the experimental problems are not very formidable. On the other hand interpretation is often difficult and because the nature of X-ray diffraction evidence is not well understood in general, it is worth drawing attention to one or two points.

At the heart of interpretation lies the mathematical entity, the *Fourier Transform*, which provides the link between the structure under investigation and the diffraction pattern which is observed. In particular if the electron density in an atom is represented as $\rho\ (\underline{r})$, where $\underline{r}$ is the distance from the nucleus, then the Fourier

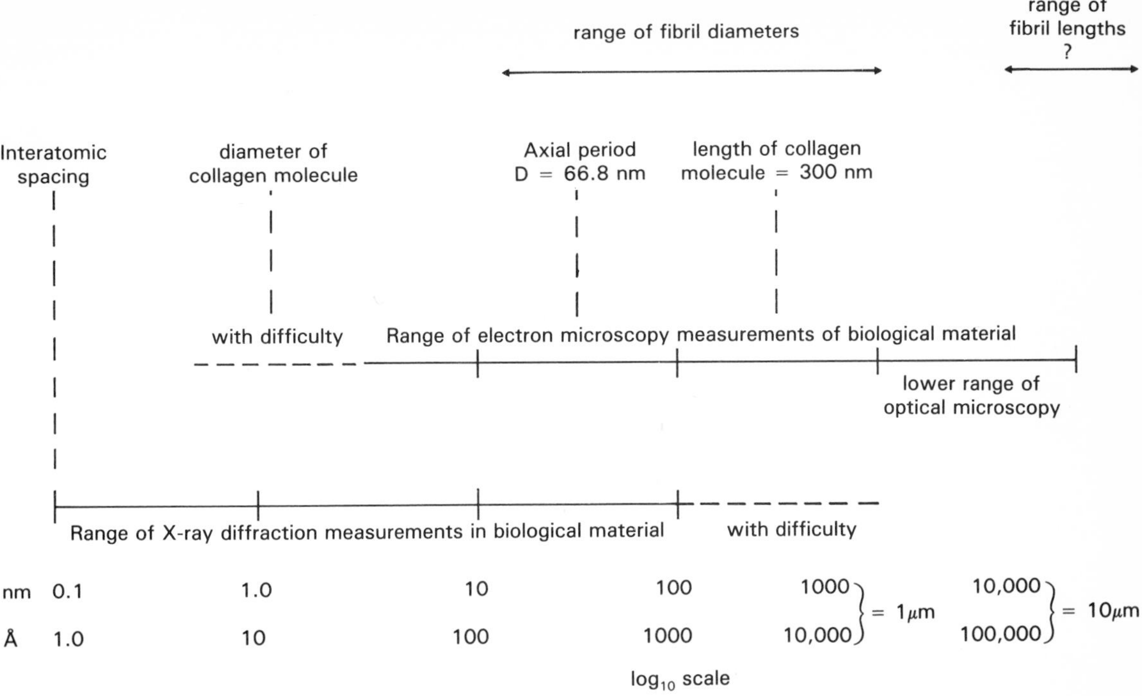

Fig. 3.1 Diagram to show the degree of structural detail accessible to X-ray diffraction and electron-microscopy.

Transform of the density is given by

$$f(\underline{K}) = \int \rho(\underline{r})\, e^{-i\underline{K}\cdot\underline{r}}\, dV \qquad (1)$$

$\underline{K}$ is a vector which defines points in 'diffraction space'. For practical purposes it is related to the wavelength, λ, of the X-rays used and the angle, ψ, through which the X-rays are diffracted and which is measurable on a diffraction photograph produced by a camera of known geometry.

$$\underline{K} = \frac{4\pi}{\lambda} \cdot \sin\theta \qquad (2)$$

Diffraction is a combination of scattering and interference among the scattered waves. Since interference involves combining waves emanating from two points simultaneously it follows that the *intensity*, I, of scattering from an assembly of N atoms is given (more or less exactly) by

$$I(\underline{K}) \propto \sum_{n}^{N} \sum_{m}^{N} f_n(\underline{K})\, f_m(\underline{K})\, e^{i\underline{K}\cdot(\underline{r}_n - \underline{r}_m)} \qquad (3)$$

The importance of this relationship can scarcely be overestimated. In 1933 Bernal and Crowfoot stated — 'the intensive analysis of X-ray diffraction patterns is one of the chief means of transformation from the classical qualitative chemistry of the 19th century to the quantum mechanical metrical chemistry of the present day'. Today this is equally true of (molecular) biology.

However the success of methods involving X-ray diffraction in chemistry, biochemistry and molecular biology — for example in the revealing of the detailed atomic structure of insulin and haemoglobin — have led to a somewhat unwarranted faith in structures proposed on the basis of the method.

Two particular points are worth noting. First, the Fourier Transform is what mathematicians call a *Functional* — in practical terms *each point*, $\underline{K}$, in the diffraction pattern involves information collected from *every point* in the specimen under observation. Thus in a pattern obtained from cartilage, say, each point in the pattern includes information about the collagen molecule, the way molecules are arranged in fibrils, the distribution of fibrils, as well as similar information for the polysaccharides and water (see Ch. 4 by D.W.L. Hukins). Second, it is true that diffraction patterns can be used diagnostically — they are very characteristic of the material being studied — but in the absence of the conceptual simplification and technological paraphernalia of single-crystal protein crystallography their interpretation in detail is difficult. A structure must be imagined, its consequences compared with the data, and a judgment made of how good is the fit between the two. At least a dozen models have been proposed for the three-dimensional structure of the

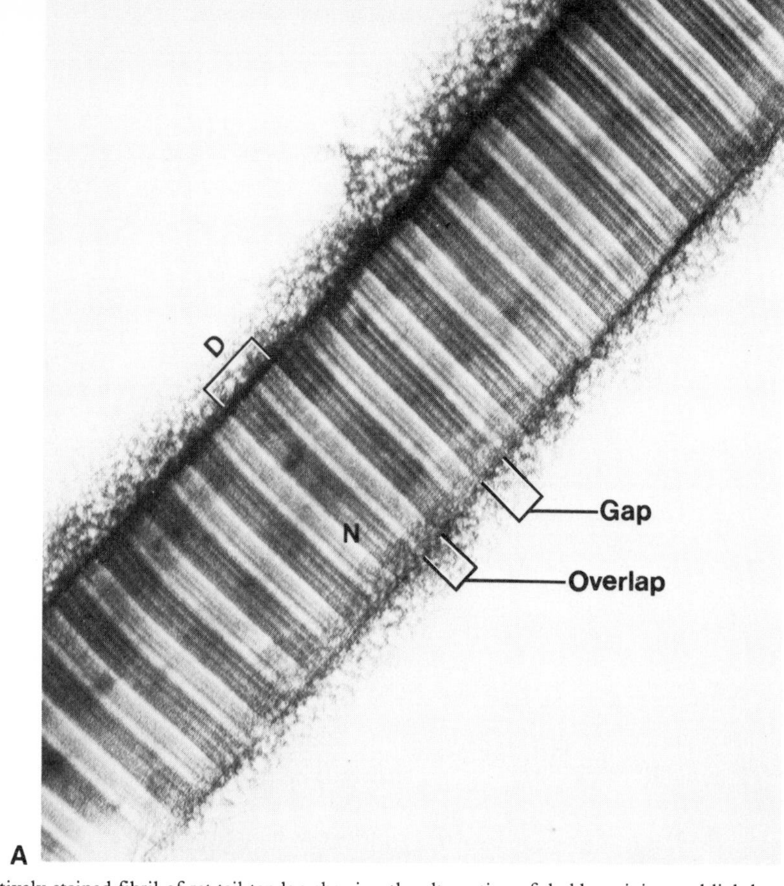

Fig. 3.2A Negatively stained fibril of rat-tail tendon showing the alternation of darkly staining and lightly staining regions, explained by the gap/overlap model of Hodge and Petruska.

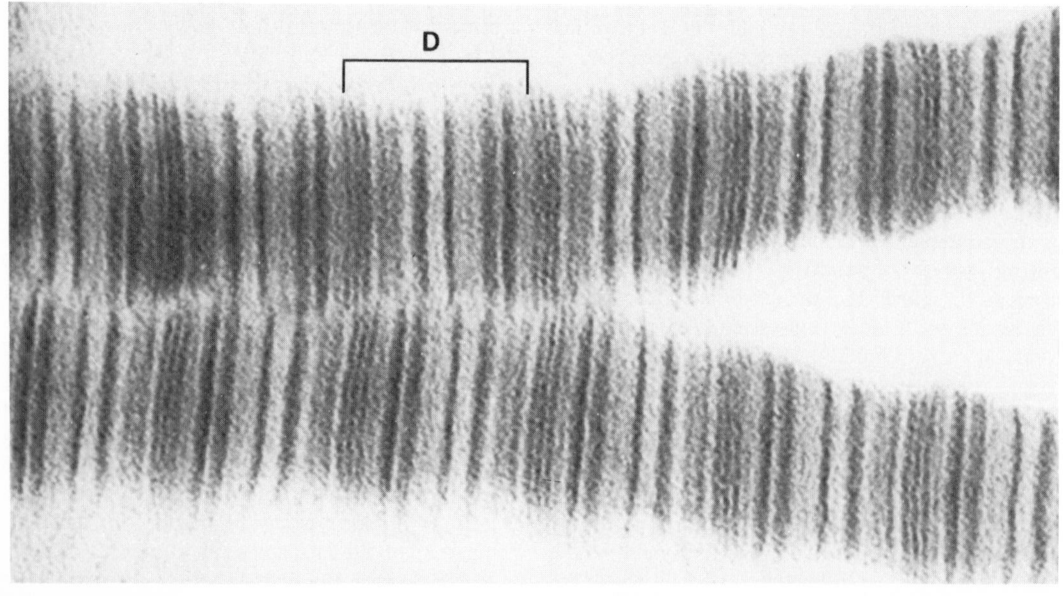

Fig. 3.2B Positively stained fibrils of rat-tail tendon showing the cross striations. (See section on the fibril in an axial projection for an explanation of these in terms of the distribution of charged residues in the collagen molecule). The two fibrils point in opposite directions illustrating the directionality of the fibrils under positive staining.

collagen fibril, most of which have claimed support from X-ray diffraction data. A model being accepted means only that at present there does not seem to exist a better one. Remember that science is the art of the provisional as well as the soluble.

It has not been my intention to depress the readers of my chapter, merely to suggest that a little scepticism is usually in order when given a solution to a problem. Nor will the story be developed historically except where there is an interesting explanatory advantage to be gained. For those interested in history, an appendix is included listing some of the events leading to our present picture of the organisation of molecules within the fibril.

THE AXIALLY-PERIODIC FIBRIL

Overwhelmingly in animal tissues, collagen is present as fibrils, threads at least some tens to hundreds of micrometres long and a few tens to hundreds of nanometres in diameter. The ceratotrichia (fin rays) of some fish each seem to consist of a single giant fibril of the order of a millimetre across.

A fibril is characterised by an (as will be seen later, *apparent*) axial period whose repeat distance of 66.8 nm is usually referred to as D. I shall suppose this feature to be of central importance. And indeed the whole of this chapter concerns its significance and explanation.

Figure 3.2 shows fibrils (in this case from rat tail tendon) as they appear negatively and positively stained (remember the previous section). In both, the axial periodicity can be seen quite clearly. The same feature is revealed in low angle X-ray diffraction patterns from tendons and some other collagens (Fig. 3.3). The set of strong equally spaced reflections near the meridian of the pattern is a consequence of the axial period.

The negative-staining pattern shows that there is a regular alternation of dense and less dense regions along the fibril axis, a feature suggested in 1963 by Hodge and Petruska (see section on Gaps and Overlaps) though anticipated on the basis of X-ray diffraction patterns by Tomlin and Worthington in 1956. Fibrils are not only periodic, they are also polar (Fig. 3.2B), possessing a unique directionality.

THE COLLAGEN MOLECULE

A collagen molecule is a triple helix of three amino acid α-chains. Its length, L, is about 295 nm. For example in type 1 collagen the α-chains have a central part, about 290 nm long, consisting of 1014 residues (338 triplets) of an average translation along the molecular length of 0.287 nm. Terminal peptides of an unknown (though often speculated about) and perhaps not well defined conformation, add about 5 nm to this. For the moment I will neglect the molecule's detailed structure, primary and secondary, and suppose that it is a simple cylinder of diameter rather more than 1 nm.

The point to observe here is that the molecule's length, L, is far greater than the axial period, D, of intact fibrils. In fact

$$\frac{L}{D} \simeq 4.4 \qquad (4)$$

This value varies a little among different collagen types, probably because of the variable length of the terminal peptides.

GAPS AND OVERLAPS

F.O. Schmitt et al, 1955, noted the relation of (4) but supposed that this was an experimental approximation to the integral relationship

$$L \neq 4D$$

(At that time in the early fifties, L and D were not known very precisely.)

They suggested that molecules are arranged parallel to the fibril axis and 'staggered' with respect to one another by a distance of $L/4$, this giving rise to the axial period.

This suggestion was refined by Hodge and Petruska in 1963 who realised that the non-integral nature of the relationship explained the appearance of the fibril when negatively-stained. Molecules are staggered by D or an integral multiple of it (Fig. 3.4) but this leaves between the end of one molecule and the next a 'gap' (see Fig. 3.5) of length

$$L_G = 5D - L \simeq 0.6\mathrm{D} \qquad (5)$$

(See Fig. 3.2A where stain has been taken up by the gaps.) The part of the D-period which is not a gap is usually referred to as the overlap (for obvious reasons) and is of length

$$L_O = L - 4D \simeq 0.4D \qquad (6)$$

Thus the speculation of Tomlin and Worthington in 1956 is seen to be correct (see Fig. 3.3A).

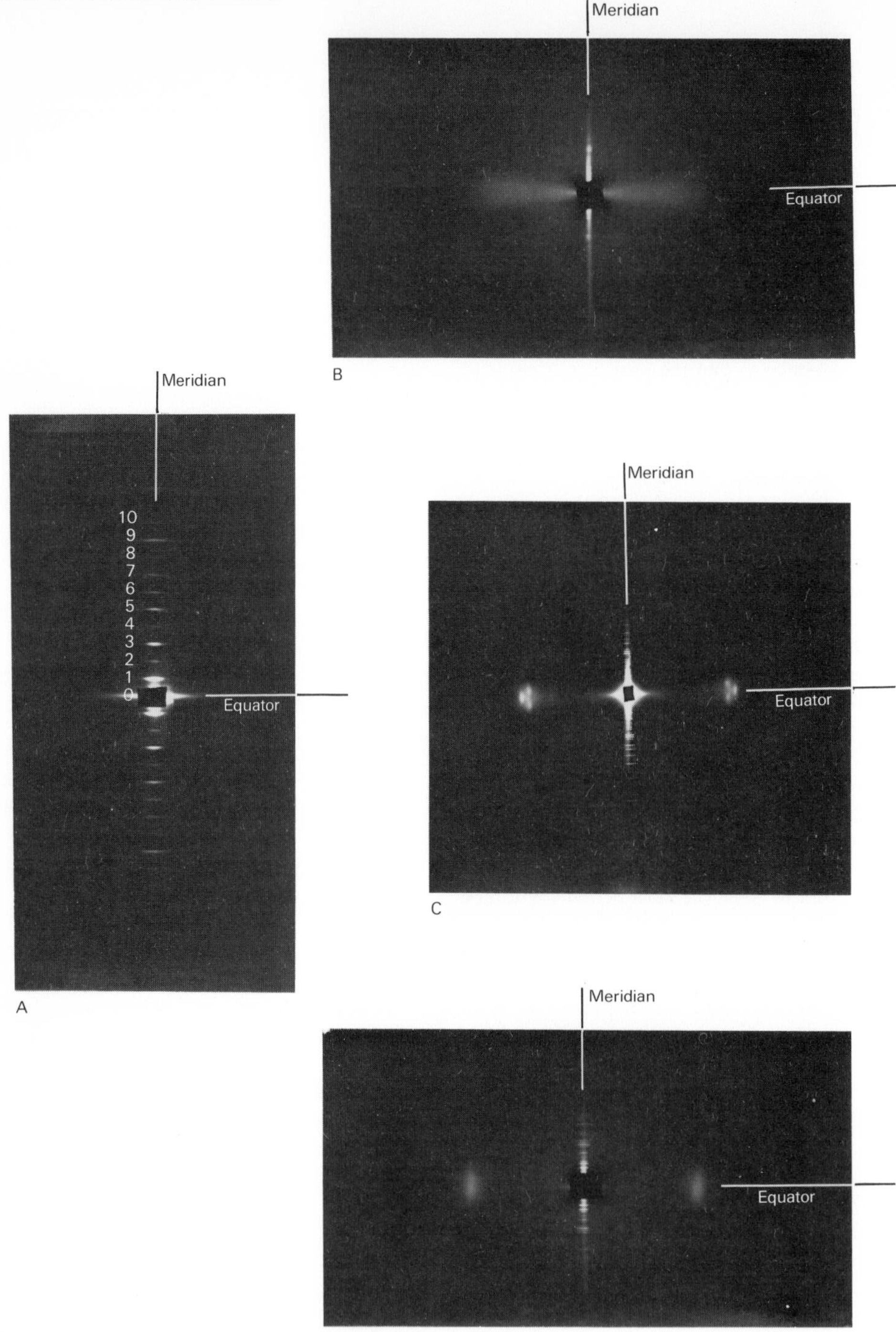

Fig. 3.3 Low angle X-ray diffraction patterns from collagens.
(A) Meridional pattern is a series of sharp equally spaced 'reflections'. The orders are numbered. The relative weakness of the second and fourth orders suggests that the D-period is a step function; a dense and a less dense region. The meridional pattern can be seen quite clearly in the other three pictures which show also the equatorial intensity.
(B) A simple continuous fan of diffuse scatter from wet elastoidin.
(C) Pattern obtained from wet rat-tail tendon. A number of discrete reflections are superposed on a diffuse fan similar to that seen in elastoidin.
(D) In this pattern from dried tendon a diffuse peak may be seen corresponding to a distance between neighbouring molecules of about 1.1 nm–1.2 nm.

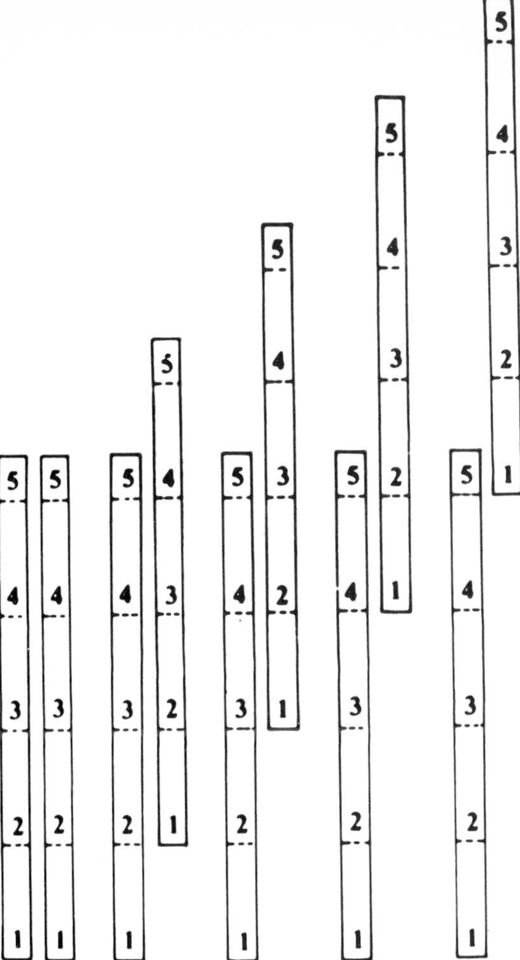

Fig. 3.4 Allowed molecular relationships implied by the Hodge-Petruska model, i.e. staggers of integral multiples of D. The molecule has been divided into five segments (numbered). Thus an intermolecular relation can be specified either by giving the degree of mutual stagger or by giving the numbers of a pair of adjacent segments (one on each molecule). In native fibrils neighbouring molecules related by a stagger of 4D allow a covalent cross-link involving a hydroxylysine in the triple helix and a lysine in the terminal peptide.

THE FIBRIL IN AN AXIAL PROJECTION

It is clear from Figure 3.5 that the true axial period of a fibril is $5D$ (= 334 nm). It is equally clear from electron microscopy and X-ray diffraction that the fibril's *apparent* period is D. How may these seemingly conflicting views be reconciled?

The meridional X-ray diffraction pattern gives information about structure in an axial projection, as though the whole electron density of the tendon were condensed (projected) on to the axis of the fibre. Equally, electron-micrographs of whole fibrils reveal no details of side to side packing of molecules, showing merely an averaged structure equivalent to an axial projection.

Figure 3.5 shows that any two molecules in the fibril must be related axially by a displacement of

$$Q5D + PD \tag{7}$$

where Q and P are integers; Q, the number of true periods intervening, may take any value within a limit set by the fibril's length; P, the remaining number of fractional true periods, is restricted to the values 0, 1, 2, 3, 4. The condition for a group of molecular strands to possess a true axially projected D-period is that between any one molecule and all the others the relationships corresponding to the five values of P must occur with equal frequency. This condition is equivalent to, within any single D-period, the five molecular segments of Figure 3.4 appearing with equal frequency.

This may be achieved in three quite distinct ways. First a fibril may be an assembly of unitary objects which are themselves D-periodic — the microfibril concept (Smith, 1968). I do not propose to discuss this option further here, but see the section on self assembly, the acknowledgements and the historical summary.

The remaining two options illustrated in Figures 3.5A and 3.5B may be called, respectively, deterministic and probabilistic models.

In the deterministic model the relation of each molecule to its neighbours, preceding and following, is fixed. The structure is built up by repetition of a single operation. Notice that this has the consequence of producing *local D*-periodicity. Any group of five strands possesses D-periodicity in an axial projection. On the other hand unless the assembly possesses an exact multiple of five strands the whole assembly is not D-periodic, and in particular the surface of a fibril may well not be.

In the probabilistic model the relationship of any strand to its predecessor is decided randomly. p_i is the probability of any of the five relationships and is equal to 1/5. Then the possible configurations of a group of N strands are given by expanding the multinomial

$$(p_0 + p_1 + p_2 + p_3 + p_4)^N \tag{8}$$

The expected value of each relationship is $Np_i = N/5$ so the statistical expectation for a whole fibril is that it is D-periodic. Any particular fibril would not be exactly D-periodic and roughly speaking such departures from a true periodicity are distributed normally with a standard deviation $\sim \sqrt{N}$. Nor in a model like this is D-periodicity a local property. The smaller the group of molecules, N, the greater is its coefficient of variation

$$\frac{\text{S.D.}}{\text{mean}} \quad \frac{5}{\sqrt{N}} \tag{9}$$

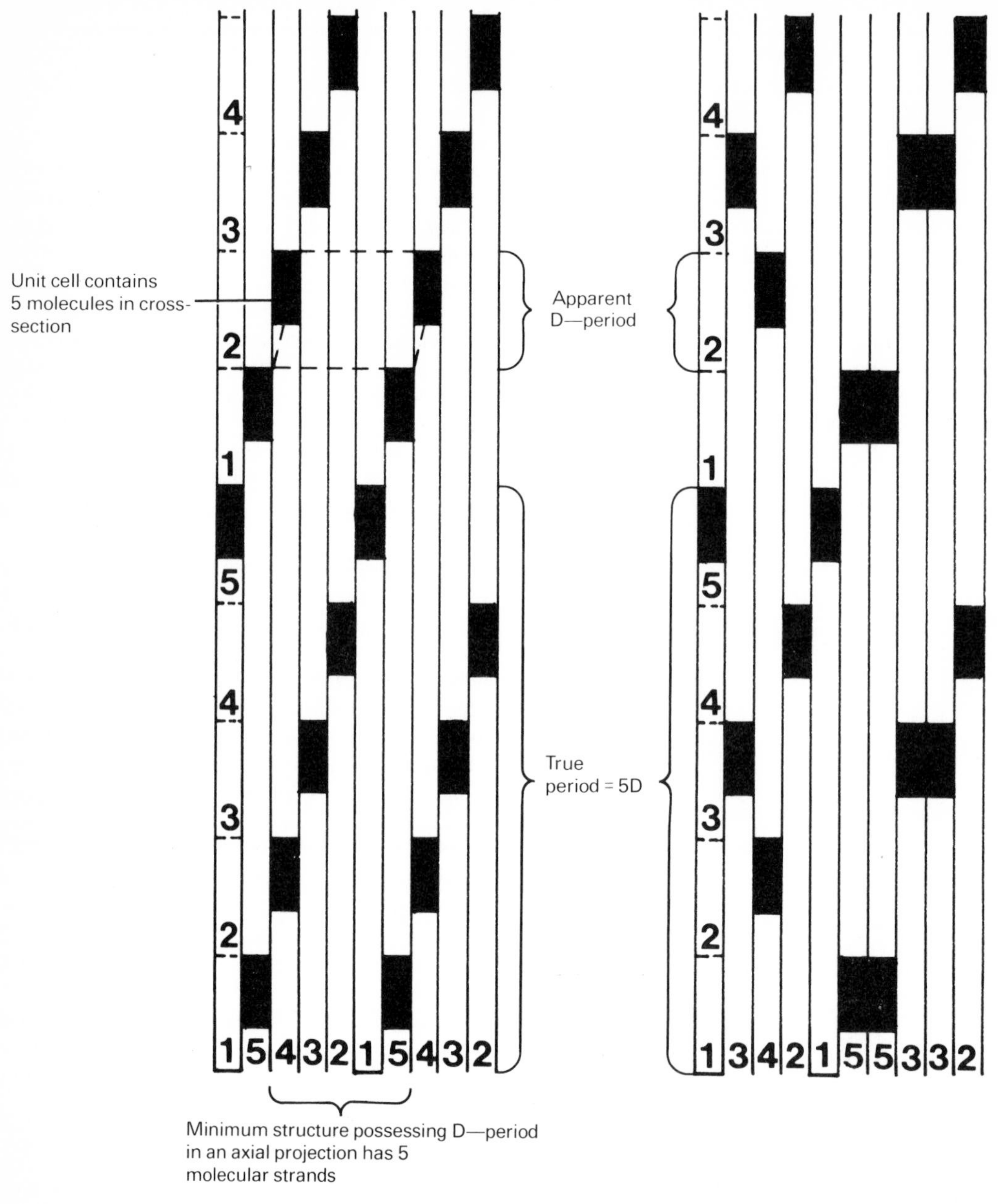

Fig. 3.5 Schematic idealised arrangements of molecules in fibrils using the allowed molecular relationships implied by the Hodge-Petruska model (Fig. 3.4), *viz* staggers of integral multiples of the observed axial period, 66.8 nm(D). Notice that the true axial period of the fibril is 5D = 5 × 66.8 nm = 334 nm. The molecules have been divided into five segments which are numbered 1-5. Thus the intermolecular relationships can be specified either by giving the degree of stagger *or* by specifying the numbers of a single pair of adjacent segments (one on each molecule).
(A) A deterministic scheme: a simple regular structure generated by a single repeated operation. The structure can be described in terms of a crystallographic unit cell containing one molecule. (B) A probabilistic scheme. The simple invariant generating operation of 3.5A is replaced by one in which molecules are added, staggered by randomly generated integral multiples of D. There is no crystallographic unit cell. *NB* Both schemes lead to fibrils which are D-periodic in axial projection.

The equal frequency condition has been assumed in a number of investigations, when attempting to explain the positively-stained banding pattern. The result has always been a good fit between theory and experiment. Figure 3.6 summarises the procedure. The molecule is well approximated by a linear chain of molecules equally spaced and it is assumed that stain has adhered only to charged residues (lys, arg, asp, glu), producing a densitometric trace similar to that in Figure 3.6A. If this is compared with a reconstruction as in Figure 3.6C or D there is no doubt that the fit is excellent. But the effect of small departures from equal frequency has not been investigated. More particularly no one has thought to test the random model. Notice that if the molecule itself possessed a *D*-periodic distribution of charged residues the two models would predict the same positively-stained pattern — identical with that of a single *D*-period on the molecule. And the molecule is in fact approximately *D*-periodic (see section on Origins of the D-stagger).

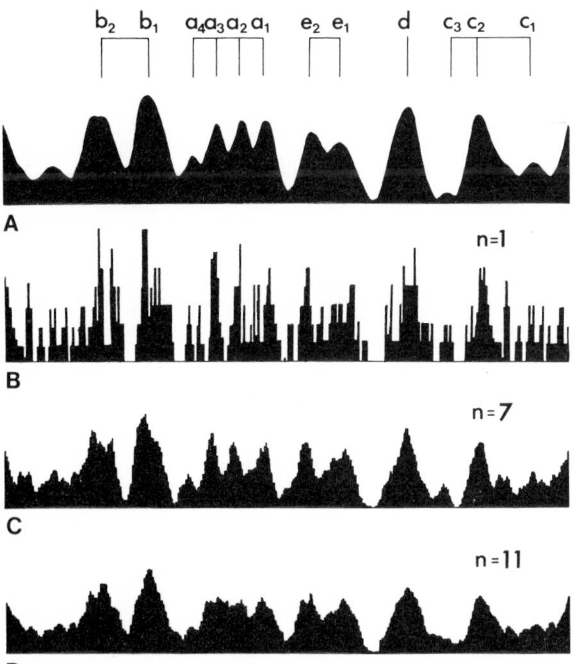

Fig. 3.6 (A) Densitometric tracing along one period of a positively stained collagen fibril from tendon. (B, C, D) attempts to reconstruct the appearance of the D-period using amino acid sequence data; assuming (i) the Hodge-Petruska model (Fig. 3.5A) and (ii) that molecules of stain stick preferentially to those residues with charged side chains. D is taken to be 234 residues. (B) The height of the histogram represents the number of charged residues out of a maximum of 15 (five molecules of three chains each).
(C, D) The density at each residue of (B) has been smeared across seven and eleven residues respectively, in an attempt to improve the match with (A).
(From Meek et al, 1979). (The lettering above is the accepted nomenclature for the observed cross-striations.)

SUBFIBRILS: INSTANCES OF LOCAL D-PERIODICITY

Electron microscopy of *native fibrils* does not permit the direct observation of the detailed arrangement of molecules. The positively-stained banding pattern in the fibril is used as evidence for an 'equal frequency model' and by implication therefore a structure in which axially projected *D*-periodicity is a local as well as a global property of fibrils — and thence a deterministic as opposed to a stochastic structure. But more disordered models have not been ruled out explicitly.

Two in vitro forms of collagen ('tactoids') are known however, where local *D*-periodicity is directly observable by the electron microscope. Examples are shown in Figure 3.7. One is a polar structure made up of *D*-periodic filaments or subfibrils; these are not in register and it is this feature that reveals them. Each is staggered with respect to its neighbour by approximately 10 nm. The other structure is more intriguing. The subfibrils alternate in their polarity giving a structure which is actually symmetrical overall.

The width of subfibrils varies greatly from tactoid to tactoid although within any one, the size is quite uniform. The widest reported are about 35 nm. Narrow subfibrils are more interesting though. We know that to possess a *D*-period a subfibril must have *at least* 5 strands. For simplicity suppose they are arranged symmetrically at the vertices of a regular pentagon then this object would have a diameter of very roughly $2.7 \times 2R$, where R is the molecular radius. There is evidence (see p. 39) that R is about 0.6 nm or rather more, so the smallest subfibril would be expected to be rather greater than 3.3 nm across. In fact *D*-periodic filaments rather less than 4.0 nm are observed which suggests that the limiting size is of 5 molecular strands.

ORIGINS OF THE D-STAGGER

Formation of the collagen fibril is a process of self-assembly. In common with other examples of this phenomenon it is presumed therefore that the 'instructions' for the correct self-assembly must be contained in the sequence of amino acid residues (for proteins). The importance of the residues, glycine, alanine, proline, hydroxyproline for the structure of the triple helix itself were recognised relatively early. However, 30 per cent of all residues in the sequence are not these four. One possibility is that they (or at least some of them) are responsible for specifying the structure of the fibril. But how?

The simple physico-chemical answer — although clearly merely a restatement of the question — is that the fibril must be an energetically favourable configuration of

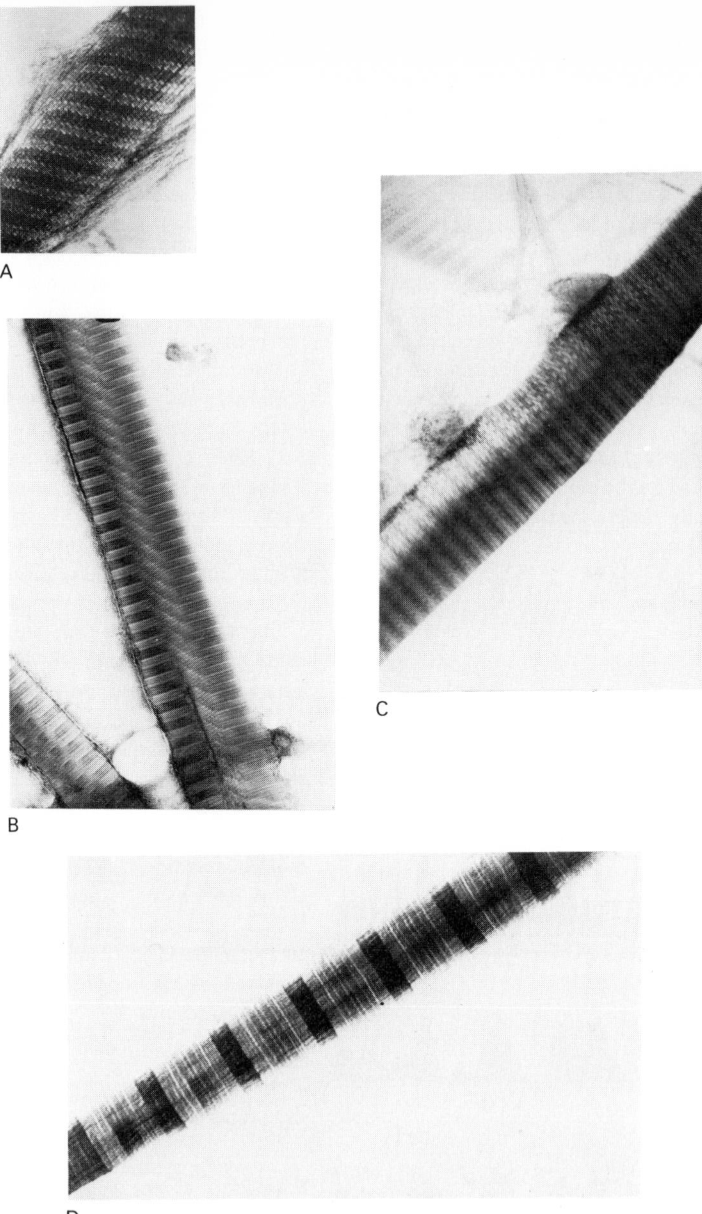

Fig. 3.7 Appearance of some forms (tactoids) of reconstituted collagen under negative staining.
(A) D-periodic sub-fibrils staggered by 10 nm to give a sheared appearance (from Bruns et al, 1973).
(B) Notice the sheared structure connecting the two D-periodic tactoids. Both sheared and normal fibrils are precipitated under the same conditions (Doyle et al, 1975).
(C) Symmetric D-periodic tactoid. Sub-fibrils alternate in polarity. This is a most interesting structure.
(D) Fibrous long spacing (FLS IV) tactoid precipitated in the presence of mucopolysaccharides. This form of collagen is *not* D-periodic. (Table 3.1 lists all known polymorphisms.)

molecules. However, scarcely any persuasive energy calculations involving biological molecules have ever been carried out. It is expedient therefore to have a more modest aim and to make two simplifying assumptions. First that the total energy of interaction of the molecules in the fibril can be accurately represented as the sum of that between pairs of neighbouring molecules. Second, that the ways in which amino acids side-chains interact with one another form a small class: strong covalent bonds; hydrogen bonds (believed to define the three-dimensional molecular structure); salt bridges — electrostatic interactions between side chains with net charges; hydrophobic interactions between large uncharged side chains — these latter involve a direct 'dispersion' contribution similar to that between neutral atoms and also an entropic contribution via the surrounding water molecules. Briefly, to put this classification in perspective: in the insulin molecule the two polypeptide chains (A and B chains) are held together by two disulphide bridges (covalent) and hydrophobic and polar side chain interactions. The dimer structure is stabilised by hydrophobic interactions and interchain hydrogen bonds.

The ultimate stability and strength of collagen fibrils relies on covalent cross links involving lysine and hydroxylysine. It seems reasonable to suppose, however, that these are not able to form until self-assembly has taken place and that this is dictated by hydrophobic and polar side chain interactions.

The simplest way in which a distribution of side chains may specify a *D*-stagger is through a pattern of appropriate residues repeating along the molecular length with a period, *D* — this of course assumes that the amino acid sequence can be analysed directly as if the molecule were one dimensional — each of the three chains is contributing alternately to all interactions. Thus if the sequence of residues is run past itself and all the hydrophobic interactions counted (i.e., an auto correlation function is computed) peaks should be observed at multiples of *D*. Similarly, peaks should be observed in a cross correlation between residues with positive and negative side chains. And this is indeed the case (Hulmes et al, 1973). Thus it seems clear that the intermolecular interactions via residue side chains are maximised (locally) when two molecules are mutually staggered by *D* or an integral multiple of it (Fig. 3.8).

A number of points are worth making about the analysis. First, it is not at all clear why the preferred configuration is not with the two molecules in register — this may be clearer when the structure of the fibril is looked at in a less naive way (see section on self assembly). Second, notice that the calculation is not in any way an energy calculation, it is simply a statistical analysis of the sequence. It is sometimes said that the fundamental law of the sciences is that any first approximation turns out to be far better than one has any right to expect. This analysis is almost certainly an instance of it.

A problem that has exercised a number of people over the years is that of the role of the terminal peptides. It has been proposed, for example, that they are involved in ensuring that all the molecules point the same way and also have a role in limiting the size of fibrils (Leibovich & Weiss, 1970; Helseth et al, 1979). However, collagen molecules, with terminal peptides, can be precipitated from solution under different conditions giving rise to an extensive polymorphism (see Table 3.1) and many of these forms are not polar but symmetric. All of these forms seem to be determined by the distribution of amino acids side chains along the *whole* length of the molecule rather than by the terminal peptides. Doyle et al, (1975), review collagen polymorphism and attempt an explanation of its origin in these terms.

Table 3.1 The observed tactoidal polymorphism of collagen (Doyle et al, 1975)

Name	*Description*
Native	Fibrils with periodic asymmetric banding pattern after positive staining, repeating every 670 Å (D)
D periodic symmetric	Same as native but with symmetric banding pattern
D/3 periodic	Fibrils with periodic banding pattern repeating every 220 Å (D/3)
Oblique striated	Tactoids composed of D-periodic polar sub-fibrils staggered with respect to nearest neighbours by about 90 Å
D/6 periodic	Tactoids with 110 Å (D/6) periodicity
Segment long spacing (SLS)	Segments equal to the molecular length with asymmetric banding patterns after positive staining
SLS symmetric	Same as SLS though with a symmetric banding pattern
SLS fibrils	Fibrils with periodic, asymmetric banding pattern after positive staining, repeating every 2680 Å (4D)
Fibrous long spacing (FLS)	A class of fibrils all produced under similar conditions, each having a periodic, symmetric banding pattern after positive staining, repeating at a distance greater than 670 Å (D)

THE QUESTION OF DENSITY

Three points have been made so far. First, that many, perhaps all, collagen fibrils have the same *D*-periodic structure in an axial projection explained by the Hodge-Petruska theory. Second, that the origins of this periodicity are long range quasi-periodicities in the sequence of amino acids in the α-chains. Third, that there is circumstantial evidence that *D*-periodicity is a local property of fibrils — there is a well defined and finite grouping of molecules which is itself *D*-periodic in projection. Any further elucidation of the fibril structure requires analysis of the side-to-side relationships among the molecules. A straightforward way to get this latter problem into perspective is through a consideration of the density of both collagen molecules and fibrils.

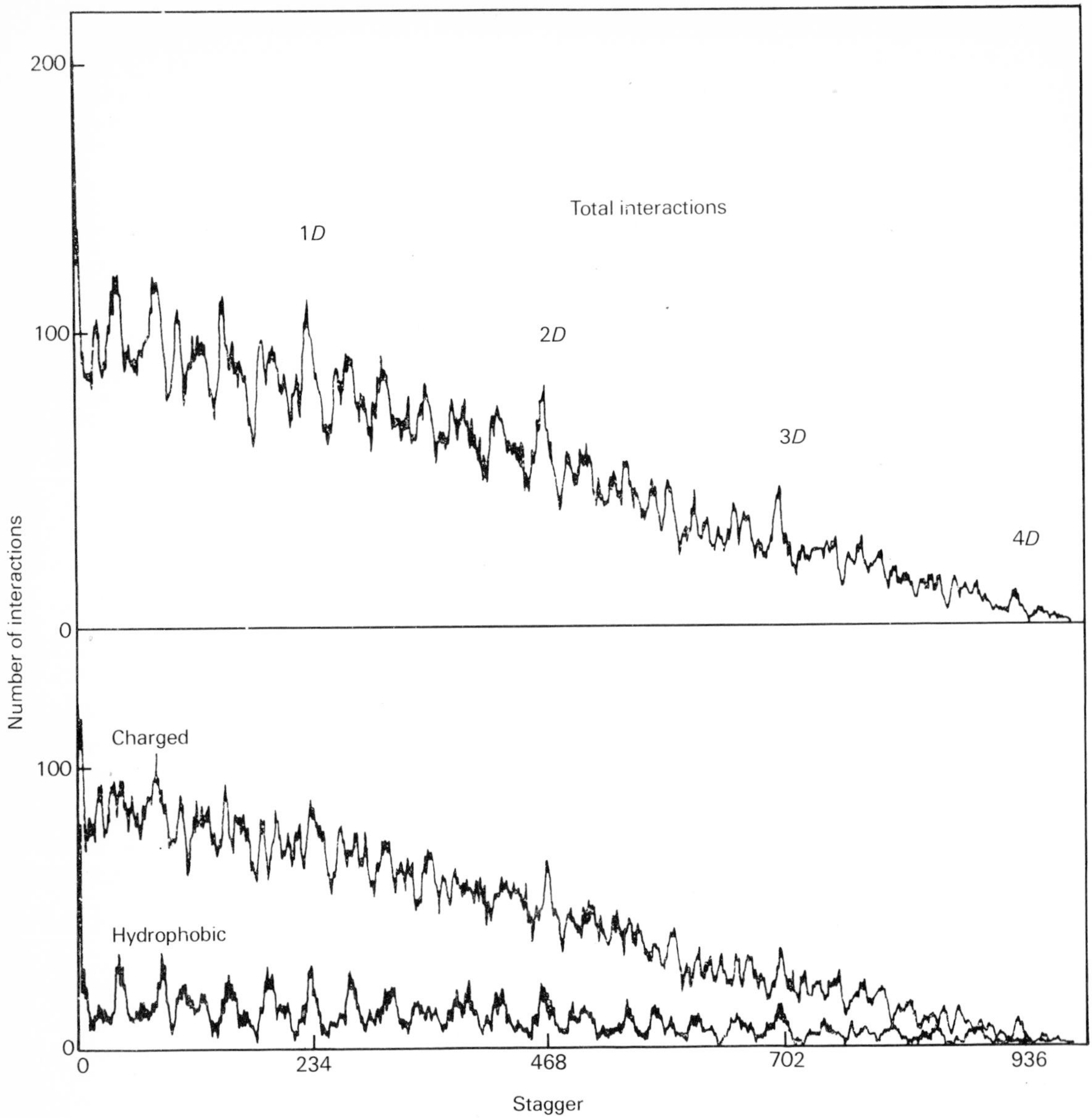

Fig. 3.8 Computer plot of the number of hydrophobic and charge interactions between two collagen molecules (ordinate) as a function of the stagger between them (abscissa). The stagger is measured in residues. There are pronounced peaks at integral multiples of 234 residues indicating a pattern of interactions repeating with this period — readily identified as the D-period (from Hulmes et al, 1973). Analysis was based on 1011 residues. It is now known that there are 1014 residues in the triple helical region — an extra triplet in the region 613—618 (see Appendix).

Consider first not the collagen molecule itself but a simplified version of it — a triple helix of the polymer (gly-pro-aln-gly-pro-pro)$_n$. Such a molecule is essentially the collagen molecule shorn of its large hydrophobic and charged side chains responsible for the *D*-staggers. Matthews, 1968, showed that the specific volume (V) of many proteins is close to 0.74 cm^3/g. Using this value and the molecular mass/triplet of this synthetic polymer (which can easily be calculated) it can be shown that if the molecule is approximated by a simple uniform cylinder its diameter would be 1.13 nm. (In fact it was discovered by Traub and his colleagues, (1969), that such a triple helix will form crystallites (small quasi-crystals) in which the molecules are packed hexagonally with an intermolecular spacing of 1.20 nm).

Next, consider the density of dried collagen; this has been measured several times, not only for tendon but also elastoidin and for artificially spun Ethicon collagen tape, used as sutures. The density of the bulk material is often measured as ~ 1.34 g/cm^3 (ie V = 0.75 cm^3/g. The molecular mass, M, of the collagen molecule is roughly 3 × 10^{5}u or 5.0 × 10^{-18}g. Thus the number density (n) of the molecules in dried collagen is 2.68×10^{18} per cm^3. The Hodge-Petruska model then shows that in a plane perpendicular to the axis the number density (n_o) of collagen molecules is 0.90 per nm^2. Assuming that the molecules are hexagonally packed their centre-to-centre spacing is again

$$\frac{1}{\sqrt{n_0 \sin 60°}} = 1.13 \text{ nm}$$

It seems reasonable to suppose that this represents the closest distance of approach of two collagen molecules and it is remarkable that it is equal to the 'diameter' of the synthetic triple helix. Perhaps the collagen molecule consists of a 'core' of gly, pro, hyp and ala with an interactive halo of charged and hydrophobic regions producing the intermolecular specificity responsible for self-assembly.

So much for the molecule. What is really of interest is the lateral packing of molecules in native fibrils. Measurements of bulk density of native wet elastoidin are not difficult to make (Woodhead-Galloway, et al, 1978) and a value of 0.458 ± 0.009 (2 SE) g/cm^3 has been quoted. The argument of the last paragraph then suggests that n_o in this case is 0.31 molecules/nm^2 and the intermolecular distance is 1.93 nm. The density of native tendons is more difficult to estimate — see for example Katz and Li (1973) who carried out a detailed analysis and gave a figure of 0.88 g/cm^3. This yields a value of 0.60 molecules/nm^2 for n_o and an intermolecular spacing (again, assuming hexagonal packing) of 1.39 nm. (See section on Self assembly).

A quantity often used to represent the density of protein crystals is the crystal volume per unit molecular mass (V_m) measured in $Å^3$ per dalton (Matthews, 1968). This is a quantity accurately estimated for crystallites of synthetic triple helix and, for $(\text{gly-pro-ala-gly-pro-pro})_n$ it is 1.535 $Å^3$/u. For wet elastoidin the corresponding quantity is close to 3.61 and Katz and Li's figures for wet reconstituted tendon suggest a value of V_m of about 1.90. The range for protein crystals is from approximately 1.6–3.6. If interest is in the solvent content of crystals or fibrils, for example, when studying mineralisation of bone then it is useful to define the fraction of crystal volume (V_{prot}) occupied by the protein

$$V_{prot} = \frac{10^{24}\,V}{NV_m} \quad \textit{where } N \textit{ is the Avagadro constant}$$

$$\simeq 1.66\ V/V_m$$

Then the fraction of volume occupied by solvent is given simply as

$$1 - V_{prot}$$

A quantity like this is not defined precisely (V_m is defined exactly of course). For collagen its precision depends on the extent to which a regular cylinder is a good approximation to the true molecular shape. Assuming it is, then the molecular radius is R and the length, L $V_{prot} = n\pi R^2L$ As it turns out the notion of packing fraction is an extremely valuable one but not quite as defined here — rather in a plane perpendicular to the fibril and molecular axes. This two dimensional packing fraction, η is given by

$$\eta = n_o\,\pi\,R^2$$

where n_o has already been defined as the number density, not of whole molecules in the fibril but of molecules in a fibril cross section. The problem is now reduced to that of packing discs in a plane, rather than cylinders in space.

DIFFUSE EQUATORIAL SCATTERING: LIQUID-LIKE LATERAL MOLECULAR PACKING

The near-equatorial fan of continuous diffuse scatter (Fig. 3.3) shows that laterally the arrangement of molecules is disordered — in fact, as will be seen, it could not be more irregular.

The combination of diffuse equatorial fan and meridional reflections is seen clearly in Figure 3.3B produced by wet elastoidin. Figure 3.3C is the pattern from wet tendon (this has been stretched) and shows in addition to the diffuse fan a pattern of more discrete reflections superimposed on it (a consideration of these is made in the next section). Upon drying tendon, the discrete reflections disappear as does the continuous diffuse scatter which is replaced by more localised peaks of diffuse intensity. Figure 3.9 is a set of densitometric tracings taken along the equators of a number of diffraction photographs — the figure caption gives details. It is the purpose of the present section to explain these curves.

At the end of the previous section it was implied that the problem of lateral packing of molecules could be considered to be that of how to pack discs in a plane. Suppose there are N such discs (molecules) scattered randomly but subject to the constraint that each disc excludes all other discs from the area it occupies itself. We need to describe this arrangement and may do so by using a probability density known as the radial distribution function $g(r)$. This assumes, quite legitimately, that the structure is isotropic.

Imagine a molecule — any one — in a central position and consider the distribution of molecules around it. Within an annulus, whose inner edge is at distance r from this molecule, and whose outer edge is at $(r + dr)$, then the probability of finding a second molecule is given by

$$n_o\,g\,(r)\,dr \tag{10}$$

And the intensity of scattered X-rays is given by

$$f^2(K')S(K') \tag{11}$$

where $f(K')$ is the Fourier Transform of a molecule in projection (remember (3)). K′ defines positions in

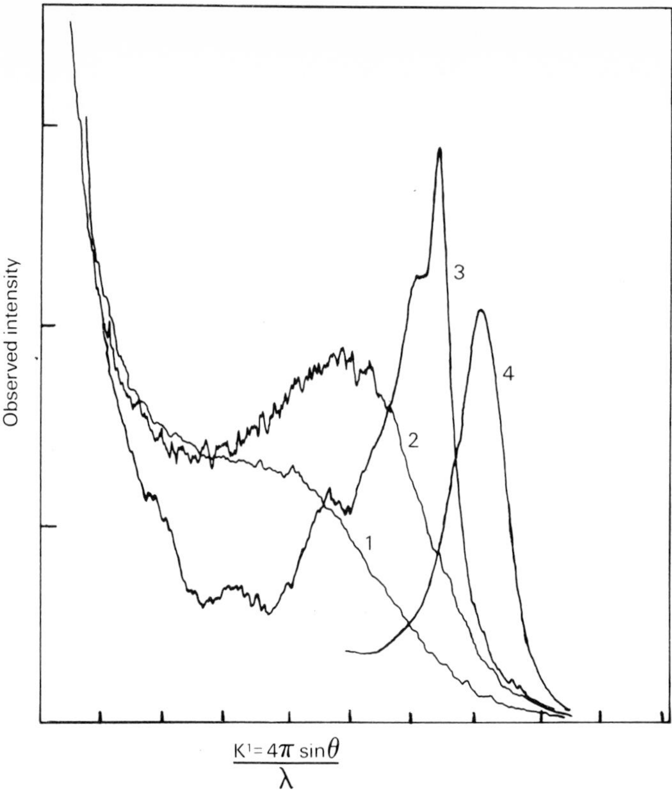

Fig. 3.9 Densitometric traces along the equators of the low angle diffraction patterns of a number of collagens.
(1) Wet elastoidin from the fin ray of *Scyliorhinus caniculus* (Fig. 3.3B).
(2) Partially dried elastoidin.
(3) Wet rat-tail tendon; note the additional peaks superposed on the diffuse scatter as in Figure 3.3C.
(4) Partially dried tendon. More thorough drying results in relatively broad thouqh discrete peaks, see Figure 3.3D.

diffraction space within the equatorial plane. $S(K')$ is essentially the Fourier Transform of *g(r)*. $f(K')$ may be calculated by recourse to the atomic co-ordinates of the model of the collagen molecule, although, in fact, in the low angle region $f(K')$ can be approximated very well by the transform of a uniform disc.

$S(K')$ is more difficult. However, if N is very large the calculation of $S(K')$ becomes equivalent to that of calculating the same quantity for a 'liquid' of hard discs through the Partition function of classical thermodynamics using a potential energy function $\phi(r)$ to describe the interaction between two discs.

Considerable success has been achieved in accounting for the diffraction patterns of simple atomic liquids (though in three dimensions, not two, of course) by assuming a simple form

$$\phi(r) = +\infty \qquad r \leqslant 2R$$
$$\phi(r) = 0 \qquad r > 2R \qquad (12)$$

Such a simplification is also made in investigating the allowed configuration of macromolecules. And there are excellent theoretical reasons why what appears to be a drastic simplification should be a good approximation.

It is important to notice that using this model $S(K')$ depends on only two parameters. R is the molecular radius which acts simply as an inverse scaling factor on $S(K')$: the larger R, the more $S(K')$ is concentrated near the origin. η, the packing fraction dictates the shape of the intensity curve for this model (Fig. 3.10B).

Before comparing this theory with experiment one further point is worth noting. It has been assumed that in the fibril, molecules are arranged parallel to the fibril axis. This is not quite true. The fanning of the diffracted intensity $I(K')$ (Fig. 3.3B and 3.3C) shows that the molecules are tilted haphazardly by up to $\sim 5°$ from the axis, then

$$I(K')_{\text{tilted}} = \frac{I(K')_{\text{untilted}}}{K'} \qquad (13)$$

Thus, before the comparison is made it is worth transforming the experimental equatorial densitometric traces in which I(K') (tilted) is plotted against K'. From (13) it can be seen that the transformation involves multiplying each experimental (tilted) value of $I(K')$ by the corresponding value of K'. Figure 3.10A shows the result of this procedure for the four curves of Figure 3.9.

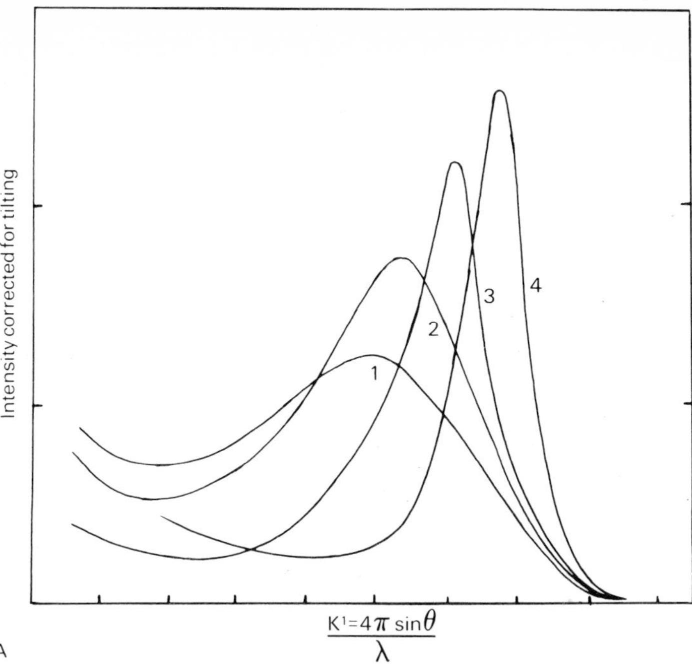

Fig. 3.10A Densitometric traces of Figure 3.9 'corrected' for random molecular tilting (see text). Notice that a peak has now appeared in the trace from wet elastoidin (curve 1). The profile has been smoothed and the discrete peaks removed from the trace produced by stretched wet rat-tail tendon (curve 3).

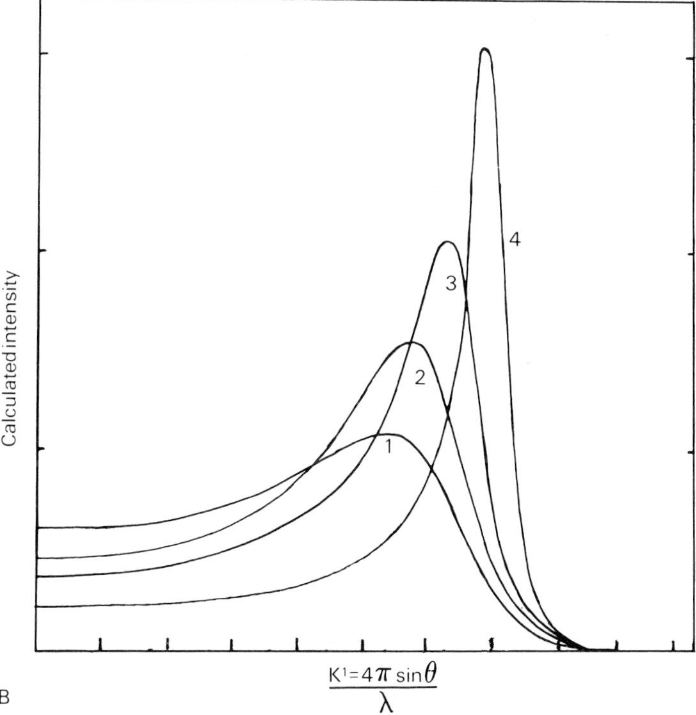

Fig. 3.10B Theoretical intensity curves predicted by two dimensional liquid-like arrays of discs, of increasing density. The four curves have been fitted to the four of (A) by varying the disc diameter, 2R and packing fraction, (see text). For each curve 2R = 1.2 nm. The values of $\eta$are: (1) η = 0.45; (2) η = 0.55; (3) η = 0.63; (4) η = 0.69.

Figure 3.10B gives four curves calculated for two dimensional hard disc liquids of differing packing fractions η the values of which have been chosen to fit the shapes of the experimental curves. It is difficult to doubt that the experimental results are accounted for by this, conceptually very simple, though technically very difficult theory. Woodhead-Galloway and Machin, (1976) and Woodhead-Galloway et al (1978), give more details of the method and list appropriate references.

The implications of this theory are not without significance. First, the fibril is an object reminiscent of a liquid crystal — it combines a high degree of order (crystalline) in the axial direction with an almost total lack of it in a plane perpendicular to the axis — retaining only the short range order forced by steric exclusion, Figure 3.11. Indeed the smectic liquid crystal does provide a good (though imperfect) structural analogy. (Hukins & Woodhead-Galloway, 1978). The sharing of characteristics with liquid crystals is also implied in the work of Nemetschek, Hosemann and their colleagues (eg Nemetschek & Hosemann, 1973).

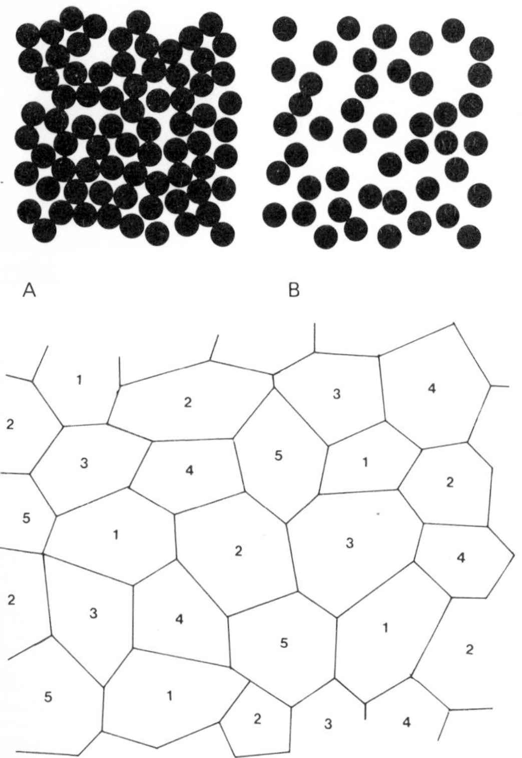

Fig. 3.11 Representations of lateral liquid-like irregularity. (A) Dense packing of discs corresponding to dried collagens (η = 0.7).
(B) Dilute packing characteristic of wet elastoidin (η = 0.4).
(C) Irregular 'statistical' geometry. Notice that it is possible to combine lateral spatial irregularity with a 'configurational' near-regularity (see section on local D-periodicity).

Second, whereas all collagens have the same axially projected structures their densities are different. Elastoidin, whose molecule may be like a type II collagen, is much less dense than tendon (remember the question of density). Bone collagen is also not very dense. Grynpas et al (1980), have suggested that fibrils obtained from cartilage show a range of densities depending on the relative proportions they contain of types I and type II collagen. It may be that the different collagen types are associated with different degrees of hydration.

LOCAL D-PERIODICITY: THE PROBLEM REVISITED

Low angle X-ray diffraction patterns from native collagens as has been seen usually possess two features. The strong, sharp, equispaced reflections on the meridian derive from a structure which in an axial projection possesses a well defined period of 66.8 nm (D). The diffuse continuous fan of scatter on the equator shows that laterally the collagen molecules form a considerably disordered assembly in two dimensions. These two projections however are not sufficient to define the local axial relationships among the rod-like collagen molecules (Fig. 3.5).

But if the diffuse scattter is a consequence of an irregular packing of single molecules it is most consistent to suppose that the pattern of Bragg reflections given by stretched tendons (Fig. 3.3C) arises in a regular arrangement of single molecules (rather than from some form of (Smith, 1968) microfibril intermediate in complexity between the molecule and the whole fibril (see section on subfibrils)). Thus the detailed pattern of reflections may solve the problem of the intermolecular relationships and consequently throw light on how the fibril assembles. What follows is an attempt to formulate systematically models which are consistent with indexing schemes suggested for the pattern of near-equatorial row lines.

Molecules in fibrils are related to one another by axial staggers of D or integral multiples of this distance. The two possible (ideal) broad schemes based on this idea (remember section on the fibril in axial projection) may be described respectively as deterministic and probabilistic (random). That is, there is an axially projected model which is deterministic (Fig. 3.5A) and one which is probabilistic (Fig. 3.5B), both of which lead to a fibril with an axially projected D-period. The latter is expected, using the word in the statistical sense, to be D-periodic only if it is very large, but the average fibril (about 150 nm in diameter) is large enough.

The probabilistic model presents an extremely interesting problem in applying the theory of diffraction — it does not however seem to account for the observed patterns from a number of different collagens (Woodhead-Galloway & Young, 1978). A priori the probabilistic scheme seems unlikely in any case. It is well established that covalent cross-links form within the shortest molecular overlap regions (Kuhn, 1969) (i.e. between segments 1 and 5 of Fig. 3.5). The arrangement of Figure 3.5a permits this, on a quite large scale; that of Figure 3.5B permits only a small, haphazard degree of such cross-linking. Deterministic means that all molecules in an equivalent axial position possess identical axial relationships with their neighbours. This need not necessarily lead to molecular arrangements as simple as that of Figure 3.5A or as a corollary be generated by such a simple algorithm — a repeated invariant operation of staggering each successive molecule by D with respect to its predecessor. Different degrees of complexity lead to crystallographic unit cells containing different numbers of molecules (see below). That shown in Figure 3.5A contains just one for example.

The pattern of diffraction spots seen in pictures Figure 3.3C does suggest a deterministic model in that it seems to be based on a crystallographic unit cell. This ought to be clear from Figure 3.5A, even though this represents matters schematically. Figure 3.5A is describable in the term of a unit cell whereas the molecular arrangement of Figure 3.5B is not so describable. The unit cell contains one molecule. The height (i.e. along the axis) of the cell is *D*. The width is 5*d* where *d* is the intermolecular spacing and in a lateral cross section the unit cell cuts through 5 molecules (in the overlap region it contains 5 molecular segments; in the gap region one segment is missing). More generally for deterministic models the unit cell contains an integral number of molecules (q = 1,2 . . .) and in a cross section the unit cell contains 5q molecular segments. Equivalently, structures possessing true axially projected D-periods must contain 5q molecular strands. Several attempts have been made to index the experimental row lines. Recently, since relatively detailed data have been available, interest has been concentrated on two schemes. (i) a unit cell square in cross section of side 3.80 nm (Miller & Parry, 1973; Woodhead-Galloway, 1977) (this has been elaborated in some accounts to a large cell of side $\sqrt{2}$ × 3.80 nm (Miller & Parry), or even 2 × 3.80 nm (Fraser et al, 1974)). An 'almost square' cell has also been proposed (Nemetschek & Hosemann, 1973) (ii) a monoclinic cell (McFarlane, 1971) the most precisely defined version of which possesses sides 3.90 nm, 2.61 nm and an internal angle of 75°25′ (Hulmes & Miller, 1979).

Consider now the problem of how a unit cell (of sides a, b and an internal angle γ may be generated. The general problem of enumerating the possible structures for arbitrary q is formidable. When q = 1 however the process is quite straightforward. Look at the fibril projected down the axis on to a plane perpendicular to it in an overlap zone in which the five molecular segments will appear. A description of the structure contains two *independent* components.

(i) a two dimensional lattice, defined by sides A, B and an internal angle Γ, on the points of which the molecules are placed.

(ii) a combinatorial feature — for given values of A, B, Γ in how many ways the molecules can be arranged.

Two *sorts* of molecular arrangement are possible other than the trivial one of merely stacking the layers in register when γ = Γ; b = B; a = 5A. These schemes are shown in Figure 3.12 and denoted I and II. Notice however that within each 'horizontal' row the molecules may be permuted in 4! = 24 distinct ways while maintaining the

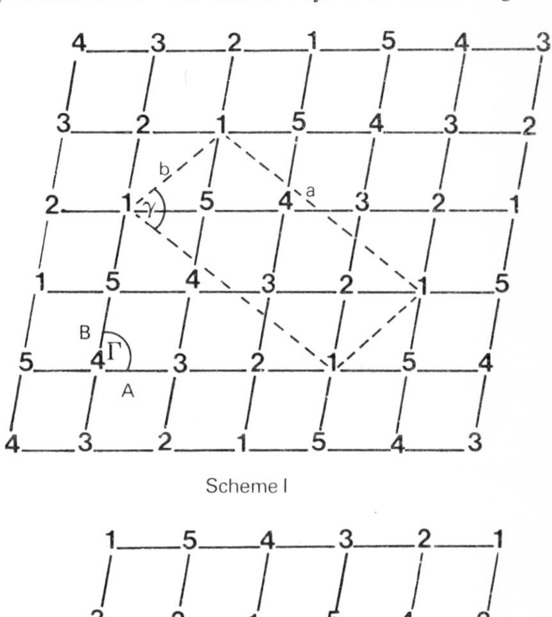

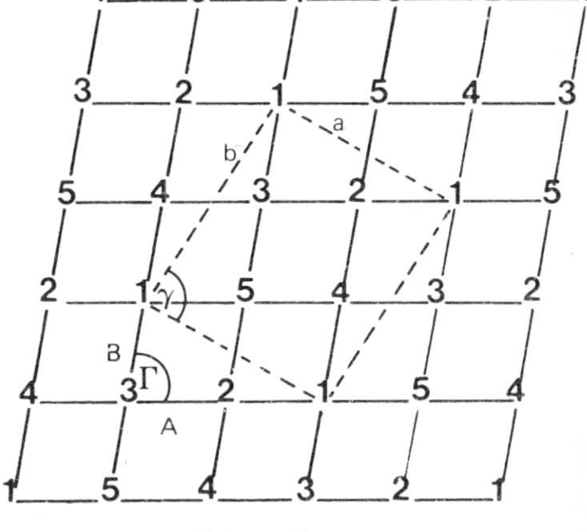

Fig. 3.12 Hypothetical lattices representing fibrils in lateral cross sections. The *only two possible non-trivial sorts of ways* of arranging single molecules on a lattice so that a crystallographic unit cell is formed containing 1 molecule. To specify the fibril's structure two features are needed. First a lattice (A, B, Γ) on the points of which the molecules are placed. Second a combinatorial aspect. Sheets of molecules of the type shown in Fig. 1A are stacked. Two types of intersheet relationship are possible — a shift of one intermolecular spacing (I) or two intermolecular spaces (II). No other algorithms are possible if the unit cell is to contain just one molecule. Within 'horizontal' sheets the molecular positions may be permuted in 4! = 24 ways without altering the size and shape of the unit cell.

same size and shape of unit cell, i.e. all of these permutations would be consistent with a particular indexing scheme.

The relationships between the two sets of lattice parameters (A, B, Γ) and (a, b, γ) are as follows:

For scheme I

$$a^2 = 9A^2 + 4B^2 - 12AB\cos\Gamma$$
$$b^2 = A^2 + B^2 + 2AB\cos\Gamma \qquad (14)$$
$$\sin\gamma = \frac{5AB\sin\Gamma}{ab}$$

and for scheme II

$$a^2 = 4A^2 + B^2 - 4AB\cos\Gamma$$
$$b^2 = A^2 + 4B^2 + 4AB\cos\Gamma \qquad (15)$$
$$\sin\gamma = \frac{5AB\sin\Gamma}{ab}$$

These two sets of equations may be used to deduce possible molecular packing schemes from the unit cell dimensions which are determined experimentally. Consider first the 'experimental' square unit cell (a = b = 3.80 nm, γ = 90°). This cell allows *only* a type II configuration, specifically when $A = B = \frac{3.80}{\sqrt{5}} = 1.70$ nm, and Γ = 90° i.e. when the underlying molecular lattice is itself square (Fig. 3.13A).

On the other hand only a type I configuration is allowed by the alternative experimental unit cell (a = 3.90 nm, b = 2.61 nm, γ = 75°25′) and this is generated by two different molecular lattice (Figs 3.13B and 3.13C):

Fig. 3.13B { A = 1.45 nm, B = 1.56 nm, Γ = 60° 18′

Fig. 3.13C { A = 1.13 nm, B = 1.92 nm, Γ = 64° 55′

Each of these three, similar schemes is superficially plausible. Those of Figures 3.13A and 3.13B have been used as the bases of detailed models for the fibril. They possess some interesting similarities in their attribution of the main features of the pattern. That of Figure 3.13C has not been used in this way. There seems little doubt now that the monoclinic almost hexagonal packing (Fig. 3.13B) of molecules provides much the neatest account of the low angle diffraction pattern.

Suppose that Figure 3.13B is essentially correct. How can the particular arrangement — out of the 24 possible — be determined? The direct way is by calculating the intensities for each and comparing them with experiment. It is not clear that with available patterns this is feasible. A possible clue to the correct configuration may be given by the constraints necessary for intermolecular cross-linking. For example the particular configuration given in Figure 3.13B (or its enantiomorph) allows covalently cross-linked structures of the sort illustrated in Figure 3.14B. Structures resembling these are frequently seen in electron micrographs of partially dissolved collagen. In general other schemes do not permit the formation of an extended cross-linked network like this.

What is the link between the analysis of this paper and that leading to the conclusion that in many collagens, and presumably even in a large proportion of stretched tendon, the molecules show only a lateral liquid-like, though static,

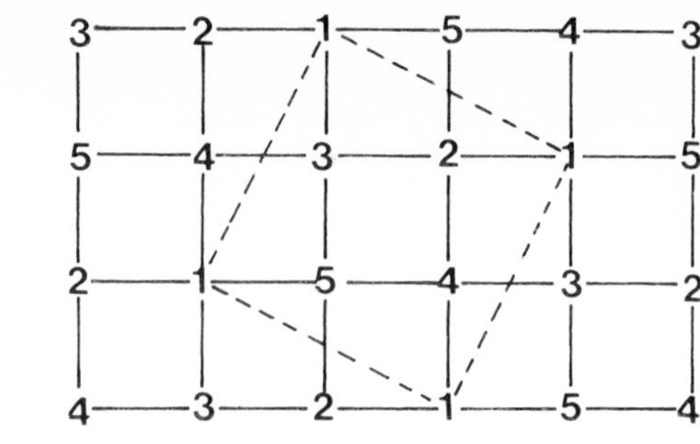

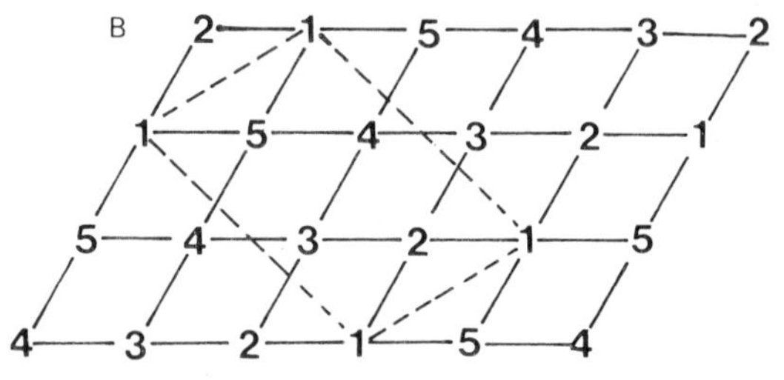

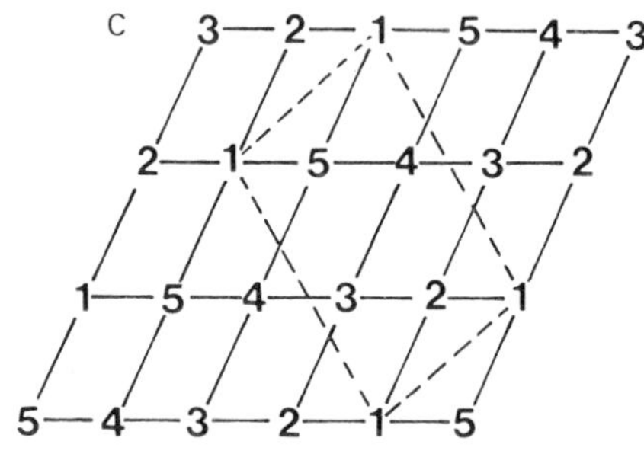

Fig. 3.13 Molecular arrangements consistent with *indexing* of row lines in X-ray diffraction patterns from stretched rat tail tendon. (A) indexing based on a square unit cell of side 3.80 nm is consistent only with a square packing of molecules using the combinatorial type shown in Fig. 2(II). (B) and (C) two molecular configurations are consistent with the indexing of Hulmes and Miller (1979) who base their detailed model on (B). Both configurations are of the sort indicated in Figure 3.2(I). In 13.B A = 1.45 nm, B = 1.56 nm, Γ = 60°18′. In 3C A = 1.13 nm, B = 1.92 nm, Γ = 64°55′.

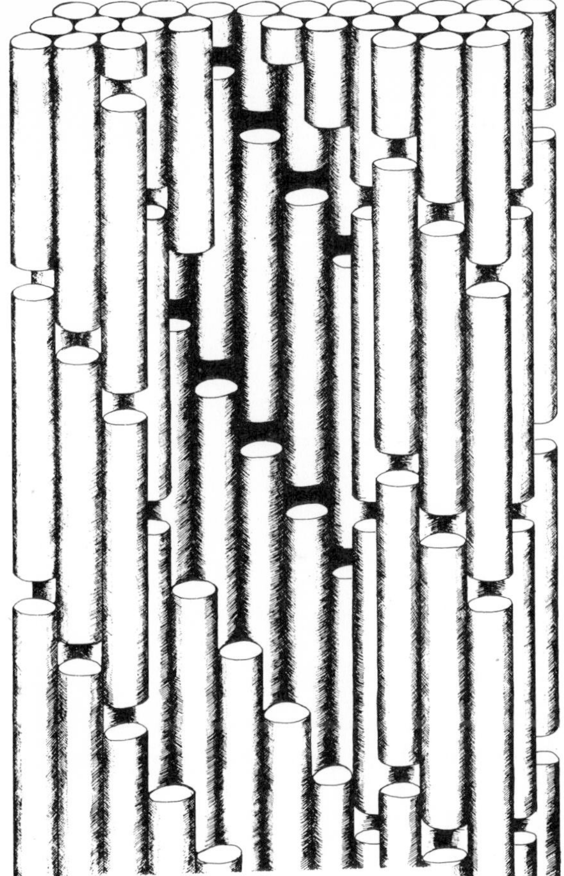

Fig. 3.14A Schematic drawing to show how collagen molecules appear to be arranged within fibrils — an attempt to combine in a single illustration the ideas of Figures 3.5A, 3.12 and 3.13B. However, remember that in fact the molecular length is 240 × the diameter and that in a native unstretched fibril there would be little lateral order.

order? The crystallographic lattices of Figures 3.12 and 3.13 must be replaced by statistical lattices of the sort sometimes used to describe liquid structure (Fig. 3.11C). The structure of the fibril while well organised possesses less simple order than the crystal model implies, a feature it shares with much structural biochemistry (Williams, 1977).

SELF ASSEMBLY

A good idea of the structure of a collagen fibril has been obtained, in the sense that relatively convincing explanations have been found for observations made by electron microscopy and X-ray diffraction. The most detailed picture has emerged from rat-tail tendon. Whether the same picture will appear for other collagens, given the differences of density, or whether other collagen types will present rather more interesting variations on the Hodge-Petruska theme remains to be seen.

Now the assembly of a structure (Fig. 3.5A) depends on *two* interactions between a pair of neighbouring molecules, an axial displacement of 1D and an axial displacement of 4D. This seemingly simple requirement presents a conceptual difficulty: how does the amino acid sequence contrive to define two axial stagger relations, one of which is an integral multiple of the other? Three possibilities are worth considering.

First the 4D-stagger might be a logical consequence of the single D-stagger. This is the solution provided by the *regular helical* microfibril model (Smith, 1968). Repeated addition of molecules staggered by 1D with respect to their preceding neighbour in a five stranded helix generates automatically and exactly the 4D-stagger relation. No explicit provision of the amino acid sequence for the 4D-stagger is needed: it is implicit in the provision of a single D-stagger.

Second, the best way to define a single D-stagger is by a pattern of amino acids with large side chains (large hydrophobics or charges occurring D-periodically (Hulmes et al, 1973)), but such a periodicity automatically generates the potentials for staggers of 2D, 3D and 4D. Notice that in the sort of models shown in Figure 3.13, neighbouring molecules are related in each of the four possible ways.

Thirdly, suppose that in this latter mechanism, the two sorts of displacement are not related as an integral multiple but only approximately so. (This is not an unreasonable supposition: the pattern of residues in the sequence of amino acids does not, in fact, repeat exactly). The relations are (for example):

$$D, 4D + \Delta$$

A regular structure assembled from these two interactions is like that shown in Figure 3.5A but is sheared through an angle.

$$\phi_S = \arctan \Delta / 2R \qquad (16)$$

In fact shearing does seem to be a feature of the structure of the fibril (Miller & Wray, 1971; Hulmes & Miller, 1979; Woodhead-Galloway, 1980).

For completeness, it should also be noticed that in general the molecular axes are not quite parallel to the fibril axes (see p. 40). An analysis of the combination of tilting and shearing is given by Woodhead-Galloway (1980).

The question of the role of the amino acid sequence in dictating structure is not fully answered. It is not clear how the one dimensional treatment (p. 37) may be elaborated to explain 'three dimensional interactions' among groups of molecules. The model of Figure 3.13B — a fairly close approximation to the truth (for tendon at least) — requires a 'hexagonal' molecule with complementary opposing faces. How the amino acid sequence contrives such a subtle structural determinism is not at present understood.

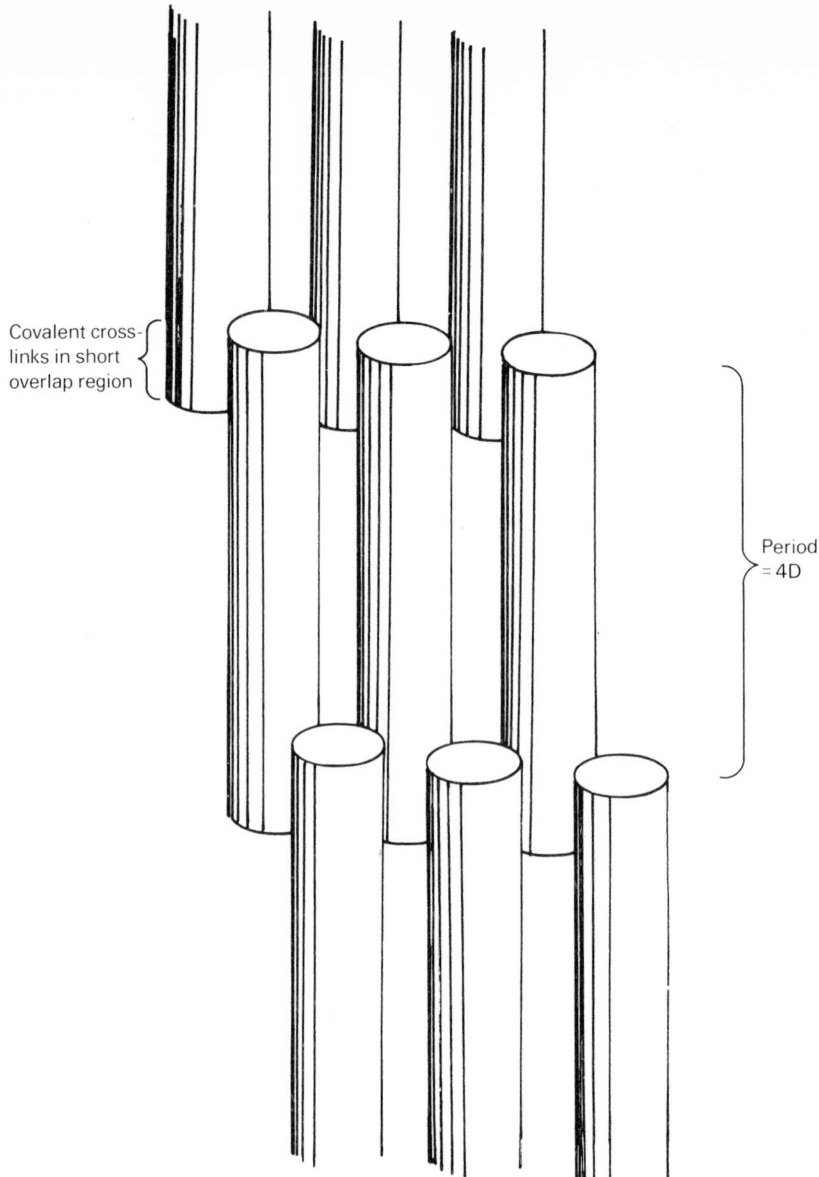

Fig. 3.14B The arrangement of Fig. 3.13B allows a network of covalent crosslinks between segments 1 and 5 giving rise to loosely packed structures of the sort illustrated here. Electron microscopy has repeatedly shown the existence of these (e.g. Kuhn 1969). In an axial projection they possess a period of 4D = 2670 nm. Each molecule is linked to its nearest neighbours at each end.

The picture of the fibril depends on the means used to observe it. Both electron microscopy and X-ray diffraction provide a static image. The work of Torchia and his colleagues using Nuclear Magnetic Resonance (e.g. Torchia & Vander Hart, 1976) shows that the fibril's structure is not specified by a rigid determinism of closely interlocking amino acid side chains. Rather the side chains remain flexible and may take part in several interactions between two collagen molecules — or perhaps more than two. This feature was anticipated in the amino acid sequence analysis of Hulmes et al, 1973.

An aspect of the problem that will attract attention in the future is that of the *dynamics* of self assembly rather than what the finished product looks like. An interesting observation made by Chapman et al, 1980, is an asymmetry between the two ends of a growing fibril which reflects a difference in the rate of accretion of molecules. However, the relationship between such in vitro experiments, interesting though they are, and what actually happens in the extra-cellular space, may be a tenuous one.

The growth of a fibril might depend on an intermediate structure, like the screw dislocation of a crystal whose energy, E, varies with the dislocation's diameter, d, according to

$$E \alpha \ln d \tag{17}$$

Boltzmann's law then suggests that the smaller the diameter, the faster the growth. This could explain how a fibril, whose ends are known to taper initially, tends towards a uniform cylinder as it grows. But this is all highly speculative.

HISTORICAL SUMMARY

What follows is a brief chronological survey of some of those events which have been important in leading to the present picture we have of the collagen fibril.

1910's

1912, W. Friedrich and P. Knipping produce X-ray diffraction pattern from a crystal of zinc sulphide. 1914, P. Debye and P. Scherrer take an analogous picture from liquid paraffin. The first pattern from a biological fibre has to wait until 1921 when M. Polanyi produces one from cellulose.

1920's

1924, L. de Broglie suggests wave-particle dualism; particles of momentum p should possess a wave-length $\lambda = h/p$ where h is Planck's constant. This is confirmed in 1927 by C.J. Davisson and L.H. Germer, and independently by G.P. Thomson, who demonstrate electron diffraction effects. Also in 1924, D. Gabor makes the first short concentrating electro-magnetic coil which *focuses* a beam of electrons.

1930's

1931, E. Ruska demonstrates two-stage magnification by an electron beam and two magnetic lenses; total magnification is 17.4, (Ruska knows nothing of de Broglie's ideas). 1934, W.T. Astbury introduces the idea of average amino acid residue weight in proteins and connects analytical data on molecular weight with the peptide hypothesis. He is working on gelatine and realises that glycine makes up $\frac{1}{3}$ the total number of residues in collagen. 1936, L. Marton takes first electron micrograph of a biological object — a section of root of the Sundew (*Drosera intermedia*). W.T. Astbury reports that high angle X-ray diffraction patterns are characteristic for different natural protein fibres. In particular he shows the pattern for collagen.

1940's

Discovery of a long period (D) in collagen in the 1930s is put on a proper basis. F.O. Schmitt, C.E. Hall and M.A. Jakus and independently C. Wolpers are using electron microscopy. R.S. Bear and independently O. Kratki and A. Sekora are using low angle X-ray diffraction.

1950's

1951, R. Hosemann points out that collagen fibrils are rather disordered molecular assemblies and describes them as para-crystals. 1954–55, F.O. Schmitt, J.A. Highberger and J. Gross isolate whole collagen molecules. They grow segment-long-spacing collagen (SLS) in which the molecules are assembled in register and show that the molecule is 300 nm long. They suggest the quarter stagger model; with a molecular length, L of 4D. 1956, S.G. Tomlin and C.R. Worthington show that the low angle diffraction pattern of meridional reflections indicate an alternation of dense with less dense zones within the D-period. This is not explained by the Quarter Stagger Model. 1955, A.C.T. North and his colleagues have collected improved high angle X-ray data and the triple-helical collagen molecule is proposed by A. Rich and F.H.C. Crick and by G.N. Ramachandran and his colleagues. 1959, negative staining is introduced by S.D. Brenner and R.W. Horne.

1960's

1963, A.J. Hodge and J.A. Petruska refine quarter stagger model pointing out that $L \neq 4D$. This explains negative staining pattern of fibril and Tomlin and Worthington's results. 1967, R.W. Cox and his colleagues demonstrate the correctness of this model in a classic experiment; SLS ribbons are grown on native fibrils and the molecule is seen to run through 4 gap regions and 5 overlap regions. 1968, J.W. Smith suggests a 4 stranded helical micro-fibril as the basic structural unit in the fibril. 1969, K. Kuhn reviews several years work supporting the idea of a covalently cross-linked proto-fibril. (1 proto-fibril = $\frac{1}{4}$ microfibril).

1970's

1971, A. Miller and J.S. Wray report improved low angle X-ray data (similar data has been collected by T. Nemetschek and his colleagues) and claim that it supports Smith's microfibril model. In the same year A.F. McFarlane suggests a model based on hexagonal packing of single molecules. His model, now known to be essentially correct, is ignored. The microfibril model, despite its wrongness being readily demonstrable, dominates structural thinking and analysis of amino acid sequence for a decade. 1973, T. Nemetschek and R. Hosemann point out that tilting within a molecular plane offers the best explanation for the off-equatorial intensity in the low angle

X-ray diffraction pattern. 1973, D.J.S. Hulmes and his colleagues show that the origins of axial specificity reside in quasi-D-periods in the distribution of residues with charged and hydrophobic side-chains. 1976, J. Woodhead-Galloway and P.A. Machin show that an analogy with a simple atomic liquid offers an explanation of the strong diffuse intensity in the X-ray diffraction pattern. 1979, D.J.S. Hulmes and A. Miller show that a combination of McFarlane's and Nemetschek's and Hosemann's ideas explain the ordered phase of *stretched* tendon extremely well.

ACKNOWLEDGEMENTS

Figure 3.3A is reproduced by kind permission of Dr H.E. Huxley. The rest of the X-ray diffraction pictures shown and the electron micrographs (with the exception of Fig. 3.7A) were taken in Professor Sir David Phillips' Laboratory of Molecular Biophysics in the University of Oxford. I am grateful to John Wray and Christopher Rodger for help with the diffraction and Barbara Brodsky and David Hulmes who collaborated in the microscopy.

Kate Fountain very kindly drew Figure 3.14A.

REFERENCES

Bernal J D 1964 The structure of liquids (Bakerian Lecture) Proceedings of the Royal Society of London A280: 299

Bruns R R, Trelstad R L, Gross J 1973 Cartilage collagen: a staggered substructure in reconstituted fibrils. Science N.Y. 181: 269

Chapman J A, Holmes D F, Meek K M, Rattew C J 1980 Electron optical studies of collagen fibril assembly. Proceedings of the Aharon Katzir-Katchalsky Conference on Structural Aspects of Recognition and Assembly in Biological Macromolecules

Cox R W, Grant R A, Horne R W 1967 Structure and assembly of collagen fibrils. Journal of the Royal Microscopical Society 87: 123

Doyle B B, Hukins D W L, Hulmes D J S, Miller A, Woodhead-Galloway J, 1975 Collagen polymorphism: its origins in the amino acid sequence. Journal of Molecular Biology 91: 79

Fraser R D B, Miller A and Parry D A D 1974 Packing of microfibrils in collagen. Journal of Molecular Biology 83: 281

Grynpas D, Eyre D R, Kirschner D A 1980 Collagen type II differs from type I in native molecular packing. Biochimica Biophysica Acta 626: 346

Helseth D L, Lechner J H, Veis A 1979 Role of amino terminal extralelical region of type I collagen in directing the 4D overlap in fibrillogenesis. Biopolymers 18: 3005

Hodge J A, Petruska A J 1963: In Aspects of protein structure Ramachandran G N (ed) 289: Academic Press

Hukins D W L, Woodhead-Galloway J 1978 Liquid crystal model for the organisation of molecules in collagen fibrils. Biochemical Society Transactions 6: 238

Hulmes D J S, Miller A, Parry D A D, Piez K A, Woodhead-Galloway J 1973 Analysis of the primary structure of collagen for the origins of molecular packing. Journal of Molecular Biology 79: 137

Hulmes D J S, Miller A 1979 Quasi-hexagonal molecular packing in collagen fibrils. Nature, (London) 282: 878

Katz E P, Li S T 1973 The intermolecular space of reconstituted collagen fibrils. Journal of Molecular Biology 73: 351

Kuhn K 1969 The structure of collagen. Essays in Biochemistry 5: 59

Leibovich S J, Weiss J B 1970 Electron microscope studies of the effects of endo and exopeptidase digestion of tropocollagen. Biochimica Biophysica Acta 214: 445

Lipson S G, Lipson H 1969 Optical Physics. Cambridge University Press

McFarlane E F 1971 Molecular packing structure of collagen. Search 2: 171

Matthews B W 1968 Solvent content of protein crystals. Journal of Molecular Biology 33: 491

Meek K M, Chapman J A, Hardcastle R A 1979 Staining pattern of collagen fibrils. Improved correlation with sequence data. Journal of Biological Chemistry 254: 10710

Miller A, Parry D A D 1973 Structure and packing of microfibrils in collagen. Journal of Molecular Biology 75: 441

Miller A, Wray J S 1971 Molecular packing in collagen. Nature (London) 230: 437

Nemetschek T, Hosemann R 1973 A kink model of native collagen. Kolloid-Z u. Z Polymere 251: 1044

Schmitt F O, Gross J, Highberger J H 1955 Tropocollagen and the properties of fibrous collagen. Experimental Cell Research Supplement 3: 326

Smith J W 1968 Molecular patterns in native collagen. Nature (London) 219: 157

Tomlin S G, Worthington C R 1956 Low-angle X-ray diffraction patterns of collagen. Proceedings of the Royal Society of London A35: 189

Torchia D A, Vander Hart D L 1976 ^{13}C magnetic resonance evidence for anisotropic molecular motion in collagen fibrils. Journal of Molecular Biology 104: 315

Traub W, Yonath A, Segal D M 1969 On the molecular structure of collagen. Nature, London 221: 914

Williams R J P 1977 Review of 'Inorganic aspects of biological and organic chemistry' by R P Hanzlik. Nature, (London) 266: 481

Woodhead-Galloway J 1977 A molecular crystal model as a basis for the structure of the collagen fibril. Acta Crystallographica B33: 1212

Woodhead-Galloway J 1980 Structure of the collagen fibril. Some variations on a theme of tetragonally packed dimers. Proceedings of the Royal Society of London B209: 275

Woodhead-Galloway J, Machin P A 1976 Modern theories of liquids and the diffuse near equatorial X-ray scattering from collagen. Acta Crystallographica A32: 368

Woodhead-Galloway J, Hukins D W L, Knight D P, Machin P A, Weiss J B 1978 Molecular packing in elastoidin spicules. Journal of Molecular Biology 118: 567

Woodhead-Galloway J, Young W H 1978 Probabilistic aspects of the structure of the collagen fibril. Acta Crystallographica A34: 12

4

Biomechanical properties of collagen

D. W. L. HUKINS

In the overwhelming majority of tissues the most obviously important function of collagen is a mechanical one — to withstand tensile stress. Collagen occurs in these tissues as microscopic fibres, known as fibrils, which typically have diameters of around 100 nm (although fibril diameter depends on age and varies from one tissue to another). The lengths of the fibrils are unknown but they are certainly many orders of magnitude greater than fibril diameters. In some tissues the fibrils could be several millimetres, or even several centimetres, long. Collagen fibril structure is described in considerable detail in Chapter 3; the aim of this present chapter is to explore the influence of the fibrils on the mechanical properties of tissues. Any fibre is able to withstand a force which tends to stretch it, provided the force is not so great as to cause breakage. Such a force will have a component along the fibre-axis direction and this component is referred to as an axial tension. Thus a collagen fibril can withstand axial tension. But, like any other fibre, it offers little resistance to bending or torsion i.e. a collagen fibril, like a fibre of wool or cotton, can be very easily bent or twisted. And it will simply crumple up under axially applied compression.

This behaviour of collagen fibrils can be illustrated by the properties of excised tendons which are readily bent, crumpled and twisted. However if the ends of the tendon are pulled it becomes taut and very difficult to stretch i.e. it withstands axial tension because considerable energy is required to stretch the tendon's constituent collagen fibrils. Although tendons provide a useful demonstration of the properties of collagen in this instance, they do not always provide a reliable model for the mechanical behaviour of the collagen fibrils themselves — the reason is that tendon is a composite material whose microstructure is far from simple (the properties of tendon will be described in detail in a later section). But if tendons can be easily bent, crumpled and twisted, their collagen fibrils must be too.

Collagen fibrils can then only confer stability on a tissue if they are arranged so that the forces acting on the tissue are transmitted to them as axial tension. How can tension stabilise a structure which is subjected to different kinds of deformation? Guy ropes supporting a vertical pole provide a very simple example. They hold the pole up simply by pulling on it i.e. by axial tension — they do not push the pole up yet they resist all but the most strenuous attempts to push it down. But the ropes have to point in opposing directions — otherwise down falls the pole! The importance of the direction of the ropes illustrates the important implications of structure for the stability of mechanical systems. Biological tissues are no exception — they must obey the rules of mechanics and their mechanical properties are consequently dependent on their structures. And in the context of this chapter structure usually means the directions in which their collagen fibrils point.

The importance of tension-withstanding components for the integrity of tissues is demonstrated by a variety of diseases in which collagen fibrils either do not form or are broken down. As we shall see later, when these vital components are defective, or not present in sufficient quantity, the tissues will tear if they are stretched or sheared. Scurvy arises when the diet contains insufficient ascorbic acid for collagen fibrils to form; the biochemistry of this failure of fibril formation is discussed in Chapter 28. Wounds do not then heal, because no mechanically stable tissue can be formed, or the new tissue soon ruptures because of its low tensile strength. Scurvy is thus characterised in its early stages by bleeding gums and loosened teeth followed, in later stages, by multiple haemorrhages. Gas gangrene results from infection of wounds by bacteria belonging to the genus *Clostridium*. The bacteria secrete enzymes which degrade the collagen in tissues as described in Chapter 1. Consequently the infected tissues are unable to withstand the tensile stresses to which they are subjected and are rapidly destroyed.

Collagen does not act alone in maintaining the structures of connective tissues when they are subjected to mechanical forces. The extracellular matrices of these tissues are composite materials; in particular the collagen fibrils are surrounded by a highly hydrated gel of glycosaminoglycans (also called mucopolysaccharides). The liquid-like gel will transmit applied pressure equally in all directions to other components of the tissue; pressure can also squeeze water out.

Glycosaminoglycans have a strong affinity for water (Maroudas, 1979) and so squeezing fluid out requires appreciable energy. Fluid flow is then one possible response to applied pressure which provides a mechanism for dissipating compressive energy; expression of fluid occurs during deformation of articular cartilage (Maroudas, 1979) and the intervertebral disc (Farfan, 1973). Another mechanism is for the incompressible fluid to transmit pressure to the collagen. If the structure of the tissue is such that pressure applied to it leads the axial tension in the collagen fibrils to increase, compressive energy will be used to stretch the fibrils and so is absorbed. A simple illustrative example of a system where applied pressure is transmitted by a liquid is provided by the brakes of a car. When the brake pedal is depressed, the pressure is transmitted by the incompressive brake fluid. Because this energy is used to prevent the wheels from rotating, i.e. it is dissipated, the driver feels the system opposing further compression of the brake pedal. If there is a leak in the system, fluid may be forced out i.e. some energy will be used to initiate fluid flow. Although this is an acceptable mechanism for many tissues to dissipate energy, it is unacceptable in a car; the function of the braking system is to stop the car — not to absorb energy from the driver!

It is clear that if we are to understand the biomechanical properties of collagen we must know the arrangement of fibrils in tissues. This relationship between the arrangement of fibrils and the function of the tissue has already been emphasised by Harkness (1968) and by Kenedi et al (1975). Thus the first section of this chapter is concerned with tissue structure. Furthermore we cannot consider the collagen in isolation but must treat it as one, albeit important, component in a composite material in which the glycosaminoglycan gel is another major component. Thus a later section is concerned with the behaviour of composite materials, in particular the so-called fibre composites of which collagenous tissues are an example. But before the behaviour of composite materials can be considered it will be necessary to introduce some simple mechanical concepts. When this background material has been covered it is possible to describe the biomechanical properties of some real collagenous tissues. The discussion is not intended to be comprehensive: rather it is intended to stress general principles with emphasis on those tissues where mechanical function is commonly impaired by degeneration and disease. Tissues will be classified into two kinds: those where bundles of fibrils function as larger fibres and the second where the arrangement of fibrils is more complex. Finally, even in a chapter on mechanical properties, it is important to remember that mechanical energy cannot be completely divorced from other forms of energy. Although energy can be neither created nor destroyed, one form of energy can be converted into another. The last section of this chapter, apart from the final conclusions, is concerned with the ability of collagen to interconvert mechanical and electrical energy.

STRUCTURAL HIERARCHIES

Three structural levels can be identified in collagen: (1) the structure of the collagen molecule, (2) the structure of the collagen fibril i.e. the arrangement of molecules in a fibril (the subject of Ch. 3) and (3) the arrangement of fibrils in a tissue. This third level, sometimes referred to as the 'microstructure' of the extracellular matrix of the tissue or its 'collagen fibril network' structure is usually the most appropriate for formulating a model for the mechanical behaviour of an intact collagenous tissue; the directions in which the collagen fibrils are aligned can be identified with the directions in which the tissue can withstand tension. Of course the structure of the collagen molecule influences the structure of the fibril which, in turn, affects its mechanical properties. But, unless they are defective, both molecular and fibril structures are very similar in all tissues. Actually our understanding of the mechanical properties of isolated fibrils is far from complete. And, since the extracellular matrix is a composite material, it is equally important to understand the properties of the glycosaminoglycan gel — including its interactions with collagen. This complication will be considered in more detail in the section on Composite Materials.

The triple-helical conformation of the collagen molecule is familiar from biochemistry textbooks. Although details of its structure continue to be debated, there is no doubt that it consists of three polypeptide chains twisted together. Thus the rope-like molecular structure reflects the mechanical function of collagen: like any other rope it is to withstand tensile stress. But, like all ropes, it can be bent or twisted and, although it is difficult to stretch, it will not withstand axial compression. There are several different types of collagen molecule. In type I collagen (found in bone, tendon, skin, ligament, fascia, arteries and uterus) two polypeptide chains are the same but the third is different; in the other types all three chains are the same (see Ch. 1). Thus there is a slight structural difference between types at the molecular level which may cause their fibrils to have slightly different properties. But any differences in mechanical properties have yet to be identified — it would be difficult to isolate them from the influence of different glycosaminoglycan compositions and tissue microstructures. Finally X-ray diffraction shows that the application of tension to a collagen fibril does not stretch the individual molecules. Their conformation does not change when rat-tail tendon is stretched by up to 20% of its original length (Rigby et al, 1959).

There is no universally accepted model for the fibril structure (see Ch. 3). But it is clear that the rope-like molecules are packed with their axes parallel to the fibril axis (at least to within a few degrees) so that the ability of the molecules to withstand tension is reflected by the properties of the fibril. Tensile strength and stiffness are conferred on the fibril by covalent cross-links between the molecules (see Ch. 9). Fibril diameter is likely to affect the mechanical properties of a tissue but in a rather complicated way — as described in the section on Composite Materials. Diameters are not the same in different tissues; they also depend on species and the age of an individual (Harkness, 1961). Unfortunately it turns out that, to determine the effect of fibril diameter experimentally, we would also have to measure several other variables, including fibril length, which have so far proved elusive. For an assembly of parallel fibrils, surrounded by a glycosaminoglycan gel, the tensile strength of the composite (as opposed to its stiffness) depends more on the proportion of collagen than on the diameters of its fibrils.

How, and to what extent, fibril structure is affected by axially applied tension is uncertain. Hosemann et al (1974) showed that the 67 nm fibril periodicity was not measurably changed when a rat-tail tendon was stretched. But their explanation of this observation ignores the fact that the first stage of tendon elongation involves straightening its 'crimp' i.e. the microstructure of the tissue is deformed before the fibril structure changes (see section on Crimped fibres). Also it ignores the contribution of the glycosaminoglycan gel. The experiments of Cowan et al (1955) are sometimes cited as evidence that stretching a tendon increases the fibril periodicity (Harkness, 1968). But Cowan et al were investigating dried rat-tail tendon in which the contribution of the glycosaminoglycan gel to the mechanical properties would have been destroyed. As we shall see, in later Sections, this gel is crucial to the proper mechanical functioning of tendons and other collagenous tissues. My own ideas on the effects of tension on fibril structure are described on p. 58.

Several inborn errors of metabolism are characterised by tissues of low tensile strength because their collagen molecules do not cross-link or cannot pack together to form stable fibrils. The biochemistry of these disorders is discussed in Chapter 16; the aim here is simply to draw attention to the effect of molecular defects on mechanical properties. It is perhaps worth noting that none of these diseases is common; they have gained prominence largely because their biochemical mechanisms can be explained. Defects in the conversion of procollagen to collagen molecules prevent the molecules packing together in the usual manner to form strong fibrils so that tissues lose tensile strength. Such defects appear in dermatosporaxis in cattle and sheep, where the skin is easily torn, and in some cases of Type VII Ehlers-Danlos syndrome. There is a tendency for failure of cross-link formation in some types of Ehlers-Danlos syndrome, Menke's kinky hair syndrome and some forms of cutis-laxa. All of these are characterised by weakening of tissues. In, for example, Type V Ehlers-Danlos syndrome the skin is easily bruised and there can be congenital heart disease involving floppy valves. Further details of these conditions are given by Prockop et al (1979). In scurvy, which is a deficiency disease and not an inborn error of metabolism, insufficient proline residues are hydroxylated for the collagen molecule to adopt its usual triple-helical conformation; consequently fibrils are not formed.

The third level of structural organisation is the arrangement of fibrils in a tissue; collagen fibrils are dispersed throughout the extracellular matrix and their directions can be identified with the directions in which the tissue can withstand tensile stress. Suppose the fibrils in a hypothetical tissue were all aligned parallel to each other. Since the fibrils can withstand only axial tension, our tissue can withstand tension if it is applied along the direction of alignment but not if it is applied at right-angles to this direction. In another hypothetical tissue the fibrils might point randomly in all directions; thus this tissue can withstand tension equally well in all directions. Although both tissues contain exactly the same components they have very different mechanical properties simply because of their differing arrangments of fibrils.

How can the arrangement of fibrils within a tissue be determined? The most obvious technique, electron microscopy, is not quite as useful as might be expected. To correlate structure with mechanical function the arrangement of fibrils must be determined in a macroscopic sample of tissue. Electron microscopy provides such a limited field of view that one has no idea of the structure in the tissue as a whole. Transmission micrographs are commonly obtained from sections which are about 100 nm thick at a magnification of around 30 000 and recorded on films whose dimensions are 8×8 cm^2. Thus the volume of tissue sampled by a single micrograph is only about 2×10^{-5} mm^3. In order to picture the arrangement in a tiny piece of tissue whose volume was only 1 mm^3 we would have to record about 50 000 micrographs — and somehow be able to measure the orientation of all of them relative to the original piece of tissue. However transmission electron microscopy can be useful when a very small area of tissue has to be examined in detail e.g. for investigating the structure of the site of crimping in tendon (Dlugosz et al, 1978). Scanning electron microscopy fares little better from the statistical point of view because, although a typical magnification might only be around 1000, it images only the very surface of the specimen. Once again, however, scanning electron microscopy has proved useful in certain specialised applications e.g. for determining whether collagenous fibres are crimped (Gathercole & Keller, 1975).

There are two different approaches to investigating the arrangement of microscopic fibrils in a macroscopic sample. One is X-ray diffraction (Aspden & Hukins, 1979); the other is polarised light microscopy (Diamant et al, 1972; Speer & Dahners, 1979). Although X-ray diffraction patterns can be obtained rapidly from some tissues (e.g. in about 10 minutes from annulus fibrosus) it can often be a very slow technique (e.g. it takes two to three days to record a diffraction pattern from articular cartilage). Polarised light microscopy is more rapid but usually less quantitative; although in some applications it is perfectly adeqate e.g. for demonstrating the structure of the crimp in rat-tail tendon (Diamant et al, 1972). However polarised light can, at least in principle, be used to obtain more quantitative results, if the arrangement of fibrils has a reasonable degree of preferred orientation, by using it to measure birefringence. When the structure of the collagen fibril network has been determined it can often be related to mechanical function of the tissue.

MECHANICAL CONCEPTS

Stress and strain

This section serves two purposes: to explain some mechanical ideas which may be unfamiliar and to draw attention to a few of the more important complications which are involved in relating the deformation of a material to an applied force. Complications include the extent to which the previous history of the tissue may affect its mechanical properties and the importance of e.g. the rate at which a force is applied. When a tissue is removed from an animal it must be subjected to some mechanical stress i.e. cutting, pulling, bending etc. How will this pre-treatment affect its behaviour in the mechanical testing apparatus? And when the tests are performed, it must be remembered that the mechanical behaviour of a collagenous tissue depends on the rate at which it is loaded. Before these complications are considered any further it will be necessary to explain some mechanical terms.

A fibre of length L can be stretched by an increment l, so that its new length is $L + l$, by a force F pulling along its axial direction. In order to stretch the fibre one end has to be tethered — otherwise the applied force would simply pull it along instead of stretching it. Tethering allows an equal and opposite reaction to the applied force i.e. a force of magnitude F acts in both directions along the stretched fibre. The value of l depends on F and the cross-sectional area, A, of the fibre as well as on the material which the fibre is made of — rubber stretches more easily than steel. Everyday experience teaches us that thick ropes are more difficult to stretch than thin strings. In the seventeenth century Robert Hooke showed that if we double the cross-sectional area of a wire of fixed length, without changing the material it is made of, we must double the force required to produce a given extension. Therefore, to compare the mechanical properties of different specimens, we do not compare the values of F required to produce a given deformation but instead consider force divided by cross-sectional area. This quantity is called *stress*, denoted here by σ, which is defined by:

$$\sigma = F/A$$

Since force is measured in newtons (N) and area in square metres (m^2), stress is measured in newtons per square metre ($N\ m^{-2}$) i.e. it has the same units as pressure. But, unlike pressure in a fluid which acts equally in all directions, stress is associated with a direction. The effect of the force, F, on the cross-sectional area, A, is often ignored. Actually this effect is rather slight but strictly the A in the equation above refers to the cross-sectional area when the force is acting; A is slightly greater when the force is removed.

Experience also teaches us that a string which is several metres long can easily be stretched by a few millimetres — but for a few centimetres of the same string this same extension is far more difficult to attain. Thus, when comparing the mechanical behaviour of specimens, we should consider not the extension, l, but this extension expressed as a fraction of the original length. This quantity is called *strain* and is denoted here by ϵ, so that

$$\epsilon = l/L.$$

Note that since l and L are both lengths, measured for example in metres, dividing one by another yields a number with no units. Since ϵ values encountered in practice are often very small, it is sometimes more convenient to express them as percentages i.e. a strain of 0.02 becomes a 2 per cent strain.

We have already seen that when a fibre is stretched it becomes slightly thinner i.e. its thickness decreases when its length increases. Thus an axial stress produces a small radial strain at the same time as the axial strain. The ratio of the radial strain to the axial strain is called the *Poisson's ratio* of the material of the fibre — although it always has a value of around 0.3 for metal wires, biological materials can exhibit a wide range of values (Gordon, 1978). However throughout this chapter 'strain' is taken to mean the strain along the direction of the applied stress.

So far we have only considered axial stress which tends to stretch a fibre, so called 'tensile stress'. In the Introduction we saw that the function of a fibre is to withstand such axial tension but it simply crumples if an axial stress which tends to compress it is applied. Collagen fibrils are unlikely to be an exception. But many collagenous tissues, such as articular cartilage, can withstand compressive stress. Consider a block of cartilage of thickness T being compressed by a piston of cross-sectional area A. The thickness of the cartilage will decrease, by a decrement t, over the compressed area so that its thickness is only T-t where it is in contact with the piston. Thus it is subjected to an uniaxial compressive stress of F/A and the axial strain which it experiences is t/T. (According to our definition of strain it is strictly $-\ t/T$ since the increase in thickness is negative; but we can overcome this difficulty simply by calling t/T the 'compressive strain' as opposed to the 'tensile strain').

The mechanical behaviour of a material can be simply

illustrated by a graph showing the stress required to produce a given strain. Figure 4.1a shows the shape of a typical stress-strain curve obtained by stretching tendon. Actually the applied force, *F*, is used in this figure as a measure of stress because of the difficulty of measuring the cross-sectional area of a tendon. Since this area does not change appreciably for the small strains shown in the figure, the shape of the curve is unaffected. Notice that as the strain becomes greater so the curve becomes steeper i.e. more force is required to produce a given increase in strain: thus the steeper the slope the stiffer the material. Figure 4.1b shows a stress-strain curve obtained by compressing articular cartilage. Once again the material becomes stiffer as the strain increases.

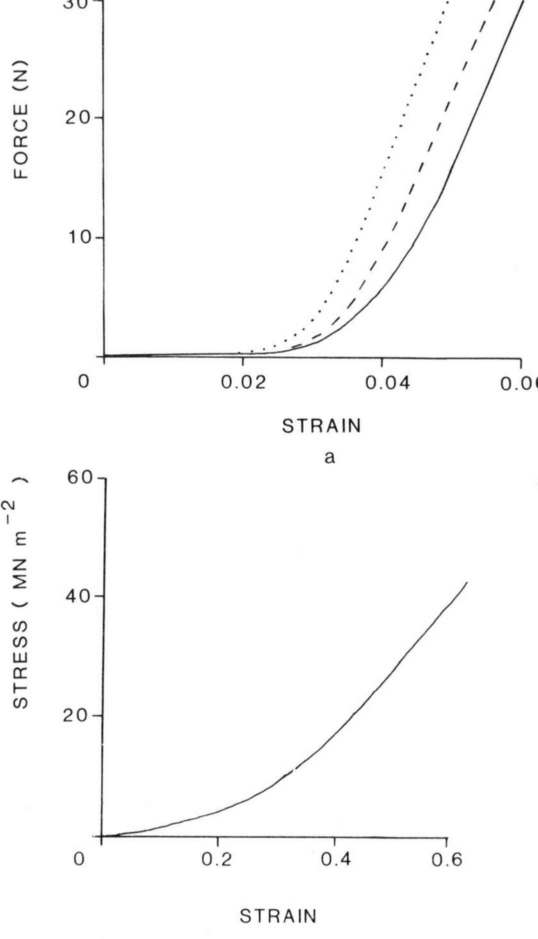

Fig. 4.1 Continuous curves show the shapes of the stress-strain curves obtained (a) by stretching tendon (data from Kenedi et al, 1975) and (b) when compressing the deep layer of articular cartilage (data from Kempson, 1979). In (a) the applied force, rather than stress, is plotted because of the difficulty of measuring the cross-sectional area of a tendon. These curves correspond to slow loading; in (a) the dotted and dashed curves correspond to strain rates of 0.01 s^{-1} and 0.001 s^{-1} respectively.

The slope of a stress-strain curve is often called the *Young's modulus* of the material, but this term can be very misleading when applied to collagenous tissues. Figure 4.1a shows that the slope of the curve is not constant for tendon i.e. there is no unique Young's modulus because its value depends on the strain. Cartilage ehibits similar behaviour in compression (see Fig. 4.1b). But one frequently encounters references to 'the Young's modulus' of tendon, implying that it has a unique value. Why? The reason is that the stress-strain curve for a metal wire is a straight line (except at strains near the breaking point) i.e. it has a unique Young's modulus. Materials which behave in this way are said to obey Hooke's law. Many physicists and engineers have an unhealthy respect for this law which is little more than an observation on the mechanical properties of metals.

In general a stress need not be confined to a single axis i.e. it need not be uniaxial. If the stress is the same in all directions and the material has the same properties in all directions (i.e. it is isotropic) then the mechanics of deformation is simple. But biological materials do not usually have the same properties in all directions — they are anisotropic e.g. the size and strength of scars in skin depends on the direction of the original incision (Kenedi et al, 1975). In general the description of the stresses acting on a body and the resulting strains is very complicated. Fortunately we can understand many of the properties of collagenous tissues simply by considering the stress propagated in the directions of the collagen fibril axes, since the function of the fibrils is to withstand axially applied tensile stress. This simple approach will be used throughout this chapter and more details on the underlying mechanical concepts can be found in an excellent book by Gordon (1978).

We have to recognise a further variety of stress — that associated with shear. Tensile and compressive stress are essentially the same idea; compression is simply tension applied in the opposite direction. But shear stress is completely different — it is associated with a force which tends to cause slippage. Fig. 4.2a shows a cube of material each of whose faces has an area A. In Fig. 4.2b a force, F, is applied which skews the cube — the shear stress is defined to be F/A.

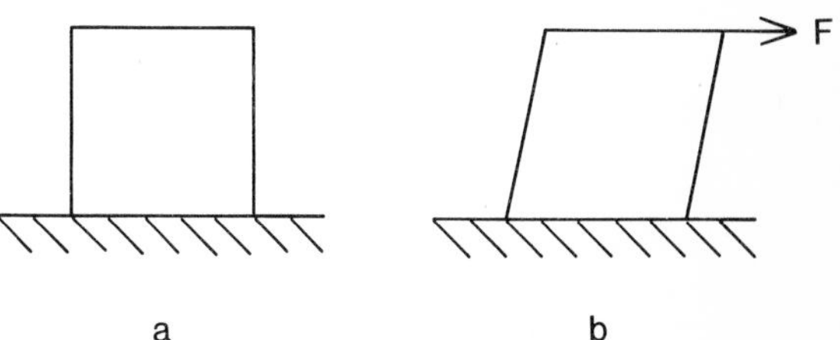

Fig. 4.2 A cube which is fixed to a base so that an applied force will not cause it to slide along or topple over is shown in (a). The same cube is sheared by a force, F, in (b).

Energy, hysteresis and creep

We have considered how an applied force deforms a material but have not considered the work done by the force. In other words the energetics of deformation has been ignored — energy being just stored work. Suppose force is applied to a fibre so as to gradually increase its length from L to $L + l$. No force is required to maintain the original length, L, and, as the applied force gradually increases, so the length gradually increases. Figure 4.3a shows the applied force needed to maintain the fibre at a given length; it increases from an initial value of zero, when the length if L, to a final value of F when the length is $L + l$. (Although the force increases linearly with length in this figure, there is no reason for it to do so in general — see Figure 4.1.) By definition the work done in stretching the fibre is the shaded area under the curve of Figure 4.3a. In Figure 4.3b we see the corresponding stress-strain curve; the strain increases from an initial value of zero to a final value of l/L. Since stress is simply force divided by cross-sectional area and strain is the fractional increase in length, the shaded area under the stress-strain curve is the work done in stretching a unit volume of the fibre. Now consider the force on a fibre, which has a stretched length of $L + l$, being gradually decreased to zero. And suppose that Figure 4.3a represents the decreasing force required to maintain a contracted length, so that when there is no applied force the length is L. Now the shaded area of Figure 4.3a represents the work done by the fibre in contracting i.e. it represents the energy which was stored by the stretched fibre. Similarly the shaded area in Figure 4.3b now represents the energy stored by a unit volume of stretched fibre.

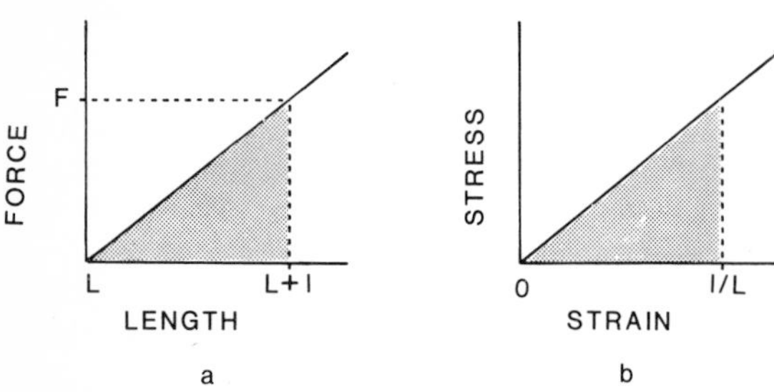

Fig. 4.3 (a)Force plotted against length for a fibre which obeys Hooke's Law. (b) Corresponding stress-strain curve.

Figure 4.4a shows the stress-strain curves obtained when a tendon is stretched (continuous line) and then allowed to relax (dashed line); the two are not the same. Thus a tendon follows a different path on the stress-strain diagram when a tensile stress is applied than when the stress is removed. Given sufficient time the tendon will relax to its original length (provided the strain does not exceed a critical value) — it is said to be *elastic*. But, because of the different paths followed in stretching and relaxation, it is also said to exhibit hysteresis. Notice that the area under the continuous curve is greater than the area under the dashed curve. Thus more work is required to stretch a unit volume of tendon than it can perform on relaxing i.e. the tendon does not store all the energy used to deform it. Its behaviour is then intermediate between that of a metal wire which (except near its breaking point) stores nearly all its deformation energy and a viscous liquid which, although it offers resistance to deformation (i.e. energy is required to deform it) does not store any of the energy. Few biological materials store most of the energy used to deform them and it is never safe to assume that their mechanical properties resemble those of the idealised metal wires which inhabit physics textbooks.

Figure 4.4 actually illustrates some experimental results obtained by Torp et al (1975a) in which a rat-tail tendon was subjected to fifty cycles of successive extension and relaxation. At no time in this particular experiment did the strain exceed the critical value above which the tendon would be incapable of returning to its original length. In Figure 4.4a the stress-strain curves are shown for the first extension and subsequent relaxation; in Figure 4.4b the fiftieth extension and relaxation curves are shown. Comparison of the two sets of data shows that this cyclic loading increases the stiffness of the tendon somewhat and, very noticeably, decreases the area between the extension and relaxation curves. Thus, after repeated loading and relaxation, the tendon stores most of its deformation energy and slightly stiffens.

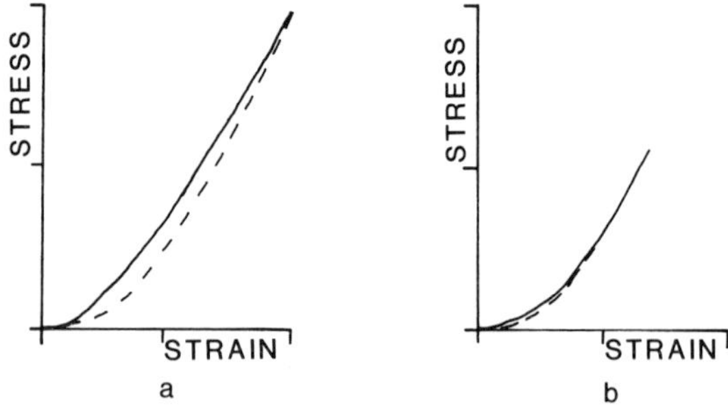

Fig. 4.4 Stress-strain curves for a rat-tail tendon which is stretched (continuous curve) and then relaxed (dashed curve): (a) initial results and (b) after 50 cycles of rapid extension and relaxation (data from Torp et al, 1975a).

How can we explain hysteresis and the effects of repeated loading? Harkness (1968) indicates that tendon behaves like 'an elastic framework with fluid in the interstices displaced by successive tests'. Some of the energy expended in stretching such a system is used to drive out fluid. Since fluids are viscous the energy used for this purpose is not stored but is dissipated as heat. Thus the system does not store all the energy used to deform it. On relaxation fluid would be absorbed to compensate for that lost in stretching — but this absorption process is not expected to be instantaneous. After many cycles of rapid loading and unloading the system has no chance to replenish all its fluid. Thus there is progressively less fluid available to be driven out in later cycles of deformation so that this mechanism is no longer available for dissipating energy. Now the system has to store most of its deformation energy and, because none of this energy can be diverted to expressing fluid, it becomes stiffer.

Figure 4.1a shows that the stress-strain curve obtained when a tendon is stretched depends on the rate at which the stress is applied. Tendon is not unique in this respect; indeed a range of collagenous tissues has been shown to exhibit this behaviour. Unfortunately stress rates are not always recorded in the literature concerned with the mechanics of collagenous tissues. This neglect has led Kenedi et al (1975) to comment that 'it is unfortunate that a large portion of the literature reporting careful and well meant work is of questionable value because of the disregard of this time factor'. It can be seen from Figure 4.1a that the stiffness of tendon increases as the rate of loading is increased.

The time dependence of mechanical behaviour is associated with the phenomenon of *creep*. When a load of 10 N was applied to a human flexor digitorum tendon the initial strain was 0.015. But after a period of 100 s under this same constant load, the strain increased to greater than 0.016 (Cohen et al, 1976). Creep is defined as the continuance of deformation with time under a constant applied stress. Materials which exhibit time dependence in their mechanical properties, i.e. which creep under a constant stress, are said to be *viscoelastic.* The rate at which a viscoelastic material creeps depends on temperature; Cohen et al performed their experiments on human digital tendons at 30°C. Note that the faster successive loads are applied to a viscoelastic material, the less time the material has to creep under that load — so the less the observed strain. Thus the stiffening of collagenous tissues as the rate of loading is increased is to be expected if they are viscoelastic and so exhibit creep.

Toughness, fracture and resilience

If increasing tensile stress is applied to a fibre it will eventually break. The tensile *strength* of a material is simply the stress required to break it in tension. Thus the tensile strength of tendon (82 MN m^{-2}) is much greater than that of muscle (0.1 MN m^{-2}). Consequently the force generated by a muscle can be applied to a much smaller cross-sectional area of tendon without breaking it — so that tendons can be much thinner than the muscles they are attached to. Notice that strength and stiffness are not the same. Gordon (1978) makes the point as follows:

> A biscuit is stiff but weak, steel is stiff and strong, nylon is flexible [opposite of stiff] and strong, raspberry jelly is flexible and weak. The two properties together describe a solid about as well as you can reasonably expect.

(Puzzled North Americans should remember that 'biscuit' and 'jelly' mean different things to the English — in American English the corresponding words are 'cookie' and 'jello'.)

In the jargon of materials science *toughness* and strength are not the same. When the tensile stress on a fibre is increased it will eventually become permanently deformed — although the resulting irreversible change could be considered as a form of damage it is not the same as breakage. Some materials can withstand high stresses even when they are already permanently deformed; they break gradually and then only after a very high stress is applied. If the stress is removed before the deformed material breaks, its original length is not recovered — it is said to be *plastically deformed* and to have acquired a *permanent set.* Such materials are said to be tough. Strong materials are very resistant to plastic deformation — they break suddenly after very little plastic deformation has occurred. High tensile steel is strong but tendon is tough and so fails gradually. There are various estimates in the literature for the strain at which tendon acquires a permanent set; the spread of values probably arises because of the difficulty of deciding what initial stress has to be applied to the tendon to remove kinks and bends without causing strain. However estimates only vary between 0.02 and 0.04; the lower figure is mentioned by Harkness (1968) although the higher seems to have been reasonably reliably established by Rigby et al (1959). Cohen et al (1976) list further references which establish that the onset of plastic deformation in tendons occurs at strains of between 0.02 and 0.04.

If we apply a sharp tug to a short length of thread it breaks but a long thread does not. Why? The idea of some critical breaking stress does not help us to understand this observation — the stress is independent of the length of the thread. In order to gain any understanding we have to consider the energy required to cause fracture. For the sake of simplicity we can consider a material which obeys Hooke's law; but the qualitative conclusions we shall reach are more general and apply to all materials. Figure 4.3a shows the force required to stretch a fibre which obeys Hooke's law from an initial length, L, to a final length, $L + l$; at this final length the applied force is F. The energy, E, expended in stretching the fibre is given by the shaded area in the figure which, since it is triangular, is

$$E = Fl/2.$$

But because the fibre obeys Hooke's law, stress divided by strain is a constant called the Young's modulus, Y, of the material. Thus

$$Y = \frac{\sigma}{\epsilon} = \frac{F}{A} \cdot \frac{L}{l}$$

where A is the cross-sectional area of the fibre. This equation can be rearranged to give

$$l = FL/YA$$

We can substitute this expression for l into the equation which gives us the energy to stretch a fibre; the result is

$$E = LF^2/2YA$$

Thus the greater the length, L, of the fibre the greater is the energy required to stretch it — even though the force, F, is the same. If we suddenly apply energy to a fibre we can stretch it. For a long fibre all the energy may be used up in stretching; energy is released as soon as tension is removed when the fibre relaxes to its original length — so a sharp tug of short duration will not cause damage. But for a short fibre less energy will be required for stretching and, if the same quantity of energy is supplied, some will be left over for breaking bonds.

Energy, which can break bonds, rather than force, is ultimately responsible for fracture. We have already seen that collagenous tissues exhibit mechanical hysteresis i.e. they do not store all their deformation energy. It seems likely that this behaviour is a mechanism for protecting against the danger of energy stored during a period under tension being used to cause fracture. Fracture can occur if the formation of two new surfaces (propagation of a crack) requires less energy than that stored. If some of the deformation energy is dissipated, instead of being stored, less will be available for causing fracture. In a tough material the energy tends to become dissipated far from the potential new surfaces so that sudden fracture does not occur — and the resulting 'ductile fracture' has the appearance of (well chewed) chewing gum which has been pulled apart. But in a strong material two new surfaces can be formed as soon as is energetically favourable, with little plastic deformation, and the resulting 'brittle fracture' is a clean break.

This energetic view of fracture is closely linked to the idea of *resilience*. Resilience is the ability to deform without fracture occurring. We have seen that the principal deformation of a stretched fibre is l, its increase in length. To simplify this discussion, consider a fibre which obeys Hooke's law; although, once again, the conclusions we shall reach are more general and apply to all materials. A little manipulation of the equations we have already obtained gives the result.

$$l = (2LE/YA)^{\frac{1}{2}}$$

i.e. if a given quantity of energy, E, is applied the deformation will be greater if the fibre is long compared with its cross-sectional area (high value of L/A) and has low stiffness (low Y value). Resilient materials are useful because they absorb energy which might otherwise be used to fracture more easily damaged materials. Thus foam rubber, which is very resilient (because of its very low stiffness) can be used in packaging to prevent damage to glassware because it absorbs the temporary sudden increases in deformation energy which a parcel is subjected to in handling.

Resilience is useful, because it guards against sudden jolts causing fracture, but it can lead to a structure which is just too floppy for its intended purpose — because high resilience implies low stiffness. Thus glass packaged in foam rubber has to be enclosed in a stiff cardboard box. But collagenous materials manage to be resilient without being too floppy. Figure 4.1 shows stress-strain curves for tendon and cartilage. At low strains these tissues have low stiffness i.e. they are resilient. But as the strain increases so does the stiffness — ensuring that they are not too floppy to transmit force from a contracting muscle (tendon) or to withstand applied pressure (articular cartilage).

COMPOSITE MATERIALS

Extracellular matrices consist of collagen fibrils surrounded by a glycosaminoglycan gel; the properties and applications of mixtures of this kind are well known to materials scientists who call them *fibre composites*. We have already seen that bulk materials fracture in tension when cracks propagate across them. Similarly a scratch on the surface of a bulk material can enlarge under tension and lead to fracture — for further details see Gordon (1978). When a sheet of glass is bent the length of the convex surface increases i.e. it is under tension. A crack can form in this stretched surface and propagate across the sheet — leading to fracture. If a scratch is introduced into this surface, before bending, it acts as an initiating site from which a crack can spread. (Scratching, followed by bending is the standard method for cutting glass.) Thus a sheet of glass is easily broken by attempts to bend it. In complete contrast glass fibres can be used to make very flexible fishing rods, vaulting poles, etc. which bend easily and whose behaviour is not greatly affected by small surface scratches. To make these flexible structures the glass fibres are surrounded by weak plastic. A crack will form in the plastic before it forms in the glass — because it is weaker. But Figure 4.5a shows that the crack will not spread across the material because it soon encounters a much stronger fibre; it may spread some distance along the length of a fibre but it does not continue to be propagated in its original direction — in complete contrast to the spread of a crack in a bent glass plate. Thus glass fibre reinforced plastics do not fracture as readily as a sheet of glass or a slab of plastic. Note that, in glass reinforced plastics, it is important, for maximum strength, that each fibre is surrounded by plastic. Similarly the individual collagen fibrils in extracellular matrices invariably seem to be surrounded by a layer of gel. Figure 4.5b shows the side-to-side spacing of fibrils in the annulus fibrosus of the intervertebral disc, as an example. If two fibrils were to touch it would be possible for a crack to spread from one to another.

Since tissues which contain collagen also contain glycosaminoglycans, it is immediately clear that we are

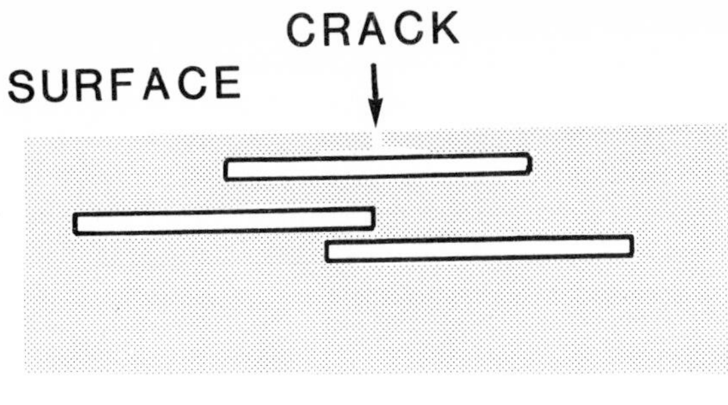

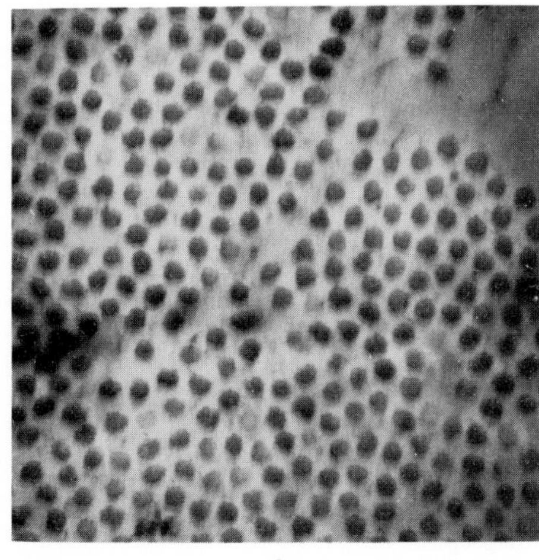

Fig. 4.5 (a) Longitudinal section of a fibre composite showing how a weak filler prevents crack propagation, from one fibre to another, compared with (b) a transverse section of annulus fibrosus of intervertebral disc, showing the collagen fibrils surrounded by glycosaminoglycan gel. The electron micrograph in (b) was taken (by D.S. Hickey) at an original magnification of 80 000.

never really concerned with the biomechanical properties of collagen alone; the mechanical properties of tissues are dictated by the behaviour of collagen in composite materials. To this extent the title of the chapter is rather a misnomer. Biophysicists often refer to the physical properties of 'collagen' when they mean 'tendon'; they assume that, because tendon contains so much collagen, the two terms are effectively synonymous. Nothing could be further from the truth. This assumption makes about as much sense as assuming that window glass has the same properties as a fibre glass fishing rod! Actually we only need to understand the mechanical properties of collagen itself in so far as it helps us to understand its properties in fibre composites. Mechanical experiments on tissues such as tendon tell us about the behaviour of such composites directly — we can only infer what the properties of the collagen alone would be.

Consider a rod consisting of a bundle of parallel fibres embedded in a weaker medium, like the plastic in fibre glass or the glycosaminoglycan gel in a tissue, which is subjected to tensile stress; we can assume, for the present, that the fibres are continuous along the length of the rod. At a critical stress, σ_m, the weaker medium will begin to flow plastically along the fibres. Friction then causes a tensile stress to be applied to them. Thus applied tensile stress is transmitted to the fibres via the surrounding medium. But the stress is not exerted uniformly along the length of a fibre. At the ends the stress is zero; it reaches its maximum value only over a critical length, L_c, which is given by

$$L_c = r\sigma_f / \tau$$

where r is the radius of a fibre which fractures at a stress of σ_f and τ is the stress exerted on it by yielding medium (Cottrell, 1964). The stress at which the rod fractures is given by

$$\sigma_c = \sigma_f V_f + \sigma_m (l - V_f)$$

where V_f is the fraction of the composite's volume occupied by fibres.

What happens if the fibres are not continuous throughout the length of the composite? This question is relevant to the properties of collagenous tissues because there is no evidence as to whether, for example, the fibrils are continuous throughout the thickness of articular cartilage coating a bone. We shall consider an example where it is particularly easy to see that a problem might arise: can a tendon withstand tensile stress if its collagen fibrils are shorter than the tendon itself? The answer is — maybe yes. If the length, L, of a fibril is much greater than its critical length, L_c, then the expression for the fracture stress of the tendon, σ_c, is expected to be unchanged, according to the theory of fibre composites (Cottrell, 1964). But if L is reduced to L_c the tensile strength of the composite is halved. And if L is much less than L_c, the fibrils will be pulled out of the gel by applied tensile stress. Thus for intrinsic strength the ratio L/L_c should be as large as possible. However the fibrils will then be evenly stressed over most of their lengths — if one breaks the others are then likely to become overloaded and the tendon would fail. For greater toughness L should be slightly smaller than L_c — and L_c should be as large as possible. Since we have already seen that tendon is a tough material, we would expect L_c for its collagen fibrils to be very high and their actual length, L, to be rather less.

What are the lengths of collagen fibrils in tissues and how do they compare with the critical lengths? Nobody knows. Fibril lengths have never been measured experimentally because no-one has yet thought of a way. And there are insufficient experimental data to calculate L_c from the expression given above. Although the radii, r, of fibrils have been measured, σ_f, the stress at which a fibril fractures, and τ, the stress exerted on a fibril by a yielding glycosaminoglycan gel, have not. Two further complications arise. One: all the fibrils in a tissue do not have the same value of r — indeed in some tissues there is a considerable spread of values. Two: τ will depend on the chemical composition of the glycosaminoglycan gel which is tissue dependent and varies with age. We can now see why the problem of relating collagen fibril diameters to the mechanical properties of a tissue, which was raised in the section on Structural Hierarchies, is far from trivial.

Despite our ignorance of the values of important parameters, the theory of fibre composites can still help us to understand a little more about collagenous tissues. We have seen that, for maximum toughness, the critical length, L_c, of a fibril should be as large as possible and that this aim can be achieved in three ways: (1) increase r, (2) increase σ_f and (3) decrease τ. Changes in cross-linking with age (Schofield & Weightman, 1978) presumably affect σ_f and in those diseases where cross-links do not form σ_f will be very low i.e. the tissue will not be as tough as normal. The most interesting result is that L_c is increased by decreasing τ — which can be achieved by weakening the gel itself and/or its interactions with fibrils (Cottrell, 1964). Paradoxically, then, weakening the gel toughens the tissue. Chemical changes occur in the glycosaminoglycan gels of aging tissues (Muir, 1978) and during development (Markwald et al, 1978). But the mechanical consequences of these chemical changes remain unknown.

Other components

Collagenous tissues contain other extracellular macromolecules besides collagen and glycosaminoglycans; elastin, in particular, is likely to have a profound effect on mechanical properties. Elastin occurs in association with collagen in very many tissues; especially large amounts occur in blood vessels and in certain ligaments. It has the remarkable property of being able to withstand a 100 per cent strain without acquiring a permanent set. Harkness (1968) believes its function is to prevent creep in tissues under prolonged stress (he cites the posterior ligament in the necks of grazing animals as an example) and to store energy with minimal loss. Energy storage might be useful in blood vessels to even out the pressure surges caused by heart beat (McNeill Alexander, 1975). Minns & Steven (1977) consider that the combination of elastin, which has low stiffness, with the relatively stiffer collagen may introduce more variety into the mechanical properties of collagenous tissues.

Calcification also affects the properties of collagenous tissues — as illustrated by the stiffness of bone. Actually we might expect bone to be stiffer than tendon simply because its collagen is not 'crimped' (Gathercole & Keller, 1975) — we shall see, in a later section, that crimping is responsible for the decreased stiffness of tendon at low strains noted in the section on Stress and strain (p. 53). Nevertheless it seems likely that the stiffness of bone is, in part, due to the presence of hydroxyapatite crystals; this view is consistent with the observation that the calcified leg tendons of turkeys are stiffer than other tendons. Furthermore Minns & Steven (1977) showed that calcification increased the stiffness of pig thoracic aorta just before rupture and that it decreased the stored deformation energy. It appeared that the collagen in the aorta, rather than the elastin, was affected by treatment with calcium and that this treatment also affected the appearance of the fracture when the aorta finally failed. According to the Section on Toughness fracture and resilience (p. 56) the latter result implies that calcification affects the mechanism of fracture.

How does calcification stiffen collagen? It has been suggested by Lees & Davidson (1977) as well as by McCutcheon (1975) that the crystals of calcium salts are actually bonded to the collagen. Some indirect evidence for this suggestion has been presented by Lees (1979). Although McCutcheon makes the unlikely assumption that collagenous tissues deform solely by extension of their collagen molecules, the idea that bonding to crystals would stiffen collagen is still valid. However, stiffening of fibrils themselves can be explained by an entirely different mechanism, without the need to postulate bonds between crystals and collagen molecules (Hukins, 1978). The molecules within a fibril are regularly staggered, to give a periodic structure in the fibril axis direction, but there appears to be far less order in their lateral arrangement (see Ch. 3). Axial extension of such systems is accompanied by a side-to-side rearrangement of molecules. Crystals within a fibril will inhibit this rearrangement and hence stiffen the fibril.

Any structural heterogeneties will affect the mechanical properties of a tissue; thus pathological calcification could affect mechanical properties even if it is only of limited extent. Figure 4.6a shows a homogeneous block of material subjected to tensile stress; because of the homogeneity the stress in the material is even distributed all over its cross-

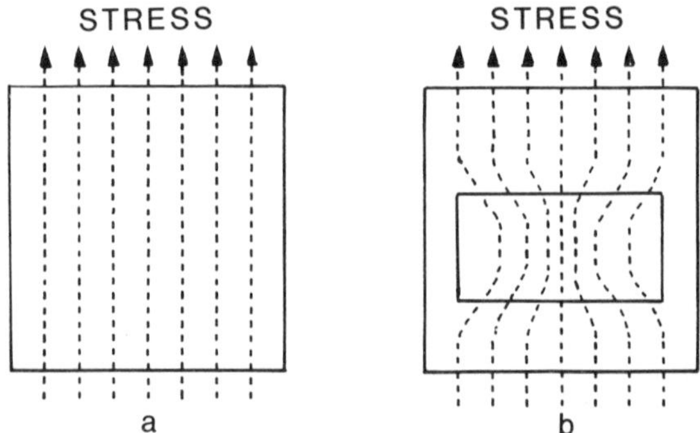

Fig. 4.6 Stress trajectories arising from tension (a) of a homogeneous material and (b) of the same material with a stiffer insert.

sectional area. The dotted lines that indicate the directions in which stresses are generated, called *stress trajectories*, are, therefore, parallel. But in Figure 4.6b a small piece of stiffer material has been inserted into the block and, in consequence, the stress trajectories are distorted. If the block is uniformly strained, i.e. if the stiff insert is firmly stuck to the surrounding material, the stress in the insert will be greater than in the less stiff surroundings. Thus the stress trajectories are redistributed as in Figure 4.6b i.e. in the original material stress is concentrated around the position of the insert. Stress concentration can be a source of mechanical damage — paradoxically a weak material can be damaged in this way by inserting a piece of stronger material into it! Thus any inserts, be they stronger or weaker than the surrounding material will redistribute stress. Stress concentrations would thus appear to have important implications in surgery. Prostheses should not cause stress concentrations which are sufficiently high to damage the surrounding tissue.

Finally it should not be forgotten that cells will influence the mechanical properties of a tissue. One way is simply to introduce stress concentrations and hence to weaken surrounding regions of tissue — Torp et al (1975b) noted that tendons tended to fracture around fibroblasts which 'seemed to act as stress concentrators'. Another way cells may influence mechanical properties is to cause a certain 'roughness' at the surface of articular cartilage (Longmore & Gardner, 1978); bumps and hollows, about 1 μm high or deep, mean that the surface is not so smooth as carefully polished metal.

FIBRES

Crimping

When tendons are examined under the light microscope they have a characteristic wavy appearance; this waviness, or *crimp*, is not confined to tendon but can be observed in the collagen of most mammalian tissues with the exception of bone and articular cartilage (Gathercole & Keller, 1975). Determination of the crimp structure is not as trivial as it might, at first sight, appear. The wavy appearance of tendon could be caused by its fibres being bent into a 'zig-zag' or by their being wound into a helix, like a corkscrew. Figures 4.7a and b illustrate these two extreme models with a strip of paper which is white on one side and black on the other; in (a) it is bent into a zig-zag and in (b) into a helix. We can describe the bending of the zig-zag.completely by drawing a side-on view as in Figure 4.8a: but the helix bends backwards and forwards as well as up and down i.e. the helical waveform is truly three-dimensional but the zig-zag structure has a planar waveform. Although it is easy to distinguish these two structures in Figure 4.7a and b, for a less flattened fibre, which is not painted different colours on different sides, it is far more difficult to make the distinction purely by inspection. And the true structure

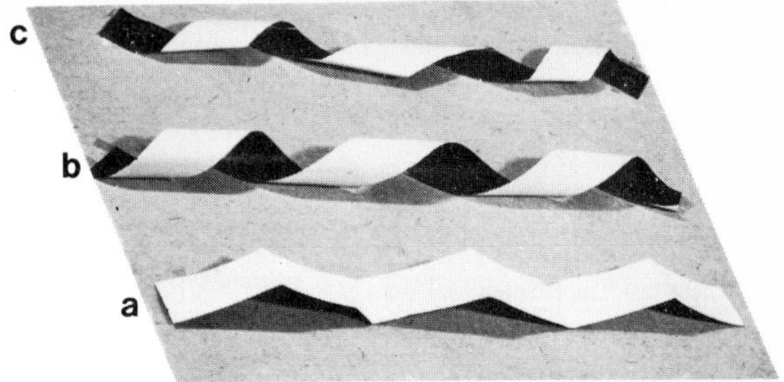

Fig. 4.7 Possible models for fibre crimp: (a) zig-zag, (b) helix and (c) flattened helix. These models were constructed from a strip of paper blackened on one side.

could be intermediate between these two extremes — like the flattened helix of Figure 4.7c.

Diamant et al (1972) showed conclusively, using polarised light microscopy, that the crimp in rat-tail tendon was planar. The period of the crimp (the peak-to-peak distance, p, of Figure 4.8a was typically about 200 μm and its angle (θ of Figure 4.8a) was in the range 15 to 20°. Although the crimp is most easily observed in fibres, of diameter around 100 μm, which can readily be dissected from the tendon, these fibres can be teased apart without destroying the crimp until, at last, it is found to be a property of the individual collagen fibrils (Diamant et al, 1972). Transmission electron micrographs show the kinks in the collagen fibrils which give rise to the crimp (Dlugosz et al, 1978). Kinks provide further evidence that, in this

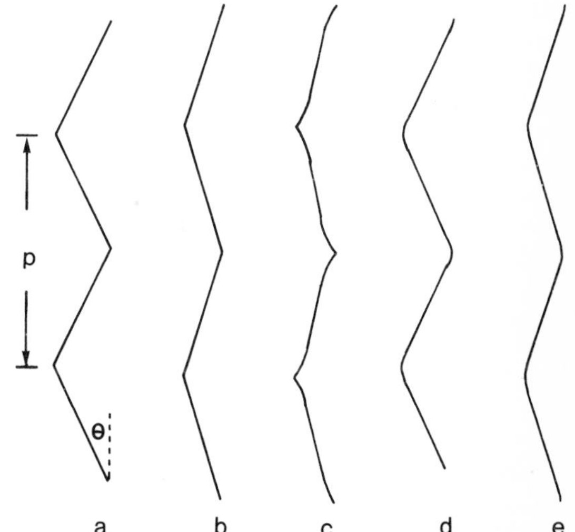

Fig. 4.8 Side views of crimp models. (a) Simple zig-zag of period p and crimp angle θ. (b) Simple zig-zag in an intermediate stage of extension, assuming flexible apices. (c) Intermediate stage of extension of a simple zig-zag recognising that the apices are infinitely stiff. (d) Modified zig-zag with slightly rounded apices. (e) Intermediate stage of extension of modified zig-zag.

tissue, the wavy appearance is not caused by the collagen fibrils being wound into helices. A fibre which is bent into a helix has a constant curvature along its length — there are no kinks in a corkscrew. But a fibre bent into a plane wave, illustrated by Figures 4.7a and 4.8a, suddenly changes direction at each peak and trough.

Millington et al (1971) referred to the fibres in a variety of collagenous tissues as being 'coiled'. Their scanning electron micrographs certainly suggest that in skin the crimp structure may be rather more complicated than in rat-tail tendon — perhaps like the flattened helix of Figure 4.7c. But Gathercole & Keller (1975) show a scanning electron micrograph of a fibre teased from skin which appears to have a planar crimp — although it is just possible that this fibre could be atypical because it was obtained from the skin of a patient suffering from Ehlers-Danlos syndrome. Nevertheless their micrographs suggest that the crimp waveform is planar in very many tissues; the planarity has been established in human spinal ligaments, as well as in rat tail tendon, by polarised light microscopy (Shah et al, 1979). There is, however, considerable variability in the period of the crimp — in bovine skin it is as low as 3 μm (Gathercole & Keller, 1975).

It has long been recognised that the first stage in the extension of a tendon simply involves straightening out its crimp (Rigby et al, 1959; Elliott, 1965). The ease of straightening accounts for the low stiffness of tendon when it is first stretched. But, when the crimp is removed, further extension becomes very difficult and the tendon is much stiffer as shown by the characteristic shape of its stress-strain curve in Figure 4.1 a. In the initial stages of extension, i.e. for strains of up to about four per cent, the length of the tendon increases simply because straightening the crimp increases its angle (θ of Figure 4.8 a) and hence the crimp period (p in Figure 4.8 a).

Diamant et al (1972) appeared to have formulated a quantitative theory of the initial stages of tendon deformation based on straightening the crimp; but recent results show that their theory is not so successful as it seemed (Buckley et al, 1980). Such a theory requires a detailed knowledge of crimp geometry. Diamant et al assumed the simple plane wave of Figure 4.8a — a zig-zag whose segments are straight lines. They treated each area of the zig-zag as a cantilever so that Figure 4.8b represented an intermediate stage of crimp straightening. The simplicity of this model is especially appealing because it corresponds very closely to the observed crimp shape while requiring few parameters for its description. Furthermore the mechanical behaviour of this cantilever depends on the cross-sectional area of its tension-bearing elements — the collagen fibrils. Diamant et al (1972) calculated the fibril diameters solely from mechanical properties, using their theory, and compared the results with those obtained by electron microscopy — the agreement was excellent. However they realised that if the apices of the crimped tendon were infinitely stiff (i.e. if they could never bend), an intermediate stage in fibre deformation would resemble Figure 4.8c rather than Figure 4.8b. Buckley et al (1980) showed that the apices of the simple zig-zag must be infinitely stiff i.e. the assumption that a crimp with this geometry would straighten via the form shown in Figure 4.8b was invalid. But tendon does not change its shape as shown in Figure 4.8c when it is stretched — so the crimp geometry must be rather more complicated than Figure 4.8a suggests. More complicated planar crimps can be described by a single further parameter and the effect of changing its value on the mechanical properties of a crimped fibre found by computer simulation. Buckley et al (1980) changed this shape parameter until they were able to reproduce the mechanical properties of tendon; their results for the initial crimp shape and an intermediate stage of straightening are illustrated, schematically, in Figures 4.8d and e, respectively. Unfortunately their model considerably overestimates the diameters of the collagen fibrils in rat-tail tendon. And when they treated the zig-zag model rigorously, by considering that it deformed as shown in Figure 4.8c, it underestimated the diameters to about the same extent. Models of this kind are bound to be unsuccessful for tendon because they ignore the viscoelasticity which was shown, in the section on Energy, hysteresis and creep (p. 55) to be an important feature of the mechanical behaviour of tendon. Nevertheless the results of both Diamant et al (1972) as well as those of Buckley et al (1980) have provided valuable insights into the way in which tissues containing crimped collagen fibrils respond to applied tensile stress.

The function of the crimp appears to be to produce a stress-strain curve with the shape shown in Figure 4.1a; tendon is then resilient without being too floppy as described in a previous section p. 56. This 'shock-absorbing' function of the crimp was recognised by Rigby et al (1959) and will be discussed further in a later Section p. 61.

All the evidence suggests that collagen fibrils are crimped (except in bone and articular cartilage) and that in most tissues the crimp resembles the planar zig-zag of Figure 4.7a but it might sometimes look more like the flattened helix of Figure 4.7c; the first stage in the deformation of collagen fibrils is the straightening of the crimp and this accounts for the relatively low stiffness of tendon when it is first stretched. Fibre crimping is not unique to collagen but has been exploited in textiles and, more recently, in synthetic composite materials; experimental tests have been made on the theory of deformation of crimped steel wires (further details and references are given by Buckley et al, 1980). Unfortunately simple theories based only on crimp straightening do not provide a quantitative description of the behaviour of collagenous tissues which are composite materials with viscoelastic properties i.e. their mechanical properties are extremely complicated.

Tendons and ligaments

Tendon has been used throughout this chapter to illustrate the properties of collagenous tissues; the reason is simply that so much is known about its mechanical behaviour. One reason why it is a favourite subject for experiments is almost certainly the mistaken belief that its mechanical properties are very nearly those of pure collagen — but, as explained previously tendon is a composite material whose mechanical properties depend to a large extent on the glycosaminoglycan gel surrounding its collagen fibrils as well as on its elastin and cellular content. Nevertheless the high proportion of collagen in tendon (70 per cent of the dry mass, 30 per cent when wet; Harkness, 1968) reflects its function of transmitting tensile stress. In tendon the collagen fibrils are bundled together to form fibres whose diameters may be as high as 300 μm; the 'fibres' are also called 'bundles', 'fibre bundles' and 'sub-fibres' — which can cause confusion! Similar bundles occur in other tissues — in skin, for example, they are between 10 and 40 μm in diameter. The bundles of fibrils in tendon are further grouped into secondary bundles or 'fasciculi' (about 600 μm in diameter) and then into larger tertiary bundles (Elliott, 1965). As a result of this structure, and its high collagen content, tendon is a fibrous rather rope-like tissue.

The important mechanical properties of tendon, which have been encountered at various points throughout this chapter, are: (1) its stress-strain curve is not linear — the stiffness is greater at higher strains, (2) the initial stage of tendon deformation (for strains of up to about 0.04) involves straightening its crimp, (3) it creeps under a constant applied stress, (4) its strain depends on the rate at which stress is applied, (5) it exhibits mechanical hysteresis i.e. it does not store all its deformation energy, (6) after a rapid series of extension and relaxation cycles, the stiffness increases and the hysteresis is less marked, and (7) when the strain exceeds a value of around 0.04 the tendon becomes plastically deformed. Most of these results were obtained from experiments on rat-tail tendon but other tendons appear to be reasonably similar in their composition and structure. Notice that fracture occurs at a much higher strain (typically around 0.10) than plastic deformation (Harkness, 1968). Rigby et al (1959) showed that if the temperature exceeds 37°C, by only a few degrees, rat-tail tendon breaks at strains of only 0.03 to 0.04. This observation suggests that physiological strains do not exceed this upper limit since such elevated temperatures can easily be attained in fever without tendons apparently becoming damaged. Haut & Little (1972) cite a variety of other evidence for physiological strains in tendons not exceeding 0.03. Rigby et al (1959) noted other abrupt changes in the mechanical properties of rat-tail tendon at strains exceeding 0.04. They followed the decay of stress, when the strain was kept constant, as a function of time. The temperature dependence of this stress decay, which arises because of the creep behaviour of tendon, is completely different at strains in excess of 0.04. However the usually high fracture strain means that tendon does not suddenly snap when it is overloaded — it is a tough material. It has thus been established, during the course of this chapter, that tendon is a tough, viscoelastic fibre composite.

The function of tendon is to transmit the force generated by a contracting muscle to the correct point of application in the skeletal system; there are several reasons why tendons are often preferable to direct attachments of muscle to bone. Muscles have a low tensile strength (see p. 55) and so must have a large cross-sectional area if they are to transmit force without fracturing. Around many joints there simply isn't enough room to attach a large muscle to the bone; sometimes the bones themselves are just too small for large muscles to be joined to them. Consider the fingers which have to perform a wide range of delicate manipulative movements while also exerting considerable force. The need for many large muscles surrounding the finger joints conflicts with the need for small, precise movements. Thus some of the muscles which control the fingers are situated in the arm and their contractile force is transmitted by tendons. Long tendons also guard against damage from suddenly applied forces — as explained earlier length confers resilience. Resilience is also provided by the low stiffness of tendon at low strains; but at higher strains the tendon becomes much stiffer. If stiffness did not increase, a contracting muscle would continue to stretch a tendon. Then much of the energy expended by the muscle would be used to deform tendons rather than to perform useful work; since this energy is ultimately supplied by food, insufficiently stiff tendons would then lead to a waste of resources.

There are several different ways of describing how tendons function. In this chapter their behaviour has been described by stress-strain curves; these curves can be plotted for different rates of loading and unloading. This approach is not limited to tendon — it has also been used, for example, to describe the compression of articular cartilage. An alternative description is to formulate equations which relate the stress to the strain. These equations may be purely empirical i.e. they make no presumptions about the mechanism of deformation but seek only to describe the results of experiment. An example was given by Elden (1968) who epressed the stress in rat-tail tendon by

$$\sigma = k\epsilon^2$$

where k is a constant whose value is chosen to give the best agreement with experimentally determined stress-strain curves. This equation does not allow for the effects of changing the rate of loading or of rapidly repeated loading, neither does it allow for mechanical hysteresis. Haut & Little (1972) related the stress applied to rat-tail tendon to produce a given strain by

$$\sigma = B\epsilon^A$$

where the values of A and B are chosen to give the best agreement with experimental observation. Different values of A and B were tabulated to correspond to different rates of increase of strain; at lower strain rates (less than about 0.12 min^{-1}) the rate has little influence on the values of these two coefficients — in agreement with the common observation that the mechanical behaviour of tendon is not much affected by the rate of loading at low rates, provided the strain is not too high (Diamant et al, 1972). As would be expected, from comparison with Elden's equation which attempts to explain the same experimental observations, the value of A is always very close to 2 (between 1.80 and 2.07) and B (which is similar to Elden's k) is between 1.80×10^{10} and $3.14 \times 10^{10} N\ m^{-2}$; as expected from Figure 4.1a, the higher values of B correspond to higher strain rates (about 0.5 min^{-1}). These equations are of limited usefulness although they can be handy for avoiding consulting detailed compilations of stress-strain data in simple, semi-quantitative calculations (see, e.g. Hickey & Hukins, 1980a).

Mechanical analogues are very frequently used to describe the response of biological tissues to deforming forces — such analogues are especially common in descriptions of the mechanical properties of tendons and ligaments. The idea is to design a mechanical system so that if the force required to produce a qiven extension were plotted on a graph, the resulting curve would have the same shape as that obtained from the tissue. Such systems can be designed from three separate kinds of elements: (1) a spring which obeys Hooke's Law (i.e. stress is directly proportional to strain and independent of time), (2) a dashpot (the 'Newton element') and (3) a frictional element (the 'Coulomb element'). The dashpot continues to move all the time the force is applied and deformation only ceases when the force is removed — it thus describes the tendency of the system to creep. The frictional element only moves when the applied force exceeds some critical value. There are conventions for representing each of these elements (compare electrical circuit diagrams) which are indicated in Figure 4.9. Figure 4.10a shows how springs can be combined in an attempt to give the shape of force-

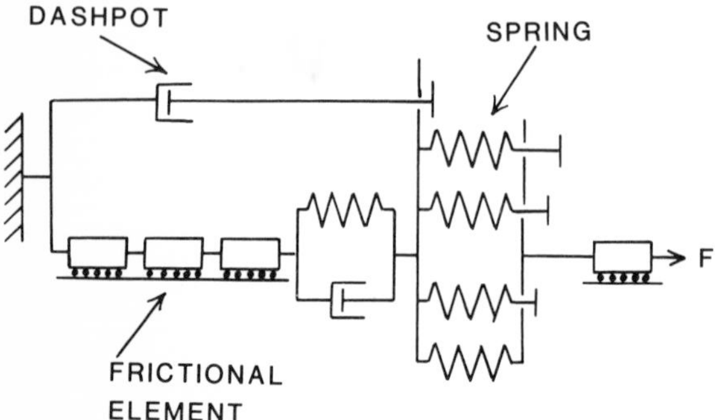

Fig. 4.9 Mechanical analogue for the behaviour of the anterior cruciate ligament (Viidik, 1973).

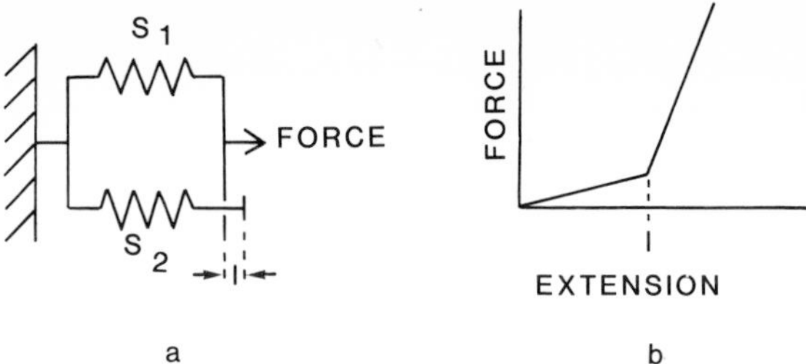

Fig. 4.10 (a) Mechanical analogue for the behaviour of tendon with (b) its force-deformation curve (Viidik, 1973).

deformation curve shown in Figure 4.1a (Viidik, 1973); at first the applied force extends only the spring S_1 but, when this has increased in length by l, the second spring, S_2, has to be stretched and the system stiffens. The resulting force-deformation curve, in Figure 4.1b, does not look much like that obtained experimentally. In order to faithfully reproduce the behaviour of an anterior cruciate ligament under certain loading conditions, a very comblicated analogue, shown in Figure 4.9, is required (Viidik, 1973). Personally, I find the more complicated mechanical analogues totally unhelpful.

Neither the empirical equations nor the mechanical analogues explain why, as opposed to how, tendons behave as they do e.g. they provide no clue that crimping is responsible for the initially low stiffness. Explanations of why tendons have particular mechanical properties are largely based on observation (e.g. the crimp can be seen to straighten when a tendon is stretched) but some progress has been made with a more theoretical approach. The idea that the stretching process for tendon has zero enthalpy of activation (Rigby et al, 1959) has been discounted, at least for human digital tendon, by experiment (Cohen et al, 1976). (Enthalpy of activation is simply the energy required to get a process going — ignoring entropy effects which describe the temperature dependence). But Hooley & Cohen (1979) formulated a model for the mechanical properties of tendon in which the parameters described the actual properties of either the collagen fibrils or the surrounding glycosaminoglycan gel. In principle, although not yet in practice, the values of these parameters could be obtained from independent experiments. The theory has been used to find the values for the parameters which lead to the best agreement with mechanical testing results. For the activation energy of viscoelastic deformation and the crimp angle (θ of Figure 4.8) there is good agreement with the results of independent experiments. Hooley and Cohen describe the advantages of their technique as: 'all the parameters in the model relate either to structural constants of the material . . . or to the usual (and, in principle, measurable) viscoelastic parameters . . . there is no reliance on an arbitrary array of springs and dashpots'. Unfortunately the resulting model is rather complicated. Cohen et al (1976) point out that straightening the crimp involves shearing the glycosaminoglycan gel. Now this gel closely resembles a liquid and consequently is likely to be viscous rather than elastic — thus little of the energy used to shear the gel will be stored by the tendon. It seems to me that this must contribute to the mechanical hysteresis of tendon; the fluid flow model described on page 54 may be a contributory factor, in the case of tendon, or it may be just a useful analogue for describing observed properties.

Ligaments transmit tension from one bone to another; although the various tendons in the body have a similar composition, structure and function, there is considerably more variety among ligaments and it is not so easy to make general comments about their properties. And much less is known about the relationship between their structures and functions — but it appears that their collagen fibrils often have a more complex pattern of preferred orientations than those of tendon (Viidik, 1973). Figure 4.11 shows that ligamentum flavum is much less stiff than tendon —

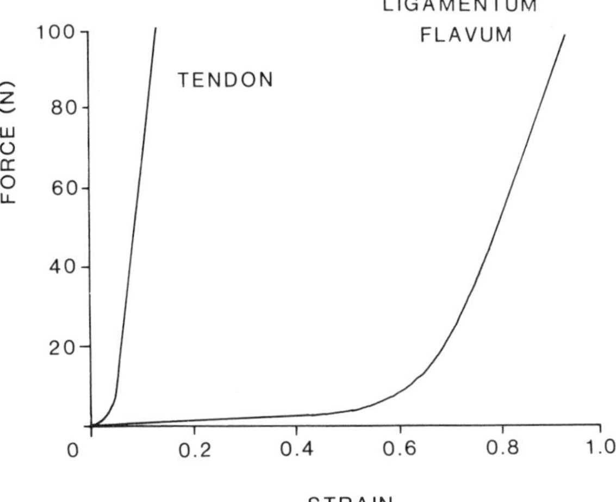

Fig. 4.11 Comparison of force-strain curves obtained for extension of tendon and ligamentum flavum (data from Kenedi et al, 1975).

presumably because of its high elastin content (Nachemson and Evans, 1968). From this figure it appears that ligamentum flavum does not stiffen until the strain reaches about 0.6 which, by comparison with the behaviour of tendon, suggests that it does not deform plastically until this strain is reached. Inspection of the experimental results published by Tkaczuk (1968) also suggests that the longitudinal ligaments of the spine do not acquire a permanent set for strains of up to 0.24; the stress on the posterior longitudinal ligament is then $4.9 \times 10^6 N\ m^{-2}$ and it fractures at $1.9 \times 10^7 N\ m^{-2}$. The posterior longitudinal ligament provides a simple example of ligament function. It joins consecutive vertebrae and becomes stretched in forward bending. It thus limits the extent to which the intervertebral disc can be bent forward and hence tends to protect it from damage.

Damage to ligaments in vivo usually occurs at their junction to bone — this junction is called an enthesis and lesions at this site are referred to as enthesopathies (Ball, 1971). According to Viidik (1973) the injuries encountered in orthopaedic surgery often involve the attachment of ligament to bone and during in vitro testing experiments this attachment usually fails before the ligament itself (Millington et al, 1972). The structural reason for this weakness appears to remain unexplained. Explanation of the mechanical properties of such systems is probably more complicated than for relatively simple fibrous systems, like tendon, and leads us naturally into the next section — complex networks of fibrils.

COMPLEX FIBRIL NETWORKS

General properties (Illustrated by skin, scars, uterine cervix and liver)

In many tissues the collagen fibrils of the extracellular matrix form a complex network; nevertheless in some of these networks the fibrils are still arranged in fibres, much like those in tendon. Scanning electron microscopy shows that skin contains collagenous fibres whose diameters are typically in the range of 10 to 40 μm but, in contrast to tendon, these fibres are far from being parallel — they have a wide range of orientations (Millington et al, 1971). The reason for skin having a more disoriented structure is that it has to withstand tensile stresses in very many directions — hence it must have a range of collagen fibril orientations. Nevertheless most mechanical tests on skin have been confined simply to uniaxial extension, although some experiments have been performed to demonstrate that the mechanical properties of skin are not the same in all directions (Millington et al, 1971), Skin structure changes under tensile stress which tends to improve the degree of fibre orientation — thus fibre reorientation is one way in which the tissue responds to mechanical deformation (Millington et al, 1971). It is an everyday observation that the mechanical behaviour of skin changes during ageing when it becomes less resilient and wrinkles over those areas of the body where it is most stretched. This observation has lead to many mechanical and structural studies of ageing skin which have been reviewed by Viidik (1973).

Incisions in skin illustrate its mechanical anisotropy; a needle inserted into the skin produces an elliptical hole, not a round one. The long axis of the ellipse lies along a so-called 'Langer's line', which can be identified with the preferred orientation for the collagen fibrils (Millington et al, 1971) and the direction of maximum skin stiffness (Kenedi et al, 1975). Since cracks travel more readily along these lines they are used by surgeons to indicate the directions in which to make incisions. An incision at right-angles to a Langer's line will not be readily propagated because it will soon encounter a collagen fibril which is perpendicular to its direction of propagation, as shown in Figure 4.5a; the fibril will then impede its progress. But an incision along a direction of preferred orientation is less likely to encounter the barrier of a fibril and will propagate readily through the weaker glycosaminoglycan gel. Of course even these incisions will not continue indefinitely because the arrangement of collagenous fibres in skin is sufficiently haphazard for a fibril to be encountered before too long. Finally there are more collagen fibrils to withstand tension along a Langer's line and so the skin is stiffer. Notice that the organisation of fibrils into fibres does not affect these arguments concerning the propagation of incisions.

The behaviour of incisions has important implications for surgical practice. It appears to be generally accepted that an elliptical wound can be closed provided its eccentricity (the ratio of its breadth to length) is not much greater than about $\frac{1}{4}$. But experiments have shown that the maximum eccentricity of a closable wound depends on whereabouts on the surface of the body the incision in the skin is made — its value can be as high as 0.6 (Kenedi et al, 1975). This variation in the anisotropy of skin is presumably a result of local differences in the degree of orientation of its collagenous fibres reflecting the different forces which are applied to skin at different sites on the body's surface. Also the strength of skin varies over the surface of the body. Harkness (1968) attributes this variability to differences in fibre arrangement and notes that it has been extensively studied because of its importance in leather manufacture.

When an incision in skin heals, the resulting scar is stiffer than the surrounding tissue. Although the tensile strength of wounded skin returns to its original value within 60 days, it remains weaker than the surrounding skin whose strength increases at the same time (Harkness, 1968). An incision is followed by the formation of an intricate pattern of collagen fibrils; in older animals the pattern is less intricate and the wound takes longer to heal (Viidik, 1973). This observation illustrates the importance of the collagen network structure in tissues. It has been suggested that scars have similar structures, and presumably similar properties, wherever they are formed — although some exceptions to this suggestion are known. As a result scar tissue is more suited to joining some tissues than others — which might explain why wounds in muscular tissue rapidly regain their original strength whereas those in more collagenous tissues (such as fascia and skin) take longer to heal (Harkness, 1968). Besides being of interest in its own right, the healing wound is a useful model system for investigating the effects of hormones on the mechanical properties of collagenous tissues (Viidik, 1973).

Hormones are presumably implicated in the changes which occur in the mechanical properties of collagenous tissues during pregnancy — the uterine cervix provides a remarkable and important example. It is a ring of collagenous tissue around the lower end of the uterus whose stiffness has to decrease sufficiently for it to expand and allow the neonate to pass from the uterus to the vagina at parturition. In the rat the stiffness of the cervical tissue decreases rapidly between the twelfth and twenty-first days of pregnancy (the gestation period of the rat is 21 to 22 days) — but it increases almost to its original value within 24 hours post partum (Harkness, 1968). The smooth muscle of the cervix is believed to contribute little to its mechanical properties (Viidik, 1973) which are, presumably, dictated largely by the arrangement of its collagen fibrils. In the non-pregnant rat the cervix swells during estrus because of its considerable water content; it appears that this change is achieved by hormonal influence on the tissue as a result of which the collagen fibrils become more dispersed (Viidik, 1973). Little is known about the mechanisms of the changes which occur in the mechanical properties of the cervix during pregnancy and at different stages in the estrus cycle — perhaps its collagen network structure needs to be investigated further.

Both skin and the uterine cervix have highly specialised mechanical functions which we might expect to be reflected in a high collagen content and specialised arrangement df fibrils; but tissues whose functions are not normally considered to be mechanical need collagen fibrils for the maintenance of structural integrity. Collagen frameworks hold the components of a tissue together in much the same way as a string bag is used to carry shopping — the weight of the individual items is supported, and they are pulled together, by the tension in the strings. Unlike the string bag, however, the collagen fibrils need be neither continuous nor knotted because they form part of a fibre composite — provided that the fibril length is, at least, comparable with the critical length as described earlier. The importance of collagen in such tissues is illustrated by comparing the proportions of collagen in the livers of different animal species. If m represents the average mass of liver in adults of a species (e.g. in mice), then the proportion of this mass which consists of collagen, c, is given by

$$c = am^{1.3}$$

where a is a constant for all species (Harkness, 1961, 1968). Thus if the mass of liver in species A is twice that in species B, the liver of A contains more than twice as much collagen as that in B. This result illustrates a common difficulty encountered when trying to 'scale up' the design of structures which are held together by tension (Gordon, 1978). Too much collagen in the liver disrupts its structure and hence its function. Disruption of hepatic function, including blood flow, by excess collagen occurs in cirrhosis (McGee & Fallon, 1978).

This section of the chapter could continue almost indefinitely — although much of its content would necessarily be both sketchy and speculative because so little is known about how collagen networks actually fulfill their mechanical functions in the vast majority of tissues. It therefore seems more profitable to consider the collagen fibril networks in two tissues where the relationship between structure and function is better understood — articular cartilage and the annulus fibrosus of the intervertebral disc.

Articular cartilage

Articular cartilage forms a resilient coating on the bones and, in conjunction with synovial fluid, leads to low friction in joints; its degeneration, in osteoarthrosis, is accompanied by impairment of joint function (Ball et al, 1978). The chemical constitution of the glycosaminoglycan gel in cartilage is responsible for its high water content of 60 to 80 per cent — the water in cartilage exerts a hydrostatic pressure which can be as high as 0.3 MN m^{-2} even in unloaded cartilage (Maroudas, 1979). This high internal pressure means that the cartilage is not easily distorted which is important if joints are to withstand loads arising not only from the weight of the body but also from the forces exerted by muscles acting on them. A car tyre illustrates how internal pressure prevents distortion — if its air pressure is too low the tyre is too easily distorted by the weight of the car and its road-holding properties are impaired.

The function of collagen fibrils in cartilage is to contain the internal pressure — just as the walls of a tyre withstand air pressure i.e. the hydrostatic pressure exerted by the water in the glycosaminoglycan gel is balanced by tension in the fibrils (Maroudas, 1979). Collagen fibrils in cartilage are not crimped (Gathercole & Keller, 1975) perhaps because they are under sufficient tension even in the unloaded tissue for any discernable crimp to be removed. According to the section on Crimping, fibrils from which the crimp has been removed are stiffened. Crimp removal could then be the mechanism which stiffens cartilage collagen and prevents the tissue from swelling when it imbibes extra fluid — in complete contrast to the behaviour of cornea or intervertebral disc (Maroudas, 1979).

There are several different models in the literature for the structure of the collagen fibril network in cartilage, although it has been recognised for a long time that it consists of four layers: (1) in the surface layer the collagen fibrils are parallel to the articular surface, (2) in an intermediate layer there is a more-or-less random arrangement of fibrils, (3) there is a deep layer where the fibrils are perpendicular to the articular surface and (4) adjacent to the subchondral bone there is a calcified layer (Meachim & Stockwell, 1979). Recently the arrangement of collagen fibrils in the layers has been described quantitatively and related to the mechanical function of the tissue (Aspden & Hukins, 1981). This description applies to articular cartilage of human patella and may differ in detail for the cartilage coating other bones — but differences are likely to be slight because the layered structure does not appear to be confined to patellar cartilage.

The preferred orientation of collagen fibrils in the surface layer, parallel to the articular surface, is essential if the tissue is to be stable i.e. if its internal pressure is not to cause it to swell perhaps until it bursts. This surface layer, like the wall of a tyre or a balloon or the soap film which encloses a bubble, is a pressure vessel. Pressure vessels work because internal pressure expands their walls — as the walls stretch the tension in the material of the walls increases. The stiffer the material, the greater the tension produced by a small deformation. Tension tends to return the wall to its original size and shape — an inflated balloon thus gets smaller when some of its air is released. A point will be reached when the pressure, tending to expand the vessel, and the tension, tending to contract it, balance i.e. the vessel is in equilibrium — unless the internal pressure is so great that the tension in the walls is sufficient to burst the vessel! A simple account of pressure vessels is given by Gordon (1978); more details are given by Higdon et al (1976) — many of the statements below, some of which are specific to 'thin-walled' pressure vessels, are justified there. Figure 4.12 shows a section through part of the wall of a pressure vessel in which an internal pressure, P, is balanced by a force, F, tangential to the wall. Why is the force tangential to the wall? Consider as an example a thin sheet of waterproof material which is being used to carry water — the weight of the water then leads to the higher internal pressure. We know, intuitively, that we have to pull on the sheet in the direction shown in Figure 4.12 to maintain the shape of the bulging waterproof sheet whilst supporting the water. Similarly surface tension is able to maintain the structure of a bubble because it acts tangentially to the surface.

Collagen fibrils in the articular surface can withstand tensile stress and their tension balances the internal

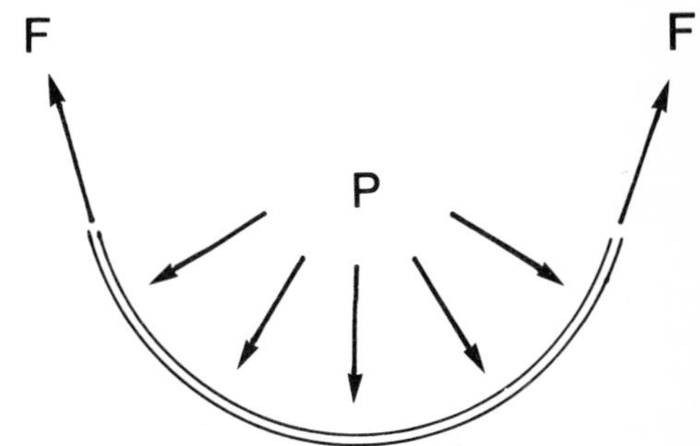

Fig. 4.12 Tangential force, F, in part of the wall of a pressure vessel balancing its internal pressure, P.

pressure of the cartilage; tangential forces arising from the tension in stretched collagen fibrils will be greatest if the fibrils are parallel to the articular surface. For a spherical vessel of radius r, the force, F, in the wall which is required to maintain equilibrium is given by

$$F = rPs/2$$

where s is the length of wall across which the force is acting. The surface layer of the articular cartilage coating the femoral head might provide an example of such a vessel. But the important point here is a general one — the greater the value of r, i.e. the flatter the surface, the greater the tangential force required for equilibrium. The force which a wall can exert in a vessel of radius r, to withstand a given pressure, P, could in principle be increased in two ways: (1) increase the proportion of collagen in the surface layer and (2) make the fibrils more highly oriented parallel to the surface. As far as I know, the proportion of collagen in the surface layer of articular cartilage has never been measured as a function of curvature. But in patellar cartilage the fibrils in the surface layer are more highly oriented where it is flatter i.e. the structure of the collagen fibril network allows it to exert higher tangential forces where they are required (Aspden & Hukins, 1981).

In the early stages of osteoarthrosis the articular surface becomes worn (Ball et al, 1978) and the cartilage swells (Maroudas, 1979); we can now see that these observations are different sides of the same coin. If the surface layer is damaged, tension in its collagen fibrils is less able to provide the necessary tangential force for stability and the internal pressure leads to swelling. But what is the first stage in the onset of osteoarthrosis? The surface layer might be directly damaged by mechanical abuse. But it could be that chemical changes in the glycosaminoglycans lead them to attract more water so that the internal pressure of the cartilage increases. The collagen fibrils of the surface layer might then be unable to exert sufficient tangential force to withstand the increased pressure and so the tissue could swell. Which comes first — damage to the surface layer or increased pressure? This question can only be answered by detailed studies of the early stages of osteoarthrosis.

The preferred directions of alignment of the collagen fibrils in the plane of the patellar cartilage surface can also be related to the function of the cartilage (Aspden & Hukins, 1981). Over most of the articular surface the fibrils are not only parallel to this surface but also tend to be aligned in the proximo-distal direction. This direction coincides with the direction of movement of the condyles of the femur over the patellar surface during normal flexion of the knee. Presumably there is sufficient friction in the joint for the cartilage to need special reinforcement in this direction. However the extra reinforcement is not great as there is an extensive spread about the preferred alignment. On a small area of surface, the extreme medial facet, the direction of preferred alignment changes to medio-lateral. This area only contacts a femoral condyle in extreme flexion — and then the direction of movement is changed so that the preferred fibril alignment still coincides with the direction of motion.

In the deep layer the perpendicular orientation of the collagen fibrils ties the cartilage to the bone while the structure of the intermediate layer allows a smooth transition from parallel to perpendicular orientation; neighbouring layers merge gradually into each other. Hydrostatic pressure pushes equally in all direction. Thus the internal pressure of the cartilage pushes against the bone as well as against the surface layer. To prevent the cartilage from lifting off the calcified tissue below, it must be tethered to it by fibrils which are perpendicular to the calcified surface — just as a balloon can be tethered to the ground by vertical ropes. Any discontinuity between the surface and deep layers would lead to their being pushed apart by the internal pressure — it would be a weak region, like a flaw in a tyre or balloon. The intermediate layer ensures that there is no such weak discontinuity. Interestingly the preferred orientations of the collagen fibrils lie along arcs much as suggested by Benninghoff in 1925 (Aspden & Hukins, 1981). But the arcs only describe directions of preferred orientation and since they also bend in different directions the appearance of the intermediate layer in scanning electron micrographs is essentially random.

Figure 4.1b shows a stress-strain curve for compression of the deep layer of articular cartilage. Results of mechanical tests on the tissue are reviewed by Kempson (1979). As explained in the Introduction, cartilage also responds to compression by fluid flow. Since the flow is slow, cartilage creeps under a constant applied load and the tissue exhibits mechanical hysteresis — further explanation, with tendon as an example, is given on p. 54. But although fluid flow may be the most important mechanism for creep and hysteresis, the response of the tissue is likely to be very complicated — for much the same reasons as given for tendon in an earlier section.

Intervertebral disc

The intervertebral disc consists of a soft centre, the *nucleus pulposus* (abbreviated here to *nucleus*), surrounded by a fibrous outer wall, the *annulus fibrosus* (abbreviated here to *annulus*). The nucleus consists largely of a highly hydrated gel of glycosaminoglycans which is liquid-like and, therefore, tends to transmit pressure applied to it equally in all directions. Before the onset of ageing changes there is very little collagen in the nucleus and the fibrils have random orientations. Even when more collagen is deposited during ageing, leading to a *fibrotic* disc, it does not form any well defined structure (Happey, 1976).

In complete contrast the annulus consists of coaxial lamellae in which there is a specific pattern of collagen fibril orientations. Crimped fibres can be teased from the annulus (Gathercole & Keller, 1975) and Figure 4.13a is an exploded view of two consecutive annular lamellae which shows how their fibres are arranged. They are tilted by an angle, marked α, with respect to the axis of the spine; the direction of tilt alternates in successive lamellae. The value of the tilt angle is not measurably different in a variety of mammals or in fetal and adult human material; in the human fetus, where the structure is likely to remain undamaged by mechanical forces, it has a value of around 70° (Hickey & Hukins, 1980b). Hickey & Hukins (1980a) have related the structure of this collagen network to the function of the disc.

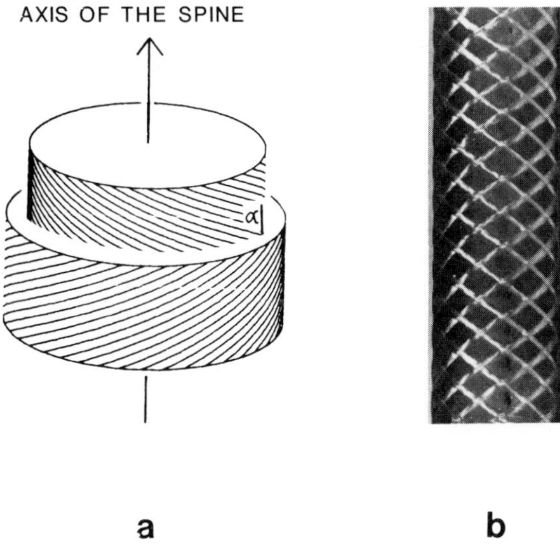

Fig. 4.13 Exploded view showing the arrangement of collagenous fibres in two consecutive lamellae of the annulus fibrosus of the intervertebral disc, in (a), compared with the fibre arrangement in a length of reinforced hose, in (b).

The function of the intervertebral disc is to allow the spine to bend and twist; as a result it must be able to withstand compressive forces. Compression of the disc arises not only from the weight of the body and any loads which are carried. When the muscles which are responsible for bending and twisting are contracted they will exert forces which have appreciable components along the direction of the axis of the spine. Contraction of these muscles then tends to compress the disc. Gordon (1978) has indicated that the resilience of the intervertebral disc may also be important. Experiments show that the cancellous bone of the vertebrae fails before the disc under compressive load (Jayson et al, 1973). And it is often supposed that the low stiffness of the discs means that they, rather than the vertebrae, are deformed by the forces which are suddenly transmitted to the spine when we land on our feet after jumping. Therefore the stronger discs are considered to absorb the potentially damaging energy which is suddenly transferred to the spine and thus protect the cancellous bone of the vertebrae i.e. they act like the shock-absorbers in a car. Actually the shock-absorbing mechanism of the spine appears to be rather more complicated than this simple model would suggest (Roaf, 1960).

When a disc is compressed the glycosaminoglycan gel which forms the nucleus and surrounds the fibres of the annulus must transmit the applied pressure — in the same way as the brake fluid in a car transmits the pressure applied to the pedal. This transmitted pressure stretches the collagenous fibres of the annulus and the tension which is generated in them balances the applied pressure. Like the collagen fibrils in the surface layer of articular cartilage, the stretched fibres of the annulus generate a force which allows the tissue to function as the wall of a pressure vessel. But because of its cylindrical shape, a better analogy to the annulus might be a length of reinforced hose. And Figure 4.13b shows that the pattern of fibres in a reinforced hose closely resembles that shown in Figure 4.13a for the intervertebral disc. A disc cannot withstand compression unless its fibres are stretched — only then are they under tension and thus able to balance the applied pressure; it can also be shown, purely by geometry, that the fibre tilt must increase when the disc is compressed i.e. compression increases the value of α in Figure 4.13a. This increase has recently been demonstrated experimentally (Klein & Hukins, 1982). Further geometry then shows that the fibres will not stretch i.e. the disc cannot withstand compression, unless the initial value of α exceeds 54.7° — fortunately it does!

Collagenous fibres are expected to reinforce the intervertebral disc in torsion even though they cannot withstand it themselves; the reason is that forces which tend to twist the disc will be transmitted to the fibre network of Figure 4.13a as axial tension in the fibres (Hickey & Hukins, 1980a). Figure 4.14a shows the fibres in a single undistorted lamella of the annulus. When the top of the disc is twisted anticlockwise with respect to the lower surface, as in Figure 4.14b, the fibres are stretched. In order to stretch the fibres the forces applied to the disc must exert appreciable tension along the direction of the fibre axes. As the fibres stretch, their tilt angle, α, will increase — compare Figures 4.14a and b. Actually Figure 4.14b exaggerates the stretching and reorientation of the fibres because the torsion angle chosen for illustration is much greater than would be encountered physiologically — the maximum value possibly does not exceed about 3° (Farfan, 1973). Nevertheless the fibres in the lamella illustrated are able to withstand the stress generated by torsion of.the disc during the course of which they become slightly reoriented. In the next lamella the fibres are angled in the opposite direction and so are able to withstand clockwise, but not anticlockwise, torsion. Only half the

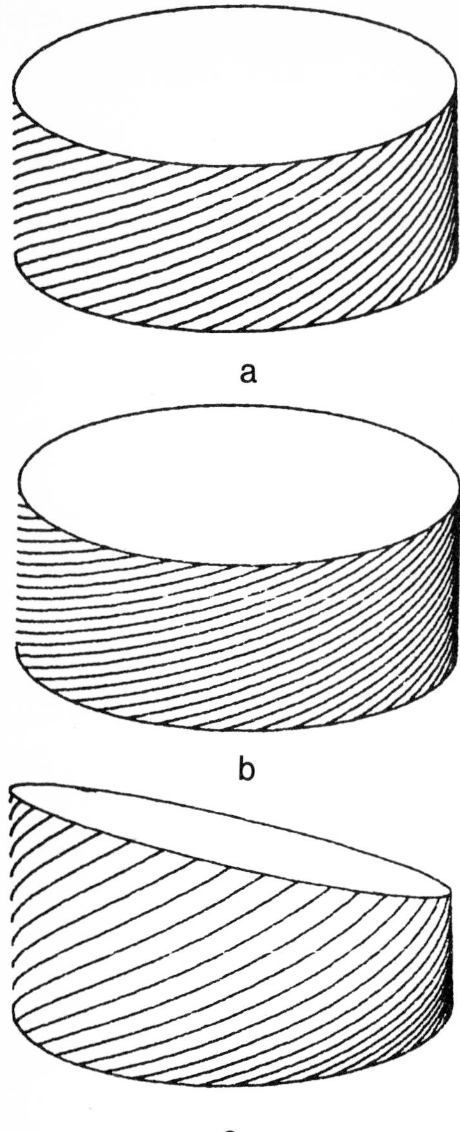

Fig. 4.14 Computer drawings of a single lamella from the annulus fibrosus (a) undistorted, (b) twisted and (c) bent, obtained with a programme written by J.A. Klein. The degree of twisting and bending is much greater than would be encountered physiologically in order to exaggerate the predicted fibre extension and reorientation for the sake of illustration.

fibres in the annulus have their fibres tilted to withstand torsion in a given direction.

Similarly, although the fibres themselves are easily bent, they are expected to reinforce the disc in bending — because forces which tend to bend the disc will be transmitted to some of them as tension along their axes (Hickey & Hukins, 1980a). Bending tilts the top surface of the disc with respect to the lower surface; Figure 4.14c then shows that forward bending will stretch the posterior but not the anterior fibres. Thus only the posterior fibres are subject to tensile stress and able to strengthen the disc in forward bending; as these fibres stretch their tilt angle, α, decreases. Once again, Figure 4.14c illustrates the geometry of a physiologically unreasonable bending angle to exaggerate these effects. Actually the disc structure is rather more complicated than these simple figures suggest and incorporates features which protect it in forward bending — including the posterior longitudinal ligament whose function was described previously (Hickey & Hukins, 1980a). These protective features are important because, as seen in Figure 4.14c, bending tends to concentrate tensile stress on a few fibres and is thus potentially very damaging.

Hysteresis and creep of the disc are associated with fluid flow just as they were for articular cartilage (Farfan, 1973) i.e. they are considered to be properties of the disc itself rather than just of the annular fibres. But the fibres are so like those in tendon that they are also expected to exhibit these phenomena for themselves — as described on p. 61. Thus both fluid flow and the intrinsic properties of the fibres may contribute to hysteresis and creep of the intact disc. Furthermore the similarity to tendon suggests that the strain in the fibres should not exceed about 0.04 otherwise they will acquire a permanent set — any deformation of the disc which leads the fibre strain to exceed this critical value is likely to impair function (Hickey & Hukins, 1980a).

PIEZOELECTRICITY

A material is said to be piezoelectric if mechanical stress can lead to the creation of an electric field across it; piezoelectricity is reversible in the sense that if an electric field is applied to the material it will contract or elongate just as it would under mechanical stress i.e. it exhibits a strain. In many experiments on collagen piezoelectricity a pulsed stress or a pulsed electric field is applied; the rate of application is characterised by the frequency which is the number of deformations produced in a second. The unit of frequency is the hertz (abbreviated to Hz) so that a pulsed stress of 60 Hz represents sixty deformations per second. Until the 1940's piezoelectricity was considered to be a property of crystals. But not all crystals exhibit the piezoelectric effect — some are so symmetric that the effect in opposing directions cancels itself out.

Now piezoelectricity is understood to be a property of anisotropic materials whose structures need not be as regular as those of crystals but must not be so disordered that their structures are effectively the same in all directions. Collagen fibrils have an anisotropic structure and their axial periodicity does not exhibit the symmetry which would preclude their being piezoelectric materials (see Chapter 3). Nevertheless a sample of collagenous tissue would be isotropic if its fibrils had perfectly random orientations. But we have seen that in many tissues the fibrils have definite preferred orientations so that the anisotropy of the fibril structure is reflected by a structural and mechanical anisotropy of the tissue which might then be expected to exhibit the piezoelectric effect.

There is a wealth of experimental evidence for collagen and collagenous tissues being piezoelectric materials. Early experiments established that bone, skin, tendon, cartilage, arteries and ligaments could all exhibit piezoelectricity which was, at least in part, attributable to collagen (Shamos & Lavine, 1967; Bassett, 1968). Unfortunately these experiments were performed on dried material whose properties might be expected to differ from those of the hydrated native tissue. Typical experiments involved applying a 60 Hz pulsed stress to the material and measuring the electric output. Although a potential difference of only about 2 mV may be set up across a macroscopic sample, it is likely that much higher local potential differences are set up within the material (Bassett, 1968). The frequency of the applied mechanical pulse in many experiments is higher than a tissue might be expected to encounter in normal usage but such experiments do demonstrate that the material is piezoelectric. More recent experiments show that hydrated tissues exhibit piezoelectricity and that this behaviour is also a property of reasonably pure, hydrated collagen. Netto & Zimmerman (1975) showed that the presence of water decreased the piezoelectric effect in bone and tendon; but this decrease was considerably less marked for bone. Fukada et al (1976) extracted collagen, used it to prepare oriented films and measured the piezoelectricity as a function of water content and temperature. The piezoelectric effect was detectable at temperatures and hydration levels which would be encountered physiologically.

Several attempts have been made to formulate a quantitative theory for the piezoelectric effect in bone. There are several theoretical analyses in the literature (some of the more recent are Williams & Breger, 1975; Martin, 1979; Korostoff, 1979) but no generally accepted, definitive theory. Fortunately the absence of such a theory does not detract from this discussion which is concerned with establishing that the effect does indeed exist, in order to consider its biological implications and possible clinical applications. It is worth noting that the published theories seek to explain bone piezoelectricity solely in terms of the piezoelectric effect in collagen. Although the hydroxyapatite in bone is crystalline it might not be expected to contribute to the piezoelectricity because the symmetry of macroscopic, perfect crystals of apatites precludes their exhibiting the effect (Shamos & Lavine, 1967). Bassett (1968) has indicated that this expectation might be an over simplification because a very small crystal might not be perfectly symmetric and because a large number of dislocations in the crystal might affect its electrical properties. Recent X-ray diffraction studies show that the hydroxyapatite crystals in bone are far from perfect (Wheeler & Lewis, 1977); also the crystals have preferred orientations (Bacon et al, 1979) so that any electrical anisotrophy in the crystals might be reflected in the properties of the tissue as a whole.

Ideas about the biological implications of collagen piezoelectricity are essentially speculative; there appears to be no direct evidence for its having any function. Speculations stem from the, not unreasonable, expectation that such an apparently useful physical property of collagen is likely to be exploited biologically. It is now well established that cells respond to applied electric fields — a relevant example is the stimulation of DNA synthesis in cartilage cells (Rodan et al, 1978). Thus, when a mechanical stress is applied to a collagenous tissue, the resulting electric field could affect the metabolism of its cells i.e. collagen fibrils could act as sensors which convey information to the cells about the stress applied to the tissue. It has been suggested that the piezoelectric effect could then be implicated in such processes as bone remodelling and fracture healing (Shamos & Lavine, 1967; Bassett, 1968).

Conveying information about mechanical stress to the cells in collagenous tissues could be especially important because the function of such tissues is often primarily mechanical. It has been suggested that mechanical stress leads to increased deposition of the tension-withstanding collagen fibrils by connective tissue cells (Pickup, 1978). Such hypotheses require cells to be aware of the stresses being applied to their tissue. As we have seen, the function of collagen fibrils is to be oriented so that stress applied to a tissue is transmitted as tensile stress along their fibril axes. This tensile stress might produce an electric field which could transmit the stress information to the cells.

Experiments on the effects of electric currents on collagenous tissues may well prove to be of considerable practical value. Already applied currents have been used in the clinical treatment of bone fractures (Brighton, 1977). Such experiments are merely suggestive of the biological importance of the piezoelectric effect — they do not demonstrate that the transduction of a mechanical signal into an electrical signal, or vice versa, has any natural function. But they do demonstrate the remarkable effects which electric currents can have on metabolism in collagenous tissues. And the practical value of the experiments is the development of new techniques for accelerating the repair of fractures.

CONCLUSIONS

The theme of this chapter is that the most important function of collagen fibrils in the majority of tissues is to withstand tensile stress. Although tissues may be subjected to many different kinds of deformation, such as compression, twisting and bending, their collagen fibrils are so arranged that the deforming forces are applied to these fibrils as axial tension. Of course collagen is involved in other processes (see e.g. Chapters 10, 11 and 13) and the arrangement of fibrils in a tissue may be subject to other constraints e.g. the cornea must be transparent (Cox et al, 1970). The emphasis throughout the chapter has been on human tissues — particularly those where the collagen fibril network is commonly affected by degeneration and disease. But the principles involved can sometimes be illustrated more simply by the tissues of lower animals (Woodhead-Galloway, 1980). I have avoided any description of the experimental methods involved in determining the mechanical properties of tissues; this topic is covered by Viidik (1973).

Collagenous tissues are viscoelastic — their mechanical properties are intermediate between those of ideal solids and viscous liquids. Thus they do not store all the energy which is used to deform them, their response to an applied stress depends on its rate of application and they continue to deform even though the applied stress remains constant. Also they can withstand increased stress even when they are already deformed — a much higher stress is needed to cause breakage which occurs gradually.

Other components of collagenous tissues help to determine their mechanical properties — the hydrated glycosaminoglycan gel which surrounds the fibrils is particularly important. These tissues can be considered as fibre-reinforced gels which are actually strengthened by the weak gel because it prevents crack propagation from one collagen fibril to another. In such a material there is no stress transmitted to the ends of the fibres. And so collagen fibril lengths need not be continuous throughout a tissue for them to withstand the tensile stresses which are applied to it i.e. collagen fibrils in a tendon need not be as long as the tendon itself. Mechanical properties of collagenous tissues can be further modified by elastin (which is more flexible than collagen) and by calcification (which stiffens the collagen). Even small calcified deposits could affect mechanical properties because of the phenomenon of stress concentration. Collagenous tissues appear to be weakened around their cells for the same reason.

In most tissues the collagen fibrils are crimped — removal of the crimp is the initial structural response to tensile stress. The function of the crimp appears to be to act as a 'shock absorber' protecting the fibrils against suddenly applied loads; fibrils stiffen as soon as the crimp is removed. Often crimped fibrils aggregate into fibres; there are parallel bundles of these fibres in tendon. When an applied stress increases a tendon length by more than about 4 per cent it becomes permanently deformed — almost all this length increase arises from straightening the crimp. Physiological length increases in tendon are not expected to exceed this value. Many ligaments can be stretched to a considerably greater extent — presumably because of their more complex collagen fibril networks and sometimes also high elastin content. Damage to ligaments usually occurs at their junction to bone.

The arrangement of collagen fibrils in the majority of tissues is far more complicated than in tendon — although in some, such as skin, the fibrils are still organised into fibres. In articular cartilage fibrils which are oriented parallel to the surface are stretched by the internal hydrostatic pressure of the tissue. The resulting tension in the fibrils, which acts tangentially to the cartilage surface, then opposes the swelling effects of the internal pressure conferring stability on the tissue. When the surface structure is damaged by osteoarthrosis, the tissue swells because the collagen fibril network is not strong enough to withstand the internal pressure. Deeper in the tissue the preferred orientation of collagen fibrils gradually changes so that they are perpendicular to the surface of the subchondral bone. This perpendicular orientation of fibrils ties the cartilage to the bone and prevents the internal pressure from lifting it off.

Despite the inability of collagen fibrils themselves to withstand twisting and bending, they are able to reinforce the intervertebral disc. Forces which tend to twist and bend the disc are transmitted to the fibrils as axial tension because of the way they are arranged in the annulus fibrosus. This arrangement, which resembles the structure of a reinforced hose, allows the disc to withstand applied pressure which is transmitted to the fibril network via the virtually incompressible glycosaminoglycan gel.

Collagen exhibits piezoelectricity; application of mechanical stress to an oriented array of collagen fibrils leads to the creation of an electric field. Although water decreases the piezoelectric effect, it is still observable in hydrated tissues — particularly bone. Piezoelectricity might provide a mechanism for conveying information about the mechanical forces acting on a collagenous tissue to its cells; experiments on the electrical properties of collagenous tissues have led to the development of methods for accelerating the repair of fractures.

Collagen is thus able to hold tissues together because of the tension in its fibrils; this statement is equally true of tissues like liver as well as the more obviously 'mechanical' tissues like tendon and cartilage. Tissues are 'tension structures' like the rigging on a sailing ship. Engineers tend to avoid such structures because of the inherent design problems (Gordon, 1978) and we are, therefore, more familiar with structures consisting of beams and pillars. Nature appears able to overcome design problems with ease and favours extracellular matrices which hold tissues together because their collagen fibrils can withstand tensile stress. The importance of these tension-withstanding 'ropes' in such structures cannot be overemphasised.

ACKNOWLEDGEMENTS

Many of the ideas in this chapter arose in the course of research carried out in collaboration with Richard Aspden, Steve Hickey and Jeremy Klein. I thank them and Irene Hartley, who typed the manuscript.

REFERENCES

Aspden R M, Hukins D W L 1979 Determination of the direction of preferred orientation and the orientation distribution function of collagen fibrils in connective tissues from high-angle X-ray diffraction patterns. Journal of Applied Crystallography 12: 306

Aspden R M, Hukins D W L 1981 Collagen organisation in articular cartilage determined by X-ray diffraction and its relationship to tissue function. Proceedings of the Royal Society B 212: 299

Bacon G E, Bacon P J, Griffiths R K 1979 Neutron diffraction studies of lumbar vertebrae. Journal of Anatomy 128: 277

Ball J 1971 Enthesopathy of rheumatoid and ankylosing spondylitis. Annals of the Rheumatic Diseases 30: 213

Ball J, Sharp J, Shaw N E 1978 Osteoarthrosis. In: Scott J T (ed) Copemann's Textbook of the Rheumatic Diseases, 5th Edn. Churchill Livingstone, Edinburgh. Ch 25, p 595

Bassett C A L 1968 Biologic significance of piezoelectricity. Calcified Tissue Research 1: 252

Brighton C T (ed) 1977 Bioelectric effects on bone and cartilage. Clinical Orthopedics and Related Research 124: 1

Buckley C P, Lloyd D W, Konopasek M 1980 On the deformation of slender filaments with planar crimp: theory, numerical solution and applications to tendon and textile materials. Proceedings of the Royal Society A372: 33

Cohen R E, Hooley C J, McCrum N G 1976 Viscoelastic creep of collagenous tissue. Journal of Biomechanics 9: 175

Cottrell A H 1964 Strong solids. Proceedings of the Royal Society A 282: 2

Cowan P M, North A C T, Randall J T 1955 X-ray diffraction studies of collagen fibres. Symposia of the Society for Experimental Biology 9: 115

Cox J L, Farrell R A, Hart R W, Langham M E 1970 The transparency of the mammalian cornea. Journal of Physiology 210: 601

Diamant J, Keller A, Baer E, Litt M, Arridge R G C 1972 Collagen; ultrastructure and its relationship to mechanical properties as a function of ageing. Proceedings of the Royal Society B 180: 293

Dlugosz J, Gathercole L J, Keller A 1978 Transmission electron microscope studies and their relation to polarizing optical microscopy in rat tail tendon. Micron 9: 71

Elden H R 1968 Physical properties of collagen fibres. International Review of Connective Tissue Research 4: 283

Elliott D H 1965 Structure and function of mammalian tendon. Biological Reviews 40: 392

Farfan H F 1973 Mechanical disorders of the low back. Lea and Febiger, Philadelphia

Fukada E, Ueda H, Rinaldi R 1976 Piezoelectric and related properties of hydrated collagen. Biophysical Journal 16: 911

Gathercole L J, Keller A 1975 Light microscopic waveforms in collagenous tissues and their structural implications. In: Atkins E D T, Keller A (eds) Structure of Fibrous Biopolymers, Butterworth, London. Ch 11, p 153

Gordon J E 1978 Structures or why things don't fall down. Penguin Books, Harmondsworth, Middlesex

Happey F 1976 A biophysical study of the human intervertebral disc. In: Jayson M (ed) The Lumbar Spine and Back Pain, Sector, London. Ch 13, p 293

Harkness R D 1961 Biological functions of collagen. Biological Reviews 36: 399

Harkness R D 1968 Mechanical properties of collagenous tissues. In: Gould B S (ed) Treatise on Collagen, Vol 2, Part A. Academic Press, London and New York. Ch 6, p 248

Haut R C, Little R W 1972 A constitutive equation for collagen fibres. Journal of Biomechanics 5: 423

Hickey D S, Hukins D W L 1980a Relation between the structure of the annulus fibrosus and the function and failure of the intervertebral disc. Spine 5: 106

Hickey D S, Hukins D W L 1980b X-ray diffraction studies of the arrangement of collagenous fibres in human fetal intervertebral disc. Journal of Anatomy 131: 81

Higdon A, Ohlsen E H, Stiles W B, Weese J A, Riley W F 1976 Mechanics of Materials, 3rd edn. Wiley, London

Hooley C J, Cohen R E 1979 A model for the creep behaviour of tendon. International Journal of Biological Macromolecules 1: 123

Hosemann R, Bonart R, Nemetschek T 1974 The inhomogenous stretching process of collagen. Colloid and Polymer Science 252: 912

Hukins D W L 1978 Bone stiffness explained by the liquid crystal model for the collagen fibril. Journal of Theoretical Biology 71: 661

Jayson M I V, Herbert C M and Barks J S 1973 Intervertebral discs, nuclear morphology and bursting pressures. Annals of the Rheumatic Diseases 32: 308

Kempson G E 1979 Mechanical properties of articular cartilage. In: Freeman M A R (ed) Adult Articular Cartilage, 2nd Edn. Pitman Medical, Tunbridge Wells. Ch 6, p 333

Kenedi R M, Gibson T, Evans J H, Barbenel J C 1975 Tissue mechanics. Physics in Medicine and Biology 20: 699

Klein J A, Hukins D W L 1982 Intervertebral disc: reorientation of collagen fibres during compression demonstrated by X-ray diffraction. Biochimica et Biophysica Acta, submitted

Korostoff E 1979 A linear piezoelectric model for characterising stress generated potentials in bone. Journal of Biomechanics 12: 335

Lees S 1979 A model for the distribution of HAP crystallites in bone — an hypothesis. Calcified Tissue International 27: 53

Lees S, Davidson C L 1977 The role of collagen in the elastic properties of calcified tissue. Journal of Biomechanics 10: 473

Longmore R B, Gardner D L 1978 The surface structure of ageing human articular cartilage: a study by reflected light interference microscopy. Journal of Anatomy 126: 353

Markwald R R, Fitzharris T P, Bank H, Bernanke D H 1978 Structural analyses on the matrical organization of glycosaminoglycans in developing endocardial cushion. Developmental Biology 62: 292

Maroudas A 1979 Physicochemical properties of articular cartilage. In: Freeman M A R (ed) Adult Articular Cartilage, 2nd Edn. Pitman Medical, Tunbridge Wells. Ch 4, p 215

Martin R B 1979 Theoretical analysis of the piezoelectric effect in bone. Journal of Biomechanics 12: 55

McCutchen C W 1975 Do mineral crystals stiffen bone by strait jacketing its collagen? Journal of Theoretical Biology 51: 51

McGee J O'D, Fallon A 1978 Hepatic cirrhosis — a collagen formative disease? Journal of Clinical Pathology 31: Supplement (Royal College of Pathologists) 12: 150

McNeill Alexander R 1975 Biomechanics. Chapman and Hall, London

Meachim G, Stockwell R A 1979 The matrix. In: Freeman M A R (ed) Adult Articular Cartilage, 2nd Edn. Pitman Medical, Tunbridge Wells. Ch 1, p 1

Millington P F, Gibson T, Evans J H, Barbenel J C 1971 Structural and mechanical aspects of connective tissue. Advances in Biomedical Engineering 1: 189

Minns R J, Steven F S 1977 The effect of calcium on the mechanical behaviour of aorta media elastin and collagen. British Journal of Experimental Pathology 58: 572

Muir H 1978 Proteoglycans of cartilage. Journal of Clinical Pathology 31: Supplement (Royal College of Pathologists) 12: 67

Nachemson A L, Evans J H 1967 Some mechanical properties of the third lumbar interlaminar ligament (ligamentum flavum). Journal of Biomechanics 1: 211

Netto T G, Zimmerman R L 1975 Effect of water on piezoelectricity in bone and collagen. Biophysical Journal 15: 573

Pickup A J 1978 Collagen and behaviour: a model for progressive debilitation. IRCS Medical Science 6: 499

Prockop D J, Kivirikko K I, Truderman L, Guzman N A 1979 The biosynthesis of collagen and its disorders (second of two parts). New England Journal of Medicine 301: 77

Rigby B J, Hirai N, Spikes J D, Eyring H 1959 The mechanical properties of rat tail tendon. Journal of General Physiology 43: 265

Roaf R 1960 A study of the mechanics of spinal injuries. Journal of Bone and Joint Surgery 42B: 810

Rodan G N, Bourret L A, Norton L A 1978 DNA synthesis in cartilage cells is stimulated by oscillating electric fields. Science 199: 690

Schofield J D, Weightman B 1978 New knowledge of connective tissue ageing. Journal of Clinical Pathology 31: Supplement (Royal College of Pathologists) 12: 174

Shah J S, Jayson M I V, Hampson W G J 1979 Mechanical implications of crimping in collagen fibres of human spinal ligaments. Engineering in Medicine 8: 95

Shamos M H, Lavine L S 1967 Piezoelectricity as a fundamental property of biological tissues. Nature 213: 267

Speer D P, Dahners L 1979 The collagenous architecture of articular cartilage: correlation of scanning electron microscopy and polarized light microscopy observations. Clinical Orthopedics and Related Research 139: 267

Tkaczuk H 1968 Tensile properties of human lumbar longitudinal ligaments. Acta Orthopaedica Scandinavica Supplementum No. 115

Torp S, Arridge R G C, Armeniades C D, Baer E 1975a Structure-property relationships in tendon as a function of age. In: Atkins E D T, Keller A (eds) Structure of Fibrous Biopolymers. Butterworth, London. Ch 13, p 197

Torp S, Baer E, Friedman B 1975b Effects of age and of mechanical deformation on the ultrastructure of tendon. In: Atkins E D T, Keller A (eds) Structure of Fibrous Biopolymers. Butterworth, London. Ch 14, p 223

Viidik A 1973 Function properties of collagenous tissues. International Review of Connective Tissue Research 6: 127

Wheeler E J, Lewis D 1977 An X-ray study of the paracrystalline nature of bone apatite. Calcified Tissue Research 24: 243

Williams W S, Breger L 1975 Piezoelectricity in tendon and bone. Journal of Biomechanics 8: 407

Woodhead-Galloway J 1980 Collagen: the anatomy of a protein. Arnold, London

5

Procollagen genes and messenger RNAs

K. S. E. CHEAH and M. E. GRANT

INTRODUCTION

The discovery that collagen occurs in vertebrate tissues in several genetically distinct forms has added a new dimension to the biology of connective tissues. Although structure-function relationships remain to be defined for the different collagen types, it is clear that regulation of the expression of the different collagen genes is basic to the development and differentiation of vertebrates and is also relevant to a number of diseases associated with defective or altered collagen molecules (for review see Prockop et al, 1979). In this chapter we initially outline how the recently developed techniques of recombinant DNA technology have revolutionised ideas of eukaryotic gene structure and mRNA processing. We review the studies carried out to date on the isolation and characterization of procollagen mRNAs and discuss how the messengers are being used both directly and indirectly to probe the structure, organization and control of the collagen genes.

On the basis of the unique amino acid sequences of collagen polypeptides, it can be predicted that the mRNAs, and hence their respective genes, must exhibit very distinctive characteristics. Thus, a messenger coding for pro-α chains of approximately 1500 amino acids must comprise at least 4500 nucleotides corresponding to a minimum molecular weight of 1.5×10^6 and an expected sedimentation coefficient in the region of 26–28 S. As well as being one of the largest mRNAs in eukaryotic cells, the collagen mRNA will also have an unusual base composition to code for a polypeptide rich in glycine (over 330 residues/mol) and the imino acids, proline and hydroxyproline (over 220 residues/mol). The codons for glycine and proline contain at least two residues of guanine (G) and cytosine (C) per triplet respectively and, hence, procollagen mRNAs should be readily distinguished from the majority of other eukaryotic mRNAs on account of their unusually high contents of G and C residues. Base sequences in the collagen genes will likewise be distinguished by high contents of C and G residues and the regions coding for the triplet sequence -Gly-X-Y- in the helical domains of the collagen polypeptides should be easily recognised in DNA base sequence analyses. These predictions are based on our understanding of the genetic code and both the composition and amino acid sequences of the collagen species. Other predictions of the structure and organization of collagen genes and messengers can be made on the basis of extensive studies on other eukaryotic genes and mRNAs. The general methodology used in such studies is discussed in a later section and the application of these procedures predominantly to the study of type I collagen suggests that collagen genes fit into the general pattern emerging for the organization of eukaryotic genes and their transcription.

Eukaryotic gene structure

The concept of one gene — one polypeptide which was embodied in the original hypothesis of one gene — one enzyme has found widespread support, and data obtained with prokaryotes provided direct evidence that the mRNA which determines the primary sequence of a protein is copied directly from a colinear gene sequence. However, in animal cells and some viruses it has become apparent that the cistron, the genetic unit of function that was thought to correspond in its entirety to a single polypeptide chain, does not exist as such, and the dogma of one gene — one polypeptide is not directly applicable to eukaryotic systems. The notion of the cistron is now replaced by that of a transcription unit, for in studies on a number of genes in higher organisms and in DNA viruses infecting vertebrates, it has been found that the coding sequences in DNA, ie. the regions that will ultimately be translated into an amino acid sequence, are not continuous but are broken up by stretches of 'silent' DNA. Thus, eukaryotic genes contain intervening sequences, termed *introns* by Gilbert (1978), interspersed between the 'sense' sequences, termed *exons,* which contain the regions expressed in the translated polypeptide. This view of eukaryotic genes as 'split genes' with their non-continguous arrangement of coding sequences is now widely accepted (for reviews see Abelson, 1979; Crick, 1979; Doel, 1980) but the term gene itself is no longer so clearly defined and is therefore used in its loosest sense throughout this chapter.

As the gene is now known to consist of dispersed sections of DNA, the mRNA is essentially a mosaic of regions (exons) of the gene and the synthesis of eukaryotic mRNA becomes, therefore, a complex mechanism of linking together the transcribed RNA coding sequences (Darnell, 1979). In studies on the genes of several vertebrate proteins it has been possible to demonstrate that the coding sequences (exons) are frequently much shorter than the intervening sequences (introns) which are of considerable but varying length running from under a hundred base pairs to more than a thousand (Fig. 5.1). In certain immunoglobulin light chains (Tonegawa et al, 1978) and various haemoglobin chains (Jeffreys & Flavell, 1977a; Tilghman et al, 1978a, b; Smithies et al, 1978; Kinniburgh et al, 1978; Konkel et al, 1978; van der Berg et al, 1978) two introns occur whereas seven occur in chick ovalbumin (Dugaiczyk et al, 1979) and chick ovomucoid (Lai et al, 1979) and a startling 33 intervening sequences have been described in the vitellogenin gene (Wahli et al, 1980). Where specific genes eg. for rabbit haemoglobin (Jeffreys & Flavell, 1977b) or chick ovalbumin (Breathnach et al, 1977), have been investigated in cells specialised in their expression and in a variety of other non-specific tissues not making haemoglobin or ovalbumin, the same array of non-continguous DNA sequences complementary to each of the specific mRNAs has been found. Thus, split genes would seem to be a stable feature of the eukaryotic genome and, with the special exception of the immunoglobulin genes (Davis et al, 1980; Maki et al, 1980; Molgaard, 1980), there is no experimental support for DNA rearrangement for the purpose of transcription. As indicated above, split genes also occur in eukaryotic DNA viruses (Berget et al, 1977; Klessig, 1977; Nevins & Darnell, 1978; Reddy et al, 1978), and the presence of introns has been demonstrated in genes with no protein product such as the tRNA genes of yeast (Goodman et al, 1977; Valenzuela et al, 1978; Knapp et al, 1978) and the rRNA genes in *Drosophila* (Glover & Hogness, 1977) and *Tetrahymena pigmentosa* (Wild & Gall, 1979).

A further feature of eukaryotic gene structure is the occurrence of distinctive base sequences in the regions immediately flanking the genes. Thus, a region rich in repeating TA sequences has been found at a position about 20–30 nucleotides from the 5′ end of several genes (Konkel et al, 1978; Bernard et al, 1978; Sures et al, 1978; Lai et al, 1979; Tsujimoto & Suzuki, 1979; Thimmappaya et al, 1979) whereas the region just beyond the 3′ end of genes may contain TTTT (Korn & Brown, 1978; Konkel et al,

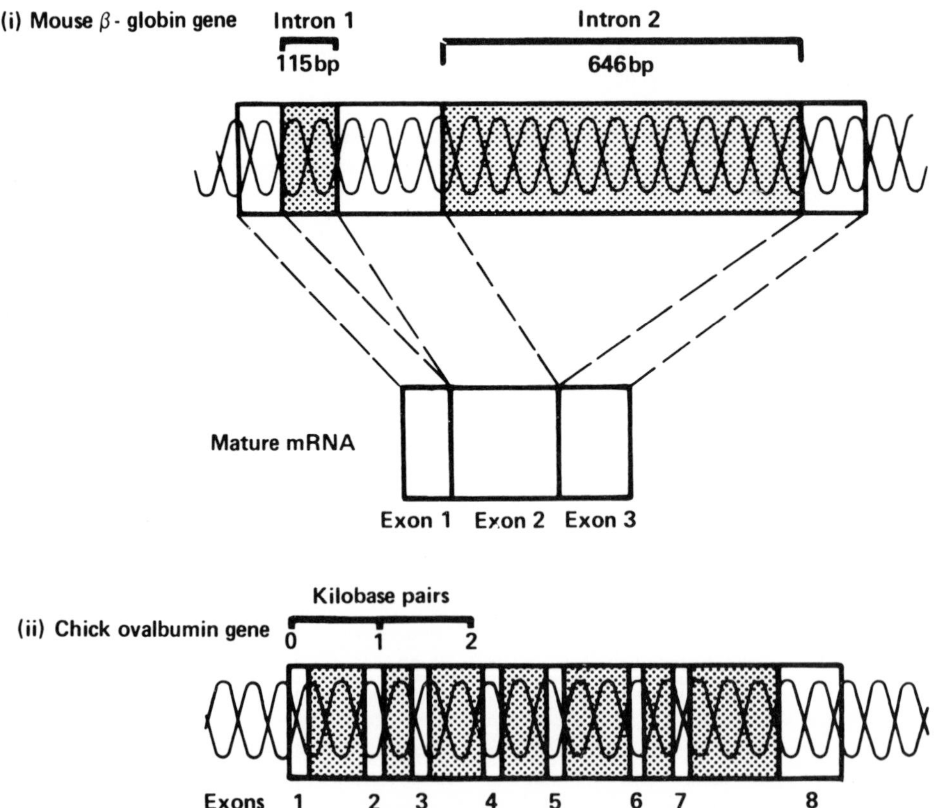

Fig. 5.1 Schematic representations of the structures of (i) the mouse β-globin gene containing two intervening sequences (shaded), and (ii) the chick ovalbumin gene containing seven intervening sequences.

1978) or TTGT sequences (Efstratiatis et al, 1979; Lai et al, 1979). The possibility that these sequences denote the signals for initiation and termination of transcription respectively has some experimental support (Corden et al, 1980) although there is evidence that in some genes the control of initiation is dependent on a specific base sequence occurring at an intra-gene position (Sakonju et al, 1980; Bogenhagen et al, 1980).

The transcriptional process occurring within the nucleus of eukaryotic cells appears to involve the synthesis of a primary transcript of the whole gene or transcription unit (for review see Darnell, 1979). The large mRNA precursor containing both exons and introns must then undergo a process described as 'RNA splicing' in which the removal of introns and the ligation of exons occurs to produce the single functional RNA molecule. The mechanisms of splicing are as yet ill-defined but some insight into the specificity required of enzymes promoting these events has been sought by determining the base sequences of introns and particularly those sequences corresponding to intron-exon boundaries. Detailed analyses of the ovalbumin gene (Breathnach et al, 1978; Catterall et al, 1978) show some conservation of the base sequence near the beginning and near the end of an intron (Fig. 5.2); and together with similar investigations on introns of other protein-coding genes (reviewed by Lerner et al, 1980) it appears that every intron could begin with GT and end with AG. The sequence homologies which exist at these intron-exon junctions, although not extensive, have allowed Kourilsky & Chambon (1978) to propose prototype sequences (Fig. 5.2) which might define the cutting site.

The intron sequences at the intron-exon junction have recently been shown to exhibit extensive complementarity with base sequences at the 5′-terminal region of a small RNA species found in the nuclei of eukaryotic cells (Lerner et al, 1980). The presence of small nuclear RNAs (snRNAs) ranging in size from 90 to 220 nucleotides has been known for over a decade (Weinberg & Penman, 1968) although their function has remained obscure. The most abundant snRNAs exist as a closely-related set of RNA-protein complexes (snRNPs) each of which may contain the same set of seven polypeptides (Lerner & Steitz, 1979). It is of interest to note that snRNPs are the antigens recognized by antibodies from some patients with systemic lupus erythematosus (SLE), the autoimmune rheumatic disease (Notman et al, 1975; Provost, 1979). When the sequence of the major snRNA (UIA) precipitated by the antibodies from lupus sera was determined, it was found that at the 5′ end there were adjacent sequences which exactly matched sequences at the 5′ and 3′ end of intervening sequences (Lerner et al, 1980; Rogers & Wall, 1980). Thus, it was proposed (Fig. 5.3) that the snRNAs might interact with the terminal sequences of introns and serve a template function by correctly aligning the sequences to be spliced by the proteins associated with the snRNA (Murray & Holliday, 1979; Lerner et al, 1980; Richards, 1980). Enzymes responsible for the splicing process have been detected in yeast cells (Knapp et al, 1978; O'Farrell et al,

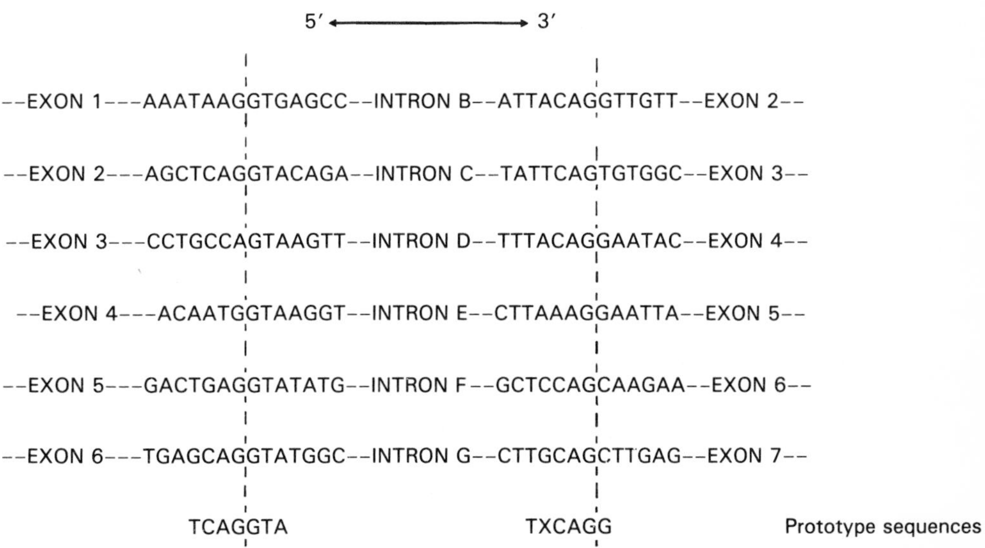

Fig. 5.2 Comparison of the DNA sequences at the intron-exon junctions of the ovalbumin gene with the 'prototype' sequences proposed by Chambon.

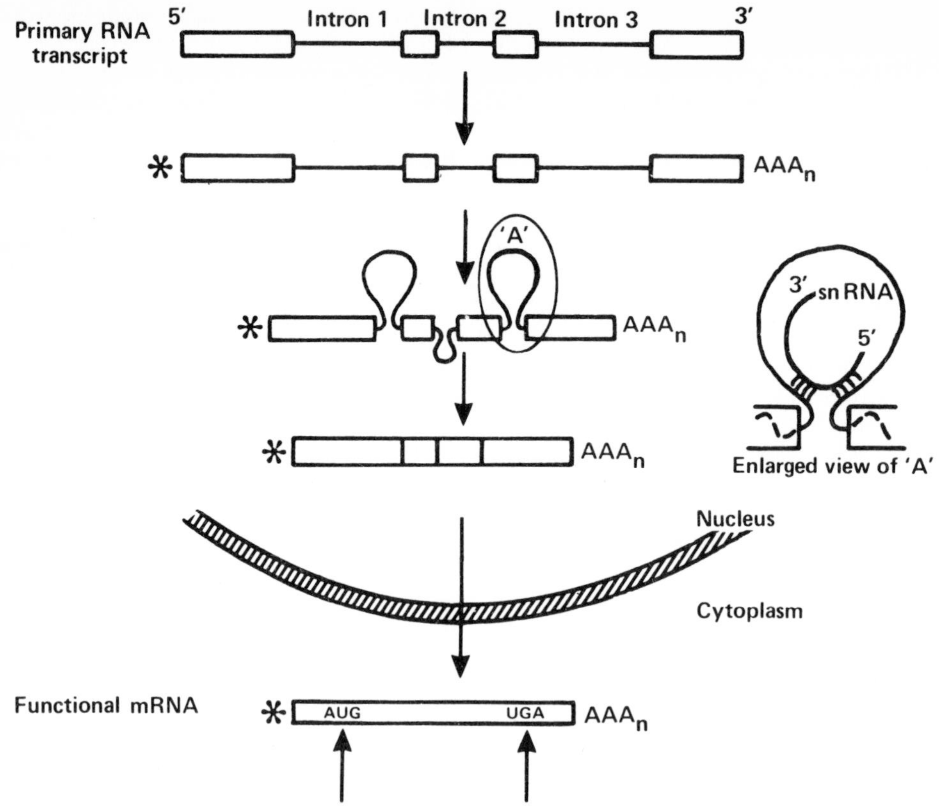

Fig. 5.3 Diagrammatic representation of the processing of a hypothetical mRNA precursor containing three intervening sequences. After synthesis of the primary RNA transcript the following post-transcriptional events occur: 1, Addition of a cap (*) at the 5′ end and a polyA tail at the 3′ end; 2, Splicing out of the introns in which snRNA molecules are implicated; 3, Ligation of the exons, and 4, Transport of the functional mRNA into the cytoplasm.

1978) but the fate of the excised introns is unknown. Indeed, the function(s) of introns is unknown although they appear to have a critical role in the production of functional mRNA (Lai & Khoury, 1979; Gruss et al, 1979; Hamer et al, 1979; Hamer & Leder, 1979; Wickens et al, 1980). The significance of the evolution of split genes and the possible role of splicing in the control of gene expression at the transcriptional level remain to be established (for reviews see Darnell, 1978, 1979; Crick, 1979; Abelson, 1979).

General features of eukaryotic mRNAs

In contrast to prokaryotes where transcription of genes and translation of mRNA are linked, in eukaryotes these processes are physically separated by the nuclear membrane. For many years it has been considered that a multistep process is involved in the flow of information from the eukaryotic genome to the site of translation in the cytoplasm. A large proportion of the RNA isolated from nuclei consists of large molecules some 10 to 20 times the size of mRNAs and much of this material (known as heterogeneous nuclear RNA, HnRNA) has a very short half-life. These observations led to the concept that HnRNA might be a pre-mRNA; and the evidence for a precursor-product relationship between RNA transcripts in the nucleus and cytoplasmic mRNA is now widely accepted (for reviews see Perry, 1976; Revel & Groner, 1978; Darnell, 1979; Scherrer et al, 1979).

The nuclear processing of the primary RNA transcripts involves several post-transcriptional steps (Fig. 6.3) including the removal of the intervening sequences as described above. One of the most unexpected findings in the characterization of eukaryotic messengers and their precursors was the discovery of 'cap' — structures at their 5′ ends. These caps comprise a 7-methyl guanosine residue linked by a 5′-5 triphosphate group to the first coded nucleotide of the RNA; the latter and subsequent nucleotide in the sequence can also be methylated giving rise to structures of the type $m^7G(5')ppp(5')X^mpY^m$. The mechanism of cap synthesis is well documented (for reviews see Shatkin, 1976; Filipowicz, 1978) and this process occurs soon after transcription and probably before splicing (Fig. 5.3). In addition, methylated adenosine residues (m^6A) are found at internal positions of some eukaryotic cellular and viral mRNAs. The functional significance of m ^{6}A residues is unknown but the 5′ cap structure appears to have at least two roles. The cap protects the mRNA from 5′-exonucleolytic degradation and the m^{7}G seems to be important in the initiation of protein synthesis being involved in mRNA-ribosome interactions (Clemens, 1979; Paterson & Rosenberg, 1979; Rosenberg & Paterson, 1979).

Another important post-transcriptional event involves the stepwise addition of adenylate residues to the 3′-OH terminus of the mRNA precursors to form long (180–200 nucleotide) tracts of polyA (Darnell et al, 1973). The finding that polyA occurs in HnRNA supported the hypothesis that polyA(+)HnRNA is the precursor of mRNA with the polyA segment being conserved in the processing (Fig. 5.3), although there are also indications that polyadenylation can take place after processing of HnRNA and in some cases may occur in the cytoplasm. One of the functions attributed to the polyA tail is that it may be essential for the nuclear processing mechanism for cordycepin (3′-deoxy-adenosine) which inhibits polyA synthesis, inhibits the appearance of mRNA in the cytoplasm. Histone mRNA is an exception to the general rule and contains no polyA but it is nevertheless synthesized and transported to the cytoplasm although it does turn over faster than polyA-containing messengers. The polyA segment is known to shorten as the mRNA ages and although not a requirement for translation of the message in the cytoplasm, the polyA may confer stability on eukaryotic mRNAs (Greenberg, 1975; Marbaix et al, 1977; Revel & Groner, 1978).

The 5′-cap and the polyA segments are not translated during protein synthesis but even after allowing for these regions, the sizes of eukaryotic mRNAs are usually much greater than that required to code for their specific protein products. The extra nucleotides, which can constitute a significant portion of the total mRNA molecule, are located on each side of the coding sequence and are defined as the 5′- and 3′- non-coding regions. One might speculate that the role(s) of non-coding regions will involve interaction of mRNA and rRNA, ribosomal proteins and factors participating in the initiation and termination of protein synthesis. It is also important to remember that neither mRNAs nor their precursors exist as free nucleic acid molecules but occur as ribonucleoprotein complexes (mRNPs and HnRNPs respectively) (for reviews see Williamson, 1973; Billings & Martin, 1978). Thus, in a wide variety of eukaryotic cells, polysomal mRNA has been found to be tightly associated with a few, apparently similar, non-ribosomal proteins. Two major polypeptides of approximate molecular weight 50 000 and 78 000 appear to be common to the majority of mRNAs investigated and a small number of other polypeptides in the range 40 000–100 000 are also detected in some mRNP particles. The functions of the protein components is unclear although the polyA tail may serve as a binding site for the major proteins (see for example Blobel, 1973; Schwartz & Darnell, 1976) which may influence the long-term stability of the mRNA by affording protection against degradation of the polyA tail in vivo. A role for polyA-binding proteins in the transport of mRNA from the nucleus to the cytoplasm has also been suggested (Schwartz & Darnell, 1976).

PROCOLLAGEN MESSENGER RNAs

Over the past decade considerable advances have been made in our understanding of the biochemistry of collagen and its precursor procollagen with respect to molecular structure, assembly and post-translational processing (for reviews see Grant & Jackson, 1976; Fessler & Fessler, 1978; Prockop et al, 1979; Heathcote & Grant, 1980). In contrast little is known of the factors influencing transcription, post-transcriptional events and translation of procollagen mRNAs. At least five genetically distinct collagen types have been described for which a minimum of eight genes must exist to code for their constituent αchains (Bornstein & Sage, 1980; Gay et al, 1980) and it is clear that the regulation of the expression of these collagen genes in vertebrates must be a complex and finely coordinated process. The isolation and characterization of mRNAs for procollagen and the construction of gene probes are first prerequisites in any evaluation of the mechanism(s) by which procollagen biosynthesis may be controlled at the level of transcription or translation.

mRNA for procollagen I

Type I collagen has been studied in greatest detail both chemically and biosynthetically and it is therefore natural that the majority of investigations in this field have concentrated on type I procollagen messenger RNA.

Detection and cell-free translation

The ability to achieve complete translation of a specific mRNA in cell-free protein-synthesizing systems is a necessary first step in both the detection and isolation of mRNAs in cell or tissue extracts. Authenticity of the polypeptides synthesized in vitro is of importance in assessing both the integrity of the mRNA and the nature of the primary translation product.

In this respect considerable difficulties were experienced initially in the cell-free translation of procollagen mRNA into complete pro-αchains (reviewed by Harwood, 1979). Thus, in early stages the synthesis of pro-αchains was achieved only when isolated polyribosomes were allowed to complete their nascent polypeptides in vitro (Kerwar et al, 1972, 1973). The use of RNA, extracted directly from cells or tissues synthesizing type I collagen, to programme cell-free protein-synthesizing systems derived from Krebs II ascites cells (Benveniste et al, 1973; Wang et al, 1975a) or wheat germ (Neufang et al, 1975; Benveniste et al, 1976; Zeichner & Rojkind, 1976) generally resulted in the synthesis of collagenous polypeptides mainly of αchain size or smaller. Even where some polypeptides the size of pro-αchains were detected by cell-free synthesis in untreated reticulocyte-lysates (Boedtker et al, 1974) yields were extremely low, probably because translation was hampered by the high level of endogenous messenger activity.

The above difficulties experienced in achieving complete pro-αchains were probably attributable to partial degradation of mRNA during extraction and more particularly to the deficiencies of the translation systems used. For example, cell-free systems from Krebs II ascites cells have the disadvantage of endogenous collagen synthesizing abilities (Benveniste et al, 1976); and the efficiency of the wheat germ system has been found to be vary variable among batches of wheat germ (Marcu & Dudock, 1974; Carlier & Peumans, 1976) especially in the translation of large mRNAs (Shih & Kaesburg, 1976; Davies et al, 1977). Some success has been reported with the wheat-germ system which does have the advantage of very low levels of endogenous mRNA and the cell-free synthesis of pro-αchains was achieved with mRNA from embryonic chick tendon cells, embryonic chick calvaria and fibroblasts in culture (Harwood et al, 1975a; Boedtker et al, 1976; Adams et al, 1977; Frischauf et al, 1978; Cheah et al, 1979a). It is noteworthy, however, that a high background of lower molecular weight polypeptides was usually observed and the synthesis of pro-α2 chains predominated over that of pro-α1. Since the pro-α1 chain is believed to be slightly longer than the pro-α2 chain (Fessler & Fessler, 1978) any restricted ability of the cell-free system to complete the translation of large mRNAs would result in the synthesis of more of the shorter pro-α2 chains despite the potential for synthesis of pro-α1 and pro-α2 chains in a 2:1 ratio.

Latterly, workers have adopted the mRNA-dependent reticulocyte-lysate system of Pelham & Jackson (1976) and have obtained high yields of both pro-α1 and pro-α2 chains (Rowe et al, 1978; Howard et al, 1978; Monson & Goodman, 1978; Cheah et al, 1979a; Palmiter et al, 1979; Paglia et al, 1979; Sandell & Veis, 1980). In a comparative study of the wheat germ and the mRNA-dependent reticulocyte-lysate systems, it was demonstrated that although the same chick tendon cell mRNA preparation directed the synthesis of mostly pro-α2 chains in the wheat-germ system, pro-α1 and pro-α2 chains were synthesized in a 2:1 ratio in the reticulocyte-lysate system (Cheah et al, 1979a). The 2:1 ratio achieved in the translation in vitro of procollagen I mRNA (Cheah et al, 1979a; Paglia et al, 1979) correlates well with the synthesis of type I collagen polypeptides in a 2:1 ratio in calvaria (Fessler et al, 1975), tendon cells (Harwood et al, 1977) and in studies with collagen-synthesising polysomes (Kerwar et al, 1972; Vuust, 1975). Such studies suggest that translatable mRNA species for pro-α1 and pro-α2 chains are also present in a 2:1 ratio.

The identification of collagenous polypeptides on the basis of size alone (as judged by SDS/polyacrylamide gel electrophoresis or gel filtration chromatography) is not in itself definitive. Other criteria are also necessary for a rigorous identification of pro-αchains among cell-free translation products. Hence, specific susceptibility to highly purified bacterial collagenase, immunoprecipitation by specific antibodies to procollagen (Rowe et al, 1978; Monson & Goodman, 1978; Palmiter et al, 1979; Paglia et al, 1979; Sandell & Veis, 1980) and the ability of the cell-free product to act as a substrate for prolyl hydroxylase (Boedtker et al, 1976; Wilczek et al, 1978; Cheah et al, 1979a, b) have been used to identify collagenous cell-free products. Of these criteria, only immunoprecipitation by procollagen antibodies and hydroxylation of proline residues may be considered as specific demonstrations of the collagenous nature of the translation products. Susceptibility to purified bacterial collagenases cannot be taken as an unambiguous means of identifying collagenous polypeptides. This enzyme cleaves peptide bonds which are found most commonly in collagen (Weiss, 1976) but which may also occur in a few other proteins rich in glycine and proline e.g. tropoelastin (Sandberg, 1976) and chondroitin sulphate proteoglycan core protein (Muir & Hardingham, 1975). Thus, tropoelastin from embryonic chicks has been found to be degraded by highly purified bacterial collagnease (Cheah et al, 1980) and the polypeptide of approximately 65 000 molecular weight synthesized in cell-free extracts of Chinese hamster lung cells probably corresponds to this protein, although it was tentatively designated a collagenous product on the basis of bacterial collagenase susceptibility (Haralson et al, 1979).

A further characteristic of collagenous polypeptides useful in their identification among cell-free translation products relates to their capacity for hydroxylation and their corresponding electrophoretic mobility. Compared to globular protein standards collagen is known to migrate anomalously in SDS/polyacrylamide gels (Furthmayr & Timpl, 1971; Weber & Osborn, 1975; Sandell & Veis, 1980) and a difference in mobility of pro-αchains has been observed depending on the extent of hydroxylation of these polypeptides (Harwood et al, 1977; Cheah et al, 1979a, b). Since the post-translational hydroxylation of proline residues in collagen does not occur in cell-free systems (Rowe et al, 1978; Cheah et al, 1979a) the choice of unhydroxylated pro-αchains as molecular weight standards is important both in the identification and in the sizing of the primary translation products of procollagen mRNAs. In addition, when products of cell-free synthesis are incubated with exogenous prolyl hydroxylase, a decrease in electrophoretic mobility of pro-αchains as a result of hydroxylation provides a simple and specific means of identification of collagenous polypeptides among the spectrum of translation products (Cheah et al, 1979a, b).

Nature of the primary translation product

Studies on the assembly of proteins destined for secretion have revealed that cell-free translation of the appropriate mRNA species results in the synthesis of polypeptides of slightly higher molecular weight than the corresponding precursors normally detected in vivo owing to the occurrence of an additional 15–30 amino acid residues at the N-terminus of the translation products. Such observations formed the basis of the 'Signal Hypothesis' (for review see Blobel, 1977) which proposed that the initiation of protein synthesis always commences on free ribosomes but for secretory proteins there exists very close to the N-terminus a signal sequence of predominantly hydrophobic amino acid residues which interacts with the membrane of the endoplasmic reticulum to cause the association of several ribosome acceptor proteins which form a tunnel through the membrane. In this way the protein destined for secretion (Fig. 5.4) is directed into the lumen of the endoplasmic reticulum where an enzyme, signal peptidase, cleaves the signal peptide or pre-sequence from the uncompleted remainder of the nascent chain. The 'processed' nascent chain continues to elongate and after polypeptide termination and release will be entirely segregated within the cisternal space. Evidence in support of the initial predictions of Blobel & Dobberstein (1975a, b) have come from studies on a large number of secreted proteins (for review see Harwood, 1980) although some refinements of the hypothesis have become necessary with the discovery of internal signal sequences in ovalbumin (Lingapaa et al, 1979).

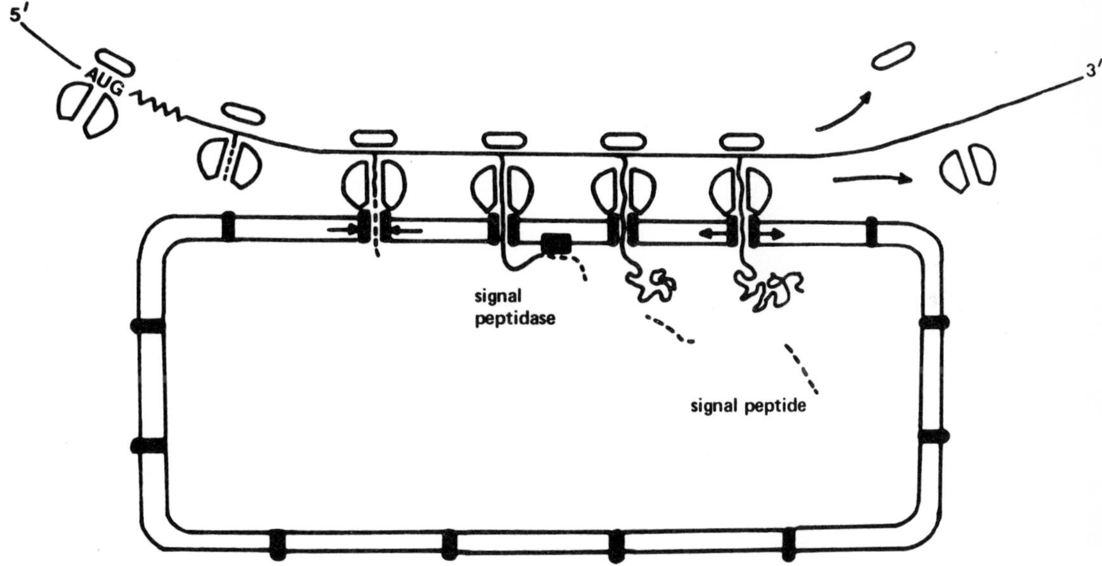

Fig. 5.4 Schematic illustration of the signal hypothesis. For details, see text.

It is generally accepted that procollagen is synthesised on membrane-bound polyribosomes (Harwood, 1979; Oborotova et al, 1979; Martinell & Lukens, 1980) and follows the classical route of secretion (Grant & Jackson, 1976). In addition, cell-free translation studies of the mRNAs associated with subcellular fractions from chick tendon cells (K.S.E. Cheah & M.E. Grant, unpublished observations) indicate that the mRNAs for pro-α1 and pro-α2 are associated with membrane bound polysomes and not with free polysomes (Fig. 5.5). These observations together with studies on the products of cell-free translation indicate that the assembly of procollagen polypeptides is consistent with the signal hypothesis. Thus, the synthesis of a precursor form of pro-α1 chains (pre-pro-α1) has been demonstrated in analyses of the primary translation product of embryonic chick proα1(I) mRNA (Cheah et al, 1979a; Graves et al, 1979; Palmiter et al, 1979; Sandell & Veis, 1980). The pre-peptide of pro-α1 is rich in phenylalanine and leucine and is cleaved off in the presence of microsomal membranes (Palmiter et al, 1979; Sandell & Veis, 1980). A tentative sequence containing many hydrophobic amino acids has been put forward by Palmiter et al (1979):

Met-phe-ser-phe-val-X-ser-arg-leu-leu-leu-leu-
ile-ala-ala-X-X-leu-leu- . . .

Estimates of the size of the pre-peptide of pre-pro-α1 have varied, most probably because of the difficulties involved in obtaining accurate molecular weight values for polypeptides with both globular and collagenous domains. Palmiter et al (1979) estimate that pre-pro-α1 is 5500 daltons larger than pro-α1 whereas Graves et al (1979) suggest that the pre-sequence has a molecular weight of 10 000. The data of Sandell & Veis (1980) indicate a difference of 20 000 between pre-pro-α1 and pro-α1. The technical difficulties in making these molecular weight determinations suggest that the above discrepancy may be more apparent than real but it is certain that the size of the signal peptide of pro-α1(I) exceeds that expected for a sequence of 15–30 residues at the N-terminus and could be as large as 100 amino acids. The significance of a pre-sequence larger than the signal peptides found in other secreted proteins is unclear but it may be a feature of the chick protein for the pre-pro-α1(I) of human fibroblasts is not correspondingly large (M. L. Chu, personal communication). As yet, no evidence for a pre-pro form of pro-α2 chains has been presented, for gel electrophoretic analyses of the translation product of pro-α2 mRNA have not revealed any substantially larger precursor than unhydroxylated pro-α2 chains (Cheah et al, 1979a; Palmiter et al, 1979a; Sandell & Veis, 1980).

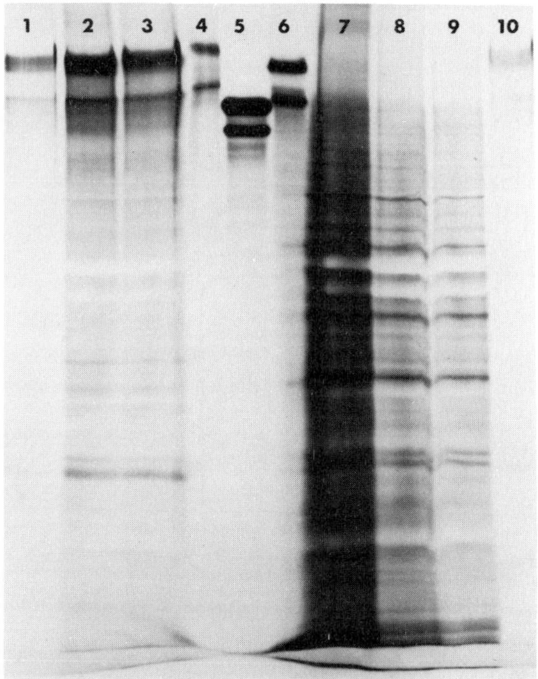

Fig. 5.5 Cell-free translation of mRNAs associated with free and membrane-bound polyribosomes isolated from embryonic chick tendon cells.

Polysomes were prepared from matrix-free cells from 17-day old chick embryos. Free and membrane-bound polysomes were separated on sucrose density gradients and the two fractions were collected by centrifugation through a sucrose cushion (40% w/v and 1.0M respectively) containing 50mM-Tris-HC1 buffer, pH 7.6, 25mM KC1, 5mM-magnesium acetate and 0.2 vols guinea pig liver RNAase inhibitor [for details see Craig et al (1979)]. Membranes were not solubilised in the membrane-bound fraction. Both fractions were resuspended in 0.5mM-Tris-HC1 buffer, pH 7.6, 96mM-KC1, 0.5mM-magnesium acetate and after translation of the associated mRNA in a reticulocyte-lysate cell-free system containing [^{35}S]methionine, the translation products were analysed by polyacrylamide gel electrophoresis and fluorography (Cheah et al, 1979a).

Tracks 1, 2, 3 and 10 show products of cell-free translation obtained with 0.1, 0.2, 0.3 and 0.15 A_{260} units of membrane-bound polysomes respectively. Tracks 7, 8 and 9 show products of cell-free translation obtained with 0.34, 0.17 and 0.08 A_{260} units of free polysomes. Tracks 4, 5 and 6 contain the following standards: pro-α1(I) and pro-α2(I) chains, α1(I) and α2(I) chains, and unhydroxylated pro-α1(I) and pro-α2(I) chains respectively.

Characterization of the mRNAs

Virtually all the studies on the mRNA for procollagen I have been carried out on preparations extracted from the cells of embryonic chick tissues. In some instances whole embryos have been used and the assumption implicit in such studies is that procollagen I mRNA is likely to represent the predominant collagen messenger present (Neufang et al, 1975; Wang et al, 1975a, b; Salles et al, 1976; Brentani et al, 1977). However, the majority of studies have used leg tendons (Harwood et al, 1974, 1975a; Rowe et al, 1978; Cheah et al, 1979a) or calvaria (Benveniste et al, 1973, 1976; Boedtker et al, 1974, 1976; Breitkreutz et al, 1978; Monson & Goodman, 1978; Frischauf et al, 1978; Rowe et al, 1978) each of which contains only one major cell type whose considerable collagen-synthesising activity is devoted exclusively to procollagen I. Other systems used for the isolation of procollagen I mRNA include neonatal rat calvaria (Diaz de Leon et al, 1977), foetal calf tendon (Tolstoshev et al, 1979), foetal calf skin (Kaufmann et al, 1980) and fibroblasts in culture (Rowe et al, 1978).

Because of the high molecular weight of pro-αchains, it has long been recognised that the mRNA for procollagens must be among the largest in nature and, accordingly, many investigations have been directed towards the identification of a large RNA species having the characteristics of such a messenger. The studies based on the size of collagen-synthesising polysomes which suggested that procollagen mRNA might be polycistronic (Kretsinger et al, 1964; Fernandez-Madrid, 1967; Manner et al, 1967; Park et al, 1975) have not been substantiated by subsequent investigations in which it has been demonstrated that collagen synthesis occurs on polysomes comprised of 30–40 ribosomes (Lazarides & Lukens, 1971; Lazarides et al, 1971; Kerwar et al, 1973; Harwood et al, 1974, 1975b; Pawlowski et al, 1975; Vuust, 1975; Cutroneo et al, 1977; Diaz de Leon et al, 1977; Nwagu & Reid, 1977). Thus, it is generally accepted that procollagen mRNA is monocistronic and exhibits electrophoretic, chromatographic and sedimentation characteristics consistent with an RNA species in the range 26–30s depending on the method of analysis (Boedtker et al, 1974,

1976; Harwood et al, 1975c; Zeichner & Stern, 1977; Breitkreutz et al, 1978; Frischauf et al, 1978; Tolstoshev et al, 1978; Rowe et al, 1978; Adams et al, 1979; Rave et al, 1979). In those experiments where procollagen mRNA preparations containing major species of 22s to 25s were reported (Harwood et al, 1974; Benveniste et al, 1974; Wang et al, 1975b; Zeichner & Rojkind, 1976), it is now apparent that some degradation of the procollagen mRNA had probably occurred in the isolation procedures, an observation consistent with the difficulties in achieving cell-free translation of these species into polypeptides of pro-αchain size (for review see Harwood, 1979).

In the majority of procedures adopted for the isolation of procollagen mRNAs, a preliminary separation of mRNAs from rRNAs and tRNAs has been achieved by affinity chromatography on columns of cellulose (Harwood et al, 1974), oligo(dT)-cellulose (Boedtker, 1974, 1976; Wang et al, 1975b; Rowe et al, 1978; Cheah et al, 1979a), polyU-sepharose (Breitkreutz et al, 1978), and on polyU-coated filters (Zeichner & Rojkind, 1976). The success of these procedures are all consistent with the occurrence of a polyA tail in procollagen mRNA; and the lengths of the polyA extensions of the mRNAs isolated from chick tendon membrane-bound polysomes (Harwood et al, 1975c) and from a 22s procollagen mRNA from chick embryos (Salles et al, 1976) have been estimated by electrophoretic analyses to be in the region of 140–150 nucleotides. However, in neither of these studies was the anomalous behaviour of polyA molecules on polyacrylamide gels considered (Burness et al, 1975) and these values are probably inaccurate. Further insight into the 3′-untranslated region of collagen mRNAs has come from analyses of procollagen cDNA clones (see section on Procollagen genes). Sequences of 133 and 300 nucleotides, rich in A + T residues, have been demonstrated in the chicken pro-α1(I) and pro-α2(I) mRNAs respectively beyond the termination codons; and within these regions of both mRNAs occurs an oligo(dC)-tract of 7–8 nucleotides (Fuller & Boedtker, 1981). The significance of this sequence is unknown.

Estimates of the molecular weight of procollagen mRNA based on electrophoretic studies of the 28s mRNA species (Boedtker et al, 1974; Harwood et al, 1975c) suggested a molecular weight of $1.6–1.7 \times 10^6$. Similar values have been obtained in experiments in which recombinant DNA techniques have been used to generate cDNA clones which hybridise to polyA-containing RNA from embryonic chick calvaria (Adams et al, 1979; Rave et al, 1979). The major RNA species isolated in this way have been identified as procollagen mRNAs of approx. 5000 nucleotides corresponding to an MW of 1.7×10^6; but also present were higher molecular weight species in the range 5600 to 7100 nucleotides which probably represent nuclear precursors of procollagen mRNAs (Adams et al, 1979; Rave et al, 1979). A surprising observation arising from these studies is the fact that the pro-α2 mRNA is slightly larger than the pro-α1 mRNA although the pro-α2 chain is believed to be shorter than the pro-α1 chain (Fessler & Fessler, 1978). In contrast, Tolstoshev et al (1979) have obtained data suggesting that the pro-α1 mRNA is significantly larger than the pro-α2 mRNA. However, the basis on which their separation and specific identification of the two messengers was achieved, ie. on formamide-sucrose gradients, is probably dependent more on differences in secondary structure than on actual size differences, and is in any case less accurate than denaturing gel electrophoresis as a means of estimating the molecular weight of nucleic acids.

Secondary structure is a feature attributed more to ribosomal RNAs than to messenger RNAs but the anticipated high G and C content of procollagen mRNA is likely to contribute to considerable potential for base pairing and hairpin loop formation (Brentani et al, 1977). The fact that procollagen mRNA and 28s rRNA exhibit similar properties when chromatographed (Boedtker et al, 1974) or electrophoresed (Harwood et al, 1975c) under conditions in which RNA is denatured by formamide treatment suggests that procollagen mRNA possesses a degree of secondary structure similar to rRNA. Whether or not the secondary structure of procollagen mRNA has any influence on protein-RNA interactions or on translation is unknown. It is noteworthy, however, that removal of secondary structure in mRNA has been shown to result in enhanced cell-free translation of chick ovalbumin and conalbumin mRNAs (Payvar & Schimke, 1979).

It should not be forgotten that in vivo there is always a close association of mRNAs with proteins (see p. 77) which may play a crucial role in transport and function. Little information is available on the proteins associated with procollagen mRNA but mRNPs have been obtained from embryonic chick tendon cells (Standart & Harwood, 1978) and non-ribosomal proteins of 45 000, 60 000, 80 000 and 100 000 have been detected in mRNPs associated with membrane-bound polysomes from these cells (Standart, 1979). The demonstrations that the synthesis of procollagen occurs on membrane-bound polysomes (see Harwood, 1979; Oborotova et al, 1979), and the fact that procollagen mRNA is the major messenger present in such preparations from chick tendon cells (Fig. 6.5) suggest that the proteins isolated in the membrane-bound mRNPs by Standart (1979) are likely to be associated predominantly with procollagen mRNA. As interest moves from the structural aspects of mRNAs to the control of their synthesis and translation, it is clear that a consideration of the protein components of these ribonucleoprotein particles will be necessary.

Studies on mRNAs for pro-α1(II) and pro-α1(III)

Investigations on the mRNAs for the other collagen types have not progressed at the same rate as for procollagen I mRNA. Several laboratories have experienced difficulties in extracting and translating the type II procollagen mRNA, presumably due to the presence of ribonuclease in cell homogenates (Upholt et al, 1979); and only one report tentatively identifying pro-α1(III) polypeptides in cell-free translation products of foetal calf skin mRNA has appeared (Kaufman et al, 1980). However, using matrix-free chondrocytes released from embryonic chick sternal cartilage by enzymic digestion it has been possible to extract a polyA-rich fraction which when translated in a reticulocyte-lysate yields a high molecular weight collagenous polypeptide. This component was identified as the unhydroxylated precursor of type II collagen on the basis of its electrophoretic mobility, its susceptibility to bacterial collagenase, and its ability to act as a substrate for prolyl hydroxylase (Cheah et al, 1979b). Similar results have also been obtained with a total RNA fraction isolated from 8-day chick embryo limb buds and 17-day embryonic sternae (Upholt et al, 1979), and with a 26s polyA-containing RNA fraction from a murine chondrosarcoma (Diaz de Leon et al, 1980).

These studies provide the basis for future investigations of the type II collagen gene and the potential analysis of cell systems in which collagen gene expression can be modulated. For example, during the differentiation of mesenchymal cells to cartilage a switch in synthesis of type I to type II collagen synthesis occurs whereas the reverse is frequently observed when chondrocytes are maintained in culture for extended periods (for review see von der Mark & Conrad, 1979). The availability of probes for the mRNAs and genes of procollagens I and II will offer the opportunity to study these changes in collagen gene expression at the level of transcription and translation.

PROCOLLAGEN GENES

Chromosomal location of collagen genes

Although the numbers of known genes specifying collagen α-chains number at least nine, the total membership of the collagen gene family may extend to 15–16 if proteins with collagenous domains i.e. repeating triplets of -gly-X-Y-, are also included (Solomon, 1980). Evidence that there is only one copy of each of the type I collagen genes has been reported by Frischauf et al (1978) but almost nothing is known of the structure, location, interaction and linkage of collagen genes. However, determination of the chromosomal location of genes is important, not only with respect to the effect of gene linkage and interaction in developmental processes, but also to the diagnosis and understanding of genetic diseases characterized by abnormal gene expression.

The ability to form viable hybrids between two different somatic cell types, e.g. mouse and human cells, has been used in the assignment of genes to specific chromosomes. In particular, the preferential loss of human chromosomes from mouse-human cell hybrids, the ability to identify individual chromosomes by specific staining methods, and the availability of purified species-specific antibodies to individual proteins have aided precise localisation of many human genes (see Giles & Ruddle, 1973; McKusick & Ruddle, 1977; Evans et al, 1979; for reviews). Using these techniques, attempts have been made to assign human collagen genes to specific chromosomes.

Studies by Church and coworkers (Sundar-Raj et al, 1977; Church et al, 1980) have resulted in the assignment of type I procollagen genes to a specific site on chromosome 17; and tentative evidence for the mapping of the gene for collagen type III on chromosomes 18 and 4 has also been obtained (Church, 1981). In contrast, it has been proposed that the genes for the three collagen chains, α1(I), α2(I) and α1(III) are located on chromosome 7 (Sykes & Solomon, 1978; Solomon & Sykes, 1978, 1979). These inconsistencies remain as yet unresolved but may in part be attributable to difficulties in obtaining pure chain-specific and species-specific anti-collagen antibodies. The data in both studies were obtained by biochemical analyses of the gene products of somatic cell hybrids carrying either human chromosome 7 or 17 and it is unlikely that the inconsistencies are due to incorrect identification of the chromosomes involved. It can be anticipated that in future studies the availability of specific DNA probes for collagen genes, as discussed below, will provide a more accurate and direct means of chromosome assignment and therefore will help to resolve this controversy.

Recombinant DNA technology as applied to the study of procollagen genes

With the isolation and partial purification of the mRNAs for procollagen I, the first steps have been taken towards exploiting recombinant DNA techniques in the investigation of the genes for pro-α(I) and pro-α2(I) collagen chains. The principal strategies and methods used in such studies are discussed briefly before considering the data obtained on the structural organisation of collagen genes. For more detailed information about recombinant DNA techniques the reader is referred to several excellent reviews (Sinsheimer, 1977; Old & Primrose, 1980; Wu, 1980).

The basic approach involves the isolation of specific genes or pieces of genes and the subsequent insertion of this foreign DNA into suitable vectors (or cloning vehicles) which can be introduced into a bacterial host. Small plasmids or bacteriophages are the most suitable vectors as they undergo replication in their own right, their maintenance does not necessarily require integration into the host genome, and their DNA can be isolated readily in an intact form. Gene manipulation involving the construction of such composite or artificial recombinant DNA molecules is often referred to as molecular or gene cloning because a line of genetically identical organisms, all containing the composite molecule, can be propagated and grown in bulk thereby amplifying the recombinant DNA and any gene product whose synthesis it directs. The principles of genetic engineering are, therefore, very simple but the insertion of a piece of foreign DNA into a vector requires mechanisms for cutting and joining DNA molecules from different sources as well as a means of introducing the vectors into (i.e. transforming) bacteria such as E. coli. Subsequently it becomes necessary to have techniques to recognize and characterize the amplified DNA sequences of specific genes.

Restriction endonucleases

DNA technology is totally dependent on the use of bacterial endonucleases (restriction enzymes) which cleave double stranded DNA (dsDNA) at highly specific sites. A

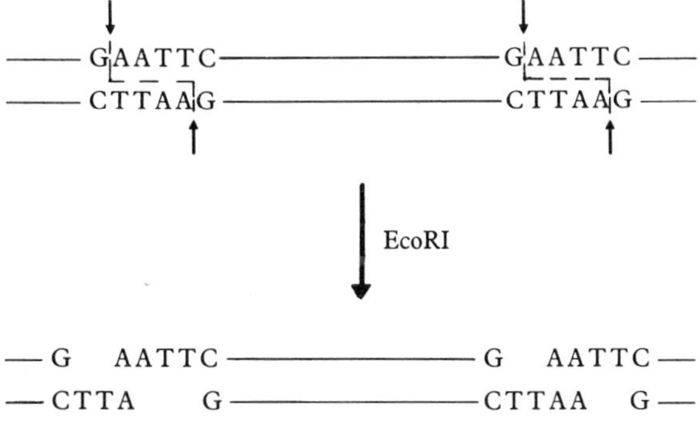

striking feature of these target sequences is their symmetry as shown above in the cleavage of DNA at two sites by the restriction enzyme EcoRI from E. coli. The products of cleavage include a length of dsDNA with cohesive (sticky) ends which can be annealed to complementary ends of foreign DNA cleaved by the same enzyme (see Fig. 5.6). The sequences recognized by some of the restriction endonucleases used to probe procollagen genes are displayed in Table 5.1. Using a variety of such enzymes permits the construction of restriction maps of DNA sequences which is equivalent to the peptide mapping procedure used in the study of protein structure.

Table 5.1 Target sites of some restriction endonucleases used in the study of procollagen DNA

Source	*Enzyme*	*Target Sequence* (5′——3′)
Escherichia coli RY13	Eco RI	G AATTC
Bacillus amyloliquefaciens H	Bam HI	G GATCC
Haemophilus aegyptius	Hae III	GG CC
Haemophilus influenzae Rd	Hind III	A AGCTT
Haemophilus parainfluenzae	Hpa I	GTT AAC
	Hpa II	C CGG
Klebsiella pneumoniae	Kpn I	GGTAC C

Construction of cDNA and genomic clones

Two different types of recombinant DNA clones have been constructed in studies of the procollagen genes — cDNA clones which can be used to probe the coding regions of the genes, and genomic clones which are complementary to the entire gene (or part thereof) including its introns.

The procedures used in the construction of procollagen cDNA clones (Lehrach et al, 1978; Sobel et al, 1978) are summarised in Figure 5.6. Initially, a complementary DNA copy (cDNA) to partially purified procollagen mRNA was synthesised using reverse transcriptase and then the complementary strand to single-stranded cDNA was synthesized using DNA polymerase I. The double stranded cDNA molecules were inserted into plasmids which, being circular DNA molecules, had first to be cleaved using one or two restriction endonucleases so that the resulting linear molecule had single-stranded 'tails' at both 5′ and 3′ ends. Single-stranded sequences (cohesive ends) complementary to the plasmid tails were created at the ends of the ds cDNA molecules and these fragments were then annealed to the plasmid DNA and ligated by DNA ligase. In the construction of procollagen cDNA clones, the plasmid pBR322 was used as the vector and the recombinant plasmid propagated in the enfeebled bacterium E. coli χ1776.

The construction of genomic clones requires the generation by cloning of a random collection of DNA fragments large enough in size so as to contain representative portions of every gene. Such a collection of DNA fragments comprise a gene library from which it is possible to purify structural genes present only as single copies in the genome. The construction of a gene library from complex eukaryotic genomes using λ phage as a cloning vehicle is described by Maniatis et al (1978) and its use in the construction of a procollagen genomic clone is outlined in Figure 5.7.

Bacteriophage λ (Charon 4A) is useful as a cloning vector for the formation of gene libraries because over a third of its DNA, forming a continuous block within the genome, can be removed and replaced by a foreign DNA fragment of approximately the same size without the phage losing its ability to replicate in its host (Blattner et al, 1977). The DNA piece is excised from an asymmetric location to yield one larger and one smaller fragment referred to as the left (5′ end) and right (3′ end) arms respectively. The difference in size between these two arms is particularly useful in determining the 5′–3′ orientation of heteroduplexes formed between DNA and mRNA as observed by electron microscopy. Eukaryotic DNA fragments approximately 20 kilobases (kb) in length are annealed and ligated to the right and left arms of λ, the recombinant λ molecules packaged into phage particles in vitro (Sternberg et al, 1977; Hohn & Murray, 1977; Maniatis et al, 1978) and amplified in E. coli to establish a library of genes which may be stored permanently and repeatedly screened for appropriate gene fragments.

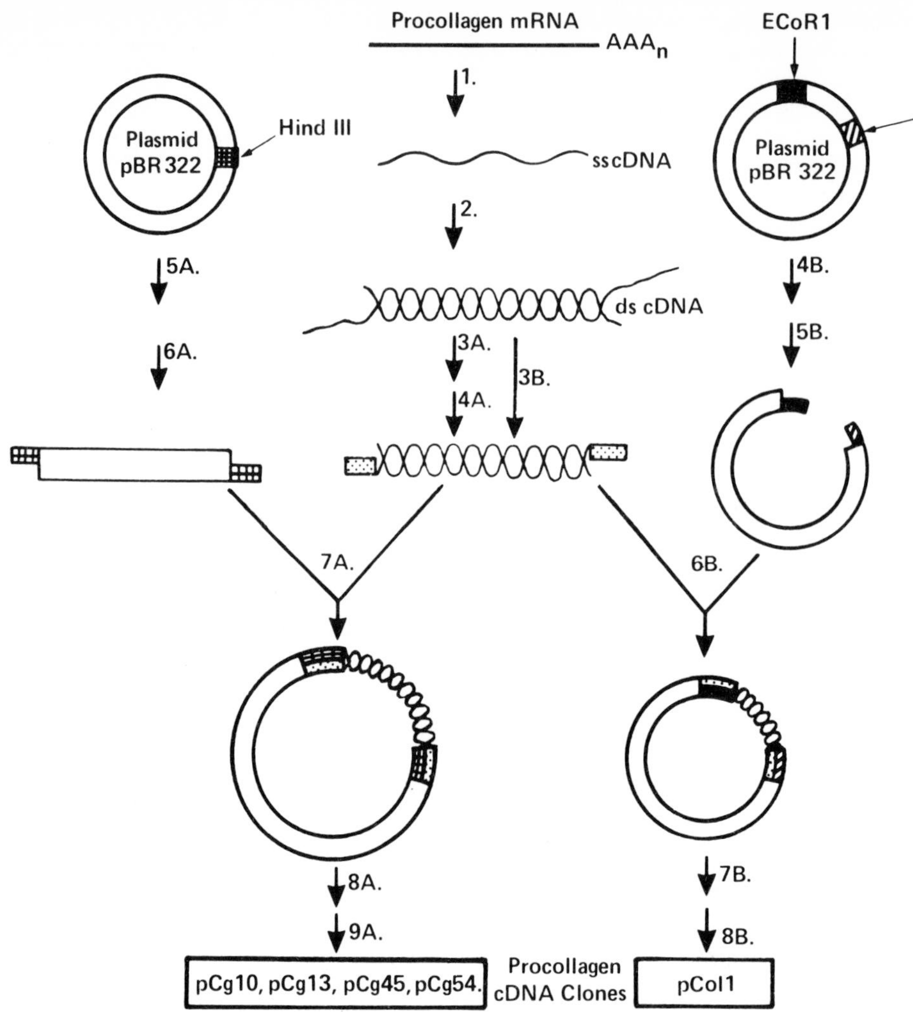

Fig. 5.6 Outline of the steps involved in the construction of procollagen cDNA clones.

1. Synthesis of single-stranded complementary DNA (ss cDNA) on a partially purified procollagen mRNA template using reverse transcriptase.
2. Synthesis of complementary strand to ss cDNA using DNA polymerase I to yield ds cDNA.

(A) *Summary of procedures used by Lehrach et al (1978, 1979)*
(3A) Conversion of ds cDNA molecules to perfect duplexes with S1 nuclease. (4A) Ligation of ds cDNA to synthetic ^{32}P-labelled Hind III linkers. Digestion with Hind III to create Hind III half-sites and separation from unligated linkers on sucrose density gradients. (5A) Digestion of plasmid pBR322 with Hind III. (6A) Removal of terminal phosphates to prevent self-ligation. (7A) Ligation of pBR322 and ds cDNA to yield recombinant plasmids. (8A) Transformation of E.Coli$_x$1776 with recombinant plasmids. (9A) Selection of procollagen cDNA clones by colony hybridisation to [^{32}P]cDNA followed by isolation of inserted and cloned procollagen cDNA excised by Hind III digestion.

(B) *Summary of procedures used by Sobel et al (1978)*
(3B) Double digestion of ds cDNA with ECoRI and BamHI to yield 200 bp cDNA fragments (BR200) with ECoRI and BamHI half sites which are recovered by elution from an excised section of polyacrylamide gels after electrophoresis. (4B) Double digestion of pBR322 with ECoRI and BamHI. (5B) Isolation of large fragment by gel-filtration chromatography. (6B) Ligation of plasmid DNA to BR200 to yield recombinant plasmid. (7B) Transformation of E.Coli$_x$1776 with recombinant plasmid. (8B) Selection of colonies carrying BR200 by tetracycline sensitivity and ampicillin resistance since tetracycline resistance has been removed from pBR322 by BamHI digestion. Recovery of cloned BR200 fragments by digestion of plasmids with ECoRI and BamHI.

Detection of intervening sequences

The presence of introns in cloned DNA sequences can usually be detected when restriction endonuclease maps of a cDNA clone and its corresponding genomic clone selected by screening of gene libraries are compared. Thus, introns are indicated when specific restriction sites present in the segment of the genomic derived DNA clone are not present in its complementary cDNA cloned fragment. The lengths and numbers of introns may also be estimated by hybridising the λ recombinant DNA molecules carrying the genomic clone to purified mRNA and then examining the DNA–RNA hybrids in the electron microscope. In this method, known as 'R-looping' (Thomas et al, 1976), the introns form loops on either side of the DNA–RNA hybrids because they do not contain complementary sequences capable of base pairing with the mRNA. The size and number of loops corresponding to introns can be measured, with their 5′–3′ orientation determined by their location with respect to the left and right arms of λ DNA.

Using these methods of analysis, it was possible to determine the total size and intron number of a particular gene by employing one genomic clone to isolate by successive screenings of gene libraries a series of overlapping clones covering the entire gene and its flanking regions.

Structural organisation of procollagen I genes

Procollagen cDNA clones

The construction of cDNA clones requires the initial preparation of cDNA to procollagen mRNA and two approaches have been taken to isolate cDNA copies specific to chicken procollagen sequences. One procedure has involved the extensive purification of RNA to yield a procollagen mRNA preparation (80% pure) which was used as a template for the synthesis of double-stranded blunt-ended cDNA molecules (Frischauf et al, 1978; Lehrach et al, 1978) (see Fig. 5.6). These ds cDNA molecules were annealed and ligated to the plasmid pBR322 via synthetic DNA links to yield recombinant plasmids which were cloned in E. coli. Bacterial colonies carrying collagen DNA sequences were identified by colony hybridisation to procollagen[^{32}P]cDNA. By this method three pro-α2(I) cDNA clones [pCg 10, pCg 13 and pCg 45 ranging in size from 1200–2550 bp (Lehrach et al, 1978)] and two pro-α1(I) cDNA clones (pCg 1 and pCg 54 of 850bp and 1100bp respectively) have been isolated (Lehrach et al, 1979).

Using a different approach to select for procollagen cDNA sequences, Howard et al (1978) started with a much less pure procollagen mRNA as their template for cDNA synthesis. In order to select procollagen coding sequences from this impure fraction these workers exploited (a) the specificity of two restriction enzymes (Hap II and Hae III) which cleave sequences (Table 5.1) likely to be very common in the collagen gene by virtue of the abundance of G- and C-rich codons for proline and glycine residues, and (b) the fact that collagen synthesis in chick embryo fibroblasts is decreased on transformation with Rous sarcoma virus (RSV). A comparison was therefore made of the Hpa II and Hae III fragments derived from the cDNA prepared from mRNA fractions from normal and transformed cells. A decrease in the amount of any fragment as a result of viral transformation was taken as an indication that the fragment was probably a collagen-coding sequence and in this way the necessity to start with highly purified mRNA could be avoided. Using a similar strategy, Sobel et al (1978) selected for a transformation-sensitive restriction fragment of cDNA in the construction of a procollagen cDNA clone and isolated a recombinant plasmid with a 200 bp DNA insert (pCOL 1) carrying pro-α2(I) sequences.

A disadvantage of this method for the general preparation of collagen cDNA clones as opposed to the procedures used by Lehrach et al (1978) is that the DNA fragment cloned was much smaller (200 bp compared to 2550 bp) and the application of this method is relevant only to systems where collagen synthesis can be manipulated e.g. by viral transformation. In addition the assumption that a reduction in quantity of certain restriction fragments corresponds to non-expression of collagen genes may not necessarily be valid, for such fragments could derive from cDNA synthesized to mRNAs of other transformation sensitive proteins such as fibronectin (Adams et al, 1977). However this method was useful as a preliminary means to select for procollagen cDNA clones and it is of interest that Yamamoto et al (1980) starting with an impure procollagen mRNA fraction were able to use a combination of the above two approaches to isolate a recombinant plasmid containing an 800 bp insert (pCOL 3) with pro-α1 DNA sequences.

Several methods have been used to correlate cloned cDNA sequences to the procollagen gene. Hybridisation of DNA in bacterial colonies to partially purified [^{32}P]cDNA is a useful but not unambiguous means of identifying procollagen cDNA clones; and an alternative procedure used involves the demonstration of resistance to S1 nuclease of hybrids formed between cloned cDNA and partially purified procollagen mRNA. This enzyme exhibits specificity for single stranded nucleic acids and Lehrach et al (1979) were able to show that 90% of their pro-α1 cDNA clone, pCg 54, was protected from SI nuclease by purified procollagen mRNA. However, since the RNA preparation was at best only 80% pure and was used as the template for cDNA synthesis in the first place, this method served more as a test of reverse transcriptase fidelity and a demonstration that little sequence alteration in the cDNA occurred during cloning. Perhaps the most definitive means of identifying procollagen DNA sequences is the comparison of the known amino acid sequence with that derived from reading the DNA base sequences.

Because the amino acid sequence of the entire pro-α1 chain is not available this method is to a large extent restricted to the helical regions whose repeating triplet sequences should be readily recognised. Thus, the base sequence of part of the pCg 45 and pCg 54, the largest of the pro-α1 and pro-α2 cDNA clones (Lehrach et al, 1978; 1979), could be correlated with known stretches of 48 amino acids of α1(I) and 21 amino acids of α2(I) respectively. From the size of the pCg 54 and pCg 45 and the DNA base sequence obtained from restriction fragments, it was also concluded that these cDNA clones contained sequences which were complementary to the 3′-half of the pro-α1 and pro-α2 mRNAs respectively and that pCg 45 extended to the polyA tail of the mRNA. More recently a 2.2kb human cDNA clone has been constructed using a 28s polyA-rich RNA fraction and shown to contain α2(I) sequences (Myers et al, 1981).

Where a putative procollagen cDNA clone does not contain base sequences which can be correlated with known amino acid sequences, hybridisation of the cDNA insert to total polyA-RNA and cell-free translation of the hybridised mRNA provides an alternative means of identification. Thus, Sobel et al (1978) and Yamamoto et al (1980) linked the pro-α2 and pro-α1 cDNA clones, pCOL 1 and pCOL 3, to diazobenzyloxymethyl-cellulose (DBM-cellulose) and applied total polyA-RNA from chick calvaria and long bones to these affinity media. The RNA species which hybridised to the respective cDNA clones were translated in a reticulocyte-lysate and shown to direct the synthesis of bacterial collagenase-sensitive polypeptides corresponding in size to pro-α2 and pro-α1 chains respectively. Although these procedures cannot assign the cDNA sequences to a particular region of the mRNAs they have the advantage of indirectly testing for the broad fidelity of reverse transcription and cloning for they result in the isolation of functional mRNA. The fidelity of reverse transcription is especially important in the context of procollagen cDNA synthesis for the mRNA probably has considerable secondary structure which could predispose towards errors which reverse transcriptase can make (Falvey et al, 1976; Gopinathan et al, 1979; Fagan et al, 1980). Indeed there is evidence that reverse transcription or the subsequent amplification of the cDNA in E. coli did not faithfully reproduce the pro-α1 mRNA sequence of clone pCOL 3 (Showalter et al, 1980).

Construction of procollagen genomic clones

Only regions of the procollagen gene which are expressed in mature mRNA, ie. exons, may be probed by cDNA. In order to study the organisation of the entire procollagen gene and determine the regions responsible for gene regulation it is, therefore, necessary to obtain other probes, genomic clones, which also contain the non-expressed intervening sequences (introns). The isolation of such genomic clones coding for regions of the whole procollagen genes involves the screening of gene libraries (Fig. 5.7) with cDNA probes derived from procollagen mRNA. Thus, a library of chicken genomic DNA fragments has been screened using the chick pro-α2 cDNA clone pCOL 1 as a hybridisation probe. A 6.8 kb pro-α2 genomic clone, λgCOL 204, covering one third of the coding region towards the 3′ end of the α2 gene was thereby isolated (Vogeli et al, 1980a). Similarly the chick cDNA clone pCg 45 has been used to isolate a 33 kb pro-α2 genomic clone spanning the 3′ end of the gene (Wozney et al, 1981). Subsequently the genomic clone λgCOL 204 has been employed as a hybridisation probe to isolate an overlapping pro-α2 genomic fragment and the process further extended using one clone to isolate another. In this fashion successive screenings of the chicken library has resulted in the isolation of a series of overlapping genomic clones spanning the entire collagen α2(I) gene (Vogeli et al, 1980b; Ohkubo et al, 1980).

The establishment of coidentity of each individual clone with a procollagen gene is an important step in these procedures and several criteria were used to define the clone λgCOL 204 as a pro-α2 gene probe. Thus the RNA species which hybridised to this genomic clone was shown to be similar in size to procollagen mRNA (approx. 5 kb) and also directed the cell-free synthesis of a high molecular weight polypeptide with similar electrophoretic mobility to pro-α2 chains. In addition this RNA species could not be isolated by hybridization to λgCOL 204 from polyA-RNA from RSV-transformed fibroblasts. More definitively, the DNA sequence of part of a 1.7 kb long Hind III restriction fragment of λgCOL 204 corresponded to an amino acid sequence specific to the triple helical region of α2 (Vogeli et al, 1981).

Genomic clones to sheep pro-α2 have also been isolated. Boyd et al (1980) used [^{32}P]cDNA synthesised from a 28s polyA-RNA fraction from foetal sheep tendons to isolate two pro-α2 genomic clones, designated SpC3 and SpC7, from a sheep gene library. The identity of these species was also established by experiments in which the cell-free translation of hybridization-selected mRNA gave rise to a bacterial collagenase-sensitive polypeptide with similar electrophoretic mobility to pro-α2 (Boyd et al, 1980). The sheep genomic clones, SpC3 and most of SpC7, were also shown to hybridise to chick pro-α2 cDNA clone pCg45 confirming the relative conservation of amino acid sequences within the triple helical region of procollagens. Because of the importance of the helical sequences in terms of collagen structure and function, considerable conservation between species of amino acid sequences in the helical regions is not too suprising and is indeed confirmed by amino acid sequence analyses (Fietzek & Kuhn, 1976). However, there may be significant differences in the amino- and carboxy-terminal propeptides and, therefore, the use of chicken procollagen cDNA clones complementary to the 5′ and 3′ coding regions to probe for genomic clones from other species may be limited.

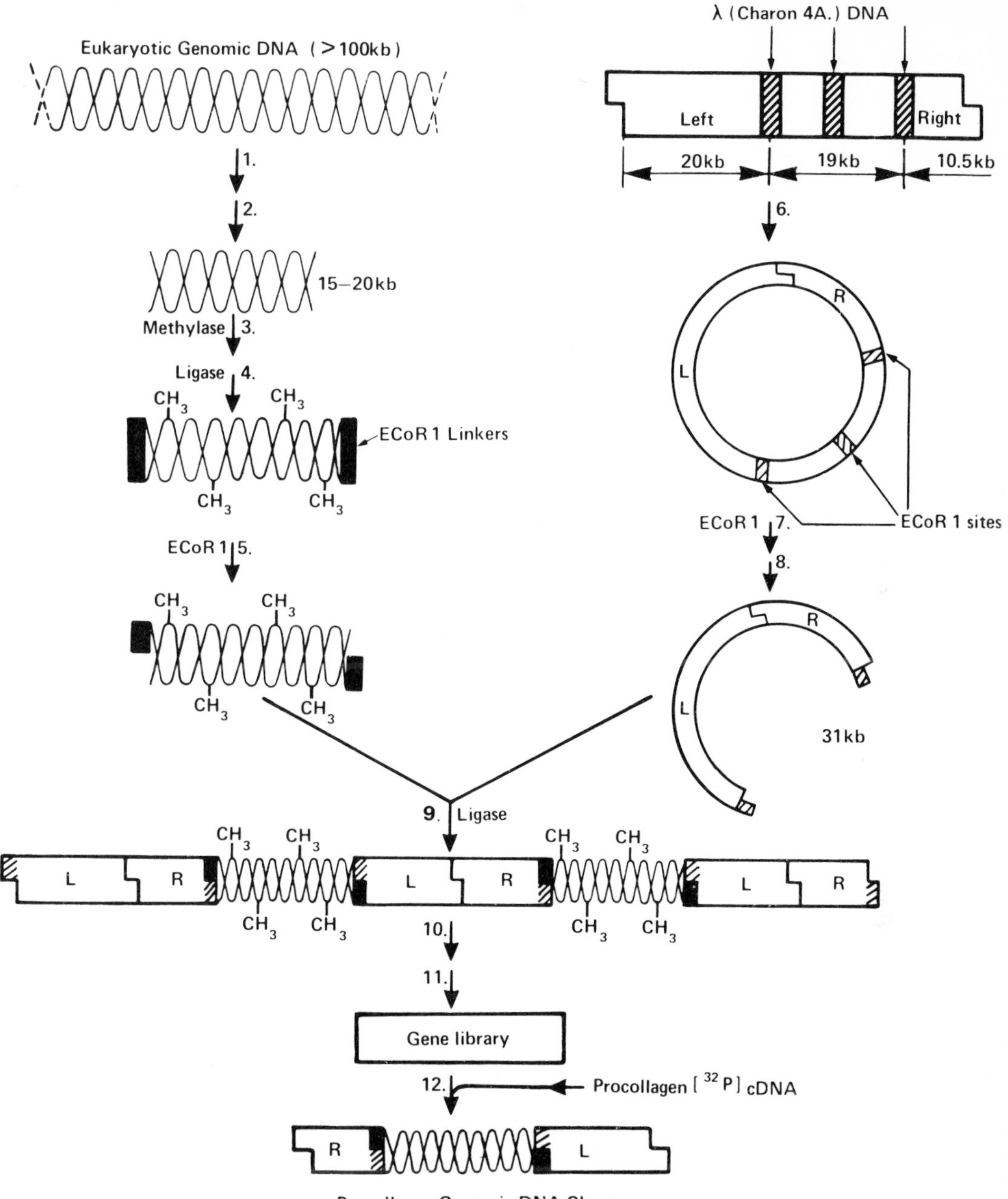

Fig. 5.7 Outline of the steps involved in the construction of procollagen genomic clones.
(1) High mol. wt. DNA is fragmented by a non-limit restriction endonuclease digestion to yield a spectrum of blunt-ended DNA molecules of varying size. (2) DNA fragments of approx. 20kb are selected by sucrose density gradient centrifugation. (3) Fragments are methylated thereby rendering potential cleavage sites resistant to ECoRI. (4) Synthetic DNA linkers with ECoRI recognition sequences are covalently attached to the ends. (5) Digestion with ECoRI creates cohesive ends. (6) Cohesive ends of λDNA are annealed and ligated to give a circular DNA molecule. (7) Digestion with ECoRI cleaves at three sites (arrowed) and removes a 19 kb sequence to yield a linear molecule with ECoRI cohesive ends which consist of the left arm, L (20 kb from 5′ end), cohered to the right arm, R (10.5 kb from 3′ end). (8) Isolation of 31 kb fragment on sucrose gradients. (9) The genomic DNA fragments and the λ-derived molecules are annealed and ligated to form concatameric DNA recombinants. (10) Recombinant phage DNA is packaged into phage particles. (11) Phage is propagated in E.coli thereby amplifying (cloning) eukaryotic DNA insert. (12) Selection of procollagen genomic clones by colony hybridisation to [^{32}P]cDNA.

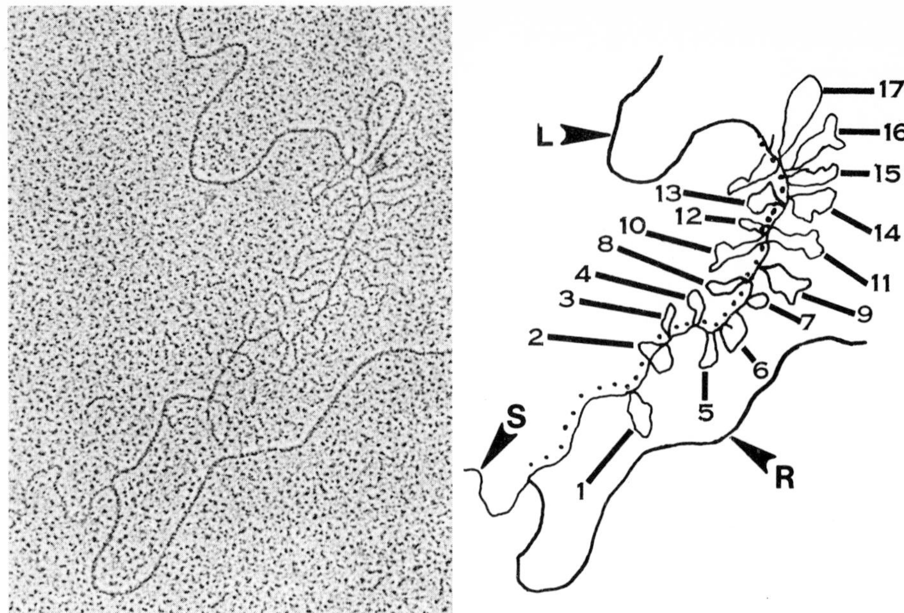

Fig. 5.8 Electron microscopic visualization of all 17 introns and 18 exons from hybrid molecules formed between recombinant clone SpC3 DNA and foetal sheep tendon pro-α2 mRNA. The diagrammatic representation on the right indicates the location of the double-stranded segments of the right arm (R) and left arm (L) of Charon 4A; the displaced single-stranded DNA segment of the insert S; single-stranded DNA loops representing introns sequentially labelled 1 to 17 in the 3′ to 5′ direction; and 18 regions of insert DNA sequences hybridised to pro-α2 mRNA (----). Reproduced with permission from Schafer et al (1980).

Primary structure of the collagen pro-α2 gene

The isolation and characterisation of the pro-α2 genomic clones from both the sheep and the chicken have revealed that the collagen pro-α2 gene is extremely large and has the greatest number of intervening sequences (introns) of any gene studied to date. A number of studies have led to this somewhat startling conclusion.

The overlapping sheep genomic DNA fragments SpC3 and SpC7 have been found to cover 17 kb of the pro-α2 gene representing just over one half of the 3′ portion of the gene; and hence, by extrapolation, it can be calculated that the complete pro-α2 collagen gene is likely to be dispersed throughout a 30 kb DNA segment (Schafer et al, 1980). The DNA region required for coding the interspersed 5 kb of pro-α2 genetic information appears, therefore, to be at least 6-fold longer than the corresponding translatable cytoplasmic mRNA. Electron microscopic (R-looping) analysis of hybrids formed between SpC3 and partially-purified procollagen mRNA revealed that the non-coding region within the 3′ half of the sheep pro-α2 gene is distributed in 17 introns (Fig. 5.8) varying in size from 340 bp to 1540 bp (Schafer et al, 1980). The distribution of introns and exons is not random, however, but a clustering of the smaller introns and larger exons (up to 900 bp) is found at the 3′ end of the gene whereas exons are small (approx. 50–100 bp) and introns large (approx. 1000 bp) within the region corresponding to the triple helical domain of collagen (Fig. 5.9).

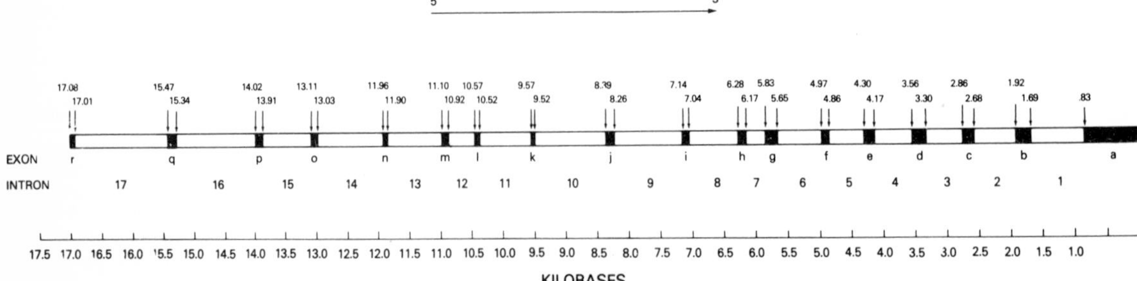

Fig. 5.9 Organisation of the 3′ end of the sheep pro-α2 collagen gene, showing the exon and intron order as determined by R loop analysis of SpC3 DNA-pro-α2 mRNA hybrid molecules. Arrows represent the approximate location of intron-exon junctions and all values are presented as kilobase pairs. Reproduced with permission from Schafer et al (1980).

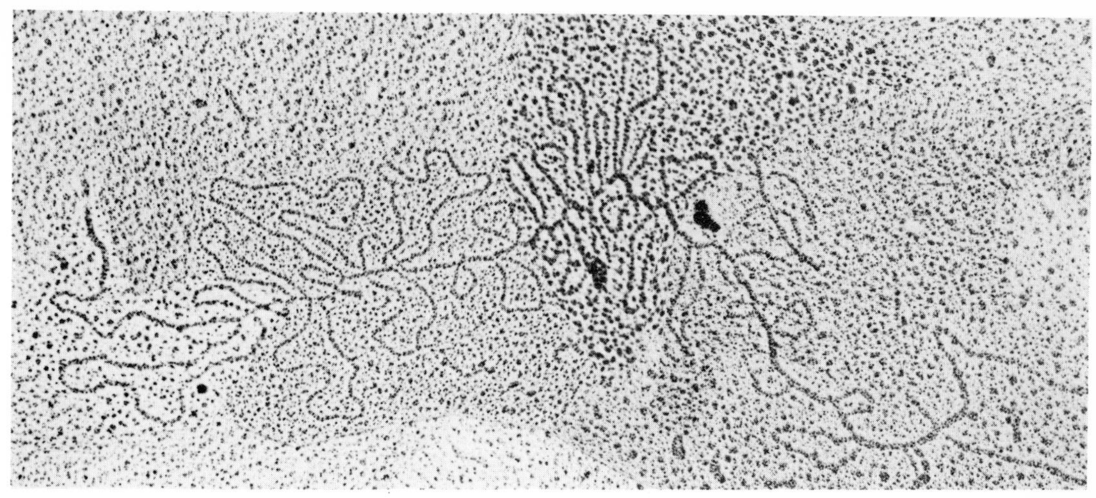

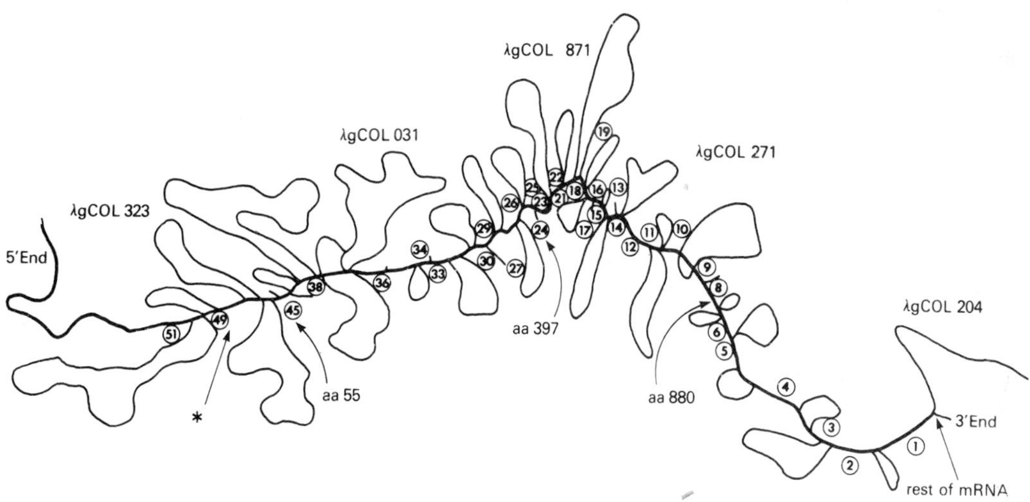

Fig. 5.10 Composite electron micrograph of the chick pro-α2 collagen gene assembled from photographs of hybrids between pro-α2 mRNA and the DNAs of the overlapping clones COL 204, 271, 871, 031 and 323. In the diagrammatic representation below the coding regions (exons) are numbered. (* Between exon 48 and 49 there is an additional intervening sequence of 1.5 kb which was omitted during the photographic reconstruction). Reproduced with permission from Vogeli et al (1980b).

Similar conclusions have been reached in the more extensive studies on the primary structure of the chicken pro-α2 gene for which clones covering 55 kb of contiguous chick genomic DNA have been isolated (Vogeli et al, 1980b; Ohkubo et al, 1980). Analyses of DNA-mRNA hybrids indicate that the coding information for chick pro-α2 is distributed over a DNA sequence of at least 38 kb containing more than 50 exons with introns varying in size from less than 100 bp to greater than 3000 bp (Figs. 5.10 and 5.11). As with the sheep pro-α2 gene, introns in the chick pro-α2 gene were largest and exons smallest within the region coding for the triple helical portion of the collagen polypeptide. A remarkable finding was the observation that the sizes of 7 exons in this major part of the gene were identical, comprising 54 bp (Vogeli et al, 1980b; Yamada et al, 1980). It should be noted that the numbers of exons and introns determined may be underestimates of the absolute values for the technique of R-looping requires considerable expertise and yields only an overall picture of the gene — some coding sequence can be lost and most small intervening sequences are not detectable. Such studies do, however, reveal the immense size and extraordinarily split nature of the collagen pro-α2 gene, and the fact that similar conclusions are being

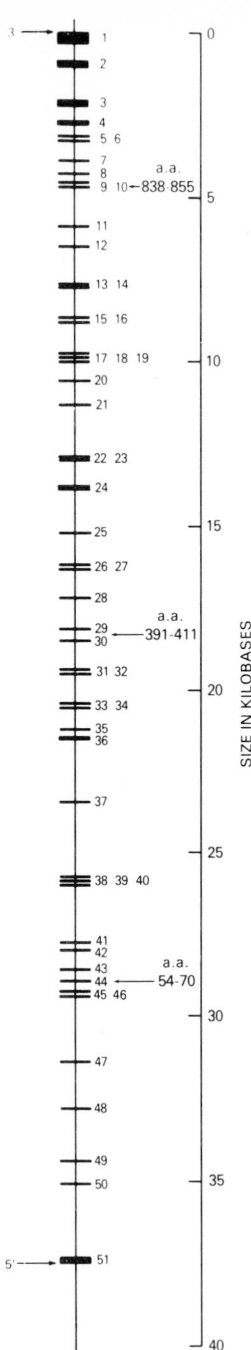

Fig. 5.11 Diagram of the chick pro-α2 collagen gene. The numbered horizontal bars represent coding regions (exons) beginning from the 3′ end of the gene, and the vertical lines connecting the bars represent intervening sequences (introns). The gene spans around 38 kb and sequence information has been obtained for 3 small DNA segments which are indicated with the position of the amino acids in the collagen protein for which they code. Reproduced with permission from Vogeli et al (1980b).

reached in studies on the sheep and chick genomes suggest these observations may reflect a general feature of collagen genes.

Collagen gene structure: implications for procollagen structure, synthesis and evolution

DNA sequence data and primary protein structure

Determination of the nucleotide sequences in cDNA clones provides a very useful means of obtaining the primary structure of polypeptides and has the great advantage that DNA sequencing is much more rapid than the conventional peptide sequencing procedure which is tedious and requires significant amounts of purified peptide. Thus, sequence analysis of the chick pro-α1 cDNA clone, pCOL 3, (Showalter et al, 1980) and the pro-α1 and pro-α2 cDNA clones pCg 1, pCg 26, pCg 54, pCg 13 and pCg 45 (Fuller & Boedtker, 1981) have provided the first amino acid sequences of the C propeptides of both pro-α1 and pro-α2 chains. An important feature of this approach in relation to collagen structure is the fact that DNA-derived peptide sequences are likely to give a more accurate estimation of molecular weights of procollagen peptides, e.g. CNBr peptides (see Showalter et al, 1980), for the post-translational hydroxylation and glycosylation modifications often hinder precise size measurement, particularly those made by electrophoretic procedures. On this basis it has been deduced from the number of nucleotides in clones of pCg 54 and pCg 45 which cover the 3′ ends of pro-α1 and pro-α2 mRNAs respectively that the size of the carboxy-terminal propeptides might be smaller than anticipated (Lehrach et al, 1979).

It is important to recognise that determination of DNA base sequences as the sole means of amino acid sequencing may not be entirely reliable. Although the CNBr peptides of the pro-α1 C propeptide were shown to have N terminal sequences identical to those predicted by the nucleotide sequences of pCOL3, some inconsistencies were detected (Showalter et al, 1980). Approximately 40 amino acid residues present in a CNBr peptide could not be located in the DNA base sequence and certain amino acids specified by the DNA were absent from the peptide. These anomalies could have been caused by errors in reverse transcription and/or deletion and rearrangement of sequences during cloning or alternatively could have arisen if the cyanogen bromide peptide sample sequenced was not absolutely pure. In the absence of a complete amino acid sequence for the procollagen C propeptide, Fuller & Boedtker (1981) have attempted to quantify the extent of such errors in the construction of the cDNA clones. Their data indicate that the process of cDNA synthesis and amplification in E. coli is only moderately faithful with an error rate of 1.5×10^{-3}, though such an error frequency is unlikely to result in the differences observed between the cDNA and protein sequences. Some sequence rearrangements in the pro-α1 cDNA clones did occur however and could have contributed to the discrepancies observed. In addition, determining amino acid sequences within the triple helical domain of procollagen from nucleotide sequences presents some technical difficulties because of the electrophoretic anomalies caused by the high G & C content (Fuller & Boedtker, 1981).

One may now wonder whether DNA sequencing technology will render obsolete the determination of amino acid sequences by conventional protein chemistry. While it is clear that it will no longer be necessary to determine primary protein structure by extensive amino acid sequencing there are limitations on the extent to which DNA sequences may be the sole source from which amino acid sequences are derived (Prockop, 1981). For example complete cDNA copies may not always be obtainable especially where large proteins are concerned and sequence determination from genomic clones covering the entire gene may be time-consuming if numerous long introns are present. The existence of 'pseudogenes' i.e. unexpressed genes which are very closely similar to expressed genes, also require that at least part of the primary protein structure be determined by a method other than from DNA sequencing. In addition, it should be noted that nucleotide sequences can provide no information on specific enzyme cleavage sites nor on post-translational modifications although it may be possible to predict the location of potential carbohydrate-attachment sites (Pesciotta et al, 1981).

Codon usage in collagen biosynthesis

The concept of a regulatory role of tRNA in controlling protein sythesis by allowing optimal translation of the mRNAs present was suggested a number of years ago (Ames & Hartman, 1963; Stent, 1964). There is now considerable evidence that the pattern of tRNA species within cells is adapted to the needs of the protein synthesizing system (Smith & MacNamara, 1971; Mäenpää & Ahonen, 1972; Garel, 1974; Garel et al, 1974; Sprague et al, 1977), and changes during embryogenesis, development and oncogenesis (Littauer & Inouye, 1973; Soffer, 1973). The adaptation of tRNA species to fit the amino acid requirements of a particular protein synthesizing pattern appears to be related also to the isoaccepting species cognate to the ratio of codons in mRNA. For example, the two major alanyl-tRNA species in the silk gland of *Bombyx mori* correspond to the codons used for alanine in fibroin mRNA (Sprague et al, 1977). In addition, tRNAs have been found to participate in the regulation of transcription of mRNAs for enzymes associated with amino acid biosynthesis in both prokaryotes and eukaryotes (Brenchley & Williams, 1975; Simpson et al, 1975).

Tissues active in collagen synthesis have been shown to have proportionately elevated levels of the tRNAs for glycine, proline, alanine (the most abundant amino acids in collagen) and lysine, which is important for crosslinking of collagen fibrils (Lanks & Weinstein, 1970; Maenpaa & Ahonen, 1972; Christner & Rosenbloom, 1976; Carpousis et al, 1977a, b; Drabkin & Lukens, 1978). No marked preferential usage of particular tRNA isoacceptor species could be detected for proline, alanine or lysine (Drabkin & Lukens, 1978) but a clear preference for $tRNA^{Gly}$ specific for GGU and GGC codons was demonstrated (Carpousis et al, 1977a, b; Drabkin & Lukens, 1978). This latter phenomenon may be a reflection of the ratio of specific glycine codons present in procollagen mRNA but the possibility of specific glycyl-tRNAs exerting a translational control on collagen synthesis in vivo cannot as yet be ruled out.

The relationship between codon usage and levels of individual tRNA isoaccepting species may be assessed by determination of the DNA sequence of the collagen genes. Studies on the cDNA clones for chicken pro-α1 and pro-α2 chains (Fuller & Boedtker, 1981) have revealed that, of the 4 possible codons for proline, CCU and CCC predominate. In addition the majority of codons for glycine are GGU and GGC which obviously correlates well with the $tRNA^{Gly}$ species predominating in collagenous tissues but their relative frequencies are significantly reversed between pro-α1 and pro-α2. A similar difference between the two chains was also found for the two preferred alanine codons (Fuller & Boedtker, 1981). It is interesting that such preferences in codon usage should be seen in codons for amino acids which are most abundant in collagens. However, the signifiance, if any, of these observations and their relationship to any regulatory role tRNAs may play in collagen synthesis cannot be fully assessed for the cDNA clones sequenced correspond only to approximately half the length of the mRNA for pro-α1 and pro-α2.

Collagen gene structure and pre-mRNA processing

The logistics of processing the primary transcripts of the collagen genes are awesome by virtue of their immense size alone. The excision of 49 introns from a transcript of the 38 kb pro-α2 gene requires a minimum of 50 processing steps to yield a 5 kb functional mRNA. Little is known of the exact mechanism of splicing but small nuclear RNAs (snRNA) have been implicated as already discussed (see page 75). Investigations of the processing of a procollagen mRNA precursor by isolation of the entire pre-mRNA and intermediate products of splicing presents considerable difficulties. However, Avvedimento et al (1980) have obtained some insight into these mechanisms by analysing two separate small DNA restriction fragments of 256 bp and 156 bp, from the chick pro-α2 gene, containing two short introns of 215 bp and 93 bp. Nucleotide sequences of these introns and of parts of their adjacent exons revealed a relative conservation of sequences at both ends of the introns. In addition, there was complementarity between these sites and the 5′ end of U1 RNA, the snRNA postulated to be involved in the splicing mechanism

(Lerner et al, 1980; Rogers & Wall, 1980). These putative splicing sites were not restricted to the ends of the introns but separate stretches of sequences complementary to U1 RNA were discovered within the 215 bp intron. These complementarities predict three potential internal splicing sites and evidence for stepwise excision at these sites with a 3′ to 5′ polarity was obtained (Avvedimento et al, 1980). This occurrence of internal splicing sites within introns is not unique to the procollagen gene for multi-step excision of intervening sequences has also been demonstrated in the processing of the mouse β-globin gene (Kinniburgh & Ross, 1979) and in an adenovirus gene (Chow & Broker, 1978).

Many questions still remain unanswered as to the precise manner in which the primary RNA transcripts are processed to yield cytoplasmic procollagen mRNA. Whether internal splicing sites in introns are widespread in the procollagen genes with the consequent existence of multiple intermediate mRNA precursors remains to be ascertained. It might be anticipated that a method of proof-reading such enormous transcripts will be required to check that correct splicing has been achieved, but the presence of a termination codon a short distance into the beginning of an intron sequence in the same reading frame found by de Crombrugghe and co-workers (personal communication) could be one way to ensure that incorrectly spliced mRNAs are not translated into faulty protein. In this context it is conceivable that the products of incomplete translation of such aberrant mRNAs could account for the observed high intracellular degradation of collagenous polypeptides (Bienkowski et al, 1978).

The primordial collagen gene

Collagen is an exceedingly ancient molecule being found in all invertebrate and vertebrate phyla studied including primitive organisms such as fresh water sponges and sea anemones (Bornstein & Traub, 1979). While at present it is only possible to speculate on the mechanism by which collagen genes evolved (Solomon & Cheah, 1981) it is generally accepted that proteins with repetitive or periodic amino acid sequences e.g. silk fibroin and collagen, probably arose by duplication of a primordial sequence (Ycas, 1972; McLachlen, 1976; Barker et al, 1978). It has been proposed that in evolution the primordial collagen gene duplicated to specify enormous collagenous polypeptides (approx. 500 000 MW) as found in some invertebrates, and evolutionary modifications have been suggested whereby sequences coding for non-collagenous regions arose within the collagenous domains (Tanzer, 1978). This could be one way of generating a gene for the procollagen molecule with a triple helical collagenous domain and globular extensions at both N- and C-termini. In this context it would be tempting to speculate that the short non-collagenous sequences interspersed between the triple helical domains of type IV collagen (Schuppan et al, 1980) represent relics of such an ancestral collagen molecule.

Any model proposing an origin of a protein by internal gene duplication would predict the existence of homologies within the polypeptide. Until recently detection of such homologies have relied on complex statistical analysis of amino acid sequences (Ycas, 1972; Barker et al, 1978). Using this approach, McLachlen (1978) obtained evidence to suggest that the primordial collagen gene consisted of DNA sequences coding for 78 triplets of -gly-X-Y- (i.e. 234 amino acids). This repeat length, designated D, has also been found by Hofman et al (1980) in their amino acid sequence analyses of interchain homology between the α1(I), α2(I) and α1(III) chains. In addition smaller repeats of D/3, D/6, D/11 and D/13 were observed, particularly in α1(I) and α1(III). Interestingly, the data also revealed that the homology within one repeat was more conserved between chains in different species than from one repeat to another within the chain. This finding could imply that intrachain duplication occurred before duplication of the entire chain. Many questions remain to be answered as to the events leading to the existence of at least 9 different collagen αchains. The observation that the conservation of sequence of each type of vertebrate αchain is far greater across the species than it is between different chains within a species (Mathews, 1980; Hofman et al, 1980) indicates an early divergence of types. The pathway from a primordial gene to a point of divergence is however more difficult to predict from amino acid sequence data alone. With the development of recombinant DNA technology and the consequent ability to determine DNA sequences of entire genes, more definitive predictions and tests may be made for the hypothetical origin of vertebrate collagens. Such analysis of nucleotide sequences have already been used to support proposals of gene duplication during the evolution of the chick X, Y and ovalbumin gene families (Chambon et al, 1979; Royal et al, 1979; Heilig et al, 1980).

DNA sequence analyses of 7 exons of the chick collagen pro-α2 gene corresponding to the triple helical region reveal that these exons always end at a position corresponding to the Y position of the -gly-X-Y- sequences and never in the middle of a triplet (Vogeli et al, 1980*b*; Yamada et al, 1980). Measurements of the lengths of 8 exons suggest, with one exception, a minimum size of 54 bp i.e. a coding capacity for 18 amino acids, with the other exon of 99 bp (i.e. 54 and 45) specifying 33 amino acids (Yamada et al, 1980; Vogeli et al, 1980b). Five additional exons have now been sequenced by these workers — three of 54 bp and two of 108 bp (B. de Crombrugghe, personal communication). On the basis of such analyses, these authors have proposed that the first collagen gene arose by amplification of a single coding unit of 54 bp embedded in a genetic unit containing non-coding sequences of more variable size. In this context it is interesting that 54 bp or

18 amino acids also corresponds to the D/13 repeat found by Hofman et al (1980).

During evolution various recombinational and mutational events involving the deletion or addition of 9 bp (corresponding to one gly-X-Y- triplet) gave rise to exons longer or shorter than the 54 bp unit. They predict that this unit is likely to represent the basic exon length for all collagen genes from sponges to man. This primordial short collagen gene may have played an important functional role in a primitive cell and small collagenous regions found in other proteins such as C19 and acetylcholinesterase could therefore be relics of such a function.

Wozney et al (1981) have arrived at a similar hypothesis based on their analyses of 7 exons derived from genomic clones covering 33 kb of the chick pro-α2 gene and they also propose that the ancestral gene could have been 54 bp. A total of 14 exons from these clones have now been sequenced, of which 7 were 54 bp, 2 were 45 bp, 3 were 99 bp and 2 were 108 bp (H. Boedtker, personal communication). To accommodate the exons of size 45 bp, 99 bp and 108 bp, Wozney et al (1981) also suggest that during evolution duplication of this gene was accompanied by the addition or deletion of 9 base pairs. Most interestingly, one of the exons they studied was found to contain the coding sequences covering the end of the triple helical region and part of the non-helical carboxy terminal domain of the proα2 chain (including the procollagen peptidase cleavage site). This observation is somewhat surprising since according to the concept of introns separating different functional domains (Gilbert, 1978), one would have expected to find an intron separating sequences specifying helical and globular regions of the procollagen molecule and also the recognition site for procollagen peptidase. It is clear therefore that any hypothesis involving the duplication of a 54 bp (or some other multiple of 9 bp) primordial collagen sequence must also involve a means by which a gene specifying the procollagen molecule could have arisen, e.g. perhaps by loss of an intron.

Attractive though the hypothesis of evolution of collagen may be, it must be remembered that this proposal is based solely on the α2(I) gene. Further analyses of more exons from the α2 gene and the other 8 genes for the different αchains are awaited. It also cannot be discounted that the distribution of coding sequences into small exons may be more a reflection of a means to protect the repetitive GC sequences (required in the -gly-pro-Y- and -gly-X-pro- sequences of the triple helical conformation) from an increased susceptibility to recombination. However, the presence of only one intron in the silk fibroin gene (Tsujimoto & Suzuki, 1979) which also contains repetitive sequences rich in G and C residues would argue against such an interpretation.

Finally, it has been suggested that in proteins exhibiting internal periodicity, amino acids in the same position of a repeating unit would be specified by the same codons depending on the antiquity of the protein (Ycas, 1972). Preferential codon usage for glycine, proline and alanine as discussed earlier (p. 91) would correlate well with such a hypothesis. Accordingly, it may be tempting to postulate that the difference in codon usage for proline and alanine observed in pro-α1(I) and pro-α2(I) may reflect the duplication of independent coding units in the evolution of the pro-α1(I) and pro-α2(I) genes.

THE CONTROL OF PROCOLLAGEN SYNTHESIS

There is little doubt that collagen gene expression, synthesis and secretion are complex processes that are finely controlled during growth and differentiation. As yet, investigations of the mechanisms by which these processes are modulated have been to a large extent restricted to the study of overall changes in collagen synthesis in a number of biological systems. In the majority of studies, collagen synthesis has been determined by measurement of the incorporation of [^{14}C]proline into either non-diffusible hydroxy[^{14}C]proline-containing peptides or into ^{14}C-peptides rendered diffusible by bacterial collagenase digestion. Assessment of changes in the rates of synthesis using these methods depend on accurate measurement of amino acid pool sizes and of radioactive precursor uptake, and interpretation of the data may be complicated by the high level and variable rates of intracellular degradation of collagen (Bienkowski et al, 1978). This approach suffers from the further disadvantage that the site of control cannot be identified whereas direct measurements of procollagen mRNA levels under conditions of increased or decreased collagen synthesis can be used to probe for control at the levels of transcription, post-transcription or translation.

A system to which such an approach is readily applicable is the developing membranous cranial bones (calvaria) of the embryonic chick which undergo marked morphological and biochemical changes between days 10 and 17 of development. During this period the relative rate of procollagen synthesis increases from about 10 per cent of total protein synthesis to approximately 60 per cent on day 17 (Diegelmann & Peterkofsky, 1972). Determination of procollagen mRNA levels by cell-free translation into collagenous polypeptides provides a means of measuring functional mRNA and suggests that in the calvarial system the levels of procollagen synthesis can be correlated with the amount of procollagen mRNA (Breitkreutz et al, 1978; Moen et al, 1979). However, assessment of mRNA levels by cell-free translation are subject to the potential problems of variable degradation of messengers during extraction and to changes in translational efficiency which may be influenced by a variety of factors, including rates of initiation of protein synthesis (Lodish, 1976) and mRNA secondary structure (Payvar & Schimke, 1979). Tests for degradation of RNA during extraction of calvaria were conducted by Moen et al (1979) who also used a more direct means of measuring mRNA levels i.e. by hybridisation of total mRNA to a cDNA fraction synthesised from a mRNA-fraction enriched in procollagen mRNA. It should be pointed out that the validity of this more direct procedure is dependent on the purity of the cDNA probe and the assumption that no self-annealing of internal complementary sequences occurs. This latter study on calvarial development revealed that after the initial increase in collagen and procollagen mRNA synthesis during days 10 to 12, further increases in collagen synthesis from day 12 to 17 could be attributed to a decrease in the synthesis of non-collagenous protein while the rate of collagen production and procollagen mRNA levels remained constant (Moen et al, 1979). Thus, collagen synthesis was found to be a direct reflection of mRNA levels and no evidence was obtained to suggest that procollagen synthesis during development is modulated via mRNA translation.

Several detailed studies of the decrease in collagen synthesis associated with viral transformation of fibroblasts in culture have also been undertaken. Cell-free translation of the mRNAs extracted from normal and transformed cells (Adams et al, 1977), and hybridisation studies of total polyA-RNA to procollagen cDNA probes (Rowe et al, 1978; Sandmeyer & Bornstein, 1979) have suggested that the decrease in collagen synthesis is associated with reduced transcription of procollagen mRNA. This conclusion is also supported by the data of Howard et al (1978) discussed already. Further convincing evidence in favour of a transcriptional control of collagen synthesis in chick fibroblasts on viral transformation has been obtained by measuring levels of procollagen mRNA (Adams et al, 1979) and their nuclear precursors (Avvedimento et al, 1981) using the two cloned pro-α1(I) and pro-α2(I) cDNA fragments for the former (Sobel et al, 1978; Yamamoto et al, 1980) and the chick α2(I) genomic clones (Vogeli et al, 1980) for the latter. It is also noteworthy that studies on procollagen metabolism during the cell cycle of 3T6 mouse fibroblasts also ascribe fluctuating levels of collagen synthesis to changes in the amount of procollagen mRNA present (Parker & Fitschen, 1980) although the data were obtained only by cell-free translation of RNA.

Little is known of hormonal effects on the regulation of collagen synthesis but the application of low concentrations of insulin, parathyroid hormone and vitamin D to organ cultures of foetal rat calvaria significantly alters collagen production (Raisz et al, 1978). Insulin and vitamin D increase collagen synthesis; and procollagen mRNA levels, as measured by cell-free translation of total RNA, are correspondingly elevated (Kream et al, 1979, 1980). Parathyroid hormone, conversely, causes a decrease in procollagen synthesis and procollagen mRNA levels are similarly depressed (Kream et al, 1980). It appears, therefore, that in all the systems discussed above, collagen synthesis is modulated at the level of transcription and/or post-transcription. However, the effect of the amino terminal propeptides of pro-αchains in inhibiting both collagen synthesis in cultured cells (Weistner et al, 1979) and cell-free translation of procollagen mRNA (Paglia et al, 1979) suggest that translational control mechanisms probably do exist.

The relevance of the above findings, which have in the main been obtained with cells or tissues in culture, to the control of collagen synthesis in vivo remains an open question. However, the systems studied so far have provided an opportunity to manipulate collagen synthesis and develop methodology by which changes in procollagen mRNA levels can be detected. The success of these procedures stems from the ability to isolate mRNAs for type I procollagen, synthesise cDNA probes, and apply the rapidly progressing techniques of recombinant DNA technology to this field of connective tissue research. The basis has now been established for the future extension of these techniques to the isolation and characterisation of the messengers and genes for the other collagen types. This exciting work can be expected to provide a greater understanding of the structure and organisation of the various collagen genes and give an insight into the coordinated controls exerted on their expression during vertebrate development. The construction of cloned DNA probes to the range of human collagen types can be anticipated in the near future and it will then become possible to investigate in greater detail a wide variety of connective tissue diseases, both genetic and acquired, in which the primary defect may involve collagen structure or synthesis. The progress made in studies of the haemoglobinopathies (Weatherall & Clegg, 1979) provides the impetus to this approach but the huge size of collagen messengers and genes and the heterogeneous and non-specific nature of collagen-related genetic defects will continue to pose a formidable challenge to molecular biologists seeking to unravel the complexities of collagen gene expression in health and disease.

ACKNOWLEDGEMENTS

We should like to thank the following who allowed us to read manuscripts in press at the time of writing: H. Boedtker, B. de Crombrugghe, R. G. Crystal, D. W. Rowe, M. P. Schafer and G. Vogeli. We should also like to thank Mrs Carol Hardman for typing the manuscript and Miss J. Jeffries for assistance in the collation of references. Original contributions from this laboratory were supported by grants from the Science Research Council and the Arthritis and Rheumatism Council.

REFERENCES

Abelson J 1979 RNA processing and the intervening sequence problem. Annual Review of Biochemistry 48: 1035

Adams S L et al 1977 Levels of translatable mRNAs for cell surface protein, collagen precursors, and two membrane proteins are altered in Rous sarcoma virus-transformed chick embryo fibroblasts. Proceedings of the National Academy of Sciences USA 74: 3399

Adams S L, Alwine J C, de Crombrugghe B, Pastan I 1979 Use of recombinant plasmids to characterise collagen RNAs in normal and transformed chick embryo fibroblasts. Journal of Biological Chemistry 254: 4935

Ames B N, Hartman P E 1963 The histidine operon. Cold Spring Harbor Symposia on Quantitative Biology 28: 349

Avvedimento V E, Vogeli G, Yamada Y, Maixel J V Jr, Pastan I, de Crombrugghe B 1980 Correlation between splicing sites within an intron and their sequence complementary with u_1RNA. Cell 21: 689

Avvedimento E, Yamada Y, Lovelace E, Vogeli G, de Crombrugghe B, Pastan I 1981 Decrease in levels of nuclear RNA precursors for alpha 2 collagen in Rous sarcoma virus-transformed fibroblasts. Nucleic Acids Research 9: 1123

Barker W C, Ketcham L K, Dayhoff M O 1978 A comprehensive examination of protein sequences for evidence of internal gene duplication. Journal of Molecular Evolution 10: 265

Benveniste K, Wilczek J, Stern R 1973 Translation of collagen mRNA from chick embryo calvaria in a cell-free system derived from Krebs II ascites cells. Nature 246: 303

Benveniste K, Wilczek J, Stern R 1974 Translation of collagen messenger RNA in ascites and wheat germ cell free systems. Federation Proceedings 33: 1541

Benveniste K, Wilczek J, Ruggieri A, Stern R 1976 Translation of collagen messenger RNA in a cell-free system derived from wheat germ. Biochemistry 15: 830

van der Berg J et al 1978 Comparison of cloned rabbit and mouse β-globin genes showing strong evolutionary divergence of two homologous pairs of introns. Nature 276: 37

Berget S M, Moore C, Sharp P A 1977 Spliced segments at the 5′ terminus of adenovirus 2 late mRNA. Proceedings of the National Academy of Sciences USA 74: 3171

Bernard O, Hoxumi N, Tonegawa S 1978 Sequence of mouse immunoglobulin light chain genes before and after somatic changes. Cell: 1133

Bienkowski R S, Baum B J, Crystal R G 1978 Fibroblasts degrade newly-synthesised collagen within the cell before secretion. Nature 276: 413

Billings P B, Martin T E 1978 In: Stein G, Stein J, Kleinsmith L J (eds) Methods in Cell Biology. Academic Press, New York, p 349

Blattner F R et al 1977 Charon phages: safer derivatives of bacteriophage λ for DNA cloning. Science 196: 161

Blobel G 1973 A protein of molecular weight 78 000 bound to the polyadenylate region of eukaryotic messenger mRNAs. Proceedings of the National Academy of Sciences USA 70: 924

Blobel G, Dobberstein B 1975a Transfer of proteins across membranes: Presence of proteolytically processed and unprocessed nascent immunoglobulin light chains on membrane-bound ribosomes of murine myeloma. Journal of Cell Biology 67: 835

Blobel G, Dobberstein B 1975b Transfer of proteins across membranes: Reconstitution of functional rough microsomes from heterologous components. Journal of Cell Biology 67: 852

Blobel G 1977 Synthesis and segregation of secretory proteins: the signal hypothesis. In: Brinkley R R, Porter K R (eds) International Cell Biology. Rockefeller University Press, New York, p 318

Boedtker H, Crkvenjakov R B, Last J A, Doty P 1974 The identification of collagen messenger RNA. Proceedings of the National Academy of Sciences USA 71: 4208

Boedtker H, Frischauf A M, Lehrach H 1976 Isolation and translation of calvaria procollagen messenger ribonucleic acids. Biochemistry 15: 4765

Bogenhagen D F, Sakonju S, Brown D D 1980 A control region in the center of the 5S RNA gene directs specific initiation of transcription: II The 3′ border of the region. Cell 19: 27

Bornstein P, Sage H 1980 Structurally distinct collagen types. Annual Review of Biochemistry 49: 957

Bornstein P, Traub W 1979 The chemistry and biology of collagen In: Neurath H, Hill R (eds) The Proteins 3rd edn. Academic Press, New York, 4: 411

Boyd C D et al 1980 Isolation and characterization of a 15-kilobase genomic sequence coding for part of the pro-α2 chain of sheep type I collagen. Journal of Biological Chemistry 255: 3212

Breathnach R, Mandel J L, Chambon P 1977 Ovalbumin gene is split in chicken DNA. Nature 270: 314

Breathnach R, Benoist C, O'Hare K, Gannon F, Chambon P 1978 Ovalbumin gene: evidence for a leader sequence in mRNA and DNA sequence at the exon-intron boundaries. Proceedings of the National Academy of Sciences USA 75: 4853

Breitkreutz D, Diaz de Leon L, Pagli L, Zeichner M, Wilczek J, Stern R 1978 The synthesis of presumptive procollagen messenger ribonucleic acid in the calvaria of the developing chick embryo. Biochimica et Biophysica Acta 517: 349

Brenchley J E, Williams L S 1975 Transfer RNA involvement in the regulation of enzyme synthesis. Annual Review of Microbiology 29: 251

Brentani M, Salles J M, Brentani R 1977 Determination of the extent of secondary structure in chick embryo procollagen messenger RNA. Biochemistry 16: 5145

Burness A T H, Pardoe I U, Goldstein N O 1975 Overestimates of the size of poly(A) segments. Biochemical and Biophysical Research Communications 67: 1408

Carlier A R, Peumans W J 1976 The rye embryo system as an alternative to the wheat system from protein synthesis in vitro. Biochimica et Biophysica Acta 447: 436

Carpousis A, Christner P, Rosenbloom J 1977a Preferential usage of glycyl-tRNA isoaccepting species in collagen synthesis. Journal of Biological Chemistry 252: 2447

Carpousis A, Christner P, Rosenbloom J 1977b Preferential usage of tRNA isoaccepting species in collagen synthesis. Journal of Biological Chemistry 252: 8023

Catterall J F, O'Malley B W, Robertson M A, Staden R, Tanaka Y, Brownlee G G 1978 Nucleotide sequence homology at 12 intron-exon junctions in the chick ovalbumin gene. Nature 275: 510

Chambon P et al 1979 Structure and expression of ovalbumin and closely-related chicken genes. In: Axel R, Maniatis T, Fox C F (eds) ICN–UCLA Symposia on Molecular and Cellular Biology, 14, Eucaryotic Gene Regulation. Academic Press, New York, p 259

Cheah K S E, Grant M E, Jackson D S 1979a Translation of embryonic-chick tendon procollagen messenger ribonucleic acid in two cell-free protein-synthesizing systems. Biochemical Journal 182: 81

Cheah K S E, Grant M E, Jackson D S 1979b Translation of type II procollagen mRNA and hydroxylation of the cell-free product. Biochemical and Biophysical Research Communications 91: 1025

Cheah K S E, Grant M E, Jackson D S 1981 Identification of the primary translation product of elastin mRNA. Connective Tissue Research, 8: 205

Chow L T, Broker T R 1978 The spliced structures of adenovirus 2 fiber message and the other late mRNAs. Cell 15: 497

Christner P J, Rosenbloom J 1976 A comparison of tRNA isoaccepting species between collagenous and non-collagenous tissues in the embryonic chick. Archives of Biochemistry and Biophysics 172: 399

Church R L, Sundar Raj N, McDougall J K 1980 Regional chromosome mapping of the human skin type 1 procollagen gene using adenovirus 12-fragmentation of human mouse somatic cell hybrids. Cytogenetics and Cell Genetics 27: 24

Church R L 1981 Chromosome mapping of connective tissue protein genes. International Review of Connective Tissue Research, 9: 99

Clemens M J 1979 Why do messengers wear caps? Nature 279: 673

Corden J, Wasylyk B, Buchwalder A, Sassone-Corsi P, Kedviger C, Chambon P 1980 Promoter sequences of eukaryotic protein-coding genes. Science 180: 1406

Craig R K, Boulton A R, Harrison O S, Parker D, Campbell P N 1979 Studies on the intracellular segregation of polyribosome-associated messenger ribonucleic acid species in the lactating guinea-pig mammary gland. Biochemical Journal 181: 737

Crick F 1979 Split genes and RNA splicing. Science 204: 264

Cutroneo K R, Newman R A, Prichard P M, Guzman N A, Sharawy M M 1977 Localization of collagen-synthesising ribosomes on the dense segments of the endoplasmic reticulum. International Journal of Biochemistry 8: 421

Darnell J E, Jellinek W R, Molloy G R 1973 Biogenesis of mRNA: genetic regulation in mammalian cells. Science 181: 1215

Darnell J E 1978 Implications of RNA–RNA splicing in evolution of eukaryotic cells. Science 202: 1257

Darnell J E 1979 Transcription units for mRNA production in eukaryotic cells and their DNA viruses. In: Cohn W E (ed) Progress in Nucleic Acid Research and Molecular Biology. Academic Press, London, Vol 22, p 327

Davies J W, Aalbers A M J, Stuik E J, Van Kammen A 1977 Translation of cowpea mosaic virus RNA in a cell-free extract from wheat germ. FEBS Letters 77: 265

Davis M, Kim S K, Hood L E 1980 DNA sequences mediating class switching in α-immunoglobulins. Science 209: 1360

Diaz de Leon L, Paglia L, Breitkreutz D, Stern R 1977 Evidence that the messenger RNA for collagen is monocistronic. Biochemical and Biophysical Research Communications 77: 11

Diaz de Leon L, Breitkreutz D, Zeichner M, Stern R, Paglia L 1980 Partial characterization of procollagen messenger ribonucleic acid in a murine chondrosarcoma. Connective Tissue Research 7: 135

Diegelmann R F, Peterkofsky B 1972 Collagen biosynthesis during connective tissue development in chick embryo. Developmental Biology 28: 443

Doel M T 1980 Gene inserts. Introns and exons, a condensed review. Cell Biology International Reports 4: 433

Drabkin H J, Lukens L N 1978 Preferential use in collagen synthesis of the same glycyl-tRNA species that is elevated in collagen-synthesizing tissues. Journal of Biological Chemistry 253: 6233

Dugaiczyk A, Woo S L C, Cobert D A, Lai E C, Mace M L, O'Malley 1979 The ovalbumin gene: cloning and molecular organization of the entrie natural gene. Proceedings of the National Academy of Sciences USA 76: 2253

Efstratiatis A et al 1979 The structure and transcription of rat prepoinsulin gene. Eukaryotic gene regulation, 8th ICN–UCLA Symposium. Academic Press, New York. In press

Evans J H, Hamaton J L, Klingex H P, McKusick V A (eds) Human Gene Mapping 5 Edinburgh Conference (5th International Workshop on Human Gene Mapping). S. Karger, Basel

Fagan J B, Pastan I, de Crombrugghe B 1980 Sequence rearrangement and duplication of double stranded fibronectin cDNA probably occurring during cDNA synthesis by AMV reverse transcriptase and E. Coli DNA polymerase 1. Nucleic Acid Research 8: 3055

Falvey A K, Weiss B, Kreuger L S, Kantor J A, Anderson W F 1976 Transcription of single base oligonucleotides by ribonucleic acid-directed deoxyribonucleic acid polymerase. Nucleic Acid Research 3: 79

Fernandez-Madrid F 1970 Collagen biosynthesis: a review. Clinical Orthopaedics 68: 163

Fessler J H, Fessler L I 1978 Biosynthesis of procollagen. Annual Review of Biochemistry 47: 129

Fessler L I, Morris N P, Fessler J H 1975 Procollagen: biological scission of amino and carboxyl extension peptides. Proceedings of the National Academy of Sciences USA 72: 4905

Fietzek P P, Kuhn K 1976 The primary structure of collagen. International Review of Connective Tissue Research 7: 1

Filipowicz A 1978 Functions of the 5′-terminal m^7G cap in eucaryotic mRNA. FEBS Letters 96: 1

Frischauf A M, Lehrach H, Rosner C, Boedtker H 1978 Procollagen complementary DNA, a probe for messenger RNA purification and the number of type I collagen genes. Biochemistry 17: 3243

Fuller F, Boedtker H 1981 Sequence determination and analysis of the 3′ region of chicken pro α1(I) and pro α2(I) collagen mRNAs including the carboxy terminal propeptide sequences. Biochemistry: 20: 996

Furthmayr H, Timpl R 1971 Characterization of collagen peptides by sodium dodecyl sulfate — polyacrylamide electrophoresis. Analytical Biochemistry 41: 510

Garel J-P 1974 Functional adaptation of tRNA population. Journal of Theoretical Biology 43: 211

Garel J-P, Hentzen D 1974 Codon responses of $tRNA^{Ala}$, $tRNA^{Gly}$ and $tRNA^{Ser}$ from the posterior part of the silk gland of Bombyx Mori L. FEBS Letters 39: 359

Gay S, Gay R E, Miller E J 1980 The collagens of the joint. Arthritis and Rheumatism, 23: 937

Gilbert W 1978 Why genes in pieces? Nature 271: 501

Giles R E, Ruddle F H 1973 Production and characterisation of proliferating somatic cell hybrids. In: Kruse P F, Patterson M K (eds) Tissue Culture Methods and Applications. Academic Press, New York, p 475

Glover D M, Hogness S 1977 A novel arrangement of the 18s and 28s sequences in a repeating unit of Drosophila melanogaster rDNA. Cell 10: 167

Goodman H M, Olson M V, Hall B D 1977 Nucleotide sequence of a mutant eukaryotic gene. The yeast tyrosine-inserting ochre suppressor SUP4-0. Proceedings of the National Academy of Sciences USA 74: 543

Gopinathan K P, Weymouth L A, Kunkel T A, Loeb L A 1979 Mutagenesis in vitro by DNA polymerase from an RNA tumour virus. Nature 278: 857

Grant M E, Jackson D S 1976 The biosynthesis of procollagen. Essays in Biochemistry 12: 77

Graves, P N, Olsen B R, Fietzek P P, Monson J M, Prockop D J 1979 Type I pre-procollagen chains synthesised in a messenger RNA dependent reticulocyte lysate. Federation Proceedings 38: 620

Greenberg J R 1975 Messenger RNA metabolism of animal cells. Possible involvement of untranslated sequences and mRNA-associated proteins. Journal of Cell Biology 64: 269

Gruss P, Lai C, Dhar R, Khoury G 1979 Splicing as a requirement for biogenesis of functional 16s mRNA of simian virus 40. Proceedings of the National Academy of Sciences USA 76: 4317

Hamer D H, Leder P 1979 Splicing and the formation of stable RNA. Cell 18: 1299

Hamer D H, Smith K D, Boyer S H, Leder P 1979 SV40 recombinants carrying rabbit β-globin gene coding sequences. Cell 17: 725

Haralson M A, Frey K L, Mitchell W M 1978 Collagen biosynthesis by cultured chinese hamster lung cells. Cell-free synthesis of procollagen αchains. Biochemistry 17: 864

Harwood R, Connolly A D, Grant M E, Jackson D S 1974 Presumptive mRNA for procollagen: occurrence in membrane-bound ribosomes of embryonic chick tendon fibroblasts. FEBS Letters 41: 85

Harwood R, Grant M E, Jackson D S 1975a Translation of type I and type II procollagen messengers in a cell-free system derived from wheat germ. FEBS Letters 57: 47

Harwood R, Bhalla A K, Grant M E, Jackson D S 1975b The synthesis and secretion of cartilage procollagen. Biochemical Journal 148: 129

Harwood R, Grant M E, Jackson D S 1975c Further characterization of procollagen messenger RNA from embryonic chick tendon cells. Biochemical Society Transactions 3: 916

Harwood R, Merry A H, Woolley D E, Grant M E, Jackson D S 1977 The disulphide-bonded nature of procollagen and the role of the extension peptides in the assembly of the molecule. Biochemical Journal 161: 405

Harwood R 1979 Collagen polymorphism and messenger RNA. International Review of Connective Tissue Research 8: 159

Harwood R 1980 Signal sequences and signal peptidease. In: Freedman R, Hawkins H (eds) The Enzymology of Post-Translational Modifications of Proteins. Academic Press, London, p. 3

Heathcote J G, Grant M E 1980 Extracellular modification of connective tissue proteins. In: Freedman R, Hawkins H (eds) The Enzymology of Post-Transcriptional Modifications of Proteins. Academic Press, London, p 457

Heilig R, Perrin F, Gannon F, Mandel J L, Chambon P 1980 The ovalbumin gene family: structure of the X gene and evolution of duplicated split genes. Cell 20: 625

Hofman H, Fietzek P P, Kuhn K 1980 Comparative analysis of the sequences of the three collagen chains α1(I), α2 and α1(III). Journal of Molecular Biology 141: 293

Hohn B, Murray K 1977 Packaging recombinant DNA molecules into bacteriophage particles in vitro. Proceedings of the National Academy of Sciences USA 74: 3259

Howard B H, Adams S L, Sobel M E, Pastan I, de Crombrugghe B 1978 Decreased levels of collagen mRNA in rous sarcoma-transformed chick embryo fibroblasts. Journal of Biological Chemistry 253: 5869

Jeffreys A J, Flavell R A 1977a A physical map of the DNA regions flanking the rabbit β-globulin gene. Cell 12: 429

Jeffreys A J, Flavell R A 1977b The rabbit β-globin gene contains a large insert in the coding sequence. Cell 12: 1097

Kaufmann R, Belayew A, Nusgens B, Lapière C M, Gielen J E 1980 Extraction and translation of collagen mRNA from fetal calf skin. European Journal of Biochemistry 106: 593

Kerwar S S, Kohn L D, Lapière C M, Weissbach H 1972 In vitro synthesis of procollagen on polysomes. Proceedings of the National Academy of Sciences USA 69: 2727

Kerwar S S, Cardinale G J, Kohn L D, Spears C L, Stassen F L H 1973 Cell-free synthesis of procollagen: L–929 fibroblasts as a cellular model for Dermatosparaxis. Proceedings of the National Academy of Sciences USA 70: 1378

Kinniburgh A J, Ross J 1979 Processing of the mouse β-globin mRNA precursor: at least two cleavage-ligation reactions are necessary to excise the larger intervening sequence. Cell 17: 915

Kinniburgh A J, Mertz J E, Rars J 1978 The precursor of mouse β-globin messenger RNA contains two intervening RNA sequences. Cell 14: 681

Klessig D F 1977 Two adenovirus mRNAs have a common 5′ terminal leader sequence encoded at least 10 kb upstream from their main coding regions. Cell 12: 9

Knapp G, Beckman J S, Johnson P F, Fuhrman S A, Abelson J 1978 Transcription and processing of intervening sequences in yeast tRNA genes. Cell 14: 221

Konkel D, Tilghman S M, Leder P 1978 The sequence of the chromosomal mouse β-globin major gene: homologues in capping, splicing and poly A sites. Cell 15: 1125

Korn L J, Brown D D 1978 Nucleotide sequences of Xenopus borealis oocyte 5S DNA: comparison of sequences that flank several related eukaryotic genes. Cell 15: 1145

Kourilsky P, Chambon P 1978 The ovalbumin gene: an amazing gene in eight pieces. Trends in Biochemical Sciences 3: 244

Kream B E, Rowe D W, Gworek S C, Raisz L G 1979 Insulin and parathyroid hormone alter collagen synthesis and procollagen messenger RNA levels in fetal rat bone in vitro. Calcified Tissue Research 28: 148

Kream B E, Rowe D W, Gworek S C, Raisz L G 1980 Parathyroid hormone alters collagen synthesis and procollagen mRNA levels in fetal rat calvaria. Proceedings of the National Academy of Sciences USA 77: 5654

Kretsinger R H et al 1964 Synthesis of collagen on polyribosomes. Nature 202: 438

Lai E C et al 1979 Molecular structure and flanking nucleotide sequences of the natural chicken ovomucoid gene. Cell 18: 829

Lai C-J, Khoury G 1979 Deletion mutants of simian virus 40 defective in biosynthesis of late viral mRNA. Proceedings of the National Academy of Sciences USA 76: 71

Lanks K W, Weinstein I B 1970 Quantitative differences in proline tRNA content of rat liver and granulation tissue. Biochemical and Biophysical Research Communications 40: 708

Lazarides E, Lukens L N 1971 Collagen synthesis on polysomes in vivo and in vitro. Nature New Biology 232: 37

Lazarides E, Lukens L N, Infante A A 1971 Collagen polysomes: site of hydroxylation of proline residues. Journal of Molecular Biology 58: 831

Lehrach H et al 1978 Construction and characterisation of a 2.5-kilobase procollagen clone. Proceedings of the National Academy of Sciences USA 75: 5417

Lehrach H, Frischauf A M, Hanahan D, Wozney J, Fuller F, Boedtker H 1979 Construction and characterisation of pro αI collagen complementary deoxyribonucleic acid clones. Biochemistry 18: 3146

Lerner M R, Steitz J A 1979 Antibodies to small nuclear RNAs complexed with proteins are produced by patients with systemic lupus erythematosus. Proceedings of the National Academy of Sciences USA 76: 5495

Lerner M R, Boyle J A, Mount S M, Wolin S L, Steitz J A 1980 Are SnRNPs involved in splicing? Nature 283: 220

Lingappa V R, Lingappa J R, Blobel G 1979 Chicken ovalbumin contains an internal signal sequence. Nature 281: 117

Littauer U Z, Inouye H 1973 Regulation of tRNA. Annual Review of Biochemistry 42: 439

Lodish H F 1976 Translational control of protein synthesis. Annual Review of Biochemistry 45: 39

Mäenpää P H, Ahonen J (1972) tRNA changes in rat granulation tissue possibly related to collagen synthesis. Biochemical and Biophysical Research Communications 49: 179

Maki R, Kearney J, Paige C, Tonegawa S 1980 Immunoglobulin gene rearrangement in immature β cells. Science 209: 1366

Maniatis T et al 1978 The isolation of structural genes from libraries of eukaryotic DNA. Cell 15: 687

Manner G et al 1967 The polyribosomal synthesis of collagen. Biochimica et Biophysica Acta 134: 411

Marbaix et al 1977 What is the role of polyA on eucaryotic messengers? Trends in Biochemical Sciences 2: N106

Marcu K, Dudock B 1974 Characterization of a highly efficient protein synthesizing system derived from commercial wheat germ. Nucleic Acids Research 1: 1385

von der Mark K, Conrad G 1979 Cartilage cell differentiation. Clinical Orthopaedics and Related Research 139: 185

Martinell J, Lukens L N 1980 Collagen proα_1 polysomes appear to sediment more rapidly than polyα_2 polysomes. FEBS Letters 115: 105

Mathews M 1980 Coevolution of collagen. In: Vidik A, Vuust J (eds) Biology of Collagen. Academic Press, London, p 173

McKusick V A, Ruddle F H 1977 The status of the gene map of the human chromosomes. Science 196: 390

McLachlen A D 1976 Evidence for gene duplication in collagen. Journal of Molecular Biology 107: 159

Moen R C, Rowe D W, Palmiter R D 1979 Regulation of procollagen synthesis during the development of chick embryo calvaria. Journal of Biological Chemistry 254: 3526

Molgaard H V 1980 Assembly of immunoglobulin heavy chain genes. Nature 286: 657

Monson J M, Goodman H M 1978 Translation of chick calvarial procollagen messenger RNAs by a messenger RNA-dependent reticulocyte lysate. Biochemistry 17: 5122

Muir H, Hardingham T E 1975 In: Whelan W J (ed) Medical and Technical Publishing Company, Biochemistry Series 1: Biochemistry of Carbohydrates. Butterworth's, London, Volume 5, p 153

Murray V, Holliday R 1979 Mechanism for RNA splicing of gene transcripts. FEBS Letters 106: 5

Myers J C, Chu M-L, Faro S H, Clark W J, Prockop D J, Ramirez F 1981 Cloning a cDNA for the proα2 chain of human type I collagen. Proceedings of the National Academy of Sciences USA 78: 3516

Neufang O, Tiedmann H 1975 Stimulation of collagen synthesis in a cell-free system by mRNA from chick embryos. Hoppe-Zeyler's Zeitschrift fur Physiologisches Chemie 356: 1445

Nevins J R, Darnell J E 1978 Steps in the processing of Ad2 mRNA: poly $(A)^+$ nuclear sequences are conserved and poly (A) addition precedes splicing. Cell 15: 1477

Notman D D, Kurata N, Tan E M 1975 Profiles of antinuclear antibodies in systemic rheumatic diseases. Annals of Internal Medicine 83: 464

Nwagwu M, Reid S A 1977 Collagen synthesis in the muscle of developing chick embryos. Biochemical Journal 166: 199

Oborotova T A, Berman A E, Mazurov V I 1979 Biosynthesis of collagen and other proteins on tightly and loosely bound polyribosomes from chick embryos. Biokhimaya 44: 1715

O'Farrell P Z, Cordell B, Valenzuela P, Rutter W J, Goodman H M 1978 Structure and processing of yeast precursor tRNAs containing intervening sequences. Nature 274: 438

Ohkubo H, Vogeli G, Mudryj M, Avvedimento V E, Sullivan M, Pastan I, de Crombrugghe B 1980 Isolation and characterization of overlapping genomic clones covering the chick α2 (type) collagen gene. Proceedings of the National Academy of Sciences USA 77: 7059

Old R W, Primrose S B 1980 Principles of gene manipulation. An introduction to genetic engineering. Studies in Microbiology Vol. 2. Blackwell Scientific Publications, Oxford

Paglia L, Wilczek J, Diaz de Leon L, Martin G R, Hörlein D, Müller P 1979 Inhibition of procollagen cell-free synthesis by amino-terminal extension peptides. Biochemistry 18: 5030

Palmiter R D, Davidson J M, Gagnon J, Rowe D W, Bornstein P 1979 NH_2-terminal sequence of the chick proα1(I) chain synthesised in the reticulocyte lysate system. Journal of Biological Chemistry 254: 1433

Park E, Tanzer M L, Church R L 1975 Procollagen synthesis in cell culture: nascent chain population consistent with polycistronic mRNA. Biochemical and Biophysical Research Communications 63: 1

Parker I, Fitschen W 1980 Procollagen mRNA metabolism during the fibroblast cell cycle and its synthesis in transformed cells. Nucleic Acids Research 8: 2823

Pesciotta D M et al 1981 Primary structure of the carbohydrate-containing region of the carboxyl propeptides of type I procollagen. FEBS Letters 125: 170

Paterson B M, Rosenberg M 1979 Efficient translation of prokaryotic mRNAs in a eukaryotic cell-free system requires addition of a cap structure. Nature 279: 692

Pawlowski P J, Gillette M T, Martinell J, Lukens L N 1975 Identification and purification of collagen-synthesizing polysomes with anti-collagen antibodies. Journal of Biological Chemistry 250: 2135

Payvar F, Schimke R T 1979 Methylmercury hydroxide enhancement of translation and transcription of ovalbumin and conalbumin mRNAs. Journal of Biological Chemistry 254: 7636

Pelham H R B, Jackson R J 1976 An efficient mRNA-dependent translation system from reticulocyte lysates. European Journal of Biochemistry 67: 247

Perry R P 1976 Processing of RNA. Annual Review of Biochemistry 45: 605

Prockop D J 1981 Recombinant DNA and collagen research. Is amino acid sequencing obsolete? Can we study diseases involving collagen by analysis of the genes. Collagen and Related Research 1: 129

Prockop D J, Kivirikko K I, Tuderman L, Guzman N A 1979 The biosynthesis of collagen and its disorders. New England Journal of Medicine 301: 13 & 77

Provost T T 1979 Subsets in systemic lupus erythematosus. Journal of Investigative Dermatology 72: 110

Raisz L G, Canalis E M, Dietrich J W, Kream B E, Gworek S C 1978 Hormone regulation of bone formation. Recent Progress in Hormone Research 34: 335

Rave N, Crkvenjakov R, Boedtker H 1979 Identification of procollagen mRNAs transferred to diazobenzyloxymethyl paper from formaldehyde agarose gels. Nucleic Acids Research 6: 3559

Reddy V B et al 1978 The genome of simian virus 40. Science 200: 494

Revel M, Groner Y 1978 Post-transcriptional and translational controls of gene expression in eukaryotes. Annual Review of Biochemistry 47: 1079

Richards R 1980 Small RNAs and splicing. Nature 283: 132

Rogers J, Wall R 1980 A mechanism for RNA splicing. Proceedings of the National Academy of Sciences USA 77: 1877

Rosenberg M, Paterson B M 1979 Efficient cap-dependent translation of polycistronic prokaryotic mRNAs is restricted to the first gene in the operon. Nature 279: 696

Rowe D W, Moen R C, Davidson J M, Byers P H, Bornstein P, Palmiter R D 1978 Correlation of procollagen mRNA levels in normal and transformed chick embryo fibroblasts with different rates of procollagen synthesis. Biochemistry 17: 1581

Royal A et al 1977 The ovalbumin gene region: common features in the organisation of three genes expressed in chicken oviduct under hormonal control. Nature 279: 125

Sakonju S, Bogenhagen D F, Brown D D 1980 A control region in the center of the 5S RNA gene directs specific initiation of transcription: 1. The 5′ border of the region. Cell 19: 13

Salles J M, Sonohara S, Brentani R 1976 Further studies on collagen mRNA: partial chemical characterisation and polyadenylic acid sequence. Molecular Biology Reports 2: 517

Sandberg L B 1976 Elastin structure in health and disease. In: Hall D A, Jackson D S (eds) International Review of Connective Tissue Research vol 7. Academic Press, London, p 160

Sandell L, Veis A 1980 The molecular weight of the cell-free translation product of αI(I) procollagen mRNA. Biochemical and Biophysical Research Communications 92: 554

Sandmeyer S, Bornstein P 1979 Declining procollagen mRNA sequences in chick embryo fibroblasts infected with Rous Sarcoma virus. Journal of Biological Chemistry 254: 4950

Schafer M P, Boyd C D, Tolstoshev P, Crystal R G 1980 Structural organisation of a 17KB segment of the $\alpha2$ collagen gene: evaluation by R loop mapping. Nucleic Acid Research 8: 2241

Scherrer K, Imaizumi-Scherrer M-T, Reynaud C-A, Therwath A 1979 On pre-mRNA and transcriptions — a review. Molecular Biology Report 5:

Schuppan D, Timpl R, Glanville R W 1980 Discontinuities in the tiple helical sequence Gly-X-Y of basement membrane (type IV) collagen. FEBS Letters 115: 297

Shatkin A J 1976 Capping of eucaryotic mRNAs. Cell 9: 645

Shih D S, Kaesberg P 1976 Translation of the RNAs of Brome Mosaic Virus: the monocistrionic nature of RNA1 and RNA2. Journal of Molecular Biology 103: 77

Showalter A M et al 1980 Nucleotide sequence of a collagen cDNA-fragment coding for the carboxyl end of proα1(I)-chains. FEBS Letters 111: 61

Schwartz H, Darnell J E 1976 The association of protein with the polyadenylic acid of HeLa cell messenger RNA: evidence for a 'transport' role of a 75 000 molecular weight polypeptide. Journal of Molecular Biology 104: 833

Simpson D R, Arfin S M, Wesley Hatfield G 1975 A role for asparaginyl-tRNA in the repression of asparagine synthetase in chinese hamster ovary cells. Federation Proceedings 34: 586

Sinsheimer R L 1977 Recombinant DNA. Annual Review of Biochemistry 46: 416

Smith D W E, McNamara A L 1971 Specialization of rabbit reticulocyte transfer RNA content for hemoglobin synthesis. Science 171: 577

Smithies O et al 1978 Cloning human fetal γ-globin and mouse α-type globin DNA: characterization and partial sequencing. Science 202: 1284

Sobel M E et al 1978 Construction of a recombinant bacterial plasmid containing a chick pro-$\alpha2$ collagen gene sequence. Proceedings of the National Academy of Sciences USA 75: 5846

Soffer R L 1973 Post-translational modification of proteins catalysed by aminoacyl-tRNA-protein transferases. Molecular and Cellular Biochemistry 2: 3

Solomon E, Cheah K S E 1981 Collagen evolution. Nature 291: 450

Solomon E, Sykes B 1978 Assignment of a structural gene for type I collagen to chromosome 7. Cytogenetics and Cell Genetics 22: 281

Solomon E, Sykes B 1979 Assignment of $\alpha1$(I), $\alpha2$ and possibly α_1(III) chains of human collagen to chromosome 7. In: Evans J H, Hamaton J L, Klingex H P, McKusick V A (eds) Human Gene Mapping 5 Edinburgh Conference (5th International Workshop on Human Gene Mapping). S. Karger, Basel, p 205

Solomon E 1980 The collagen gene family. Nature 286: 656

Sprague K U, Hagenbüchle O 1977 The nucleotide sequence of two silk gland alanine tRNAs: Implications for fibroin synthesis and for initiator tRNA structure. Cell 11: 561

Standart N M, Harwood R 1977 Isolation and partial characterization of polyribosomal messenger ribonucleoproteins from embryonic-chick tendon cells. Biochemical Society Transactions 5: 1389

Standart N M 1979 Polysomal mRNP particles in embryonic chick tendon cells. Ph.D. thesis, University College, Cardiff

Stent G S 1964 The operon: on its third anniversary. Science 144: 816

Sternberg N, Tiemeier D, Enquist L 1977 In vitro packaging of a λDam vector containing ECoR1 DNA fragment of Escherischia coli and phage P1. Gene 1: 255

Sundar-Raj C V, Church R L, Klobutcher L A, Ruddle F H 1977 Genetics of the connective tissue proteins: assignment of the gene for human type I procollagen to chromosome 17 by analysis of cell hybrids and microcell hybrids. Proceedings of the National Academy of Sciences USA 74: 4444

Sures I, Lowry J, Kedes L H 1978 The DNA sequence of sea urchin (S. purpuratus) H2A, H2B and H3 histone coding and spacer regions. Cell 15: 1033

Sykes B, Solomon E 1978 Assignment of a type I collagen structural gene to human chromosome 7. Nature 272: 548

Tanzer M L 1978 The biological diversity of collagenous proteins. Trends in Biochemical Sciences 3: 15

Thimmappaya B, Jones N, Shenk T 1979 A mutation which alters initiation of transcription by RNA polymerase III on the Ad 5 chromosome. Cell 18: 947

Thomas M, White R L, Daws R W 1976 Hybridisation of RNA to double stranded DNA: formation of R-loops. Proceedings of the National Academy of Sciences USA 73: 2294

Tilghman S M et al 1978a Intervening sequence of DNA identified in the structural portion of a mouse β-globin gene. Proceedings of the National Academy of Sciences USA 75: 725

Tilghman S M, Curtis P J, Tiemeier D C, Leder P, Weissman C 1978b The intervening sequence of a mouse β-globin gene is transcribed within the 15S β-globin mRNA precursor. Proceedings of the National Academy of Sciences USA 75: 1309

Tolstoshev P, Haber R, Crystal R G 1979 Procollagen $\alpha2$ mRNA is significantly different from procollagen $\alpha1$(I) mRNA in size or secondary structure. Biochemical and Biophysical Research Communications 87: 818

Tonegawa S, Maxam A M, Tizard R, Berhard O, Gilbert W 1978 Sequence of a mouse germ-line gene for a variable region of an immunoglobulin light chain. Proceedings of the National Academy of Sciences USA 75: 1485

Tsukimoto Y, Suzuki Y 1979 Structural analysis of the fibroin oocyte 5S DNA: comparison of sequences that flank several related eukaryotic genes. Cell 15: 1145

Upholt W B, Vertel B M, Dorfman A 1979 Translation and characterization of messenger RNAs in differentiating chicken cartilage. Proceedings of the National Academy of Sciences USA 76: 4847

Valenzuela P, Venegas A, Weinburg F, Bishop R, Rutter W J 1978 Structure of yeast phenylalanine-tRNA genes: an intervening DNA segment within the region coding for the tRNA. Proceedings of the National Academy of Sciences USA 75: 190

Vogeli G et al 1980a Isolation and characterization of genomic DNA coding for α2 type I collagen. Nucleic Acids Research 8: 1823

Vogeli G, Ohkubo H, Avvedimento V E, Sullivan M, Yamada Y, Mudryj M, Pastan I, de Crombrugghe B 1980b A repetitive structure in the chick α2-collagen gene. Cold Spring Harbour Symposium, 45: 777

Vuust J 1975 Procollagen biosynthesis by embryonic-chick-bone polysomes. European Journal of Biochemistry 60: 41

Wahli W, Dawid I B, Wyler T, Weber R, Ryffel G U 1980 Comparative analysis of the structural organization of two closely-related vitellogenin genes in X. laevis. Cell 20: 107

Weatherall D J, Clegg J B 1979 Recent developments in the molecular genetics of human haemoglobin. Cell 16: 467

Wang L et al 1975a Isolation and characterization of collagen messenger RNA. Nucleic Acids Research 2: 655

Wang L, Andrade H F, Silva S M F, Simoes C L, D'Abronzo F H, Brentani R 1975b Isolation and characterization of collagen synthesising polysomes from chick embryos. Preparative Biochemistry 5: 45

Weber K, Osborn M 1975 In: Neurath H (ed) The Proteins 3rd edn. Vol 1, Academic Press, New York, p 179

Weinberg R, Penman S 1968 Small molecular weight monodisperse nuclear RNA. Journal of Molecular Biology 38: 289

Weiss J B 1976 Enzymic degradation of collagen. In: Hall D A, Jackson D S (eds) International Review of Connective Tissue Research, Vol 7. Academic Press, London, p 102

Wickens M P, Woo S, O'Malley B W, Gurdon J B 1980 Expression of a chicken chromosomal ovalbumin gene injected into frog oocyte nuclei. Nature 285: 628

Wiestner M, Krieg T, Hörlein D, Glanville R W, Fietzek P, Müller P K 1979 Inhibiting effect of procollagen peptides on collagen biosynthesis in fibroblast culture. Journal of Biological Chemistry 254: 7016

Wilczek J, Diaz de Leon L, Breitkreutz D, Stern R 1978 Translation of procollagen messenger RNA in a cell free system derived from wheat germ: hydroxylation of polyl residues in the product. Connective Tissue Research 6: 93

Wild M A, Gall J G 1979 An intervening sequence in the gene coding for 25S ribosomal RNA of Tetrahymena pigmentosa. Cell 16: 565

Williamson R 1973 The protein moieties of animal messenger ribonucleoproteins. FEBS Letters 37: 1

Wozney J, Hanahan D, Morimoto R, Boedtker H, Doty P 1981 Fine structure analysis of the chicken pro α2 collagen gene. Proceedings of the National Academy of Sciences 78: 712

Wu R 1980 Recombinant DNA. In: Colowick S P, Kaplan N O (eds) Methods in Enzymology Vol 68. Academic Press, New York

Yamada Y et al 1980 The collagen gene: evidence for its evolutionary assembly by amplification of a DNA segment containing an exon of 54 bases. Cell 22: 887

Yamamoto T et al 1980 Construction of a recombinant bacterial plasmid containing pro-α1(I) collagen DNA sequences. Journal of Biological Chemistry 255: 2612

Ycas M 1972 De novo origin of periodic proteins. Journal of Molecular Evolution 2: 17

Zeichner M, Rojkind M 1976 RNA biosynthesis in the chick embryo during development and its relation to collagen synthesis. Connective Tissue Research 4: 169

Zeichner M, Stern K 1977 Resolution of ribonucleic acids by sepharose 4B column chromatography. Biochemistry 16: 1378

Note added in proof

Since this chapter was prepared the assignment of the human α2(I) gene to chromosome 7 has been confirmed by Junien et al (1982) using an α2(I) cDNA probe. The human α1(I) gene (Weiss et al, 1982) and mouse α1(I) gene (Monson & McCarthy, 1981) have been studied and both have a similar basic 54bp exon structure. Comparison of the structure of the human α1(I) gene with the chicken α2(I) gene (Wozney et al, 1981) and the mouse α1(I) gene reveal the interesting fact that the positions and sizes of a number of exons have been conserved in the α1(I) and α2(I) genes.

REFERENCES

Junien C et al 1982 Assignment of human proα2(I) collagen structural gene to chromosome 7 by molecular hybridization. VIth International Workshop on Human Gene Mapping. Birth Defects: Original Article Series (in press); The National Foundation, New York; also in Cytogenetics and Cell Genetics: in press

Monson J M, McCarthy B J 1981 Identification of a Balb/C mouse proα1(I) procollagen gene: evidence for insertions or deletions in gene coding sequences. Recombinant DNA 1: 59

Weiss E H, Cheah K S E, Grosveld F G, Dahl H H, Solomon E, Flavell R A 1982. Isolation and characterization of a human collagen α1(I)-like gene from a cosmid library. Nucleic Acid Res 10: in press

Wozney J, Hanahan D, Tate V, Boedtker H, Doty P 1981 Structure of the proα2(I) collagen gene. Nature 294: 129

6

Post-translational modifications

K. I. KIVIRIKKO and R. MYLLYLÄ

INTRODUCTION

Collagen biosynthesis is characterised by the presence of a large number of post-translational modifications which occur after the assembly of the amino acids into the peptide linkages. Many of these modifications are unique to collagens and a few other proteins with collagen-like amino acid sequences. The purpose of this review is to summarise current information on the post-translational modifications and their regulation; the changes taking place in disease states will be reviewed elsewhere in this book. Since there is a voluminous literature concerning these modifications, it is not possible to cite all the original contributions, and therefore the references include in the main only work published during the last few years. For more detailed references the reader is referred to recent reviews on various aspects of these modifications and collagen biosynthesis in general (Bailey & Robins, 1976; Grant & Jackson, 1976; Kivirikko & Risteli, 1976; Miller, 1976; Fessler & Fessler, 1978; Bornstein & Traub, 1979; Prockop et al, 1979; Bornstein & Sage, 1980; Eyre, 1980; Minor, 1980) or on the intracellular modifications (Prockop et al, 1976), hydroxylations (Adams & Frank, 1980; Kivirikko & Myllylä, 1980), glycosylations (Kivirikko & Myllylä, 1979) and lysyl oxidase (Siegel, 1979).

Fig 6.1 Post-translational modifications in the biosynthesis of collagen and their main functions

Modification	*Biological significance*
Intracellular modifications	
Removal of pre-protein sequences	Unknown
4-Hydroxylation of prolyl residues	Essential for triple helix at 37°C
3-Hydroxylation of prolyl residues	Unknown
Hydroxylation of lysyl residues	Essential for hydroxylysyl glycosylations Essential for stable cross-links
Glycosylation of hydroxylysyl residues	Possibly affects fibril morphology
Glycosylation of propeptides	Unknown
Chain association and disulphide bonding	Essential for triple helix formation
Triple helix formation	Essential for normal rate of procollagen secretion Various properties of the collagen molecules
Extracellular modifications	
Conversion of procollagen to collagen	Essential for normal fibril formation
Aggregation of collagen molecules	Fibril formation
Cross-link formation	Essential for stability of fibrils

GENERAL FEATURES OF THE MODIFICATIONS

The post-translational modifications of collagen can be regarded as occurring in two stages. Intracellular modifications, together with the synthesis of the polypeptide chains, result in the formation of the procollagen molecule, and extracellular processing converts this molecule into collagen and incorporates it into a stable, cross-linked fibril. The main modifications and their basic functions are summarized in Table 6.1.

Intracellular modifications and secretion of procollagen

Removal of pre-protein sequences

Many secretory proteins are synthesized in a precursor form with an additional hydrophobic amino-terminal 'pre-protein' (or 'signal' or 'leader') sequence. This sequence probably binds to the membrane of the rough endoplasmic reticulum and leads the nascent polypeptide chain into the membrane (see Blobel et al, 1979; Davis & Tai, 1980). The newly-synthesized collagen polypeptide chains have similar pre-protein sequences, although these may be significantly longer than those of most other proteins (Palmiter et al, 1979; Sandell & Veis, 1980; Graves et al, 1981).

The pre-protein sequences are cleaved within the membrane during the translation, a single enzyme being probably involved in the removal of these sequences from a number of proteins. One such protease, which cleaves pre-placental lactogen, has been solubilized and in part characterised from dog pancreas membranes (Strauss et al,

1979). This enzyme removes the pre-peptide in one step and is inhibited by high concentrations of chymostatin and by some serine protease inhibitors. The pre-protein sequence of the chick proα1(I) chain synthesized in the reticulocyte lysate system (see Chapter 5) is also cleaved by the dog pancreas membranes (Palmiter et al, 1979), but it has not been demonstrated whether the pre-proα chains are cleaved by the same enzyme that is involved in the case of the pre-placental lactogen. It is not known how the specific cleavage site is recognized by the protease(s), as the amino acid sequences at the cleavage site vary greatly from one protein to another.

Hydroxylations of prolyl and lysyl residues

The hydroxylation of prolyl and lysyl residues is catalyzed by three separate enzymes, prolyl 4-hydroxylase (E.C. 1.14.11.2., usually termed prolyl hydroxylase), prolyl 3-hydroxylase (E.C. 1.14.11.?) and lysyl hydroxylase (E.C. 1.14.11.4.). All three hydroxylate peptide-bound prolyl or lysyl residues. The products of their reactions, 4-hydroxyproline, 3-hydroxyproline and hydroxylysine (Fig. 6.1), are found in vertebrate proteins almost exclusively in collagens and a few other proteins with collagen-like amino acid sequences (see Adams & Frank, 1980; Kivirikko & Myllylä, 1980; and Ch. 2).

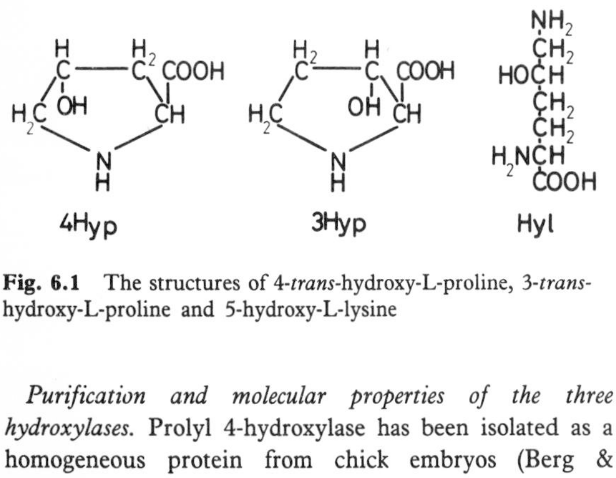

4Hyp 3Hyp Hyl

Fig. 6.1 The structures of 4-*trans*-hydroxy-L-proline, 3-*trans*-hydroxy-L-proline and 5-hydroxy-L-lysine

Purification and molecular properties of the three hydroxylases. Prolyl 4-hydroxylase has been isolated as a homogeneous protein from chick embryos (Berg & Prockop, 1973; Tuderman et al, 1975), new-born rats (J. Risteli et al, 1976), the skin of new-born rats (Chen-Kiang et al, 1977), human fetal tissues (Kuutti et al, 1975) and cultured L-929 fibroblasts (Kao & Berg, 1979). The active enzyme from all these sources is a tetramer with a molecular weight of about 240 000, and consists of two different types of enzymatically inactive monomer with molecular weights of about 64 000 and 60 000, having a subunit structure $\alpha_2\beta_2$. Distinct differences are found between the two monomers in amino acid and peptide map analysis (Chen-Kiang et al., 1977; Berg et al, 1979). Electron microscopy indicates that both monomers are rod-shaped, and the tetramer probably consists of two V-shaped dimers which are interlocked (see Prockop et al, 1976; Kivirikko & Myllylä, 1980). Intra-chain disulphide bonds seem essential for the monomers to maintain the native structure necessary for their association, whereas the presence of inter-chain disulphide bonds does not seem likely (see Prockop et al, 1976).

Lysyl hydroxylase has been purified to homogeneity from chick embryos and human placentas and to near homogeneity from human foetal tissues (Turpeenniemi-Hujanen et al, 1980, 1981). The molecular weight of the enzyme from both sources is about 190 000 by gel filtration and the active enzyme appears to be a dimer consisting of only one type of monomer with a molecular weight of about 85 000. Lysyl hydroxylase purification has also been reported from porcine foetal skin (Miller & Varner, 1979), but the specific activity of this enzyme preparation is about 100 times lower than that of the chick-embryo enzyme, and hence the purity and properties of this porcine skin enzyme require additional studies.

Prolyl 3-hydroxylase has been purified up to about 5000-fold from an ammonium sulphate fraction of chick-embryo extract (Tryggvason et al, 1979b). This enzyme has a molecular weight of about 160 000 by gel filtration, but its subunit structure is not known.

Prolyl 4-hydroxylase (Guzman et al, 1976), lysyl hydroxylase (Ryhänen, 1976; Turpeenniemi et al, 1977) and prolyl 3-hydroxylase (Tryggvason et al, 1979b) are probably all glycoproteins. The main sugar of prolyl 4-hydroxylase is mannose and most or all of the carbohydrate is located on the larger monomer (Chen-Kiang et al, 1977; Berg et al, 1979).

Many observations suggest that lysyl hydroxylase and prolyl 3-hydroxylase may have collagen type-specific or tissue-specific isoenzymes. The extents of lysyl hydroxylation and prolyl 3-hydroxylation vary markedly between different collagen types and within the same collagen type from different tissues (see Regulation below). The deficiency in lysyl hydroxylase activity encountered in the type VI variant of the Ehlers-Danlos syndrome causes hydroxylysine deficiency, which also shows a wide variation in its degree from tissue to tissue (see Krane, 1980). On the other hand, lysyl hydroxylase purified to homogeneity from extract of whole chick embryos consists of only one type of subunit, at least with respect to its molecular weight (Turpeenniemi-Hujanen et al, 1980). Furthermore, antiserum prepared to pure chick embryo lysyl hydroxylase gives a line of identity with the enzyme from a number of chick-embryo tissues in immunodiffusion, and approximately similar amounts of the antiserum are required for a 50 per cent inhibition of the same amount of enzyme units from various tissues (Turpeenniemi-Hujanen, 1981). The latter observations argue against the presence of tissue-specific isoenzymes with significantly different specific activities. Nevertheless, additional studies are required to elucidate either the presence or absence of such isoenzymes.

Requirements for the peptide substrates. None of the three enzymes hydroxylates free proline or free lysine, and they all require that the residue to be hydroxylated must be in a peptide linkage (see Kivirikko & Myllylä, 1980). Studies with a number of peptides have indicated that the minimum sequence requirement for interaction with vertebrate prolyl 4-hydroxylase is fulfilled by an -X-Pro-Gly- triplet, and that for interaction with lysyl hydroxylase by an -X-Lys-Gly- triplet, but both enzymes appear to hydroxylate certain other triplets in some cases (see Kivirikko & Myllylä, 1980). In agreement with these sequence requirements, 4-hydroxyproline and hydroxylysine have been identified in collagens and other vertebrate proteins with collagen-like amino acid sequences almost exclusively in the Y positions of -X-Y-Gly- triplets. The only reported exceptions are two sequences of -X-4Hyp-Ala- in the subcomponent Clq of complement (Reid, 1977; Reid & Thompson, 1978), and one sequence of -X-Hyl-Ser- or -X-Hyl-Ala- in some collagens in the short non-triple-helical sequences at the ends of the α-chains (see Gallop & Paz, 1975; Fietzek & Kühn, 1976; Piez, 1976). 3-Hydroxyproline has been identified in collagens only in the sequence -Gly-3Hyp-4Hyp-Gly- (Gryder et al, 1975; Fietzek & Kühn, 1976), and in agreement with this, prolyl 3-hydroxylase appears to require a -Pro-4Hyp-Gly- triplet, whereas a -Pro-Pro-Gly- triplet is probably not hydroxylated (Tryggvason et al, 1977).

The interaction with prolyl 4-hydroxylase and lysyl hydroxylase is further affected by the amino acid in the X position of the -X-Y-Gly- triplet to be hydroxylated, and interaction with all three enzymes is influenced by amino acids in other parts of the peptide, by peptide chain length and by the peptide conformation (see Cardinale & Udenfriend, 1974; Prockop et al, 1976; Risteli et al, 1977; Kivirikko & Myllylä, 1980). The effect of the nature of the amino acid in the X position of the same triplet is seen in most cases in the maximal velocity (V) of the prolyl 4-hydroxylase or lysyl hydroxylase reaction, whereas the main effect of an increasing chain length is a decrease in the K_m of the peptide (see Prockop et al, 1976; Kivirikko & Myllylä, 1980). The conformation of the substrate has a marked effect, in that triple-helical peptides do not serve as substrates for any of the three hydroxylases. This indicates that the hydroxylations in the cell must occur before triple helix formation in the proα chains.

Co-substrates and reaction mechanisms. Prolyl 4-hydroxylase, lysyl hydroxylase and prolyl 3-hydroxylase all require Fe^{2+}, 2-oxoglutarate, 0_2 and ascorbate. They all decarboxylate 2-oxoglutarate, one atom of the 0_2 molecule being incorporated into the succinate while the other is incorporated into the hydroxyl group (see Cardinale & Udenfriend, 1974; Prockop et al, 1976; Risteli et al, 1977; Kivirikko & Myllylä, 1980). These reactions can thus be described by the following equation:

$$\text{Substrayte-H} + O_2 + \begin{array}{c} COOH \\ | \\ CH_2 \\ | \\ CH_2 \\ | \\ CO \\ | \\ COOH \end{array} \xrightarrow[\text{Ascorbate}]{Fe^{2+}} \text{Substrate-OH} + \begin{array}{c} COOH \\ | \\ CH_2 \\ | \\ CH_2 \\ | \\ COOH \end{array} + CO_2$$

The kinetic constants of the three enzymes for their co-substrates are very similar (see Kivirikko & Myllylä, 1980), and the catalytic-centre activities of about 3–6 mol/mol/s determined for pure prolyl 4-hydroxylase (Berg & Prockop, 1973; Kuutti et al, 1975; Tuderman et al, 1975; Berg et al, 1977; Nietfeld & Kemp, 1980) and lysyl hydroxylase (Turpeenniemi-Hujanen et al, 1980, 1981) are likewise similar. Several bivalent cations, citric acid cycle intermediates and certain other compounds inhibit the hydroxylations competitively with respect to some of the co-substrates, the inhibition constants of these compounds for prolyl 4-hydroxylase and lysyl hydroxylase again being very similar (Rapaka et al, 1976; Ryhänen, 1976; Murray et al, 1977; Tuderman et al, 1977a; Vistica et al, 1977; Myllylä et al, 1979b; Puistola et al, 1980b). Extensive kinetic studies and other data on the mechanisms of the prolyl 4-hydroxylase and lysyl hydroxylase reactions are consistent with an ordered binding of Fe^{2+}, 2-oxoglutarate, 0_2 and the peptide substrate to the enzyme in this order, and an ordered release of the hydroxylated peptide, CO_2, succinate and Fe^{2+}, in which Fe^{2+} need not leave the enzyme during every catalytic cycle and in which the order of release of the hydroxylated peptide and CO_2 is uncertain (Hobza et al, 1973; Tuderman et al, 1977a; Myllylä et al, 1977b; Puistola et al, 1980a, b). The oxygen must evidently be activated, probably to superoxide (Myllylä et al 1979b). The activated oxygen is capable of catalyzing an uncoupled decarboxylation of 2-oxoglutarate at a low rate in the absence of the polypeptide substrate (Cardinale & Udenfriend, 1974; Tuderman et al, 1977a; Counts et al, 1978; Rao & Adams, 1978; Puistola et al, 1980a), but the details of this reaction are not known.

Ascorbate is a quite specific requirement for pure prolyl 4-hydroxylase and highly purified lysyl hydroxylase, but dithiothreitol, L-cysteine and some reduced pteridines in high concentrations can partially replace this vitamin (Myllylä et al, 1978; Kivirikko & Myllylä, 1980; Puistola et al, 1980a). A low rate of hydroxylation has also been found in several cultured cells in the complete absence of ascorbate (see Evans & Peterkofsky, 1976; Kao et al, 1976; Nolan et al, 1978a), and evidence has been presented to suggest that this is due to an unidentified reductant rather than cysteine or tetrahydropteridine (Peterkofsky et al, 1980). Ascorbate is not consumed stoichiometrically during the hydroxylation, and prolyl 4-hydroxylase and lysyl hydroxylase can catalyze their reactions for a number of catalytic cycles in the complete absence of this vitamin

(Tuderman et al, 1977a; Myllylä et al, 1978; Puistola et al, 1980a; Nietfeld & Kemp, 1981). These findings together with the kinetic data suggest that the ascorbate reaction is required to reduce either the enzyme-iron complex or the free enzyme, which may be oxidized by a side-reaction during some catalytic cycles, but not the majority (Myllylä et al, 1978; Puistola et al, 1980b). Additional studies are nevertheless required to elucidate the role of ascorbate in these reactions.

Functions. The hydroxyl groups of the 4-hydroxyprolyl residues have an important function in collagens in that they stabilize the triple helix under physiological conditions (see Prockop et al, 1976, 1979; Fessler & Fessler, 1978; Bornstein & Traub, 1979). Non-hydroxylated proα chains can fold into a triple helix at low temperatures, but the transition temperature (T_m) for the unfolding of such molecules is only about 24°C, a value about 15°C lower than the T_m for molecules consisting of hydroxylated proα chains. Accordingly, non-hydroxylated proα chains cannot form triple-helical molecules at body temperature, and an almost complete 4-hydroxylation of prolyl residues in the Y positions of the -X-Y-Gly- triplets is required for the formation of a molecule which is stable at 37°C. It seems probable that 4-hydroxyproline has a similar function in other proteins which have a collagen-like primary structure. The role of the 3-hydroxyproline is not known.

The hydroxyl groups of the hydroxylysyl residues have two important functions: they serve as sites of attachment for carbohydrate units and they are essential for the stability of the intermolecular collagen cross-links (see below). The significance of lysyl hydroxylation is clearly seen in patients with the type VI variant of the Ehlers-Danlos syndrome, in which genetic lysyl hydroxylase deficiency leads to a connective tissue disorder with profound changes in the mechanical properties of the tissues (Ch. 16).

Glycosylation of hydroxylysyl residues

The only carbohydrate prosthetic groups in mammalian interstitial collagens are present in O-glycosidic linkage to hydroxylysyl residues. Part of the carbohydrate is found as the monosaccharide galactose and part as the disaccharide glucosylgalactose, the structure of the disaccharide unit with its peptide attachment being 2-O-α-D-glucopyranosyl-O-β-D-galactopyranosylhydroxylysine (Fig. 6.2), thus involving an unusual $\alpha 1 \rightarrow$ 2-O-glycoside bond between the glucose and galactose (see Kivirikko & Myllylä, 1979). The formation of these carbohydrate units is catalyzed by two specific enzymes, first hydroxylysyl galactosyltransferase (E.C. 2.4.1.50), transferring galactose to hydroxylysyl residues, and then galactosylhydroxylysyl glucosyltransferase (E.C. 2.4.9.66.), transferring glucose to galactosylhydroxylysyl residues (see Kivirikko & Myllylä, 1979).

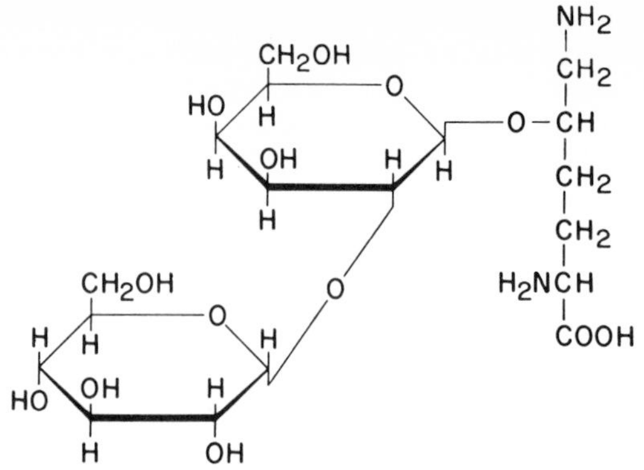

Fig. 6.2 The structure of 2-O-α-D-glucopyranosyl-O-β-D-galactopyranosylhydroxylysine

Purification and molecular properties of the hydroxylysyl glycosyltransferases. The highest degrees of purification for both transferases have been reported from extract of whole chick embryo homogenate, the galactosyltransferase having been purified about 1000-fold (L. Risteli et al, 1976b) and the glucosyltransferase having been isolated as a homogeneous protein (Myllylä et al, 1977a; Anttinen et al, 1978a). Lower degrees of purification for the latter enzyme have been obtained from several other sources, including chick embryo cartilage (Myllylä, et al, 1976), bovine arterial tissue (Henkel & Buddecke, 1975), human foetal tissues (Anttinen et al, 1977a) and human plasma and platelets (Leunis et al, 1980). No significant differences have been found in the properties of the enzymes from various sources. Recent studies with antiserum to pure chick-embryo galactosylhydroxylysyl glucosyltransferase and enzyme from a number of chick-embryo tissues have given results similar to those described above for lysyl hydroxylase, and thus do not support the concept that this enzyme may have tissue-specific isoenzymes with markedly different specific activities (Myllylä, 1981). The possible existence of isoenzymes of the hydroxylysyl glycosyltransferases nevertheless requires further elucidation.

The activity of the partially purified galactosyltransferase is found in gel filtration to fall into two major species, with apparent molecular weights of about 450 000 and 200 000 (L. Risteli et al, 1976a). The glucosyltransferase consists of only one polypeptide chain and has a molecular weight of about 70 000 (Myllylä et al, 1977a). Both transferases, like the three hydroxylases (see above), are probably glycoproteins (Anttinen et al, 1977a; Myllylä et al, 1977a; Risteli, 1978), and their activities require the presence of free sulphydryl groups, probably at the catalytic sites (see Menashi et al, 1976; Myllylä et al, 1976; L. Risteli et al, 1976a).

Requirements for the peptide substrates. Hydroxylysyl galactosyltransferase does not act on free hydroxylysine, whereas galactosylhydroxylysyl glucosyltransferase can act on free galactosylhydroxylysine, although such a reaction apparently does not occur in vivo (for references on substrate requirements, see Kivirikko & Myllylä, 1979). Presence of the free ϵ-amino group in the hydroxylysyl residue seems to be an absolute requirement for both transferases, since its N-acetylation or deamination completely prevents galactose transfer to hydroxylysyl residues and glucose transfer to galactosylhydroxylysyl residues. The reactions with both enzymes are further influenced by the peptide chain length, longer peptides being better substrates than shorter ones, and possibly by the amino acid sequence around the hydroxylysyl residue. The latter factor may only be a relative one, however, as most of the hydroxylysyl residues have the disaccharide unit in some collagens. The reaction with both hydroxylysyl glycosyltransferases is completely prevented by the triple-helical conformation in the substrate (Myllylä et al, 1975; L. Risteli et al, 1976a; Menashi et al, 1976; Anttinen et al, 1977b), indicating that these two glycosylations, like the three hydroxylations (above), must occur before triple helix formation in the cell.

Co-substrates and reaction mechanism. The preferential sugar donor for both hydroxylysyl glycosyltransferases is the corresponding UDP-glycoside, and both reactions require the presence of a bivalent cation. The cation requirement is best fulfilled by manganese (see Kivirikko & Myllylä, 1979), but Fe^{2+} and Co^{2+} can also serve as metal cofactors for highly purified glucosyltransferase in vitro (Myllylä et al, 1979a). It is possible that Fe^{2+} can also act as a physiological cofactor in vivo in addition to Mn^{2+} (Myllylä et al, 1979a), but the metal requirements of both transferases can be fulfilled in isolated cells even in the absence of Fe^{2+} (Anttinen & Hulkko, 1980). By contrast, Co^{2+} does not show any activity in concentrations comparable to its tissue levels (Myllylä et al, 1979a). The reaction product, UDP, several other nucleotides and several bivalent cations are inhibitors of the hydroxylysyl glycosyltransferases (see Kivirikko & Myllylä, 1979; Myllylä et al, 1979a).

Galactosylhydroxylysyl glucosyltransferase probably operates predominantly through an ordered mechanism: Mn^{2+}, UDP-glucose and collagen are bound to the enzyme in this order, and the products are released in the order glycosylated collagen, UDP and Mn^{2+}, in which Mn^{2+} need not leave the enzyme during every catalytic cycle (Myllylä, 1976; D. F. Smith et al, 1977; Myllylä et al, 1979a). There seem to be at least two Mn^{2+} binding sites on the enzyme, with dissociation constants of 3–5 μM (site I) and 50–70 μM (site II), and at high Mn^{2+} concentrations the enzyme appears to bind successively two Mn^{2+} ions before the binding of UDP-glucose (Myllylä et al, 1979a). Both hydroxylysyl glycosyltransferases can catalyze their reactions in the absence of any lipid in vitro, and attempts to detect a possible lipid intermediate in tissue extracts or crude enzyme preparations have given no evidence for its presence (see Kivirikko & Myllylä, 1979).

Functions. The functions of the hydroxylysyl-linked carbohydrate units are uncertain. These form the most extrusive groups in the collagen molecule, and it has therefore been speculated that they may have some role in the organization of the fibrils. This suggestion is supported by the findings that there is an inverse relationship between carbohydrate content and fibril diameter (see Kivirikko & Myllylä, 1979), and that native fibrils of type II collagen are more swollen with water than those of type I (see Eyre, 1980). Hydroxylysyl residues participating in collagen cross-links can be glycosylated (see Kivirikko & Myllylä, 1979), but it is not known whether the glycosylation has any effect on cross-link formation or the properties of the cross-links. A partial deficiency in galactosylhydroxylysyl glucosyltransferase activity has recently been found in one family in association with dominantly-inherited generalized epidermolysis bullosa simplex, a disease characterized by serous non-scarring blistering of the skin after minor trauma (Savolainen et al, 1981). Detailed studies on these patients may give information on the role of the glucosyl units in collagen.

Glycosylation of the propeptides

The propeptides of procollagen contain asparaginyl-linked oligosaccharide units which are not found in the collagen domain of the molecule (Murphy et al, 1975; Clark & Kefalides, 1976, 1978). In type I procollagen the majority, if not all, of these carbohydrates are present in the carboxy-terminal propeptides (Duksin & Bornstein, 1977; Clark & Kefalides, 1978; Clark, 1979), whereas in type II procollagen such units are found in both the carboxy-terminal and amino-terminal propeptides (Guzman et al, 1978). The carboxy-terminal propeptides of both the proα1(I) and proα2(I) chains appear each to contain a single oligosaccharide unit, linked to an asparaginyl residue and consisting of two residues of N-acetylglucosamine and about 10 residues of mannose (Olsen et al, 1977; Clark, 1979). This asparaginyl residue is present in the chick proα1(I) chain in the sequence -Asn-Val-Thr- (Showalter et al, 1980), agreeing with the general requirement of a sequence -Asn-X-Ser/Thr- for the glycosylation of a number of proteins at an asparaginyl residue (see Hart et al, 1979).

The biosynthesis of asparaginyl-linked carbohydrate units in other proteins is initiated by the en bloc transfer of a pre-formed oligosaccharide from a lipid carrier to the nascent polypeptide chain. This oligosaccharide may then be processed further within the rough and smooth endoplasmic reticulum and the Golgi complex (see Waechter & Lennarz, 1976; Li et al, 1978; Kornfeld et al, 1978; Tabas & Kornfeld, 1978). The glycosylation of procollagen likewise involves a lipid intermediate (Duksin

& Bornstein, 1977; Tanzer et al, 1977) and occurs within the rough endoplasmic reticulum (Anttinen et al, 1978b; Clark & Kefalides, 1978; Guzman et al, 1978), but it is not known whether in this case further processing occurs within other cell compartments.

The functions of the asparaginyl-linked oligosaccharide units of procollagen are unknown. Some studies suggest that this glycosylation is required for a normal rate of procollagen secretion from the cell (Tanzer et al, 1977; Housley et al, 1980), whereas others do not support this suggestion (Duksin & Bornstein, 1977; Olden et al, 1978).

Chain association, disulphide bonding and triple helix formation

The propeptides of procollagen contain cysteine, which is not found in type I and II collagens. The cysteine forms only intra-chain disulphide bonds in the amino-terminal propeptides of these collagen types, whereas in the carboy-terminal propeptides it is also involved in the inter-chain disulphide bonds (Fig. 6.3). In type III procollagen both the amino-terminal and carboxy-terminal propeptides are linked by inter-chain disulphide bonds, and this collagen type also contains two inter-chain disulphide bridges at the carboxy-terminal end of the triple-helical region of the collagen domain (for reviews on procollagen structure, see Prockop et al, 1979; Fessler & Fessler, 1978; Bornstein & Traub, 1978; Eyre, 1980).

Freedman, 1978; Brockway et al, 1980), but there is no direct evidence to demonstrate whether it is involved in the formation of the disulphide bonds of procollagen.

The triple helix formation appears to have two requirements: at least about 100 prolyl residues per proα chain must have been 4-hydroxylated (see function of 4-hydroxyproline, above) and probably the inter-chain disulphide bonds must have been formed between the carboxy-terminal propeptides (when studied in type I and II procollagens). Evidence for the latter requirement was obtained from the finding that the reduction of disulphide bonds in intact cells prevents triple helix formation in a reversible manner (see Prockop et al, 1976). Model studies on collagen triple helix formation in vitro also indicate an inter-chain disulphide bond requirement for rapid helix formation (Bruckner et al, 1978). It has further been demonstrated that a close correlation exists between the time required for disulphide bonding and triple helix formation in isolated chick embryo tendon and cartilage cells (Prockop et al, 1976). The time required for these processes varies greatly from one cell type to another, being shortest, only few minutes, in tendon cells synthesizing type I collagen, intermediate in cartilage cells synthesizing type II collagen, and longest, of the order of one hour, in various cells synthesizing basement membrane collagens (see Grant & Jackson, 1976; Kivirikko & Risteli, 1976; Prockop et al, 1976, 1979; Fessler & Fessler, 1978). At low

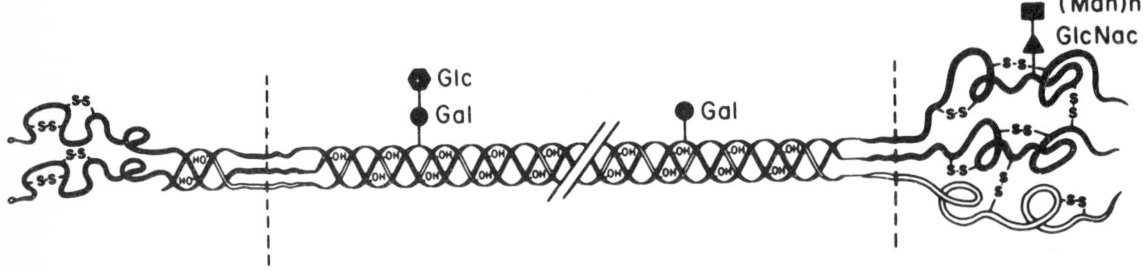

Fig. 6.3 Schematic presentation of the structure of the procollagen molecule. Abbreviations: Glc, glucose; Gal, galactose; Man, mannose, GlcNac, N-acetylglucosamine. Reproduced from Prockop et al (1979) by permission of the publisher.

It seems likely that the propeptides begin to fold into their appropriate secondary and tertiary structure soon after synthesis, and their conformations then determine the association of the three polypeptide chains (see Prockop et al, 1976). The inter-chain disulphide bonds are formed after the association of the propeptides, but, as with other proteins containing disulphide bonds, it is not known whether the synthesis of these linkages requires an enzyme or whether it occurs spontaneously. An enzyme, protein-disulphide isomerase, catalyzes the rearrangement of random 'incorrect' pairs of half-cystine residues, and may function to ensure a rapid attainment of native-disulphide bonds during protein synthesis (see Freedman, 1979). This enzyme activity is found in microsomal fractions of isolated cells or tissues actively synthesizing collagen (Harwood &

temperatures the slow *cis* → *trans* isomerization of the peptide bonds may restrict the rate of triple helix formation considerably, but at 37°C isomerization seems to occur at a rate comparable with that of translation (Bächinger et al, 1978).

Intracellular sites of the modifications

The pre-proα chains are synthesized on membrane-bound ribosomes (Fig. 6.4), and while being assembled pass through the membranes into the cisternae of the rough endoplasmic reticulum (see Chapter 6 and Grant & Jackson, 1976; Prockop et al, 1976, 1979; Fessler & Fessler, 1978; Bornstein & Traub, 1979). The pre-protein sequences are cleaved within the membrane at an early stage of biosynthesis (see above).

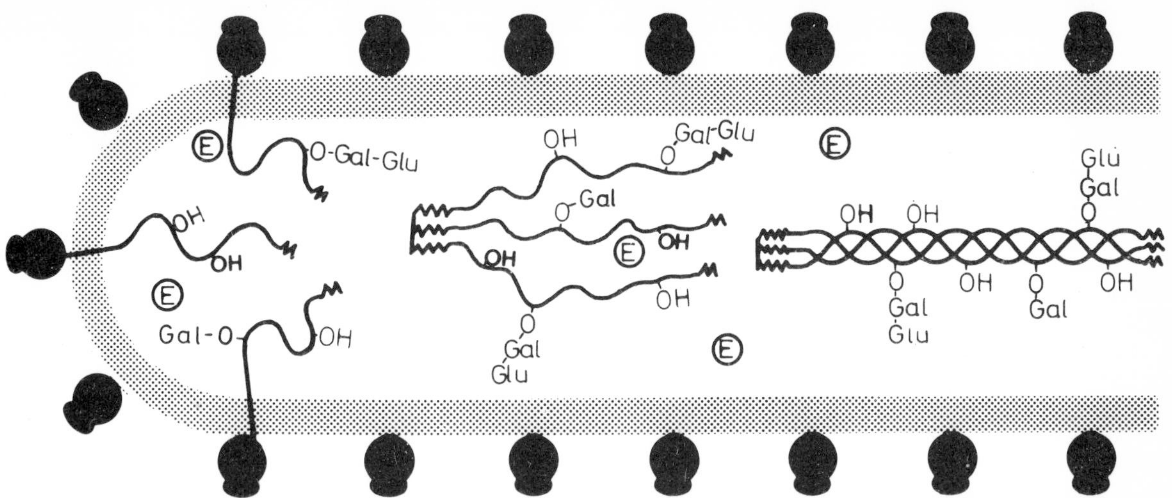

Fig. 6.4 Schematic presentation of the intracellular events in collagen biosynthesis. The figure does not show the presence of the amino-terminal pre-protein sequences and their cleavage within the membrane at an early stage of biosynthesis (see text). The scheme indicates that the hydroxylations of prolyl and lysyl residues and the glycosylations of the hydroxylysyl residues are initiated while the polypeptide chains are being assembled on the ribosomes and continue after the synthesis of complete proα chains up to formation of the triple helix. The formation of the inter-chain disulphide bonds between the carboxy-terminal propeptides is also shown. E = enzyme. Reproduced from Kivirikko & Myllylä, (1979) by permission of the publisher.

Prolyl 4-hydroxylase and lysyl hydroxylase have been located within the cisternae of the rough endoplasmic reticulum, prolyl 4-hydroxylase being either free within the cisternae or loosely bound to the inner membrane, and lysyl hydroxylase probably being in part either free or loosely bound and in part tightly bound (see Prockop et al, 1976; Ryhänen, 1976; Peterkofsky & Assad, 1979; Kivirikko & Myllylä, 1980). Prolyl 3-hydroxylase (Risteli et al, 1977) and the two hydroxylysyl glycosyltransferases (see Kivirikko & Myllylä, 1979) are probably likewise located within the cisternae. Most of the hydroxylations of prolyl and lysyl residues and the glycosylations of hydroxylysyl residues takes place while the polypeptide chains are growing on the ribosomes, but these reactions are continued after the release of complete proα chains from the ribosomes, until triple helix formation prevents any further hydroxylation and hydroxylysyl glycosylations (see Kivirikko & Myllylä, 1979, 1980; Anttinen & Hulkko, 1980; Majamaa, 1981, Pihlajaniemi et al, 1981). In some experimental cases, however, all the hydroxylation and hydroxylysyl glycosylation has been found to take place after the release of the completed polypeptide chains from the ribosomes. Such a situation has been demonstrated by incubating cells or tissues under conditions in which the hydroxylations are inhibited, and subsequently reversing this inhibition. During the inhibition period the cells synthesize non-hydroxylated proα chains, which accumulate within the cisternae of the rough endoplasmic reticulum, and which are hydroxylated and glycosylated during the reversal (see Prockop et al, 1976; Kivirikko & Myllylä, 1979, 1980). The glycosylation of the propeptides likewise occurs within the rough endoplasmic reticulum, but it is not known whether further processing of these oligosaccharide units takes places within the smooth endoplasmic reticulum and the Golgi complex (see above).

Translocation and secretion of procollagen

Procollagen follows the classical route of secretion taken by other extracellular proteins, and passes through the Golgi complex (see Prockop et al, 1976). The conformation of the procollagen markedly affects the secretion rate. If triple helix formation is prevented, the non-helical proα chains first accumulate within the cisternae of the rough endoplasmic reticulum and are then secreted at a delayed rate (see Prockop et al, 1976; Kao et al, 1977, 1979; Jimenez & Yankowski, 1978). Such a situation has been demonstrated in a number of studies with isolated cells or tissues by excluding some of the co-substrates of the hydroxylases. For example, the cells can be incubated under conditions in which intracellular iron is chelated or the supply of oxygen is limited or ascorbate is absent. Another technique for demonstrating this situation is to incubate cells or tissues with certain proline analogues such as *cis*-4-hydroxyproline or azetidine-2-carboxylic acid, which are incorporated into protein. The proα chains synthesized under all these conditions are normal in size and are disulphide bonded, but they do not become triple-helical (see Prockop et al, 1976, 1979). It is not known why the non-helical proα chains are secreted at a delayed rate, but it seems possible that the secretion is influenced by an interaction of procollagen with prolyl hydroxylase and other post-translational enzymes (see Kao et al, 1977, 1979; Jimenez & Yankowski, 1978). These bind to non-helical proα chains but do not interact with triple-helical procollagen (see above), and thus the non-helical protein may remain in equilibrium with the post-translational enzymes within the cisternae of the rough endoplasmic reticulum.

The secretion of procollagen requires metabolic energy in the form of ATP (Kruse & Bornstein, 1975; Harwood et al, 1976). Studies on the inhibition of secretion by colchicine, vinblastine and other agents suggest that microtubuli and microfilaments are involved in the secretory process (see Bornstein & Traub, 1979; Prockop et al, 1979).

The form in which procollagen is secreted is not known, but a number of observations suggest that it may be packed into structured aggregates inside the cell, carried to the cell surface and exocytosed in the form of such aggregates (e.g. Weinstock & Leblond, 1974; Trelstadt et al, 1976; Weinstock, 1977; Bruns et al, 1979; Trelstadt & Hayashi, 1979). Aggregation would probably also increase the thermal stability of the procollagen, and thus protect individual molecules against denaturation at body temperature. This may be important, as the transition temperature (T_m) for the unfolding of monomeric procollagen is only about 40°C (Hayashi et al, 1979; Peltonen et al, 1980). One study gave no evidence for the existence of such aggregates in the medium of chick embryo fibroblasts, but did not exclude the possibility that procollagen within the cells and associated with the cells could be in an aggregated form (Hayashi et al, 1979).

Extracellular modifications

Conversion of procollagen to collagen

The conversion of procollagen to collagen requires at least two enzymes, one to remove the amino-terminal propeptides and the other the carboxy-terminal propeptides.

Purification and properties of procollagen proteases. The amino-terminal protease has been purified about 300 to 2000-fold from chick embryo tendon extract (Tuderman et al, 1978; L. Tuderman and D. J. Prockop, unpublished) and to a lower extent from calf tendons (Kohn et al, 1974). The molecular weight of the chick-embryo tendon enzyme is about 200 000 by gel filtration (Tuderman et al, 1978). The carboxy-terminal protease has been shown to have a lower molecular weight, but this enzyme has been characterized only preliminarily (Leung et al, 1979). Both proteases are probably glycoproteins (Duksin et al, 1978; Tuderman et al, 1978).

Procollagen proteases are endopeptidases. They act at a neutral pH and require the presence of a bivalent cation such as calcium (Kohn et al, 1974; Goldberg et al, 1975; Uitto, 1977; Tuderman et al, 1978; Leung et al, 1979). Both enzymes can act on both monomeric and aggregated procollagen molecules (Leung et al, 1979). Heat-denaturation of procollagen markedly reduces the rate of cleavage by the amino-terminal protease, indicating a triple-helical substrate conformation requirement (Kohn et al, 1974; Tuderman et al, 1978). Certain synthetic peptides with sequences similar to the cleavage site in the proα1(I) chain are inhibitors of this enzyme (Morikawa et al, 1980). The chick-embryo tendon amino-terminal protease, isolated from a system synthesizing only type I procollagen, cleaves both type I and type II procollagens (Tuderman et al, 1978), whereas a separate enzyme is involved in the processing of type III procollagen (Fessler & Fessler, 1979; Nusgens et al, 1980; L. Tuderman and D. J. Prockop, unpublished).

Processing of various procollagens by intact tissues or cells. The conversion of procollagen to collagen probably occurs in the extracellular space. This assumption is based on kinetic data indicating that the cleavage of procollagen occurs coincident with or subsequent to secretion (e.g. Davidson et al, 1975; Morris et al, 1975; Leung et al, 1979; Uitto et al, 1979) and on observations demonstrating that in freshly-isolated or cultured fibroblasts intact procollagen molecules are secreted by the cells and subsequently processed (e.g. Taubman & Goldberg, 1976; Uitto & Lichtenstein, 1976; Goldberg 1977; Uitto, 1977). Furthermore, incubation of tissues with an iron chelator, proline analogues or colchicine, agents which delay procollagen secretion, also inhibits the conversion (Uitto et al, 1979).

In many systems synthesizing type I procollagen, the amino-terminal propeptides are cleaved before the carboxy-terminal propeptides (Davidson et al, 1975; 1977; Fessler et al, 1975; Uitto et al, 1976). In the biosynthesis of type II procollagen in chick-embryo sterna, however, some conversion occurs in the opposite order (Uitto et al, 1979), and in the case of type III procollagen synthesized by chick-embryo blood vessels, the carboxy-terminal propeptides are cleaved off first (Fessler & Fessler, 1979). It seems likely that there is no preferential sequence of cleavage, the order being at least in part determined by the ratio of various procollagen protease activities in the tissue.

There are differences between type I and III procollagens in their rates of conversion by the same cultured cells (Benya et al, 1977; Goldberg, 1977; Wu et al, 1978; Limeback & Sodek, 1979) or intact tissue (B. D. Smith et al, 1977; Fessler & Fessler, 1979), type III procollagen being processed at a slower rate. In the case of type IV collagen, no processing of the newly-synthesized polypeptide chains has been observed in vitro (Minor et al, 1976; Heathcote et al, 1978; Kefalides et al, 1979; Alitalo et al, 1980; Crouch et al, 1980; Tryggvason et al, 1980a), but conversion to shorter chains may take place in vivo (Tryggvason et al, 1980a, b).

Functions. The conversion of procollagen to collagen appears to be necessary for the formation of native-type collagen fibrils (see Bornstein & Traub, 1979; Prockop et al, 1979). Evidence for this requirement has been obtained especially in animals with dermatosparaxis and patients with the type VII variant of the Ehlers-Danlos syndrome, in which a genetic defect in the removal of the amino-terminal propeptides results in impaired fibril formation (Ch. 16). The amino-terminal propeptides, after they have been cleaved off from the procollagen, may also act as feedback regulators for cellular collagen synthesis. This suggestion is based on observations that amino-terminal propeptides reduce the rate of procollagen synthesis when added to either cells in culture (Krieg et al, 1978; Wiestner et al, 1979) or to procollagen mRNA in a cell-free system (Paglia et al, 1979).

Ordered aggregation of collagen molecules into collagen fibrils

The collagen molecules formed by removal of the propeptides assemble spontaneously in a specific manner to form collagen fibrils. This process does not require any enzyme and will occur easily in a collagen solution in vitro. Such fibrils are indistinguishable from those found in intact tissues on electron optical and X-ray diffraction criteria, with the exception of the fibril diameter and length. It has seemed likely, therefore, that physical chemical studies in vitro will give useful information on fibril formation. The assembly is a multi-step process, involving at least initiation, linear growth and lateral growth (e.g. Gelman et al, 1979; Silver & Trelstadt, 1979; Silver et al, 1979).

The non-helical ends of the collagen molecule affect both the kinetics of the assembly and the morphology of the product (see Comper & Veis, 1977a, b; Gelman et al, 1979).

It is not known, however, to what extent the results of the in vitro studies can be applied to the situation in vivo, as the other connective tissue components may affect the rate of the process and the length and diameter of the fibrils. Also, if procollagen is secreted in the form of ordered aggregates (see above), it is possible that processing may lead to structures that are incorporated into the fibrils directly.

Cross-link formation

The newly-formed collagen fibrils are cross-linked by a series of co-valent bonds. This process requires oxidative deamination of ϵ-amino groups in certain lysyl and hydroxylysyl residues catalyzed by lysyl oxidase (see Siegel, 1979) to give reactive aldehydes (Fig. 6.5).

Purification and properties of lysyl oxidase. Lysyl oxidase has been purified to near homogeneity or homogeneity from several sources (e.g. Harris et al, 1974; Narayanan et al, 1974; Shieh & Yasunobu, 1976; Siegel & Fu, 1976; Stassen, 1976; Siegel et al, 1978; Han & Tanzer, 1979; Kagan et al, 1979). Preparations of the enzyme from all tissues studied to date are heterogeneous, with multiple peaks of activity in DEAE chromatography, the molecular weight of most species being approximately 30 000 or a multiple thereof (above references and Siegel, 1979). The

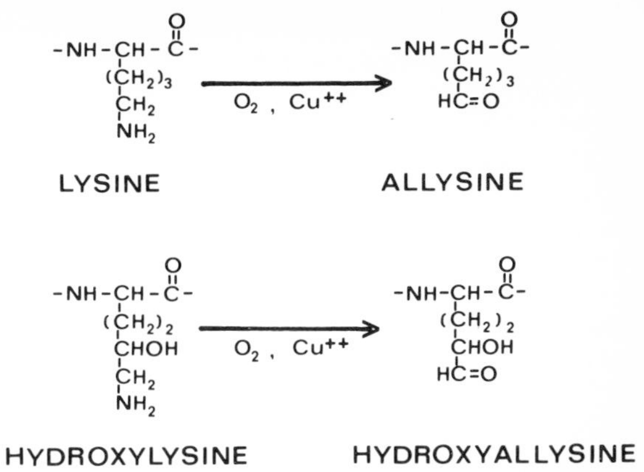

$$-NH-CH(-(CH_2)_3-CH_2-NH_2)-C(=O)- \xrightarrow{O_2,\ Cu^{++}} -NH-CH(-(CH_2)_3-HC{=}O)-C(=O)-$$

LYSINE ALLYSINE

$$-NH-CH(-(CH_2)_2-CHOH-CH_2-NH_2)-C(=O)- \xrightarrow{O_2,\ Cu^{++}} -NH-CH(-(CH_2)_2-CHOH-HC{=}O)-C(=O)-$$

HYDROXYLYSINE HYDROXYALLYSINE

Fig. 6.5 Schematic presentation of the lysyl oxidase reaction.

reasons for the multiple forms are unknown, but they may be related to limited degradation of the enzyme during purification or to variable aggregation (Siegel, 1979).

Lysyl oxidase is a copper-containing protein (see Siegel, 1979), this cation probably being in the cupric form (Shieh & Yasunobu, 1976). The enzyme requires molecular oxygen (see Siegel, 1979) and possibly pyridoxal (Murray & Levene, 1977), but the evidence for the latter is not definitive (Siegel, 1979). The activity is inhibited by copper chelators, by carbonyl reagents such as phenyl hydrazine, isoniazid and hydroxylamine and by lathyrogens such as β-aminopropionitrile (see Siegel, 1979). The lathyrogens are irreversible, non-competitive inhibitors that probably become covalently bound to the enzyme during inactivation (Siegel, 1979).

Lysyl oxidase catalyzes the initial reaction in the synthesis of cross-links of both collagen and elastin. Highly purified enzymes from several tissues utilize both of these proteins as substrates, there being no difference in the substrate specificity between the multiple enzyme forms (Siegel & Fu, 1976; Stassen, 1976; Siegel, 1979). The highest activity is seen with reconstituted collagen fibrils (Siegel & Fu, 1976), coacervates of elastin or certain synthetic peptides, and possibly other ordered molecular aggregates of soluble elastin (Narayanan et al, 1978; Siegel, 1979; Kagan et al, 1980). A single enzyme acts on both lysyl and hydroxylysyl residues, the activity being greater with hydroxylysyl residues (Siegel, 1976).

Formation of co-valent cross-links. The aldehydes generated in the lysyl oxidase reaction can form either intramolecular cross-links by aldol condensation of two of the aldehydes or intermolecular cross-links by condensation between an aldehyde and an ϵ-amino group from a second lysyl, hydroxylysyl or glycosylated hydroxylysyl residue (see Bailey et al, 1974; Tanzer, 1976; Ranta, 1978; Bornstein & Traub, 1979; Eyre, 1980). The cross-links built up of a hydroxylysine-derived aldehyde are more stable than those built up of a lysine-derived aldehyde, possibly due to the migration of the double bond to a stable keto form. Most cross-linking amino acids have been identified after chemical reduction by tritiated sodium borohydride, which stabilizes them during acid hydrolysis and labels them with tritium for isolation. The reducible cross-links of collagen and their formation are summarized in Figure 6.6. It should be noted that there is controversy over whether histidine participates in the cross-links in vivo or whether the histidine-containing cross-links are artefacts of borohydride reduction (Robins & Bailey, 1977). The presence of hydroxymerodesmosine as a collagen cross-link has likewise been debated (Robins & Bailey, 1977).

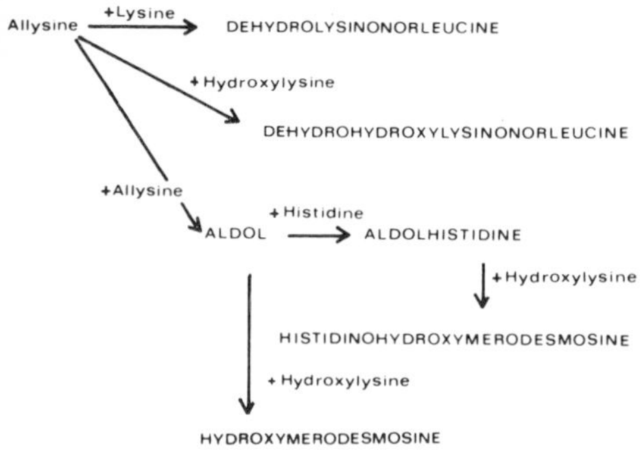

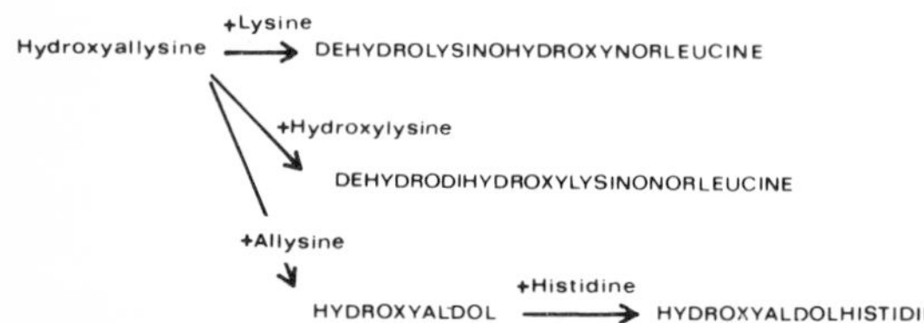

Fig. 6.6 Reducible collagen cross-links and their formation. It should be noted that there is controversy over whether hydroxymerodesmosine and the histidine-containing cross-links are present in collagen in vivo (see text).

The reducible cross-links gradually disappear from adult collagen, suggesting that they are long-lived intermediates which can react further (Bailey et al, 1974; Eyre, 1980). The possibility of in vivo reduction has been studied intensively, but this mode of stabilization does not seem to take place in collagen (see Eyre, 1980). Other stabilization mechanisms have been presented more recently, one involving oxidation to yield a peptide bond (Bailey et al, 1977), one formation of a multivalent cross-link of unknown structure (Light & Bailey, 1979, 1980) and one involving interaction of two residues of hydroxylysino-5-oxo-norleucine to give a 3-hydroxy-pyridimin compound derived from three of the hydroxylysyl residues (Fujimoto et al, 1977, 1978; Fujimoto & Moriguchi, 1978; Eyre, 1980). The presence of the last-mentioned compound in collagen is controversial, however (Elsden et al, 1980). (See Ch. 9.)

Functions. The newly formed collagen fibrils do not have the necessary tensile strength until the cross-links are formed. This has been demonstrated in numerous studies on experimental osteolathyrism, an acquired molecular disease characterized by a marked fragility of growing connective tissues (Barrow et al, 1974; Kivirikko & Risteli, 1976; Bornstein & Traub, 1979; Minor, 1980). This disease can be induced by the administration of β-aminopropionitrile or other lathyrogens that inhibit lysyl oxidase activity (see above) and block the cross-linking of collagen and elastin. Impaired cross-linking is also found in animals with copper deficiency, in aneurysm-prone mice and in patients with an X-linked form of cutis laxa, the two latter diseases being due to a genetic deficiency in lysyl oxidase activity (Ch. 16).

REGULATION OF THE RATES AND EXTENTS OF THE MODIFICATIONS

A large number of events or factors can affect the rates of the individual modifying reactions and the extent to which the collagen is modified. In some cases, such as when triple helix formation is prevented, the synthesis of collagen fibrils is inhibited completely. In others there may be no effect on the overall rate of synthesis of collagen fibrils, but the properties of the fibrils may be affected profoundly. The review on the regulation aspect begins with a summary of some of the variability in the extents to which the collagens are modified.

Variability in the extents of the modifications

The genetically distinct collagen types (Chapter 2) have relatively small but distinct differences in their extents of prolyl 4-hydroxylation, whereas the extents of prolyl 3-hydroxylation, lysyl hydroxylation and the hydroxylysyl glycosylations and the ratio of galactosylhydroxylysyl to glucosylgalactosylhydroxylysyl residues show a marked variation (see Kivirikko & Myllylä, 1979, 1980). The modifications occur to the highest extents in type IV collagens from basement membranes, and to the lowest extent in type I collagen from adult tissues (Table 6.2).

An additional variation is found within the same collagen type from different tissues and even the same tissue in many physiological and pathological states (see Kivirikko & Myllylä, 1979, 1980). The term quality is used to indicate the variation in the extent of modification of a single collagen type. The 4-hydroxyproline content of a given collagen type varies only within narrow limits, apparently because of the function of 4-hydroxyproline (see above), whereas a marked variation is found in 3-hydroxyproline, total hydroxylysine, galactosylhydroxylysine and glucosylgalactosylhydroxylysine. The changes in the extent of lysyl hydroxylation are further reflected in changes in the ratios of hydroxylysyl to lysyl-derived cross-links.

Table 6.2 Variability in the extents of prolyl and lysyl hydroxylation and hydroxylysyl glycosylation between genetically distinct collagen types[a]

	Residues/1000 amino acid residues						
Type[b]	4-hyp	3-hyp	Pro	Total Hyl	Gal-Hyl	Glu-Gal-Hyl	Lys
I: chain $\alpha 1$	99	1	131	5	0.6	0.3	30
I: chain $\alpha 2$	89	1	113	8	1.5	0.3	24
II	100	2	122	23	4	5	13
III	128	1	109	5	0.1	0.8	30
IV[b, c]	130	11	61	45	2	32	10
V: chain αA[c]	109	3	97	24	3	5	18
V: chain αB[c]	109	3	118	35	5	29	20

[a] for references, see Kivirikko & Myllylä (1979, 1980) and Chapter 2.
[b] Type IV collagen consists of at least two genetically distinct polypeptide chains.
[c] Pepsin-solubilized type IV or V collagen.

High contents of hydroxylysine and glycosylated hydroxylysine in type I and/or III collagens in vivo have been reported in tissues of embryos or young animals (e.g. Barnes et al, 1974; Murai et al, 1975; Royce & Barnes, 1977), in scars (Bailey et al, 1975; Shuttleworth et al, 1975), in vitamin D or dietary calcium deficiency (see Royce & Barnes, 1977; Dickson et al, 1979) and in tissues of patients with osteogenesis imperfecta (see Trelstadt et al, 1977, and Ch. 16). A low content of 3-hydroxyproline in type IV collagen is found in the glomerular basement membrane of patients with congenital nephrotic syndrome of the Finnish type (Tryggvason et al, 1978), while a specific decrease in one of the modifications is present in patients or animals with lysyl hydroxylase, galactosylhydroxylysyl glucosyltransferase, procollagen amino-terminal protease or lysyl oxidase deficiency (Ch. 16).

A marked variability in collagen quality has also been demonstrated in experiments with freshly isolated or cultured cells. Type I collagen synthesized by freshly isolated chick embryo tendon cells, for example, contains 17 total hydroxylysyl residues per 1000, about 3.5 of these having the disaccharide and 1.5 the monosaccharide unit (Oikarinen et al, 1976; Oikarinen et al, 1977). Similarly, type I collagen synthesized by cultured fibroblasts during cell attachment contains five 3-hydroxyprolyl residues per 1000 (Lembach et al, 1977; Schwartz et al, 1979). All these values are markedly higher than those given above for type I collagen from adult tissues.

Regulation of intracellular modifications

Changes in the concentrations of the active enzymes

Prolyl 4-hydroxylase activity has been found in a number of cultured cell types, both fibroblastic and non-fibroblastic, including cells of non-mesenchymal origin (Kivirikko & Myllylä, 1980). Some cells have prolyl 4-hydroxylase activity even though they do not synthesize any collagenous protein, some have this enzyme activity and produce collagenous polypeptide chains, but do not convert prolyl residues to 4-hydroxyproline, and some have relatively high prolyl 4-hydroxylase activity even though they synthesize only traces of collagenous polypeptide chains (Bates, 1976; Anttinen et al, 1977b; Kelleher et al, 1977; Chen-Kiang et al, 1978; Myllylä & Seppä, 1979). In all these cases prolyl 4-hydroxylase activity is clearly present in the cell in a large excess. In a number of other situations, however, the levels of prolyl 4-hydroxylase activity in cultured cells and intact tissues increase and decrease with the rates of collagen biosynthesis, there being marked differences in this enzyme activity between different cell types (Table 6.3) and even in the same cell type under various experimental conditions (see Kivirikko & Myllylä, 1980; Myllylä et al, 1981). Due to the good correlation between the level of prolyl 4-hydroxylase activity and the rate of collagen biosynthesis, assays of this enzyme activity have been used in numerous studies for estimating the rate of collagen biosynthesis in many experimental models and in patients with various diseases (for references, see Kivirikko & Myllylä, 1980). Prolyl 4-hydroxylase activity and immunoreactive enzyme protein are also present in human serum (see Kivirikko & Myllylä 1980), and assays of the latter have been suggested to be of value for estimating the rate of collagen synthesis in patients with liver and some other diseases (Tuderman et al, 1977c; Kuutti-Savolainen, 1979; Kuutti-Savolainen et al, 1979, 1980).

An interesting aspect of the regulation of prolyl 4-hydroxylase activity is that this enzyme protein is present in cells in two forms: the active enzyme tetramers and an inactive form which corresponds to the smaller subunit of the enzyme (i.e. the 60 000-molecular-weight β-subunit) both in size and in amino acid and peptide map analysis (see Chen-Kiang et al, 1977; Tuderman et al, 1977b; Kao & Berg, 1979; Majamaa et al, 1979; Berg et al, 1980). The concentration of the active enzyme tetramers in most cells and tissues is much lower than that of the β-subunit-related protein, and the ratio of active enzyme tetramers to total enzyme protein varies markedly between tissues and even in the same cell type or tissue in various conditions (e.g.

Table 6.3 Comparison of prolyl 4-hydroxylase, lysyl hydroxylase, hydroxylysyl galactosyltransferase and galactosylhydroxylysyl glucosyltransferase activities in different cell types.

Activities are expressed per unit extractable cell protein as relative values, taking the activity in freshly isolated chick-embryo tendon cells as 100. The values are obtained from the papers of Myllylä & Seppä (1979), Risteli et al (1979) and Myllylä et al (1981).

	Relative enzyme activity			
Cell type	Prolyl 4-hydroxylase	Lysyl hydroxylase	Galactosyl-transferase	Glucosyl-transferase
Freshly isolated				
Chick embryo tendon cell	100	100	100	100
Chick embryo cartilage cell	91	168	175	105
Rat peritoneal macrophage	3	4	32	24
Rat peritoneal mast cell	<0.1	<0.1	<1	<1
Cultured, non-transformed				
3T6, early log phase	4	7	36	41
late log phase	14	15	35	41
Chick-embryo tendon cell, late log phase	24	43	55	58
Human skin fibroblast[a], late log phase	12	15	66	66
Human lung fibroblast (WI-38)[b], late log phase	11	17	122	75
Cultured, transformed				
SV-40 transformed WI-38 cell[c], late log phase	4	9	62	35
Human rhabdomyosarcoma (RD) cell, late log phase	3	11	77	61

[a] Fibroblasts from adult human skin
[b] Fibroblasts from embryonic human lung
[c] Simian virus 40 transformed fibroblasts from embryonic human lung

Stassen et al, 1974; Kao et al, 1975; Tuderman, 1976; Tuderman & Kivirikko, 1977; Risteli et al, 1978; Kuutti-Savolainen & Kero, 1979). Usually a higher percentage of total prolyl 4-hydroxylase protein is in the form of the active tetramers under conditions in which the rate of collagen synthesis is increased.

Experiments involving labelling of the two forms of the enzyme protein in freshly isolated or cultured cells (Tuderman et al, 1977b; Berg et al, 1980; Kao & Chou, 1980) and in chick-embryo (Majamaa et al, 1979) or rabbit (Chichester et al, 1976, 1979) tissues in vivo have demonstrated that at least one function of the β-subunit related protein is to serve as a precursor of the β-subunits in the assembly of the prolyl 4-hydroxylase tetramer. The α-subunit seems to be utilized immediately to form the active enzyme, whereas the β-subunit is synthesized in an excess and enters a precursor pool of this subunit before being incorporated into the tetramer (Kao & Berg, 1979; Majamaa et al, 1979; Berg et al, 1980; Kao & Chou, 1980). Data demonstrating that the subunits can be assembled into the tetramer after their release from the ribosomes (Stassen et al, 1973; Tuderman et al, 1977b) are consistent with this mechanism. The synthesis of the α-subunit is probably regulated more effectively than that of the β-subunit, and this may explain the large variation in the ratio of the active tetramers to the total enzyme protein. It seems very likely that the β-subunit-related protein is processed in some way before being converted into the final subunit (Berg et al, 1980), an assumption supported by some minor but distinct differences found between these two proteins in peptide map analysis (Chen-Kiang et al, 1977; Berg et al, 1980).

The biological significance of the β-subunit-related protein has not been fully elucidated, however. It has been reported very recently that while the active prolyl 4-hydroxylase tetramers are located only within the cisternae of the rough endoplasmic reticulum (see above), the β-subunit-related protein is also found in association with the plasma membrane (Kao & Chou, 1980). It is not known whether this protein is an integral part of the plasma membrane or just associated with the membrane through some unknown mechanism, neither is it known whether the β-subunit-related protein is exclusively related to prolyl 4-hydroxylase or whether it also has some additional functions. The latter question is raised especially by demonstrations that the β-subunit-related protein is present in most cells in a very large excess, forming up to 99 per cent of the total prolyl 4-hydroxylase protein (see Kivirikko & Myllylä, 1980).

Lysyl hydroxylase and the two hydroxylysyl glycosyltransferases are also present in a number of different cell types, and, like prolyl 4-hydroxylase activity, these enzyme activities are in a distinct excess over the synthesis of only traces of collagenous protein or none at all in some cells (Anttinen et al, 1977b; Myllylä & Seppä, 1979). Prolyl 3-hydroxylase, lysyl hydroxylase and the two hydroxylysyl glycosyltransferases further resemble prolyl 4-hydroxylase in that their activities show marked differences between various cell types (Table 5.3) and tissues, and in the same cell type or tissue under many experimental or clinical conditions (Risteli & Kivirikko, 1976; Kivirikko & Myllylä, 1979, 1980; Myllylä & Seppä, 1979; Risteli et al, 1979; Myllylä et al, 1981). The ratios of the intracellular enzyme activities of collagen synthesis are not constant, however, but vary markedly, and this appears to explain many of the differences in the extents of various modifications between the genetically distinct collagen types or in the same collagen type in various conditions. For example, the ratio of prolyl 3-hydroxylase to prolyl 4-hydroxylase activity in rat kidney cortex is about 15 times that in the skin (Tryggvason et al, 1979a), a finding that agrees with the abundance of the 3-hydroxyproline-rich type IV collagen in this tissue (Man & Adams, 1975).

Other factors

The rates and/or extents of the intracellular modifications depend not only on the amounts of active enzymes (discussed above), but also on the amounts of the co-factors and co-substrates required by the enzymes, the rate of procollagen synthesis and the rate at which the proα chains fold into the triple-helical conformation.

The modifying enzymes require several co-factors or co-substrates. Exclusion of any of these will inhibit the corresponding reactions, as has been demonstrated in the case of the hydroxylases in a number of experiments with isolated cells or tissues (Kivirikko & Myllylä, 1980). It has not been shown directly whether the concentrations of the reactants limit the rates of the corresponding reactions in vivo, but it seems very likely that such a situation exists in the case of the hydroxylysyl glycosyltransferases even under normal conditions (Myllylä et al, 1979a; Anttinen & Hulkko, 1980), and in the case of the three hydroxylases at least in certain pathological states. For example, the K_m of oxygen in the hydroxylation reactions is of about the same magnitude as the O_2 tensions measured in several kinds of wounds, suggesting that changes in O_2 tension may influence the rate of these reactions (see Kivirikko & Myllylä, 1980). Scurvy provides an example of the effect of the ascorbate concentration, since the decreased rate of collagen biosynthesis in this disease is probably due to a lack of ascorbate for the hydroxylations (see Barnes, 1975; Myllylä et al, 1978). It is of interest that in cultured cells a deficiency in this vitamin affects the 4-hydroxylation of prolyl residues much more readily than the hydroxylation of lysyl residues (see Quinn & Krane, 1979; Anttinen et al, 1981), even though the K_m values for ascorbate in these two reactions are very similar (Puistola et al, 1980a; Anttinen et al, 1981).

Changes in the rate of procollagen synthesis influence the ratio of the modifying enzymes to their substrate in the cell. It thus seems likely that a marked decrease in the rate of procollagen synthesis can in itself increase the extent to which the proα chains are modified. Such a situation has been demonstrated in several kinds of transformed cells in culture: the rate of procollagen synthesis is markedly decreased and the extents of the modifications in the newly synthesized proα chains are distinctly increased, even though the corresponding enzyme activities are unchanged or even decreased (Myllylä et al, 1981).

The rate at which the proα chains fold into the triple-helical conformation influences the time available for the modifications, as none of the five enzymes can act on triple-helical substrates (see above). It is possible to manipulate isolated cells so that the triple helix formation becomes either inhibited or accelerated. Such studies have indicated that when triple helix formation is inhibited, the prolyl 3-hydroxylation, lysyl hydroxylation and hydroxylysyl glycosylations in newly synthesized procollagen increase in extent, while the opposite changes take place if triple helix formation is accelerated (Uitto & Prockop, 1974; Oikarinen et al, 1976, 1977; Uitto et al, 1978; Majamaa, 1981). This factor may in part explain the differences in the extents of the modification between various genetically distinct collagens, as large differences are found in the time required for triple helix formation between cells synthesizing various collagen types (see above).

Regulation of extracellular modifications

The activities of procollagen amino-terminal protease and lysyl oxidase vary in the culture medium of human fibroblasts, with a maximal value towards the end of the logarithmic phase of growth, at about the same time as prolyl 4-hydroxylase has its maximal activity (see Kivirikko & Risteli, 1976; Siegel 1979). These findings indicate that regulation of the enzyme activities responsible for the extracellular modifications takes place, although little specific information is currently available on the nature of this regulation.

Lysyl oxidase activity has been measured in tissues in many physiological and pathological states. These studies should be evaluated with caution, however, as a number of technical problems are encountered in the measurement of this enzyme activity (see Siegel, 1979). Lysyl oxidase activity is nevertheless known to correlate with development of increased wound tensile strength in implanted sponges (see Siegel, 1979) and collagen deposition in liver fibrosis (Siegel et al, 1978), while it is low in copper deficiency, being restored by administration of trace amounts of this cation (see Rayton & Harris, 1979; Siegel, 1979). The latter phenomenon appears to involve an induction of new enzyme synthesis rather than an activation of pre-existing enzyme protein (Rayton & Harris,

1979). Hypophysectomy markedly reduces the enzyme activity and also reduces the aldehyde content of soluble collagen and the process of cross-link formation (Shoshan & Finkelstein, 1976, Siegel, 1979).

CONCLUSIONS

Collagen biosynthesis is unusual in that it involves a large number of post-translational modifications, many of which are unique to collagens and a few other proteins. The unique reactions are hydroxylation of appropriate prolyl and lysyl residues to 4-hydroxyprolyl, 3-hydroxyprolyl and hydroxylysyl residues, glycosylation of certain hydroxylysyl residues to galactosylhydroxylysyl and glucosylgalactosylhydroxylysyl residues, folding of proα chains into a triple-helical conformation, ordered aggregation of collagen molecules into collagen fibrils, and oxidative deamination of ϵ-amino groups in certain lysyl and hydroxylysyl residues to give reactive aldehydes. The conversion of procollagen to collagen is also unique in that it requires specific enzymes, while removal of the pre-protein sequences, glycosylation of certain asparaginyl residues in the propeptides, and formation of the inter-chain disulphide bonds between the propeptides are probably similar to those in many other proteins.

The main features of most of these reactions are now well defined, and many of the enzymes involved have been characterized. The unique reactions are catalyzed by at least eight different enzymes. Four of these, prolyl 4-hydroxylase, lysyl hydroxylase, galactosylhydroxylysyl glucosyltransferase and lysyl oxidase have been purified to homogeneity, and three additional ones, prolyl 3-hydroxylase, hydroxylysyl galactosyltransferase and procollagen amino-terminal protease have been purified to a high extent, while procollagen carboxy-terminal protease has been purified only preliminarily. Several important aspects require additional studies, however. It is not known, for example, whether any of these enzymes has tissue-specific or collagen type-specific isoenzymes.

The functions of many of the modifications have been elucidated in great detail. Prolyl 4-hydroxylation is required for the formation of a triple-helical molecule at body temperature, lysyl hydroxylation is essential for hydroxylysyl glycosylations and the formation of stable cross-links, disulphide bonding between the propeptides is probably likewise required for triple helix formation and a triple-helical molecule is necessary for a normal rate of procollagen secretion and various properties of the collagen molecule. The conversion of procollagen to collagen is required for normal fibril formation and the lysyl oxidase reaction is necessary for cross-linking which gives collagen fibrils their tensile strength. The functions of the other modifications are either uncertain or unknown.

Some information is available on the regulation of the rates and extents of many of the modifications. These depend in many cases both on the amounts of active enzyme present and also on the amounts of the co-factors and co-substrates required by the enzyme, the rate of procollagen synthesis, and the rate at which the proα chains fold into the triple-helical conformation. The regulation data which are now rapidly accumulating will form a basis for an understanding of the marked differences that are found in the extent of some of the modifications between the genetically distinct collagen types and even within the same collagen type in various physiological and pathological states.

ACKNOWLEDGEMENTS

The original research in the laboratory of the authors was supported in part by grants from the Medical Research Council of the Academy of Finland.

REFERENCES

Adams E, Frank L 1980 Metabolism of proline and the hydroxyprolines. Annual Review of Biochemistry 49: 1005

Alitalo K, Vaheri A, Krieg T, Timpl R 1980 Biosynthesis of two subunits of type IV procollagen and of other basement membrane proteins by a human tumor cell line. European Journal of Biochemistry 109: 247

Anttinen H, Hulkko A 1980 Regulation of the glycosylations of collagen hydroxylysine in chick embryo tendon and cartilage cells. Biochimica et Biophysica Acta 632: 417

Anttinen H, Myllylä R, Kivirikko K I 1977a Hydrophobic and carbohydrate-recognition chromatographies of collagen glucosyltransferase. European Journal of Biochemistry 78: 11

Anttinen H, Tuderman L, Oikarinen A, Kivirikko K I 1977b Intracellular enzymes of collagen biosynthesis in human platelets. Blood 50: 29

Anttinen H, Myllylä R, Kivirikko K I 1978a Further characterization of galactosylhydroxylysyl glucosyltransferase from chick embryos. Biochemical Journal 175: 737

Anttinen H, Oikarinen A, Ryhänen L, Kivirikko K I 1978b Evidence for the transfer of mannose to the extension peptides of procollagen within the cisternae of the rough endoplasmic reticulum. FEBS Letters; Federation of European Biochemical Societies 87: 222

Anttinen H, Puistola U, Pihlajaniemi T, Kivirikko K I 1981 Differences between proline and lysine hydroxylations in their inhibition by zinc or by ascorbate deficiency during collagen synthesis in various cell types. Biochimica et Biophysica Acta, 674: 336

Bächinger H P, Bruckner P, Timpl R, Engel J 1978 The role of cis-trans isomerization of peptide bonds in the coil-triple helix conversion of collagen. European Journal of Biochemistry 90: 605

Bailey A J, Robins S P 1976 Current topics in the biosynthesis, structure and function of collagen. Science Progress (Oxford) 63: 419

Bailey A J, Bazin S, Sims T J, LeLous M, Nicoletis C, Delaunay A 1975 Characterization of the collagen of human hypertrophic and normal scars. Biochimica et Biophysica Acta 405: 412

Bailey A J, Ranta M H, Nicholls A C, Partridge S M, Elsden D F 1977 Isolation of α-aminoadipic acid from mature dermal collagen and elastin. Evidence for an oxidative pathway in the maturation of collagen and elastin. Biochemical and Biophysical Research Communications 78: 1403

Bailey A J, Robins S P, Balian G 1974 Biological significance of the intermolecular crosslinks of collagen. Nature (London) 251: 105

Barnes M J 1975 Function of ascorbic acid in collagen metabolism. Annals of the New York Academy of Sciences 258: 264

Barnes M J, Constable B J, Morton L F, Royce P M 1974 Age-related variations in hydroxylation of lysine and proline in collagen. Biochemical Journal 139: 461

Barrow M V, Simpson C F, Miller E J 1974 Lathyrism: a review. Quarterly Review of Biology 49: 101

Bates C J 1976 Prolyl hydroxylase in platelets. FEBS Letters; Federation of European Biochemical Societies 72: 235

Benya P D, Padilla S R, Nimni M E 1977 The progeny of rabbit articular chondrocytes synthesize collagen types I and III and type I trimer, but not type II. Verifications by cyanogen bromide peptide analysis. Biochemistry 16: 865

Berg R A, Prockop D J 1973 Affinity column purification of protocollagen proline hydroxylase from chick embryos and further characterization of the enzyme. Journal of Biological Chemistry 248: 1175

Berg R A, Kao W W-Y, Kedersha N L 1980 The assembly of tetrameric prolyl hydroxylase in tendon fibroblasts from newly synthesized α-subunits and from preformed cross-reacting protein. Biochemical Journal 189: 491

Berg R A, Kedersha N L, Guzman N A 1979 Purification and partial characterization of the two nonidentical subunits of prolyl hydroxylase. Journal of Biological Chemistry 254: 3111

Berg R A, Kishida Y, Sakakibara S, Prockop D J 1977 Hydroxylation of $(\text{Pro-Pro-Gly})_5$ and $(\text{Pro-Pro-Gly})_{10}$ by prolyl hydroxylase. Evidence for an asymmetric active site in the enzyme. Biochemistry 16: 1615

Blobel G, Walter P, Chang C N, Goldman B M, Erickson A H, Lingappa V R 1979 Translocation of proteins across membranes: The signal hypothesis and beyond. Symposia of the Society for Experimental Biology 33: 9

Bornstein P, Sage H 1980 Structurally distinct collagen types. Annual Review of Biochemistry 49: 957

Bornstein P, Traub W 1979 The chemistry and biology of collagen. In: Neurath H, Hill R L (eds) Proteins Volume IV. Academic Press, New York, p 411

Brockway B E, Forster S J, Freedman R B 1980 Protein disulphide isomerase activity in chick embryo tissues — correlation with the biosynthesis of procollagen. Biochemical Journal 191: 873

Bruckner P, Bächinger H P, Timpl R, Engel J 1978 Three conformationally distinct domains in the aminoterminal segment of type III procollagen and its rapid triple helix $\rightleftarrows$ coil transition. European Journal of Biochemistry 90: 595

Bruns R R, Hulmes D J S, Therrien S F, Gross J 1979 Procollagen segment-long-spacing crystallites: their role in collagen fibrillogenesis. Proceedings of the National Academy of Sciences of the United States of America 76: 313

Cardinale G J, Udenfriend S 1974 Prolyl hydroxylase. Advances in Enzymology 41: 245

Chen-Kiang S, Cardinale G J, Udenfriend S 1977 Homology between a prolyl hydroxylase subunit and a tissue protein that crossreacts immunologically with the enzyme. Proceedings of the National Academy of Sciences of the United States of America 74: 4420

Chen-Kiang S, Cardinale G J, Udenfriend S 1978 Expression of collagen biosynthetic activities in lymphocytic cells. Proceedings of the National Academy of Sciences of the United States of America 75: 1379

Chichester C O, Fuller G C, Cardinale G J 1976 In vivo labeling and turnover of prolyl hydroxylase and a related immunoreactive protein. Biochemical and Biophysical Research Communications 73: 1056

Chichester C O, Fuller G C, Mo Cha C-J 1979 Turnover of prolyl hydroxylase and an immunologically related protein in rabbit tissue. Biochimica et Biophysica Acta 586: 341

Clark C C 1979 The distribution and initial characterization of oligosaccharide units on the COOH-terminal propeptide extensions of the pro-α1 and pro-α2 chains of type I procollagen. Journal of Biological Chemistry 254: 10798

Clark C C, Kefalides N A 1976 Carbohydrate moieties of procollagen: incorporation of isotopically labelled mannose and glucosamine into propeptides of procollagen secreted by matrix-free chick embryo tendon cells. Proceedings of the National Academy of Sciences of the United States of America 73: 34

Clark C C, Kefalides N A 1978 Localization and partial composition of the oligosaccharide units on the propeptide extensions of type I procollagen. Journal of Biological Chemistry 253: 47

Comper W D, Veis A 1977a The mechanism of nucleation for in vitro collagen fibril formation. Biopolymers 16: 2113

Comper W D, Veis A 1977b Characterization of nuclei in in vitro collagen fibril formation. Biopolymers 16: 2133

Counts D F, Cardinale G J, Udenfriend S 1978 Prolyl hydroxylase half reaction: peptidyl prolyl-independent decarboxylation of α-ketoglutarate. Proceedings of the National Academy of Sciences of the United States of America 75: 2145

Crouch E, Sage H, Bornstein P 1980 Structural basis for apparent heterogeneity of collagens in human basement membrane: Type IV procollagen contains two distinct chains. Proceedings of the National Academy of Sciences of the United States of America 77: 745

Davidson J M, McEneany S G, Bornstein P 1975 Intermediates in the limited proteolytic conversion of procollagen to collagen. Biochemistry 14: 5188

Davidson J M, McEneany S G, Bornstein P 1977 Intermediates in the conversion of procollagen to collagen. Evidence for stepwise limited proteolysis of the COOH-terminal peptide extensions. European Journal of Biochemistry 81: 349

Davis D B, Tai P-C 1980 The mechanism of protein secretion across membranes. Nature 283: 433

Dickson I R, Eyre D R, Kodicek E 1979 Influence of plasma calcium and vitamin D on bone collagen. Effects on lysine hydroxylation and cross-link formation. Biochimica et Biophysica Acta 588: 169

Duksin D, Bornstein P 1977 Impaired conversion of procollagen to collagen by fibroblasts and bone treated with tunicamycin, an inhibitor of protein glycosylation. Journal of Biological Chemistry 252: 955

Duksin D, Davidson J M, Bornstein P 1978 The role of glycosylation in the enzymatic conversion of procollagen to collagen: studies using tunicamycin and concanavalin A. Archives of Biochemistry and Biophysics 185: 326

Elsden D F, Light N D, Bailey A J 1980 An investigation of pyridinoline, a putative collagen cross-link. Biochemical Journal 185: 531

Evans C A, Peterkofsky B 1976 Ascorbate independent proline hydroxylation resulting from viral transformation of Balb 3T3 cells and unaffected by dibutyryl cAMP treatment. Journal of Cellular Physiology 89: 355

Eyre D R 1980 Collagen: Molecular diversity in the body's protein scaffold. Science 207: 1315

Fessler J H, Fessler L J 1978 Biosynthesis of procollagen. Annual Review of Biochemistry 47: 129

Fessler L J, Fessler J H 1979 Characterization of type III procollagen from chick blood vessels. Journal of Biological Chemistry 254: 233

Fessler L J, Morris N P, Fessler J H 1975 Procollagen: biological scission of amino and carboxyl extension peptides. Proceedings of the National Academy of Sciences of the United States of America 72: 4905

Fietzek P P, Kühn K 1976 The primary structure of collagen. International Review of Connective Tissue Research 7: 1

Freedman R B 1979 How many distinct enzymes are responsible for the cellular processes involving thiol: protein-disulphide interchange? FEBS Letters; Federation of European Biochemical Societies 97: 201

Fujimoto D, Moriguchi T 1978 Pyridinoline, a non-reducible crosslink of collagen. Quantitative determination, distribution and isolation of a crosslinked peptide. Journal of Biochemistry 83: 863

Fujimoto D, Akiba K-Y, Nakamura N 1977 Isolation and characterization of a fluorescent material in bovine Achilles tendon collagen. Biochemical and Biophysical Research Communications 76: 1124

Fujimoto D, Moriguchi T, Ishida T, Hayashi H 1978 The structure of pyridinoline, a collagen crosslink. Biochemical and Biophysical Research Communications 84: 52

Gallop P M, Paz M A 1975 Posttranslational protein modifications, with special attention to collagen and elastin. Physiological Reviews 55: 418

Gelman R A, Poppke D C, Piez K A 1979 Collagen fibril formation in vitro. The role of the nonhelical terminal regions. Journal of Biological Chemistry 254: 11741

Goldberg B 1977 Kinetics of processing of type I and type III procollagens in fibroblast cultures. Proceedings of the National Academy of Sciences of the United States of America 74: 3322

Goldberg B, Taubman M B, Radin A 1975 Procollagen peptidase: its mode of action on the native substrate. Cell 4: 45

Grant M E, Jackson D S 1976 The biosynthesis of procollagen. Essays in Biochemistry 12: 77

Graves P N, Olsen B R, Fietzek P P, Prockop D J, Monson J M 1981 Comparison of the NH_2-terminal sequences of chick type I preprocollagen chains synthesized in a mRNA-dependent reticulocyte lysate. European Journal of Biochemistry 118: 363

Gryder R M, Lamon M, Adams E 1975 Sequence position of 3-hydroxyproline in basement membrane collagens. Isolation of glycyl-3-hydroxyprolyl-4-hydroxyproline from swine kidney. Journal of Biological Chemistry 250: 2470

Guzman N A, Berg R A, Prockop D J 1976 Concanavalin A binds to purified prolyl hydroxylase and partially inhibits its activity. Biochemical and Biophysical Research Communications 73: 279

Guzman N A, Graves P N, Prockop D J 1978 Addition of mannose to both the amino- and carboxyterminal propeptides of type II procollagen occurs without formation of a triple helix. Biochemical and Biophysical Research Communications 84: 691

Han S, Tanzer M L 1979 Collagen cross-linking. Purification of lysyl oxidase in solvents containing nonionic detergents. Journal of Biological Chemistry 254: 10438

Harris E D, Gonnerman W A, Savage J E, O'Dell B L 1974 Connective tissue amine oxidase. Purification and partial characterization of lysyl oxidase from chick aorta. Biochimica et Biophysica Acta 341: 332

Hart G W, Brew K, Grant G A, Bradshaw R A, Lennarz W J 1979 Primary structural requirements for the enzymatic formation of the N-glycosidic bond in glycoproteins. Journal of Biological Chemistry 254: 9747

Harwood R, Freedman R B 1978 Protein disulphide isomerase activity in collagen-synthesizing tissues of the chick embryo. FEBS Letters; Federation of European Biochemical Societies 88: 46

Harwood R, Grant M E, Jackson D S 1976 The route of secretion of procollagen: The influence of $\alpha\alpha'$-bipydiryl, colchicine and antimycin A on the secretory process in embryonic-chick tendon and cartilage cells. Biochemical Journal 156: 81

Hayashi T, Curran-Patel S, Prockop D J 1979 Thermal stability of the triple helix of type I procollagen and collagen. Precautions for minimizing ultraviolet damage to proteins during circular dichroism studies. Biochemistry 18: 4182

Heathcote G J, Sear C H J, Grant M E 1978 Studies on the assembly of the rat lens capsule. Biosynthesis and partial characterization of the collagenous components. Biochemical Journal 176: 283

Henkel W, Buddecke E 1975 Purification and properties of UDP-glucose galactosylhydroxylysine collagen glucosyltransferase (EC 2.4.1.?) from bovine arterial tissue. Hoppe-Seyler's Zeitschrift für Physiologische Chemie 356: 921

Hobza P, Hurych J, Zahradnik R 1973 Quantum chemical study of the mechanism of collagen proline hydroxylation. Biochimica et Biophysica Acta 304: 466

Housley T J, Rowland F N, Ledger P W, Kaplan J, Tanzer M L 1980 Effects of tunicamycin on the biosynthesis of procollagen by human fibroblasts. Journal of Biological Chemistry 255: 121

Jimenez S A, Yankowski R 1978 Role of molecular conformation on secretion of chick tendon procollagen. Journal of Biological Chemistry 253: 1420

Kagan H M, Tseng L, Trackman P C, Okamoto K, Rapaka R S, Urry D W 1980 Repeat polypeptide models of elastin as substrates for lysyl oxidase. Journal of Biological Chemistry 255: 3656

Kagan H M, Sullivan K A, Olsson T A, Gronlund A L 1979 Purification and properties of four species of lysyl oxidase from bovine aorta. Biochemical Journal 177: 203

Kao W W-Y, Chou K-L L 1980 CRP, Immunologically cross-reacting protein of prolyl hydroxylase. Its role in assembly of active prolyl hydroxylase and cellular localization in L-929 fibroblasts. Archives of Biochemistry and Biophysics 199: 147

Kao W W-Y, Berg R A 1979 Cell density-dependent increase in prolyl hydroxylase activity in cultured L-929 cells requires de novo protein synthesis. Biochimica et Biophysica Acta 586: 528

Kao W W-Y, Berg R A, Prockop D J 1975 Ascorbate increases the synthesis of procollagen hydroxyproline by cultured fibroblasts from chick embryo tendons without activation of prolyl hydroxylase. Biochimica et Biophysica Acta 411: 202

Kao W W-Y, Berg R A, Prockop D J 1977 Kinetics for the secretion of procollagen by freshly isolated tendon cells. Journal of Biological Chemistry 252: 8391

Kao W W-Y, Flaks J G, Prockop D J 1976 Primary and secondary effects of ascorbate on procollagen synthesis and protein synthesis by primary cultures of tendon fibroblasts. Archives of Biochemistry and Biophysics 173: 638

Kao W W-Y, Prockop D J, Berg R A 1979 Kinetics for the secretion of nonhelical procollagen by freshly isolated tendon cells. Journal of Biological Chemistry 254: 2234

Kefalides N A, Alper R, Clark C C 1979 Biochemistry and metabolism of basement membranes. International Review of Cytology 61: 167

Kelleher P C, Thanassi N M, Moehring J M 1977 Prolyl hydroxylase in pulmonary alveolar macrophages. FEBS Letters; Federation of European Biochemical Societies 81: 125

Kivirikko K I, Myllylä R 1979 Collagen glycosyltransferases. International Review of Connective Tissue Research 8: 23

Kivirikko K I, Myllylä R 1980 Hydroxylation of prolyl and lysyl residues. In: Freedman R B, Hawkins H A (eds) The Enzymology of Post-Translational Modification of Proteins Academic Press, London, p 53

Kivirikko K I, Risteli L 1976 Biosynthesis of collagen and its alterations in pathological states. Medical Biology 54: 159

Kohn L D, Isersky C, Zupnik J, Lenaers A, Lee G, Lapiere C M 1974 Calf tendon procollagen peptidase: its purification and endopeptidase mode of action. Proceedings of the National Academy of Sciences of the United States of America 71: 40

Kornfeld S, Li E, Tabas J 1978 The synthesis of complex-type oligosaccharides. II Characterization of the processing intermediates in the synthesis of the complex oligosaccharide units of the vesicular stomatitis virus G protein. Journal of Biological Chemistry 253: 7771

Krane S M 1980 Genetic diseases of collagen. In: Prockop D J, Champe P C (eds) Gene Families of Collagen and Other Proteins, Elsevier, New York, p. 57

Krieg T, Hörlein D, Wiestner M, Müller P K 1978 Aminoterminal extension peptides from type I procollagen normalize excessive collagen synthesis of scleroderma fibroblasts. Archives of Dermatological Research 263: 171

Kruse N J, Bornstein P 1975 The metabolic requirements for transcellular movement and secretion of collagen. Journal of Biological Chemistry 250: 4841

Kuutti E-R, Tuderman L, Kivirikko K I 1975 Human prolyl hydroxylase. Purification, partial characterization and preparation of antiserum to the enzyme. European Journal of Biochemistry 57: 181

Kuutti-Savolainen E-R 1979 Enzymes of collagen biosynthesis in skin and serum in dermatological diseases. II Serum enzymes. Clinica Chimica Acta 96: 53

Kuutti-Savolainen E-R, Kero M 1979 Enzymes of collagen biosynthesis in skin and serum in dermatological diseases. I. Enzymes of the skin. Clinica Chimica Acta 96: 43

Kuutti-Savolainen E-R, Kivirikko K I, Laitinen O 1980 Serum immunoreactive prolyl hydroxylase in inflammatory rheumatic diseases. Annals of the Rheumatic Diseases 39: 217

Kuutti-Savolainen E-R, Risteli J, Miettinen T A, Kivirikko K I 1979 Collagen biosynthesis enzymes in serum and hepatic tissue in liver disease. I Prolyl hydroxylase. European Journal of Clinical Investigation 9: 89

Lembach K J, Branson R E, Hewgley P P, Cunningham L W 1977 The synthesis of macromolecular 3-hydroxyproline by attaching and confluent cultures of human fibroblast. European Journal of Biochemistry 72: 379

Leung M K K, Fessler L I, Greenberg D B 1979 Separate amino and carboxyl procollagen peptidases in chick embryo tendon. Journal of Biological Chemistry 254: 224

Leunis J C, Smith D F, Nwokoro N, Fishback B L, Wu C, Jamieson G A 1980 The distribution of collagen: glucosyltransferase in human blood cells and plasma. Biochimica et Biophysica Acta 611: 79

Li E, Tabas I, Kornfeld S 1978 The synthesis of complex-type oligosaccharides. I Structure of the lipid-linked oligosaccharides of the vesicular stomatitis virus G protein. Journal of Biological Chemistry 253: 7762

Light N D, Bailey A J 1979 Changes in crosslinking during ageing in bovine tendon collagen. FEBS Letters; Federation of European Biochemical Societies 97: 183

Light N D, Bailey A J 1980 The chemistry of the collagen cross-links. Purification and characterization of cross-linked polymeric peptide material from mature collagen containing unknown amino acids. Biochemical Journal 185: 373

Limeback H F, Sodek J 1979 Procollagen synthesis and processing in periodontal ligament *in vivo* and *in vitro*. A comparative study using slab-gel flurography. European Journal of Biochemistry 100: 541

Majamaa K 1981 Effect of prevention of procollagen triple-helix formation on proline 3-hydroxylation in freshly isolated chick-embryo tendon cells. Biochemical Journal 196: 203

Majamaa K, Kuutti-Savolainen E-R, Tuderman L, Kivirikko K I 1979 Turnover of prolyl hydroxylase tetramers and the monomer-size protein in chick-embryo cartilaginous bone and lung in vivo. Biochemical Journal 178: 313

Man M, Adams E 1975 Basement membrane and interstitial collagen content of whole animals and tissues. Biochemical and Biophysical Research Communications 66: 9

Menashi S, Harwood R, Grant M E 1976 Native collagen is not a substrate for the collagen glucosyltransferase of platelets. Nature (London) 264: 670

Miller E J 1976 Biochemical characteristics and biological significance of the genetically-distinct collagens. Molecular & Cellular Biochemistry 13: 165

Miller R L, Varner H H 1979 Purification and enzymatic properties of lysyl hydroxylase from fetal porcine skin. Biochemistry 18: 5928

Minor R R 1980 Collagen metabolism. A comparison of diseases of collagen and diseases affecting collagen. American Journal of Pathology 98: 225

Minor R R, Clark C C, Strause E L, Koszalka T R, Brent R L, Kefalides N A 1976 Basement membrane procollagen is not converted to collagen in organ cultures of parietal yolk sac endoderm. Journal of Biological Chemistry 251: 1789

Morikawa T, Tuderman L, Prockop D J 1980 Inhibitors of procollagen N-protease. Synthetic peptides with sequences similar to the cleavage site in the proα1(I) chain. Biochemistry 19: 2646

Morris N P, Fessler L I, Weinstock A, Fessler J H 1975 Procollagen assembly and secretion in embryonic chick bone. Journal of Biological Chemistry 250: 5719

Murai A, Miyahara T, Shigeo S 1975 Age-related variations in glycosylation of hydroxylysine in human and rat skin collagens. Biochimica et Biophysica Acta 404: 345

Murphy W H, Mark K, McEneany L S G, Bornstein P 1975 Characterization of procollagen-derived peptides unique to the precursor molecule. Biochemistry 14: 3243

Murray J C, Levene C J 1977 Evidence for the role of vitamin B-6 as a cofactor of lysyl oxidase. Biochemical Journal 167: 463

Murray J C, Cassell R H, Pinnell S R 1977 Inhibition of lysyl hydroxylase by catechol analogs. Biochimica et Biophysica Acta 481: 63

Myllylä R 1976 Studies on the mechanism of collagen glucosyltransferase reaction. European Journal of Biochemistry 70: 225

Myllylä R 1981 Preparation of antibodies to chick-embryo galactosylhydroxylysyl glucosyltransferase and their use for an immunological characterization of this enzyme of collagen synthesis. Biochimica et Biophysica Acta, 658: 299

Myllylä R, Seppä H 1979 Studies on enzymes of collagen biosynthesis and the synthesis of hydroxyproline in macrophages and mast cells. Biochemical Journal 182: 311

Myllylä R, Alitalo K, Vaheri A, Kivirikko K I 1981 Regulation of collagen post-translational modification in transformed human and chick embryo cells. Biochemical Journal, 196: 683

Myllylä R, Anttinen H, Risteli L, Kivirikko K I 1977a Isolation of collagen glucosyltransferase as a homogenous protein from chick embryos. Biochimica et Biophysica Acta 480: 113

Myllylä R, Anttinen H, Kivirikko K I 1979a Metal activation of galactosylhydroxylysyl glucosyltransferase, an intracellular enzyme of collagen biosynthesis. European Journal of Biochemistry 101: 261

Myllylä R, Kuutti-Savolainen E-R, Kivirikko K I 1978 The role of ascorbate in the prolyl hydroxylase reaction. Biochemical and Biophysical Research Communications 83: 441

Myllylä R, Risteli L, Kivirikko K I 1975 Glucosylation of galactosylhydroxylysyl residues in collagen *in vitro* by collagen glucosyltransferase. Inhibition by triple helical conformation of the substrate. European Journal of Biochemistry 58: 517

Myllylä R, Risteli L, Kivirikko K I 1976 Collagen glucosyltransferase. Partial purification and characterization of the enzyme from whole chick embryos and chick embryo cartilage. European Journal of Biochemistry 61: 59

Myllylä R, Schubotz L M, Weser U, Kivirikko K I 1979b Involvement of superoxide in the prolyl and lysyl hydroxylase reactions. Biochemical and Biophysical Research Communications 89: 98

Myllylä R, Tuderman L, Kivirikko K I 1977b Mechanism of the prolyl hydroxylase reaction. 2. Kinetic analysis of the reaction sequence. European Journal of Biochemistry 80: 349

Narayanan A S, Page R C, Kuzan F, Cooper C G 1978 Elastin crosslinking *in vitro*. Studies on factors influencing the formation of desmosines by lysyl oxidase action on tropoelastin. Biochemical Journal 173: 857

Narayanan A S, Siegel R C, Martin G R 1974 Stability and purification of lysyl oxidase. Archives of Biochemistry and Biophysics 162: 231

Nietfeld J J, Kemp A 1980 Properties of prolyl 4-hydroxylase containing firmly-bound iron. Biochimica et Biophysica Acta 613: 349

Nietfeld J J, Kemp A 1981 The function of ascorbate with respect to prolyl 4-hydroxylase activity. Biochimica et Biophysica Acta 657: 159

Nolan J C, Cardinale G J, Udenfriend S 1978a The formation of hydroxyproline in collagen by cells grown in the absence of serum. Biochimica et Biophysica Acta 543: 116

Nolan J C, Ridge S, Oronsky A L, Kerwar S S 1978b Studies on the mechanism of reduction of prolyl hydroxylase activity by D,L-3,4-dehydroproline. Archives of Biochemistry and Biophysics 183: 448

Nusgens B V, Goebels Y, Shinkai H, Lapiere C M 1980 Procollagen type III N-terminal endopeptidase in fibroblast culture. Biochemical Journal 191: 699

Oikarinen A, Anttinen H, Kivirikko K I 1976 Effect of L-azetidine-2-carboxylic acid on glycosylations of collagen in chick-embryo tendon cells. Biochemical Journal 160: 639

Oikarinen A, Anttinen H, Kivirikko K I 1977 Further studies on the effect of the collagen triple helix formation on the hydroxylation of lysine and the glycosylations of hydroxylysine in chick-embryo tendon and cartilage cells. Biochemical Journal 166: 357

Olden K, Pratt R M, Yamada K A 1978 Role of carbohydrates in protein secretion and turnover: effects of tunicamycin on the major cel surface glycoprotein of chick embryo fibroblasts. Cell 13: 461

Olsen B R, Guzman N A, Engel J, Condit C, Aase S 1977 Purification and characterization of a peptide from the carboxy-terminal region of chick tendon procollagen type I. Biochemistry 16: 3030

Paglia L, Wilczek J, de Leon L D, Martin G R, Hörlein D, Müller P 1979 Inhibition of procollagen cell-free synthesis by aminoterminal extension peptides. Biochemistry 18: 5030

Palmiter R D, Davidson J M, Gagnon J, Rowe D W, Bornstein P 1979 NH_2-terminal sequence of the chick proα(I) chain synthesized in the reticulocyte lysate system. Journal of Biological Chemistry 254: 1433

Peltonen L, Palotie A, Hayashi T, Prockop D J 1980 Thermal stability of type I and type III procollagens from normal human fibroblasts and from a patient with osteogenesis imperfecta. Proceedings of the National Academy of Sciences of the United States of America 77: 162

Peterkofsky B, Assad R 1979 Localization of chick embryo limb bone microsomal lysyl hydroxylase at intracisternal and intramembrane sites. Journal of Biological Chemistry 254: 4714

Peterkofsky B, Kalwinsky D, Assad R 1980 A substance in L-929 cell extracts which replaces the ascorbate requirement for prolyl hydroxylase in a tritium release assay for reducing cofactor; correlation of its concentration with the extent of ascorbate-independent proline hydroxylation and the level of prolyl hydroxylase activity in these cells. Archives of Biochemistry and Biophysics 199: 362

Piez K A 1976 Primary structure. In: Ramachandran G N, Reddi A H (eds) Biochemistry of Collagen. Plenum Press, New York, p 1

Pihlajaniemi T, Myllylä R, Alitalo K, Vaheri A, Kivirikko K I 1981 Post-translational modifications in the biosynthesis of type IV collagen by a human tumor cell line. Biochemistry 20: 7409

Prockop D J, Berg R A, Kivirikko K I, Uitto J 1976 Intracellular steps in the biosynthesis of collagen. In: Ramachandran G N, Reddi A H (eds) Biochemistry of Collagen. Plenum Press, New York, p 163

Prockop D J, Kivirikko K I, Tuderman L, Guzman N A 1979 The biosynthesis of collagen and its disorders. New England Journal of Medicine 301: 13 & 77

Puistola U, Turpeenniemi-Hujanen T M, Myllylä R, Kivirikko K I 1980a Studies on the lysyl hydroxylase reaction. I Initial velocity kinetics and related aspects. Biochimica et Biophysica Acta 611: 40

Puistola U, Turpeenniemi-Hujanen T M, Myllylä R, Kivirikko K I 1980b Studies on the lysyl hydroxylase reaction. II Inhibition kinetics and the reaction mechanism. Biochimica et Biophysica Acta 611: 51

Quinn R S, Krane S M 1979 Collagen synthesis by cultured skin fibroblasts from siblings with hydroxylysine-deficient collagen. Biochimica et Biophysica Acta 585: 589

Ranta H 1978 Age-related changes in collagen cross-linking. Proceedings of the Finnish Dental Society, 74 Supplement II 1

Rao N V, Adams E 1978 Partial reaction of prolyl hydroxylase. $(Gly\text{-}Pro\text{-}Ala)_n$ stimulates α-ketoglutarate decarboxylation without prolyl hydroxylation. Journal of Biological Chemistry 253: 6327

Rapaka R S, Sorensen K R, Lee S D, Bhatnagar R S 1976 Inhibition of hydroxyproline synthesis by palladium ions. Biochimica et Biophysica Acta 429: 63

Rayton J K, Harris E D 1979 Induction of lysyl oxidase with copper. Properties of an in vitro system. Journal of Biological Chemistry 254: 621

Reid K B M 1977 Amino acid sequence of the N-terminal forty-two amino acid residues of the C chain of subcomponent C1q of the first component of human complement. Biochemical Journal 161: 247

Reid K B M, Thompson O P 1978 Amino acid sequence of the N-terminal 108 amino acid residues of the B chain of subcomponent C1q of the first component of human complement. Biochemical Journal 173: 863

Risteli J, Kivirikko K I 1976 Intracellular enzymes of collagen biosynthesis in rat liver as a function of age and in hepatic injury induced by dimethylnitrosamine. Changes in prolyl hydroxylase, lysyl hydroxylase, collagen galactosyltransferase and collagen glucosyltransferase activities. Biochemical Journal 158: 361

Risteli J, Tryggvason K, Kivirikko K I 1977 Prolyl 3-hydroxylase: Partial characterization of the enzyme from rat kidney cortex. European Journal of Biochemistry 73: 485

Risteli J, Tuderman L, Kivirikko K I 1976 Intracellular enzymes of collagen biosynthesis in rat liver as a function of age and in hepatic injury induced by dimethylnitrosamine. Purification of rat prolyl hydroxylase and comparison of changes in prolyl hydroxylase activity with changes in immunoreactive prolyl hydroxylase. Biochemical Journal 158: 369

Risteli J, Tuderman L, Tryggvason K, Kivirikko K I 1978 Effect of hepatic injury on prolyl 3-hydroxylase and 4-hydroxylase activities in rat liver and on immunoreactive prolyl 4-hydroxylase concentrations in the liver and serum. Biochemical Journal 170: 129

Risteli L 1978 Further characterization of collagen galactosyltransferase from chick embryos. Biochemical Journal 169: 189

Risteli L, Myllylä R, Kivirikko K I 1976a Partial purification and characterization of collagen galactosyltransferase from chick embryos. Biochemical Journal 155: 145

Risteli L, Myllylä R, Kivirikko K I 1976b Affinity chromatography of collagen glycosyltransferases on collagen linked to agarose. European Journal of Biochemistry 67: 197

Risteli L, Risteli J, Salo L, Kivirikko K I 1979 Intracellular enzymes of collagen biosynthesis in 3T6 fibroblasts and chick-embryo tendon and cartilage cells. European Journal of Biochemistry 97: 297

Robins S P, Bailey A J 1977 The chemistry of the collagen cross-links. Characterization of the products by reduction of skin, tendon and bone with sodium cyanoborohydride. Biochemical Journal 163: 339

Royce P M, Barnes M J 1977 Comparative studies on collagen glycosylation in chick skin and bone. Biochimica et Biophysica Acta 498: 132

Ryhänen L 1976 Lysyl hydroxylase: Further purification and characterization of the enzyme from chick embryos and chick embryo cartilage. Biochimica et Biophysica Acta 438: 71

Sandell L, Veis A 1980 The molecular weight of the cell-free translation product of α1(I) procollagen mRNA. Biochemical and Biophysical Research Communications 92: 554

Savolainen E-R, Pihlajaniemi T, Kero M, Kivirikko K I 1981 Deficiency of galactosylhydroxylysyl glucosyltransferase, an enzyme of collagen synthesis, in a family with dominant epidermolysis bullosa simplex. New England Journal of Medicine 304: 197

Schwartz C E, Hellerqvist C G, Cunningham L W 1979 Attaching human fibroblasts secrete type I procollagen rich in 3-hydroxyproline. Biochemical and Biophysical Research Communications 90: 240

Shieh J J, Yasunobu K T 1976 Purification and properties of lung lysyl oxidase, a copper enzyme. Advances of Experimental Medical Biology 74: 447

Shoshan S, Finkelstein S, 1976 Lysyl oxidase: A pituitary hormone-dependent enzyme. Biochimica et Biophysica Acta 439: 358

Showalter A M, Pesciotta D M, Eikenberry E F, Yamamoto T, Pastan I, DeCrombrugghe B, Fietzek P P, Olsen B R 1980 Nucleotide sequence of a collagen cDNA-fragment coding for the carboxyl end of proα(I) chains. FEBS Letters; Federation of European Biochemical Societies 111: 61

Shuttleworth C A, Forrest L, Jackson D S 1975 Comparison of the cyanogen bromide peptides of insoluble guinea-pig skin and scar collagen. Biochimica et Biophysica Acta 379: 207

Siegel R C 1976 Collagen cross-linking. Synthesis of collagen cross-links *in vitro* with highly purified lysyl oxidase. Journal of Biological Chemistry 251: 5786

Siegel R C 1979 Lysyl oxidase. International Review of Connective Tissue Research 8: 73

Siegel R C, Fu J C C 1976 Collagen cross-linking. Purification and substrate specificity of lysyl oxidase. Journal of Biological Chemistry 251: 5779

Siegel R C, Chen K H, Greenspan J R, Aguiar J M 1978 Biochemical and immunological study of lysyl oxidase in experimental hepatic fibrosis in the rat. Proceedings of the National Academy of Sciences of the United States of America 75: 2945

Silver F H, Trelstadt R L 1979 Linear aggregation and the turbidimetric lag phase: type I collagen fibrillogenesis in vitro. Journal of Theoretical Biology 81: 515

Silver F H, Langley K H, Trelstadt R L 1979 Type I collagen fibrillogenesis: Initiation via reversible linear and lateral growth steps. Biopolymers 18: 2523

Smith B D, McKenney K H, Lustberg T J 1977 Characterization of collagen precursors found in rat skin and rat bone. Biochemistry 16: 2980

Smith D F, Kosow D P, Wu C, Jamieson G A 1977 Characterization of human platelet UDP-glucose-collagen glucosyltransferase using a new rapid assay. Biochimica et Biophysica Acta 483: 263

Stassen F L H 1976 Properties of highly purified lysyl oxidase from embryonic chick cartilage. Biochimica et Biophysica Acta 438: 49

Stassen F L H, Cardinale G J, Udenfriend S 1973 Activation of prolyl hydroxylase in L-929 fibroblasts by ascorbic acid. Proceedings of the National Academy of Sciences of the United States of America 70: 1090

Stassen F L H, Cardinale G J, McGee J O'D, Udenfriend S 1974 Prolyl hydroxylase and an immunologically related protein in mammalian tissues. Archives of Biochemistry and Biophysics 160: 340

Strauss A W, Zimmerman M, Boime I, Ashe B, Mumford R A, Alberts A W 1979 Characterization of an endopeptidase involved in pre-protein processing. Proceedings of the National Academy of Sciences of the United States of America 76: 4225

Tabas I, Kornfeld S 1978 The synthesis of complex-type oligosaccharides. III Identification of an α-D-mannosidase activity involved in a late stage of processing of complex-type oligosaccharides. Journal of Biological Chemistry 253: 7779

Tanzer M L 1976 Cross-linking In: Ramachandran G N, Reddi A H (eds) Biochemistry of Collagen. Plenum Press, New York, p 137

Tanzer M L, Rowland F N, Murray L W, Kaplan J 1977 Inhibitory effects of tunicamycin on procollagen biosynthesis and secretion. Biochimica et Biophysica Acta 500: 187

Taubman M B, Goldberg B 1976 The processing of procollagen in cultures of human and mouse fibroblasts. Archives of Biochemistry and Biophysics 173: 490

Trelstadt R L, Hayashi K 1979 Tendon collagen fibrillogenesis: Intracellular subassemblies and cell surface changes associated with fibril growth. Developmental Biology 71: 228

Trelstadt R L, Derba R, Gross J 1977 Osteogenesis imperfecta congenita. Evidence for a generalized molecular disorder of collagen. Laboratory Investigation 36: 501

Trelstadt R L, Hayashi K, Gross J 1976 Collagen fibrillogenesis: intermediate aggregates and suprafibrillar order. Proceedings of the National Academy of Sciences of the United States of America 73: 4027

Tryggvason K, Gehron Robey P, Martin G R 1980a Biosynthesis of type IV procollagens. Biochemistry 19: 1284

Tryggvason K, Majamaa K, Kivirikko K I 1979a Prolyl 3-hydroxylase and 4-hydroxylase activities in certain rat and chick-embryo tissues and age-related changes in their activities in the rat. Biochemical Journal 178: 127

Tryggvason K, Majamaa K, Risteli J, Kivirikko K I 1979b Partial purification and characterization of chick-embryo prolyl 3-hydroxylase. Biochemical Journal 183: 303

Tryggvason K, Pihlajaniemi T, Liotta L A, Foidart J M, Martin G R, Kivirikko K I 1980b Processing of proα(I) and proα2(IV) collagen chains in vivo and in vitro. Abstracts of VII European Symposium on Connective Tissue Research, Prague, p. 29

Tryggvason K, Risteli J, Kivirikko K I 1977 Separation of prolyl 3-hydroxylase and 4-hydroxylase activities and the 4-hydroxyproline requirement for synthesis of 3-hydroxyproline. Biochemical and Biophysical Research Communications 76: 275

Tryggvason K, Risteli J, Kivirikko K I 1978 Glomerular basement membrane collagen and activities of the intracellular enzymes of collagen biosynthesis in congenital nephrotic syndrome of the Finnish type. Clinica Chimica Acta 82: 233

Tuderman L 1976 Developmental changes in prolyl hydroxylase activity and protein in chick embryo. European Journal of Biochemistry 66: 615

Tuderman L, Kivirikko K I 1977 Immunoreactive prolyl hydroxylase in human skin, serum and synovial fluid: changes in the content and components with age. European Journal of Clinical Investigation 7: 295

Tuderman L, Kivirikko K I, Prockop D J 1978 Partial purification and characterization of a neutral protease which cleaves the N-terminal propeptides from procollagen. Biochemistry 17: 2948

Tuderman L, Kuutti E-R, Kivirikko K I 1975 An affinity-column procedure using poly(L-proline) for the purification of prolyl hydroxylase. Purification of the enzyme from chick embryos. European Journal of Biochemistry 52: 9

Tuderman L, Myllylä R, Kivirikko K I 1977a Mechanism of the prolyl hydroxylase reaction. Role of co-substrates. European Journal of Biochemistry 80: 341

Tuderman L, Oikarinen A, Kivirikko K I 1977b Tetramers and monomers of prolyl hydroxylase in isolated chick embryo tendon cells. The association of inactive monomers to active tetramers and a preliminary characterization of the intracellular monomer-size protein. European Journal of Biochemistry 78: 547

Tuderman L, Risteli J, Miettinen T, Kivirikko K I 1977c Serum immunoreactive prolyl hydroxylase in liver disease. European Journal of Clinical Investigation 7: 537

Turpeenniemi T M, Puistola U, Anttinen H, Kivirikko K I 1977 Affinity chromatography of lysyl hydroxylase on concanavalin A-agarose. Biochimica et Biophysica Acta 483: 215

Turpeenniemi-Hujanen T M 1981 Immunological characterization of lysyl hydroxylase, an enzyme of collagen synthesis. Biochemical Journal 195: 669

Turpeenniemi-Hujanen T M, Puistola U, Kivirikko K I 1980 Isolation of lysyl hydroxylase, an enzyme of collagen synthesis, from chick embryos as a homogeneous protein. Biochemical Journal 189: 247

Turpeenniemi-Hujanen T M, Puistola U, Kivirikko K I 1981 Human lysyl hydroxylase: Purification to homogeneity, partial characterization and comparison of catalytic properties with those of a mutant enzyme from Ehlers–Danlos syndrome type VI fibroblasts. Collagen and Related Research Clinical and Experimental 1: 355

Uitto J 1977 Biosynthesis of type II collagen. Removal of amino- and carboxy-terminal extensions from procollagen synthesized by chick embryo cartilage cells. Biochemistry 16: 3421

Uitto J, Prockop D J 1974 Synthesis and secretion of under-hydroxylated procollagen at various temperatures by cells subject to temporary anoxia. Biochemical and Biophysical Research Communications 60: 414

Uitto J, Lichtenstein J R 1976 Removal of amino-terminal and carboxy-terminal extension peptides from procollagen during synthesis of chick embryo tendon collagen. Biochemical and Biophysical Research Communications 71: 60

Uitto J, Allan R E, Polak K L 1979 Conversion of type II procollagen to collagen. Extracellular removal of the amino-terminal and carboxyterminal extensions without a preferential sequence. European Journal of Biochemistry 99: 97

Uitto J, Lichtenstein J R, Bauer E A 1976 Characterization of procollagen synthesized by matrix-free cells isolated from chick embryo tendons. Biochemistry 15: 4935

Uitto V-J, Uitto J, Kao W W-Y, Prockop D J 1978 Procollagen polypeptides containing cis-4-hydroxy-L-proline are over-glycosylated and secreted as nonhelical pro-α-chains. Archives of Biochemistry and Biophysics 185: 214

Vistica D T, Ahrens F A, Ellison W R 1977 The effect of lead upon collagen synthesis and proline hydroxylation in the swiss mouse 3T6 fibroblasts. Archives of Biochemistry and Biophysics 179: 15

Waechter C J, Lennarz W J 1976 The role of polyprenol-linked sugars in glycoprotein synthesis. Annual Review of Biochemistry 45: 95

Weinstock M 1977 Centrosymmetrical crossbanded structures in the matrix of rat incisor predentin and dentin. Journal of Ultrastructural Research 61: 218

Weinstock M, Leblond C P 1974 Synthesis, migration and release of precursor collagen by odontoblasts as visualized by radioautography after [^{3}H]proline administration. Journal of Cellular Biology 60: 92

Wiestner M, Krieg T, Hörlein D, Glanville R W, Fietzek P, Müller P K 1979 Inhibiting effect of procollagen peptides on collagen biosynthesis in fibroblast cultures. Journal of Biological Chemistry 254: 7016

Wu C H, Rojkind M, Rifas L, Seifter S 1978 Biosynthesis of type I and type III collagens by cultured uterine smooth muscle cells. Archives of Biochemistry and Biophysics 188: 294

7

Degradation of collagen

Z. WERB

INTRODUCTION

Collagens are complex fibrous proteins that function as the major structural proteins of animals because of their characteristic rigidity and resistance to proteolytic attack. In adult organisms most intact collagen fibres turn over slowly. However, the orderly degradation of interstitial and basement membrane collagens is one of the fundamental processes governing growth, development, morphogenesis, remodelling, and repair under both normal and pathological conditions. The degradative mechanisms that operate under one set of conditions may not apply to different tissues or conditions. The differing primary structures of the genetically distinct collagen types may require distinct enzymes. The extent and type of intermolecular cross-links and the assembly of the collagen types and other connective tissue proteins into supramolecular structures may also influence the susceptibility of collagens to proteolysis. Collagen degradation may take place at extracellular sites, in the pericellular zone within 30 nm of the plasma membrane, and in the vacuolar system within cells.

ENZYMATIC MECHANISMS FOR COLLAGEN DEGRADATION

The mechanisms by which collagen molecules are removed from their extracellular structures and degraded are only now being elucidated. Few direct data favouring participation of any enzyme system in collagen degradation in vivo have been obtained despite perhaps one thousand publications on this subject during the past twenty years (Woolley & Evanson, 1980). Nevertheless, from circumstantial evidence we can assign putative roles for various enzymatic processes in collagen degradation (Table 7.1).

Table 7.1 Enzymatic mechanisms for collagen degradation

Process	*Enzymes*	*Sites of action*
A. *Degradation related to collagen synthesis*		
1. Degradation of signal sequences, newly synthesized collagen chains, and underhydroxylated collagen	Unknown	Intracellular, by membrane-bound enzymes in endoplasmin reticulum or by lysosomal hydrolases
2. Procollagen NH_2- and COOH-terminal peptide cleavage	Procollagen peptidases	Intracellular, cell surface, or extracellular, at neutral pH
B. *Degradation related to turnover of extracellular collagens*		
1. Breakdown of insoluble polymeric collagen fibrils	Depolymerases, including nonspecific proteinases, granulocyte elastase, and limited action of collagenase	Extracellular, at neutral pH
2. Cleavage of native collagen fibrils and monomers through the helical portion of individual molecules into large fragments	Type-specific collagenases, granulocyte elastase	Extracellular and cell surface, at neutral pH
3. Degradation of large collagen fragments after thermal denaturation to gelatin	Numerous 'gelatinases' and nonspecific tissue and plasma proteinases	Extracellular and cell surface
	Collagenolytic cathepsin	Intralysosomal, after endocytosis
4. Final degradation to oligopeptides and amino acids	Pz-peptidase, exopeptidases	Extracellular fluids and intralysosomal

Gross & Lapiere (1962) first described a proteinase that was released into the tissue culture medium of tissue explants from tadpole tails undergoing morphogenesis. This metalloproteinase, called collagenase, cleaved helical type I collagen molecules in solution at neutral pH in a unique way, giving rise to two fragments (Fig. 7.1).

Fig. 7.1 Diagrammatic representation of the helical type I collagen molecule (TC) and its cleavage into three-quarter (TC^A) and one-quarter (TC^B) fragments by vertebrate collagenase (Kang et al, 1966). In this particular molecule there is an intramolecular cross-link near the NH_2-terminal end between one $\alpha 1$ chain and the $\alpha 2$ chain, which after denaturation would form a $\beta 1$, 2 dimer subunit; the cross-link may also occur between two $\alpha 1$ chains, giving rise to the $\beta 1$, 1 dimer. The native TC molecule denatures at $> 37°C$, but after digestion with collagenase the TC^A fragment denatures at $> 33°C$ and the TC^B fragment at $> 28°C$, giving rise to $\beta 1$, 2^A, $\alpha 1^A$, $\alpha 1^B$, and $\alpha 2^B$ chains. The native and denatured collagen chains and their fragments resulting from cleavage by collagenase are shown in Figs. 7.3 and 7.4.

Since those original experiments, a number of collagenolytic proteinases have been obtained from tissue and cell cultures and from a wide range of tissues in which collagen is degraded under both physiological and pathological conditions.

Degradation related to collagen synthesis

Although it is widely recognised that newly synthesized collagen is degraded more readily than mature collagen, it has only recently been suggested that a significant proportion of collagen (about 30 per cent) is degraded within minutes of its synthesis, probably intracellularly (Bienkowski et al, 1978). Although this may appear to be a wasteful process, collagen synthesis is already known to be rather wasteful, considering that degradation of precursor sequences is involved in intracellular compartmentalization and in secretion (see Chapter 6). One possible explanation is that intracellular processes 'edit' collagens so that abnormal molecules containing synthetic errors generated at the transcriptional, translational, or post-translational levels can be destroyed (Berg et al, 1980; Tolstoshev et al, 1981). Another possibility is regulation of the proper ratio of $\alpha 1(I)$ to $\alpha_2(I)$ chains during synthesis of type I collagen.

Degradative mechanisms may also control the proportion of collagen types secreted into interstitial spaces; this is supported by evidence that cells synthesise two types of collagen intracellularly but secrete only one of them (see Chapter 6). The processing of procollagens to collagens by cleavage of the amino (NH_2) and carboxyl (COOH) terminal extension peptides by specific procollagen peptidases is another example of a requirement for specialized enzymes to effect proteolysis during collagen synthesis and assembly (see Chapter 6).

Degradation related to turnover of extracellular collagens

Depolymerization of cross-linked collagen fibres.

The degradation of collagens becomes more complex once they are in place extracellularly. Polymeric collagen fibrils containing intermolecular cross-links are, in general, much more resistant to degradation than soluble collagens (Leibovich & Weiss, 1971; Harris & Farrell, 1972; Vater et al, 1979). It is not known whether the amino or carboxy terminal cross-link regions of the collagen molecule must be cleaved before the helical portion of the molecules can be attacked; however, a number of enzymes cleave the terminal peptides of type I collagen in vitro (Fig. 7.2) and may have similar actions on collagens of types II, III, and IV.

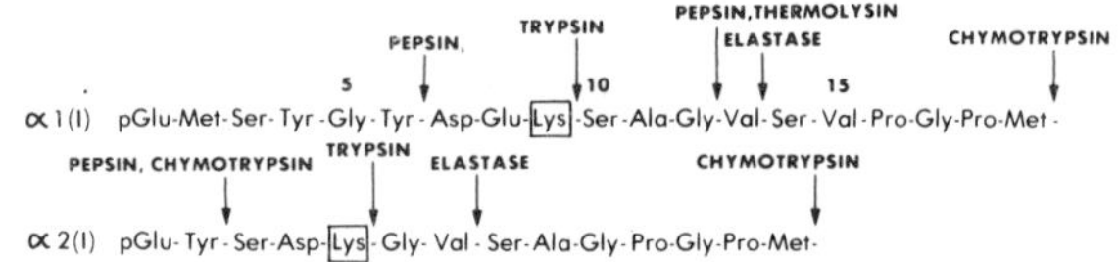

Fig. 7.2 Primary structure of the non-helical NH_2-terminal region of the rat type I collagen molecule showing enzyme cleavage sites. The lysine residues that are involved in intra- and intermolecular cross-links are shown in the boxes (Kang et al, 1967; Furthmayr & Timpl, 1972; Fietzek et al, 1974; Becker et al, 1975). Cathepsin B also cleaves the $\alpha 1(I)$ chain between residues 12 and 13 and between residues 14 and 15 (Etherington, 1976).

These enzymes are unlikely to be present in tissue spaces, and thus are not likely to play a role in collagen degradation in vivo. Specific collagenases can solubilize some peptides even from highly cross-linked collagen (Vater et al, 1979). Enzymes with depolymerase activity at neutral pH that could be present in vivo include granulocyte elastase, cathepsin G, and some less well characterized proteinases (Stevens et al, 1975; Burleigh, 1977; Burleigh et al, 1977; Mainardi et al, 1980a, b). Thiol proteinases, such as cathepsins B, N, H, and L, that are active at acid pH and also cleave the telopeptides of collagen types I and II (Etherington, 1976; Burleigh, 1977) could depolymerize insoluble collagen fibres within lysosomes and in pericellular spaces where the local pH is acidified by metabolic products such as lactic acid.

Cleavage of the helical portion of collagen

The triple helix of collagen endows the molecules with their property of resistance to proteolysis. One group of collagenolytic enzymes attacks the native collagen molecule, cleaving all three subunits at a specific locus characteristic of each enzyme. The vertebrate collagenases discussed at greater length subsequently have a high degree of substrate specificity and a strong preference for collagen in its native form; denatured collagen (gelatin) and peptides containing the cleaved sequence are poor substrates by comparison. The other proteinases that degrade the helical sequences, such as granulocyte elastase, may also degrade other proteins. The cleavage products of specific collagenases are resistant to further proteolysis unless they denature.

Enzymes of a second group cleave the native collagen molecules at numerous sites. The bacterial proteinase clostridiopeptidase A degrades the collagen molecule sequentially inward from the ends (reviewed by Weiss, 1976), and it is possible that the vertebrate collagenolytic thiol cathepsins act by a similar mechanism (Etherington, 1976; Burleigh, 1977).

Phagocytosis of collagen fibres

During rapid collagen breakdown, such as in the involuting uterus post partum, collagen fibrils are found within cells enclosed in membrane-bounded vesicles, presumably secondary lysosomes (Parakkal, 1969; Padykula, 1976). The fibrils are probably cleaved from an intact fibre by the combined action of specific and nonspecific collagenolytic enzymes. Once within lysosomes, cathepsins B, N, H, and L may cleave the collagen fibrils (Etherington, 1976; Barrett, 1980).

Degradation of denatured collagens

Once the collagen fibril is attacked by collagenase or one of the other enzymes making limited cleavage in the helical portion of molecule, fragments dissociate from the fibril and at 37°C immediately denature into gelatin (Fig. 7.1). At sites of collagen degradation numerous enzymes are present that may further degrade the gelatin to amino acids and oligopeptides. Neutral proteinases with activity against gelatin are produced along with collagenase in a number of systems (Ryan & Woessner, 1974; Steven et al, 1975; Weiss, 1976). Proteinases derived from plasma, such as plasmin, may also play an important role in the degradation of gelatin. Other distinct peptidases active against the collagen-like Pz-peptide are found in tissue fluids, culture supernatants, and plasma (Weiss, 1976). There are also a number of other exopeptidases in extracellular fluids and within cells (Barrett, 1980). As an alternative to extracellular degradation by neutral proteinases and peptidases, the large fragments derived from the primary collagenolytic event may be endocytosed and degraded by lysosomal enzymes within connective tissue and inflammatory cells. The collagenolytic cathepsins B, N, H, and L are, in fact, much more active against gelatin than against native collagen (Burleigh, 1977).

Degradation of proteins with collagen-like sequences

In addition to the genetically distinct collagens of types I, II, III, IV, and V, a number of other proteins have been found to have helical collagen sequences in their primary structure. These proteins include the complement component C1q, the synaptic membrane-bound form of acetylcholinesterase, and the neurophysins. The enzymes involved in the degradation of these proteins have not been studied. The collagenous sequences of these proteins appear to be resistant to the action of vertebrate collagenases, but the biological activities of the proteins are altered by incubation with clostridiopeptidase A (Lwebuga-Mukasa et al, 1976; Katayama et al, 1978; Reid, 1979).

MODE OF ACTION OF TISSUE COLLAGENASES

Hundreds of papers have been written on the production of specific collagenases that have the capacity for collagen degradation. Despite these many studies, surprisingly little is understood about the molecular structure and biological function of these enzymes. That they have a biological role has been inferred from their association with tissues undergoing collagenolysis, from their ability to degrade collagen in test situations, and from the demonstration of their specific cleavage products in extracellular fluids during collagen degradation. Only cells secreting collagenases are able to degrade a collagen matrix in culture (Werb & Aggeler, 1978; Werb et al, 1980a, b). In addition, collagenases have been directly demonstrated in tissues immunologically (Woolley & Evanson, 1980).

Properties of vertebrate collagenases

The classic vertebrate collagenases are defined as enzymes with a strong preference for native collagen rather than gelatin that have the property of cleaving collagen molecules in their helical region into fragments three-quarters and one-quarter the size of the original molecule. These enzymes, which have specificity toward type I collagen, are widely distributed. In a number of vertebrate species, collagenases are found in culture medium or lysates of a wide variety of tissues, including the rheumatoid synovium, tumors, corneal tissues, periodontal tissue, the gastrointestinal tract, granulomas, uterus, skin, and several cell types, including polymorphonuclear leucocytes, macrophages, fibroblasts, endothelial cells, and melanoma cells (Woolley & Evanson, 1980). Nearly all the collagenases studied to date are of molecular weight ranging from 25 000 to 60 000 and are metalloproteinases as defined by their requirement for calcium and, most likely, zinc ions for their catalytic activity. Their activity is

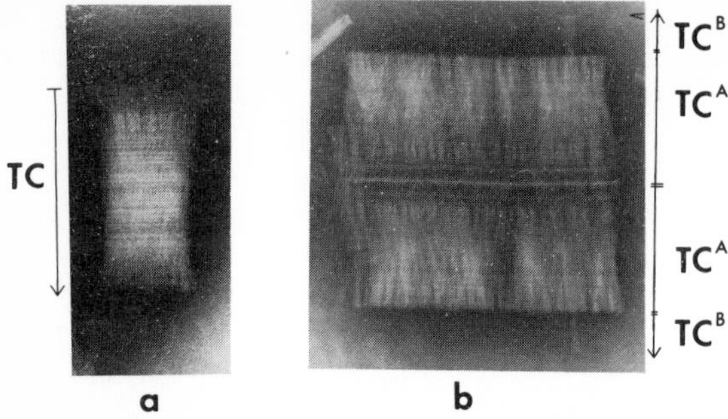

Fig. 7.3 Segment-long spacing crystallites of (a) rabbit skin collagen type I (TC) and (b) its three-quarter (TC^A) fragment arising from the NH_2-terminal end and its one-quarter (TC^B) fragment arising from the COOH-terminal end. After dialysis against acetic acid and addition of adenosine 5′-triphosphate, the collagen molecules aggregate into ribbons side-to-side with NH_2-terminal ends all together; the segment-long spacing fragments are then negatively stained and examined by electron microscopy (Werb & Burleigh, 1974).

inhibited by chelators such as EDTA and 1,10-phenanthroline, and by compounds with reactive sulfhydryl groups such as cysteine, dithiothreitol, and D-penacillamine in the 1–10 mM range. Most of the detailed studies of this class of enzymes have dealt with their behaviour against collagen substrates rather than with their molecular properties. They are obtained in exceedingly small amounts from cell and tissue cultures. One striking feature of the collagenases studied is their appearance in inactive forms in cell culture and tissue extracts. It is still hotly debated whether these inactive forms are inactive precursor forms (zymogens) or enzyme-inhibitor complexes (Birkedal-Hansen et al, 1975, 1976; Eeckhout & Vaes, 1977; Murphy et al, 1977a, b; Sellers et al, 1977; Werb et al, 1977; Valle & Bauer, 1979; Woessner, 1979; Woolley & Evanson, 1980). Further information on the molecular properties of collagenase is needed to understand these issues as well as the interrelationships of collagenases from different tissues.

Cleavage of native collagens

The unusual specificity of vertebrate collagenases is clearly demonstrated when they react with native collagen in solution at neutral pH at temperatures below that required to denature the substrate and the cleavage products of the substrate (<27°C) (Fig. 7.1). Gel electrophoresis of the collagen solution at the end of the incubation period reveals the presence of three new pairs of bands in addition to the pairs of intact α-chains and the β-dimer components (Fig. 7.3). When the soluble collagen and cleaved collagen molecules are assembled into segment-long spacing aggregates, stained, and examined by electron microscopy, the distinct cleavage site giving rise to the three-quarter fragment and the one-quarter fragment can be seen (Fig. 7.4).

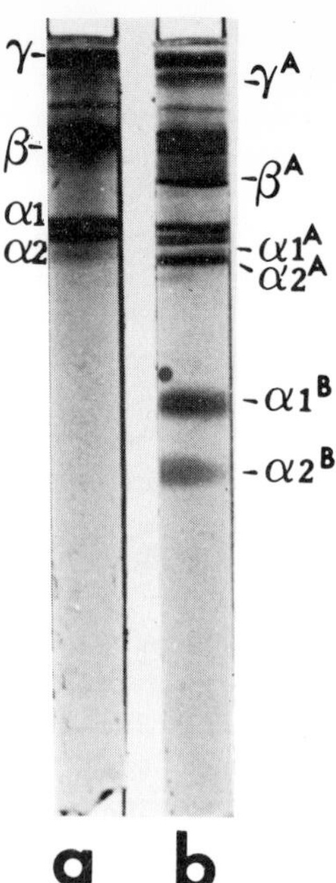

Fig. 7.4 Polyacrylamide gel electrophoretic separation of denatured rabbit skin collagen type I into collagen subunits at pH 3.5. (a) Undigested collagen contains β1, 1 and β1, 2 cross-linked dimer components, α1 and α2 monomers, as well as some trimers (γ) and higher-order aggregates from intermolecular cross-links. (b) After digestion with rabbit fibroblast collagenase, β1, 1^A, β1, 2^A, α1^A, and α2^A fragments arising from the three-quarter-length cleavage product and α1^B and α2^B fragments from the one-quarter-length product are seen (Werb & Burleigh, 1974).

The three-quarter fragment has three COOH-terminal glycine residues and the one-quarter fragment has three NH_2-terminal isoleucine residues for type I collagen; a Gly-Ile bond is also cleaved by vertebrate collagenases in type II and III collagen (Fig. 7.5). Thus it appears that collagenase recognizes certain Gly-Ile bonds. In its 1000 residues the type I collagen chain contains three Gly-Ile bonds, yet only one of these is cleaved by collagenase and none of the 18 chemically similar Gly-Leu bonds are cleaved. Purified

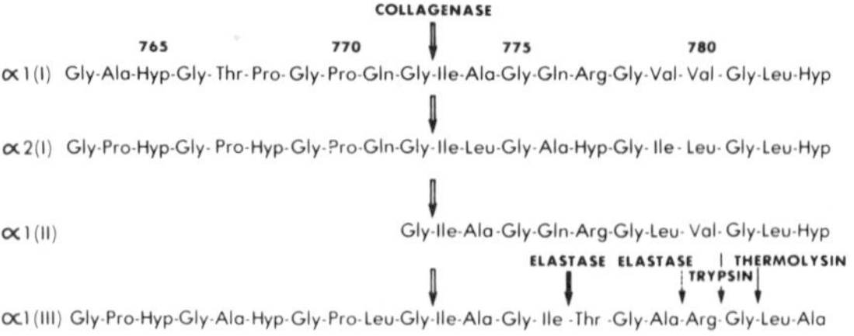

Fig. 7.5 Primary structure of the collagenase cleavage site region of interstitial collagen chains. The sequence and cleavage sites of α1(I) are from Highberger et al (1975), α2(I) from Dixit et al (1979), α1(II) from Miller et al (1976b), and α1(III) from Miller et al (1976a), Mainardi et al (1980b), Seyer et al (1980), and Wang et al (1978). Cleavage sites for collagenase are shown for all four chains. The cleavage sites in α1(III) for granulocyte elastase, trypsin, and thermolysin are also shown.

collagenase also cleaves the appropriate Gly-Ile bond in the α_1 CB7 peptide from the cleavage site region. There are reports of additional limited cleavage in the COOH-terminal region of the three-quarter fragment with the use of partially purified preparations of several of the collagenases. Whether these cleavage sites represent the action of collagenase or of contaminating proteinases has not been determined. Collagens of types IV and V are resistant to the action of the classic vertebrate collagenases; thus, it may be predicted that these collagens do not contain a Gly-Ile bond in the homologous region of their sequence.

One striking feature of the collagenase cleavage region of the collagen molecule is that this region may be only semi-helical. Although glycine is present at every third residue, there is a paucity of proline and hydroxyproline residues in this sequence (Fig. 7.5). The exact nature of the specificity of this site remains unknown. Further evidence that the specificity of collagenase cleavage to this site is limited by the conformation of the collagen is the finding that trypsin and thermolysin also attack near the cleavage site in the native type III molecule (Fig. 7.5). Thermolysin and very high concentrations of trypsin also cleave the intact type I collagen molecule close to the cleavage site, although the details are not yet known (Wang et al, 1978).

Collagen-type specificity of collagenases

Although the classic vertebrate collagenases attack the same peptide bond locus of type I collagen, there is emerging evidence for differences in the rate of attack of the same substrate by enzymes from different sources, and for collagen-type specificity of collagenolytic enzymes. Vertebrate collagenases from human skin fibroblasts and macrophages have about the same rate and extent of cleavage of both type I and III collagens; however, the collagenase extracted from human polymorphonuclear leucocytes attacks type I collagen about 15 times more effectively than type III (Horwitz et al, 1977) (Table 7.2).

Table 7.2 Collagen-type specificity of collagenolytic proteinases

Enzyme	*Collagen-type specificity**
Vertebrate collagenase	I = III > II IV, V no reaction
Granulocyte collagenase	I > III
Granulocyte elastase	III, IV II > I, V non-helical peptides only
Mast cell proteinase	IV>I
Tumour type IV collagenase	IV I, II, III, V no reaction
Macrophage type V collagenase	V I, III, IV no reaction
Trypsin	III, IV, V
Collagenolytic cathepsins	I, II

* Where known

A collagenolytic enzyme extracted from a highly invasive, rapidly growing mouse fibrosarcoma degrades type IV collagen (Liotta et al, 1979). A collagenolytic enzyme specific for type V collagen has been found in the supernatants of rabbit alveolar macrophages; this enzyme cleaves the helical region of type V collagen and can be separated from the classic vertebrate collagenase secreted by the same cells (Mainardi et al, 1980c). Tumour cells also produce a type V collagenolytic enzyme (Liotta et al, 1981).

Although the collagens of types IV and V are resistant to cleavage by vertebrate collagenase and appear to require the newly described type-specific collagenases, other enzymes of broad specificity are able to attack the helical portion of these basement membrane collagen molecules. For example, granulocyte elastase appears to have a major pathological role in the degradation of these proteins. Granulocyte elastase specifically cleaves collagens of types III and IV (Mainardi et al, 1980a, b) (Table 7.2) and is able to cleave the non-helical peptides and possibly to nibble somewhat at the ends of the molecule in types I, II, and IV. Because this enzyme may be prevalent in inflammatory sites, e.g., in glomerulonephritis, its potent collagenolytic activities must be reckoned with.

Although trypsin is not found in normal sites of collagen degradation, it is able to degrade collagens of types III, IV, and V (Miller et al, 1976a; Liotta et al, 1979; Mainardi et al, 1980a). Trypsin is one of a large family of arginine- and lysine-specific serine proteinases, and it is possible that the cleavage specificities for collagen degradation are properties of trypsin-like enzymes (e.g., plasmin and other enzymes of the coagulation and fibrinolytic systems) that are present in interstitial fluids.

The collagenolytic cathepsins, active at acid pH, degrade collagens of types I and II, but their specificity for other collagen types has not been determined. However, because their mechanism of action is more like that of the bacterial collagenases, it is probable that these enzymes are able to degrade the whole spectrum of collagen types.

Differential susceptibility of collagen types to cleavage

In addition to collagen-type specificity of collagenolytic enzymes, the various collagen types seem to differ in their susceptibility to collagenolytic attack. In general, cartilage collagen (type II) in solution and in fibril form is more resistant to attack by a variety of specific collagenases than are types I and III. It is not clear whether the greater extent of glycosylation of type II collagen may be responsible for this difference. Collagen type III appears to be the most susceptible to attack by a large variety of nonspecific and specific collagenases that all hydrolyze peptide bonds near the cleavage site for specific collagenases. However, it is interesting to note that granulocyte elastase is able to cleave the non-helical peptides of type II collagen much more rapidly than those of type I (Burleigh, 1977). Liotta et al (1979) demonstrated that the type IV-specific collagenase extracted from a mouse tumour was unable to cleave collagens of types I, II, III, and V, and that the classic specific collagenase from human skin cleaved types I, II, and III, but not types IV and V. The macrophage type V-specific collagenase is unable to cleave collagens of types I, III, and IV (Mainardi et al, 1980c). Thus, there is a marked difference in susceptibility of native substrates to a particular collagenase.

Other factors influencing the rates of degradation of collagen include its state of aggregation and cross-linking. Collagens from older human individuals are more resistant to degradation by bacterial collagenase, and the introduction of formaldehyde- or lysyl oxidase-generated cross-links into reconstituted collagen fibrils and gels simultaneously decreases solubility and increases resistance to collagenolysis by both bacterial and specific collagenase (Harris & Farrell, 1972; Vater et al, 1979).

In tissues, collagens are assembled into complex fibrillar patterns containing more than one type of collagen. These mixtures of collagen types may produce constraints on the rate of degradation. Other components of the extracellular matrix, including fibronectins, proteoglycans, and elastin bundled together into complex connective tissue, may also play an important role in regulating the rate of collagen degradation in tissues. Glycoproteins may regulate the degradation of collagen (Anderson, 1976) and of native elastin fibrils (Werb et al, 1980a, b; Jones & Werb, 1980). Additionally, the rate of glycosaminoglycan degradation may be reduced in the presence of collagen (David & Bernfield, 1979).

Influence of temperature on collagen degradation

Because peripheral tissues such as skin and joints have normal temperatures of 30°C to 33°C, and these temperatures are increased by inflammation, the altered susceptibility of collagen by temperature may have important consequences in the degradation of collagen. The rate of degradation of collagen fibrils of types I and II is influenced markedly by temperature (Harris & McCroskery, 1974; Burleigh et al, 1977). An increase of 2° in the range of 30°C to 37°C increases the rate of collagen degradation about four-fold. At temperatures above 33°C the cleavage fragments produced by the primary collagenolytic event denature (Fig. 7.1). In the form of gelatin polypeptides, they become susceptible to many proteinases.

REGULATION OF COLLAGENASE ACTIVITY

The first observation and subsequent isolation of collagenases from vertebrate tissues depended on the fact that these enzymes appear not to be stored for subsequent release but are synthesized de novo and secreted from cells in culture in either an inactive or active form. Subsequently, there have been a number of reports of collagenase in homogenates of tissue. These observations have led to speculations about the form in which collagenases are released from cells and how collagenase activity is regulated.

Cellular regulation of collagenase

Origins of collagenolytic enzymes

The specific collagenases and the enzymes responsible for collagen-type-specific degradation originate in a number of different cells of mesenchymal, endothelial, and epithelial origin (Table 7.3). Fibroblasts and stromal cells from a variety of tissues including synovium, cornea, skin, and gingiva can, when appropriately triggered, produce prodigious amounts of specific collagenase that degrades collagens of types I, II, and III (Werb & Burleigh, 1974; Birkedal-Hansen et al, 1975, 1976; Werb & Aggeler, 1978; Newsome & Gross, 1979; Valle & Bauer, 1979). The collagenases produced by fibroblasts are in latent form and

Table 7.3 Cellular origins of collagenolytic enzymes active at neutral pH

Cell type	*Collagen type degraded**	*Range of collagenase activity produced†*
Fibroblast, stromal cell	I, II, III	0–150
Macrophage	I, III	0–0.5
	V	2.5
Chondrocyte	I, II	0–5
Corneal epithelial cell	I	0–20
Polymorphonuclear leucocyte (collagenase)	I	1–10
Polymorphonuclear leucocyte (elastase)	III, IV	1–10
Endothelial cell	I	0–0.5
Tumour cell	I, III	1
	IV	1
	V	—
Rheumatoid synovial cell	I, II, III	0–250

* Where known

† μg collagen degraded per min at 37°C produced from 10^6 cells in 24h

require subsequent activation. Macrophages have also been shown to produce collagenolytic activity; however, the amount of type I- and type III-specific collagenase produced by these cells is exceedingly small (Wahl et al, 1975, 1977; Horwitz et al, 1976; Werb, 1978; Werb et al, 1980a, b). More recently, macrophages have been shown to secrete a proteinase capable of specific cleavage of type V collagen in quantities that, though small, are significant because type V collagen is resistant to degradation by virtually all other collagenolytic enzymes (Mainardi, C. L., personal communication). Chondrocytes can be stimulated to produce collagenolytic activity against type I and II collagens (Deshmukh-Phadke et al, 1978). Rheumatoid synovial cells, which are of mesenchymal origin, can produce very large amounts of collagenase, and this specific collagenase is active against collagen of types I, II, and III (Dayer et al, 1976, 1977; Werb et al, 1977). Endothelial cells also produce minute amounts of a collagenase active against type I collagen (Moscatelli et al, 1980).

Collagenases have also been found in the extracts or culture supernatants of tumours. It is difficult to know whether these enzymes originate in the tumour cells or in normal cells, such as macrophages and stromal cells, that are interspersed in the tumour. Homogeneous cultures of tumour cells have also been shown to degrade collagens. Collagenases active against type I and III collagen and both type IV-specific and type V-specific collagenases (Liotta et al, 1979, 1981) have been isolated. In addition, tumour cells in culture have been shown to have the capacity to degrade extracellular matrix that contains a complex mixture of glycoproteins, elastin, and collagens of types I, III, IV, and V (Jones & DeClerck, 1980); however, no extracellular enzyme was secreted by these cells, and no collagenolytic enzyme was recovered from cell lysates.

Polymorphonuclear leucocytes contain within their granules two distinct collagenolytic systems. They have been shown to contain a small amount of a specific collagenase that is likely to be different from the specific collagenases secreted by other cells, such as fibroblasts and macrophages. This collagenase is present in the specific granules and degrades soluble type I collagen (Horwitz et al, 1977; Murphy et al, 1977b). The second collagenolytic system of the polymorphonuclear leucocyte is the elastase present in its azurophil granules. This serine proteinase has a wide variety of substrates among plasma and interstitial proteins, including collagens of types III and IV, which it cleaves specifically (Mainardi et al, 1980a, b). Interestingly, the polymorphonuclear leukocyte appears to lack enzymes that degrade type V collagen appreciably and it is not particularly active against type II collagen (Mainardi, C. L., personal communication). Granulocyte elastase is active in depolymerizing cross-linked fibrils of type I collagen, thus making them susceptible to the type I-specific collagenase.

Factors regulating collagenase production

Although a range of collagenolytic potential is exhibited by a variety of cells (Table 7.3), many cells secrete little if any collagenolytic enzyme unless appropriately triggered. Factors involved in the stimulation or suppression of collagenolytic activity in tissue or cell culture are well described and appear to act directly on the enzyme-producing cells (Table 7.4).

Table 7.4 Factors affecting production of vertebrate collagenases

A. *Stimulatory factors*	B. *Inhibitory factors*
Cell-cell interactions	Glucocorticoids
Lymphokines	Retinoids
Macrophage factors	Increased production of endogenous inhibitors
Proteinases	Hormones (oestrogens, progesterone)
Phagocytosis	Indomethacin
Formation of multinucleate giant cells	
Prostaglandin E	
Phorbol diester tumour promoters	
Cytochalasin B	
Bacterial toxins	
Colchicine	
Soluble collagen	

Most of the experiments on the regulation of collagenolytic activity are designed to study stimulation of collagenase production by cells that are producing little or no enzyme. Cell-cell interactions have been implicated in a number of systems. Epithelial cells isolated from alkali-burned rabbit corneal epithelium stimulated the production of collagenase in mixed cultures of these epithelial cells and cells derived from the corneal stroma (Johnson-Muller & Gross, 1978). Similarly, macrophages stimulated the degradation of cartilage collagen by fibroblasts (Huybrechts-Godin et al, 1979). Mononuclear cells stimulated the production of collagenase and prostaglandin E_2 by rheumatoid synovial cells in culture (Dayer et al, 1977). In all three of these cases it was subsequently shown that direct cell-cell interaction was not required, but that medium conditioned by epithelial cells in the case of the cornea (Newsome & Gross, 1979), by macrophages or T-lymphocytes in the case of the rheumatoid synovium (Dayer et al, 1977), and by macrophages in the case of the cartilage (Deshmukh-Phadke et al, 1978) were responsible. Factors produced by lymphocytes (so-called lymphokines) also induce collagenase production in macrophage cultures, but in this case it is possible that the production of collagenase by a small number of fibroblasts has been initiated indirectly.

Proteolytic enzymes can induce secretion of specific collagenase by fibroblasts (Werb & Aggeler, 1978); this induction is dependent on the ability of the proteinase to induce a morphologic change in the fibroblasts, and is independent of the ability of the proteinase to activate the latent form of collagenase. Phagocytosis of particles and their storage within lysosomes also induce secretion of collagenase by fibroblasts (Werb & Reynolds, 1974) and by macrophages (Werb & Gordon, 1975). The mechanism governing the secretion of collagenase after phagocytosis is not known, but prolonged lysosomal storage of materials appears to be necessary. Not all cells respond to the phagocytic stimulus alone, although the phagocytic stimulus coupled with an additional stimulant such as lymphocyte supernatants, proteinases, or pharmacologic agents appears to work in a two-stage manner to stimulate collagenase secretion. Fusion of fibroblasts into multinucleate giant cells, which are often found in sites of rapid collagen degradation, can also induce the production of collagenase (Brinckerhoff & Harris, 1978).

Prostaglandins of the E-series (PGE) are associated with the production of collagenase in several systems, including the macrophage (Wahl et al, 1975; Dayer et al, 1976, 1977). Under some conditions it appears that the micromolar concentrations of these prostaglandins that can be found in vivo and in tissue culture medium are able to induce the secretion of collagenase by macrophages and synovial cells. The response of cells to exogenous PGE, which is intimately connected with cellular concentrations of cyclic AMP, may be variable because of the transient increases in cyclic AMP. In addition, responses of cells to PGE and cyclic AMP may exhibit the phenomenon of down regulation, in which exposure to a hormone results in a state of refractoriness during which no response to the hormone can be elicited. It is also possible that the response of cells to mononuclear factors, lymphokines, and possibly some of the other stimulating factors may be mediated indirectly by an increase in PGE concentration of cells (Woolley & Evanson, 1980).

Bacterial toxins (lipo-polysaccharide) have also been shown to induce the production of collagenase by macrophages (Wahl et al, 1975). One curious finding is the observation that collagen in solution may induce collagenase production by fibroblasts (Biswas & Dayer, 1979) in view of the fact that fibroblasts normally produce collagens of type I and III as part of their differentiated function, and fibroblasts growing on insoluble collagen fibrils or extracellular matrix do not secrete collagenase until triggered by another factor such as a proteinase (Werb & Aggeler, 1978).

A number of pharmacologic agents also induce the secretion of collagenases. Cytochalasin B is one of the most potent of these inducers (Harris et al, 1975). This compound, like proteinases, produces a morphologic alteration in cells by interfering with the assembly of cytoskeletal proteins. Cytocholasin B may not work alone but may induce secretion of collagenase in cells triggered by another mechanism. Thus, cells that were filled with secondary lysosomes secreted more collagenase when triggered with cytochalasin B (Harris et al, 1975). Cytochalasin B did not itself induce collagenase secretion in corneal stromal cells, but acted synergistically with a factor from epithelial cells (which also did not trigger collagenase secretion appreciably) to induce secretion of a large quantity of collagenase (Johnson-Muller & Gross, 1978; Newsome & Gross, 1979). Colchicine, another agent that interferes with the cytoskeleton of cells, also induced secretion of collagenase by macrophages that was accompanied by an alteration in cell shape (Gordon & Werb, 1976). The tumour-promoting phorbol diesters are also extremely potent inducers of collagenase secretion. Like colchicine and cytochalasin B, these compounds alter the shape of fibroblasts and endothelial cells (Aggeler et al, 1979; Moscatelli et al, 1980). The tumour-promoting 12-0-tetradecanoylphorbol-13-acetate is by far the most potent inducer of collagenase discovered to date for rabbit fibroblasts (Aggeler et al, 1979), although nothing is known about the mechanism by which tumour-promoting phorbol diesters act.

Few substances have been reported to inhibit the production of collagenases by cells that are already triggered to secrete these enzymes. Glucocorticoids at concentrations of 1 to 1000 nM (within the range for binding affinity of the glucocorticoid receptors) are potent inhibitors of collagenase secretion (Werb et al, 1977; Werb, 1978). These compounds also decrease the secretion of PGE by cells; however, it appears that the action of glucocorticoids on secretion of collagenase is direct, because the addition of PGE along with glucocorticoids to the culture medium of macrophages or synovial cells does not affect the inhibitory activity of glucocorticoids. On the other hand, indomethacin, a compound that inhibits PGE production directly, may decrease production of collagenase by macrophages and synovial cells in other situations (Wahl et al, 1977). Collagenase production may also be hormonally regulated by estrogens and progesterone, particularly in hormone-responsive tissues such as the uterus (Ryan & Woessner, 1974; Koob & Jeffrey, 1974; Woessner, 1979).

Retinoic acid and its derivatives may also inhibit the secretion of collagenase (Brinckerhoff et al, 1980). This observation presents a dilemma because, although vitamin A deficiency leads to destruction of the cornea through increased collagenolysis, hypervitaminosis A leads to increased degradation of connective tissues such as cartilage. Whether there is cell and tissue specificity in the responses to these compounds remains to be determined.

Another source of inhibitory factors may be increased production of endogenous inhibitors of collagenases by cells during various stages of growth and development or during culture (Sellers et al, 1977; Murphy et al, 1977a). In view of the newly discovered irreversible inhibitors of collagenase (discussed subsequently), it is possible that apparent stimulation or inhibition of the production of collagenases may be linked not to alteration of the synthesis of the collagenase molecule itself, but to the production of inhibitors. Both these points require detailed structural and molecular studies on the collagenolytic enzymes and the inhibitors of collagenase.

Extracellular regulation of collagen degradation

One of the key factors in our understanding of connective tissue catabolism is the regulation of the activity of collagenases. As already described, one mechanism of regulation is the variation in susceptibility to collagenases by the genetic type of collagen in the tissue, as well as the degree of cross-linking of the collagen. Other proteinases may also be involved in the breakdown of collagen in vivo by removing proteoglycans and glycoproteins surrounding collagen fibrils, and by breaking collagen cross-links before the action of collagenase and the further degradation of the products of the initial cleavage. A second mechanism involved in the local control of collagenase activity is that of inhibitors and activators. Collagenase inhibitors, as well as latent enzyme forms and putative activators, have been found in association with connective tissue.

Activation of latent collagenase

It is well established that collagenases are present in inactive form in media from both cells and tissues in culture and in tissue extracts. These have been explained as either proenzymes (Birkedal-Hansen et al, 1976; Eeckhout & Vaes, 1977; Valle & Bauer, 1979) or reversible complexes of inhibitors with enzymes (Sellers et al, 1977; Vater et al, 1978). The interpretation of latent collagenases as proenzymes is based on the observation that limited digestion with trypsin caused a marked activation of collagenase accompanied by a decrease in apparent molecular weight, as judged by gel filtration (Woessner, 1977). Without detailed protein sequence analysis, however, it is not at all clear whether this alteration in molecular weight can be ascribed to activation of a proenzyme form. More significantly, a number of endogenous proteinases have been described as efficient collagenase activators (Table 7.5). Eeckhout and Vaes (1977) have presented evidence that the collagenase and its endogenous activator found in the medium from mouse bone cultures are present in latent form activatable by plasmin, kallikrein, and lysosomal proteinases, including cathepsin B, as well as by trypsin. A number of other collagenases are also activated by proteinases, including trypsin and plasmin (Werb et al, 1977; Dayer et al, 1977; Werb & Aggeler, 1978). Endogenous proteinases appear to be of diverse specificity. The rabbit alveolar macrophage secretes both latent collagenase and an endogenous metalloproteinase responsible for activating it (Horwitz et al, 1976), whereas an endogenous serine proteinase activator can be found in uterine tissue (Woessner, 1977, 1979) and a mast cell serine proteinase is also capable of activating collagenases (Birkedal-Hansen et al, 1976). The latent forms of collagenase can be activated not only by limited proteolysis by trypsin and other enzymes but also by chemical treatment with a number of thiol-binding reagents and chaotropic agents (4-aminophenylmercuric acetate, 4-chloromercuribenzoate, Mersalyl, and sodium iodide or sodium thiocyanate) (Werb & Burleigh, 1974; Sellers et al, 1977; Shinkai & Nagai, 1977; Vater et al, 1978). Interestingly, no synergism between trypsin and these organomercurial activators has been observed (i.e., either trypsin or one of the organomercurials activates the same amount of collagenase). It has been proposed that these reagents dissociate a collagenase inhibitor from the latent enzyme. Latent collagenases also bind to collagen (Vater et al, 1978). Thus, once secreted in an inactive form, collagenase may bind to collagen and remain in sites of potential collagenolysis until activated by a proteinase or thiol-binding compound.

Table 7.5 Activators of vertebrate collagenases

Plasmin
Trypsin
Kallikrein
Cathepsin B
Endogenous metalloproteinase
Endogenous serine proteinase
Mast cell serine proteinase
4-Chloromercuribenzoate
4-Aminophenylmercuric acetate
Mersalyl
3 M sodium iodide or sodium thiocyanate
Dental plaque

Inhibitors of specific collagenase

Our understanding of the nature of latent collagenases and of the regulation of collagenase activity (Table 7.6) has been complicated by the identification of a number of inhibitors of collagenase in plasma, tissue extracts, and culture medium. α_2-Macroglobulin (α_2M) is the major plasma inhibitor of collagenase (Werb et al, 1974). This molecule interacts stoichiometrically with nearly all known proteinases, usually binding 2 mol of proteinase per mol of α_2M. Only active endopeptidases interact with α_2M, forming essentially irreversible complexes. Saturation of an α_2M molecule with a proteinase prevents the subsequent binding of other proteinase molecules. The bound enzyme is inhibited against high molecular weight substrates and is protected from other high molecular weight inhibitors. α_2M-enzyme complexes are removed rapidly from tissue fluids by binding to specific α_2M receptors on macrophages followed by endocytosis (Kaplan & Nielsen, 1979). Limited reactivation of α_2M-collagenase complexes has been described after dialysis against 3 M sodium thiocyanate (Werb et al, 1974). However, such complexes are unlikely to be the source of active enzyme in vivo because native α_2M is extremely resistant to proteolytic breakdown.

Trypsin-activatable latent collagenases do not bind to α_2M. Although α_2M is present in plasma at concentrations of about 200 μg/ml, its concentration in tissue fluids is considerably lower.

Woolley et al (1976) have described a lower molecular weight inhibitor, β_1-anticollagenase, that is specific for vertebrate collagenase and present at very low concentrations in plasma. Complexes of this inhibitor with collagenase could be the source of some latent collagenases because they are reactivated to some extent by trypsin and plasmin.

Collagenase inhibitors have also been extracted from connective tissues and from the culture medium of connective tissue fragments and cells (Kuettner et al, 1976; Sellers et al, 1977; Murphy et al, 1977a). These inhibitors are all cationic glycoproteins and, where investigated, the collagenase-inhibitor complexes can be reactivated with proteinases and organomercurials, and thus may give rise to latent collagenases. Interestingly, the inhibitor from rabbit bone apparently inhibits other neutral metalloproteinases produced by connective tissue cells, including gelatinase and proteoglycanase, but does not inhibit serine proteinases (Sellers et al, 1979). Platelet factor 4, a protein stored in platelet granules, also has collagenase-inhibitory activity (Hiti-Harper et al, 1978).

More recently, a new class of collagenase inhibitor has been described. The prototype inhibitor has been isolated from human amniotic fluid (Aggeler et al, 1981; Murphy, G., Cawston, T. E., Reynolds, J. J., personal communication). This inhibitor is a glycoprotein that binds to gelatin-agarose (and thus contaminates some fibronectin preparations) and shares many of the properties of other tissue inhibitors (e.g., that from bone, Sellers et al, 1979). The collagenase-amniotic fluid inhibitor complex cannot be reactivated by any of the known activators (Table 7.5). Such an inhibitor therefore could regulate the extracellular activity of tissue metalloproteinases, including collagenase. Because this inhibitor is irreversible, it may regulate the production of demonstrable collagenase (active and latent) by cells and tissues in culture and the amount of extractable collagenase from tissues. Existing data on the production of collagenase, its regulation, and its localization must be re-evaluated in light of this new inhibitor.

Fibronectin binds to gelatin and collagen in the region of the collagenase cleavage site (see Chapter 9). Although it is possible that this blockade may represent a physiological control mechanism of collagen degradation, and it has been observed that agents such as proteinases that remove cell surface fibronectin induce collagenase secretion (Werb & Aggeler, 1978; Aggeler et al, 1979), direct investigation of the degradation of type I collagen in the presence of fibronectin has indicated that fibronectin does not alter the rate of collagenolysis. The inhibitory activity of some fibronectin preparations appears to be due to contaminating lower molecular weight protein inhibitors (Aggeler et al, 1981). Whether fibronectin affects the rate of degradation of other collagen types by vertebrate collagenases or degradation of collagens by type-specific collagenolytic enzymes remains to be studied.

A discussion of the inhibition of specific collagenases is incomplete without mentioning nonprotein inhibitors. The specific collagenases are all metalloproteinases, and are thus inhibited by metal-ion chelating agents including EDTA and 1,10-phenanthroline. A number of sulphhydryl-containing molecules that may be present in tissue fluids also inhibit collagenases effectively at 1 to 10 mM concentrations, presumably by chelating calcium and zinc ions. These compounds include cysteine and related molecules, such as D-penicillamine (Werb & Burleigh, 1974; Woolley & Evanson, 1980).

Inhibition of other collagenolytic enzymes

Little is known about the regulation of the activity of the type-specific collagenases from granulocytes, macrophages, and tumour cells. The type I-specific granulocyte collagenase, a metalloproteinase, is more resistant to inhibition than the other vertebrate collagenases. It appears to bind very slowly to α_2M (Werb et al, 1974) and is inhibited by the bone-derived tissue inhibitor of

Table 7.6 Polypeptide inhibitors of vertebrate collagenases

Inhibitor	*Molecular weight*	*Source*	*Collagenase/ inhibitor complex reactivating agents*
α_2-Macroglobulin	725 000	Plasma	Chaotropic agents
β_1-Anticollagenase	40 000	Plasma	Trypsin, plasmin
Cationic glycoproteins	12 000	Cartilage, aorta, bone	Trypsin, plasmin
	30 000	Cell culture	Organomercurials, chaotropic agents
Platelet factor 4		Platelets	Not determined
Amniotic fluid inhibitor	30 000	Amniotic fluid	Irreversible

metalloproteinases (Sellers et al, 1979). The inhibition of the type IV- and type V-specific collagenases of tumour cells and macrophages has not yet been explored. Granulocyte elastase that is active against type III and IV collagens is a serine proteinase inhibited by α_2M and α_1-proteinase inhibitor from plasma. It is not affected by the tissue inhibitors of metalloproteinases.

The gelatin-degrading metalloproteinases that may act as accessory enzymes after the initial collagenolytic cleavage are inhibited by both α_2M and the tissue inhibitors of metalloproteinases (Sellers et al, 1979).

Specific localization of collagenolytic enzymes

Several factors may influence the limiting of collagenolytic enzymes to specific sites of collagen breakdown. Cell- and tissue-specific collagenolytic enzymes may help achieve selective functions. Human granulocytes contain both a distinct collagenase and an elastase within granules (Burleigh, 1977; Mainardi et al, 1980a, b), and mast cells contain a granule-bound proteinase that activates collagenase (Birkedal-Hansen et al, 1976). Selective mobilization of these granule enzymes may be associated with localized collagenolysis. Through recruitment of specific cells by selective induction of collagenase secretion or by attraction of specific cells to sites of collagen degradation by chemoattractants, additional specificity may be achieved. Collagen peptides are chemotactic for fibroblasts and monocytes (Postlethwaite & Kang, 1976). To fulfill specific proteolytic functions, organelles and membranes may be equipped with their own collagenases. Fibroblast-derived matrix vesicles that may be involved in basal lamina degradation and calcification of cartilage to bone in epiphyseal plates have been shown to contain a collagenolytic enzyme (Sorgente et al, 1977). Collagenolytic enzymes may also be associated with the cell surface, which would restrict collagen degradation to areas of contact (Jones & DeClerck, 1980).

Locally, high concentrations of collagenolytic enzymes may be achieved by binding to collagen fibrils near sites of secretion. The rate of extracellular diffusion of molecules of molecular weight similar to that of collagenase is quite slow (Zigmond, 1980). When macrophages are grown on extracellular matrix, localized areas of connective tissue degradation can be seen around individual cells (Werb et al, 1980a, b).

It is likely that collagenolytic enzymes are secreted concomitantly with inhibitors. Collagenolytic activity would then be limited to the immediate vicinity of secretion of an active collagenase or the site of activation of a latent collagenase. Such mechanisms are involved in limiting the cascade systems of enzymes of complement and coagulation.

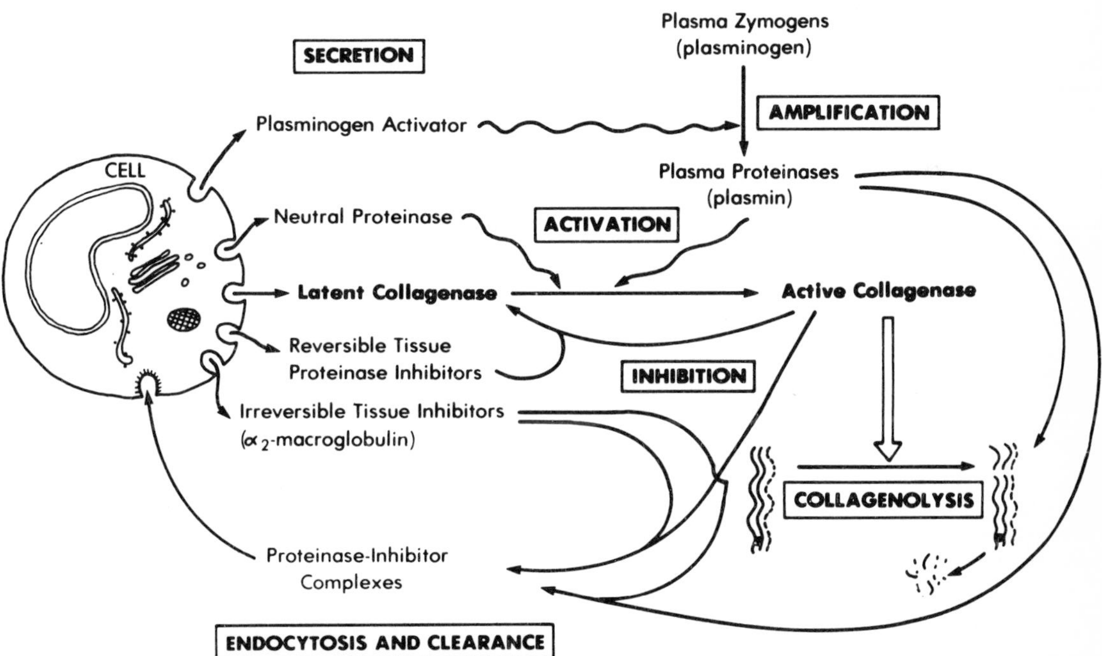

Fig. 7.6 Factors regulating the extracellular expression of collagenolytic activity. The collagenase activity available to degrade collagen is the net result of (a) secretion of collagenase, (b) activation of its zymogen and inhibitor-complex latent forms by tissue neutral proteinases, lysosomal proteinases, or plasma proteinases, (c) inhibition of active collagenase by tissue and plasma inhibitors, and (d) clearance of collagenase-inhibitor complexes.

MECHANISMS CONTROLLING THE RATE OF COLLAGEN DEGRADATION IN VIVO

It is still not clear whether any or all of the enzymes described in this chapter have any function in collagen degradation during physiologic or pathologic processes. Assuming that they are involved in collagenolysis, the rate of collagen degradation would be governed by the same properties controlling proteolysis in general: availability of substrates and substrate-specific enzymes, modification of substrates, modulation of proteinase activity, specific localization of proteinase, and availability of vesicles or particles containing proteinase (Holzer & Heinrich, 1980). These factors, as they apply to collagen degradation, are summarized in Table 7.7.

The rate of collagen degradation would be the net result of the production of enzymes and inhibitors of the collagenolytic system, activation and inhibition of collagenases, clearance of enzymes and inhibitors, and additional modulation of the availability of enzymes by binding of collagenolytic enzymes to collagen and influx of zymogens of proteolytic enzymes from plasma (Fig. 7.6). These stringent conditions may explain the difficulty in pinpointing a function for any collagenase in collagen degradation in vivo. The prospect of elucidating these processes is exciting and central to understanding the mechanisms underlying development and disease.

Table 7.7 Factors controlling the rate of collagen proteolysis in vivo

1. Specificity of susceptibility of collagen types to actions of collagenolytic enzymes.
2. Modulation of the susceptibility of collagen to degradation by mineralization, cross-linking (aging), and interaction with other connective tissue components.
3. Induction or repression of production of collagenolytic enzymes.
4. Sequestration of latent collagenases on collagen fibres.
5. Activation of latent collagenases by limited proteolysis by cellular and plasma zymogens.
6. Control by tissue and interstitial inhibitors of collagenases and of accessory proteinases.
7. Variation of tissue temperature during inflammation.
8. Alteration in rate of endocytosis of collagen fragments.
9. Limited tissue distribution and concentration of collagenases by sequestration in vesicles, by cell surface localization, and by rate of diffusion.
10. Recruitment of cells with collagenolytic potential.

ACKNOWLEDGEMENTS

This work was supported by the U.S. Department of Energy. I thank my colleagues for sharing unpublished data and data from papers in press.

REFERENCES

Aggeler J, Engvall E, Werb Z 1981 An irreversible tissue inhibitor of collagenase in human amniotic fluid: Characterization and separation from fibronectin. Biochemical and Biophysical Research Communications 100: 1195

Aggeler J, Mainardi C, Kramer J L, Werb Z 1979 Regulation of collagenase and plasminogen activator secretion by phorbol esters and cytochalasin B: Correlation of biochemistry and morphology. Journal of Cell Biology 83: 435a

Anderson J C 1976 Glycoproteins of the connective tissue matrix. International Review of Connective Tissue Research 7: 251

Barrett A J 1980 The many forms and functions of cellular proteinases. Federation Proceedings 39: 9

Becker U, Fietzek P P, Furthmayr H, Timpl R 1975 Nonhelical sequences of rabbit collagen: Correlation with antigenic determinants detected by rabbit antibodies in homologous regions of rat and calf collagen. European Journal of Biochemistry 54: 359

Berg R A, Schwartz M L, Crystal R G 1980 Regulation of the production of secretory proteins: Intracellular degradation of newly synthesized 'defective' collagen. Proceedings of the National Academy of Sciences USA 77: 4746

Bienkowski R S, Cowan M J, McDonald J A, Crystal R G 1978 Degradation of newly synthesized collagen. Journal of Biological Chemistry 253: 4356

Birkedal-Hansen H, Cobb C M, Taylor R E, Fullmer H M 1975 Trypsin activation of latent collagenase from several mammalian sources. Scandanavian Journal of Dental Research 83: 302

Birkedal-Hansen H, Cobb C M, Taylor R E, Fullmer H M 1976 Activation of fibroblast procollagenase by mast cell proteases. Biochimica et Biophysica Acta 438: 273

Biswas C, Dayer J-M 1979 Stimulation of collagenase production by collagen in mammalian cell cultures. Cell 18: 1035

Brinckerhoff C E, Harris E D Jr 1979 Collagenase production by cultures containing multinucleated cells derived from synovial fibroblasts. Arthritis and Rheumatism 21: 745

Brinckerhoff C E, McMillan R M, Dayer J-M, Harris E D Jr 1980 Inhibition by retinoic acid of collagenase production in rheumatoid synovial cells. New England Journal of Medicine 303: 432

Burleigh M C 1977 Degradation of collagen by non-specific proteinases. In: Barrett A J (ed) Proteinases in Mammalian Cells and Tissues. North-Holland, Amsterdam. Ch 7, p 285

Burleigh M C, Werb Z, Reynolds J J 1977 Evidence that species specificity and rate of collagen degradation are properties of collagen, not collagenase. Biochimica et Biophysica Acta 494: 198

David G, Bernfield M R 1979 Collagen reduces glycosaminoglycan degradation by cultured mammary epithelial cells: Possible mechanism for basal lamina formation. Proceedings of the National Academy of Sciences USA 76: 786

Dayer J-M, Krane S M, Russell R G G, Robinson D R 1976 Production of collagenase and prostaglandins by isolated adherent rheumatoid synovial cells. Proceedings of the National Academy of Sciences USA 73: 945

Dayer J-M, Russell R G G, Krane S M 1977 Collagenase production by rheumatoid synovial cells: Stimulation by a human lymphocyte factor. Science 195: 181

Deshmukh-Phadke K, Lawrence M, Nanda S 1978 Synthesis of collagenase and neutral proteases by articular chondrocytes: Stimulation by a macrophage-derived factor. Biochemical and Biophysical Research Communications 85: 490

Dixit S N, Mainardi C L, Seyer J M, Kang A H 1979 Covalent structure of collagen: Amino acid sequence of α2-CB5 of chick skin collagen containing the animal collagenase cleavage site. Biochemistry 18: 5416

Eeckhout Y, Vaes G 1977 Further studies on the activation of procollagenase, the latent precursor of bone collagenase. Effects of lysosomal cathepsin B, plasmin and kallikrein, and spontaneous activation. Biochemical Journal 166: 21

Etherington D J 1976 Bovine spleen cathepsin B1 and collagenolytic cathepsin. A comparative study of the properties of the two enzymes in the degradation of native collagen. Biochemical Journal 153: 199

Fietzek P P, Breitkreutz D, Kuhn K 1974 Amino acid sequence of the aminoterminal region of calf skin collagen. Biochimica et Biophysica Acta 365: 305

Furthmayr H, Timpl R 1972 Structural requirements of antigenic determinants in the aminoterminal region of the rat collagen α2 chain. Biochemical and Biophysical Research Communications 47: 944

Gordon S, Werb Z 1976 Secretion of macrophage neutral proteinase is enhanced by colchicine. Proceedings of the National Academy of Sciences USA 73: 872

Gross J, Lapiere C M 1962 Collagenolytic activity in amphibian tissues: A tissue culture assay. Proceedings of the National Academy of Sciences USA 48: 1014

Harris E D Jr, Farrell M E 1972 Resistance to collagenase: A characteristic of collagen fibrils cross-linked by formaldehyde. Biochimica et Biophysica Acta 278: 133

Harris E D Jr, McCroskery P A 1974 The influence of temperature and fibril stability on degradation of cartilage collagen by rheumatoid synovial collagenase. New England Journal of Medicine 290: 1

Harris E D Jr, Reynolds J J, Werb Z 1975 Cytochalasin B increases collagenase production by cells in vitro. Nature 257: 243

Highberger J H, Corbett C, Kang A H, Gross J 1975 The amino acid sequence of chick skin collagen α1-CB7. Biochemistry 14: 2872

Hiti-Harper J, Wohl H, Harper E 1978 Platelet factor 4: An inhibitor of collagenase. Science 199: 991

Holzer H, Heinrich P C 1980 Control of proteolysis. Annual Review of Biochemistry 49: 63

Horwitz A L, Hance A J, Crystal R G 1977 Granulocyte collagenase: Selective digestion of type I relative to type III collagen. Proceedings of the National Academy of Sciences USA 74: 897

Horwitz A L, Kelman J A, Crystal R G 1976 Activation of alveolar macrophage collagenase by a neutral protease secreted by the same cell. Nature 264: 772

Huybrechts-Godin G, Hauser P, Vaes G 1979 Macrophage fibroblast interactions in collagenase production and cartilage degradation. Biochemical Journal 184: 643

Johnson-Muller B, Gross J 1978 Regulation of corneal collagenase production: Epithelial-stromal cell interactions. Proceedings of the National Academy of Sciences USA 75: 4417

Jones P A, DeClerck Y 1980 Destruction of extracellular matrices containing glycoproteins, elastin and collagen by metastatic human tumor cells. Cancer Research in press

Jones P A, Werb Z 1980 Degradation of connective tissue matrices by macrophages. II. Influence of matrix composition on proteolysis of glycoproteins, elastin, and collagen by macrophages in culture. Journal of Experimental Medicine 152: 1527

Kang A H, Bornstein P, Piez K A 1967 The amino acid sequence of peptides from the cross-linking region of rat skin collagen. Biochemistry 6: 788

Kang A H, Nagai Y, Piez K A, Gross J 1966 Studies on the structure of collagen utilizing a collagenolytic enzyme from tadpole. Biochemistry 5: 509

Kaplan J, Nielsen M L 1979 Analysis of macrophage surface receptors. II. Internalization of α-macroglobulin trypsin complexes by rabbit alveolar macrophages. Journal of Biological Chemistry 254: 7329

Katayama S, Betheil J J, Seifter S 1978 Specific cleavage of reduced and S-carboxamidomethylated neurophysin II by the collagenase of Clostridium histolyticum. Biochimica et Biophysica Acta 524: 188

Koob T J, Jeffrey J J 1974 Hormonal regulation of collagen degradation in the uterus: Inhibition of collagenase expression by progesterone and cyclic AMP. Biochimica et Biophysica Acta 354: 61

Kuettner K E, Hiti J, Eisenstein R, Harper E 1976 Collagenase inhibition by cationic proteins derived from cartilage and aorta. Biochemical and Biophysical Research Communications 72: 40

Leibovich S J, Weiss J B 1971 Failure of human rheumatoid synovial collagenase to degrade either normal or rheumatoid arthritic polymeric collagen. Biochimica et Biophysica Acta 251: 109

Liotta L A, Abe S, Robey P G, Martin G R 1979 Preferential digestion of basement membrane collagen by an enzyme derived from a metastatic murine tumor. Proceedings of the National Academy of Sciences USA 76: 2268

Liotta L A, Lanzer W L, Garbisa S 1981 Identification of a type V collagenolytic enzyme. Biochemical and Biophysical Research Communications 98: 184

Lwebuga-Mukasa J S, Lappi S, Taylor P 1976 Molecular forms of acetylcholinesterase from Torpedo californica: Their relationship to synaptic membranes. Biochemistry 15: 1425

Mainardi C L, Dixit S N, Kang A H 1980a Degradation of type IV (basement membrane) collagen by a proteinase isolated from human polymorphonuclear leukocyte granules. Journal of Biological Chemistry 255: 5435

Mainardi C L, Hasty D L, Seyer J M, Kang A H 1980b Specific cleavage of human type III collagen by human polymorphonuclear leukocyte elastase. Journal of Biological Chemistry 255: 12006

Mainardi C L, Seyer J M, Kang A H 1980c Type-specific collagenolysis: a type V collagen degrading enzyme from macrophages. Biochemical and Biophysical Research Communications 97: 1108

Miller E J, Finch J E Jr, Chung E, Butler W T, Robertson P B 1976a Specific cleavage of the native Type III collagen molecule with trypsin. Similarity of the cleavage products to collagenase-produced fragments and primary structure at the cleavage site. Archives of Biochemistry and Biophysics 173: 631

Miller E J, Harris E D Jr, Chung E, Finch J E Jr, McCroskery P A, Butler W T 1976b Cleavage of type II and III collagens with mammalian collagenase: Site of cleavage and primary structure at the NH_2-terminal portion of the smaller fragment released from both collagens. Biochemistry 15: 787

Moscatelli D, Jaffe E, Rifkin D B 1980 Tetradecanoyl phorbol acetate stimulates latent collagenase production by cultured human endothelial cells. Cell 20: 343

Murphy G, Cartwright E C, Sellers A, Reynolds J J 1977a The detection and characterisation of collagenase inhibitors from rabbit tissues in culture. Biochimica et Biophysica Acta 483: 493

Murphy G, Reynolds J J, Bretz U, Baggiolini M 1977b Collagenase is a component of the specific granules of human neutrophil leukocytes. Biochemical Journal 162: 195

Newsome D A, Gross J 1979 Regulation of corneal collagenase production: Stimulation of serially passaged stromal cells by blood mononuclear cells. Cell 16: 895

Padykula H A 1976 Cellular mechanisms involved in cyclic stromal renewal of the uterus. III. Cells of the immune response. Anatomical Record 184: 49

Parakkal P F 1969 Involvement of macrophages in collagen resorption. Journal of Cell Biology 41: 345

Postlethwaite A E, Kang A H 1976 Collagen- and Collagen peptide-induced chemotaxis of human blood monocytes. Journal of Experimental Medicine 143: 1299

Reid K B M 1979 Complete amino acid sequences of the three collagen-like regions present in subcomponent C1q of the first component of human complement. Biochemical Journal 179: 367

Ryan J N, Woessner J F Jr 1974 Oestradiol inhibition of collagenase role in uterine involution. Nature 248: 526

Sellers A, Cartwright E, Murphy G, Reynolds J J 1977 Evidence that latent collagenases are enzyme-inhibitor complexes. Biochemical Journal 163: 303

Sellers A, Murphy G, Meikle M C, Reynolds J J 1979 Rabbit bone collagenase inhibitor blocks the activity of other neutral metalloproteinases. Biochemical and Biophysical Research Communications 87: 581

Seyer J M, Mainardi C, Kang A H 1980 Covalent structure of collagen: Amino acid sequence of $\alpha 1$ (III)-CB5 from type III collagen of human liver. Biochemistry 19: 1583

Shinkai H, Nagai Y 1977 A latent collagenase from embryonic human skin explants. Journal of Biochemistry (Tokyo) 81: 1261

Sorgente N, Brownell A G, Slavkin H C 1977 Basal lamina degradation: The identification of mammalian-like collagenase activity in mesenchymal-derived matrix vesicles. Biochemical and Biophysical Research Communications 74: 448

Steven F S, Torre-Blanco A, Hunter J A A 1975 A neutral protease in rheumatoid synovial fluid capable of attacking the telopeptide regions of polymeric collagen fibrils. Biochimica et Biophysica Acta 405: 188

Tolstoshev P, Berg R A, Rennard S I, Bradley K H, Trapnell B C, Crystal R G 1981 Procollagen production and procollagen messenger RNA levels and activity in human lung fibroblasts during periods of rapid and stationary growth. Journal of Biological Chemistry 256: 3135

Valle K -J, Bauer E A 1979 Biosynthesis of collagenase by human skin fibroblasts in monolayer culture. Journal of Biological Chemistry 254: 10115

Vater C A, Harris E D Jr, Siegel R C 1979 Native cross-links in collagen fibrils induce resistance to human synovial collagenase. Biochemical Journal 181: 639

Vater C A, Mainardi C L, Harris E D Jr 1978 Binding of latent rheumatoid synovial collagenase to collagen fibrils. Biochimica et Biophysica Acta 539: 238

Wahl L M, Olsen C E, Sandberg A L, Mergenhagen S E 1977 Prostaglandin regulation of macrophage collagenase production. Proceedings of the National Academy of Sciences USA 74: 4955

Wahl L M, Wahl S M, Mergenhagen S E, Martin G R 1975 Collagenase production by lymphokine-activated macrophages. Science 187: 261

Wang H-M, Chan J, Pettigrew D W, Sodek J 1978 Cleavage of native type III collagen in the collagenase susceptible region by thermolysin. Biochimica et Biophysica Acta 533: 270

Weiss J B 1976 Enzymic degradation of collagen. International Review of Connective Tissue Research 7: 101

Werb Z 1978 Biochemical actions of glucocorticoids on macrophages in culture. Specific inhibition of elastase, collagenase, and plasminogen activator secretion and effects on other metabolic functions. Journal of Experimental Medicine 147: 1695

Werb Z, Aggeler J 1978 Proteases induce secretion of collagenase and plasminogen activator by fibroblasts. Proceedings of the National Academy of Sciences USA 75: 1839

Werb Z, Burleigh M C 1974 A specific collagenase from rabbit fibroblasts in monolayer culture. Biochemical Journal 137: 373

Werb Z, Gordon S 1975 Secretion of a specific collagenase by stimulated macrophages. Journal of Experimental Medicine 142: 346

Werb Z, Reynolds J J 1974 Stimulation by endocytosis of the secretion of collagenase and neutral proteinase from rabbit synovial fibroblasts. Journal of Experimental Medicine 140: 1482

Werb Z, Bainton D F, Jones P A 1980a Degradation of connective tissue matrices by macrophages. III. Morphological and biochemical studies on extracellular, pericellular, and intracellular events in matrix proteolysis by marcophages in culture. Journal of Experimental Medicine 152: 1537

Werb Z, Banda M J, Jones P A 1980b Degradation of connective tissue matrices by macrophages. I. Proteolysis of elastin, glycoproteins, and collagen by proteinases isolated from macrophages. Journal of Experimental Medicine 152: 1340

Werb Z, Burleigh M C, Barrett A J, Starkey P M 1974 The interaction of α_2-macroglobulin with proteinases. Binding and inhibition of mammalian collagenases and other metal proteinases. Biochemical Journal 139: 359

Werb Z, Mainardi C L, Vater C A, Harris E D Jr 1977 Endogenous activation of latent collagenase by rheumatoid synovial cells: Evidence for a role of plasminogen activator. New England Journal of Medicine 296: 1017

Woessner J F Jr 1977 A latent form of collagenase in the involuting rat uterus and its activation by a serine proteinase. Biochemical Journal 161: 535

Woessner J F Jr 1979 Total, latent and active collagenase during the course of post-partum involution of the rat uterus. Biochemical Journal 180: 95

Woolley D E, Evanson J M (ed) 1980 Collagenase in normal and pathological connective tissues. John Wiley & Sons, Chichester

Woolley D E, Roberts D R, Evanson J M 1976 Small molecular weight β_1 serum protein which specifically inhibits human collagenases. Nature 261: 325

Zigmond S H 1980 Gradients of chemotactic factors in various assay systems. In: van Furth R (ed) Mononuclear Phagocytes-Functional Aspects. Martinus Nijhoff, The Hague. p 461

8

Degradation of collagen: pathology

R. PEREZ-TAMAYO

DEGRADATION OF COLLAGEN: PATHOLOGY

One of the few things that may be said with confidence about the pathology of collagen degradation is that it is a 'new field'. Perusal of current text-books of pathology fails to reveal other than passing references to collagen breakdown. In the present revival of interest on collagen diseases, redefined at the molecular level (Pérez-Tamayo, 1974a; Pérez-Tamayo, 1974b; Uitto & Prockop, 1975; Kivirikko & Risteli, 1976; Lapiére & Nusgens, 1976; Uitto & Lichtenstein, 1976; Gay & Miller, 1978; Prockop et al, 1979), disturbances in collagen degradation occupy a modest place. Specialized publications contain a few recent reviews (Harris & Cartwright, 1977; Bauer & Uitto, 1979; Pérez-Tamayo, 1979a). The publication of the first monograph on the subject has been announced (Woolley & Evanson, 1979). And yet, the literature on the subject is growing at such a fast rate and covers such a wide variety of tissues, organs, and diseases, that this may well be the last time to attempt a complete (though by no means exhaustive) general review of the pathology of collagen degradation.

Like other general pathological processes, such as inflammation or neoplastic growth, abnormal collagen degradation may represent the major pathogenetic mechanism of some diseases, or else it may be only one among several processes contributing to tissue damage in other diseases. Regardless of how they are encountered in pathology, many instances of abnormal collagen degradation reveal a variety of features in common; in other words, it is both possible and convenient to build a general pathology of collagen degradation. On the other hand, in different organs and tissues abnormal collagen breakdown shows unique or specific aspects, so that a special pathology of collagen degradation is equally justified. In order to avoid repetitions and for the sake of clarity the present chapter has been organized following the division just mentioned, namely 'general' and 'special' pathology of collagen degradation. The first part contains a brief summary of the normal mechanisms of collagen degradation; the interested reader should consult Chapter 7, contributed by Werb, for a more detailed treatment of the subject.

CLASSIFICATION

A satisfactory classification of disturbances of collagen degradation should probably be based on precise knowledge of all mechanisms involved in each pathological instance included. Unfortunately, this is not possible today. Several alternatives for a useful classification are left, such as primary (disturbances in the degradative mechanisms) and secondary (abnormal changes in the susceptibility of the substrate), or congenital and acquired, reversible and irreversible, etc. Again, the information available appears inadequate to support any one of those taxonomic schemes. The next step down would be the grouping of abnormalities in collagen degradation by tissues, organs, and systems involved, a valid but almost certainly boring classification. Finally, the least attractive choice is no classification but simply an alphabetical listing of all recognized disturbances in collagen degradation. It must be admitted that currently we are almost reduced to an excercise of this type. Nevertheless, to ease the feeling of phonebook writing (and reading!) two real and hopefully not unwise categories are introduced, namely excessive and deficient collagen degradation. The result (Table 8.1) may not be very appealing but is probably the best we can have, given our current limited knowledge in the field.

Table 8.1 A Classification of abnormal collagen degradation

Excessive	*Deficient*
Corneal ulcers	Fibrosis and cirrhosis of the liver
Rheumatoid (and other) Arthritis	Scleroderma
Epidermolysis bullosa	Idiopathic pulmonary fibrosis
Chronic periodontal disease	Osteopetrosis
Tumours	Others
Others	

GENERAL PATHOLOGY OF COLLAGEN DEGRADATION

Collagen degradation represents a special instance of a general biological phenomenon, namely the catabolic phase of the metabolic turnover of all tissue components.

Collagen is just one (albeit the more abundant) of the many extracellular substances that contribute structural support, and perhaps other functions, to the elaborate make-up of the different tissues and organs of multicellular organisms. In addition to its extracellular location, collagen has at least three other properties that make it unique as a substrate for degradation: (a) it displays a complex, paracrystalline, and mostly fibrillar structure in normal tissues, (b) under physiological conditions native collagen is resistant to the proteolytic action of almost all endogenous and non-specific proteases (the exceptions are some almost theoretical 'depolymerases' and mammalian collagenase); (c) collagen is no longer the specific name of a single chemical substance but rather a generic term encompassing a family of genetically different proteins, four of which (Types I to IV) are reasonably well characterized (see Ch. 2 p. 000) and there are several other molecular species waiting to be generally accepted. Furthermore, deep in the physiological intimacy of normal tissues collagen is never alone; many other substances are more or less closely associated with it, such as proteoglycans, elastin, fibronectin, a variety of 'serum' proteins, and many other components.

All known collagens are proteins and their specific degradation is primarily an enzymatic process (Fullmer, 1970; Pérez-Tamayo, 1973; Gross 1974; Gross, 1976; Weiss, 1976). Collagen breakdown may be considered at two different levels of biological organization: (a) as a test-tube phenomenon, where the two components of the isolated system (enzyme and substrate) are ideally in a molecular state of purity and all pertinent variables, such as relative concentrations, incubation time, temperature, ionicity, pH, etc., may be experimentally controlled; (b) as a physiological or pathological tissue process, where local circumstances probably prevail and include all variables mentioned above plus many additional parameters, such as specific enzyme activators and inhibitors, hormonal influences, cellular participation, substrate susceptibility and/or topographic accessibility, therapeutic intervention, etc. Needless to say, most of the available information on collagen degradation has been obtained through the careful study of 'in vitro' models. Extrapolation of such data to pathological conditions observed in living animals or man should be done with parsimony, to say the least.

Collagen breakdown 'in vivo'

Collagen breakdown 'in vivo' is probably not the effect of a single hydrolytic enzyme (Nordwig, 1971; Harris & Cartwright, 1977; Pérez-Tamayo, 1979b). Several degradation schemes have been proposed which include at least three or four different steps (Woessner, 1968; Nordwig, 1971; Burleigh, 1977; Harris & Cartwright, 1977; Pérez-Tamayo, 1979b), which may be summarized as follows:

(a) Depolymerisation of collagen fibres

An initial step considered necessary (Milson et al, 1972; Strauch, 1975; Weiss, 1976; Harris & Cartwright, 1977) before significant cleaving along the triple helical chain can occur. There is 'in vitro' evidence (Leibovich & Weiss, 1971) that insoluble polymeric collagen fibres (Steven, 1970) are totally resistant to partially purified human synovial collagenase, under conditions in which soluble collagen is degraded. Leibovich & Weiss (1971) proposed that a preliminary attack on the cross-link regions was essential prior to true collagenolysis. A good candidate for this initial collagen-depolymerising role would be the elastase derived from polymorphonuclear leucocytes (Janoff, 1972; Burleigh, 1977; Starkey, 1977) although cathepsin G, obtained from the same cells, was found to have a similar effect on cartilage collagen (Starkey et al, 1977), but not on skin or tendon collagen, which are predominantly type I. On the other hand, the need for a depolymerising step prior to specific collagenolysis has been disputed (Gross, 1976) on the basis of similar 'in vitro' experiments with insoluble polymeric collagen fibres but employing semipurified tadpole collagenase; degradation of the substrate occurred to the extent of 50 per cent but without cleavage of cross-links. Furthermore, several instances of physiological and pathological collagen degradation are not characterized by the presence of abundant polymorphonuclear leucocytes, such as the post partum rat uterus (Luse & Hutton, 1964; Parakkal, 1972; Padykula & Campbell, 1976; Padykula, 1976; Tansey & Padykula, 1978), or the carrageenin granuloma (Williams, 1957). The issue obviously requires further examination, not only 'in vitro' and with collagenases purified to homogeneity, but also in experiments that attempt to reproduce the complex conditions prevailing in 'in vivo' situations.

(b) True or physiological collagenolysis

This term is generally accepted to mean cleavage along the triple helical polypeptide chains of the native substrate (Gross, 1970; Gross, 1976). The provision that it should occur 'under physiological conditions' fits this review rather poorly; 'in a milieu found in vivo' (Harris & Cartwright, 1977) is certainly more adequate. The definition of physiological collagenolysis has two components which should be briefly examined:

(i) the breakdown of tissue collagen requires the dismantling of highly complex, extracellular, insoluble, and paracrystalline fibres which preserve their native state through wide physiological variations in their local physico-chemical environment. Nature found the more efficient way to physiologically degrade collagen in a combination of a single specific enzymatic clip, which renders the reaction products susceptible to denaturation at physiological temperature, followed by non-specific proteolysis of the denatured collagen fragments (Sakai &

Gross, 1967; Eisen et al, 1970; Seifter & Harper, 1970; Evanson, 1971; Nordwig, 1971; Pérez-Tamayo, 1973; Gross, 1974; Harris & Krane, 1974; Gross, 1976). The single peptide cleavage *must* occur somewhere along the triple helical polypeptide chain, which is the molecular stretch resistant to all other known animal proteases; in fact, it has been established (Gross et al, 1974) that both mammalian and amphibian collagenases have the same specificity. Further aspects of physiological collagenolysis are presented in Part a of this Chapter (page 000).

(ii) The other component of true collagenolysis is that the substrate should be in a native state i.e., resistant to degradation by any proteases other than collagenase. This requirement is central to the definition of physiological collagenolysis since it has been abundantly documented that denatured collagen is susceptible to many non-specific proteases. Pathologists, however, may feel slightly uncomfortable here, since disease may locally change physico-chemical microenvironments beyond the wildest dreams of biochemists. In addition, it has been shown (Miller et al, 1976) that trypsin at neutral pH and below the substrate denaturation temperature will cleave native type III collagen in solution making one scission in the triple helical chain at the -ala-arg-bond, seven peptides beyond the collagenase cleavage site toward the COOH terminus of the molecule. In summary, physiological collagenolysis is the specific enzymatic transformation of native collagen fibres into denatured collagen fragments; this is brought about by a specific enzyme through a single peptide scission along the triple helical chain of the native substrate. The extent (if any) to which pathological conditions may alter and/or circumvent the suggested mechanisms of physiological collagenolysis is undetermined.

(c) Further extracellular breakdown of collagen-derived peptides.

This step is usually attributed to nonspecific proteinases of which several types have been detected in tissue cultures and extracts (Harper & Gross, 1970; Harris & Krane, 1972; Aswanikumar & Radakrishnan, 1973; Sopata & Dancewicz, 1974; Werb & Reynolds, 1974; Deshmukh-Phadke et al, 1978; Pettigrew et al, 1978; Sellers et al, 1978; Vaes et al, 1978). It was stated by Nordwig (1971) that degradation of denatured fragments containing regions of the molecule rich in polar residues by endo- and exopeptidases of the tissues is quite feasible, but that digestion of tripeptide polymers of the nonpolar regions is more difficult due to their high content of amino acid residues; finally, cleavage of Gly-pro-X tripeptides would be accomplished by aminopeptidase and carboxypeptidase activity, such as described in microsomes (Nordwig, 1971). Although it would seem unlikely that all enzymes required for the degradation of collagen breakdown products are present in the excracellular space under physiological conditions (Gross, 1976), pathological changes certainly exist in which inflammatory cells of various types accumulate in the interstitial spaces and release many intracellular components, several proteases among them (Coombs & Fell, 1969; Page Thomas, 1969; Weissman, 1972; Poole, 1973).

(d) Intracellular breakdown of collagen fibres

Intracellular breakdown of collagen fibres has been postulated by several authors because collagen fibrils are frequently observed within cytoplasmic vacuoles of mesenchymal cells of various tissues undergoing resorption (for references see Woessner, 1968; Pérez-Tamayo, 1973; Rentería & Ferrans, 1976) The possibility that some of the ultrastructural images interpreted as intracellular collagen are artifactual and result from the presence of extracellular fibrils in deep invaginations of convoluted plasma membranes has been denied on the basis of serial section studies of fibroblasts in collagen-synthetizing tissues (Oakes, 1974) or in vitro (Svoboda et al, 1979). In addition, some authors (Brandes & Anton, 1969a; Brandes & Anton, 1969b; Deporter & Ten Cate, 1973; Ten Cate & Syrbu, 1974) have demonstrated acid and alkaline phosphatase activity within the collagen-containing vacuoles, thus establishing their true cytoplasmic (lysosomal) nature. Such observations have provided support for the 'lysosomal' theory of collagen degradation (Woessner, 1968; Pérez-Tamayo, 1973) as well as for other more recent formulations (Ten Cate & Deporter, 1975; Garant, 1976) in which intracellular breakdown of collagen plays the central role in remodelling and turnover of this extracellular substance. Lysosomes contain proteases such as cathepsin B and collagenolytic cathepsin (Burleigh et al, 1974; Etherington, 1974; Burleigh, 1977; Etherington, 1977; Etherington & Evans, 1977; Evans & Etherington, 1978) which degrade both soluble and insoluble collagen at pH 3.5–5.0 by causing both an increase in the ratio of alpha chains to higher components and the appearance of multiple products of size lower than alpha chains. The pH within phagocytic vacuoles, at least in polymorphonuclear leukocytes, may be as low as 4.0 units (Jensen & Bainton, 1973), in liver cells is approximately 5.0 units (Mego, 1971), and it is widely believed to be equally acid in all phagocytic cells. All this, however, is purely circumstantial evidence: an identical ultrastructural picture of collagen fibrils within cytoplasmic vacuoles is also present in some tumours and other abnormal conditions (Welsh, 1966; Welsh & Meyer, 1967; Azar & Lunardelli, 1969; Seifert, 1971; Allerga & Broderick, 1973; Ryan et al, 1973; Rentería & Ferrans, 1976) where the interpretation suggested has been the opposite, namely that intracellular collagen fibrils are being secreted. In addition, electron microscopic studies of tadpole tail fin (Usuku & Gross, 1965; Usuku, 1969) and carrageenin granuloma (Pérez-

Tamayo, 1970; Pérez-Tamayo, 1972) undergoing resorption revealed large numbers of extracellular collagen fibrils with many signs of disintegration, strongly suggesting that they have already been attacked by extracellular collagenolytic enzymes. Finally, immunohistochemical studies of collagenase in the post partum uterus (Montfort & Pérez-Tamayo, 1975), in cholesteatoma (Abramson & Huang, 1977), in experimental cirrhosis of the liver (Montfort & Pérez-Tamayo, 1979), in rheumatoid arthritis (Wooley et al, 1977), and in other conditions with active collagen breakdown (Grantz et al, 1978; Sakamoto et al, 1979; Woolley et al, 1979), have uniformly demonstrated the presence of the enzyme protein bound to extracellular collagen fibres. In summary, it would appear that if intracellular digestion of collagen plays any role in the breakdown of tissue fibres, it is probably secondary to extracellular enzymatic mechanisms and then only during brief periods of massive tissue loss.

Collagen-bound collagenase

It was first suggested by Gross & Lapiére (1962) that collagenase is tightly bound to extracellular collagen in normal tissues. The idea gained in likelihood when homogenates of rat uterus were incubated at 37° under sterile conditions for 24 or more hours (Ryan & Woessner, 1971) and collagen breakdown products were detected in the supernatant. Other observers (Nagai & Hori, 1972) extracted collagenase from insoluble pellets of previously frozen and thawed tissues from three different animal species (tadpole, rat, and man), also by incubation at 37° for prolonged periods. Direct extraction of collagenase from tissues without prior incubation has been achieved from embryonic chick bones (Sakamoto et al, 1973), from involuting mouse uterus and mouse skin (Wirl, 1975), from liver, kidney and involuting rat uterus (Weeks et al, 1976), from rabbit (McCroskery et al, 1975; Steven & Itzhaki, 1977) mouse (Labrosse & Liener, 1978) and human (Wirl & Frick, 1979) tumours, and from human gingiva (Uitto et al, 1978). There is evidence (Nagai, 1973; Vater et al, 1978) that purified collagenase, active or latent, added in vitro to insoluble collagen binds tightly to it and cannot be removed completely by extraction with conventional methods. Even with 1.0M NaCl solution, pH 7.5, more than 50 per cent of the collagenase remains bound to the insoluble collagen (Nagai, 1973).

The well-known instability of purified collagen solutions when stored at neutral pH in the cold for prolonged periods has been systematically examined by acrylamide gel electrophoresis (Pardo & Pérez-Tamayo, 1975) and attributed to the presence of active collagen-bound collagenase. In further studies from the same laboratory (Pardo et al, 1980) active collagenase has been isolated from several preparations of soluble collagen by acrylamide gel electrophoresis at pH 8.1. The collagens were extracted from various tissues of different animal species by a standard procedure (Gross, 1958). An antibody raised against the collagenase removed from collagen preparations gave a single precipitin band when reacted in immunodifusion against the antigen and also against 'crude' collagenase preparations obtained by the tissue explant technique, using homologous tissue fragments; there was complete identity between the two precipitin bands. The antibody was also shown to quantitatively inhibit the collagenolytic activity of the same 'crude' collagenase preparations, and to give a similar immunohistochemical staining of extracellular collagenase as the one reported in other experimental systems (Pardo et al, unpublished observations). Although no actual measurements have been made, there is no doubt that the amounts of collagenase obtained from 'purified' soluble collagen are minute. Adding the in vitro evidence for the existence of collagen-bound collagenase to the immunohistochemical demonstration of the presence of the enzyme protein universally bound to extracellular collagen in different experimental and human conditions, it seems reasonable to suggest that collagen-bound collagenase is at least one (if not the more significant) of the mollecular forms in which the enzyme is present in vivo.

Rate of collagen degradation in vivo

The rate of collagen degradation in any tissue is probably determined by two variables, namely the level of enzyme activity and the susceptibility of the substrate (Gross, 1976; Pérez-Tamayo, 1979a). Much attention has been devoted to the many factors ultimately influencing the tissue level of collagenolytic activity (Ch. 7), probably because they are easier to work with. On the other hand, it has been established that the rate of collagen degradation is influenced by the genetic type of the substrate (Harris et al, 1975; McCroskery et al, 1975; Woolley et al, 1975; Horwitz, et al, 1977), by the degree of cross-linking (Harris & Farrell, 1972; Vater et al, 1979) which is probably related to the solubility of collagen (Leibovich & Weiss, 1971) and by the accessibility of collagen to collagenase in the tridimensional architecture of tissues (Rubin et al, 1963; Rubin et al, 1965; Pérez-Tamayo & Montfort, 1980). Additional factors are mentioned by Gross (1976) as follows:

> Changes in susceptibility of collagen to collagenase degradation might also be modified as a function of time of development, anatomic location, physiologic states, and pathology because of significant differences in the types and amounts of ground-substance components, such as proteoglycans, in close association with collagen fibres. The tissue complexity is very likely manipulated by enzymatic systems having nothing to do with collagen itself, such as hyaluronidases, noncollagenolytic proteases, and factors regulating rates and types of proteoglycan synthesis.

Therefore, when building a general scheme of the

regulation of the molecular mechanisms of collagen degradation 'in vivo', it would appear unwise to ignore the potentially fundamental role of the susceptibility of the substrate (Pérez-Tamayo et al, 1980). In the general field of soluble protein catabolism in mammals, which has been more deeply explored than the area of insoluble protein breakdown, a widely held concept is that degradative enzymes are universally present and that their potential substrates oscillate continuously between susceptible and nonsusceptible molecular conformations (Grisolia, 1954; Schmike, 1975). Taking into account all the reservations derived from the insoluble, extracellular, and peculiar nature of the collagen protein as a substrate for degradation (Pérez-Tamayo, 1973), it would still seem rash to cancel everything that has been learned from the breakdown of soluble proteins in mammals.

Homeostasis of collagen

The ratio of collagen content to parenchymal elements is different in each organ and tissue of normal subjects and tends to remain constant during processes as different as growth, regeneration, and the development and involution of hypertrophy and hyperplasia (for references see Pérez-Tamayo & Montfort, 1964). Such close regulation of the collagen/parenchyma ratio is partly the result of the equilibrium between two different but complementary mechanisms: collagen synthesis and collagen degradation. In the end, the total amount of collagen present in any tissue at a given moment will necessarily be the result of the algebraic sum of those two processes. The same principle applies to pathological conditions: fibrosis, or the presence of excessive collagen in a given tissue or organ, in comparison with the normal situation, will be the consequence of a relative increase in the rate of collagen synthesis above the rate of collagen degradation, whatever their respective absolute values. Such increase need not be permanently maintained; in fact, in some pathological conditions such as cirrhosis of the liver (Pérez-Tamayo, 1979c; Pérez-Tamayo & Montfort, 1980; Rojkind et al, 1978), or scleroderma (Uitto, 1972) increased collagen synthesis is frequently observed in the active stages of the disease, whereas collagen synthesis is normal or even decreased in the more advanced, fibrotic stages. In these instances it is possible that the excessive collagen has become unsusceptible to collagenolytic attack by the presence of increased cross-linking (Harris & Farrell, 1972; Vater et al, 1979) or else that the excessive collagen has been sequestered into a compartment inaccesible to collagenase (Pérez-Tamayo & Montfort, 1980). In diseases characterized by an increased rate of collagen degradation relative to the rate of collagen synthesis, such as rheumatoid arthritis or chronic periodontal disease (for references see Pérez-Tamayo, 1979a), supportive structures are weakened and even dismantled, with catastrophic results for the maintenance of normal function. An attempt to integrate several of the factors mentioned in the local homeostasis of collagen in vivo appears in Figure 8.1; the diagram can be made much more complex by adding the information given on page 148, but the general outline will probably remain the same.

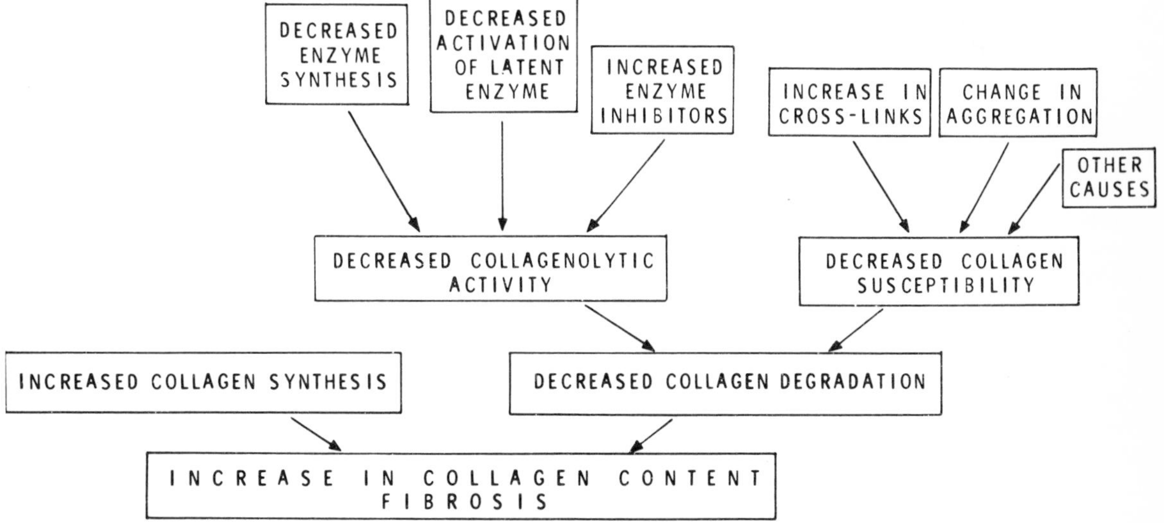

Fig. 8.1 Diagrammatic representation of the several possible ways in which decreased collagen degradation may participate in different forms of fibrosis. Increased collagen synthesis is indicated but the various mechanisms that may be responsible for it are not included because of the topic of this chapter. (Reproduced from The American Journal of Pathology, 1979, with permission of the Editor and Publisher.)

SPECIAL PATHOLOGY OF COLLAGEN DEGRADATION

Excessive collagen degradation

Corneal wounds

The cornea is formed by orthogonally arranged layers of collagen fibres covered on the outer surface by an epithelium of ectodermal origin. The perfect regularity of the alternating layers of collagen creates a quasi-crystalline structure which accounts for the translucence of the organ. Injury to the surface epithelium results in late destruction of underlying collagen, with eventual ulceration and loss of vision. This sequence of events has been known for years and is the unhappy outcome of conditions such as alkali burns, radiation or rosacea keratitis, ocular pemphigoid, scleroderma, and Steven-Johnson syndrome (Itoi et al, 1969; Brown & Weller, 1970a; Hook et al, 1971; Brown, 1972; Francis & Cambie, 1972; Lemp, 1974). Another condition associated with destruction of the cornea is vitamin A deficiency; clinically, this is characterized by dryness of the epithelium, ulceration, and finally, perforation of the cornea. This severe form is found mainly in children who are seriously malnourished but the syndrome may be reproduced in rats deficient only in vitamin A (Pirie et al, 1975).

In alkali-burned cornea, exposure to the injurious agent results in immediate death of all epithelial cells and loss of most of the proteoglycans of the organ. After approximately one week, the epithelium, accompanied by the vascularized stroma at the margin of the wound, begins a central progression. A very interesting feature of these lesions is that ulcerations are seldom seen before the end of the first week. The localization of the ulcer relative to the advancing edge of regenerating epithelium and underlying vascular stroma is also very suggestive since tissue loss is usually central to them while the peripheral area is intact.

Since the tissue undergoing necrosis and dissolution is almost pure collagen, two of the three potential sources of collagenase have been directly examined, namely corneal epithelium (Slansky et al, 1968; Brown & Weller, 1970a) and corneal cells (Hook et al, 1973; Berman et al, 1979) with positive results, i.e., both types of cells produce collagenase in vitro culture conditions. The third potential source of collagenase, polymorphonuclear leucocytes, has been implicated in principle (Brown & Hook, 1971a; Lemp, 1974; Kenyon et al, 1979) and in some indirect experiments (Rowsey et al, 1976) but their role as direct collagenase producers is still unclear. Minced whole normal human corneal tissue produced collagenase in culture (Berman et al, 1973) hence inflammatory cells are not necessary for the expression of collagenolytic activity; nevertheless, whole normal corneal tissue is not as efficient a producer of collagenase in vitro as alkali-burned corneas. Neither epithelial nor stromal cells from normal corneas nor mixtures thereof secrete detectable collagenase into the medium; however, when mixtures of these cells are co-cultured in the presence of cytochalasin B, a latent collagenase is detected in the medium which is apparently secreted by the stromal cells (Johnson-Muller & Gross, 1978) with the epithelial cells acting as inducers. In experiments in which corneal epithelium was replaced by mononuclear cells, by inflammatory cells of the anterior ocular chamber, and by culture media conditioned by these cells (Newsome & Gross, 1979), it was found that they all acted as inducers of collagenase production by corneal stromal cells.

The effect of topical applications of collagenase inhibitors (such as EDTA, cysteine, and others) to experimentally injured eyes in rabbits, and also in traumatic and other conditions in humans, has been explored (Brown et al, 1969; Itoi et al, 1969; Brown et al, 1970; Brown & Weller, 1970b; Slansky et al, 1970; Brown & Hook, 1971b; Hook et al, 1971; Slansky et al, 1971; Bohigian et al, 1974). Results of these tests showed that continuing application begun shortly after burning the cornea with alkali would prevent the development of deep ulceration and perforation in a statistically significant number of animals, and the same measures were shown to be effective in humans. Some failures, however, were also recorded, together with the need for frequent applications of collagenase inhibitors, and also some evidence of the toxicity of such compounds (Sugar & Waltman, 1973). A new approach to these problems was developed (Newsome & Gross, 1977) by reasoning that the inhibitory effect of progesterone on collagenase synthesis in post partum uteri of rats (Jeffrey et al, 1971), and rabbits (Halme & Woessner, 1978), could be used to prevent the tissue destructive action of collagenase in alkali-burn experimental corneal lesions. Newsome & Gross (1977) used medroxyprogesterone (Provera) in three different therapeutic modes, i.e., a single or twice daily instillation of one drop of the hormone solution in the subconjunctival sac, weekly subconjunctival depots of hormone and vehicle, and weekly intramuscular injections. Quantitative measurements of collagenolytic activity of treated and control corneas were performed in vitro. All three modes of administration of medroxyprogesterone were strikingly effective, since 49 of 85 corneas perforated, compared with eight of 87 treated eyes, and only four of 85 control corneas healed without serious damage, compared with 51 of 87 hormone-treated corneas that healed. Collagenolytic activity of alkali-burned corneas treated with medroxyprogesterone was reduced to less than one half of the untreated controls.

Rheumatoid (and other) arthritis

Chronic active rheumatoid arthritis is a destructive disease, often resulting in joint erosion, deformity, and partial or complete loss of function (Gardner, 1972; Fasbender, 1975; Gardner, 1978; Sokolow, 1979). One of the first events in the development of articular damage is the proliferation of synovial cells (Schumacher & Kitridou, 1972) together with inflammation and vascular neoformation in the stroma of synovial tissue. Such inflammatory reaction, or pannus, is apparently capable of eroding collagenous structures such as cartilage, bone, tendons, and ligaments (Harris et al, 1975; Harris, 1976). As the disease progresses, the proliferating synovial tissue extends over the articular cartilage and erodes from the joint surface down to and including subchondral bone. Neighbouring chondrocyte lacunae appear enlarged, and the cells may have two or more nuclei. In advanced lesions, only small islands of articular cartilage remain and there is extensive resorption of subchondral bone; synovial granulation tissue may reveal areas of proliferated synovial cells with epithelioid character (Gardner, 1972; Fasbender, 1975; Gardner, 1978; Sokolow, 1979). Polymorphonuclear leukocytes are infrequent; most inflammatory cells are mononuclear, with a predominance of lymphocytes and plasma cells (Fig. 8.2). degenerative and destructive lesion, which is probably a consequence of the invasive capabilities of the rheumatoid synovium. Loss of proteoglycans and other macromolecules different from collagen may decrease the natural resistance of cartilage to both mechanical and enzymatic disruption (Hamerman, 1969; Kempson et al, 1976) and it has been suggested that the initial damage in rheumatoid arthritis is enzymatic in nature and affects the proteoglycans (Dingle, 1978; Dingle, 1979). Even minimal degradation (1 or 2 clips) of the proteoglycan chain results in sufficient reduction of its molecular size as to allow it to diffuse out of the matrix (Morrison et al, 1973; Roughley & Barrett, 1977). This would facilitate the enzymatic attack on cartilage collagen, since proteoglycans are considered to protect it from the action of specific collagenases (Dingle, 1978; Dingle, 1979). On the other hand, however, experimental examination of this point, namely the effect of proteoglycans on the rate of collagen degradation by animal collagenase, has failed to reveal any influence of glycosaminglycans on collagen breakdown in vitro (Woolley & Evanson, 1977).

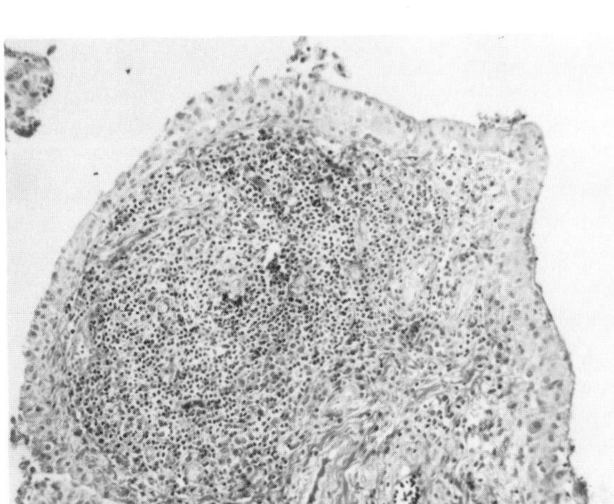

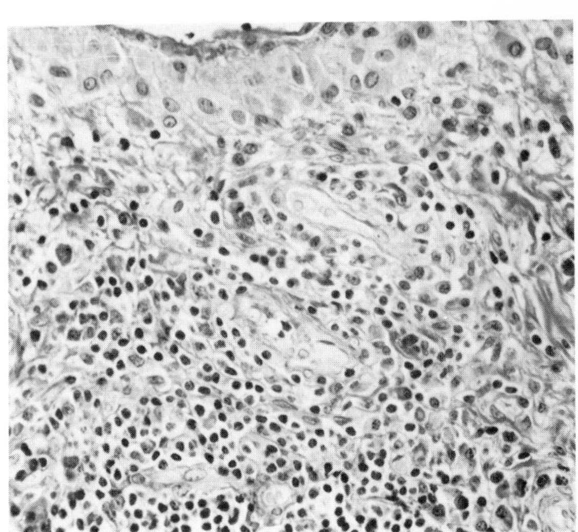

Fig. 8.2 Microscopic aspect of synovial villi in rheumatoid arthritis. (A) There is moderate hyperplasia of synovial cells, vascular neoformation, and infiltration with mononuclear cells; the nodular character of the infiltrate is apparent. (B) Higher power view of a similar field, to reveal the nature of the mononuclear cells: there are lymphocytes, macrophages and plasma cells. No polymorphonuclear leucocytes are present.

Electron microscopic study of the interface between mesenchymal cells and articular cartilage revealed a narrow band several microns wide separating cartilage from invading cells. In this zone, presumably partially degraded collagen fibres, amorphous material, and thin cytoplasmic processes of macrophage-like cells containing dilated vesicles of endoplasmic reticulum were seen (Harris et al, 1975; Harris et al, 1977).

Thus, the joint lesion in chronic active rheumatoid arthritis would seem to involve two different processes: a primary, apparently inflammatory and proliferative reaction of synovial tissue to an unknown stimulus, possibly immunologic in nature, and a secondary,

Collagenases have been demonstrated using different preparations derived from human rheumatoid joints: in vitro explants of synovium tissue, synovial fluid, frozen and thawed synovial tissue pellets, and in vitro cultures of isolated, adherent, dendritic synovial cells of obscure identity (for references see Harris & Cartwright, 1977; Krane, 1978; Pérez-Tamayo, 1979a). There is convincing evidence that the various collagenases obtained from the different sources mentioned are capable of degrading articular cartilage, used as substrate either as slices, as whole patella, or as purified soluble Type 2 collagen molecules in fibril form (Harris & Krane, 1973; McCroskery, 1974; Harris et al, 1975; Woolley et al, 1975a; Woolley et al 1975b). Synovial collagenases have been obtained in two different molecular forms, active and latent, and the latter has been claimed to be either a precursor or an enzyme-inhibitors complex. For the activation of latent rheumatoid collagenase a suggestive scheme has been proposed, involving plasminogen and a plasmin activator, although there are alternative possibilities (Wize et al, 1975). Another molecular form in which collagenase has been detected in rheumatoid synovial tissues is as enzyme-substrate complex, by means of immunohistochemical staining (Woolley et al, 1977).

In addition to the collagenases mentioned above, at least two other neutral peptidases have been described in human rheumatoid synovium. One, an endopeptidase capable of degrading gelatin to small fragments, has been found in the media from explants of rheumatoid synovial tissue (Harris & Krane, 1972). The other neutral protease has been identified in synovial fluid and shown to attack the telopeptides of fluorescein-labelled polymeric collagen fibrils in a fashion similar to trypsin, i.e., without depolymerization of the substrate (Steven et al, 1965). The possible role of these two enzymes is still uncertain but it has been suggested that the endopeptidase derived from rheumatoid synovium may be responsible for at least part of the subsequent breakdown of the primary products of collagenolysis (Harris & Krane, 1972; Gross, 1976; Krane, 1979).

In osteoarthritis small amounts of active collagenase have been found by mass culturing the synovium and subsequent concentration of the medium (Harris et al, 1969), or by culturing osteoarthritic cartilage and treating the medium with trypsin to activate latent enzyme (Ehrlich et al, 1975). The latter observation is of interest because it suggests the participation of chondrocytes in destruction of cartilage, a point also made by Dingle (1979). In septic and acute inflammatory arthritis such as gout a collagenase has been detected in synovial fluids and the activity was proportional to the concentration of polymorphonuclear leucocytes (Harris et al, 1975). In still other diseases with arthritis, such as Reiter's syndrome, pseudogout, juvenile rheumatoid arthritis and scleroderma, needle biopsies of synovial tissue have revealed collagenase activity in amounts correlated with the degree of vascular neoformation and mesenchymal proliferation (Harris et al, 1969).

Even a cursory glance at the evidence summarized above, on the existence and variety of enzymatic mechanisms capable of degrading the articular collagen in rheumatoid and other forms of arthritis, should produce in the reader an *embarrasement de richésse*. And yet, it is almost certain that this is not the whole story. Many other factors contribute to the relentless destruction of joints in chronic active rheumatoid arthritis. Many investigators will probably agree with Harris et al (1978) who comment:

> Our interests have been somewhat narrowly focussed upon the way in which collagen is degraded in rheumatoid arthritis, but we must emphasize that this is not because we view collagenase as the sun around which all other mediators of joint destruction revolve, but that it is something we know how to study!

Sufficient information has been accumulated to support the idea that, if collagenase and other neutral protease activities could be inhibited for prolonged periods in rheumatoid joints, the anatomic and functional outlook of such patients would be quite different.

Epidermolysis bullosa

This generic term designates a heterogeneous group of rare hereditary diseases characterized by the formation of blisters on minor mechanical trauma to the skin (Gedde-Dahl, 1971a; Gedde-Dahl, 1971b; Pearson, 1971). Three genetic types of dystrophic epidermolysis bullosa are recognized, which are also distinguished by several clinical parameters but have in common the dermolytic type of blister characterized by a sharp separation of the entire epithelium from the dermis below the basement membrane. In addition, anchoring fibrils are usually absent (Briggamann & Wheeler, 1975; Hashimoto et al, 1976a), there is attenuation of elastic fibres, vascular neoformation and round cell infiltration in the dermis (Fig. 8.3). An interesting feature is that phagocytosis of collagen fibrils by mesenchymal cells (called macrophages) is constantly present (Pearson, 1962).

The dominantly inherited form of the disease is less severe than the recessive, and there is a localized recessive type which may not be present at birth but develops at a later age, usually in infancy or childhood. Another recessive type is epidermolysis bullosa letalis, a widespread affection present at birth with severe involvement of all the skin but often sparing the extremities, characterized by cleavage between the basement membrane and the plasma membrane of the basal cells of the epidermis (Pearson et al, 1974). Histologic differentiation between the various types of epidermolysis bullosa is not possible; genetic and clinical evaluation, as well as electron microscopic studies of very early blisters, preferably produced by friction a few minutes before biopsy, are necessary to properly classify a new case of the disease (Hashimoto et al, 1975; Hashimoto et al, 1976a and b). This is dealt with in detail in Chapter 16.)

Chronic periodontal disease

The major structural protein of the soft and hard periodontal tissues is collagen. The attachment of the marginal gingival tissue to the calcified tooth surface is through a basement membrane and hemidesmosomes. In addition, strong bundles of collagen fibres, originating

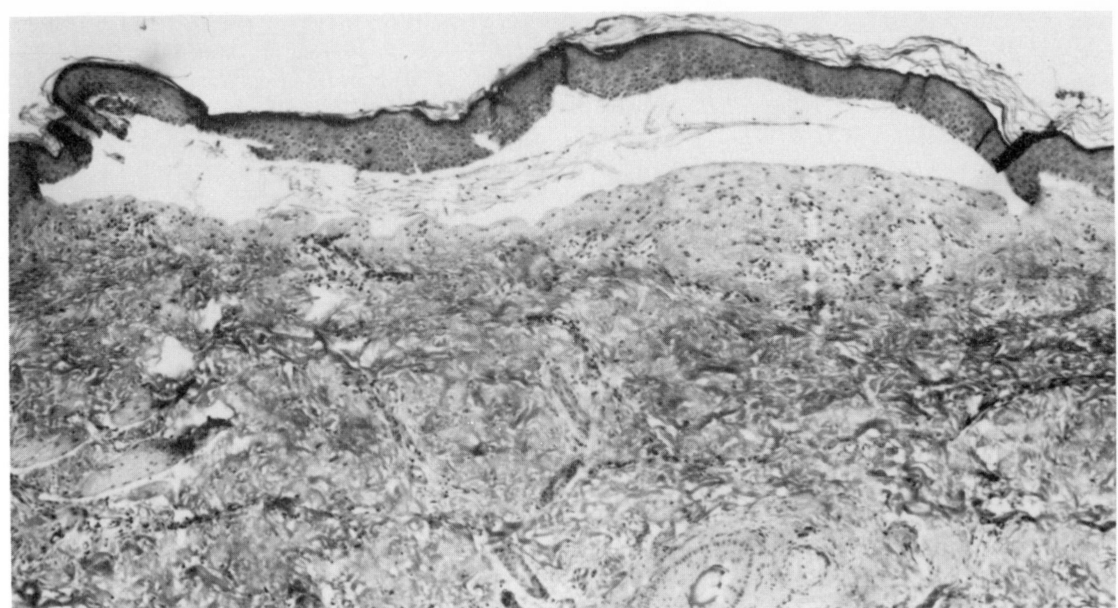

Fig. 8.3 Microscopic appearance of a bulla produced by light friction on the skin of a patient with recessive dystrophic epidermolysis bullosa. The entire epithelium is neatly lifted from the upper dermis; no inflammatory cells are present in the blister fluid. The dermis shows no changes. (Tissue courtesy of Dr Cecilia Ridaura, Insituto Nacional de Pediatría, México.)

from the cementum, just apical to the edge of the epithelium pass through the gingival chorium and terminate in the free marginal gingiva. Finally, there are also the circular and alveologingival fibre groups, completing the bulk of the connective tissue of the gingiva. Disorganization of such supporting structure, which provides tone to the tissue and a framework for the rich capillary plexus subjacent to the junctional epithelium, results in increased pocket depth, loss of gum tissue, loosening and finally loss of teeth (Page & Schroeder, 1976). Because chronic inflammation is the unfailing background of periodontal disease and also because the crevice region represents an interface between bacteria and connective tissue (a normal adult with 28 healthy teeth may still harbour about 16 mg of bacterial debris) it has been accepted for some time that bacteria initiate and perpetuate the sequence of events leading from acute and/or chronic inflammation to dental loss (Ellison, 1970; Socransky, 1970; Page & Schroeder, 1976).

Connective tissue changes in chronic periodontal disease have been documented by a variety of techniques (Schultz-Haudt, 1965; Cabrine & Carranza, 1966; Melcher, 1967). Actual decrease in the total collagen content of inflamed gingiva was suggested by microdissection followed by biochemical analysis (Flieder et al, 1966; Schroeder et al, 1973). Collagen production was found to represent 60 to 70 per cent of normal. In addition, it has been suggested (Rysky et al, 1969) that the size of the acid-soluble collagen compartment is more reduced than that of the other collagens. A marked decrease in hexosamine content has also been documented in inflamed gingivas (Rysky et al, 1969).

The heterogeneous bacteria forming the microbial plaque have been held ultimately responsible for all the connective tissue changes characteristic of chronic inflammatory gingival and periodontal disease (Russell, 1967; Ellison, 1970; Socransky, 1970). The bacterial debris in the gingival crevice fluid of patients with these disorders may increase from two- to 20-fold above normal. There are innumerable toxic substances in the microbial plaque, many of them potentially capable of producing from minimal to disastrous tissue damage (Socransky, 1970). There also are some collagenase producing bacteria, such as *B. melanogenicus* and *Cl. histolyticum*, which could easily account for the collagen loss. Nevertheless, there is much evidence that this is not the whole story and that perhaps in chronic periodontal disease there are some endogenous mechanisms that may be responsible for a few (or more) of the tissue changes. Such evidence may be listed as follows:

1. In contrast to acute necrotizing gingivitis, bacteria do not invade the gingival tissue in the commonly encountered varieties of chronic inflammatory gingival and periodontal disease (Listgarten, 1965).

2. Explants of gingival tissue are capable of degrading collagen gels (Fullmer & Gibson, 1966; Fullmer et al, 1969; Beutner et al, 1970) and this property is independent of bacteria since gingiva obtained from germ-free rats is also capable of producing collagenase 'in vitro' (Schneit & Fullmer, 1970).

3. Gingiva from alloxan and streptozotocin-diabetic rats

reveal collagenolytic activity in tissue culture (Ramamurty et al, 1973; Golub et al, 1978) whereas gingiva from normal rats is negative. Insulin treatment of alloxan-diabetic rats prevented the appearance of collagenolytic activity in gingival explants (Ramamurty et al, 1974).

4. Both epithelium and fibroblasts derived from gingival tissue have been shown to be the source of collagenase (Fullmer et al, 1969). The properties of both enzymes have been studied, together with the nature of their reaction products, and both have been shown to be indistinguishable from other animal collagenases (Fullmer et al, 1972). Of special interest is that the collagenase produced by *B. melanogenicus* is stimulated by cysteine (Gibbons & MacDonald, 1961), whereas gingival collagenase is inhibited by this reducing compound (Fullmer et al, 1972), a property shared with many other animal collagenases.

5. Gingival fibroblasts produce a latent collagenase (Birkedal-Hansen et al, 1974; Birkedal-Hansen et al, 1976a; Birkedal-Hansen et al, 1976b; Birkedal-Hansen et al, 1976c; Rosse & Robertson, 1977) which is activated by trypsin (Birkedal-Hansen et al, 1975a; Birkedal-Hansen et al, 1975b), by a mast cell factor (Simpson & Taylor, 1974); Birkedal-Hansen et al, 1975), and by a thermolabile, nondialyzable microbial plaque factor (Robertson et al, 1974).

6. Collagenase has been detected by immunohistochemical techniques in sections of human gingival tissue (Davies et al, 1979) which is considered to be an area of active collagen turnover.

7. Crevicular fluid contains a collagenolytic activity positively correlated with the severity of gingival inflammation and pocket depth (Golub et al, 1974; Golub et al, 1976). The electrophoretic pattern of the collagen breakdown products indicated its origin from tissues and not from bacteria.

In addition, it has been suggested (Page & Schroeder, 1973) that decrease in collagen content in chronic inflammatory gingival disease may also be due to inhibition of collagen synthesis, perhaps by cytopathic alterations of fibroblasts brought about by sensitized lymphoid cells.

Tumours

The invasive nature of malignant tumours makes them natural candidates for the presence of collagenolytic enzymes. 'Histolytic' substances have been postulated for a long time (Willis, 1949; Sylven, 1962) to explain the ability of malignant cells to invade the host tissues (Fig. 8.4). Hyaluronidase has been shown not to increase the invasiveness of tumours (Coman et al, 1847; Simpson, 1950). A large number of tumours have been examined for collagenolytic activity by a variety of techniques (Riley & Peacock, 1967; Robertson & Williams, 1969; Taylor et al, 1970; Dresden et al, 1972; Huang et al, 1976) with positive results, but only a few studies have attempted to characterize the enzyme and even fewer offer deffinitive proof of their origin from neoplastic cells. Collagenolytic activity in skin melanomas (Yamanishi et al, 1973; Maeyens et al, 1973) has been shown to be present in cultured neoplastic cells (Tane et al, 1978; Sauk & Witkop, 1978); on the other hand, the collagenase of basal cell carcinoma of the skin (Hashimoto et al, 1972a; Hashimoto et al, 1972b; Yamanishi et al, 1972) was identified by immunohistochemical staining to be confined to the connective tissue stroma adjacent to tumour islands (Bauer et al, 1977). Further studies (Bauer et al, 1979) with fibroblast cultures derived from human basal cell carcinomas demonstrated an increased capacity to synthesize and secrete collagenase; this phenotypic trait was lost after a few passages following primary explantation. The data suggested that the tumours probably stimulate adjacent fibroblasts to produce more collagenase, hence facilitating invasion of the surrounding connective tissue. A possible relation between enzyme content and clinical outcome has been claimed for tumours of head and neck (Huang et al, 1976) and for bladder carcinoma (Wirl & Frick, 1979); in the latter study collagenase was not detectable or low in superficially infiltrating tumours, and high in deeply invading neoplasias, Similar findings were obtained with a limited number of cervical carcinomas, and no collagenase was detected in carcinoma of the prostate and of the kidney.

Experimental tumours have also been studied extensively, such as those induced by methylcholantrene in mice (Wirl, 1977a; Wirl, 1977b; Labrose & Liener, 1978), rat (Huang et al, 1979), and the V_2-carcinoma of rabbits (Harris et al, 1972; Harris et al, 1975, Steven & Itzhaki, 1977; Biswas et al, 1978). It is interesting that when suspensions of V_2-carcinoma cells growing in rabbit muscle are used as the source material, some authors find both active and latent collagenase (Harris et al, 1972; Harris et al, 1975; Steven & Itzhaki, 1977) whereas other groups of investigators (Biswas et al, 1978) report this finding only exceptionally; if, however, the same rabbit is bearing both intramuscular and subcutaneous V_2-carcinoma tumours, extracts prepared from both tumours reveal trypsin-activatable collagenolytic activity. The well known resistance of cartilage to invasion by neoplastic cells has been attributed to an inhibitor of collagenase (Kuettner et al, 1976); in this experiment collagenase was obtained from cultures of human osteosarcoma and mammary carcinoma.

Others

There are several other pathological conditions in which excessive collagen degradation may play a pathogenetic role, but unfortunately there is little or no evidence that this is the case. Pulmonary emphysema, specially in patients deficient in alpha-l-antitrypsin, Paget's disease of bone, osteoporosis, and pressure atrophy as in bedsores or destruction of bone by a growing arterial aneurysm have

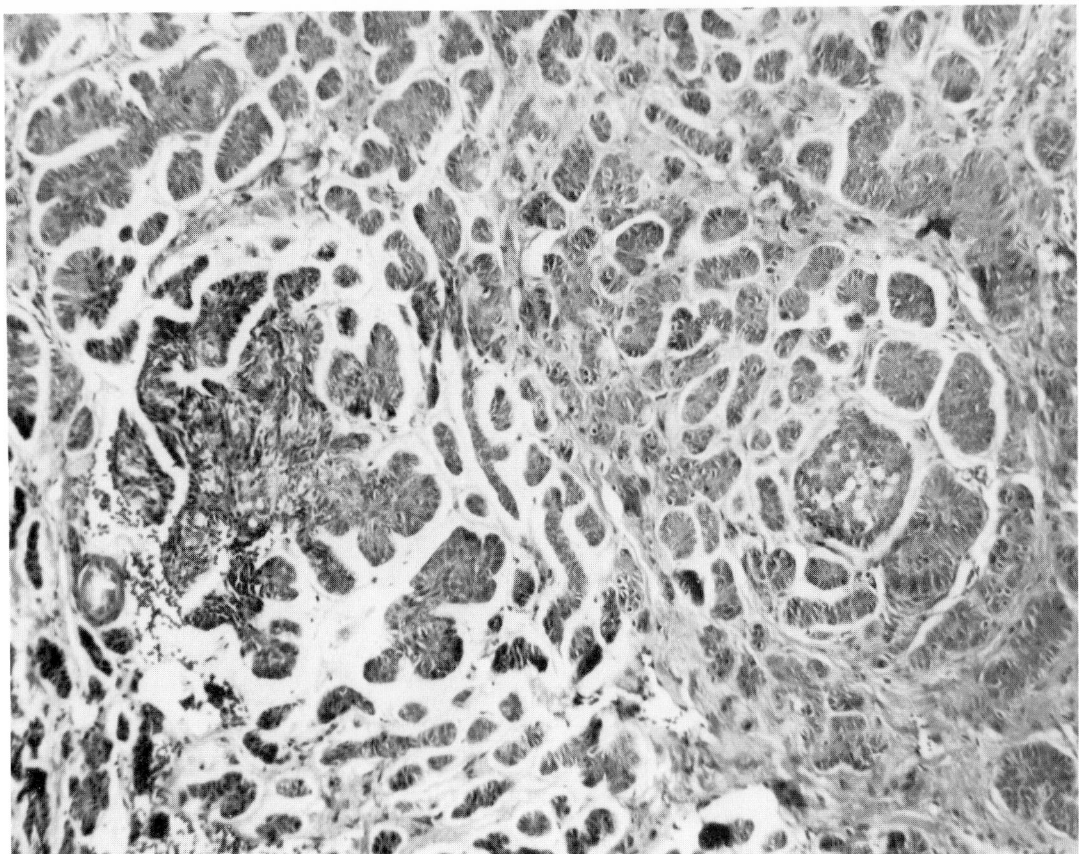

Fig. 8.4 Basal cell carcinoma of the skin. The stroma surrounding many of the cell groups appears loose and edematous, with scarce collagen fibrils. This picture, which is not frequently found in many tumours capable of invasion of surrounding tissues, is suggestive of collagen degradation.

been suggested (Pérez-Tamayo, 1973) as possible results of excessive collagen degradation. In cholesteatoma, a non neoplastic, proliferative disease involving both epithelium and connective tissue in the middle ear (Fig. 8.5) the presence of neutral collagenases produced by both elements of the lesion has been established (Abramson, 1969; Abramson & Gross, 1971) and the enzyme has been localized on the areas of tissue destruction by immunohistochemistry (Abramson & Huang, 1977). This makes it very likely that bone resorption, which is common in this disorder, may be the result of enzymatic degradation of collagen. A similar finding has been claimed for keratocysts or epithelial inclusion cysts, although the collagenase has not been well characterized (Donoff et al, 1972).

There is ample evidence that collagenase production increases during experimental wound healing (Grillo & Gross, 1967; Donoff, 1970; Donoff et al, 1971; Grillo, 1971; Shoshan & Gross, 1974), which involves not just deposition of collagen but extensive remodelling of both old and new collagen fibres. For this reason, at least in theory, there may be instances of abnormal wound healing in which collagen degradation could be excessive. Experiments with colon anastomosis in rabbits suggested that between four and 10 days after surgery there is decreased collagen content in the tissues surrounding the healing wound, increased collagenase production, and a resulting decrease in the mean bursting wall pressure of the large intestine (Hawley et al, 1970).

Deficient collagen degradation

Fibrosis and cirrhosis of the liver

A wealth of information is available on different aspects of fibrosis and cirrhosis of the liver (Pérez-Tamayo, 1965; Popper, & Udenfriend, 1970; Rojkind & Kershenobich, 1976; Popper, 1977; Pérez-Tamayo, 1979c; Rojkind & Dunn, 1979), an international symposium (Popper & Becker, 1975) and an annotated report of a workshop on this subject (Popper & Piez, 1978) have been published, and there is more to come. Although excessive collagen deposition in the liver is not synonymous with cirrhosis, the irreversibility of the disease is traditionally associated

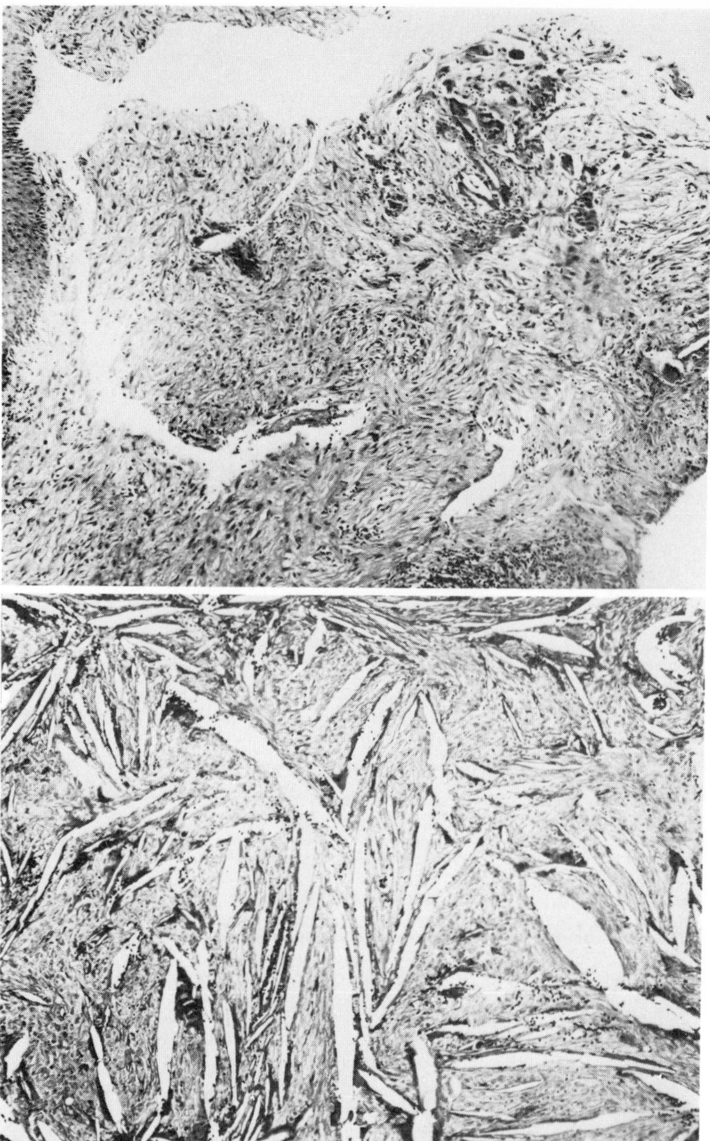

Fig. 8.5 Cholesteatoma. This is an inflammatory pseudotumour which occurs in the middle ear and is frequently accompanied by bone erosion. (A) There is some epithelium in the upper left margin of the picture, while the remaining structure corresponds to cellular fibrous tissue with neoformed vessels. Some clefts are surrounded by foreign body giant cells. (B) Another area of the same lesion, to illustrate the clefts left by cholesterol crystals (dissolved during the preparation of the slide) and the giant cells around them. (Tissue courtesy of Dr Cecilia Ridaura, Instituto Nacional de Pediatría, México.)

with it (Pérez-Tamayo, 1979c). A simple way to look at the problem suggests that if excessive fibrous tissue could be decreased or eliminated (Fig. 8.6), adequate dietary and other therapeutic measures might give better results in these unfortunate patients. Many concerned investigators subscribe to the concept that in cirrhosis of the liver, fibrosis represents a good example of reactive or secondary deposition of connective tissue (Popper, 1977). It may be suggested, however, that at least in some cases the increased collagen content characteristic of cirrhosis of the liver may be the result of a primary disturbance in the regulation of this extracellular macromolecule and, more specifically, of collagen degradation (Pérez-Tamayo & Montfort, 1964; Pérez-Tamayo, 1979a and c). The following data would support such heterodox suggestion:

1. Normal rat liver is capable of reabsorbing most or all collagen deposited as a consequence of an acute localized parenchymal injury; on the other hand, carbon tetrachloride (CCl_4)-cirrhotic rat livers preserve locally induced scars as long as the disease is present (Pérez-Tamayo & Montfort, 1964).

2. The experimental work mentioned above was

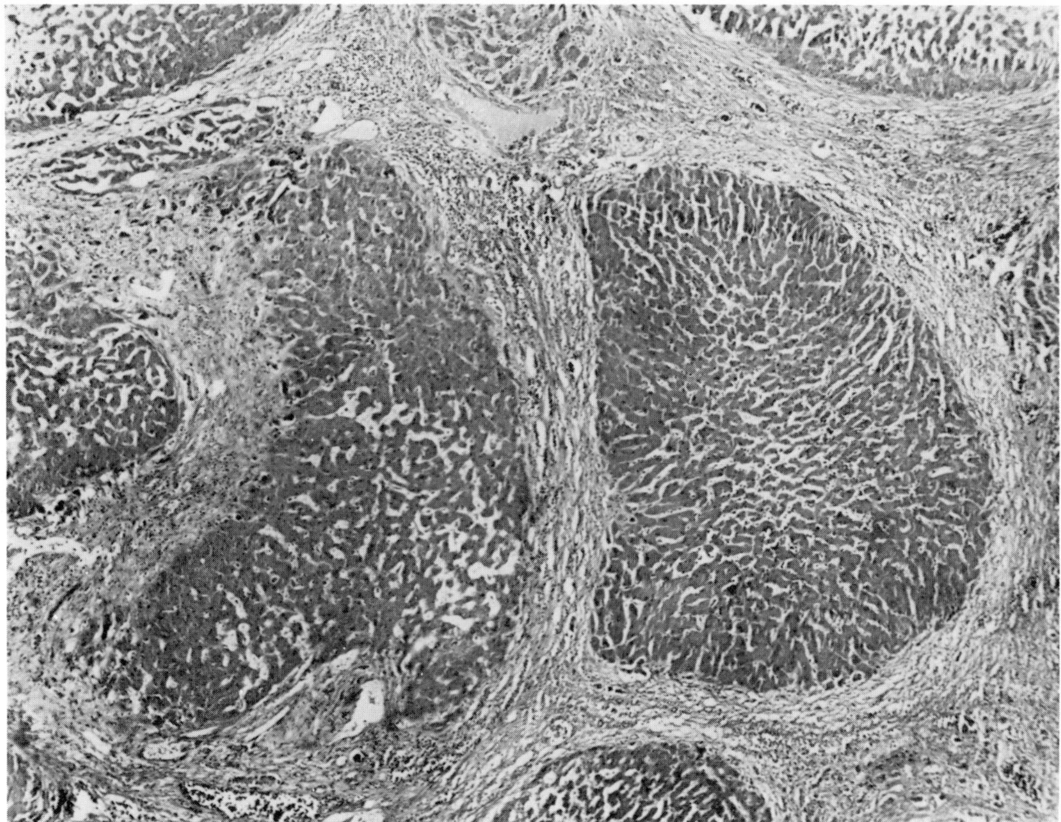

Fig. 8.6 Histologic aspect of cirrhosis of the liver. There is loss of normal architecture with nodular regeneration of the parenchyma and broad connective tissue septa separating the nodules.

stimulated by the observation that liver scars are either absent or of remarkably small size in patients with adequately documented cured amoebic abscesses of the liver in a large autopsy series (Brandt & Pérez-Tamayo, 1970).

3. Collagenolytic activity has been detected in liver explants during the early stages of CCl_4-induced cirrhosis of the liver in rats (Okazaki & Maruyama, 1974); in more advanced stages of the experimental disease, such enzymatic activity decreased. Collagenase has been detected in preparations of Kupffer cells of the rat liver (Fugiwara et al, 1973), in rat liver homogenates (Fugiwara et al, 1974), and in experimental mouse liver schistosomiasis (Takahashi et al, 1977). Quantitative determinations of collagenase in CCl_4-induced cirrhosis of the liver in rats produced conflicting results: a group of investigators reported increased collagenolytic activity during the early or reversible stage of the disease (Rojkind et al, 1979) whereas in our laboratory we found that collagenase activity is depressed throughout the development of the disease, and more so in the irreversible stage (González et al, 1980). The difference, however, may be a matter of calculation of data, since Rojkind et al (1979) expressed their findings in units of collagenase activity per gram of liver tissue, whereas we estimated the ratio of collagenase activity (also in units) to the amount of collagen present per gram of liver tissue.

4. Experimental CCl_4-induced cirrhosis of the rat liver has been shown to go through two stages: an early one, in which the process is reversible provided that the toxic substance is discontinued and the post-treatment period of observation is sufficiently prolonged (Pérez-Tamayo, 1979c), and a late one, irreversible despite discontinuation of CCl_4 administration (Cameron & Karunaratne, 1936; Hutterer et al, 1961; Rubin et al, 1963; Hutterer et al, 1964; Rubin et al, 1965), although here the duration of post-treatment observation is limited by the natural mean-survival time of the species. In some of these early studies it was suggested that the onset of irreversibility of the disease was paralleled by the appearance of a metabolically inert collagen fraction. Using different techniques, similar conclusions have been reached more recently (Rojkind et al, 1979; González et al, 1980; Pérez-Tamayo & Montfort, 1980).

5. Reversibility is not limited to the early stages of CCl_4-induced cirrhosis in the rat; it has also been observed

with almost all other toxic and dietary experimental models of the disease and in different animal species (for references, see Pérez-Tamayo, 1979c). In all other reported instances of reversibility of cirrhosis, the same two parameters appear significant for the occurrence of the phenomenon: withdrawal of the cirrhogenic agent and prolonged periods of subsequent observation. In addition, in a limited number of human cases of cirrhosis of the liver there is objective proof that the disease has disappeared (Rojkind & Dunn, 1979; Pérez-Tamayo, 1979c); again in many of those patients the etiologic agent (iron) was removed by repeated venisection, and the subsequent period of observation extended from one to many years.

6. We (Montfort & Pérez-Tamayo, 1978) have shown by immunofluorescence methods that in early, reversible CCl_4-cirrhosis in the rat liver the collagenous septums reveal collagen-bound collagenase (Pardo et al, 1980). In late, irreversible stages of the experimental liver disease, collagen-bound collagenase is no longer detectable by such techniques on the fibrous tissue (Fig. 8.7).

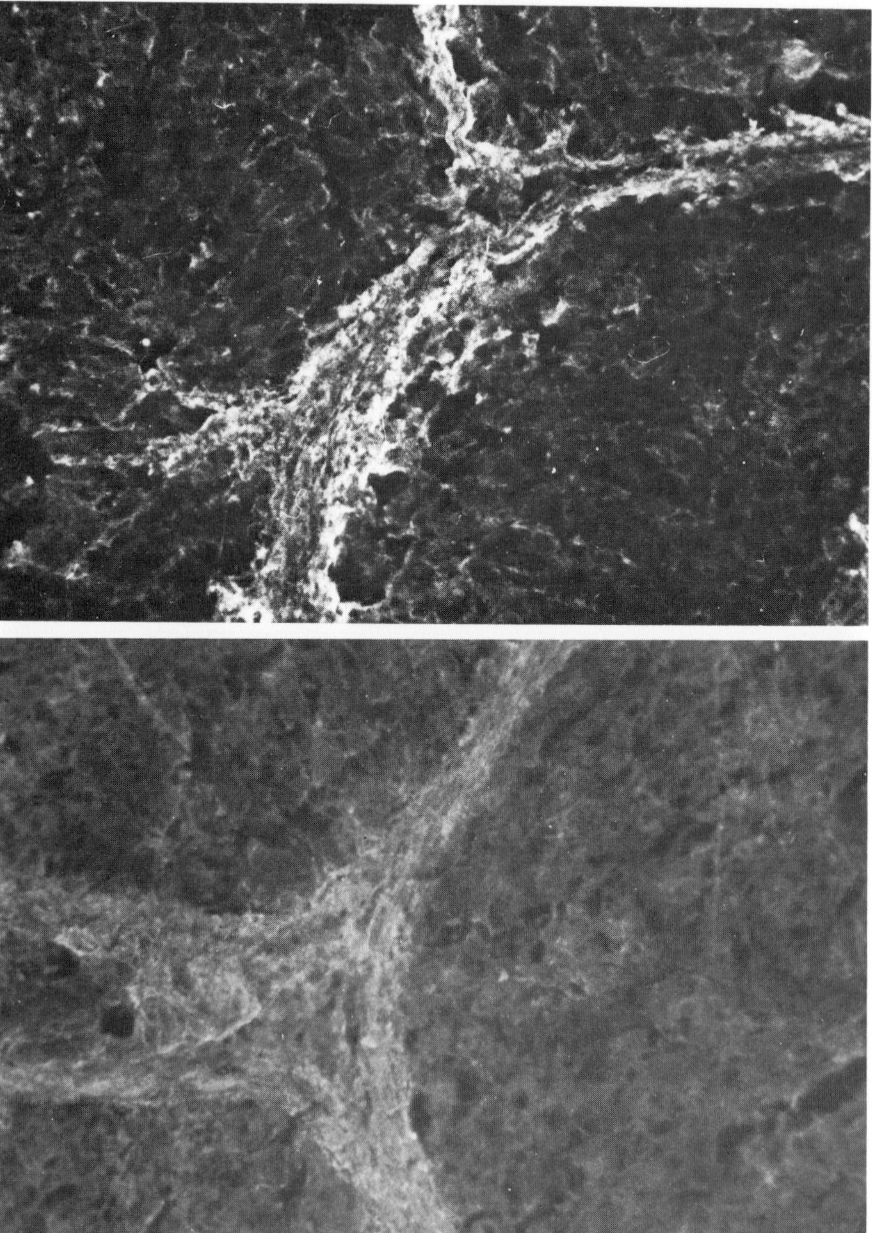

Fig. 8.7 Distribution of collagenase in experimental CCl_4 cirrhosis of the liver. The enzyme is revealed by immunohistochemical technique. (A) Connective tissue septa in reversible cirrhosis, showing the presence of collagenase probably bound to collagen fibres. (B) Connective tissue septa in irreversible cirrhosis, which fail to reveal the presence of the enzyme (from work published originally in The American Journal of Pathology, 1979; reproduced with permission of the Editor and Publisher).

7. More recently, we have studied the susceptibility of collagen to homologous collagenase in tissue sections of both CCl_4-induced cirrhosis of the liver in rats, and in human cases of the disease (Pérez-Tamayo & Montfort, 1980). The question asked was quite simple: is irreversibility in both experimental and human liver cirrhosis associated with a detectable resistance of collagen to non-limiting concentrations of their respective homologous collagenase? The answer turned out to be an unqualified no.

Thus, it appears that experimental CCl_4-induced liver cirrhosis is a reversible process as long as collagen-bound collagenase is present on fibrous tissue septums. Furthermore, irreversibility of the experimental disease is accompanied by a marked decrease or complete absence of collagenolytic activity in the liver, established by several techniques. Finally, despite some suggestions that at least part of the collagen deposited in the liver may be less susceptible to collagenase (Feinman et al, 1979), this was not substantiated under in vitro conditions and with non-limiting amounts of the enzyme (Pérez-Tamayo et al, 1980)' It has been suggested (Henley et al, 1977), on the basis of indirect data, that the collagen-increasing effect of ethanol on the livers of animals receiving a cirrhogenic diet may be due to an inhibition of collagen breakdown.

Scleroderma

Progressive systemic sclerosis or scleroderma is generally viewed as the result of excessive collagen deposition (Winkelman, 1976; Fleischmajer, 1977; Eisen et al, 1979). The outstanding pathologic feature of this disease is the increased amount of collagen in skin (Fig. 8.8),

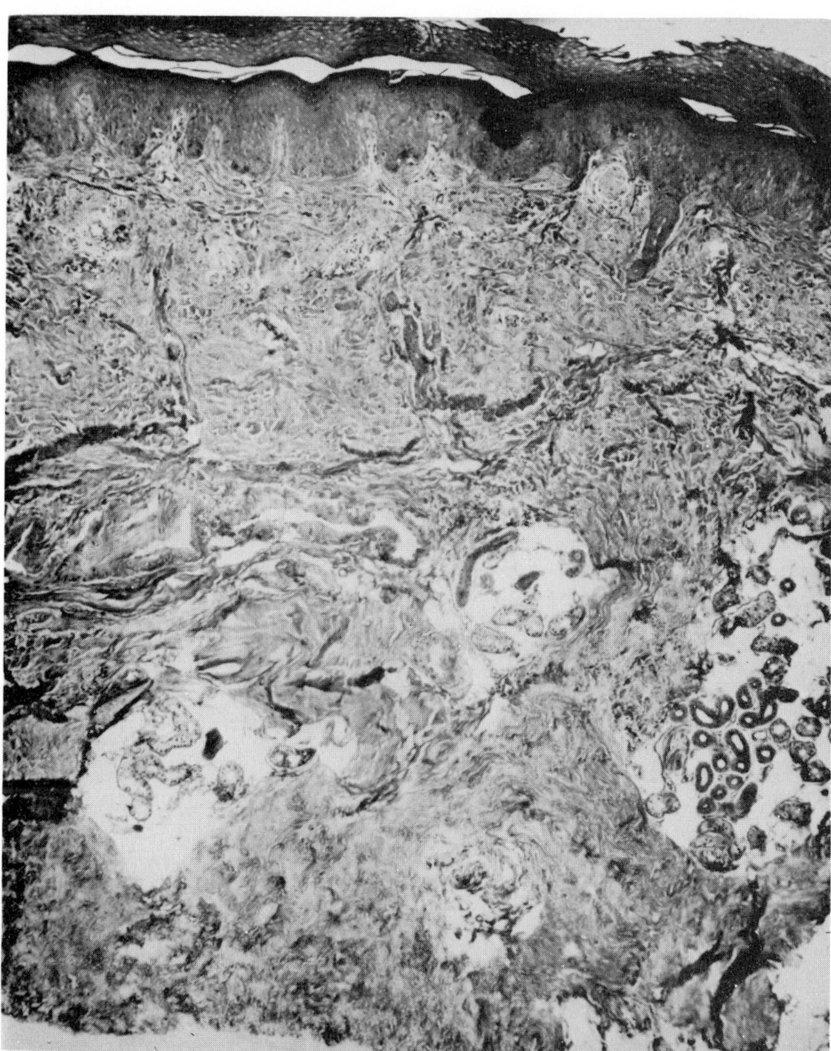

Fig. 8.8 Increased connective tissue in the dermis of a patient with scleroderma. The biopsy was taken from the skin of the third finger (lateral side). The epithelium is in the upper part of the picture and is essentially normal. The dermis shows thickening and irregularity of the collagen fibres, which penetrate deeply into the lower dermis and subcutaneous tissue below the level of the sweat glands. The latter show atrophy.

gastrointestinal tract, lungs, heart, and several other organs. Other anatomic changes, of course, are probably due to different mechanisms, such as the renal lesions (Cannon et al, 1974), or the frequent association with Sjögren's syndrome (Bloch et al, 1965). The wide range of diameters displayed by the dermal collagen fibres has been mentioned as evidence for a long-persisting synthesis (Fleischmajer & Prunieras, 1972; Kobayasi & Asboe-Hansen, 1972). Enhanced prolyl hydroxylase activity in the skin of some patients (Uitto et al, 1969; Keiser, 1971; Uitto, 1971), and increased number of reducible cross-links in the extractable collagen (Herbert et al, 1974) also support the hypothesis of increased collagen synthesis. The ultrastructural aspect of fibroblasts is compatible with hyperactivity (Fleischmajer & Prunieras, 1972), and it has been demonstrated that cultures of these cells obtained from the skin of some patients (LeRoy, 1972; LeRoy, 1974; Buckingham et al, 1978; Uitto et al, 1979) with active scleroderma synthesize larger amounts of collagen than normal controls. Contradictory results (Perlish et al, 1976) could be explained by the long standing nature of the disease, with alternating periods of quiescence and activity. In chronic cases the histologic aspect of the skin does not suggest an active process of collagen deposition: cells are very few and far between and collagen bundles are thick, hyaline, and densely arranged (Gardner, 1965; Fleischmajer et al, 1972). The urinary excretion of hydroxyproline in these patients has shown wide variations (Uitto, 1971).

The possibility that scleroderma may be due at least in part to decreased collagen breakdown has been mentioned (Pérez-Tamayo, 1973), and there is some evidence that this may be the case. Using the homogenate pellet technique of Ryan and Woessner (1971), skin biopsy specimens from 12 patients with scleroderma and nine controls were studied (Brady, 1975). In seven of those cases in which extensive involvement of the forearm and trunk existed, collagenase activity of the involved skin was minimal or absent. Moreover, in the same patient, regions of marked skin involvement showed no collagenase activity, whereas clinically uninvolved skin areas exhibited normal or nearly normal leves of enzyme activity. In other patients in whom clinical symptoms were systemic and not associated significantly with the skin, collagenase activity approximated normal levels. More recently, Uitto et al (1979) repeated these observations in two patients with scleroderma, but instead of using the homogenate pellet technique they measured collagenolytic activity in skin explants from two patients on radioactive collagen, and also in fibroblast cultures derived from eight patients with systemic scleroderma; in the latter experiments collagenase was determined both as an immunoreactive protein and also as collagenolytic activity after maximal trypsin activation of the culture medium. No differences from control values were observed in all determinations of collagenase. This discrepancy with Brady's findings (1975) may be purely a matter of technique, but even in that case it is still of great interest since it would suggest that the in vitro conditions of cell cultures and tissue explants permit the living elements to regain their 'normal' level of synthesis of collagenase, whereas tissue homogenates (in which all cells are killed) reflect more faithfully the real concentrations of the enzyme in vivo. There is some evidence that tissues that do not appear to be the site of rapid collagen degradation may produce large amounts of collagenase in culture, such as human skin (Eisen et al, 1968), bovine gingiva (Birkedal-Hansen et al, 1976), non-gravid rabbit uterus (Cartwright et al, 1977), and non-gravid rat uterus (Woessner, 1979).

Idiopathic pulmonary fibrosis

This is a progressive, generally fatal disease characterized by diffuse interstitial pulmonary fibrosis involving multiple foci in both lungs; during the early stages there is intra-alveolar and interstitial inflammation, whereas the advanced disease is characterized by severe fibrosis and minimal cellularity (Spencer, 1968; Crystal et al, 1978; Fulmer & Crystal, 1979). In the final stages the normal architecture of the lung may be so distorted and the consistency so much increased by the excessive amount of connective tissue deposited that in the older literature this condition (together with several others leading to the final 'honey-comb lung') was sometimes labelled as 'pulmonary cirrhosis' (Fig. 8.9). The current concept of the pathogenesis of idiopathic pulmonary fibrosis is that some unidentified process, probably from variable nature, initiates a chronic and repeated injury to the structures constituting the peripheral air passages which results in alveolitis. This term implies the accumulation of inflammatory cells and fluids within alveolar spaces and interstitium, as well as degenerative and proliferative reactions in the cellular components of the distal air spaces. With such profound changes in the parenchymal cell populations there is a 'derangement' of extracellular, interstitial mesenchymal elements, of which collagen is a prominent (although far from unique) one. The result is progressive increase in the amount of interstitial collagen with widening of the alveolar septa and collapse of alveolar sacs. These changes usually do not occur simultaneously throughout both lungs, but rather in a multifocal and successive pattern, so that at any given moment the involved areas may reveal different stages of the process described. Eventually, however, cellularity decreases and the picture is one of greatly thickened and sclerotic alveolar septa, surrounding small and irregular alveolar sacs with cubic, epithelial-like cell lining.

Such widespread deposition of collagen suggests that there probably is increased collagen synthesis in idiopathic pulmonary fibrosis (Fulmer & Crystal, 1979), at least during some phase of its development. But excessive

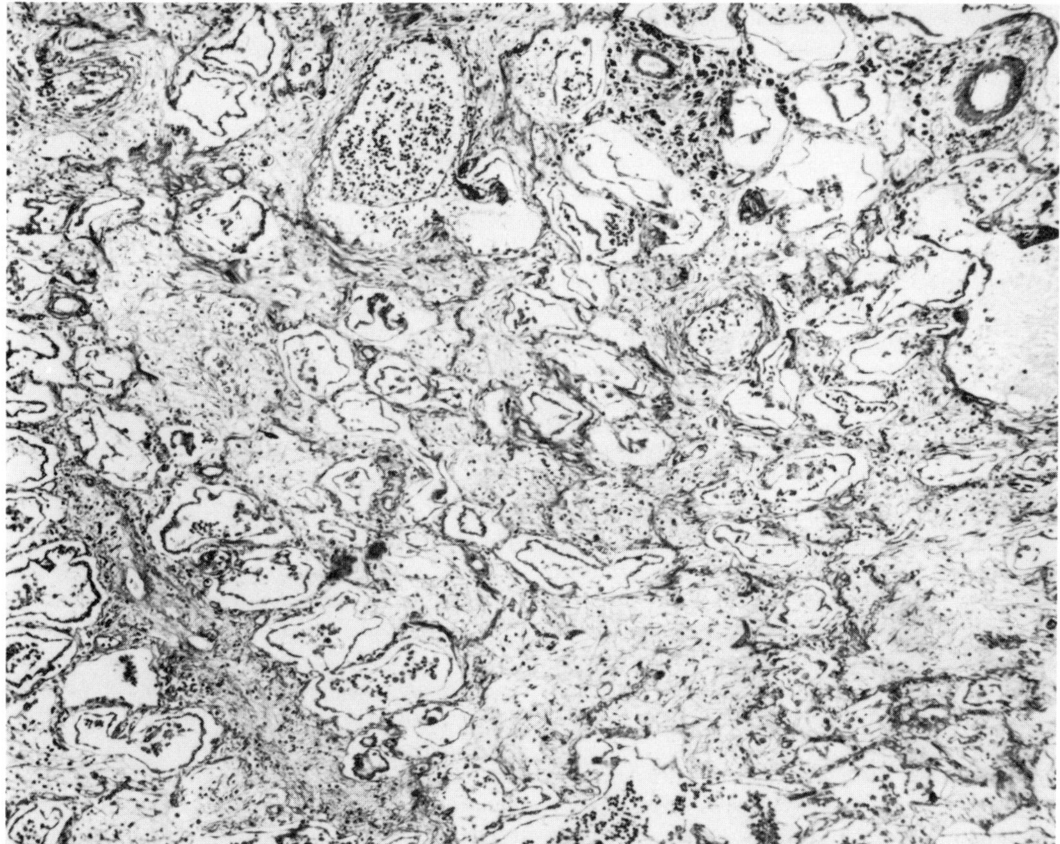

Fig. 8.9 Low power view of the lung in a human case of idiopathic interstitial pulmonary fibrosis. The alveolar septa are greatly expanded by a finely fibrillary material with very few cells. The alveolar lining appears continuous and is detached from the septa in some places (this is an artifact of the preparation of the slide); even at this low magnification it is apparent that there is cubic metaplasia of the alveolar cells. This is an early stage in the development of the lesion; in latter stages the fibrillary material is replaced by bona fide collagen fibres.

collagen deposition may also result from decreased collagen breakdown, or from a combination of both processes, regardless of how the tissues look under the light or electron microscope. No information is available on the levels of collagenolytic activity in normal and fibrotic lung parenchyma, either in experimental models or with human material. On the other hand, Gadek et al (1979) have studied collagenase and other enzymes in the fluid obtained by bronchoscopy from the lower respiratory tract of 24 patients with idiopathic pulmonary fibrosis, 18 controls, and nine patients with sarcoidosis. In this study it was found that 15 of 21 patients with idiopathic pulmonary fibrosis showed collagenolytic activity in the bronchial fluid, whereas normal controls and patients with sarcoidosis showed none. The authors suggest that since idiopathic pulmonary fibrosis is characterized by continuous disruption and replacement of normal alveolar interstitial collagen by collagen that is abnormal in location, amount, type, and form, a collagenase is required. The source of this collagenase is attributed to either (or both) macrophages and polymorphonuclear leucocytes, since both cell types have been shown to be capable of collagenase production. In this study no correlation was established between the stage of the disease (early, middle or advanced) and the presence and level of collagenolytic activity found in the bronchial fluid. It is stated (Gadek et al, 1979) that in two patients re-evaluated after eight and 24 months, collagenase was still present, but no mention is made of the stage of the disease in which these two patients were when first studied. The point here is that the authors failed to consider the possibility that their bronchial fluid collagenolytic activity may be related not to cells but to the amount of collagen bound collagenase present in the lung.

Osteopetrosis

This heritable and rare disorder occurs in many different animal species, such as mouse, rat, fowl, rabbit, and humans. The mode of hereditary transmission of the human disease is autosomal recessive in the malignant form and autosomal dominant in the benign form (McKusick, 1972). Osteopetrosis is a systemic disorder of bone in which resorption occurs at a slower rate than deposition. Curiously enough, bone explants of mice affected by the disease produce an increased amount of collagenase (Marks, 1974). Although this observation has been interpreted as indicating activation or release of a stock of latent enzyme, the evidence from other collagen-degrading systems in vitro suggests otherwise (see above). Nevertheless, using the same animal model of the human disease, it has been reported that parathormone fails to release lysosomal enzymes (Walker, 1966), which it does in explants of normal bones (Walker et al, 1974; Sakamoto et al, 1975). The current view of the major mechanism responsible for this animal type of osteopetrosis is defective activation in the release of proteases required for bone resorption.

An interesting experiment on the therapeutic effect of parabiosis in mouse osteopetrosis should be mentioned. After temporarily joining a normal mouse to one affected by the heritable bone disease, and presumably allowing the passage of competent osteolytic cells from the normal to the diseased mouse, clinical and radiological signs of osteopetrosis disappeared from the latter (Walker, 1973).

Others

In human pathology there is no dearth of conditions in which deficient collagen degradation could play a significant role. In addition to the four conditions already mentioned, many others may be listed (Pérez-Tamayo, 1973; Pérez-Tamayo, 1979a) such as chronic renal disease, diabetes, idiopathic retroperitoneal fibrosis, atherosclerosis, etc. The list could be easily extended, since fibrosis is such a widespread pathological phenomenon. But the available evidence on the role of collagen degradation, and more specifically, of collagenase, on the many conditions in which it may be implicated, stands as summarized above. A bird's eye-view of the entire field of the pathology of collagen degradation leaves the reviewer (and hopefully the reader) with the feeling that this is an area of biologic research with a few solid achievements and many potentialities open for the immediate future. The hope is that with increasing basic information we shall be able to offer better help to our patients.

SUMMARY

The degradation of collagen in animal tissues has been reviewed from the standpoint of the pathologist. Diseases in which the catabolism of this specific extracellular protein may be involved are classified and examined, first from a general viewpoint, and afterwards by specific entities, classified according to the extent to which the excessive or deficient nature (probable or possible) of the specific collagenolytic mechanisms may be involved. A preliminary list of clinico-pathological entities, experimental and human, has emerged from this review. The hope is expressed that the present exercise will contribute to the further development of the molecular pathology of connective tissues.

REFERENCES

Abramson M 1969 Collagenolytic activity in middle ear cholesteatoma. Annals of Otology, Rhinology and Laryngology 78: 112

Abramson M, Gross J 1971 Further studies on a collagenase in middle ear cholesteatoma. Annals of Otology, Rhinology and Laryngology 80: 177

Abramson M, Huang C C 1977 Localization of collagenase in human middle ear cholesteatoma. Laryngoscope 87: 771

Allegra S R, Broderick P A 1973 Desmoid fibroblastoma. Intracytoplasmic collagen synthesis in a peculiar fibroblastic tumour: light and ultrastructural study of a case. Human Pathology 4: 419

Aswanikumar S, Radkrishnan A N 1973 Studies on a peptidase acting on synthetic collagenase substrate. Development pattern in rat granuloma tissue and distribution of enzyme in the tissues of various animals. Biochimica et Biophysica Acta 292: 210

Azar H A, Lunardelli C 1969 Collagen nature of asteroid bodies of giant cells in sarcoidosis. The American Journal of Pathology 57: 81

Bauer E A 1977 Recessive dystrophic epidermolysis bullosa: Evidence for an altered collagenase in fibroblast cultures. Proceedings of the National Academy of Sciences USA 74: 4646

Bauer E A, Eisen A Z 1978 Recessive dystrophyc epidermolysis bullosa. Evidence for increased collagenase as a genetic characteristic in cell culture' The Journal of Experimental Medicine 148: 1378

Bauer E A, Uitto J 1979 Collagen in cutaneous diseases. International Journal of Dermatology 18: 251

Bauer E A, Gedde-Dahl T Jr, Eisen A Z 1977 The role of human skin collagenase in epidermolysis bullosa. The Journal of Investigative Dermatology 68: 119

Bauer E A, Gordon J M, Reddick M E, Eisen A Z 1977 Quantitation and immunocytochemical localization of human skin collagenase in basal cell carcinoma. The Journal of Investigative Dermatology 69: 363

Bauer E A, Uitto J, Walters R C, Eisen A Z 1979 Enhanced collagenase production by fibroblasts derived from human basal cell carcinoma. Cancer Research 39: 4594

Berman M B, Kerza-Kiwiatecki A P, Davison P F 1973 Characterization of human corneal collagenase. Experimental Eye Research 15: 367

Berman M, Leary R, Gage J 1979 Collagenase from corneal cell cultures and its modulation by phagocytosis. Investigative Ophthalmology and Visual Science 18: 588

Beutner E H, Triftshauser C, Hazen S P 1966 Collagenase activity of gingival tissue from patients with periodontal diseases. Proceedings of the Society for Experimental Biology and Medicine 121: 1082

Birkedal-Hansen H, Cobb C M, Taylor R E, Fullmer H M 1974 Bovine gingival collagenase: demonstration and initial characterization. Journal of Oral Pathology 3: 232

Birkedal-Hansen H, Cobb C M, Taylor R E, Fullmer H M 1975a Activation of latent bovine gingival collagenase. Archives of Oral Biology 20: 681

Birkedal-Hansen H, Cobb C M, Taylor R E, Fullmer H M 1975b Trypsin activation of latent collagenase from several mammalian sources. Scandinavian Journal of Dental Research 83: 302

Birkedal-Hansen H, Cobb C M, Taylor R E, Fullmer H M 1975c Activation of latent collagenase by mast-cell granule proteases. Journal of Dental Research 54: 66

Birkedal-Hansen H, Cobb C M, Taylor R E, Fullmer H M 1976a Procollagenase from bovine gingiva. Biochimica et Biophysica Acta 429: 229

Birkedal-Hansen H, Cobb C M, Taylor R E, Fullmer H M 1976b Synthesis and release of procollagenase by cultured fibroblasts. Journal of Biological Chemistry 251: 3162

Birkedal-Hansen H, Cobb C M, Taylor R E, Fullmer H M 1976c Fibroblastic origin of bovine gingival collagenase. Archives of Oral Biology 21: 297

Biswas C, Moran W P, Bloch K J, Gross J 1978 Collagenolytic activity of rabbit V_2-carcinoma growing at multiple sites. Biochemical and Biophysical Research Communications 80: 33

Bloch K J, Buchanan W W, Wohl M J, Bunim J J 1965 Sjögren's syndrome. A clinical, pathological and serological study of sixty-two cases. Medicine 44: 187

Bohigian G, Valenton M, Okumoto M, Caraway S L 1974 Collagenase inhibitors in pseudomonas keratitis: Adjuncts to antibiotic therapy in rabbits. Archives of Ophthalmology 91: 52

Brady A H 1975 Collagenase in scleroderma. The Journal of Clinicial Investigation 56: 1175

Brandes D, Anton E 1969a An electromicroscopic cytochemical study of macrophages during uterine involution. The Journal of Cell Biology 41: 450

Brandes D, Anton E 1969b Lysosomes in uterine involution: intracytoplasmic degradation of myofilaments and collagen. Journal of Gerontology 24: 55

Brandt H, Pérez-Tamayo R 1970 Pathology of human amebiasis. Human Pathology 1: 351

Briggaman R A, Wheeler C E 1975 Epidermolysis bullosa dystrophica recessive: A possible role of anchoring fibrils in the pathogenesis. The Journal of Investigative Dermatology 65: 203

Brown S I 1972 Collagenolytic enzymes in corneal pathology. Israel Journal of Medical Sciences 8: 1537

Brown S I, Hook C W 1971a Isolation of corneal collagenase in corneal inflammation. American Journal of Ophthalmology 72: 1139

Brown S I, Hook C W 1971b Treatment of collagen destruction with collagenase inhibitors. Transactions of the American Academy of Ophthalmology and Otolaryngology 75: 1199

Brown S I, Weller C A 1970a Cellular origin of collagenase in normal and wounded corneas. Archives of Ophthalmology 83: 74

Brown S I, Weller C A 1970b Collagenase inhibitors in prevention of ulcers of alkali-burned cornea. Archives of Ophthalmology 83: 352

Brown S I, Akiya S, Weller C A 1969 Prevention of the ulcers of the alkali-burned cornea: Preliminary studies with collagenase inhibitors. Archives of Ophthalmology 82: 95

Brown S I, Weller C A, Vidrich A M 1970 Effect of corticosteroids on corneal collagenase in rabbits. American Journal of Ophthalmology 70: 744

Buckingham R, Prince R K, Rodnan G P, Taylor F 1978 Increased collagen accumulation in dermal fibroblast cultures from patients with progressive systemic sclerosis (scleroderma). Journal of Laboratory and Clinical Medicine 92: 5

Burleigh M C 1977 Degradation of collagen by non-specific proteinases. In: Barrett A J (ed) Proteinases in mammalian cells and tissues. Elsevier/North Holland Biomedical Press, Amsterdam, p 287

Burleigh M C, Barrett A J, Lazarus G S 1974 Cathepsin B1: A lysosomal enzyme that degrades native collagen. The Biochemical Journal 137: 387

Cabrini R L, Carranza F A 1966 Histochemistry of periodontal tissues: A review of the literature. International Dental Journal 16: 466

Cameron G R, Karunaratne W A W 1936 Carbon tetrachloride cirrhosis in relation to liver regeneration. Journal of Pathology and Bacteriology 42: 1

Cannon P J, Hassar M, Case D B, Casarella W J, Sommers S C, LeRoy E C 1974 The relationship of hypertension and renal failure in scleroderma (progressive systemic sclerosis) to structural and functional abnormalities of the renal cortical circulation. Medicine 53: 1

Cartwright E, Murphy G, Sellers A, Reynolds J J 1977 Collagenase activity from cultured non-gravid rabbit uterus. Biochemical Soceity Transactions 5: 229

Comman D R, McCutcheon M, Zeidman I 1947 Failure of hyaluronidase to increase the invasiveness of neoplasms. Cancer Research 7: 383

Coombs R R A, Fell H B 1969 Lysosomes in tissue damage mediated by allergic reactions. In: Dingle J T, Fell H B (eds) Lysosomes in Biology and Pathology, vol 2. North Holland, Amsterdam, p. 3

Crystal R G, Fulmer J D, Baum B J, Bernardo J, Bradley K H, Bruel S D, Elson N A, Fells G A, Ferrans V J, Gadek J E, Hunninghake G W, Kawanami O, Kelman J A, Line B R, McDonald J A, McLees B D, Roberts W C, Rosenberg D M, Tolstoshev P, Von Gal E, Werberger S E 1978 Cells, collagen and idiopathic pulmonary fibrosis. Lung 155: 199

Davies R M, Tetlow L, Ackroyd C, Woolley D E 1979 Collagenase immunolocalization in human gingival tissue. The Journal of Dental Research 58: 1227

Deporter D A, Ten Cate A R 1973 Fine structural localization of acid and alkaline phosphatase in collagen-containing vesicles of fibroblasts. Journal of Anatomy 114: 457

Deshmukh-Phadke K, Lawrence M, Nanda S 1978 Synthesis of collagenase and neutral protease by articular chondrocytes: stimulation by a macrophage-derived factor. Biochemical and Biophysical Research Communications 85: 490

Dingle J T 1978 Articular damage in arthritis and its control. Annals of Internal Medicine 88: 821

Dingle J T 1979 Recent studies on the control of joint damage: the contribution of the Strangeways Research Laboratory. Annals of the Rheumatic Diseases 38: 201

Donoff R B 1970 Wound healing: Biochemical events and potential role of collagenase. Journal of Oral Surgery 28: 356

Donoff R B, McLennan J E, Grillo H C 1971 Preparation and properties of collagenase from epithelium and mesenchyme of healing mammalian wounds. Biochimica et Biophysica Acta 227: 639

Donoff R B, Harper E, Guralnic W G 1972 Collagenolytic activity in keratocysts. Journal of Oral Surgery 30: 879

Dresden M H, Heilman S A, Schmidt J D 1972 Collagenolytic enzymes in human neoplasms. Cancer Rsearch 32: 993

Ehrlich M G, Mankin H J, Jones H, Wright R, Crispen C 1975 Collagenase and collagenase inhibitors in osteoarthritic and normal human cartilage. The Journal of Bone and Joint Surgery 57A: 570

Eisen A Z 1969 Human skin collagenase: relationship to the pathogenesis of epidermolysis bullosa dystrophica. The Journal of Investigative Dermatology 52: 449
Eisen A Z, Jeffrey J J, Gross J 1968 Human skin collagenase. Isolation and mechanism of attack on the collagen molecule. Biochimica et biophysica Acta 161: 137
Eisen A Z, Bauer E A, Jeffrey J J 1970 Animal and human collagenases. The Journal of Investigative Dermatology 55: 359
Eisen A Z, Uitto J, Bauer E A 1979 Scleroderma. In: Fitzpatrick T B, Eisen A Z, Austen K F, Freedberg I M, Wolff K (eds) Dermatology in General Medicine, 2nd edn. McGraw-Hill Book Company, New York, p 1305
Ellison S A 1970 Oral bacteria and periodontal disease. Journal of Dental Research 49: 198
Etherington D J 1974 The purification of bovine cathepsin B1 and its mode of action on bovine collagens. The Biochemical Journal 137: 547
Etherington D J 1977 The dissolution of insoluble bovine collagens by cathepsin B1, collagenolytic cathepsin and pepsin. Connective Tissue Research 5: 135
Etherington D J, Evans P J 1977 The action of cathepsin B and collagenolytic cathepsin in the degradation of collagen. Acta Biologica Medica Germanica 36: 1555
Evans P, Etherington D J 1978 Characterisation of cathepsin B and collagenolytic cathepsin from human placenta. European Journal of Biochemistry 83: 87
Evanson J M 1971 Mammalian collagenases and their role in connective tissue breakdown. In: Barrett A J, Dingle J T (eds) Tissue proteinases. Elsevier, New York, p 327
Feinman L, Fecher R, Lue S L, Lieber C S 1979 Aldehyde content of collagen from alcoholic cirrhotic and noncirrhotic human livers. Experimental and Molecular Pathology 30: 271
Fleischmajer R 1977 The pathophysiology of scleroderma. International Journal of Dermatology 16: 310
Fleischmajer R, Prunieras M 1972 Generalized morphea. II. Electron microscopy of collagen, cells, and the subcutaneous tissue. Archives of Dermatology 106: 515
Fleischmajer R, Damiano V, Nedwith A 1972 Alteration of subcutaneous tissue in systemic scleroderma. Archives of Dermatology 105: 59
Flieder D E, Sun C N, Schneider B C 1966 Chemistry of normal and inflamed human gingival tissues. Periodontics 4: 302
Francois J, Cambie E 1972 Collagenase and collagenase inhibitors in torpid ulcers of the cornea. Ophthalmological Research 3: 145
Fugiwara K, Sakai T, Oda T, Igarashi S 1973 The presence of collagenase in Kupffer cells of the rat liver. Biochemical and Biophysical Research Communications 54: 531
Fugiwara K, Sakai T, Oda T, Igarashi S 1974 Demonstration of collagenase activity in rat liver homogenates. Biochemical and Biophysical Research Communications 60: 166
Fulmer J D, Crystal R G 1979 Interstitial lung disease. In: Simmons D H (ed) Current pulmonology, vol 1. Houghton, Mifflin and Company, Boston, p 1
Fullmer H M 1970 Metabolic hydrolysis of collagen. In Fishman W H (ed) Metabolic conjugation and metabolic hydrolysis, vol 2. Academic Press, New York, p 301
Fullmer H M, Gibson W A 1966 Collagenolytic activity in gingivae of man. Nature 209: 728
Fullmer H M, Gibson W A, Lazarus G S, Bladen H A, Whedon K A 1969 The origin of collagenase in periodontal tissues of man. Journal of Dental Research 48: 646
Fullmer H M, Taylor R E, Guthrie R W 1972 Human gingival collagenase: Purification, molecular weight, and inhibitor studies. Journal of Dental Research 51: 349
Gadek J E, Kelman J E, Fells G, Winberger S E, Horwitz A L, Reynolds H Y, Fulmer J D, Crystal R G 1979 Collagenase in the lower respiratory tract of patients with idiopathic pulmonary fibrosis. The New England Journal of Medicine 301: 737
Gantz B J, Abramson M, Huang C C 1978 Localization of collagenase in chronically inflamed guinea pig temporal bone. Annals of the Academy of Ophthalmology and Otolaryngology 86: 236
Garant P R 1976 Collagen resorption by fibroblasts: A theory of fibroblastic maintenance of the periodontal ligament. Journal of Periodontology 47: 380
Gardner D L 1965 Pathology of the connective tissue diseases. Edward Arnold, London
Gardner D L 1972 The pathology of rheumatoid arthritis. Edward Arnold, London
Gardner D L 1978 Pathology of rheumatoid arthritis. In: Scott J T (ed) Copeman's textbook of the rheumatic diseases, 5th edn. Churchill Livingstone, London, p 273
Gay S, Miller E J 1978 Collagen in the physiology and pathology of connective tissue. Fischer, Stuttgart
Gedde-Dahl T 1971a Epidermolysis bullosa: A clinical, genetic, and epidemiological study, Johns Hopkins University Press, Baltimore
Gedde-Dahl T 1971b Phenotype-genotype correlations in epidermolysis bullosa. Birth Defects 7: 107
Gibbons R J, MacDonald J B 1961 Degradation of collagenous substances by *Bacteroides melanogenicus*. Journal of Bacteriology 81: 614
Golub L M, Stakiw J E, Singer D L 1974 Collagenolytic activity of human gingival crevice fluid. Journal of Dental Research 53: 1501
Golub L M, Siegel K, Ramamurthy N S, Mandel I D 1976 Some characteristics of collagenase activity in gingival crevicular fluid and its relationship to gingival diseases in humans. Journal of Dental Research 55: 1049
Golub L M, Schneir M, Ramamurthy N S 1978 Enhanced collagenase activity in diabetic rat gingiva: in vitro and in vivo evidence. Journal of Dental Research 57: 520
González E, Montfort I, Pérez-Tamayo R 1980 Collagenase in experimental cirrhosis of the liver. In preparation
Grillo H C 1971 The healing of cutaneous wounds. In: Fitzpatrick T B, Arndt K A, Clark W H Jr, Eisen A Z, Van Scott E J, Vaughan J H (eds) Dermatology in general medicine. McGraw-Hill Book Co., New York, p 000
Grillo H C, Gross J 1967 Collagenolytic activity during mammalian wound repair. Developmental Biology 15: 300
Grisolia S 1964 The catalytic environment and its biological implications. Physiological Review 44: 657
Gross J 1958 Studies on the formation of collagen. I. Properties and fractionation of neutral salt extracts of normal guinea pig connective tissue. The Journal of Experimental Medicine 107: 247
Gross J 1970 The animal collagenases. In: Balasz E A (ed) Chemistry and molecular biology of the intercellular matrix, vol 3. Academic Press, New York, p 1623
Gross J 1974 Collagen biology: structure, degradation, and disease. Harvey Lectures, 68: 351
Gross J 1976 Aspects of the animal collagenases. In: Ramachandran G N, Reddi A H (eds) Biochemistry of collagen. Plenum Press, New York, p 1975
Gross J, Lapiére C M 1962 Collagenolytic activity in amphibian tissues: A tissue culture assay. Proceedings of the National Academy of Sciences U.S.A. 58: 1014
Gross J, Harper E, Harris E D Jr, McCroskery P A, Highberger J H, Corbett C, Kang A H 1974 Animal collagenases: Specificity of action, and structure of substrate cleavage site. Biochemical Biophysical Research Communications 61: 605

Hance A J, Crystal R G 1975 The connective tissue of the lung. American Review of Respiratory Disease 112: 657
Halme J, Woessner J F Jr 1975 Effect of progesterone on collagen breakdown and tissue collagenolytic activity in the involuting rat uterus. The Journal of Endocrinology 66: 357
Hammerman D 1969 Cartilage changes in the rheumatoid joint. Clinical Orthopaedics 64: 91
Harris E D Jr 1976 Recent insights into the pathogenesis of the proliferative lesion in rheumatoid arthritis. Arthritis and Rheumatism 19: 68
Harris E D Jr, Farrell M E 1972 Resistance to collagenase: A characteristic of collagen fibrils cross-linked by formaldehyde. Biochimica et Biophysica Acta 278: 133
Harris E D Jr, Krane S M 1972 An endopeptidase from rheumatoid synovial tissue culture. Biochimica et Biophysica Acta 258: 566
Harris E D Jr, Krane S M 1973 Cartilage collagen: Substrate in soluble and fibrillar form for rheumatoid collagenase. Transactions of the Association of American Physicians 86: 82
Harris E D Jr, Krane S M 1974 Collagenases. The New England Journal of Medicine 291: 557, 605, 652
Harris E D Jr, McCroskery P A 1974 The influence of temperature and fibril stability on degradation of cartilage collagen by rheumatoid synovial collagenase. The New England Journal of Medicine 290: 1
Harris E D Jr, Cohen G L, Krane S M 1969 Synovial collagenase: its presence in cultures from joint diseases of diverse etiology. Arthritis and Rheumatism 12: 92
Harris E D Jr, Faulkner C S, Wood S Jr 1972 Collagenase in carcinoma cells. Biochemical and Biophysical Research Communications 48: 1247
Harris E D Jr, Faulkner C S II, Brown F E 1975 Collagenolytic systems in rheumatoid arthritis. Clinical Orthopaedics 110: 303
Harris E D Jr, Cartwright E C 1977 Mammalian collagenases. In: Barrett A J (ed) Proteinases in mammalian cells and tissues. Elsevier/North Holland Biomedical Press, Amsterdam, p 249
Harris E D Jr, Glauert A M, Murley A H G G 1977 Intracellular collagen fibres at the pannus-cartilage junction in rheumatoid arthritis. Arthritis and Rheumatism 20: 657
Harris E D Jr, Vater C A, Mainardi C L, Werb Z 1978 Cellular control of collagen breakdown in rheumatoid arthritis. Agents and Actions 8: 36
Harper E, Gross J 1970 Separation of collagenase and peptidase activity of tadpole tissues in culture. Biochimica et Biophysica Acta 198: 286
Hashimoto K, Yamanishi Y, Dabbous M K 1972a Collagenolytic activities of basal cell epithelioma. The Journal of Investigative Dermatology 58: 251
Hashimoto K, Yamanishi I, Dabbous M K 1972b Electron-microscopic observations of collagenolytic activity of basal cell epithelioma of skin in vivo and in vitro. Cancer Research 32: 2561
Hashimoto I, Anton-Lamprecht I, Gedde-Dahl T, Schnyder U W 1975 Ultrastructural studies in epidermolysis bullosa hereditaria. I. Dominant dystrophic type of Pasini. Archiv fur Dermatologishes Forschung 252: 167
Hashimoto I, Gedde-Dahl T, Schnyder U W, Anton-Lamprecht I 1976a Ultrastructural studies in epidermolysis bullosa hereditaria. II. Dominant dystrophic type of Cockayne and Touraine. Archiv fur Dermatologisches Forschung 255: 285
Hashimoto I, Schnyder U W, Anton-Lamprecht I, Gede-Dahl T, Ward S 1976b Ultrastructural studies in epidermolysis bullosa hereditaria. III. Recessive dystrophic types with dermolytic blistering. Archives of Dermatological Research 256: 137
Hawley P R, Faulk W P, Hunt T K, Dunphy J E 1970 Collagenase activity in the gastrointestinal tract. The British Journal of Surgery 57: 896
Henley K S, Laughrey E G, Appelman H D, Flecker K 1977 Effect of ethanol on collagen formation in dietary cirrhosis in the rat. Gastroenterology 75: 502
Herbert C M, Lindberg K A, Jayson M I V, Bailey A J 1974 Biosynthesis and maturation of skin collagen in scleroderma and effect of D-penicillamine. Lancet 1: 187
Hook R M, Hook C W, Brown S I 1973 Fibroblast collagenase: Partial purification and characterization. Investigative Ophthalmology and Visual Science 12: 771
Hook C W, Brown S I, Iwanij W, Nakanishi I 1971 Characterization and inhibition of corneal collagenase. Investigative Ophthalmology and Visual Science 10: 496
Horwitz A L, Hance A J, Crystal R G 1977 Granulocyte collagenases: Selective digestion of type I relative to type III collagen. Proceedings of the National Academy of Sciences USA 74: 897
Huang C O, Abramson M, Schilling R W, Salome R G 1976 Collagenase activity in tumours of head and neck. Transactions of the American Academy of Ophthalmology and Otolaryngology 82: 138
Huang C C, Wu C-H, Abramson M 1979 Collagenase activity in cultures of rat prostate carcinoma. Biochimica et Biophysica Acta 570: 149
Hutterer F, Rubin E, Singer E J, Popper H 1961 Quantitative relation of cell proliferation and fibrogenesis in the liver. Cancer Research 21: 205
Hutterer F, Rubbin E, Popper H 1964 Mechanism of collagen resorption in reversible hepatic fibrosis. Experimental and Molecular Pathology 3: 215
Itoi M, Gnadiger M C, Slansky H H, Dohlman C H 1969 Prévention d'ulcéres du stroma de la cornée grace a l'utilisation d'un sel de calcium d'EDTA. Archives de Ophthalmologie (Paris) 29: 389
Itoi M, Gnadiger M C, Slansky H H, Freeman M I, Dohlman C H 1969 Collagenase in the cornea. Experimental Eye Research 8: 369
Janoff A 1972 Human granulocyte elastase. The American Journal of Pathology 68: 579
Jeffrey J J, Coffey R J, Eisen A Z 1971 Studies on uterine collagenase in tissue culture. II. Effect of steroid hormones on enzyme production. Biochimica et Biophysica Acta 252: 143
Jensen M S, Bainton D F 1973 Temporal changes in pH within the phagocytic vacuole of the polymorphonuclear neutrophilic leukocyte. The Journal of Cell Biology 56: 379
Johnson-Muller B, Gross J 1978 Regulation of corneal collagenase production: Epithelial-stromal cell interactions. Proceedings of the National Academy of Sciences USA 75: 4417
Keiser H R, Stein H D, Sjoerdsma A 1971 Increased procollagen proline hydroxylase activity in sclerodermatous skin. Archives of Dermatology 104: 57
Kempson G E, Tuke M A, Dingle J T, Barrett A J, Horsfield P H 1976 The effects of proteolytic enzymes on mechanical properties of human articular cartilage. Biochimica et Biophysica Acta 428: 741
Kenyon K R, Berman M, Rose J, Gage J, 1979 Prevention of stromal ulceration in the alkali-burned rabbit cornea by glued-on contact lens. Evidence for the role of polymorphonuclear leukocytes in collagen degradation. Investigative Ophthalmology and Visual Science 18: 570
Kivirikko K I, Risteli L 1976 Biosynthesis of collagen and its alterations in pathological states. Medical Biology 54: 159
Kobayasi T, Asboe-Hansen G 1972 Ultrastructure of generalized scleroderma. Acta Dermatovener (Stockholm) 52: 81

Krane S M 1979 Mechanisms of tissue destruction in rheumatoid arthritis. In: McCarty D J (ed) Arthritis and allied conditions, 9th edn. Lea & Febiger, Philadelphia, p 449

Kuettner K L, Soble L, Croxen R L, Marczynska B, Hiti J, Harper E 1977 Tumour cell collagenase and its inhibition by a cartilage derived protease inhibitor. Science 196: 653

Labrosse K R, Liener I E 1978 Collagenolytic activities in methylcholantrene-induced fibrosarcomas of mice. Molecular and Cellular Biochemistry 19: 181

Lapiére C M, Nusgens B 1976 Collagen pathology at the molecular level. In: Ramachandran G N, Reddi A H (eds) Biochemistry of collagen. Plenum Press, New York, p 377

Laxarus G S 1972 Collagenase and connective tissue metabolism in epidermolysis bullosa. The Journal of Investigative Dermatology 58: 242

Leibovich S J, Weiss J B 1971 Failure of human rheumatoid synovial collagenase to degrade either normal or rheumatoid arthritic polymeric collagen. Biochimica et Biophysica Acta 251: 109

LeRoy E C 1972 Connective tissue synthesis by scleroderma skin fibroblasts in cell culture. The Journal of Experimental Medicine 135: 1351

LeRoy E C 1974 Increased collagen synthesis by scleroderma skin fibroblasts in vitro: A possible defect in the regulation of activation of the scleroderma fibroblasts. Journal of Clinical Investigation 54: 880

Lemp M A 1974 Cornea and sclera' Archives of Ophthalmology 92: 158

Listgarten M A 1965 Electron microscopic observations on the bacterial flora of acute necrotizing ulcerative gingivitis. Journal of Periodontology 36: 328

Luse S, Hutton R 1964 An electronmicroscopic study of the fate of collagen in the post-partum rat uterus. The Anatomical Record 148: 308

Maeyens E, Yamanishi I, Dabbous M K, Hashimoto K 1973 Collagenolytic activity in melanoma. The Journal of Investigative Dermatology 60: 243

McCroskery P A, Richards J F, Harris E D Jr 1975 Purification and characterization of a collagenase extracted from rabbit tumours. The Biochemical Journal 152: 131

McKusick V A 1972 Heritable disorders of connective tissue, 4th edn. C.V. Mosby Co, St. Louis

Marks S C 1974 A discrepancy between measurements of bone resorption in vivo and in vitro in newborn osteopetrotic rats. American Journal of Anatomy 141: 329

Mego J L 1971 The effect of pH on cathepsin activities in mouse liver heterolysosome' The Biochemical Journal 122: 445

Melcher A H 1967 Some histological and histochemical observations on connective tissue of chronically inflamed human gingiva. Journal of Periodontal Research 2: 127

Michaelson J D, Schmidt J D, Dresden M H, Duncan C 1974 Vitamin E treatment of epidermolysis bullosa. Archives of Dermatology 109: 67

Milsom D W, Steven F S, Hunter J A, Thomas H, Jackson D S 1972 Depolymerisation of human and bovine polymeric collagen fibrils. Connective Tissue Research 1: 251

Miller E J, Finch J E, Chung E, Butler W T 1976 Specific cleavage of native type III collagen with trypsin. Similarity of the cleavage products to collagenase cleavage site. Archives of Biochemistry and Biophysics 173: 631

Montfort I, Pérez-Tamayo R 1975 The distribution of collagenase in the rat uterus during postpartum involution: An immunohistochemical study. Connective Tissue Research 3: 245

Montfort I, Pérez-Tamayo R 1978 Collagenase in experimental carbon tetrachloride cirrhosis of the liver. The American Journal of Pathology 92: 411

Morrison R I G, Barrett A J, Dingle J T, Prior D 1973 Cathepsin B1 and D: Action on human cartilage proteoglycan. Biochimica et Biophysica Acta 302: 411

Nagai Y 1973 Vertebrate collagenase: Further characterization and the significance of its latent form in vivo. Molecular and Cellular Biochemistry 1: 137

Nagai Y, Hori H 1972 Vertebrate collagenase: direct extraction from animal skin and human synovial membrane. Journal of Biochemistry 72: 1147

Newsome D A, Gross J 1977 Prevention by medroxyprogesterone of perforation of the alkali-burned rabbit cornea: Inhibition of collagenolytic activity. Investigative Ophthalmology and Visual Science 16: 21

Newsome D A, Gross J 1979 Regulation of corneal collagenase production: stimulation of serially passaged stromal cells by blood mononuclear cells. Cell 16: 895

Nordwig A 1971 Collagenolytic enzymes. Advances in Enzymology 34: 155

Oakes B W 1974 Intracellular collagen — phagocytosis or intracellular aggregation? In: Electron Microscopy 1974 (Eighth International Congress of Electron Microscopy), vol 2. Australian Academy of Sciences, Canberra, p 368

Okazaki I, Maruyama K 1974 Collagenase activity in experimental hepatic fibrosis. Nature 252: 49

Padykula H A 1976 Cellular mechanism involved in cyclic stromal renewal of the uterus. III. Cells of the immune response. The Anatomical Record 184: 49

Padykula H A, Campbell A G 1976 Cellular mechanisms involved in cyclic stromal renewal of the uterus. II. The albino rat. The Anatomical Record 184: 27

Page R C, Schroeder H E 1973 Biochemical aspects of the connective tissue alerations in inflammatory gingival and periodontal disease. The International Dental Journal 23: 455

Page R C, Schroeder H E 1976 Pathogenesis of inflammatory periodontal disease. Laboratory Investigation 33: 235

Page Thomas D P 1969 Lysosomal enzymes in experimental and rheumatoid arthritis. In: Dingle J T, Fell H B (eds) Lysosomes in biology and pathology North-Holland, Amsterdam, p 87

Parakkal P F 1969 Involvement of macrophages in collagen resorption. The Journal of Cell Biology 41: 345

Pardo A, Pérez-Tamayo R 1975 The presence of collagenase in collagen preparations' Biochimica et Biophysica Acta 389: 121

Pardo A, Soto H, Montfort I and Pérez-Tamayo R 1980 Collagen-bound collagenase. Connective Tissue Research 7: 253-261

Pearson R W 1962 Studies on the pathogenesis of epidermolysis bullosa. The Journal of Investigative Dermatology 49: 551

Pearson R W 1971 The mechanobullous diseases. In: Fitzpatrick T B, Arndt K A, Clark W H Jr, Eisen A Z, Van Scott E J, Vaughan J M (eds) Dermatology in general medicine, McGraw-Hill, New York, p 000

Pearson R W, Potter B, Strauss F 1974 Epidermolysis bullosa hereditaria letalis. Archives of Dermatology 109: 349

Pérez-Tamayo R 1965 Some aspects of connective tissue of the liver. In: Popper H, Schaffner F (eds) Progress in liver disease, vol 2. Grune & Stratton, New York, p 183

Pérez-Tamayo R 1970 Collagen resorption in carrageenin granuloma. II. Ultrastructure of collagen resorption. Laboratory Investigation 22: 142

Pérez-Tamayo R 1972 The occurrence and significance of SLS crystallites in vivo. Connective Tissue Research 1: 55

Pérez-Tamayo R 1973 Collagen degradation and resorption: physiology and pathology. In: Pérez-Tamayo R, Rojkind M (eds) Molecular pathology of connective tissues. Marcel Dekker, New York, p 229

Pérez-Tamayo R 1974a Patología molecular de la colágena. In: Mora J, Estrada-O E, Martuscelli J (eds) Los perfiles de la bioquímica en México. UNAM, México, p 495

Pérez-Tamayo R 1974b Tres variaciones sobre la muerte. Prensa Médica Mexicana México, p 79

Pérez-Tamayo R 1979a Pathology of collagen degradation. The American Journal of Pathology 92: 509

Pérez-Tamayo R 1979b The degradation of collagen. Bulletin on the Rheumatic Diseases 30: 1012

Pérez-Tamayo R 1979c Cirrhosis of the liver: a reversible disease? In: Sommers S C, Rosen P P (eds) Pathology Annual 1979, part 2. Appleton-Century-Crofts, New York, p 183

Pérez-Tamayo R, Montfort I 1964 Homeostasis of connective tissue. In: Thomas L, Uhr J W, Grant L (eds) Injury, inflammation and immunity. Williams & Wilkins, Baltimore, p 1

Pérez-Tamayo R, Montfort I 1980 The susceptibility of collagen to homologous collagenase in experimental and human cirrhosis of the liver (Submitted for publication)

Pérez-Tamayo R, Montfort I, Pardo A 1980 What controls collagen degradation in vivo? Medical Hypothesis 6: 711

Perlish J S, Bashey R I, Stephens R E, Fleischmajer R 1976 Connective tissue synthesis by cultured scleroderma fibroblasts. I. In vitro collagen synthesis by normal and scleroderma fibroblasts. Arthritis and Rheumatism 18: 891

Pettigrew D W, Ho G H, Sodek J, Brunette D M, Wang H M 1978 Effect of oxygen tension and indomethacin on production of collagenase and neutral proteinase enzymes and their latent forms by porcine gingival explants in culture. Archives of Oral Biology 23: 767

Pirie A, Werb Z, Burleigh M C 1975 Collagenase and other proteinases in the cornea of the retinol-deficient rat. British Journal of Nutrition 34: 297

Poole A R 1973 Tumour lysosomal enzymes and invasive growth. In: Dingle J T (ed) Lysosomes in biology and pathology, vol 3. North-Holland, Amsterdam, p 303

Popper H, Undenfriend S 1970 Hepatic fibrosis: correlation of biochemical morphologic investigations' The American Journal of Medicine 49: 707

Popper H, Becker K 1975 Collagen metabolism in the liver. Stratton Intercontinental Medical Book Corporation, New York

Popper H 1977 Pathologic aspects of cirrhosis. The American Journal of Pathology 87: 227

Popper H, Piez K A (eds) 1978 Collagen metabolism in the liver. Digestive Diseases 23: 641

Prockop D J, Kivirikko K I, Tuderman L, Guzman N A 1979 The biosynthesis of collagen and its disorders. The New England Journal of Medicine 301: 13, 77

Ramamurthy N S, Zebrowski E J, Golub L M 1973 Collagenolytic activity of gingivae from albxan-diabetic rat. Diabetes 22: 272

Ramamurthy N S, Zebrowski E J, Golub L M 1974 Insulin reversal of alloxan-diabetes induced changes in gingival collagen metabolism of the rat. Journal of Periodontal Research 9: 199

Rentería V G, Ferrans V J 1976 Intracellular collagen fibrils in cardiac valves of patients with the Hurler syndrome. Laboratory Investigation 34: 263

Riley W B Jr, Peacock E E Jr 1967 Identification, distribution, and significance of a collagenolytic enzyme in human tissues. Proceedings of the Society for Experimental Biology and Medicine 124: 207

Robertson D M, Williams D C 1969 In vitro evidence of neutral collagenase activity in an invasive mammalian tumour. Nature 221: 259

Robertson P B, Cobb C M, Taylor R E, Fullmer H M 1974 Activation of latent collagenase by microbial plaque. Journal of Periodontal Research 9: 81

Robertson P B, Simpson J W, Levy B M 1975 Lymphocyte mediated release of latent collagenase activity. Journal of Dental Research 54: 123

Rojkind M, Kershenobich D 1976 Hepatic fibrosis. In: Popper H, Schaffner F (eds) Progress in liver disease, vol 5. Grune & Straton, New York, p 294

Rojkind M, Takahashi S, Giambrone M-A 1978 Collagenase and reversible hepatic fibrosis in the rat. Gastroenterology 75: 984

Rojkind M, Dunn M A 1979 Hepatic fibrosis. Gastroenterology 76: 849

Rose G C, Robertson P B 1977 Collagenolysis by human gingival fibroblast cell lines. Journal of Dental Research 56: 416

Roughley P J, Barrett A J 1977 The degradation of cartilage proteoglycans by tissue proteinases. The Biochemical Journal 167: 629

Rowsey J J, Nisbet R M, Swedo J L, Katona L 1976 Corneal collagenolytic activity in rabbit polymorphonuclear leukocytes. Journal of Ultrastructure Research 57: 10

Rubin E, Hutterer F, Popper H 1963 Cell proliferation and fiber formation in chronic carbon tetrachoride intoxication. A morphologic and chemical study. The American Journal of Pathology 42: 715

Rubin E, Hutterer F, Popper H 1965 Reversibility of cirrhosis related to collagen and interstitial cel turnover. Gastroenterology 48: 504

Russell A L 1967 Epidemiology of periodontal disease. International Dental Journal 17: 282

Ryan J N, Woessner J F Jr 1971 Mammalian collagenase: Direct demonstration in homogenates of involuting rat uterus. Biochemical and Biophysical Research Communications 44: 144

Ryan G B, Cliff W J, Gabbiani G, Irlé C, Statkov P R, Majno G 1973 Myofibroblasts in an avascular fibrous tissue. Laboratory Investigation 29: 197

Rysky S, Cattaneo V, Montanari M C 1969 Determination quantitative des hexoseamines et de l'hydroxyproline dans les inflammations gingivales chroniques. Bulletin de le Group Internationale de Recherche Scientifique de la Stomatologie 12: 359

Sakai T, Gross J 1967 Some properties of the products of reaction of tadpole collagenase with collagen. Biochemistry 6: 518

Sakamoto S, Sakamoto M, Goldhaber P, Glimcher M J 1973 Isolation of tissue collagenase from homogenates of embryonic chick bones. Biochemical and Biophysical Research Communications 53: 1102

Sakamoto S, Sakamoto M, Goldhaber P, Glimcher M J 1975 Studies on the interaction between heparin and mouse bone collagenase. Biochimica et Biophysica Acta 385: 41

Sakamoto M, Sakamoto S, Goldhaber P, Glimcher M J 1978 Immunocytochemical studies of collagenase: Localization in normal mouse tissue, with special reference to cartilage and bone. Calcified Tissue Research Suppl: 441

Sauk J J, Witkop C J Jr 1978 Expression of melanoma neutral proteinase and collagenase potential by endocytosis. Biochemical and Biophysical Research Communications 83: 144

Schimke R T 1975 On the properties and mechanisms of protein turnover. In: Schimke R T, Katunuma N (eds) Intracellular protein turnover. Academic Press, New York, p 173

Schneit A W, Fullmer H M 1970 Specific collagenase from germ-free rat gingivae. Proceedings of the Society for Experimental Biology and Medicine 135: 436

Schroeder H E, Munzel-Pedrazzoli S, Page R C 1973 Correlated morphometric and biochemical analysis of gingival tissues in early chronic gingivitis in man. Archives of Oral Biology 18: 899

Schultz-Haudt S D 1965 Connective tissue and periodontal disease. International Review of Connective Tissue Research 3: 77

Schumacher H R, Kitridou R C 1972 Synovitis of recent onset. A clinicopathologic study during the first month of the disease. Arthritis and Rheumatism 15: 465

Seifert K 1971 Elektronemikroskopische Untersuchungen am juvenilen Nasenrachenfibrom. Archiv Für Klinische und Experimentelle Ohren, Nasen in Kehlkopfheilkund 198: 215

Seifter S, Harper E 1970 Collagenases. Methods in Enzymology 19: 613

Sellers A, Reynolds J J, Meikle M C 1978 Neutral metalloproteinases of rabbit bone. Separation in latent forms of distinct enzymes that when activated degrade collagen, gelatin and proteoglycans. The Biochemical Journal 171: 493

Shoshan S, Gross J 1974 Biosynthesis and metabolism of collagen and its role in tissue repair processes. Israel Journal of Medical Sciences 10: 537

Simpson W L 1950 Mucolytic enzymes and invasion by carcinomas. Annals of the New York Academy of Sciences 52: 1125

Simpson J W, Taylor A C 1974 Regulation of gingival collagenases: Possible role for a mast cell factor. Proceedings of the Society for Experimental Biology and Medicine 145: 42

Slansky H H, Freeman M I, Itoi M 1968 Collagenolytic activitiy in bovine corneal epithelium. Archives of Ophthalmology 80: 496

Slansky H H, Berman M B, Dohlman C M, Rose J 1970 Cysteine and acetylcysteine in the prevention of corneal ulcerations. Annals of Ophthalmology 2: 488

Slansky H H, Dohlman C H, Berman M B 1971 Prevention of corneal ulcers. Transactions of the American Academy of Ophthalmology and Otolaryngology 75: 1208

Socransky S S 1970 Relationship of bacteria to the etiology of periodontal disease. Journal of Dental Research 49: 203

Sokolow L 1979 Pathology of rheumatoid arthritis and allied disorders. In: McCarty D J (ed) Arthritis and allied conditions, 9th edn. Lea & Febiger, Philadelphia, p 429

Sopata I, Dancewicz A M 1974 Presence of a gelatin-specific proteinase and its latent form in human leucocytes. Biochimica et Biophysica Acta 370: 510

Spencer H 1968 Chronic interstitial pneumonia. In: Liebow A A, Smith D E (eds) The Lung. The Williams and Wilkins Company, Baltimore, p 134

Strauch L 1975 Possible mechanisms of collagen breakdown in higher animals. In: Peeters H (ed) Proceedings of the Twenty-Second Colloquium on Protides of the Biological Fluids. Pergamon Press, Oxford, p 373.

Sugar A, Waltman S R 1973 Corneal toxicity of collagenase inhibitors. Investigative Ophthalmology and Visual Science 12: 779

Svoboda E L A, Brunette D M, Melcher A H 1979 In vitro phagocytosis of exogenous collagen by fibroblasts from the periodontal ligament: an electron microscopic study. Journal of Anatomy 128: 301

Sylven B E G V 1962 The host-tumour interzone and tumour invasion. In: Brennan M J, Simpson W L (eds) Biological interactions in normal and neoplastic growth. Little, Brown & Co, Boston, p 635

Starkey P M, Barret A J, Burleigh M C 1977 The degradation of articular collagen by neutrophil proteinases. Biochimica et Biophysica Acta 483: 386

Steven F S 1970 Polymeric collagen fibrils: An example of substrate mediated steric obstruction of enzymic digestion. Biochimica et Biophysica Acta 452: 151

Steven F S, Itzhaki S 1977 Evidence for a latent form of collagenase extracted from rabbit tumour cells. Biochimica et Biophysica Acta 496: 241

Steven F S, Torre-Blanco A, Hunter J A A 1975 A neutral protease in rheumatoid synovial fluid capable of attacking the telopeptide regions of polymeric collagen fibrils. Biochimica et Biophysica Acta 405: 188

Takahashi S, Dunn M A, Seifter S 1977 Collagenolytic and elastolytic activities in liver from mice with schistosomiasis. Federation Proceedings 36: 677

Tane N, Hashimoto K, Kanzaki T, Ohyama H 1978 Collagenolytic activities of cultured human malignant melanoma cells. Journal of Biochemistry 84: 1171

Tansey T R, Padykula H A 1978 Cellular responses to experimental inhibition of collagen degradation in the postpartum rat uterus. The Anatomical Record 191: 287

Taylor A C, Levy B M, Simpson J W 1970 Collagenolytic activity of sarcoma tissues in culture. Nature 228: 366

Ten Cate A R, Syrbu S 1974 A relationship between alkaline phosphatase activity and the phagocytosis and degradation of collagen by the fibroblast. Journal of Anatomy 117: 351

Ten Cate A R, Deporter D A 1975 The degradative role of the fibroblasts in the remodeling and turnover of collagen in soft connective tissue. The Anatomical Record 182: 1

Uitto J 1971 Collagen biosynthesis in human skin. A review with emphasis on scleroderma. Annals of Clinical Research 3: 250

Uitto J, Prockop D J 1975 Molecular defects in collagen and the definition of 'collagen disease'. In Good R A, Day S B, Yunis J J (eds) Molecular Pathology. Charles C Thomas, Springfield, p 670

Uitto J, Lichtenstein J R 1976 Defects in the biochemistry of collagen in diseases of connective tissue. The Journal of Investigative Dermatology 66: 59

Uitto J, Bauer E A, Eisen A Z 1979 Scleroderma. Increased biosynthesis of triple-helical type I and type III procollagens associated with unaltered expression of collagenase by skin fibroblasts in culture. The Journal of Clinical Investigation 64: 921

Uitto J, Halme J, Hannuksela M, Peltockallio P, Kivirikko K I 1969 Protocollagen proline hydroxylase activity in the skin of normal and human subjects and of patients with scleroderma. Scandinavian Journal of Clinical and Laboratory Investigation 23: 241

Uitto V-J, Turto H, Saxén L 1978 Extraction of collagenase from human gingiva. Journal of Periodontal Research 13: 207

Usuku G, Gross J 1965 Morphologic studies of connective tissue resorption in the tail fin of metamorphosing bullfrog tadpole. Developmental Biology 11: 352

Usuku G 1968 Studies on the collagen formation and resorption. Bulletin of the Institute of Constitutional Medicine, Kunamoto University 18: Supplement, 1

Vaes G, Eeckhout Y, Lenaers-Claeys G, Francois Gillet Ch, Druetz J-E 1978 The simultaneous release by bone explants in culture and the parallel activation of procollagenase and of a latent neutral proteinase that degrades cartilage proteoglycans and denatured collagen. The Biochemical Journal 172: 261

Vater C A, Mainardi C L, Harris E D Jr 1978 Binding of latent rheumatoid synovial collagenase to collagen fibrils. Biochimica et Biophysica Acta 539: 238

Werb Z, Reynolds J J 1974 Stimulation by endocytosis of the secretion of collagenase and neutral proteinase from rabbit synovial fibroblasts. The Journal of Experimental Medicine 140: 1482

Williams G 1957 A histological study of the connective tissue reaction to carrageenin. Journal of Pathology and Bacteriology 73: 557

Willis R A 1953 Pathology of Tumours, 2nd edn. Butterworth, London, p 000

Winkelmann R K 1976 Pathogenesis and staging of scleroderma. Acta Dermato-Venereologica 56: 83

Wirl G 1975 Extraction of collagenase from the 6000 × g sediment of uterine and skin tissues of mice. A comparative study. Hoppe-Seyler's Zeitschrift fur Physiologische Chemie 356: 1289

Wirl G 1977a Extractable collagenase and carcinogenesis of the mouse skin. Connective Tissue Research 5: 171

Wirl G 1977b Kollagenaseaktivitat in einem tierischen und einem menschlichen Karzinom. Wiener Klinische Wochenschrift 89: 766

Wirl G, Frick J 1979 Collagenase — A marker enzyme in human bladder cancer? Urological Research 7: 103

Wize J, Sopata I, Wottecka E, Ksiezny S, Dancewicz A M 1975 Isolation, purification and properties of a factor from synovial fluid activating latent forms of collagenolytic enzymes' Acta Biochimica Polonnica 22: 239

Vater C A, Harris E D Jr, Siegel R C 1979 Native cross-links in collagen fibrils induce resistance to human synovial collagenase. The Biochemical Journal 181: 639

Walker D G 1966 Elevated bone collagenolytic activity and hyperplasia of parafollicular light cells of the thyroid gland in parathormone-treated grey-lethal mice' Zeitschrift fur Zellforschung und Mikroskopische Anatomie 72: 100

Walker D G 1973 Osteopetrosis cured by temporary parabiosis. Science 180: 875

Walker D G, Lapiére C M, Gross J 1964 A collagenolytic factor in rat bone promoted by parathyroid extract. Biochemical and Biophysical Research Communications 15: 397

Weeks J G, Halme J, Woessner J F Jr 1976 Extraction of collagenase from the involuting rat uterus. Biochimica et Biophysica Acta 445: 205

Weiss J B 1976 Enzymic degradation of collagen. International Review of Connective Tissue Research 7: 101

Weissman G 1972 Lysosomal mechanisms of tissue injury in arthritis. The New England Journal of Medicine 286: 141

Welsh R A 1966 Intracytoplasmic collagen formations in desmoid fibromatosis. The American Journal of Pathology 49: 515

Welsh R A, Meyer A T 1967 Intracellular collagen fibres in human mesenchymal tumours and inflammatory states. Archives of Pathology 84: 354

Woessner J F Jr 1968 Biological mechanisms of collagen degradation. In: Gould B S (ed) Treatise on Collagen, vol 2, part B. Academic Press, New York, p 253

Woessner F Jr 1979 Total, latent and active collagenase during the course of post-partum involution of the rat uterus. The Biochemical Journal 180: 95

Woolley D E, Glanville R W, Crossley M J, Evanson J M 1975a Purification of rheumatoid synovial collagenase and its action on soluble and insoluble collagen. European Journal of Biochemistry 54: 611

Woolley D E, Lindberg K A, Glanville R W, Evanson J M 1975b Action on rheumatoid synovial collagenase on cartilage collagen. Different susceptibilities of cartilage and tendon collagen to collagenase attack 50: 437

Woolley D E, Evanson J M 1977 Effect of cartilage proteoglycans on human collagenase activity. Biochimica et Biophysica Acta 497: 144

Woolley D E, Crossley M J, Evanson J M 1977 Collagenase at sites of cartilage erosion in the rheumatoid joint. Arthritis and Rheumatism 20: 1231

Woolley D E, Evanson J M 1980 Collagenase in normal and pathological connective tissues. In press

Yamanishi Y, Dabbous M K, Hashimoto K 1972 Effect of collagenolytic activity in basal cell epithelioma of skin on reconstituted collagen and physical properties and kinetics of crude enzyme. Cancer Research 32: 2551

Yamanishi I, Maeyens E, Dabbous M K, Ohyama H, Hashimoto K 1973 Collagenolytic activity in malignant melanoma: physicochemical studies. Cancer Research 33: 2507

9

Turnover and cross-linking of collagen

S. P. ROBINS

Collagen turnover has received comparatively little attention over the past three decades. Following the pioneer studies of Neuberger and his colleagues (Neuberger et al, 1951; Neuberger & Slack, 1953), the concept was established that the collagen matrix is inert and, once laid down, remains almost throughout life. In recent years, however, there has been a rapid expansion in our knowledge of collagen metabolism, particularly with respect to its biosynthesis, the nature of the stabilizing cross-links and the existence of different isomorphic forms of collagen. In addition, the limitations of some of the techniques used have now become apparent. The purpose of this chapter is primarily to discuss the relevance of these recent developments to our appreciation of collagen turnover.

As the balance between collagen synthesis and degradation represents collagen accretion (or resorption), the rates of turnover can be determined by measuring two of these three parameters. Although the mechanism of collagen degradation is discussed elsewhere in this volume (see Chapter 7), the rate of this process is highly dependent on the presence of intermolecular cross-links, the nature of which will be discussed in some detail. Measurements of both collagen synthesis and degradation rates have generally been performed for individual tissues by using isotopic labelling techniques. As an alternative approach, estimation of whole-body turnover of collagen has been attempted by measuring the urinary excretion of collagen metabolites.

URINARY EXCRETION OF COLLAGEN METABOLITES

Hydroxyproline excretion

The measurement of urinary 4-hydroxyproline as an index of total body collagen degradation has been widely used (for review see Kivirikko, 1970). The method is convenient as a number of rapid automated techniques have been developed that are suitable for clinical application (e.g. Blumenkrantz & Asboe-Hansen, 1974). There are, however, a number of problems in interpreting the results of urinary hydroxyproline measurements that result mainly from the high proportion of this imino acid that is metabolized and from the presence of hydroxyproline in the extension peptides of procollagen and in other proteins. These aspects are summarized in Figure 9.1 and will be discussed separately in more detail.

Proportion of hydroxyproline metabolized

There is efficient renal tubular reabsorbtion of free hydroxyproline which is oxidised in the liver (Adams, 1970) and the carbon skeleton is ultimately lost as expired CO_2. Consequently, most of the urinary output of this imino acid is in the form of small peptides that are not reabsorbed. These peptides, however, represent a relatively small proportion of the total hydroxyproline released from protein catabolism. Estimates of the proportion of released hydroxyproline that is metabolized in rats have varied from 75 per cent determined by ^{14}C-gelatin injections (Weiss & Klein, 1969) to over 90 per cent inferred from labelling studies with ^{14}C-proline (Prockop, 1964). In a study of patients deficient in the enzyme that oxidises free hydroxyproline, Efron et al (1965) found that 80 per cent of the urinary hydroxyproline was free and 20 per cent was in peptide form. The proportion of hydroxyproline that is metabolized may not be consistent as, under some conditions involving increased collagen degradation such as uterine involution, no increase in urinary hydroxyproline is observed (Woessner. 1962). These possible inconsistencies render the use of urinary excretion of hydroxyproline as a quantitative index of collagen degradation somewhat limited. In addition, even if the commonly assumed figure of 90 per cent metabolism of hydroxyproline is universally valid, the small proportion that is excreted makes the method rather insensitive, as relatively large differences in collagen breakdown are necessary to produce a measureable effect on the amounts of urinary hydroxyproline.

Hydroxyproline in extension peptides of procollagen

Collagen is synthesized as a precursor molecule containing at each end extension peptides that are removed by extracellular proteases (see Chapter 6). The N-terminal extension peptides of the pro-α1 chains of type I

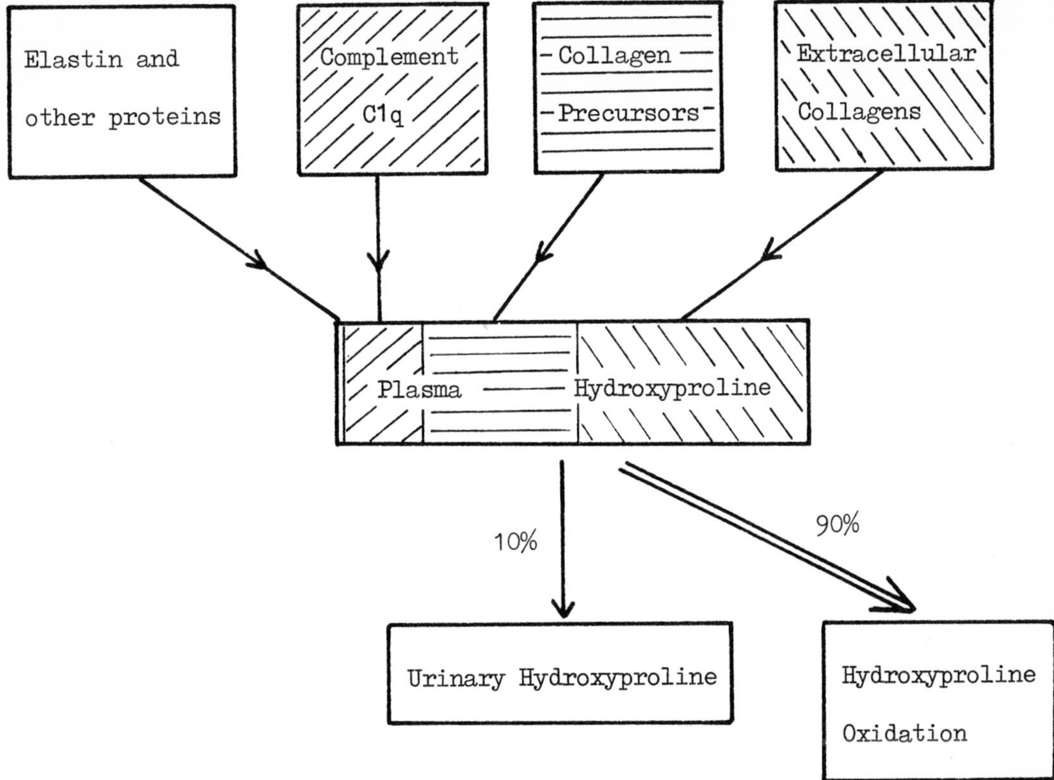

Fig. 9.1 A simplified schematic representation of the sources of plasma hydroxyproline indicating approximate quantitative contributions to the flow of this imino acid through the blood: these proportions may alter under particular circumstances. As discussed in the text, the precursor fraction includes an estimate of hydroxyproline derived from both the release of procollagen extension peptides and intracellular degradation of collagen precursors.

procollagen have been shown to contain short helical segments of about 80 residues of which seven are hydroxyproline (Hörlein et al, 1978). Thus, of the total collagen hydroxyproline, about 5 per cent is present in the extension peptides and is released during normal biosynthesis and fibre formation. This hydroxyproline could, therefore, make a considerable contribution to urinary excretion of this imino acid, especially in situations where rates of collagen synthesis are high, such as during rapid growth. Indeed, hydroxyproline from degraded extension peptides may partly explain the high urinary excretion in children (Smiley & Ziff, 1964; Uitto et al, 1968) that has often been assumed to be the result of tissue remodelling. In support of this interpretation, the excretion of hydroxyproline is higher in children than in adults relative to the excretion of hydroxylysine and its derivatives (Krane et al, 1977); the latter components are not present in the extension peptides.

More recently, an additional problem has arisen with the proposal that a large proportion (20–40 per cent) of procollagen is degraded intracellularly before secretion (Steinberg, 1978; Bienkowski et al, 1978a, b). This aspect will be discussed in more detail later in this Chapter (p. 170).

Hydroxyproline in other proteins

Until comparatively recently, the presence of hydroxyproline was thought to be restricted to collagen and, to a lesser extent, elastin. There are now known to be a number of proteins whose function apparently requires the rigid, rod-like structure afforded by a collagen-like triple helix. Of these, the sub-unit of the first component of complement, C1q, is the best characterized (see Chapter 2). The collagen-like sequences contain both hydroxyproline and hydroxylysine residues. Even though C1q constitutes only 0.3 per cent of total plasma protein, turnover studies have indicated that about two-thirds of the total plasma pool of this protein is catabolized per day (Kohler & Müller-Eberhard, 1972). From these data and the amino acid composition of C1q (Reid et al, 1972), it can be calculated that, for normal individuals, the hydroxyproline released from complement protein could account for about half of the total urinary hydroxyproline excretion (Krane et al, 1977). However, assuming that the proportion of released hydroxyproline that is oxidised is similar to the value for the collagen-derived imino acid, it is probable that the normal contribution of C1q to urinary hydroxyproline excretion is about 10–15 per cent, as proposed by Nimni (1974).

Approximately one per cent of the amino acids in elastin are hydroxyproline but, owing to the slow turnover of this protein, this source is unlikely to make a significant contribution to urinary output. There is little information about the turnover of acetylcholinesterase, another protein containing collagen-like sequences (Anglister et al, 1976).

3-Hydroxyproline excretion

Measurements of urinary 3-hydroxyproline have been made (Adams et al, 1978) with the primary aim of assessing the turnover of basement membrane collagens, in which this imino acid is prevalent. Most of the urinary excretion of 3-hydroxyproline can, however, be accounted for by the single residue present in the $\alpha1$ chain of type I collagen (Szymanowicz et al, 1979).

Excretion of hydroxylysine glycosides

Galactosyl-(Hyl-gal) and glucosyl-galactosyl-hydroxylysine (Hyl-gal-glc) are formed during collagen biosynthesis by enzymatic addition of the hexoses to the hydroxyl group of hydroxylysine residues (see Chapter 6). These derivatives were identified in normal human urine (Segrest & Cunningham, 1970; Kakimoto & Akazawa, 1970) and were proposed as a better quantitative index of collagen degradation as they appeared to be less extensively metabolized than hydroxyproline (Segrest & Cunningham, 1970). Direct evidence that hydroxyproline glycosides are metabolically inert was obtained by intravenous injection of ^{3}H-labelled derivatives into rabbits: for both the mono- and di-saccharide compounds, recovery in urine was virtually complete within 48 hours after the injections (Robins, 1980).

The analysis of hydroxylysine glycosides is less amenable to automation than that for hydroxyproline and, although procedures involving the use of a single chromatographic column have been described for direct analysis of protein hydrolysates (Odell et al, 1974; Peczon et al, 1979) and urine samples (Askenasi, 1973), a preliminary fractionation step is often deemed necessary (Isemura et al, 1976; Krane et al, 1977). For clinical studies, these difficulties of analysis are offset to some extent by the fact that gelatin-free diets are unnecessary as the contribution of dietary hydroxylysine glycosides to the urine is minimal (Segrest & Cunningham, 1970; Askenasi, 1975). Dietary control is essential for measuring total hydroxyproline excretion (Kivirikko, 1970; Gasser et al, 1979).

Measurement of the ratio, Hyl-gal-glc/Hyl-gal, in urine has been proposed as a means of differentiating between the rates of collagen degradation in different tissues. This emanated from the observation that the Hyl-gal-glc/Hyl-gal ratio was consistent for a particular tissue but that there were marked differences between these tissues. The major differences were between skin, in which the Hyl-gal-glc/Hyl-gal ratio is about 2, and bone in which this ratio is less than 0.5 (Segrest & Cunningham, 1970; Pinnell et al, 1971; Royce & Barnes, 1977). Reported variations with age in the relative proportions of mono- and disaccharide units in skin collagen (Murai et al, 1975) have not been confirmed (Isemura et al, 1976; Royce & Barnes, 1977). The normal Hyl-gal-glc/Hyl-gal ratio in urine is about 1.5 (Askenasi, 1973), a fact that led to the suggestion that degradation of skin collagen is a major contributor to urinary hydroxylysine glycosides. Although a relatively large proportion of disaccharide units is present in basement membrane collagens (see Chapter 17), their turnover rate is probably slow (Walker, 1972; Price & Spiro, 1977; Cohen & Surma, 1980). As mentioned previously, the complement component, C1q, contains hydroxylysine residues of which about 90 per cent are glycosylated, almost exclusively by disaccharide units (Calcott & Müller-Eberhard, 1972; Campbell et al, 1979; Shinkai et al, 1979). From the data for C1q turnover determined by measuring the disappearance of injected ^{125}I-labelled protein (Kohler & Müller-Eberhard, 1972), it can be calculated that catabolism of this complement protein could account for almost all of the urinary excretion of Hyl-gal-glc. Thus, even though the radioiodine labelling method for measuring protein turnover may lead to a slight overestimate of catabolism (Opresko et al, 1980), it is evident that turnover of C1q has a dramatic effect on hydroxylysine glycoside excretion (Krane et al, 1977). Indeed, it is likely that under normal conditions very little urinary Hyl-gal-glc is derived from skin collagen breakdown. In agreement with this interpretation is the fact that hydroxylysine glycoside excretion was normal in patients with lysyl hydroxylase deficiency (Ehlers-Danlos, type VI), a disease in which hydroxylysine is virtually absent from skin collagen (Pinnell et al, 1972) but where the hydroxylysine content of C1q is normal (Hanauske-Abel & Röhm, 1980). Increased turnover of complement protein should also be considered in conditions where elevated urinary Hyl-gal-glc excretion was attributed to skin collagen breakdown, such as acute granuloma (Askenasi et al, 1976b) and adjuvant-induced arthritis (Orloff et al, 1979).

As C1q contains very little monosaccharide derivative (Campbell et al, 1979; Shinkai et al, 1979), the use of Hyl-gal as a measure predominantly of bone collagen turnover appears to be valid. Certainly, in Paget's disease of bone, there is a decrease in the urinary Hyl-gal-glc/Hyl-gal ratio which is restored to normal values after treatment of the disease with calcitonin (Askenasi, 1974; Krane et al, 1977; Kelleher, 1979). Recently, however, an additional complication has been introduced by the discovery of a specific α-glucosidase in rat kidney cortex that converts Hyl-gal-glc to Hyl-gal (Sternberg & Spiro, 1979). Clearly, if this enzyme is widespread in other tissues, it could have a considerable effect on the composition of urinary hydroxylysine glycosides.

As discussed for hydroxyproline excretion, the amounts

of hydroxylysine glycosides in urine would also be greatly affected if a large proportion of collagen were degraded intracellularly, since glycosylation is generally believed to occur in the same cellular compartment as hydroxylation (Harwood et al, 1975; Oikarinen et al, 1977).

It must be concluded, therefore, that urinary excretion of hydroxylysine glycosides offers few real advantages over hydroxyproline as a quantitative index of collagen degradation. Nevertheless, provided the possible ambiguities are borne in mind, both hydroxyproline and hydroxylysine derivatives can provide useful clinical information, particularly in the classification and management of certain bone disorders (Gielen et al, 1976; Kelleher, 1979).

COLLAGEN CROSS-LINKING

Intermolecular cross-linking plays a major role in providing the mechanical strength of fibrous collagens and in determining their physical and chemical stability. The initial step in the formation of collagen cross-links is conversion of specific lysine or hydroxylysine residues situated at each end of the molecule by a copper-dependent enzyme, lysyl oxidase (for review see Siegel, 1979). This enzymatic step is believed to occur at the surface of collagen fibrils during their assembly and gives rise to the aldehydes, allysine and hydroxyallysine:

$$\begin{array}{lcl} | & & | \\ \mathrm{CO} & & \mathrm{CO} \\ | & & | \\ \mathrm{CH{-}CH_2{-}CH_2{-}CH_2{-}CH_2{-}NH_2} & \xrightarrow[\text{oxidase}]{\text{lysyl}} & \mathrm{CH{-}CH_2{-}CH_2{-}CH_2{-}CHO} \\ | & & | \\ \mathrm{NH} & & \mathrm{NH} \\ | & & | \\ \text{Lysine} & & \text{Allysine} \end{array}$$

$$\begin{array}{lcl} | & & | \\ \mathrm{CO} \qquad\quad \mathrm{OH} & & \mathrm{CO} \qquad\quad \mathrm{OH} \\ | \qquad\qquad\quad | & & | \qquad\qquad\quad | \\ \mathrm{CH{-}CH_2{-}CH_2{-}CH{-}CH_2{-}NH} & \xrightarrow[\text{oxidase}]{\text{lysyl}} & \mathrm{CH{-}CH_2{-}CH_2{-}CH{-}CHO} \\ | & & | \\ \mathrm{NH} & & \mathrm{NH} \\ | & & | \\ \text{Hydroxylysine} & & \text{Hydroxyallysine} \end{array}$$

These groups spontaneously condense with reactive amino groups on adjacent molecules. Generally, these condensations result in the formation of Schiff base compounds containing labile aldimine links (–CH=N–) that require stabilization by reduction with borohydride to facilitate isolation of the compounds from collagen (Bailey, 1968; Tanzer, 1968). The large number of compounds that have been isolated from borohydride-reduced collagen (Fig. 9.2) has been extensively reviewed (Tanzer, 1973; Bailey et al, 1974; Gallop & Paz, 1975).

The first aldehyde-derived cross-link to be identified was the aldol condensation product (Bornstein & Piez, 1966), an intramolecular cross-link that appears to be present only at the amino terminal end of the molecule (Bailey & Robins, 1976). As shown in Figure 9.2, it was proposed that this cross-link reacts with histidine and hydroxylysine residues on adjacent molecules to form the compounds, histidinohydroxymerodesmosine (Tanzer et al, 1973a), aldolhistidine (Fairweather et al, 1972) and hydroxymerodesmosine (Tanzer et al, 1973b) that have been isolated from reduced collagen. It is probable, however, that these compounds are formed only during the reduction step with borohydride and, hence, that their respective non-reduced forms are not present in the native fibres (Robins & Bailey 1973a, 1977a). These compounds involving the aldol condensation product are unlikely, therefore, to play any role in stabilizing the collagen fibril.

Thus, there are two major cross-links present in borohydride-reduced collagen, hydroxylysinonorleucine and dihydroxylysinonorleucine (Fig. 9.2). Hydroxylysinonorleucine is produced mainly by condensations of allysine with hydroxylysine residues to form a Schiff base that is stabilized by reduction (Bailey et al, 1970). Some lysinonorleucine is produced through condensation of lysine residues with allysine but this represents a minor cross-linking component in collagen (Tanzer & Mechanic, 1970; Bailey & Peach, 1971). When the aldehyde from hydroxylysine is involved in cross-linking, the Schiff base initially produced undergoes an Amadori rearrangement to a keto-imine form (Robins & Bailey, 1973b) that is more stable than its aldimine counterpart. Condensation of a lysine residue with hydroxyallysine yields lysino-5-oxo-norleucine which, on reduction, gives an identical product to that from the Schiff base formed from hydroxylysine and allysine (Fig. 9.2). The separate derivation of hydroxylysinonorleucine can, however, be distinguished chemically by using radioisotopic labelling techniques (Robins & Bailey, 1975). The product of condensations between hydroxylysine residues and hydroxyallysine is hydroxylysino-5-oxo-norleucine, the non-reduced precursor of dihydroxylysinonorleucine (Fig. 9.2). The stability of the keto-amine linkages has facilitated the isolation of cross-link peptides without reduction of the collagen (Miller & Robertson, 1973). This fact provided direct evidence that dihydroxylysinonorleucine at least was derived from a real cross-link in vivo and, unlike the aldol-derived compounds, was not merely an artefact of the reduction procedure.

Glycosylated hydroxylysine has been shown to participate in the cross-linking reaction (Robins & Bailey, 1974; Eyre et al, 1974) giving rise to a number of glycosylated derivatives of the cross-links that are detectable after alkaline hydrolysis of reduced collagens (Robins, 1976). The amounts of these components varies between different tissues depending on the extent and

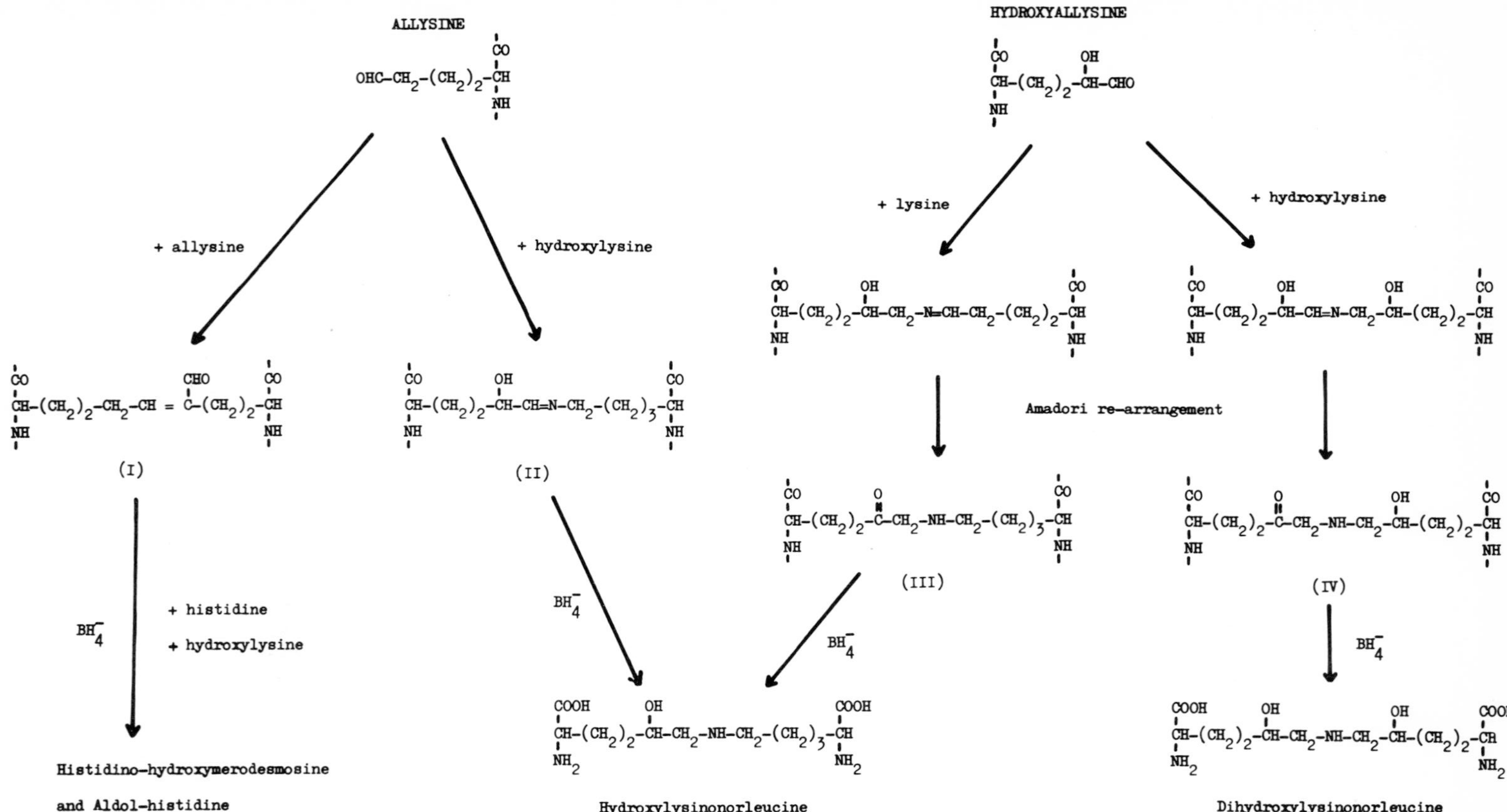

Fig. 9.2 Formation of collagen cross-links from the lysyl oxidase-produced aldehydes, allysine and hydroxyallysine. Condensation of allysine with a similar residue on an adjacent chain gives the intramolecular aldol (I) that participates in addition reactions during reduction of the tissue with borohydride (see text). Compounds derived from hydroxyallysine undergo rearrangement to form the non-reduced cross-links, hydroxylysino-5-oxo-norleucine (IV) or lysino-5-oxo-norleucine (III). The latter compound, after reduction with borohydride, gives rise to the same product as that obtained from the aldimine cross-link (II).

precise location of the glycosylated hydroxylysine residues. Whether glycosylation affects the formation or functional properties of the cross-links is unknown.

Tissue specificity in relation to properties

As indicated in Figure 9.2, the presence of hydroxylated lysine residues in the telopeptides has a profound effect on the type of cross-link formed. The degree of lysine hydroxylation within the telopeptides is generally consistent for a particular tissue in adults but various tissues are characterized by very different levels of hydroxylation giving rise to the differences in cross-link type. Thus, skin collagen contains predominantly labile aldimine bonds which render the fibres insoluble to extraction with neutral salt solutions but which are cleaved by dilute organic acids. Skin collagen, therefore, contains a relatively large oroportion that is soluble in acetic or citric acid. In bone and cartilage, the high degree of hydroxylation of telopeptide lysine results in the formation almost exclusively of the more stable keto-imine cross-links that undoubtedly contribute to the very low solubility of these collagens even after decalcification. Other tissues present a spectrum between these two extremes. In embryonic skin, there is a high degree of hydroxylation that rapidly approaches the adult values after birth (Barnes et al, 1974), resulting in a change from keto-imine to aldimine cross-links (Bailey & Robins, 1972). The collagen of acute granuloma shows similar changes in cross-link type during development and resorption (Bailey et al, 1973). The changes of cross-link type in embryonic tissue were not a result of the parallel change-over from type III to type I collagen that occurs post-natally as type III collagen showed the same pattern of reducible cross-links to that of type I collagen (Bailey & Sims, 1976). Similar results were obtained for bovine amnion (Cannon & Davison, 1978) but Fujii et al (1976) found that lysinonorleucine was the major cross-link in reduced type III collagen.

Changes in cross-linking with age

It became clear even before the structure of the reducible cross-links was fully elucidated that their amounts decreased with age. This led to the hypothesis that the reducible components are only intermediates that are converted during maturation to a more stable, non-reducible form (Bailey, 1968), thus accounting not only for the smaller amounts of reducible compounds present in adult tissue but also for the increased stability of mature tissue. The presence of relatively large amounts of reducible cross-links in young, rapidly growing tissue and the subsequent decline during maturation has been confirmed in many tissues from a number of different species (Bailey & Shimokomaki, 1971; Robins et al, 1973; Fujii & Tanzer, 1974; Shiozawa et al, 1979).

Proposed forms of stable cross-links

The mature forms of collagen cross-links have eluded identification for many years and although there are now several proposed structures, none has yet been fully authenticated. In accordance with the maturation hypothesis discussed in the previous section, most of these proposals are based on modification of the known reducible compounds.

One of the first proposals, based entirely on mass spectral data, was that reduction in vivo occurs (Mechanic et al, 1971) as was shown to occur for lysinonorleucine in elastin (Lent & Franzblau, 1967). An extensive investigation showed no trace of any naturally reduced cross-links in collagen (Robins et al, 1973) and this conclusion has subsequently been verified by many other groups. A non-reducible compound, hydroxyaldol-histidine, was characterised after isolation from calf skin (Housley et al, 1975). The proposed mechanism of formation of this non-reducible compound from allysine, hydroxyallysine and histidine residues is difficult to envisage as it involves a reductive step. Also the paucity of hydroxyallysine residues in skin collagen indicates that hydroxyaldol-histidine is a very minor constituent. The presence of this component in other tissues has not been reported and possible changes with age in the amounts of hydroxyaldol-histidine are also unknown. Davis et al, (1975) suggested that addition of lysyl or hydroxylysyl residues to the aldimine or keto-imine bonds occurred but no evidence was obtained for the proposed gem-diamine products.

A more recent suggestion for the fate of aldimine-type reducible cross-links is that they undergo oxidative modification. This followed experiments in vitro indicating an apparent acceleration of the collagen maturation process by high oxygen concentrations (Mitchell & Rigby, 1975; Robins & Bailey, 1977b, Rigby et al, 1977). Based on the detection of larger amounts of α-amino adipic acid in hydrolysates of mature collagen compared with young tissue, Bailey et al (1977) proposed that oxidation of the Schiff base cross-links in skin collagen occured to yield an isopeptide bond. The amounts of adipic acid recovered were, however, small and this proposed mechanism may not represent a major pathway.

Pyridinoline. Recently a non-reducible, fluorescent compound has been isolated from bovine Achilles tendon and partially characterized by nuclear magnetic resonance spectroscopy as a 3-hydroxypyridinium compound (Fujimoto et al, 1977, 1978). It was postulated that the compound (Fig. 9.3) could be derived from two hydroxyallysine and one hydroxylysine residue, thus giving potentially a trifunctional cross-link. Consistent with the involvement of hydroxyallysine, pyridinoline was not present in human skin but was detected in hypertrophic scar tissue (Moriguchi & Fujimoto, 1979). The amounts of pyridinoline was shown to increase with age (Moriguchi & Fugimoto, 1978).

Material with the same fluorescence characteristics has been isolated from cartilage, dentine and mature bone

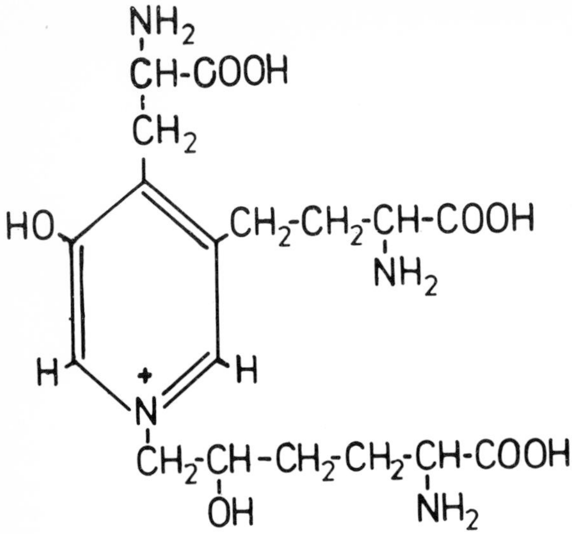

Fig. 9.3 Structure of pyridinoline. The number of methylene groups in substituents at the 4 and 5 positions are assumed from the proposed derivation of the compound (Fujimoto et al, 1978).

collagens (Eyre & Oguchi, 1980). A formative pathway involving reaction between two reducible keto-imine cross-links was envisaged (Eyre, 1980) which, although lacking experimental evidence, would account for the decrease in reducible cross-links during maturation. Doubt as to whether pyridinoline actually represents a collagen cross-link has been expressed by Elsden et al (1980) following their experiments which showed that the fluorescent material could be removed from mature bovine Achilles tendon by mild washing procedures. Elsden et al proposed that pyridinoline was an artefact produced during acid hydrolysis by the reaction of contaminating proteins with collagen. These findings were, however, disputed by Fujimoto (1980) in a report that also detailed the isolation of a small peptide containing pyridinoline from a thermolysin digest of collagen. Whether pyridinoline constitutes a collagen cross-link has not, therefore been demonstrated unequivocally. That this component is entirely an artefact seems unlikely as it is also present after hydrolysis in alkali and increases in amount during 'ageing' of collagen fibres in vitro (Robins, 1981a).

Inhibition of collagen cross-linking

Control of collagen cross-linking is potentially of great clinical significance as there are many disorders such as scleroderma, rheumatoid arthritis, osteoarthrosis, liver cirrhosis, hypertrophic scar and keloids in which the symptoms can be alleviated by softening and mobilizing the rapid proliferations of collagen that characterize these conditions. Decreasing the number of cross-links not only reduces the tensile strength of the collagen fibres but also increases their susceptibility to degradation by collagenase (Harris & Farrell 1972; Vater et al, 1979). Significant resistance to collagenase was apparently induced by as little as 0.1 bifunctional cross-links per molecule (Vater et al, 1979), but this figure may be slightly misleading as analyses were performed after lysyl oxidase-mediated crosslinking of preformed fibres in vitro which presumably, therefore, had much higher concentrations of cross-links at their periphery.

Inhibition of cross-linking can be effected at various points in the sequence of events leading to insoluble collagen summarized in Figure 9.4. Whether the cross-links are derived from allysine or its hydroxylated derivative is of paramount importance in understanding the effects of the various inhibitory agents, owing to the added stability of the cross-links derived from hydroxyallysine (see p. 163).

Catechol analogues have been shown to inhibit the activity of lysyl hydroxylase in vitro (Murray et al, 1977) which prevents the formation of stable keto-imine cross-links and alters the type of Schiff-base linkages. Inhibition of lysine hydroxylation also results in a decrease in the number of hydroxylysine glycosides which may in itself have some effect on fibril formation and stability. This may contribute to the increased solubility properties of skin collagen in a heritable disorder involving hydroxylysine deficiency (Pinnell et al, 1972).

Historically, the first clues as to the mechanism of collagen cross-linking were provided by the lathyrogen, β-aminoproprionitrile (BAPN), which is the active ingredient present in the flowering sweet pea, *L. odoratus*. BAPN is now known to act by irreversible inhibition of the enzyme, lysyl oxidase (Narayanan et al, 1972), thus preventing the formation of both allysine and hydroxyallysine (Fig. 9.4). As might be expected, this compound is highly toxic producing in animals severe skeletal lessions and dissecting aneurysms of the aorta (Barrow et al, 1974), and clinical applications are very limited. Of wider application in clinical situations are the amino-thiol compounds, of which D-penicillamine has received most attention.

Action of D-penicillamine

The mechanisms of action of penicillamine on collagen metabolism appear to be dependent on the level of administration. At low dosages, the main effect is to block the aldehyde group of allysine. This is believed to occur initially through formation of a Schiff base which is then stabilized by thiazolidine ring formation (Deshmukh & Nimni, 1969). The Schiff base cross-links in collagen that are in equilibrium with allysine are not stabilized by cyclization and removal of this aldehyde by penicillamine effects cleavage of all the aldimine-type bonds in collagen (Fig. 9.5). This is consistent with the observed increase in the proportions of salt soluble collagen in soft tissues after treatment with penicillamine (Nimni, 1968; Nimni et al, 1969). Unlike soft tissues, bone and cartilage are virtually unaffected by penicillamine treatment (Herbert et al, 1973;

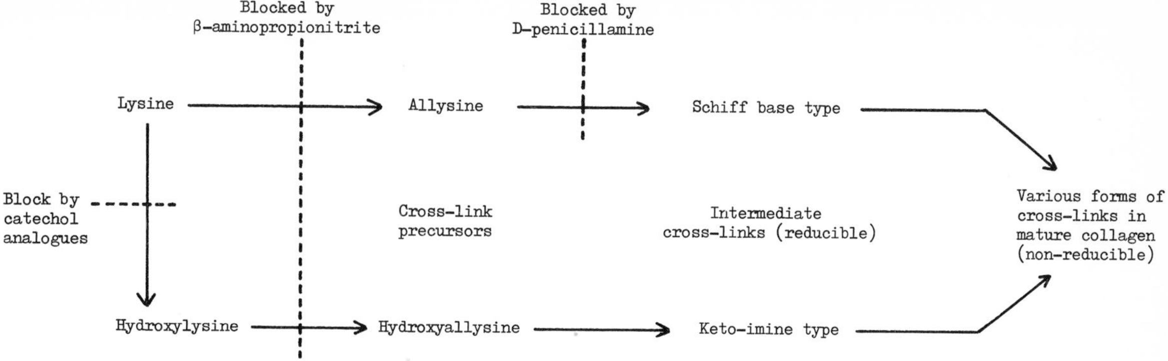

Fig. 9.4 Sites of inhibition of collagen cross-linking.

Nimni, 1977). This can now be explained by the fact that intermolecular cross-links involving hydroxyallysine, which predominate in these tissues, are stabilized by keto-imine formation (Fig. 9.4). The lack of effect of penicillamine in mobilizing acute granulation tissue (Nakagawa et al, 1976), can similarly be attributed to the presence of keto-imine cross-links in this collagen (Bailey et al, 1973). In a study of the effects of D-penicillamine on lysyl oxidase-mediated cross-link formation in bone collagen in vitro, Siegel (1977) confirmed that blocking of allysine but not hydroxyallysine occurred. A slight increase with penicillamine treatment in the amounts of bifunctional cross-links noted by Siegel (1977) could indicate an alteration in the rate of conversion to mature cross-links (see Fig. 9.5). A study of articular cargilage in vivo, however, showed no increase in keto-imine cross-links with penicillamine (Amiel et al, 1977).

At higher doses of D-penicillamine, other mechanisms of action also become operative. These include inhibition of lysyl oxidase, probably through chelation of its copper cofactor (Nimni et al, 1972). Some inhibition of the apparent rate of collagen synthesis in vitro may occur in the presence of penicillamine but this was not a consistent finding (Herbert et al, 1974; Lovell et al. 1978).

At suitable doses, therefore, penicillamine is selective in its effect by blocking the maturation of Schiff base cross-links present in certain forms of newly-synthesized collagen. In situations where maturation to stable types of cross-links has proceded, such as the inactive form of scleroderma (Herbert et al, 1974), penicillamine is ineffective. Effects of penicillamine other than on collagen metabolism undoubtedly contribute to some of its therapeutic action as is probably the case, for example, in rheumatoid arthritis where the efficacy of treatment with

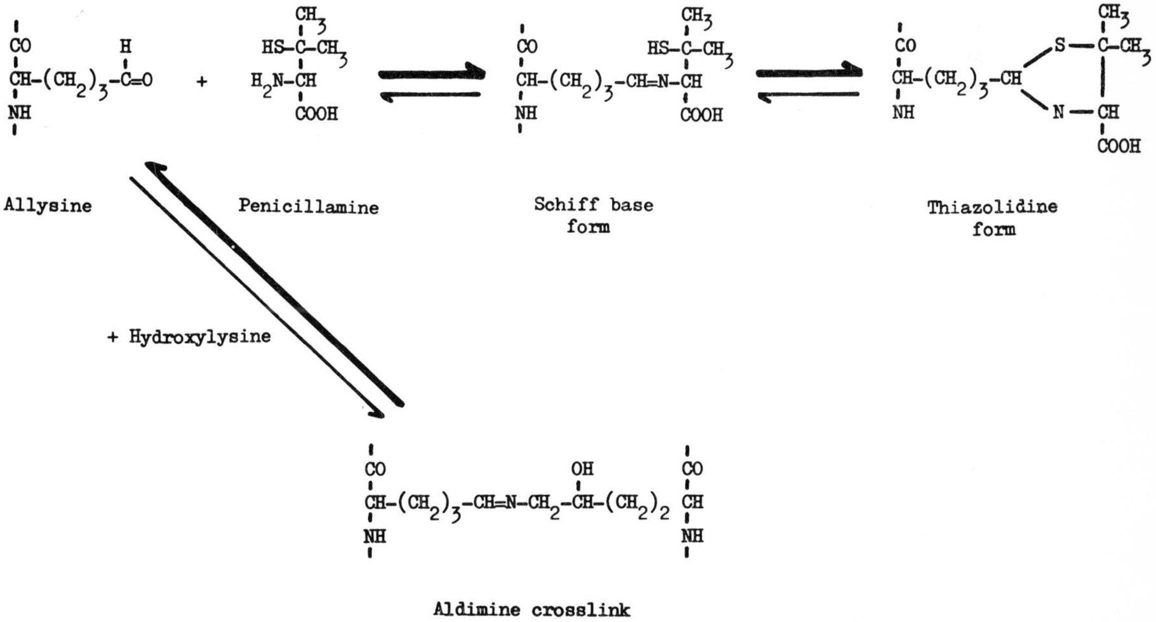

Allysine Penicillamine Schiff base form Thiazolidine form

+ Hydroxylysine

Aldimine crosslink

Fig. 9.5 Reaction of D-penicillamine with allysine to form a thiazolidine complex with consequent cleavage of aldimine crosslinks.

the drug is not accompanied by a decrease in cross-linking of synovial collagen (Lovell et al, 1978).

TISSUE LABELLING STUDIES

As discussed in the previous section (p. 165), the formation and maturation of collagen cross-links during biosynthesis gives rise to a number of soluble and insoluble fractions. Each of these fractions are theoretically susceptible to degradation and the evidence for the turnover rates of each fraction will be considered separately.

Turnover of mature, insoluble collagen

The initial experiments of Neuberger and his colleagues (Neuberger et al, 1951; Neuberger & Slack, 1953) that indicated very slow turnover rates of rat skin collagen were confirmed by several other studies (Gerber et al, 1960; Kao et al, 1961; Popenoe & Van Slyke, 1962; Nimni & Bavetta, 1964). These investigations were all based on a long-term, pulse-decay technique in which the rate of decline of specific radioactivity of protein-bound amino acid was measured following a single injection of a radioactive tracer amino acid. This technique is now known to be inaccurate unless precautions are taken to avoid or account for the recycling of labelled amino acid. Recycling occurs when labelled amino acid derived from catabolism of recently synthesized proteins is reutilized for the synthesis of new protein. Clearly the problem of label recycling becomes more pronounced for proteins with slow turnover as there is then more protein contributing labelled amino acid into the body free pools. Indeed, Nissen et al (1978) found that after a single injection of ^{3}H-proline into rats, the specific radioactivities of free proline in the plasma remained much higher than those of collagen hydroxyproline in the tissue for several weeks.

Initially, the phenomenon of label recycling was wrongly attributed to re-utilization of collagen monomers derived from de-polymerization of fibrous collagen (Klein & Weiss, 1966; Klein, 1969; Jackson & Heininger, 1971). This was based on experiments in which skin granulomas were induced in rats that had been prelabelled with ^{3}H-proline; the specific radioactivity of soluble collagen in granuloma was found to be similar to that of soluble collagen in the surrounding skin (Klein, 1969). Jackson & Heininger (1973) showed, however, that this was due to re-utilization of labelled amino acid rather than large segments of collagen by an isotope ratio method using two different labelled amino acids. These conclusions were subsequently confirmed by using a non-reutilizable label (Jackson & Heininger, 1974).

In recent years much attention has been focused on general methods of measuring protein turnover that avoid the effects of label recycling.

Free pool correction. In a study of liver protein turnover, Poole (1971) attempted to correct mathematically for label recycling using amino acid free pool specific radioactivities determined at time points corresponding to those for the proteins. The method is impracticable for proteins with half-lives longer than a few days.

Double-isotope method. Schimke and co-workers developed a double-isotope method involving injection of a ^{3}H-labelled amino acid followed at some time later by the ^{14}C-labelled form so that the second isotope was present for such a short time as to be virtually free from recycling effects; the isotope ratio in the isolated protein is proportional to its half-life (Arias et al, 1971). This method is, however, mainly comparative and for proteins with relatively long half-lives, the timing of label injections is crucial (Zak et al, 1977).

Label dilution. An in vivo pulse-chase technique has been used by a number of groups, although some doubts as to the efficacy of this procedure were expressed from experiments in vitro (Klevecz, 1971). Administration of large quantities of unlabelled proline following injection of ^{14}C-proline into rabbits was shown to cause a rapid decline in the specific radioactivity of free proline in serum (Nimni et al, 1967). In a similar experiment, Nissen et al, (1978) noted an increased renal clearance of ^{3}H-proline in rats during an 11-day dietary treatment with unlabelled proline, together with negligible residual free pool radioactivity in tissues at the end of this period compared with controls. This technique therefore appears to be effective in minimizing the effects of label recycling, although the possibility of disturbing normal metabolism with such high amino acid concentrations should be borne in mind (Rojkind & Diaz de Lion, 1970; Airhart et al, 1974).

Non-reutilizable label. A novel approach to the study of collagen turnover was devised by Jackson & Heininger (1974, 1975) involving use of the stable isotope $^{18}O_2$ as a non-reutilizable label. The method is based on the fact that the enzymatic hydroxylation reaction of proline (and lysine) uses molecular oxygen. Incorporation of ^{18}O into the hydroxyl group of hydroxyproline therefore completely irradicates label recycling as this amino acid cannot be re-used for protein synthesis. In addition, turnover of the free oxygen pool is sufficiently rapid for recycling of the ^{18}O label to be negligible. In practical terms, the method is less straightforward than those involving radioactive isotopes, both in obtaining sufficient incorporation of $^{18}O_2$ and in measuring isotope abundance by mass spectrometry. In a pulse-decay experiment in rats, the measured decrease in the abundance of [^{18}O]-hydroxyproline in skin collagen gave a calculated half-life of 27 days compared with 53 days calculated from the data for ^{3}H-proline that was administered concurrently (Jackson & Heininger, 1975). This unique experiment therefore gave a clear indication of the degree to which label recycling leads to an overestimate of collagen half-life. In common with other long-term labelling techniques, however, the method does depend on adequate correction being made for growth. Jackson & Heininger (1975) concluded from their data that the recycling of ^{3}H-proline from degraded collagen is highly efficient but their proposed model neglected the possibility that labelled proline from other body proteins was reincorporated into collagen. Nevertheless, other evidence suggests that considerable recycling of connective tissue proline does occur, as collagen abnormalities were present in a case where proline release was blocked by a prolidase deficiency (Jackson et al, 1975). Further evidence for collagen resorption by fibroblasts has been advanced from electron microscope studies apparently showing ingested collagen fibres (Ten Cate, 1972; Garant, 1976; Hentzer & Kobayasi, 1979).

Repeated labelling techniques. Klein and his colleague attempted to overcome label recycling by repeated injections of radioactive proline into young animals over an extended period during their period of rapid growth (Klein & Weiss, 1969). This procedure was designed to give an even distribution of radioactivity and prevent aberrations arising from the presence of a population of highly-labelled molecules. The animals were then grown to maturity at which time most of the label should have entered the insoluble collagen pool. As discussed previously (p. 168), in initial experiments insufficient time was allowed for the effects of amino acid recycling to completely dissipate leading to erroneous conclusions (Klein & Weiss, 1969; Klein, 1969), but more recently the animals were maintained for up to two years after labelling (Klein et al, 1977). At this stage, measurement of changes in total unlabelled hydroxyproline and total radioactive hydroxyproline in the tissues allowed calculation of collagen turnover in terms of the loss of mature, radioactive collagen and replacement by new, unlabelled material. The procedure is particularly useful for studying the effects on collagen turnover of specific manipulations such as denervation (Klein et al, 1977) or tendon grafting (Klein et al, 1972) where contralateral tissue is available as controls. In general, however, the low levels of radioactivity present in the tissues may cause considerable practical difficulties.

To summarize, most studies of the turnover of mature collagen have overestimated its half-life because of the effects of label recycling. In studies where this has been taken into account, the half-life of skin collagen was found to be 27 days in young rats (Jackson & Heininger, 1975) and about 60 days for more mature animals (Nissen et al, 1978). Thus the original conclusion that mature collagen is relatively inert remains unaltered.

Turnover of soluble collagen

Many of the early studies showed that the collagen extractable in neutral salt solution appeared to have a much higher turnover rate than the less soluble collagen mass. As indicated in Figure 9.6, turnover of the soluble forms could

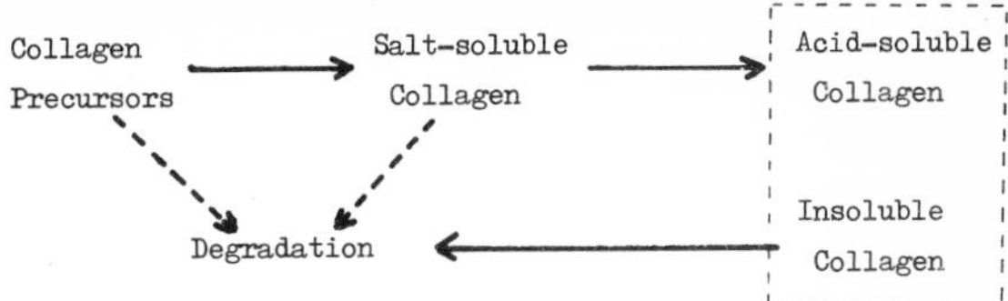

Fig. 9.6 Possible degradative pathways for collagen during biosynthesis and maturation of the fibre. The (NaCl) salt-soluble fraction comprises extracellular collagen molecules that are not cross-linked. Definition of the (acetic) acid-soluble fraction is less precise although this fraction does contain material released by cleavage of aldimine bonds. The relative rates of turnover of the different fractions are discussed in the text.

be the result solely of natural transformation into more insoluble forms (metabolic turnover): alternatively, an additional pathway could exist whereby a portion of the soluble collagen is degraded before stabilization within the fibre. Several studies have attempted to distinguish between these possibilities.

In an investigation of the turnover of rabbit skin collagen, Nimni et al (1967) determined radioactive hydroxyproline in various collagen fractions at different times up to five days after injections of ^{14}C-proline. This was performed as a serial slaughter experiment in which identical amounts of radioactivity (proportional to body weight) were administered to a series of animals which were then killed at intervals to provide data at the various time points. The results showed that radioactivity in the 0.5 M-NaCl-soluble fraction reached its maximum value five hours after the injection and that progressive increases in collagen labelling in the citrate-soluble and insoluble fractions occurred in the succeeding five-day period. As measurements of total radioactivity in the soluble and insoluble fractions at five days was only 65 per cent of that at five hours, Nimni et al (1967) concluded that about 35 per cent of the NaCl-soluble fraction of skin collagen does not form stable fibres and is presumably degraded. This conclusion is, however, unjustified as the experimental procedure is entirely dependent on achieving identical incorporation of radioactivity into skin collagen in all of the animals used to obtain the composite data.

A similar approach to determining the efficiency of transformation of soluble to insoluble collagen was adopted by Sodek (1976) using a micro-assay designed mainly for analysis of small samples of periodontal ligament. After injection of ^{3}H-proline into rats, individual animals were killed at various times up to 27 hours; this relatively short period was used to minimise the effects of label recycling. By equating changes in hydroxyproline radioactivity in the soluble and insoluble fractions over the same time period, transformation of salt-soluble collagen into insoluble material in periodontal ligament appeared to be fully efficient (Sodek, 1976). In skin an efficiency of only 32 per cent was calculated suggesting that over two-thirds of the collagen is degraded. This value, however, can be discounted as it was based on very small changes in specific radioactivity during the experimental period: also the fraction of skin collagen extracted with acetic acid appears to have been neglected in the calculations (Sodek, 1976, 1977).

As applied to skin collagen, therefore, these types of kinetic experiments do not overcome the practical problem resulting from the very small size of the NaCl-soluble collagen pool in relation to the total mass of insoluble collagen. In addition, the use of a serial slaughter type of experiment assumes the absence of any inter-animal variation which is unlikely to be the case. This aspect will be discussed further in the Section on measuring collagen synthesis rates (p. 173).

It must be concluded, therefore, that there is no firm evidence in any tissue for appreciable extracellular degradation of collagen α-chains before incorporation into fibres.

Turnover of collagen precursors

As the initial synthesis product, procollagen contains large globular extensions at each end of the molecule that are removed enzymatically in a number of discrete steps during processing, giving rise to several collagen precursor intermediates (see Chapter 6). The term collagen precursor, once used to denote any salt-soluble form of collagen, now generally refers only to material larger than α-chains. This definition will be adhered to so that the collagen precursor fraction comprises procollagen and the intermediates formed during processing.

Initial experiments carried out in vitro showed that the conversion of type I procollagen into collagen was very rapid, with a half-time of 10–30 mins (Bellamy & Bornstein, 1971; Morris et al, 1975). The processing time was therefore similar to the time required for secretion of the molecule (Dehm & Prockop, 1972; Weinstock & Leblond, 1974) leading to the conclusion that excision of procollagen extension peptides occurs very soon after extrusion from the cell. The metabolic turnover of collagen precursors in vivo is similarly rapid as shown for rabbit skin using a double-isotope, constant infusion technique; the calculated half-life of type I procollagen was less than 30 mins (Robins, 1979). From pulse-chase studies in vitro using tendon cells, Kao et al (1979) proposed a more complex model involving a main secretory pool of procollagen with a half-life of two hours. The apparently complete inhibition of labelled collagen production during the chase period, upon which the kinetic analysis is entirely dependent, is in contrast to the results of Steinberg (1973) for fibroblasts.

Type III collagen precursors appear to be processed more slowly than those of type I collagen, resulting in the extraction of relatively large amounts of type III collagen precursors from tissues (Lenears & Lapiére, 1975; Timpl et al, 1975; Smith et al, 1977). The total type III collagen precursor fraction in rabbit skin, a large proportion of which consisted of intermediates, exhibited an apparent half-life of about four hours (Robins, 1979). The intermediates that were also shown to be present in fibroblast cultures (Goldberg, 1977), may contain partially cleaved extensions at each end of the molecule (Fessler & Fessler, 1979). The presence of these intermediates that are closely associated with type III collagen fibres throughout the tissue (Meigel et al, 1977) may have important functions in controlling fibre size and in modulating the affinity of type III collagen fibres for other connective tissue constituents.

Despite the differences in processing of precursors, the overall turnover rate of type I and type III collagen appear to be similar. Thus, in the skin of rats pre-labelled in utero with ^{3}H-proline, similar losses of radioactivity from type I and type III collagens were observed during their growth from two to six-weeks-old (Klein & ChandraRajan, 1977). Similar conclusions were drawn for periodontal ligament from the fact that the type I/type III ratio for newly synthesized (radioactive) collagen was similar to that in the mature tissue (Sodek & Limeback, 1979).

Degradation of collagen prcursors

As indicated in Figure 9.6 (p. 169), a situation analogous to that for the salt-soluble fraction could exist whereby a proportion of collagen precursors is degraded before passing into the extracellular salt-soluble collagen pool. Although the relatively short half-life of the precursors might be expected to preclude this, recent evidence (Bienkowski et al, 1978a, b) corroborating the earlier work of Steinberg (1973) has suggested that considerable intracellular degradation of procollagen occurs. These conclusions were based on the observation that during labelling in vitro with ^{3}H-proline, radioactive hydroxyproline in free or small peptide form accumulates rapidly in the medium. In lung explants, 20–40 per cent of the newly synthesized collagen was degraded; this proportion was the same using very short labelling times as in extended pulse-chase experiments indicating that degradation occurred intracellularly, probably at a particular stage of secretion (Bienkowski et al, 1978b). Similar results were obtained for labelled hydroxylysine after incorporation of ^{14}C-lysine (Bienkowski et al, 1978a, b).

For cultured fibroblasts, the apparent degradation of newly-synthesized collagen was greater during the early logarithmic growth phase than at confluence (Steinberg, 1978). Alteration of the stability of procollagen affected the proportion that was degraded. Thus, incorporation of the proline analogue azetidine-2-carboxylate which partially inhibited helix formation, doubled the proportion of collagen precursors that were degraded, as determined by formation of dialysable ^{14}C-hydroxylysine (Bienkowski et al, 1978a). The degradation of newly-synthesized collagen in normal cells was interpreted either as a mechanism for controlling the amounts of collagen secreted or as a means of removing aberrant or structurally unsound molecules. In support of the former hypothesis, elevation of cyclic AMP levels in fibroblasts by treatment with either prostaglandin E_1 or cholera toxin appeared to bring about a decrease in the proportion of collagen produced by increasing the intracellular degradation of newly-synthesized collagen (Baum et al, 1980). By contrast, in studies where the culture conditions of human skin fibroblasts were systematically optimized, intracellular degradation of newly-synthesized collagen was claimed to represent only a minor pathway (Booth et al, 1980).

In a study of developing mouse limbs, Holmes & Trelstad (1979) found that the production in vivo of low-molecular-weight peptides containing hydroxyproline was much greater during the initial stages of formation than for fully developed limbs, suggesting a possible role of these peptides in morphogenesis. Some doubt as to the origin of the labelled hydroxyproline was cast by a preliminary report of an experiment in vitro performed with the iron chelator, $\alpha\alpha$-dipyridyl, in the culture medium. This removal of the cofactor for proline hydroxylation was accompanied by the expected decrease in amounts of labelled collagen but labelling of the small hydroxyproline-containing peptides was unaffected (Holmes & Trelstad, 1979). Some degradation of newly-synthesized collagen does occur in vivo (Bienkowski et al, 1978b) but at a much lower level than that determined in vitro (Holmes & Trelstad, 1979). More recently, Trelstad and his co-workers have extended their investigation of the origins of the low-molecular-weight hydroxyproline peptides by demonstrating the ability of reduced oxygen derivatives to hydroxylate both free and peptide-bound proline and lysine in vitro (Trelstad et al, 1981). These effects were partially inhibited in the presence of free radical scavengers. Whether the production of hydroxyproline or hydroxylysine peptides by a non-enzymatic mechanism occurs in vitro remains to be established. Preliminary kinetic data suggests, however, that in lung and skin tissue of rapidly growing rabbits, newly synthesized collagen is not the major source of hydroxyproline in the tissue free pools (Robins, 1981b).

There is, therefore, conflicting evidence as to the magnitude and physiological function of intracellular collagen degradation and further studies of the kinetics of labelled hydroxyproline formation in vivo are necessary. Also, it is not known whether different collagen types are degraded to the same extent.

In terms of whole-body collagen turnover, high levels of intracellular collagen degradation would have a drastic effect on the urinary excretion of collagen metabolites. Indeed, if the total body accretion of collagen represented only two-thirds of that which is synthesized, it can be calculated assuming normal metabolism of the released hydroxyproline that excretion of this imino acid from intracellular degradation alone would exceed the total normal urinary output. As glycosylation of hydroxylysine occurs very soon after polypeptide chain synthesis (Harwood et al, 1975; Myllylä et al, 1975; Oikarinen et al, 1977), a similar effect on excretion of hydroxylysine glycosides would be apparent. The high levels of collagen precursor degradation proposed by Bienkowski et al, (1978a, b) are, therefore, unlikely to occur normally in all tissues.

MEASUREMENT OF COLLAGEN SYNTHESIS RATES

The incorporation of radioactive proline into collagen as labelled hydroxyproline has been widely used to measure collagen synthesis rates. This often involves some assumptions as to the consistency and predictability of the degree of proline hydroxylation. More importantly, however, this technique is subject to the same drawback as any other radioactive tracer technique for measuring rates of protein synthesis, namely, the need to define the amino acid precursor pool (see Waterlow et al, 1978). The latter is the pool of amino acid from which t-RNA molecules are charged before insertion of their amino acid residue into the polypeptide chain. The specific radioactivity of this pool is, therefore, of primary importance in quantifying the incorporation of radioactive amino acid into protein. The pool of free amino acid that can be extracted from tissues represents the average of a number of intracellular and extracellular pools: even for cells in culture, the total intracellular free pool cannot be equated with the amino acid precursor pool used for protein synthesis owing to compartmentalization within the cells (Ward & Mortimore, 1978). Proportionate increases in the specific radioactivity of proline in synthesized collagen and in the total intracellular free pool (Breul et al, 1980) does not provide evidence that the latter approximates to prolyl-tRNA values, but merely demonstrates that the precursor proline pool rapidly equilibrates with the total free pool.

One method to overcome this problem is to measure directly the specific radioactivity of the relevant tRNA-bound amino acid (Regier & Kafatos, 1977; McKee et al, 1978). As aminoacyl-tRNA's have turnover times of only a few seconds this method does present some practical difficulties. Measurement of the specific radioactivities of nascent polypeptides removed from ribosomes provides an alternative approach (Ilan & Singer, 1975) but this requires isolation of less well-defined products. A recent innovation for measuring protein synthesis in vivo is to administer large amounts of unlabelled amino acid with the radioactive tracer so that all amino acid pools should attain the same specific radioactivity (McNurlan & Garlick, 1980).

For secreted proteins, the relatively rapid turnover of

their precursor forms ensures that, under appropriate conditions, these pro-proteins represent the specific radioactivity of their amino acid precursor pool. This concept has been applied to measurements of collagen synthesis in vivo using radioactive proline (Robins, 1979) with implications for free proline pools that will be discussed in more detail. A similar technique using pro-albumin has recently been used to define leucine precursor pools in hepatoma cells (Baker & Shiman, 1979).

Proline precursor pools

For experiments in vivo, continuous intravenous infusion of radioactive amino acid allows isotopic equilibrium to be set up within the tissue free pools at a measurable rate that approximates to first order kinetics (Gan & Jeffay, 1967; Waterlow & Stephen, 1967). This avoids the complex multi-exponential terms necessary to describe changes in specific radioactivity after single injections of tracer. As shown in Figure 9.7 continuous infusion of both ^{3}H- and

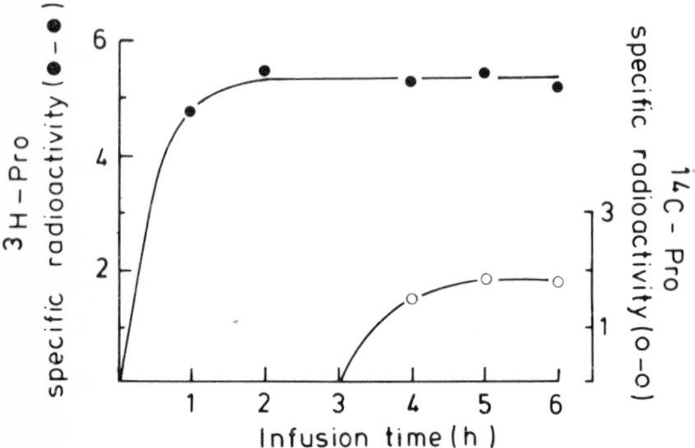

Fig. 9.7 Continuous intravenous infusion of labelled proline into a rabbit. The changes in specific radioactivity of free proline in serial blood samples are shown for infusion of ^{3}H-proline at a constant rate for 6 h; isotopic equilibrium or 'pseudo-plateau' was established within 2 h. At 3 h of infusion, the solution was changed to one that also contained ^{14}C-proline so that at the end of the infusion period, a constant ^{3}H/^{14}C ratio in blood was maintained. This ratio characterized the state of equilibrium and could be used to determine the rate of equilibration in other pools.

^{14}C-proline into rabbits results in rapid equilibration of the free proline in blood giving a pseudo-plateau that is characterized by a particular ^{3}H/^{14}C ratio. Determination of the isotope ratio in procollagen or any other amino acid pools could therefore be used to ascertain whether equilibrium in these other pools was established (Robins, 1979; Lobley et al, 1980). By using these techniques, the measured specific radioactivities of proline precursor pools in the skin of a series of young rabbits showed a remarkably wide variation in proportion to the corresponding values for blood (Table 9.1). Thus, the specific radioactivity of the

Table 9.1 Relative specific radioactivities of proline free pools. The specific radioactivities in blood and skin homogenate are equilibrium values for a series of growing rabbits given continuous intravenous infusions of ^{3}H-proline for between 5 and 10 h. The precursor pool was defined by the specific radioactivity of type I procollagen that was shown to have reached equilibrium by a double-isotope procedure (see Fig. 9.7).

Blood (S_B)	*Skin* (S_H)	*Skin precursor* pool(S_{PC})	S_{PC}/S_B	S_{PC}/S_H
Free proline specific radioactivity (dpm/nmol)			(× 100)	(× 100)
448	244	90	20	37
957	189	89	9	47
1660	829	138	8	17
995	308	53	5	17
543	264	134	25	50
580	230	69	12	30
771	450	182	24	40
632	294	74	12	25

proline pool for collagen synthesis varied from 25 per cent to as little as five per cent of the corresponding blood values; in addition, there was no consistent relationship with the total tissue free pool.

These variations can be rationalized by considering the various contributors to the free proline precursor pool that are schematically presented in Figure 9.8. In addition to active transport of proline (see Christensen, 1969) into the cell there are two intracellular sources of proline, from synthesis de novo and from protein degradation. For relatively short-term labelling procedures the intracellular sources contribute unlabelled amino acid. As a non-essential amino acid, proline can be synthesized either from

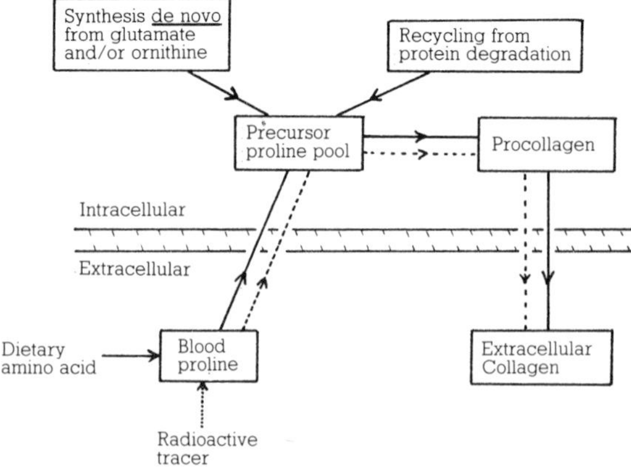

Fig. 9.8 Schematic representation of the derivation of the precursor pool of free proline for collagen synthesis. The precursor proline pool cannot be measured directly and may constitute a small proportion of the total intracellular proline. The amount of labelled proline incorporated into collagen (broken line) is governed not only by the rate of synthesis of procollagen but also by the relative amounts of unlabelled proline contributed from intracellular sources.

glutamate (Shen & Strecker, 1975) or from ornithine (Adams, 1970), although the relative importance of these pathways varies in different tissues. In cartilage about 20 per cent of proline used for collagen synthesis in vitro was derived from ornithine even in the presence of relatively high concentrations of exogenous proline (Smith & Phang, 1978). During conditions involving rapid rates of protein synthesis and turnover such as fibrotic lesions of the liver (Kershenobich et al, 1970; Dunn et al, 1977) or stretch-induced hypertrophy of muscle (Laurent et al, 1978) there are large increases in total tissue pool of free proline. For liver cirrhosis, this coincided with an increased synthesis of proline from glutamate compared to normal liver tissue (Rojkind & Diaz de Lion, 1970). There is no direct indication of the quantitative importance of recycled proline from protein degradation. The results obtained for the rabbit (Table 9.1) are consistent with the high degree of proline reutilization proposed for rat skin (Jackson & Heininger, 1974; Jackson et al, 1975).

For measurements of collagen synthesis by incorporation of labelled proline, therefore, the relative contributions from extracellular and intracellular sources to the proline precursor pool have a large effect on the apparent rate of incorporation. Disturbance of this balance is especially important where only a small proportion of extracellular (labelled) proline flows into the pool for collagen synthesis, as apparently in the case for rabbit skin. The result in Table 9.1 presumably reflects physiological variation between animals at one or a number of points in the transport, synthesis, recycling or metabolism of proline.

These findings are relevant to studies of collagen turnover using serial slaughter techniques that were referred to previously (p. 170). This type of experiment is dependent on achieving identical incorporation of labelled proline into each of a series of animals. If the animals referred to in Table 9.1 were used for this form of experiment then, even after normalization of the blood proline specific radioactivities, variations in the proline precursor pool could result in a five-fold difference in the incorporation of labelled hydroxyproline into skin collagen. Unless a suitable number of animals are used for each time-point to eradicate inter-animal variation, the serial slaughter technique is unreliable for studying collagen metabolism using radioactive tracers.

CONCLUSIONS

The excretion of hydroxyproline as a measure of collagen degradation is a guide only for gross changes in collagen metabolism owing mainly to the large proportion of this imino acid that is metabolized. Although a more sensitive index, measurement of urinary hydroxylysine glycosides is complicated by the large contributions of disaccharide derivative from the complement component, C1q. This has led to some ambiguities in interpreting mono- to di-saccharide ratios in urine (Askenasi et al, 1976a). Urinary elimination of galactosyl-hydroxylysine, however, appears to provide an index of bone collagen turnover.

Most studies of the turnover of mature collagen have over-estimated the half-life due to the effects of amino acid recycling. Nevertheless, the turnover of this fraction is relatively slow. Caution should be exercised in interpreting the results of labelling with radioactive proline as the apparent rates of incorporation into collagen are susceptible to relatively small changes in proline metabolism.

There is no firm experimental basis for the contention that a large proportion of skin collagen is degraded during transformation into soluble fibres. This is unlikely, therefore, to contribute significantly to the urinary excretion of collagen metabolites. In addition, increasing the size of the soluble collagen pool by inhibition of cross-linking does not consistently result in increased urinary hydroxyproline (Trnavská et al, 1968; Nimni et al, 1969). The proposed degradation of soluble collagen extracellularly is distinct from the recently described phenomenon of degradation of collagen precursors, which was determined by completely different techniques. A significant degree of intracellular collagen degradation probably does not occur normally in vivo but may be increased in response to special stimuli.

With current knowledge of the number of genetically distinct collagens that exist, turnover studies have acquired a new emphasis; namely, investigation of the relative turnover rates of different types of collagen and the mechanisms by which their relative proportions in the tissue are controlled during normal growth and in pathological conditions. At present, these studies are at a comparatively early stage but provide a challenging prospect for the future.

REFERENCES

Adams E 1970 Metabolism of proline and of hydroxyproline. International Review of Connective Tissue Research 5: 1-91

Adams E, Ramaswamy S, Lamon M 1978 3-Hydroxyproline content of normal urine. Journal of Clinical Investigation 61: 1482-1487

Airhart J, Vidrich A, Khairallah E A 1974 Compartmentation of free amino acids for protein synthesis in rat liver. Biochemical Journal 140: 539-548

Amiel D, Akeson W H, Harwood F L, Schmidt D A, Mechanic G L 1977 Effect of low dosage schedule of D-penicillamine on collagen cross-linking in a nine week immobilized rabbit knee. Connective Tissue Research 5: 179-183

Anglister L, Rogozinski S, Silman I 1976 Detection of hydroxyproline in preparations of acetylcholinesterase from the electric organ of the electric eel. FEBS Letters 69: 129-132

Arias I M, Doyle D, Schimke R T 1969 Studies on the synthesis and degradation of proteins of the endoplasmic reticulum of rat liver. Journal of Biological Chemistry 224: 3303-3315

Askenasi R 1973 A new rapid method for measuring hydroxylysine and its glycosides in hydrolysates and physiological fluids. Biochimica Biophysica Acta 304: 375-383

Askenasi R 1974 Urinary hydroxylysine and hydroxylysyl glycoside excretion in normal and pathological states. Journal of Laboratory and Clinical Medicine 83: 673-679

Askenaski R, De Backer M, Devos A 1976a The origin of urinary hydroxylysyl glycosides in Paget's disease of bone and in primary hyperparathyroidism. Calcified Tissue Research 22: 35-40

Askenasi R, Le Lous M, Bazin S, Rao V H 1976b Urinary excretion of hydroxylysyl glycosides during acute inflammation in the rat. Clinical Science and Molecular Medicine 50: 195-197

Bailey A J 1968 Intermediate labile intermolecular crosslinks in collagen fibres. Biochimica et Biophysica Acta 160: 447-453

Bailey A J, Peach C M 1971 The chemistry of the collagen cross-links: absence of reduction of dehydrolysinonorleucine and dehydrohydroxylysine in vivo. Biochemical Journal 121: 257-259

Bailey A J, Robins S P 1972 Embryonic skin collagen. Replacement of the type of aldimine crosslinks during the early growth period. FEBS Letters 21: 330-334

Bailey A J, Robins S P 1976 Current topics in the biosynthesis, structure and function of collagen. Science Progress (Oxford) 63: 419-444

Bailey A J, Shimokomaki M 1971 Age-related changes in the reducible crosslinks of collagelen. FEBS Letters 16: 86-88

Bailey A J, Sims T J 1976 Chemistry of the collagen crosslinks. Nature of the cross-links in the polymorphic forms of dermal collagen during development. Biochemical Journal 153: 211-215

Bailey A J, Bazin S, Delaunay A 1973 Changes in the nature of the collagen during development and resorption of granulation tissue. Biochimica et Biophysica Acta 328: 383-390

Bailey A J, Peach C M, Fowler L J 1970 The chemistry of the collagen crosslinks: isolation and characterization of two intermediate crosslinks in collagen. Biochemical Journal 117: 819-831

Bailey A J, Robins S P, Balian G 1974 Biological significance of the intermolecular cross-links of collagen. Nature (London) 251: 105-109

Bailey A J, Ranta M H, Nicholls A C, Partridge S M, Elsden D F 1977 Isolation of α-aminoadipic acid from mature dermal collagen and elastin. Evidence for an oxidative pathway in the maturation of collagen and elastin. Biochemical and Biophysical Research Communications 78: 1403-1410

Baker R E, Shiman R 1979 Measurement of phenylalanine hydroxylase turnover in cultured hepatoma cells. Journal of Biological Chemistry 254: 9633-9639

Barnes M J, Constable B J, Morton L F, Royce P M 1974 Age-related variations in hydroxylation of lysine and proline in collagen. Biochemical Journal 139: 461-468

Barrow M V, Simpson C F, Miller E J 1974 Lathyrism: A review. Quarterly Review of Biology 49: 101-128

Baum B J, Moss J, Breul S D, Berg R A, Crystal R G 1980 Effect of cyclic AMP on the intracellular degradation of newly synthesized collagen. Journal of Biological Chemistry 255: 2843-2847

Bellamy G, Bornstein P 1971 Evidence for procollagen, a biosynthetic precursor of collagen. Proceedings of the National Academy of Sciences of the United States of America 68: 1138-1142

Bienkowski R S, Baum B J, Crystal R G 1978a Fibroblasts degrade newly synthesized collagen within the cell before secretion. Nature (London) 276: 413-416

Bienkowski R S, Cowan M J, McDonald J A, Crystal R G 1978b Degradation of newly synthesized collagen. Journal of biological Chemistry 253: 4356-4363

Blumenkrantz N, Asboe-Hansen G 1974 An automated procedure for quantitative determination of hydroxyproline. Clinical Biochemistry 7: 251-257

Booth B A, Polak K L, Uitto J 1980 Collagen biosynthesis by human skin fibroblasts. I Optimization of the culture conditions for synthesis of type I and type III orocollagens. Biochimica Biophysicia Acta 607: 145-160

Bornstein P, Picz K A 1966 The nature of the intramolecular crosslink in collagen. Biochemistry 5: 3460-3473

Breul S D, Bradley K H, Hance A J, Schafer M P, Berg R A, Crystal R G 1980 Control of collagen production by human diploid lung fibroblasts. Journal of Biological Chemistry 255: 5250-5260

Calcott A, Müller-Eberhard H J 1972 C1q protein of human complement. Biochemistry 11: 3443-3450

Campbell R D, Booth N A, Fothergill J E 1979 Purification and characterization of subcomponent C1q of the first component of bovine complement. Biochemical Journal 177: 531-540

Cannon D J, Davison P F 1978 Crosslinking in type III collagen of fetal tissue. Biochemical and Biophysical Research Communications 85: 1373-1378

Christensen H N 1969 Some special kinetic problems of (amino acid) transport. Advances in Enzymology 32: 1-20

Cohen M P, Surma M 1980 Renal glomerular basement membrane: in vivo biosynthesis and turnover in normal rats. Journal of Biological Chemistry 255: 1767-1770

Davis N R, Risen O M, Pringle G A 1975 Stable, nonreducible cross-links of mature collagen. Biochemistry 14: 2031-2036

Dehm P, Prockop D J 1972 Time lag in the secretion of collagen by matriz-free tendon cells and inhibition of the secretory process by colchicine and vinblastine. Biochimica et biophysica acta 264: 375-382

Deshmukh K, Nimni M E 1969 A defect in the intramolecular and intermolecular cross-linking of collagen caused by penicillamine II Functional groups involved in the interaction process. Journal of Biological Chemistry 244: 1787-1795

Dunn M A, Rojkind M, Warren K S, Hait L R, Seiffer S 1977 Liver collagen synthesis in murine schistosomiasis. Journal of Clinical Investigation 59: 666-674

Efron M L, Bixby E M, Pryles C V 1965 Hydroxyprolinaemia II A rare metabolic disease due to deficiency of the enzyme hydroxyproline oxidase. New England Journal of Medicine 272: 1299-1309

Elsden D F, Light N D, Bailey A J 1980 An investigation of pyridinoline, a putative collagen cross-link. Biochemical Journal 185: 531-534

Eyre D R 1980 Collagen: molecular diversity in the body's protein scaffold. Science 207: 1315-1322

Eyre D R, Glimacher M J 1973 Analysis of a cross-linked peptide from calf bone collagen: evidence that hydroxylysyl glycoside participates in the crosslink. Biochemical and Biophysical Research Communications 52: 663-671

Eyre D R, Oguchi H 1980 The hydroxypyridinium crosslinks of skeletal collagens: their measurement, properties and a proposed pathway of formation. Biochemical and Biophysical Research Communications 92: 403-410

Fairweather R B, Tanzer M L, Gallop P M 1972 Aldol-histidine, a new trifunctional collagen crosslink. Biochemical and Biophysical Research Communications 48: 1311-1315

Fessler L I, Fessler J H 1979 Characterization of type III procollagen from chick embryo blood vessels. Journal of Biological Chemistry 254: 233-239

Fujii K, Tanzer M L 1974 Age-related changes in the reducible crosslinks of human tendon collagen. FEBS Letters 43: 300-302

Fujii K, Tanzer M L, Nusgens B V, Lapiére C M 1976 Aldehyde content and cross-linking of type III collagen. Biochemical and Biophysical Research Communications 69: 128-134

Fujimoto D 1980 Evidence for natural existence of pyridinoline crosslink in collagen. Biochemical and Biophysical Research Communications 93: 948-953

Fujimoto D, Moriguchi T 1978 Pyridinoline, a non-reducible crosslink of collagen. Quantitative determination, distribution and isolation of a crosslinked peptide. Journal of Biochemistry (Tokyo) 83: 863-867

Hanauske-Abel H M, Röhm K-H 1980 The collagenous part of C1q is unaffected in the hydroxylysine-deficient collagen disease. FEBS Letters 110: 73-76

Harris E D, Farrell M E 1972 Resistance of collagenase: a characteristic of collagen fibrils cross-linked by formaldehyde. Biochimica et Biophysica Acta 278: 133-141

Harwood R, Grant M E, Jackson D S 1975 Studies on the glycosylation of hydroxylysine residues during collagen biosynthesis and the sub-cellular localization of collagen galactosyl-transferase and glucosyl-transferase in tendon and cartilage cells. Biochemical Journal 152: 291-302

Hentzer B, Kobayasi T 1979 Intracellular collagen fibrils in cultured human skin. Acta Dermatovener (Stockholm) 59: 477-486

Herbert C, Jayson M I V, Bailey A J 1973 Joint capsule collagen in osteoarthrosis. Annals of the Rheumatic Diseases 32: 510-514

Herbert C M, Lindberg K A, Jayson M I V, Bailey A J 1974 Biosynthesis and maturation of skin collagen in sscleoderma, and effect of D-penicillamine. Lancet 1: 187-192

Holmes L B, Trelstad R L 1979 Identification of rapidly labelled, small molecular weight hydroxyproline-containing peptides in developing mouse limbs in vitro and in vivo. Developmental Biology 72: 41-49

Hörlein D, Fietzek P P, Kühn K 1978 Pro-gln: the procollagen peptidase cleavage site in the $\alpha 1(I)$ chain of dermatosparactic calf skin procollagen. FEBS Letters 89: 279-282

Housley T, Tanzer M L, Henson E, Gallop P M 1975 Collagen cross-linking: isolation of hydroxyaldol-histidine, a naturally-occurring cross-link. Biochemical and Biophysical Research Communications 67: 824-830

Fujimoto D, Akiba K-Y, Nakamura N 1977 Isolation and characterization of a fluorescent material in bovine Achilles tendon collagen. Biochemical and Biophysical Research Communications 76: 1124-1129

Fujimoto D, Moriguchi T, Ishida T, Hayashi J 1978 The structure of pyridinoline, a collagen cross-link. Biochemical and Biophysical Research Communications 84: 52-57

Gallop P M, Paz M A 1975 Post-translational protein modifications, with special attention to collagen and elastin. Physiological Reviews 55: 418-487

Gan J C, Jeffay H 1967 Origins and metabolism of the intracellular amino acid pools in rat liver and muscle. Biochimica et Biophysica Acta 148: 448-459

Garant P R 1976 Collagen resorption by fibroblasts. A theory of fibroblastic maintenance of the periodontal ligament. Journal of Periodontology 47: 380-390

Gasser A, Celada A, Courvoisier B, Depierre D, Hulme P M, Rinsler M, Williams D, Wootton R 1979 The clinical measurement of urinary total hydroxyproline excretion. Clinica Chimica acta 95: 487-491

Gerber G, Gerber G, Altman K I 1960 Studies on the metabolism of tissue proteins I Turnover of collagen labelled with proline-U-C^{14} in young rats. Journal of Biological Chemistry 235: 2653-2656

Gielen F, Dequeker J, Drochmans A, Wildiers J, Merlevede M 1976 Relevance of hydroxyproline excretion to bone metastasis in breast cancer. British Journal of Cancer 34: 279-285

Goldberg B 1977 Kinetics of processing of type I and type III procollagens in fibroblast cultures. Proceedings of the National Academy of Sciences of the United States of America 74: 3322-3325

Ilan J, Singer M 1975 Sampling of the leucine pool from the growing peptide chain: differences in leucine specific activity of peptidyl tRNA from free and bound polysomes. Journal of Molecular Biology 91: 39-51

Isemura J, Takahashi K, Ikenaka T 1976 Comparative study of carbohydrate-protein complexes. II Determination of hydroxylysine and its glycosides in human skin and scar collagens by an improved method. Journal of Biochemistry (Tokyo) 80: 653-658

Jackson S H, Heininger J A 1971 Collagen reutilization in normal and hypersomatotrophic rats. Clinica chimica acta 33: 179-185

Jackson S H, Heininger J A 1973 A reassessment of the collagen reutilization theory by an isotope ratio method. Clinica chimica acta 46: 153-160

Jackson S H, Heininger J A 1974 A study of collagen reutilization using an $^{18}O_2$ labelling technique. Clinica chimica acta 51: 163-171

Jackson S H, Heininger J A 1975 Proline recycling during collagen metabolism as determined by concurrent $^{18}O_2$ and ^{3}H-labelling. Biochimica et biophysica acta 381: 359-367

Jackson S H, Dennis A C O, Greenberg M 1975 Iminodipeptiduria: a genetic defect in recycling collagen; a method for determining prolidase in erythrocytes. Canadian Journal of Medicine 113: 759-763

Kakimoto Y, Akazawa S 1970 Isolation and identification of N^G, N^G and N^G, N^{IG}-dimethylarginine, N^{ϵ}-mono- di- and trimethyllysine, and glucosyl-galactosyl and galactosyl-δ-hydroxylysine from human urine. Journal of Biological Chemistry 245: 5751-5758

Kao K-Y T, Hilker D M, McGauack T H 1961 Connective tissue IV. Synthesis and turnover of proteins in tissues of rats. Proceedings of the Society for Experimental Biology and Medicine 106: 121-124

Kao W W-Y, Berg R A, Prockop D J 1977 Kinetics for the secretion of procollagen by freshly isolated tendon cells. Journal of Biological Chemistry 252: 8391-8397

Kelleher P C 1979 Urinary excretion of hydroxyproline, hydroxylysine and hydroxylysyl glycosides by patients with Paget's disease of bone and carcinoma with metastases in bone. Clinica Chimica Acta 92: 373-379

Kershenobich D, Fierro F J, Rojkind M 1970 The relationship between the free pool of proline and collagen content in human liver cirrhosis. Journal of Clinical Investigation 49: 2246-2249

Kivirikko K I 1970 Urinary excretion of hydroxyproline in health and disease. International Review of Connective Tissue Research 5: 93-163

Klein L 1969 Reversible transformation of fibrous collagen to a soluble state in vivo. Proceedings of the National Academy of Sciences of the United States of America 62: 920-927

Klein L, ChandraRajan J 1977 Collagen degradation in rat skin but not in intestine during rapid growth: effect on collagen types I and III from skin. Proceedings of the National Academy of Sciences of the United States of America 74: 1436-1439

Klein L, Weiss P H 1966 Induced connective tissue metabolism in vivo: reutilization of pre-existing collagen. Proceedings of the National Academy of Sciences of the United States of America 56: 277-284

Klein L, Dawson M H, Heiple K G 1977 Turnover of collagen in the adult rat after denervation. Journal of Bone and Joint Surgery 59A: 1065-1067

Klein L, Lunseth P A, Aadalen R J 1972 Comparison of functional and non-functional tendon grafts. Journal of Bone and Joint Surgery 54A: 1745-1753

Klevecz R R 1971 Rapid protein catabolism in mammalian cells is obscured by reutilization of amino acids. Biochemical and Biophysical Research Communications 43: 76-81

Kohler P F, Müller-Eberhard H J 1972 Metabolism of human C1q: studies in hypogammaglobulinemia, myeloma and systemic lupus erythematosus. Journal of Clinical Investigation 51: 868-875

Krane S M, Kantrowitz F G, Byrne M, Pinnell S R, Singer F R 1977 Urinary excretion of hydroxylysine and its glycosides as an index of collagen degradation. Journal of Clinical Investigation 59: 819-827

Laurent G J, Sparrow M P, Millward D J 1978 Turnover of muscle protein in the fowl. II Changes in rates of protein synthesis and breakdown during hypertrophy of the anterior and posterior latissimus dorsi muscles. Biochemical Journal 176: 407-418

Lenaers A, Lapiére C M 1975 Type III procollagen and collagen in skin. Biochimica et Biophysica Acta 400: 121-131

Lent R, Franzblau C 1967 Studies on the reduction of bovine elastin: evidence for the presence of 6,7-dehydrolysinorleucine. Biochemical and Biophysical Research Communications 26: 43-50

Lobley G E, Robins S P, Palmer R M, McDonald I 1980 Measurement of the rates of protein synthesis in rabbits. A method for the estimation of rates of change in the specific radioactivities of free amino acids during continuous infusions. Biochemical Journal in press

Lovell C R, Nicholls A C, Jayson M I V, Bailey A J 1978 Changes in the collagen of synovial membrane in rheumatoid arthritis and effect of D-penicillamine. Clinical Science and Molecular Medicine 55: 31-40

McKee E E, Cheung J Y, Rannels D E, Morgan H E 1978 Measurement of the rate of protein synthesis and compartmentation of heart phenylalanine. Journal of Biological Chemistry 253: 1030-1040

McNurlan M A, Garlick P J 1980 Contribution of rat liver and gastrointestinal tract to whole-body protein synthesis in the rat. Biochemical Journal 186: 381-383

Mechanic G, Gallop P M, Tanzer M L 1971 The nature of crosslinking in collagen from ineralized tissue. Biochemical and Biophysical Research Communications 45: 644-653

Meigel W N, Gay S, Weber L 1977 Dermal architecture and collagen type distribution. Archives for Dermatological Research 259: 1-10

Miller E J, Robertson P B 1973 The stability of collagen cross-links when derived from hydroxylysyl residues. Biochemical and Biophysical Research Communications 54: 432-439

Mitchell T W, Rigby B J 1975 In vivo and in vitro aging of collagen examined using an isometric melting technique. Biochimica et Biophysica Acta 393: 531-541

Moriguchi T, Fujimoto D 1978 Age-related changes in the content of the collagen cross-link, pyridinoline. Journal of Biochemistry (Tokyo) 84: 933-935

Moriguchi T, Fujimoto D 1979 Crosslink of collagen in hypertrophic scar. Journal of Investigative Dermatology 72: 143-145

Morris N P, Fessler L I, Weinstock A, Fessler J H 1975 Procollagen assembly and secretion in embryonic chick bone. Journal of Biological Chemistry 250: 5719-5726

Murai A, Miyahara T, Shiozawa S 1975 Age-related variations in glycosylation of hydroxylysine in human and rat skin collagens. Biochimica et Biophysica Acta 404: 345-348

Murray J C, Lindberg K A, Pinnell S R 1977 In vitro inhibition of collagen cross-links by catechol analogues. Journal of Investigative Dermatology 68: 146-150

Myllylä R, Risteli L, Kivirikko K I 1975 Glucosylation of galactosylhydroxylysyl residues in collagen in vitro by collagen glucosyltransferase. Inhibition by triple helical conformation of the substrate. European Journal of Biochemistry 58: 517-521

Nakagawa H, Ohkoshi K, Tsurufuji S 1976 Effect of D-penicillamine and β-aminopropionitrite on collagen breakdown of carrageen in granuloma in rats. Biochemical Pharmacology 25: 1129-1132

Narayanan A S, Siegel R C, Martin G R 1972 On the inhibition of lysyl oxidase by β-aminopropionitrile. Biochemical and Biophysical Research Communications 46: 745-751

Neuberger A, Slack H G B 1953 The metabolism of collagen from liver, bone, skin and tendon in the normal rat. Biochemical Journal 53: 47-52

Neuberger A, Perrone J C, Slack H G B 1951 The relative metabolic inertia of tendon collagen in the rat. Biochemical Journal 49: 199-204

Nimni M E 1968 A defect in the intramolecular and intermolecular crosslinking of collagen caused by penicillamine. I Metabolic and functional abnormalities in soft tissues. Journal of Biological Chemistry 243: 1457-1466

Nimni M E 1974 Collagen: its structure and function in normal and pathological connective tissues. Seminars in Arthritis and Rheumatism 4: 95-150

Nimni M E 1977 Mechanism of inhibition of collagen cross-linking by penicillamine. Proceedings of the Royal Society of Medicine 70 suppl. 3: 65-72

Nimni M E, Bavetta L A 1964 Collagen synthesis and turnover in the growing rat under the influence of methyl prednisolone. Proceedings of the Society for Experimental Biology and Medicine 117: 618-623

Nimni M E, DeGuia E, Bavetta L A 1967 Synthesis and turnover of collagen precursors in rabbit skin. Biochemical Journal 102: 143-147

Nimni M E, Deshmukh K, Gerth N 1972 Collagen defect induced by penicillamine. Nature New Biology 240: 220-221

Nimni M E, Deshmukh K, Gerth N, Bavetta L A 1969 Changes in collagen metabolism associated with the administration of penicillamine and various amino and thiol compounds. Biochemical Pharmacology 18: 707-714

Nissen R, Cardinale G J, Udenfriend S 1978 Increased turnover of arterial collagen in hypertensive rats. Proceedings of the National Academy of Sciences of the United States of America 75: 451-453

Odell V, Wegener L, Peczon B, Hudson B G 1974 A rapid automatic analysis of hydroxylysine, hydroxlysine glycosides and methionine sulphoxide in collagen and basement membrane. Journal of Chromatography 88: 245-252

Oikarinen A, Anttinen H, Kivirikko K I 1977 Further studies on the effect of triple-helix formation on hydroxylation of lysine and glycosylation of hydroxylysine in chick-embryo tendon and cartilage cells. Biochemical Journal 166: 357-362

Opresko L, Wiley H S, Wallace R A 1980 Proteins iodinated by the chloramine-T method appear to be degraded at an abnormally rapid rate after endocytosis. Proceedings of the National Academy of Sciences of the United States of America 77: 1556-1560

Orloff S, Rao V H, Verbruggen L 1979 Urinary excretion of hydroxyproline and hydroxylysyl glycosides in adjuvant-induced arthritis. Italian Journal of Biochemistry 28: 173-182

Peczon B D, Antreasian R, Bucay P 1979 Chromatographic analysis of hydroxylysine glycosides and acid hydrolysates. Journal of Chromatography 169: 351-356

Pinnell S R, Fox R, Krane S M 1971 Human collagens: differences in glycosylated hydroxylysines in skin and bone. Biochimica et Biophysica Acta 229: 119-122

Pinnell S R, Krane S M, Kenzora J E, Glimcher M J 1972 A heritable disorder of connective tissue: hydroxylysine-deficient collagen disease. New England Journal of Medicine 286: 1013-1020

Poole B 1971 The kinetics of disappearance of labelled leucine from the free leucine pool of rat liver and its effects on the apparent turnover of catalase and other hepatic proteins. Journal of Biological Chemistry 246: 6587-6591

Popenoe E A, VanSlyke D D 1962 The formation of collagen hydroxylysine. Journal of Biological Chemistry 237: 3491-3494

Price R G, Spiro R G 1977 Studies on the metabolism of the renal glomerular basement membrane. Turnover measurements in the rat with the use of radiolabelled amino acids. Journal of Biological Chemistry 252: 8597-8602

Prockop D J 1964 Isotopic studies on collagen degradation and the urine excretion of hydroxyproline. Journal of Clinical Investigation 43: 453-460

Regier J C, Kafatos F C 1977 Absolute rates of protein synthesis in sea urchins with specific activity measurements of radioactive leucine and leucyl-tRNA. Developmental Biology 57: 270-283

Reid K B M, Lowe D M, Porter R R 1972 Isolation and characterization of Clq, a subcomponent of the first component of complement, from human and rabbit sera. Biochemical Journal 130: 749-763

Rigby B J, Mitchell T W, Robinson M E 1977 Oxygen participation in the in vivo and in vitro aging of collagen fibres. Biochemical and Biophysical Research Communications 79: 400-405

Robins S P 1976 The separation of cross-linking components from collagen. In: Hall D A (ed) Methodology of Connective Tissue Research, Joynson-Bruvvers, Oxford, pp 37-52

Robins S P 1979 The metabolism of rabbit skin collagen. Differences in the apparent turnover rates of type I and type III collagen precursors determined by constant intravenous infusion of labelled amino acids. Biochemical Journal 181: 75-82

Robins S P 1980 Turnover of collagen and its precursors. In Vidiik A, Vuust J (eds) Biology of Collagen, Academic Press, London, pp 135-151

Robins S P 1981a Analysis of the cross-linking components in collagen and elastin. Methods of Biochemical Analysis 28: 329-379

Robins S P 1981b Evaluation of the degradation of newly-synthesized collagen in vivo by an isotope-ratio method. Biochemical Society Transactions 9: 259P

Robins S P, Bailey A J 1973a The chemistry of the collagen cross-links: the characterization of Fraction C (histidinhydroxymerodesmosine), a possible artefact produced during the reduction of collagen fibres with borohydride. Biochemical Journal 135: 756-665

Robins S P, Bailey A J 1973b Relative stabilities of the intermediate reducible crosslinks present in collagen fibres. FEBS Letters 33: 167-171

Robins S P, Bailey A J 1974 Isolation and characterization of glycosyl derivatives of the reducible cross-links in collagens. FEBS Letters 38: 334-336

Robins S P, Bailey A J 1975 The chemistry of the collagen crosslinks: mechanism of stabilization of the reducible intermediate crosslinks. Biochemical Journal 149: 381-385

Robins S P, Bailey A J 1977a The chemistry of the collagen crosslinks: characterization of the products of reduction of skin, tendon and bone with sodium cyanoborohydride. Biochemical Journal 163: 339-346

Robins S P, Bailey A J 1977b Some observations on the ageing in vitro of reprecipitated collagen fibres. Biochimica et Biophysica Acta 492: 408-414

Robins S P, Shimokomaki M, Bailey A J 1973 The chemistry of the collagen cross-links: age-related changes in the reducible components of intact bovine collagen fibres. Biochemical Journal 131: 771-780

Rojkind M, Diaz de Lion, D L 1970 Collagen biosynthesis in cirrhotic rat liver slices. A regulatory mechanism. Biochimica et Biophysica Acta 217: 512-522

Royce P M, Barnes M J 1977 Comparative studies on collagen glycosylation in chick skin and bone. Biochimica et Biophysica Acta 498: 132-142

Segrest J P, Cunningham L W 1970 Variations in human urinary O-hydroxylysyl glycoside levels and their relationship to collagen metabolism. Journal of Clinical Investigation 49: 1497-1509

Shen T F, Strecker H J 1975 Synthesis of proline and hydroxyproline in human lung (WI-38) fibroblasts. Biochemical Journal 150: 453-461

Shiozawa S, Tanaka T, Migahara T, Murai A, Kameyama M 1979 Age-related change in the reducible cross-links of human skin and aorta collagens. Gerontology 25: 247-254

Siegel R C 1977 Collagen cross-linking: effect of D-penicillamine on cross-linking in vitro. Journal of Biological Chemistry 252: 254-259

Siegel R C 1979 Lysyl oxidase. International Review of Connective Tissue Research 8: 73-118

Shinkai H, Yonemasu K 1979 Hydroxylysine-linked glycosides of human complement subcomponent C1q and of various collagens. Biochemical Journal 177: 847-852

Smiley J D, Ziff M 1964 Urinary hydroxyproline excretion and growth. Physiological Reviews 44: 30-44

Smith B D, McKenney K H, Lustberg T J 1977 Characterization of collagen precursors found in rat skin and rat bone. Biochemistry 16: 2980-2985

Smith J R, Phang J M 1978 Proline metabolism in cartilage: the importance of proline biosynthesis. Metabolism 27: 685-694

Sodek J 1976 A new approach to assessing collagen turnover by using a micro-assay. A highly efficient and rapid turnover of collagen in rat periodontal tissues. Biochemical Journal 160: 243-246

Sodek J 1977 A comparison of the rates of synthesis and turnover of collagen and non-collagen proteins in adult rat periodontal tissues and skin using a microassay. Archives of Oral Biology 22: 655-665

Sodek J, Limeback H F 1979 Comparison of the rates of synthesis, conversion and maturation of type I and type III collagens in rat periodontal tissues. Journal of Biological Chemistry 254: 10496-10502

Steinberg J 1973 The turnover of collagen in fibroblast cultures. Journal of Cell Science 12: 217-234

Steinberg J 1978 Collagen turnover and the growth state in 3T6 fibroblast cultures. Laboratory Investigation 39: 491-496

Sternberg M, Spiro R G 1979 Studies on the catabolism of the hydroxylysine-linked disaccharide units of basement membrane and collagens. Isolation and characterization of a rat kidney α-glucosidase of high specificity. Journal of Biological Chemistry 254: 10329-10336

Szymanowicz A, Malgras A, Randoux A, Borel J P 1979 Fractionation and structure of several hydroxyproline-containing urinary peptides, with special reference to some 3-hydroxyproline-containing peptides. Biochimica et Biophysica Acta 576: 253-262

Tanzer M L 1968 Intermolecular crosslinks in reconstituted collagen fibrils. Journal of Biological Chemistry 243: 4045-4054

Tanzer M L 1973 Cross-linking of collagan. Science 180: 561-566

Tanzer M L, Mechanic G 1970 Isolation of lysinonorleucine from collagen. Biochemical and Biophysical Research Communications 39: 183-189

Tanzer M L, Housley T, Berube L, Fairweather R, Franzblau C, Gallop P M 1973a Structure of two histidine-containing cross-links from collagen. Journal of Biological Chemistry 248: 393-402

Tanzer M L, Fairweather R, Gallop P M 1973b Isolation of the crosslink, hydroxymerodesmosine, from borohydride-reduced collagen. Biochimica et Biophysica Acta 310: 130-136

Ten Cate A R 1972 Morphological studies of fibrocytes in connective tissue undergoing rapid remodelling. Journal of Anatomy 112: 401-414

Timpl R, Glanville R W, Nowack H, Wiedermann H, Fietzek P P, Kühn K 1975 Isolation, chemical and electron microscopical characterization of neutral-salt-soluble type III collagen and procollagen from fetal bovine skin. Hoppe-Seyler's Zeitschrift für Physiologische Chemie 356: 1783-1792

Trnavská Z, Trnavsky, Kühn K 1968 The influence of sodium salicylate on the metabolism of collagen in the lathrytic rat. Biochemical Pharmacology 17: 1501-1509

Trelstad R L, Lawley K R, Holmes L B 1981 Nonenzymatic hydroxylations of proline and lysine by reduced oxygen derivatives. Nature (London) 289: 310-312

Uitto J, Laitinen O, Lamberg B-A, Kivirikko K I 1968 Further evaluation of the significance of urinary hydroxyproline in the diagnosis of thyroid disorders. Clinica Chimica Acta 22: 583-591

Vater C A, Harris E D, Siegel R C 1979 Native crosslinks in collagen fibrils induce resistance to human synovial collagenase. Biochemical Journal 181: 639-645

Walker F 1972 Basement membrane turnover in the rat. Journal of Pathology 107: 119-122

Ward W F, Mortimore G E 1978 Compartmentation of intracellular amino acids in rat liver: evidence for an intralysosomal pool derived from protein degradation. Journal of Biological Chemistry 253: 3581-3587

Waterlow J C, Stephen J M L 1967 The measurement of total lysine turnover in the rat by intravenous infusion of L-[U-^{14}C] lysine. Clinical Science 33: 489-506

Waterlow J C, Garlick P J, Millward D J 1978 Measurement of the rate of incorporation of labelled amino acids into tissue protein. In Protein turnover in mammalian tissues and in the whole body, North-Holland, Amsterdam, pp 339-370

Weinstock M, Leblond C P 1974 Formation of collagen. Federation Proceedings. Federation of American Societies for Experimental Biology 33: 1205-1217

Weiss P H, Klein L 1969 The quantitative relationship of urinary peptide hydroxyproline excretion to collagen degradation. Journal of Clinical Investigation 48: 1-10

Woessner J F Jr 1962 Catabolism of collagen and non-collagen protein in the rat uterus during post-partum involution. Biochemical Journal 83: 304-314

Zak R, Martin A F, Prior G, Rabinowitz M 1977 Comparison of turnover of several myofibrillar proteins and critical evaluation of double isotope method. Journal of Biological Chemistry 252: 3430-3435

10

The collagen-platelet interaction

M. J. BARNES *

INTRODUCTION

In addition to their well-known supportive or mechanical role, collagens also exhibit a number of other important biological functions. Thus some collagens are specifically associated with basement membranes and are thought thereby to play an essential role in the filtration function and other properties of these structures. Collagens also appear to be involved in cell–cell and cell–matrix interactions important for example in development and differentiation. These aspects of collagen function will be described elsewhere in this book. In this chapter a further important role, namely the interaction of collagens with blood platelets, leading to platelet aggregation, will be considered. Collagen-induced platelet aggregation is a key event in haemostasis and is regarded as the likely cause of thrombosis, the pathological expression of the haemostatic process that frequently culminates in death through pulmonary embolism or through the occurrence of a stroke or heart attack. Collagen-induced platelet aggregation may also represent an important early event in the development of arterial plaques, the focalised vascular lesions of atherosclerosis that occlude the vessel lumen and can lead thereby to coronary heart disease, for example.

It is not the author's intention to review here in detail the earlier studies appertaining to this subject that served, in particular, to identify fibrous collagen as the active constituent of the extracellular matrix responsible for the aggregation of platelets when the latter came in contact with connective tissues. The reader is referred to various previous reviews by others (Jaffe, 1976; Gastpar et al, 1978; Beachey et al, 1979). Rather will this chapter emphasise certain aspects of the collagen-platelet interaction that have been the subject of recent work, in particular, following the recognition of the existence of a number of different, genetically-distinct, collagen subtypes, the comparative platelet reactivity of the various collagens so far identified. Relevant to this particular aspect of the subject, recent studies on the role of collagen quaternary structure in the platelet response to collagens, and of specific amino acid residues within the collagen primary structure as platelet recognition sites, will be considered. Recent knowledge of the complex sequence of events occurring in platelets in the course of their response to collagen and of the significance of these events in the context of the treatment of vascular disorders will be presented. An attempt will also be made to consider the question of platelet adhesion as a distinct, physiologically significant, response occurring independently of the aggregatory response rather than simply as a forerunner of the latter.

* Member of the External Scientific Staff of the Medical Research Council.

THE SIGNIFICANCE OF THE COLLAGEN-PLATELET INTERACTION

Haemostasis

As related below, it has long been appreciated that interaction between elements of the blood and constituents of the extracellular matrix exposed to the blood after injury to the vessel wall is of fundamental importance in initiating the haemostatic mechanism. The latter process involves not only the aggregation of platelets which serves to form the initial haemostatic plug but also the activation of the coagulation pathway. Coagulation also facilitates the arrest of bleeding. In addition, fibrin, the end-product of the coagulation sequence of reactions, acts to stabilize the platelet plug. The reader is referred to the publication edited by Thomas (1977) and the article by Zucker (1980) for a general consideration of the subject of haemostasis.

Formation of platelet aggregates as a consequence of injury to the blood vessel wall is a phenomenon the existence of which has been recognised for a century or more. For example Wharton-Jones, in 1851, studying the effect of mild injury induced by temporarily pressing a blunt point upon an artery or vein in the web of a frog's foot, observed that 'an agglomeration of colourless corpuscles . . . held together, apparently by coagulated fibrin, occurs, adheres to the wall of the vessel, and more or less completely obstructs it at the place' of injury (Wharton-Jones, 1851). It was established very much later that collagen fibres were the constituents in the extracellular matrix responsible for the induction of platelet aggregation following injury. The in vitro aggregation of platelets following addition of a suspension of collagen fibres was demonstrated around the same time (Bounameaux, 1959; Hugues, 1960; Kjaerheim & Hovig, 1962; Zucker & Borelli, 1962; Hovig, 1963).

Concomitant with the aggregatory response of platelets consequent to their exposure to collagen after injury, the coagulation mechanism, as already mentioned, is also activated and these two events, leading to the arrest of bleeding, are intimately related, the one process augmenting the other. Activation of platelets leads to the exposure or release of specific coagulation factors facilitating coagulation. Coagulation results in the formation of thrombin which not only serves to convert fibrinogen to fibrin but is also a potent platelet-aggregating agent. Its formation therefore leads to increased platelet aggregation.

In addition to its role in haemostasis through its effect on platelets, tissue collagen may directly initiate the intrinsic pathway of coagulation by the activation of factor XII (Niewiarowski et al, 1966; Wilner et al, 1968). This particular role of collagen has however been disputed (Zacharski and Rosenstein, 1977). Evidence has also been presented that collagen may initiate this pathway independently of the activation of factor XII, by the activation of platelet-associated factor XI to XIa (Walsh, 1972) but again this evidence has been questioned (Osterud, 1979). Osterud and co-workers (Osterud et al, 1977) have reported that collagen specifically increases platelet-associated factor V activity. They conclude that collagen induces conformational changes on the surface of the platelet that permits binding of plasma factor V to the platelet surface, and that the effect of collagen upon platelets also leads to the exposure of activated factor V contained within the platelets.

As related in more detail later (p. 182), the stimulation of platelets exposed to collagen leads to the secretion of a number of platelet constituents including ADP, a substance that, unlike collagen, has the ability to induce platelet aggregation directly (primary aggregation, independent of platelet secretion or prostaglandin synthesis), and also the coagulation factors, factor VIII and fibrinogen. In addition to its role in coagulation, factor VIII appears to be involved in the adhesion of platelets to collagen (see p. 192). Fibrinogen, in addition to its conversion to fibrin, also acts as an essential co-factor in primary aggregation induced by ADP, for instance (Zucker, 1980).

These inter-relationships between platelet activation and coagulation and the involvement of collagen therein are represented diagrammatically in Figure 10.1.

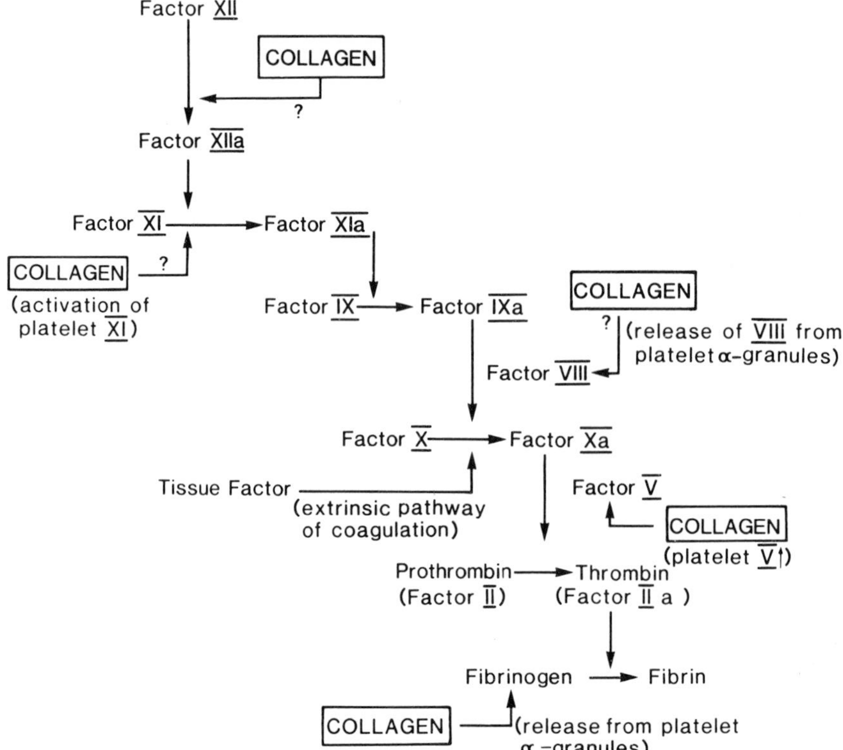

Fig. 10.1 (a) An outline of the sequence of reactions occurring during coagulation with an indication of the various places where collagen may have some involvement.

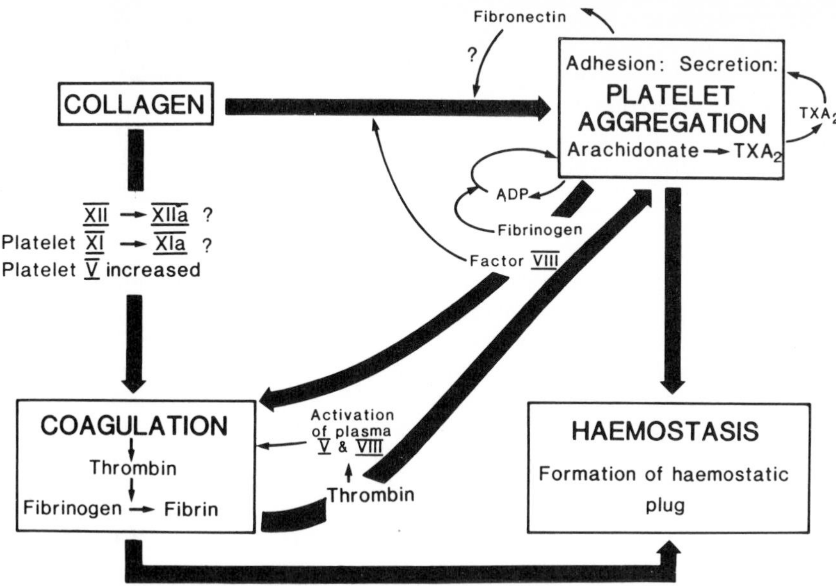

Fig. 10.1 (b) Diagrammatic illustration of the interrelationships between platelet aggregation and coagulation as occurring during haemostasis, with an indication of the nature of the collagen involvement.

Thrombosis

In addition to and arising from its role in haemostasis as indicated above, collagen(s) may also be centrally involved in thrombosis. Thrombosis can be regarded as the pathological equivalent of haemostasis: it has been described as 'haemostasis in the wrong place' (McFarlane, 1977). Stimulation of platelets by collagen is again regarded as a key event at least in some forms of the disease.

The factors involved that permit the formation of a thrombus on the surface of the vessel wall are far from being completely understood. The endothelium normally presents a non-thrombogenic surface and thrombus formation is thought to reflect alterations in this surface that may result, for example, in the exposure of underlying collagens that can thereby stimulate platelets. The relative importance in thrombosis of the basement membrane-associated collagens located in the vascular basement membrane immediately underlying the endothelium compared to the interstitial collagens located either beneath the basement membrane or immediately beneath the endothelium where the basement membrane is discontinuous or absent is, however, undefined. It is also unclear how far an alteration in normal platelet reactivity, of basement membrane for example, may be involved in the disease. Thus thrombosis may occur as a consequence of platelet interaction with a (collagenous) surface not normally exposed to platelets or from an alteration in platelet response to a surface normally only permitting adhesion but in the disease allowing aggregation.

For a wider consideration of the various aspects of thrombus formation the reader is referred to the publications edited by Thomas (1978) and Nordoy (1979) and to a short review by Wall & Harker (1980).

Atherosclerosis

The activation of platelets by vessel wall collagens has also been considered to be an important early event in atherosclerosis. As summarised by Ross and his colleagues (Ross & Glomset, 1976), the sequence of events leading to this disease is proposed as follows. Endothelial damage or denudation either as a consequence of mechanical injury, e.g. haemodynamic forces, or chemical injury, e.g. hypercholesterolaemia, results in the exposure of the underlying subendothelial connective tissue. Platelets in the circulation adhere to and become activated by collagen fibres at the site of injury. Smooth muscle cells migrate from the media into the intimal space at the site of the lesion and undergo proliferation in response to a growth factor released from the stimulated platelets. Extracellular matrix is synthesised contributing to the occlusion of the vessel lumen by the developing plaque. Plasma lipoproteins (particularly LDL) accumulate, especially in the event of repetitive injury, within the lesion which proceeds eventually to an advanced form, the complicated lesion, exhibiting calcification, ulceration and thrombus formation.

Direct experimental evidence for the involvement of platelets in the response of the vessel wall to endothelial injury has been presented. Thus experimentally-induced thrombocytopenia has been shown, in the rabbit, to inhibit the development of lesions or intimal thickening in response to endothelial injury (Moore, 1979). Also Harker and co-workers have succeeded in producing atherosclerotic lesions in primates by the use of homocysteine and were able to prevent the occurrence of these lesions by means of the anti-platelet drug dipyridimole which inhibits platelet adhesion (Wall & Harker, 1980).

Inflammation

As a consequence of stimulation by agents such as collagen, platelets are thought to be able to play a role in the acute inflammatory response following tissue trauma. Stimulated platelets release a number of specific constituents including substances regarded as mediators of inflammation, e.g. specific prostaglandins that increase vascular permeability (e.g. PGE_2) as well as other factors increasing vascular permeability and others that exhibit chemotactic activity towards polymorphonuclear neutrophils. However, the significance of platelet intervention in acute inflammation is still a question of some speculation (Nachman et al, 1972; Braunstein et al, 1980).

THE NATURE OF THE PLATELET RESPONSE TO COLLAGEN(S)

When platelets are exposed to a collagen surface, there occurs within the platelets a complex series of events, the precise relationship amongst which is still not fully understood but which culminates in platelet aggregation. These events can be studied in vitro. Aggregation can for example be examined in a platelet suspension by measuring the changes in light transmittance in an aggregometer (Born, 1962). Thus if a suspension of platelets, such as platelet-rich plasma, is mixed with a suspension of collagen fibres, aggregation rapidly ensues and there is a sharp increase in light transmittance as the platelets clump together.

Upon exposure to collagen, platelets first attach to the surface of the collagen fibre (the process of platelet adhesion). The platelets undergo a shape-change, spreading flat upon the collagen surface. Secretion of specific platelet products then follows as platelets undergo degranulation. The contents of the so-called dense granules, such as ADP and serotonin (a vasoconstrictor that thereby facilitates the haemostatic process), of the lighter α-granules, such as the platelet-derived growth factor and the coagulation factors (e.g. factor V, factor VIII, fibrinogen) already alluded to, and of the lysosomal granules, are released into the surrounding milieu. Some factors, for example fibrinogen and factor V, bind to the platelet surface altered during stimulation (Zucker, 1980).

Concomitant with these events, synthesis of the compound thromboxane A_2 (TXA_2) is induced. The interaction of collagen with the platelet surface causes the release by the platelet enzyme phospholipase A_2 (an enzyme inhibited by the steroidal anti-inflammatory drugs) of arachidonate from phospholipids occurring in platelet membranes. Arachidonate is converted by the enzyme, cyclo-oxygenase, to endoperoxides (prostaglandins G_2 and H_2) which are then converted to thromboxanes by the enzyme, thromboxane synthetase. TXA_2 is a powerful vasoconstrictor and an extremely potent platelet stimulator, causing secretion and aggregation (Moncada & Vane, 1978; Moncada & Amezcua, 1979; Mustard & Kinlough-Rathbone, 1980).

As a consequence of these events occurring within the platelets adhering to the collagen surface, other neighbouring platelets are stimulated, undergoing shape-change and the release-reaction and then attaching to each other and to the platelets already adhering to collagen (the process of platelet aggregation).

The shape-change in a suspension of stimulated platelets can generally be observed in an aggregometer as a small decrease in light transmittance immediately preceding the sharp increase that occurs as a result of aggregation (see Fig. 10.4 for example). The rate of increase in transmittance can be regarded as an indication of the rate of aggregation and the total change in transmittance as an indication of the extent of aggregation. These values are related to the concentration of the fibrous collagen (see Fig. 10.5, for example).

The relative importance of secreted ADP and the production of TXA_2 to the ultimate aggregatory process is uncertain (see Lages & Weiss, 1980). It has been maintained that the primary role of TXA_2 is the induction of secretion of ADP which serves as the direct mediator of collagen-induced aggregation (see Claesson & Malmsten, 1977). However, evidence also exists that secretion of ADP alone is not sufficient to account for all aggregation (Nunn, 1979). Furthermore TXA_2 is apparently able to induce aggregation directly in the absence of platelet secretion (Charo et al, 1977). It is also clear, however, that there exists one or more pathways of aggregation that are independent of the synthesis of TXA_2. Thus aspirin which (along with other non-steroidal anti-inflammatory drugs, e.g. indomethacin) has been shown to inhibit the enzyme cyclo-oxygenase, will prevent collagen-induced aggregation at relatively low collagen concentrations but not at higher concentrations (Kinlough-Rathbone et al, 1977; Nyman, 1977a; Best et al, 1980).

In contrast to the synthesis of TXA_2 by stimulated platelets, the vessel wall converts arachidonate to a different prostaglandin, termed PGI_2 (prostacyclin), that is a powerful vasodilator and an extremely potent inhibitor of platelet aggregation and can also cause the disaggregation of pre-existing platelet aggregates (Moncada & Vane, 1978; Moncada & Amezcua, 1979). PGI_2 is produced primarily by the endothelium (Weksler et al, 1977; MacIntyre et al,

1978; Nordoy et al, 1978; Baenziger et al, 1979). It is considered to play a crucial role in the non-thrombogenic nature of the normal endothelium (Moncada et al, 1976) and it has been proposed that disturbance in the relative levels of PGI_2 from the vessel wall on the one hand and TXA_2 from platelets on the other may be important in relation to thrombosis and atherosclerosis (Moncada & Vane, 1978; Moncada & Amezcua, 1979). In support of these views, the activity of PGI_2 has been reported to be diminished in atherosclerosis (Dembinska-Kiec et al, 1977; D'Angelo et al, 1978; Sinzinger et al, 1980). Increased platelet TXA_2 activity has been reported in some patients surviving myocardial infarction (Szczeklik et al, 1978). Increased sensitivity of platelets to TXA_2 and decreased sensitivity to PGI_2 associated with coronary artery and ischaemic heart disease has also been reported (Szczeklik et al, 1978; Mehta & Mehta, 1980). Furthermore Larrue et al, (1980) have observed a decreased formation of PGI_2 by smooth muscle cells cultured from atherosclerotic rabbit aorta in comparison to like cells from undiseased aorta. It should be noted, however, that no decrease in PGI_2 activity was observed by Mysliwiec et al (1980) in rat veins during the induction of experimental thrombosis and others have presented evidence that PGI_2 production is not a critical factor in the normal thromboresistance of the intact endothelial surface (Curwen et al, 1980; Mustard et al, 1980).

The production of PGI_2, like that of TXA_2, is aspirin-inhibited and this fact has been held to be possibly responsible for the inconclusive results with aspirin as an anti-thrombotic agent (Moncada & Amezcua, 1979; Mustard et al, 1980).

Endothelial cells are stimulated to produce PGI_2 under a number of different circumstances, e.g. in response to mechanical stimuli or to agents such as thrombin but the possible influence of collagen(s) on PGI_2 production has not so far been investigated.

THE ROLE OF COLLAGEN QUARTERNARY STRUCTURE IN PLATELET AGGREGATION

Observations made by a number of different groups all point to the same conclusion that monomeric collagen (tropocollagen) is unable to induce platelet aggregation and that some degree of polymerisation between collagen molecules is a prerequisite for aggregation to occur (Baumgartner & Muggli, 1973; Brass & Bensusan, 1974; Jaffe & Deykin, 1974; Simons et al, 1975). Exposure of tropocollagen solutions to platelet suspensions leads to aggregation of platelets only after a lag period appreciably prolonged in comparison to that observed when aggregation is induced with fibrous collagen, consistent with the notion that fibrillogenesis must precede aggregation and that its occurrence prior to aggregation is responsible for the extended lag period. The presence of inhibitors of fibrillogenesis either prevents aggregation by collagen solutions or greatly extends the lag period preceding aggregation. Perhaps the one inconsistency with the above concept of the essential role of collagen quaternary structure in platelet aggregation is the observation of Kang and his colleagues that the α1-chain from chick skin collagen (but not other collagens) and a peptide fragment, α1-CB5, derived from the chain by cyangen bromide cleavage, can induce platelet aggregation (Beachey et al, 1979). It should be noted however, that relatively high concentrations (0.1%) were required.

Although there appears little doubt then that collagen must adopt some form of quaternary structure in order to stimulate platelets to aggregate, the precise architectural requirement in terms of the degree of order needed within the polymerised structure and the minimal size of assembly that can induce aggregation are still questions of some uncertainty. The interstitial collagens (types I, II, and III) are known to form highly-ordered aggregates in vivo yielding fibrils with a characteristic banding pattern (as observed by electron microscopy) of 67 nm periodicity arising from the unipolar, 'quarter-staggered' assembly of the molecules within the fibril (Fig. 10.2). This native-type fibril can be formed in vitro from tropocollagen solutions by incubation at 37°C for example or by dialysis against 0.02M disodium hydrogen phosphate and is a potent inducer of platelet aggregation. However other ordered molecular assemblies can be produced in vitro, segment-long-spacing (SLS) polymers for example in which the collagen molecules align alongside in a 'head-to-head' and 'tail-to-tail' arrangement (Fig. 10.2) or alternatively, the fibrous long spacing (FLS) form in which there is end-to-end aggregation of molecules laterally associated in a 'head-to-tail' alignment as indicated in Figure 10.2. These different structures have also been found to be able to induce platelet aggregation thus implying that the native-

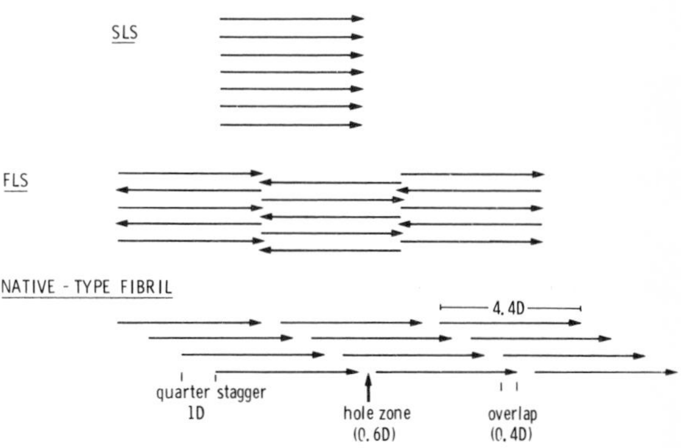

Fig. 10.2 Diagrammatic illustration of the various ordered assemblies of the collagen molecule as occurring in the native-type fibril (of interstitial collagens), segment-long-spacing aggregates (SLS) and fibrous-long-spacing aggregates (FLS).

type quaternary structure is not an essential requirement for aggregation (Muggli, 1978; Wang et al, 1978a; Barnes & MacIntyre, 1979a; Barnes et al, 1980; Santoro & Cunningham, 1980).

The same conclusion has been reached by Balleisen et al (1976), who produced a variety of active fibrillar products from type I tropocollagen by chemical modification of the molecule prior to inducing fibrillogenesis by suitable procedures. Furthermore the platelet aggregation produced by non-striated fibrils of type I collagen (Muggli, 1978), of type IV collagen (Barnes et al, 1980) and of vitreous collagen (Swann et al, 1974), fibrils in which presumably the molecules are randomly associated, suggests that a high degree of order in assembly is not an absolute requirement for aggregation. This notion is supported by the data of Santoro & Cunningham (1980), who demonstrated that tropocollagen, randomly cross-linked with glutaraldehyde to yield an amorphous precipitate, could induce platelet aggregation. The latter authors propose that the collagen-platelet interaction involves the participation of multiple sites on the platelet surface interacting simultaneously with an equivalent number of sites on the collagen surface which are not necessarily displayed in any specific repetitive pattern but which are contained within the confines of a specific topography defined by the collagen quaternary structure and fixed by virtue of the rigidity (arising from the quaternary structure) of the collagenous surface presented to the platelet. Santoro & Cunningham suggest that the degree of specificity between individual sites on platelet and collagen surfaces may be relatively low, the specificity being governed more by the need for multiple interactions. This can only be met, in view of the rigidity of the collagen fibre surface, as a result of the flexibility of the opposing platelet surface, allowing the platelet to alter its shape and spread over the fibre thereby permitting multiple interactions over a wide area between platelet and collagen surfaces. Similar thoughts have been expressed by Wang et al (1978b) and by the author and his colleagues (Gordon, 1979; Barnes et al, 1980).

It should be noted that not all forms of collagen aggregates can stimulate platelets. Thus collagen precipitated in amorphous form by addition of salt to acid solutions is inactive (Katzman et al, 1973; Jaffe & Deykin, 1974; Barnes et al, 1976a; Wang et al, 1978a; Santoro & Cunningham, 1980).

Of particular interest in the context of the preceding discussion is the observation of Meyer and his colleagues (Meyer, 1980) that tropocollagen, when attached to fine glass fibres, can induce platelet aggregation. Aggregation will only occur when the fibre diameter is less than that of the platelet. They reach conclusions entirely compatible with those advanced above, namely that as regards the ability to induce platelet aggregation the physical geometry of the collagen surface (i.e. its precise curvature) is highly important but that the degree of order of assembly of individual collagen molecules within fibres is very much less so.

As regards the question of the minimal size of assembly of collagen molecules required to produce platelet aggregation some studies (e.g. Muggli & Baumgartner, 1973) have suggested aggregation by very small fibrils (microfibrils) of the type that are found early in the course of fibrillogenesis and which occur before any increase in opacity of collagen solutions undergoing fibrillogenesis can be detected (Williams et al, 1978; Gelman et al, 1979). Wang et al (1978a) have presented evidence that a minimal fibril length equivalent to the length of three collagen molecules is required to initiate aggregation. Single bundles of SLS polymers (equivalent to one molecular length) are inactive. In the author's studies with SLS forms (Barnes & MacIntyre, 1979a; Barnes et al, 1980), SLS preparations were cross-linked with formaldehyde to stabilise the polymeric structure prior to the removal of ATP by dialysis. This yielded end-to-end assembly of SLS bundles (F–SLS) (see Fig. 10.6) and we consider in sympathy with the data of Wang et al (1978a) that it may have been this type of SLS structure that caused platelet aggregation.

Kronick & Jimenez (1980) have suggested that the aggregation induced by polymers appearing before any detectable change in turbidity is due to the presence of a few large striated fibrils amongst the non-striated microfibrils. They showed that the latter were unable to induce platelet aggregation. Small collagen polymers (sedimenting at a sendimentation coefficient as low as 4.5S) were however able to bind to platelets.

Although various types of collagen polymer can aggregate platelets, it seems likely that the native-type fibril of 67nm periodicity represents the optimum molecular configuration. The most active preparation the author has tested is a highly polymerised but highly dispersed preparation of native-type fibres obtained directly from bovine flexor tendon (kindly donated by Ethicon Inc., Somerville, New Jersey, USA), active at around 0.2 μg/ml (Barnes et al, 1980; also see Fig. 10.5). Comparisons are, however, difficult to make because not only the type of aggregation but also its extent has to be considered. The important factor may be the fibre surface area relative to collagen mass rather than collagen concentration directly, and this will depend on the actual state of aggregation. Kronick & Jimenez (198O) indicate there is an optimum state of aggregation corresponding to a polymer species with a sedimentation co-efficient of around 10^5S.

COLLAGEN POLYMORPHISM IN RELATION TO PLATELET AGGREGATION

So far in this chapter the term collagen has been used generally in the sense of referring to a single entity.

However it is now well established that collagen exists as a number of separate, genetically-distinct subtypes, the interstitial collagens, types I, II and III, the basement membrane collagen, type IV and the as yet unclassified type V collagen (see Ch. 1). With the realisation of the existence of different collagens, their comparative platelet reactivity became a question of some importance, especially in the context of their particular contribution to haemostasis and vascular disorders.

Collagen polymorphism in the blood vessel wall

Since the original observations of Chung & Miller (1974) and of Trelstad (1974), several groups have reported on the presence of both collagen types I and III in the walls of large arteries and their distribution within the tissue has been examined by immunofluorescent techniques. The blood vessel wall appears to contain relatively large amounts of type III in comparison to most other connective tissues. In the media, type III appears to be closely associated with the surfaces of the elastic laminae, whilst type I appears more to fill the spaces between these structures (Gay et al, 1975; McCullagh et al, 1980). In the young blood vessel wall where little if any intimal thickening has occurred and the intima is likely to consist of little more than the endothelium with underlying basement membrane, type III has been reported to be present without any type I in the space immediately between the endothelium and the internal elastic lamina. This had led to the suggestion that this type of collagen might therefore be of especial importance in thrombosis (Gay et al, 1975). However, in the older vessel, there is appreciable diffuse intimal thickening and in this case collagen type I generally occurs in greater amount than type III (Morton & Barnes, 1982) as is also the case in the intimal atherosclerotic fibrous plaque (McCullagh & Balian, 1975; Morton & Barnes, 1982). The medial smooth muscle cell has been shown by several groups to be the source of these two collagens in the media (Barnes et al, 1976; Burke et al, 1977; Layman et al, 1977; Rauterberg et al, 1977; Scott et al, 1977; Mayne et al, 1978). Their origin in the intima is perhaps less certain. Endothelial cells are likely, it may be thought, to synthesise only basement membrane-associated collagens (Howard et al, 1976; Jaffe et al, 1976). However they have also been shown to synthesise collagens types I and III at least in culture (Barnes et al, 1978; Sage et al, 1979).

As regards basement membrane collagen, Trelstad (1974) has reported the detection by biochemical analysis of type IV in human aorta.

Type V collagen is generally regarded as containing two types of α chain, the A and B chains (see Ch. 2). In the aorta, Miller and his colleagues (Chung et al, 1976) have reported on the presence of B chains only in the media. In the intima they found neither A nor B chains but a collagenous-type peptide of 55 000 daltons (after reduction of disulphide bonds), the origin of which is uncertain but is thought to be derived from basement membrane structures (presumably the subendothelial basement membrane). In contrast, the author has detected both A and B chains in both intima and media, in a ratio of approximately 1:2 (Morton & Barnes, 1982). This collagen appears to be at a relatively high concentration in the diffusely thickened intima and particularly abundant in the atherosclerotic plaque. Immunofluorescent studies employing an antibody raised against a type V preparation containing A and B chains in a ratio of approximately 1:2 have also detected type V collagen in the intima and media (McCullagh et al, 1980).

Type V collagen is known to occur, at least in some locations, in close association with a basement membrane. The author has detected its synthesis (as B_2A) in relatively small amounts by both endothelial and smooth muscle cells in culture (Barnes M. J. and Sankey E. A., unpublished data). Others have reported on the synthesis of type V collagen by smooth muscle cells, along with a collagenous peptide of 45 000 daltons, the origin of which is uncertain (Mayne et al, 1978).

This section has only briefly reviewed collagen polymorphism in the vessel wall since the topic will be covered in more detail elsewhere in this book by Dr R. K. Rhodes (p. 376). It should suffice however to indicate that the type of collagen exposed by injury to the vessel wall could vary depending upon the precise nature of the injury and that it follows that the platelet response to vessel wall injury will depend upon the platelet reactivity of the particular collagen(s) exposed.

Platelet reactivity of interstitial collagens

A number of different groups have now made a comparison of the activity of collagens type I and III towards platelets and there is general agreement that when these two collagens are presented to platelets in solution, type III is very much more active than type I at inducing platelet aggregation (Balleisen et al, 1975; Barnes et al, 1976; Hugues et al, 1976; Santoro & Cunningham, 1977). However, if solutions are first treated by procedures known to induce the formation of native-type fibrils of 67 nm periodity, e.g. by incubation at 37°C either in platelet-poor-plasma or a phosphate buffer or by dialysis at 4°C against 0.02M disodium hydrogen phosphate, then the lag period preceding platelet aggregation is greatly reduced, the potency of each collagen type is very much enhanced and there is little if any difference in activity between the two collagens (Balleisen et al, 1975; Barnes et al, 1976a; Santoro & Cunningham, 1977). These observations, exemplified in Figures 10.3 and 10.4 are entirely consistent with the concept already considered, that collagen must be in fibrillar form to induce platelet aggregation. The reason for the much greater activity of type III collagen relative to

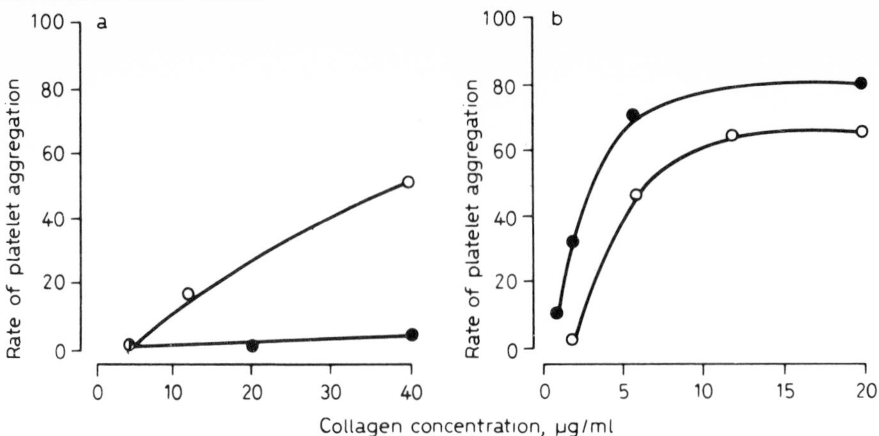

Fig. 10.3 Platelet aggregation by collagens types I and III from chick skin. Platelet aggregation was measured in 0.1 ml samples of human citrated platelet-rich plasma by observing changes in optical density following the addition of known amounts of collagen. The rate of aggregation was obtained from the maximum rate of change in light transmission. (a) Platelet responses following addition of collagen in solution (10 µl or less) in 0.1M acetic acid. Open circles = type III; closed circles, type I. (b) Responses following addition of collagen in fibrillar suspension. Collagen solutions were preincubated with an equal volume of cell-free plasma. (From Barnes et al 1976a Biochemical Journal 160: 647 with permission)

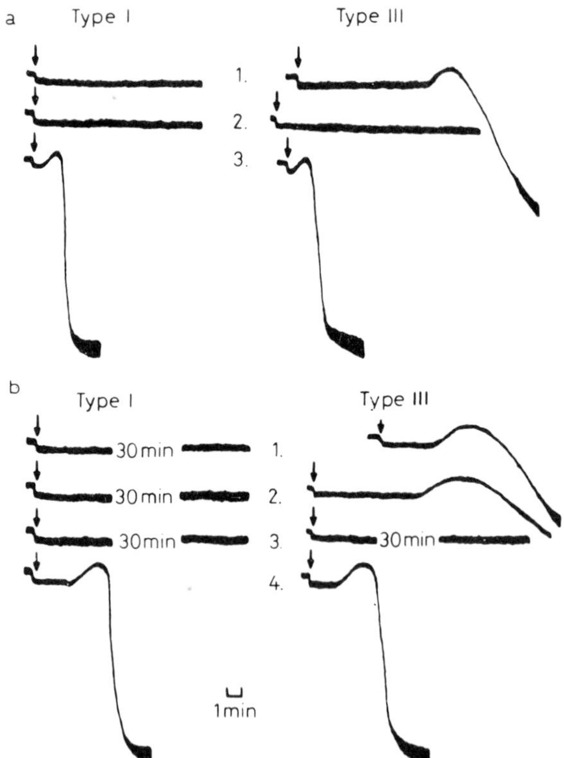

Fig. 10.4a and b Platelet aggregation by collagens types I and III from human aorta and chick skin. Platelet aggregation was measured as described in Figure 10.3. The traces shown represent actual changes in optical transmission following addition of collagen (at the arrow) to a final concentration of 20 µg/ml.

(a) Chick collagen. (1) Addition of collagen in solution in 0.1 M acetic acid. (2) Addition after preincubation in an equal volume of 0.9% sodium chloride; treatment under these conditions yields inactive precipitates. (3) After preincubation in 0.38M disodium hydrogen phosphate or cell-free plasma; preincubation under these conditions yields highly potent native-type fibrils.

(b) Human collagens: (1) As (a) 1. (2) Addition of collagen after preincubation in an equal volume of cell-free plasma; the results suggest an inhibitor of human collagen fibrillogenesis in human plasma. (3) After preincubation in an equal volume of 0.9% sodium chloride (4) After preincubation in an equal volume of 0.38M disodium hydrogen phosphate. (From Barnes et al 1976a Biochemical Journal 160: 647 with permission) that of type I when presented to platelets as a solution is unclear but presumably reflects a much more ready tendency for pepsin-isolated type III to form fibrils in the platelet-rich plasma, than pepsin-treated type I. Because of the much greater activity of type III collagen, in solution form, it was originally proposed that activity in type I preparations might in fact be due to the presence of type III as a contaminant and that type I itself had no activity towards platelets (Hugues et al, 1976). However this view seems untenable when it is considered that the two collagens in fibrillar form display a comparable order of activity. The intrinsic activity of type I collagen is borne out by the observation that the collagen $[\alpha 1(I)]_3$ prepared by isolation of $\alpha 1(I)$ chains by chromatography (which ensures removal of all type III chains) and renaturation of the isolated chains, is able to adhere to platelets (Fauvel et al, 1978a) and induce aggregation (Balleisen et al, 1976). Furthermore the use of monospecific antibodies to inhibit the collagen-platelet interaction has confirmed the activity of type I collagen (Balleisen et al, 1979). In any event it has been demonstrated that type II collagen fibrils can induce platelet aggregation (Balleisen et al, 1975), as is also the case for types IV and V collagens (see below) and it is therefore now well established that any collagen type, if in appropriate fibrillar form, will exhibit platelet activity.

The author concludes that in the blood vessel wall, types I and III collagens are both likely to be extremely potent inducers of platelet aggregation.

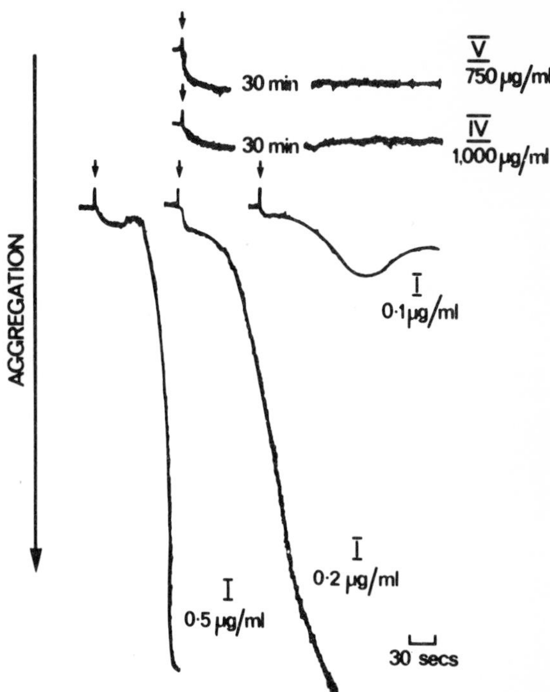

Fig. 10.5 Lack of platelet aggregation by collagens type IV (from bovine anterior lens capsule) and type V (from human placenta). Solutions were first preincubated for 30 min at 37°C in an equal volume of platelet-poor-plasma in an attempt to encourage fibrillogenesis prior to testing at the concentration specified. For comparison the aggregatory activity (at the concentrations indicated) of type I collagen as native type fibrils (isolated directly as such from bovine tendon) is shown. The point of addition of sample to platelets is indicated by an arrow. (From Barnes et al 1980 Thrombosis Research 18: 375 with permission)

Platelet reactivity of types IV and V collagens

In preliminary studies to investigate the possible platelet reactivity of collagens types IV and V, the author and his colleagues observed that solutions of type IV (from bovine anterior lens capsules) or type V (from human placenta or bovine lung parenchyma) revealed no platelet aggregatory activity (Barnes & MacIntyre, 1979a and b). This was true even if solutions were first subjected to procedures known in the case of the interstitial collagens to yield highly-potent fibrils of 67 nm periodicity, such as incubation at 37°C or dialysis at 4°C against low ionic strength phosphate buffer. Activity was absent even if concentrations as high as 1mg/ml were tested. This contrasts with the marked activity of type I fibres from bovine tendon at a concentration as low as 0.2 µg/ml (Fig. 10.5). Furthermore no activity could be detected in dispersions of whole lens capsule containing 'intact' type IV collagen. Trelstad & Carvalho (1979) observed the same phenomenon. However it has become increasingly apparent (see for example, Trelstad & Lawley, 1977) that these collagens fail, under standard in vitro conditions, to form fibrils comparable to those of types I, II and III collagens (of 67 nm periodicity). In view of the known importance of the quaternary structure of collagen in relation to its ability to induce platelet aggregation (p. 183), we decided to attempt to produce from solutions of types IV and V collagens other polymeric structures of defined nature, namely SLS structures (see Fig. 10.2). We found (Barnes & MacIntyre, 1979a; Barnes et al, 1980) that both collagens types IV and V produced SLS polymers when dialysed against an acidic solution of ATP (Fig. 10.6). These forms proved to be able, like those of type I, to induce platelet aggregation (Fig. 10.7). Prior to testing for platelet activity, it was necessary to remove ATP (since this inhibits the platelet reaction) and therefore SLS structures were first stabilised by cross-linking with formaldelyde before removing ATP by dialysis. This procedure yielded assemblies or aggregates of SLS bundles (F–SLS) (see Fig. 10.6) which we consider may be the active species of SLS forms inducing platelet aggregation. Some degree of variation we observed in platelet activity of different batches of SLS preparations is probably related to a variable degree of association of SLS bundles to yield F–SLS structures.

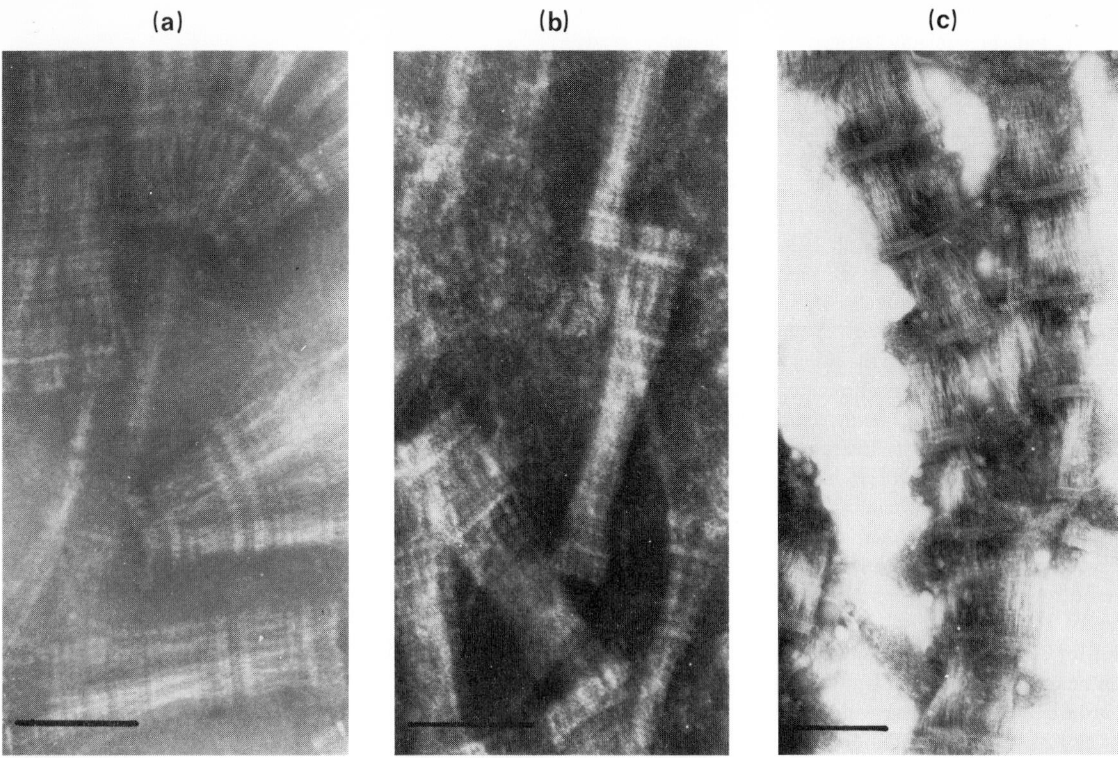

Fig. 10.6 Electron micrographs of SLS aggregates of (a) type V (b) type IV and (c) type I collagen from human placenta. The type I preparation was examined after treatment with the cross-linking agent formaldehyde and shows the end-to-end polymerisation of SLS aggregates into F–SLS form resulting from this treatment. SLS aggregates of types IV and V collagens showed similar end-to-end polymerisation when treated with formaldehyde. The bar represents O.1 μm in (a) and (b) and 0.25 μm in (c). From Barnes et al 1980 Thrombosis Research 18: 375 with permission)

We were subsequently able to produce from type V solutions fibrils of 67 nm periodicity (Fig. 10.8) by prolonged dialysis at 25°C against 0.9 per cent sodium chloride adjusted to pH 7.2 with sodium hydroxide. These fibrils were also active at inducing platelet aggregation (Barnes et al, 1980), with an order of activity comparable to that of type I fibrils produced by the same procedure (Fig. 10.9). Solutions of type IV collagen from human placenta (but not apparently from bovine lung or bovine anterior lens capsule) when dialysed against 0.02M disodium hydrogen phosphate at 4°C produced a variable quantity of non-striated fibrils (Fig. 10.8) which, as shown in Figure 10.9, proved to be potent inducers of platelet aggregation (Barnes et al, 1980). It was thus apparent that when collagens types IV and V were presented to platelets in appropriate fibrillar form, they could elicit platelet aggregation. The platelet reactivity of type V collagen fibres of 67 nm periodicity has also been reported by Chiang et al (1980). Clearly the quaternary structure of collagen is the over-riding factor in defining the platelet activity of collagen rather than collagen type as such.

Although from the foregoing it is clear that types IV and V collagens can induce platelet aggregation when exposed to platelets in a suitable fibrillar structure, it is still uncertain how far basement membranes in vivo exhibit this activity. Basement membranes are generally regarded as amophorous structures and certainly do not contain fibrils of 67 nm periodicity akin to those of the interstitial collagens. The author and his colleagues (Barnes et al, 1980) and Hudson and his associates (Freytag et al, 1978) have both found no platelet aggregatory activity with dispersions of intact bovine anterior lens capsules, containing type IV collagen in situ. However there is uncertainty as regards the platelet reactivity of glomerular and other basement membranes. Benditt and his co-workers (Huang et al, 1974; Huang & Benditt, 1978) have reported that these structures (from humans) permit platelet adhesion (discussed in greater detail later) but not aggregation. They attributed the adhesive properties to a non-collagenous constituent of the membranes. Suresh et al (1973) found neither aggregatory nor adhesive activity with rabbit heart valve basement membrane. Weak aggregatory activity reported for glomerular and tubular basement membranes in earlier studies (Hugues & Mahieu, 1970; Ts'ao, 1971) was attributed by Benditt (Huang et al, 1974) to the presence of contaminating interstitial collagen fibrils.

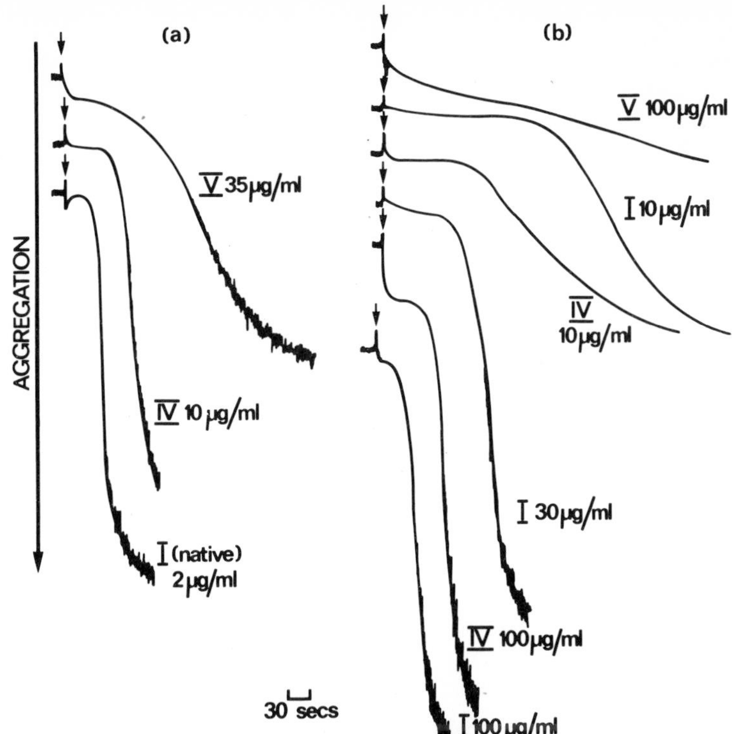

Fig. 10.7 Platelet aggregation by SLS polymers of collagens types I, IV and V. The results of two separate experiments are shown. Activity was measured at the concentrations specified. (a) Aggregation by SLS forms of types IV and V collagens (from human placenta) and by native-type fibrils of type I (from bovine tendon). (b) Aggregation by SLS forms of type IV and V collagens from human placenta and type I from rat tail tendons (SLS aggregates of type I collagen from human placenta behaved similarly to those of type I from rat tendon). (From Barnes et al 1980 Thrombosis Research 18: 375 with permission)

However, Hudson and his group (see Freytag et al, 1978) have provided evidence that bovine glomerular basement membranes have genuine platelet aggregating activity. This activity appears to be partly attributable to a non-collagenous constituent and partly to a collagenous component of the membrane. It should be noted however that the activity related to the collagenous constituent (isolated by enzymic treatment to remove the non-collagenous moiety) was only exhibited after a very appreciable lag period during which fibril formation may have been proceeding and such activity in the intact membrane may be absent.

The platelet reactivity of basement membrane in vivo, especially of vascular basement membrane, is a vital question in relation to thrombosis and the subject will be discussed further in the next section of this chapter.

PLATELET ADHESION

Platelet aggregation, of course, is unable to occur without prior platelet adhesion to or interaction with a stimulating agent such as collagen. In this section, it is intended to consider some of the factors related to adhesion and to consider in some measure the question of how far adhesion can be regarded as an event in its own right separate from aggregation, and able to occur sometimes in vivo in the absence of the latter.

Adhesion to the subendothelium

It has already been stressed that the intact endothelium presents a non-thrombogenic surface to the circulating blood. It is clear, however, that if for any reason the endothelium is disturbed and the immediate subendothelial surface thereby exposed, circulating platelets can interact with that surface. Furthermore the attachment of platelets may not necessarily lead to aggregation (or thrombus formation). Thus Tranzer & Baumgartner (1967) have observed the attachment of platelets to subendothelium filling gaps in between capillary endothelial cells induced by use of the reagent reserpine. Several other studies have also indicated similar adherence of platelets to the subendothelial surface (Majno & Palade, 1961; Movat & Fernando, 1963; Tranzer et al, 1968; Ts'ao & Glagov, 1970; Schwartz & Benditt, 1973). It has been considered that this attachment of platelets where the endothelium is interrupted may be of physiological significance, assisting in the maintenance of vascular integrity.

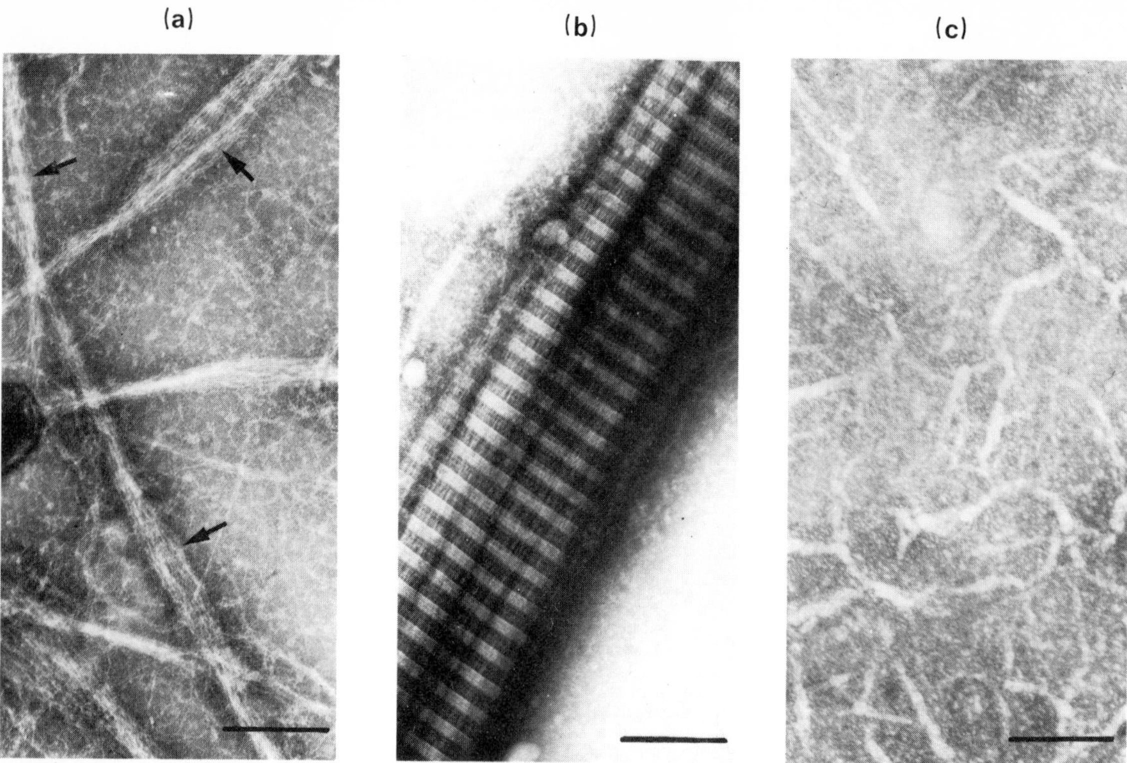

Fig. 10.8 (a) and (b) Electron micrograph of fibrils of type V collagen (from human placenta) obtained by dialysis of a solution against physiological saline at 25°C. Some fibrils appeared 'loosely-formed' with striations just becoming visible (as in (a) where examples are arrowed) whilst others appeared (as in (b)) with well-defined striations comparable to the native-type fibril of the interstitial collagens, with a 67 nm periodicity. (c) Non-striated fibrils of type IV collagen (from human placenta) formed by dialysis of a solution against 0.02M disodium hydrogen phosphate. The bar represents 0.25 μm. (From Barnes et al 1980 Thrombosis Research 18: 375 with permission)

Baumgartner and his colleagues (Baumgartner & Muggli, 1976) have made extensive studies of the interaction between platelets and the subendothelium following removal of the endothelium experimentally with a balloon catheter. They observed that platelets initially aggregated to a small degree on the exposed surface. Aggregates rapidly dispersed however leaving essentially a monolayer of platelets covering the surface. This adhesion they regarded as occurring to the basement membrane immediately underlying the endothelium. Others have considered elastin or microfibrillar elements associated with elastin to be involved (Stemerman, 1974). However adhesion studies in vitro with isolated constituents has revealed little if any adhesion to the microfibrillar protein and only slight adhesion to elastin (Ordinas et al, 1975; Barnes & MacIntyre, 1979a). Baumgartner & Muggli (1976) have observed that the interaction of platelets with interstitial collagen fibres exposed by treatment of the subendothelial surface with chymotrypsin leads to marked platelet aggregation but the total amount of adhesion i.e. the surface coverage with platelets is actually reduced in comparison to that occurring (to the basement membrane) before enzyme treatment.

The possible involvement of basement membrane and type V collagens in the adhesion of platelets to subendothelium is still uncertain. As already stated, Benditt and co-workers (Huang et al, 1974; Huang & Benditt, 1978) have demonstrated platelet adhesion to human glomerular basement membrane but present evidence that the adhesion is due to a non-collagenous glycoprotein constitutent of the membrane. In contrast, Freytag et al (1978) have reported that the collagenous component, at least in part, contributes to the adhesion (and aggregation) of platelets interacting with bovine glomerular basement membrane. The data of Barnes et al (1980) and Chiang et al (1980) clearly indicate that type IV and V collagens have the potential to interact with platelets. The possible interaction of these collagens with platelets in vivo and the question of whether an alteration in their platelet reactivity may be relevant to thrombosis, or whether thrombus formation is entirely attributable to interaction of platelets with interstitial collagens, remain important issues.

Platelet adhesion to the subendothelium and to collagen fibres appears very much less sensitive to inhibition by aspirin than platelet aggregation (Muggli et al, 1980;

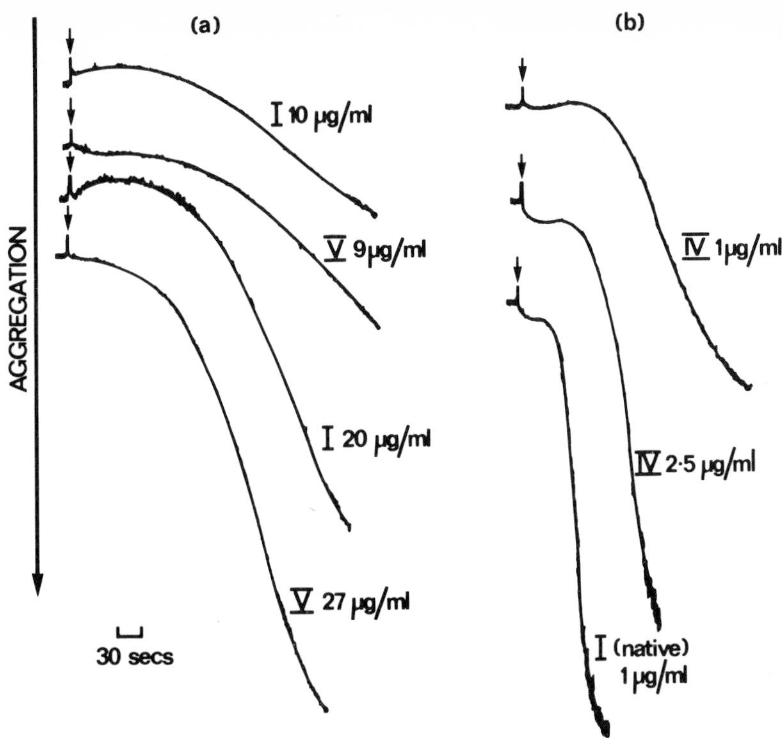

Fig. 10.9 Platelet aggregation by: (a) type I and type V collagen fibrils of 67 nm periodicity formed by dialysis of solutions of these collagens from human placenta against physiological saline at 25°C; (b) non-striated fibrils of type IV collagen (from human placenta) formed by dialysis at 4°C of a solution against 0.02M disodium hydrogen phosphate compared to native-type fibrils of type I (from bovine tendon). Activity was measured at the concentrations specified. (From Barnes et al 1980 Thrombosis Research 18: 375 with permission)

Kinlough-Rathbone et al, 1980). The same is also true for inhibition by PGI_2 and indeed it has been suggested that the production of PGI_2 may serve to permit platelet adhesion to the subendothelium without attendant aggregation (Moncada & Amezcua, 1979). These observations it may be thought, again serve to emphasize the different mechanisms operating in adhesion and aggregation.

The role of carbohydrate in the adhesion of platelets to collagen

It was originally proposed by Jamieson and his colleagues (Jamieson et al, 1971) that the interaction between platelets and collagen was mediated by the formation of an enzyme-substrate complex between the enzyme collagen glucosyltransferase on the platelet membrane and galactosylhydroxylysyl residues in collagen. However, this hypothesis has now been largely discounted for various reasons (Santoro & Cunningham, 1977; Leunis et al, 1980), particularly since only a very small proportion of the platelet enzyme is associated with the membrane and, most importantly, because the enzyme can only utilise denatured collagen as a substrate and does not interact with collagen in triple helical configuration (Menashi & Grant, 1979).

Chick skin collagen may again represent an exception (see p. 183) since the platelet aggregatory activity detected with α1-chains isolated from chick skin type I collagen appears to be associated with the carbohydrate moiety in the peptide α1–CB5 derived from the α1-chains by cyanogen bromide digestion (Beachey et al, 1979).

The collagen quaternary structure in relation to platelet adhesion

It has already been emphasised that collagen quaternary structure is of paramount importance in governing the platelet aggregatory activity of all collagens so far examined. Studies by a number of different groups indicate that it may be equally important in adhesion. Gordon & Dingle (1974), Barnes & MacIntyre (1979a) and Kronick & Jimenez (1980) have all found that tropocollagen, in contrast to fibrous collagen, does not bind to platelets. Fauvel et al (1978a) and Barnes & MacIntyre (1979a) have reported that types I and III collagens in fibrillar form bind to platelets with approximately the same affinity. However all these investigations utilised separation techniques such as centrifugation or chromatography which, in the event that the interaction between tropocollagen and platelets is relatively weak, might have prevented the detection of such an interaction. Santoro & Cunningham (1977) observed that tropocollagen did not inhibit the interaction between collagen fibres and platelets and also reached the conclusion, therefore, that tropocollagen does not adhere to platelets. In contrast, Meyer and colleagues (Meyer & Weissman, 1978; Meyer, 1980) have shown that platelets adhere to soluble (non-fibrillar) collagen coated to a flat glass surface. Adhesion was much less than to fibrils but was rather greater than to the uncoated glass surface. The adhesion to soluble collagen was unaccompanied by aggregation and these studies can again perhaps be seen to support the notion that interaction between platelets and collagen without attendant platelet aggregation may be a phenomenon that can occur in vivo.

Collagen primary structure and platelet adhesion

Although it has been stressed that the collagen quaternary structure is important in the interaction with platelets in creating perhaps an essential spatial relationship between the collagen fibre and the platelet, this is not to deny that particular chemical groupings exposed to the platelets within the confines of the specific architecture or geometry of the quaternary structure are involved in the platelet interaction. The proposed role of carbohydrate has already been discussed. Several investigations recently have attempted to define the chemical specificity of collagen in relation to the platelet reaction. Wang et al (1978b) have emphasised the importance of collagen arginyl residues and Santoro & Cunningham (1979) of collagen amino-groups. In contrast, the adhesion studies of Meyer and co-workers (Meyer, 1980) have led them to the conclusion that the relatively high content of proline and hydroxyproline represents the important specific chemical feature of the collagen molecule that distinguishes it from other platelet activators. The studies of Caen and his colleagues (Fauvel et al, 1978a and b) have implicated particular sequences of amino acids in adhesion, a sequence from the C-terminal end of the molecule in the case of type I collagen and from the central region of the molecule in the case of type III. There does not at present appear to be any obvious structural relationship between these two regions.

The role of fibronectin in platelet adhesion

Fibronectin is known to be involved in cell adhesion and to interact with collagen (Yamada & Olden, 1978; see also p. 000). It was therefore a protein that could be regarded as likely to have a role in the collagen-platelet interaction particularly since it is known to occur in platelets, and to be released in part on platelet stimulation (Zucker et al, 1979a). Bensusan and his colleagues have proposed that fibronectin does mediate the interaction between collagen and platelets mainly because they could detect the protein attached to collagen following sonication of a mixture of collagen and platelets, and also because preincubation of collagen with fibronectin inhibited the collagen-platelet interaction (Bensusan et al, 1978).

However fibronectin interacts more strongly with denatured collagen than native collagen in triple helical configuration. Evidence has also been presented that it is located in the α-granules (Zucker et al, 1979) and not on the surface of platelets (Hynes et al, 1978). For these and other reasons, such as the failure of anti-fibronectin antibody to reduce adhesion to any great extent or high concentrations of gelatin to inhibit aggregation (Santoro & Cunningham, 1979), the view has been taken that fibronectin is unlikely to be involved in any major way in mediating the collagen-platelet interaction. It should be noted however that Bensusan et al (1978) state that the fibronectin they obtained from platelets bound to collagen fibres but not to gelatin.

The role of factor VIII related-antigen in platelet adhesion

The protein factor VIII/von Willebrand factor (F VIII/VWF), occurs in both plasma and in the α-granules of platelets from which it is in part released following stimulation of platelets by collagen (Sultan et al, 1979; Zucker et al, 1979b). The plasma constituent is undoubtedly required for haemostasis since defective haemostasis in von Willebrand's disease due to a deficiency of F VIII/VWF can be corrected by an infusion of normal plasma but not of normal platelets (see Sultan et al, 1978). It is considered the platelet protein may serve to bind factor VIII coagulant activity (antihaemophiliac factor) and thereby facilitate the activation of factor X in the coagulation mechanism (see Zucker et al, 1979).

The defect in haemostasis in von Willebrand's disease appears to be due to diminished platelet adhesion. Baumgartner and his colleagues have observed that adhesion of platelets to the subendothelium and to collagen fibres is defective in von Willebrand's disease (Baumgartner et al, 1977) and that adhesion examined at blood flow rates operating normally in the microvasculative is almost completely abolished by anti-F VIII/VWF antibodies (Baumgartner et al, 1980).

Baugh et al (1979) have shown that F VIII/VWF enhances the platelet aggregatory activity of collagen fibres. Other studies have indicated that a binding between collagen and F VIII/VWF can occur (Nyman, 1977, 1980; Legrand et al, 1978). This is clearly an area that warrants further investigation particularly in the context of collagen polymorphism and quaternary structure.

Platelet membrane receptors

The protein(s) in the platelet membrane interacting with collagen(s) has yet to be defined with certainty. Meyer and his colleagues (Meyer, 1980) have reported that the three major platelet surface glycoproteins (GPI, II and III) are not involved. Lahav (see Meyer, 1980) by employing affinity chromatography techniques has detected a membrane constituent of 80 000 daltons that exhibits a high affinity for collagen.

SUMMARY

The aggregation of blood platelets following their exposure to collagen fibres in the blood vessel wall as a result of tissue injury is a central event in the haemostatic mechanism, resulting in the formation of the initial haemostatic plug. Concomitantly with platelet aggregation, coagulation occurs resulting in the formation of fibrin that serves to reinforce the platelet plug besides assisting the arrest of bleeding through coagulation. In addition to its role in the induction of platelet aggregation, collagen may also influence the coagulation process either by direct activation of the intrinsic pathway of coagulation or indirectly through its effect on platelets leading to the release or exposure of platelet-held coagulation factors which may subsequently appear on the platelet surface, able to contribute to the coagulation process. Collagen-induced platelet aggregation is also thought to be involved in thrombosis, the pathological expression of the haemostatic mechanism and may be an important early event in atherosclerosis.

Upon exposure to collagen, platelets adhere to the surface of the fibre, release specific constituents such as ADP and produce the substance thromboxane A_2 (TXA_2). Both ADP and TXA_2 are considered to play a vital role in the stimulation of neighbouring non-adherent platelets, leading to the attachment of such platelets to each other and to those already adhering to the collagen surface (the process of platelet aggregation). Prostacyclin (PGI_2) produced by the vessel wall is a potent inhibitor of platelet aggregation and it is considered a delicate balance may exist between the production of PGI_2 and TXA_2, disturbance of which may be important in the context of thrombosis and atherosclerosis.

The blood vessel wall is known to contain a number of different collagens and with the recognition of collagen polymorphism, the relative platelet reactivity of the different collagen subtypes has become a question of importance. The conclusion has been reached that collagen quaternary structure rather than collagen type per se is the important factor that determines the ability of collagen to aggregate platelets. Thus all collagens so far examined including the interstitial collagens types I, II and III and collagens, types IV and V, have been shown to induce aggregation if presented to platelets in appropriate fibrillar form. The precise requirement related to the quaternary structure in terms of the actual degree of order necessary in the assembly of collagen molecules or the minimal size of polymer needed to induce aggregation is unclear. However it has been shown that the native-type fibril of 67 nm periodicity characteristic of the interstitial collagen types is not an obligatory structural requirement. Thus aggregation has also been observed with non-striated collagen fibrils. Nevertheless, the former fibrillar structure generally appears the most effective one.

Although types IV and V collagens undoubtedly possess the ability potentially to induce the aggregation of platelets, it is not clear that these collagens normally occur in vivo in a fibrillar configuration suitable to permit such a response. They may be involved rather in the adhesion of platelets, without aggregation, when the latter, for instance attack subendothelial surface exposed following removal of loss of the vascular endothelium. This attachment is thought to be of importance in assisting the maintenance of vascular integrity and to involve the basement membrane immediately underlying the endothelium. The relative importance in thrombosis (involving platelet aggregation) of basement membrane-associated collagens (presumably of altered platelet reactivity if the contention that they normally only permit adhesion is correct) compared to the interstitial collagens remains uncertain.

The proposed role of fibronectin in mediating the adhesion of platelets to collagen has been questioned. However there is strong evidence for the participation of the protein, factor VIII/von Willebrand factor, in this process. The role of collagen quaternary structure in adhesion is less clear than in the case of collagen-induced platelet aggregation.

Note added in proof

Two reports particularly relevant to this chapter have appeared since submission of the original manuscript. In one, further evidence that fibronectin is not involved in the collagen-platelet interaction is presented (Sochynsky R A, Boughton B J, Burns J, Sykes B C, McGee J O'D 1980. The effect of human fibronectin on platelet:collagen adhesion. Thrombosis Research 18: 521). In the other, evidence for the involvement of type IV collagen in the adhesion of platelets to basement membrane is described (Balleisen L, Rauterberg J 1980 Platelet activation by basement membrane collagens. Thrombosis Research 18: 725).

Some additional references which may be of interest to the reader and which have appeared recently are appended. Please note particularly those on factor VIII.

ADDITIONAL REFERENCES

Bolhuis P A, Sakariassen K S, Sander H J, Bouma B N, Sixma J J 1981 Binding of factor VIII — von Willebrand factor to human arterial subendothelium precedes increased platelet adhesion and enhances platelet spreading. Jouranl of Laboratory and Clinical Medicine 97: 568

Harfenist E J, Izzotti M J, Packham M A, Mustard J F 1980 Plasma fibronectin is not involved in ADP-induced aggregation of rabbit platelets. Thrombosis and Haemostasis 44: 108

Jerenska M, Kopec M 1980 Blood platelets cause retraction of collagen gels. Thrombosis and Haemostasis 44: 161-4

Lahav J, Meyer F A 1981 On the role of the major platelet membrane glycoproteins in platelet adhesion to collagen. Thrombosis Research 22: 457

Legrand Y J, Karniguian A, Le Francier P, Fauvel F, Caen J P 1980 Evidence that a collagen-derived nonapeptide is a specific inhibitor of platelet-collagen interaction. Biochemical Biophysical Research Communication 96: 1579-85

Leytin V L, Ljubimova E V, Sviridov D D, Repin V S, Smirnov V N 1980 Time-response changes in the thrombogenicity of platelets spread on a collagen-coated surface. Thrombosis Research 20: 335-41

Madri J A, Dreyer B, Pitlick F A, Furthmayr H 1980 The collagenous components of the subendothelium. Laboratory Investigation 44: 303

Meyer F A, Weisman Z 1981 Collagen-induced platelet aggregation. Dependence on triple helical structure and fiber diameter. Thrombosis Research 22: 1

Morin R J, Chen A F T, Narayanan A S, Raye C, Moss R A, Srikantaiah M V, Barajas L 1980 Platelet adhesion to collagen in normal and von Willebrand's disease subjects. Thrombosis Research 17: 719-28

Sage H, Pritzl P, Bornstein P 1980 A unique, pepsin-sensitive collagen synthesized by aortic endothelial cells in culture. Biochemistry 19: 5747

Sage H, Pritzl P, Bornstein P 1981 Characterisation of cell matrix associated collagens synthesised by aortic endothelial cells in culture. Biochemistry 20: 436

Santoro S A 1981 Adsorption of von Willebrand factor/factor VIII by the genetically distinct interstitial collagens. Thrombosis Research 21: 689

Scott D M, Griffin B, Pepper D S, Barnes M J 1981 The binding of purified factor VIII/von Willebrand factor to collagens of differing type and form. Thrombosis Research 24: 467

Koteliansky V E, Leytin V L, Sviridov D D, Repin V S, Smirnov V N 1981 Human plasma fibronectin promotes the adhesion and spreading of platelets on surfaces coated with fibrillar collagen. FEBS lett 123: 59-62

Vicic W J, Lages B, Weiss H J 1980 Release of human platelet factor V activity is induced by both collagen and ADP and is inhibited by aspirin. Blood 56: 448-55

Walsh P N, Griffin J H 1981 Contributions of human platelets to the proteolytic activation of blood coagulation factors XII and XI. Blood 57: 106-18

REFERENCES

Baenzinger N L, Becherer P R, Majerus P W 1979 Characterization of prostacyclin synthesis in cultured human arterial smooth muscle cells, venous endothelial cells and skin fibroblasts. Cell 16: 967

Balleisen L, Gay S, Marx R, Kuhn K 1975 Comparative investigations of the influence of human and bovine collagen types I, II and III on the aggregation of human platelets. Klinische Wochenschrift 53: 903

Balleisen L, Marx R, Kuhn K 1976 Platelet-collagen interaction: The influence of native and modified collagen (type I) on the aggregation of human platelets. Haemostasis 5: 155

Balleisen L, Nowack H, Gay S, Timpl R 1979 Inhibition of collagen-induced platelet aggregation by antibodies to distinct types of collagen. Biochemical Journal 184: 683

Barnes M J, Gordon J L, MacIntyre D E 1976a Platelet-aggregating activity of type I and type III collagens from human aorta and chicken skin. Biochemical Journal 160: 647

Barnes M J, Morton L F, Levene C I 1976b Synthesis of collagen types I and III by pig medial smooth muscle cells in culture. Biochemical and Biophysical Research Communications 70: 339

Barnes M J, Morton L F, Levene C I 1978 Synthesis of interstitial collagens by pig aortic endothelial cells in culture. Biochemical and Biophysical Research Communications 84: 646

Barnes M J, MacIntyre D E 1979a Platelet-reactivity of isolated constituents of the blood vessel wall. Haemostasis 8: 158

Barnes M J, MacIntyre D E 1979b Collagen-induced platelet aggregation: The activity of basement membrane collagens relative to other collagen types. Frontiers of Matrix Biology 7: 246

Barnes M J, Bailey A J, Gordon J L, MacIntyre D E 1980 Platelet aggregation by basement membrane-associated collagens. Thrombosis Research 18: 375

Baugh R F, Jacoby J C, Brown J E 1979 Collagen-induced platelet aggregation is enhanced by bovine von Willebrand factor. Thrombosis Research 16: 289

Baumgartner H R, Muggli R 1976 Adhesion and aggregation: morphological demonstration and quantitation in vivo and in vitro. In: Gordon J L (ed) Platelets in biology and pathology. Elsevier/North Holland Biomedical Press, Amsterdam. ch 2, p 23

Baumgartner H R, Tschopp T B, Weiss H J 1977 Platelet interaction with collagen fibrils in flowing blood. II. Impaired adhesion-aggregation in bleeding disorders. Thrombosis and Haemostasis 37: 17

Baumgartner H R, Tschopp T B, Meyer D 1980 Shear rate dependent inhibition of platelet adhesion and aggregation on collagenous surfaces by antibodies to human factor VIII/von Willebrand factor. British Journal of Haematology 44: 127

Beachey E H, Chiang T M, Kang A H 1979 Collagen-platelet interaction. International Review of Connective Tissue Research 8: 1

Bensusan H B, Koh T L, Henry K G, Murray B A, Culp L A 1978 Evidence that fibronectin is the collagen receptor on platelet membranes. Proceedings of the National Academy of Sciences, USA 75: 5864

Best L C, Holland T K, Jones P B B, Russell R G G 1980 The interrelationship between thromboxane biosynthesis, aggregation and 5-hydroxytryptamine secretion in human platelets in vitro. Thrombosis and Haemostasis 43: 38

Born G V R 1962 Aggregation of blood platelets by adenosine diphosphate and its reversal. Nature, London 194: 927

Bounameaux V 1959 L'accolement des plaquettes fibres sousendotheliales. Comptes Rendus des Séances de la Société de Biologie, Paris 153: 658

Brass L F, Bensusan H B 1974 The role of collagen quaternary structure in the platelet collagen interaction. Journal of Clinical Investigation 54: 1480

Braunstein P W, Cuenoud H F, Joris I, Majno G 1980 Platelets, fibroblasts and inflammation. American Journal of Pathology 99: 53

Burke J M, Balian G, Ross R, Bornstein P 1977 Synthesis of types I and III procollagen and collagen by monkey aortic smooth muscle cells in vitro. Biochemistry 16: 3243

Charo I F, Feinman R D, Detwiler T C, Smith J B, Ingermann C M, Silver M J 1977 Prostaglandin endoperoxides and thromboxane A_2 can induce platelet aggregation in the absence of secretion. Nature, London 269: 66

Chiang T M, Mainardi C L, Seyer J M, Kang A H 1980 Collagen-platelet interaction. Type V (A–B) collagen induces platelet aggregation. Journal of Laboratory and Clinical Medicine 95: 99

Chung E, Miller E J 1974 Collagen polymorphism. Characterization of molecules with the chain composition $[\alpha 1(III)]_3$ in human tissues. Science 183: 1200

Chung E, Rhodes R K, Miller E J 1976 Isolation of three collagenous components of probable basement membrane origin from several tissues. Biochemical and Biophysical Research Communications 71: 1167

Claesson H E, Malmsten C 1977 On the interrelationship of prostaglandin endoperoxide G_2 and cyclic nucleotides in platelet function. European Journal of Biochemistry 76: 277

Curwen K D, Gimbrone M A, Handin R I 1980 In vitro studies of thromboresistance: The role of prostacyclin (PGI_2) in platelet adhesion to cultured normal and virally transformed human vascular endothelial cells. Laboratory Investigation 42: 366

D'Angelo V, Villa S, Mysliwiec M, Donati M B, de Gaetano G 1978 Defective fibrinolytic and prostacyclin-like activity in human, atheromatous plaques. Thrombosis and Haemostasis 39: 535

Dembinska-Kiec A, Gryglewska T, Zmuda A, Gryglewski R J 1977 The generation of prostacyclin by arteries and by the coronary vascular wall is reduced in experimental atherosclerosis in rabbits. Prostaglandins 14: 1025

Fauvel F, Legrand Y J, Caen J P 1978 Platelet adhesion to type I collagen and $\alpha 1(I)_3$ trimers: Involvement of the C-terminal $\alpha 1(I)$ CB6A peptide. Thrombosis Research 12: 273

Fauvel F, Legrand Y J, Bentz H, Fietzek P P, Kuhn K, Caen J P 1978 Platelet-collagen interaction: adhesion of human blood platelets to purified (CB4) peptide from type III collagen. Thrombosis Research 12: 841

Freytag J W, Dalrymple P N, Maguire M H, Strickland D K, Carraway K L, Hudson B G 1978 Glomerular basement membrane: studies on its structure and interaction with platelets. Journal of Biological Chemistry 253: 9069

Gastpar H, Kuhn K, Marx R (eds) 1978 Collagen-platelet interaction. Schattauer, New York

Gay S, Balleisen L, Remberger K, Fietzek P P, Adelmann B C, Kuhn K 1975 Immunohistochemical evidence for the presence of collagen type III in human arterial walls, arterial thrombi and in leucocytes, incubated with collagen in vitro. Klinische Wochenschrift 53: 899

Gelman R A, Williams B R, Piez K A 1979 Collagen fibril formation: evidence for a multistep process. Journal of Biological Chemistry 254: 180

Gordon J L 1979 Mechanism of platelet-collagen interaction. Nature, London 278: 13

Gordon J L, Dingle J T 1974 Binding of radiolabelled collagen to blood platelets. Journal of Cell Science 16: 157

Hovig T 1963 Aggregation of rabbit blood platelets produced in vitro by saline 'extract' of tendons. Thrombosis et Diathesis Haemorrhagica 9: 248

Howard B V, Macarak E J, Gunson D, Kefalides N A 1976 Characterization of the collagens synthesized by endothelial cells in culture. Proceedings of the National Academy of Science, USA 73: 2361

Huang T W, Benditt E P 1978 Mechanism of platelet adhesion to the basal lamina. American Journal of Pathology 92: 99

Huang T W, Lagunoff D, Benditt E P 1974 Nonaggregative adherence of platelets to basal lamina in vitro. Laboratory Investigation 31: 156

Hugues J 1960 Accolement des plaquettes au collagene. Comptes Rendus des Séances de la Société de Biologie, Paris 154: 866

Hugues J, Mahieu P 1970 Platelet aggregation induced by basement membranes. Thrombosis et Diathesis Haemorrhagica 24: 395

Hugues J, Herion F, Nusgens B, Lapiere C M 1976 Type III collagen and probably not type I collagen aggregates platelets. Thrombosis Research 9: 223

Hynes R O et al 1978 A large glycoprotein lost from the surfaces of transformed cells. Annals of the New York Academy of Science 312: 317

Jaffe E A, Minick C R, Adelmann B C, Becker C G, Nachmann R 1976 Synthesis of basement membrane collagen by cultured human endothelial cells. Journal of Experimental Medicine 144: 209

Jaffe R M 1976 Interaction of platelets with connective tissue. In: Gordon J L (ed) Platelets in biology and pathology. Elsevier/North Holland Biomedical Press, Amsterdam. ch 10, p 261

Jaffe R M, Deykin D 1974 Evidence for a structural requirement for the aggregation of platelets by collagen. Journal of Clinical Investigation 53: 875

Jamieson G A, Urban C L, Barber A J 1971 Enzymatic basis for platelet: collagen adhesion as the primary step in haemostasis. Nature, London 234: 5

Katzmann R L, Kang A H, Beachey E H 1973 Collagen-induced platelet aggregation: Involvement of an active glycopeptide fragment (α1–CB5). Science 181: 670

Kinlough-Rathbone R L, Packham M A, Reimers H J, Cazenave J P, Mustard J F 1977 Mechanisms of platelet shape change, aggregation and release induced by collagen, thrombin or A 23 187. Journal of Laboratory and Clinical Medicine 90: 707

Kinlough-Rathbone R L, Cazenave J P, Packham M A, Mustard J F 1980 Effect of inhibitors of the arachidonate pathway on the release of granule contents from rabbit platelets adherent to collagen. Laboratory Investigation 42: 28

Kjaerheim A, Hovig T 1962 The ultrastructure of haemostatic blood platelet plugs in rabbit mesenterium. Thrombosis et Diathesis Haemorrhagica 7: 1

Kronick P, Jimenez S A 1980 The size of collagen fibrils that stimulate platelet aggregation in human plasma. Biochemical Journal 186: 5

Lages B, Weiss H J 1980 Biphasic aggregation responses to ADP and epinephrine in some storage pool deficient platelets: relationship to the role of endogenous ADP in platelet aggregation and secretion. Thrombosis and Haemostasis 43: 147

Larrue J, Rigaud M, Daret D, Demond J, Durand J, Bricand H 1980 Prostacyclin production by cultured smooth muscle cells from atherosclerotic rabbit aorta. Nature, London 285: 480

Layman D L, Epstein E H, Dodson R F, Titus J L 1977 Biosynthesis of type I and III collagens by cultured smooth muscle cells from human aorta. Proceedings of the National Academy of Science, USA 74: 671

Legrand Y J, Rodriguez-Zeballos A, Kartalis G, Fauvel F, Caen J P 1978 Adsorption of factor VIII antigen-activity complex by collagen. Thrombosis Research 13: 909

Leunis J C, Smith D F, Nwokoro N, Fishback B L, Wu C, Jamieson G A 1980 The distribution of collagen: glucosyltransferase in human blood cells and plasma. Biochimica et Biophysica Acta 611: 79

MacIntyre D E, Pearson J D, Gordon J L 1978 Localisation and stimulation of prostacyclin production by vascular cells. Nature, London 271: 549

Majno G, Palade G E 1961 Studies on inflammation 1. The effect of histamine and serotonin on vascular permeability: an electron microscopic study. Journal of Biophysical and Biochemical Cytology 11: 571

Mayne R, Vail M S, Miller E J 1978 Characterization of the collagen chains synthesized by cultured smooth muscle cells derived from rhesus monkey thoracic aorta. Biochemistry 17: 446

McCullagh K G, Balian G 1975 Collagen characterization and cell transformation in human atherosclerosis. Nature, London 258: 73

McCullagh K G, Duance V C, Bishop K A 1980 The distribution of collagen types I, III and V (AB) in normal and atherosclerotic human aorta. Journal of Pathology 130: 45

McFarlane R G 1977 Introduction. In: Thomas D (ed) Haemostasis. British Medical Bulletin 33: 183

Mehta P, Mehta J 1980 Platelet function studies in coronary heart disease: VIII. Decreased platelet sensitivity to prostacyclin in patients with myocardial ischaemia. Thrombosis Research 18: 273

Menashi S, Grant M E 1979 Studies on the collagen glucosyltransferase activity present in platelets and plasma. Biochemical Journal 178: 777

Meyer F A 1980 Determinants for platelet adhesion and aggregation on collagen. In: Rotman A, Meyer F A, Gitler C, Silberberg A (eds) Platelets: cellular response mechanisms and their biological significance. Wiley, New York

Meyer F A, Weisman Z 1978 Adhesion of platelets to collagen: the nature of the binding site from competitive inhibition studies. Thrombosis Research 12: 431

Moncada S, Amezcua J L 1979 Prostacyclin, thromboxane A_2 interactions in haemostasis and thrombosis. Haemostasis 8: 252

Moncada S, Vane J R 1978 Unstable metabolites of arachidonic acid and their role in haemostasis and thrombosis. In: Thomas D (ed) Thrombosis, British Medical Bulletin 34: 129

Moncada S, Gryglewski R, Bunting S, Vane J R 1976 An enzyme isolated from arteries transforms prostaglandin endoperoxides to an unstable substance that inhibits platelet aggregation. Nature, London 263: 663

Moore S 1979 Endothelial injury and atherosclerosis. Experimental and Molecular Pathology 31: 182

Morton L F, Barnes M J 1982 Collagen polymorphism in the normal and diseased blood vessel wall. Investigation of collagens types I, III and V. Atherosclerosis 42: 41

Movat H Z, Fernando N V P 1963 Allergic inflammation 1. The earliest fine structural changes at the blood tissue barrier during antigens-antibody interaction. American Journal of Pathology 42: 41

Muggli R 1978 Collagen-induced platelet aggregation: native collagen quaternary structure is not an essential requirement. Thrombosis Research 13: 829

Muggli R, Baumgartner H R 1973 Collagen-induced platelet aggregation requirement for tropocollagen multimers. Thrombosis Research 3: 715

Muggli R, Baumgartner H R, Tschopp T B, Keller H 1980 Automated microdensitometry and protein assays as a measure for platelet adhesion and aggregation on collagen-coated slides under controlled flow conditions. Journal of Laboratory and Clinical Medicine 95: 195

Mustard J F, Kinlough-Rathbone R L, Packham M A 1980 Prostaglandins and platelets. Annual Review of Medicine 31: 89

Mysliwiec M, Villa S, Kornblihtt L, de Gaetano G, Donati M B 1980 Decreased plasminogen activator but normal prostacyclin activity in rat veins during development of experimental thrombosis. Thrombosis Research 18: 159

Nachman R L, Weksler B, Ferris B 1972 Characterization of human platelet vascular permeability-enhancing activity. Journal of Clinical Investigation 51: 549

Niewiarowski S, Stuart R K, Thomas D P 1966 Activation of intra-vascular coagulation by collagen. Proceedings of the Society for Experimental Biology and Medicine 123: 196

Nordoy A (ed) 1979 Blood vessel wall interactions in thrombogenesis. Haemostasis 8: 121

Nordoy A, Svensson B, Schroeder C, Hoak J C 1978 The inhibitory effect of aspirin on human endothelial cells. Thrombosis and Haemostasis 40: 103

Nunn B 1979 Collagen-induced platelet aggregation: evidence against the essential role of platelet adenosine diphosphate. Thrombosis and Haemostasis 42: 1193

Nyman D 1977a Collagen-induced platelet aggregation: evidence of several mechanisms for the induction of platelet release by collagen. Thrombosis Research 10: 743

Nyman D 1977b Interaction of collagen with the factor VIII antigen-activity-von Willebrand factor complex. Thrombosis Research 11: 433

Nyman D 1980 Von Willebrand factor dependent platelet aggregation and adsorption of factor VIII related antigen by collagen. Thrombosis Research 17: 209

Ordinas A, Hornebeck W, Robert L, Caen J P 1975 Interaction of platelets with purified macromolecules of the arterial wall. Pathologie-Biologie 23: 44

Osterud B 1979 The role of endothelial cells and subendothelial components in the initiation of blood coagulation. Haemostasis 8: 324

Osterud B, Rapoport S I, Lavine K K 1977 Factor V activity of platelets: evidence for an activated factor V molecule and for a platelet activator. Blood 49: 819

Rauterberg J, Allam S, Brehmer V, Wirth W, Hauss W H 1977 Characterization of the collagen synthesized by cultured human smooth muscle cells from foetal and adult aorta. Hoppe-Seyler's Zeitschrift fur Physiologie Chemie 358: 401

Ross R, Glomset J A 1976 The pathogenesis of atherosclerosis. New England Journal of Medicine 295: 369, 420

Sage H, Crouch E, Bornstein P 1979 Collagen synthesis by bovine aortic endothelial cells in culture. Biochemistry 18: 5433

Santoro S A, Cunningham L W 1977 Collagen-mediated platelet aggregation: evidence for multivalent interactions of intermediate specificity between collagen and platelets. Journal of Clinical Investigation 60: 1054

Santoro S A, Cunningham L W 1979 Fibronectin and the multiple interaction model for platelet-collagen adhesion. Proceedings of the National Academy of Science, USA 76: 2644

Santoro S A, Cunningham L W 1980 Collagen-mediated platelet aggregation: the role of multiple interactions between the platelet surface and collagen. Thrombosis and Haemostasis 43: 158

Schwartz S M, Benditt E P 1973 Cell replication in the aortic endothelium: a new method for study of the problem. Laboratory Investigation 28: 699

Scott D M, Harwood R, Grant M E, Jackson D S 1977 Characterization of the major collagen species present in porcine aorta and the synthesis of their precursors by smooth muscle cells in culture. Connective Tissue Research 5: 7

Simons E R, Chesney C M, Colman R W, Harper E, Samberg E 1976 The effect of the conformation of collagen on its ability to aggregate platelets. Thrombosis Research 7: 123

Sinzinger H, Clopath P, Silberbauer K, Winter M 1980 Is the variation in the susceptibility of various species to atherosclerosis due to unborn differences in prostacyclin (PGI_2) formation? Experimentia 36: 321

Stemerman M B 1974 Platelet interactions with intimal connective tissue. In: Baldini M G, Ebbe S (eds) Platelets: Production, Function, Transfusion and Storage. Grune and Stratton, New York

Sultan Y, Maisonneuve P, Angles-Caro E 1979 Release of VIII R:Ag and VIII R:WF during thrombin and collagen induced aggregation. Thrombosis Research 15: 415

Sultan Y, Jeanneau C, Lamaziere J, Maisonnauve P, Caen J P 1978 Platelet factor VIII-related antigen: studies in vivo after transfusion in patients with von Willebrand disease. Blood 51: 751

Suresh A D, Stemerman M B, Spaet T H 1973 Rabbit heart valve basement membrane: low platelet reactivity. Blood 41: 359

Swann D A, Chesney C M, Constable I J, Colman R W, Caulfield J B, Harper E 1974 The role of vitreous collagen in platelet aggregation in vitro and in vivo. Journal of Laboratory and Clinical Medicine 84: 264

Szczeklik A, Gryglewski R, Musial J, Grodzinska L, Serwonska M, Marcinkiewicz E 1978 Thromboxane generation and platelet aggregation in survivals of myocardial infarction. Thrombosis and Haemostasis 40: 66

Thomas D (ed) 1977 Haemostasis. British Medical Bulletin 33: 183

Thomas D (ed) 1978 Thrombosis. British Medical Bulletin 34: 101

Tranzer J P, Baumgartner H R 1967 Filling gaps in the vascular endothelium with blood platelets. Nature, London 216: 1126

Tranzer J P, Baumgartner H R, Studer A 1968 Ultramorphologic aspects of the early stages of experimental platelet thrombosis. Experimental Biology and Medicine 3: 80

Trelstad R L 1974 Human aorta collagens: evidence for three distinct species. Biochemical and Biophysical Research Communications 57: 717

Trelstad R L, Lawley K R 1977 Isolation and initial characterization of human basement membrane collagens. Biochemical and Biophysical Research Communications 76: 376

Trelstad R L, Carvalho A C A 1979 Type IV and Type 'A–B' collagens do not elicit platelet aggregation or the serotonium release reaction. Journal of Laboratory and Clinical Medicine 93: 499

Ts'ao C H 1971 In vitro platelet reaction with isolated glomerular basement membrane: ultrastructural comparisons with platelet-collagen reaction. Thrombosis et Diathesis Haemorrhagica 25: 507

Ts'ao C H, Glagov S 1970 Platelet adhesion to subendothelial components in experimental aortic injury: role of fine fibrils and the basement membrane. British Journal of Experimental Pathology 51: 423

Wall R T, Harker L A 1980 The endothelium and thrombosis. Annual Review of Medicine 31: 361

Walsh P N 1972 The effects of collagen and kaolin on the intrinsic coagulant activities of platelets: evidence for an alternate pathway in intrinsic coagulation not requiring factor XII. British Journal of Haematology 22: 393

Wang C H, Miyata T, Weksler B, Rubin A L, Stenzel K H 1978a Collagen-induced platelet aggregation and release II. Critical size and structural requirements of collagen. Biochimica et Biophysica Acta 544: 568

Wang C H, Miyata T, Weksler B, Rubin A L, Stenzel K H 1978b Collagen-induced platelet aggregation and release I. Effects of side-chain modifications and role of arginyl residues. Biochimica et Biophysica Acta 544: 555

Weksler B B, Marcus A J, Jaffe E A 1977 Synthesis of prostaglandin I_2 (prostacyclin) by cultured human and bovine endothelial cells. Proceedings of the National Academy of Science, USA 74: 3922

Wharton-Jones T 1851 On the state of the blood and the blood vessels in inflammation. Guy's Hospital Reports 7: 1

Williams B R, Gelman R A, Poppke D C, Piez K A 1978 Collagen fibril formation: optimal in vitro conditions and preliminary kinetic results. Journal of Biological Chemistry 253: 6578

Wilner G D, Nossel H L, LeRoy E C 1968 Activation of Hageman factor by collagen. Journal of Clinical Investigation 47: 2608

Yamada K M, Olden K 1978 Fibronectins: adhesive glycoproteins of cell surface and blood. Nature, London 275: 179

Zacharski L R, Rosenstein R 1977 Further comments on the failure of collagen to activate factor XII. Thrombosis Research 10: 771

Zucker M B 1980 The functioning of blood platelets. Scientific American 242: 70

Zucker M B, Borelli J 1962 Platelet clumping produced by connective tissue suspensions and by collagen. Proceedings of the Society for Experimental Biology and Medicine 109: 779

Zucker M B, Broekman M J, Kaplan K L 1979b Factor VIII-related antigen in human blood platelets. Journal of Laboratory and Clinical Medicine 94: 675

Zucker M B, Mosesson M W, Broekman M J, Kaplan K L 1979a Release of platelet fibronectin (cold-insoluble globulin) from alpha granules induced by thrombin or collagen: lack of requirement for plasma fibronectin in ADP-induced platelet aggregation. Blood 54: 8

11

Interaction of fibronectin with collagen

H. K. KLEINMAN and C. M. WILKES

Fibronectin and collagen are two major connective tissue proteins which have been demonstrated to have high affinity for each other. This chapter will detail what is known about fibronectin and the specificity of its interactions with collagen. In addition, the role of these two molecules in cell adhesion, tissue differentiation and growth, wound healing, and transformation will be described.

FIBRONECTIN

Serum, the cell surface of fibroblasts, and various extracellular matrices contain a large connective tissue glycoprotein now known as fibronectin (for recent reviews, Vaheri & Mosher, 1978; Yamada & Olden, 1978; Pearlstein et al, 1980). Cell surface fibronectin comprises up to 3 per cent of the total cellular protein of certain fibroblasts cultured in vitro (Yamada et al, 1977a). It is also synthesized by a variety of other cells, including chondrocytes (Hassell et al, 1979), endothelial cells (Jaffe & Mosher, 1978), some epithelial cells (Chen et al, 1977), myoblasts (Furcht et al, 1977), and astroglial cells (Vaheri et al, 1976). When localized with antibodies labelled with a fluorescent compound, it is observed in fibrillar arrays next to or on the surface of many cultured cells (for example, Vaheri et al, 1976; Chen et al, 1977; Mautner & Hynes, 1977; Bornstein & Ash, 1977). Fibronectin is concentrated in areas of cell-to-cell and cell-to-substrate contacts (Mautner & Hynes, 1977), consistent with a role in cell adhesiveness. In vivo, fibronectin is found in a variety of connective tissues including the dermis and certain basement membranes (Linder et al, 1975; Stenman et al, 1978). It is also present in the mesenchyme in developing animals but if these cells differentiate into muscle or cartilage it disappears.

Fibronectin is a high molecular weight glycoprotein containing two chains of approximately 220 000 daltons joined by disulphide bonds. After reduction, the chains from serum fibronectin electrophorese in denaturing conditions (in SDS) as two closely spaced bands, while cellular fibronectin appears as one diffuse band. The basis for this difference is not known. The molecule contains approximately six asparagine linked oligosaccharides (Fukuda & Hakomori, 1979). Alterations in the sugar content or removal of a small peptide by proteolysis could explain the differences observed. However, the molecules could also be different gene products. Fibronectin interacts with many other macromolecules and has diverse biological activities (Table 11.1). The protein was described independently in several laboratories studying a variety of phenomena and as a result, different names were assigned to the same substance, now known as fibronectin (Table 11.2). The serum form, cold insoluble globulin, was first

Table 11.1 Properties and biological activities of fibronectin

Molecules known to interact with fibronectin
Heparin
Fibrinogen
Collagens I–V, C1q and acetylcholinesterase
Transglutaminase (Factor XIII_a — of blood clotting cascade)
Fibronectin
Hyaluronic acid
Gangliosides: GD_{1a}, GT_1
Actin, DNA
Biological activities
Mediates cell adhesion and spreading to plastic and collagen substrates
Reverses transformed phenotype
Mediates opsonization activity by macrophages
Agglutinates tanned red blood cells
Promotes cell migration
Inhibits chondrogenic expression and myoblast fusion

Table 11.2 Synonyms for fibronectin

Cold insoluble globulin
Surface fibroblast antigen
Cell surface protein
Large external transformation sensitive protein
Galactoprotein a
Collagen cell attachment protein
Spreading factor
Band 1
Zeta protein
a_2-SB-opsonic glycoprotein
Anti-gelatin factor
Microfibrillar protein

described in 1948 as a component of the precipitate forming when blood was clotted in the cold (Morrison et al, 1948). Fibronectin represents 0.5–1.0 per cent of the total serum proteins. Macrophages were found to require serum fibronectin (which is called in these studies α2-SB-glycoprotein and antigelatin factor) for opsonization reactions (Hopper et al, 1976; Saba et al, 1978). Fibronectin also has a major role in promoting the adhesion of many cells. Fibroblasts, myoblasts and several other cell types, possibly including platelets, utilize fibronectin for adhesion to plastic and collagen substrates (Klebe, 1974; Pearlstein, 1976; Kleinman et al, 1978c; Chicquet et al, 1979; Santoro & Cunningham, 1979; Pearlstein et al, 1980). Fibronectin also enhances random cell migration (Ali & Hynes, 1978) and directed cell migration in a Boyden chamber (Gauss-Müller et al, 1980).

A molecule nearly identical to plasma fibronectin is also present on the cell surface (Vaheri & Mosher, 1978; Yamada & Olden, 1978; Yamada & Kennedy, 1979; Alexander et al, 1979). It has similar electrophoretic mobility, amino acid content, immunologic cross-reactivity, ability to mediate cell adhesion, and similar circular dichroism and fluorescent spectra. It is a major constituent of chick embryo fibroblasts but disappears from the surface of transformed cells (Vaheri & Mosher, 1978; Yamada & Olden, 1978). In some transformed cells, this reduction (Adams et al, 1977) is caused by a decrease in synthesis due to a decrease in transcription of the fibronectin gene. In other cells (Parry et al, 1979), synthesis is nearly normal but it is not retained on the cell surface or its degradation is increased. When added exogenously, fibronectin causes transformed cells to flatten and resemble normal cells (Ali et al, 1977; Yamada et al, 1977b). When added to cultured chondrocytes, fibronectin causes these cells to flatten and change their synthetic activities (Pennypacker et al, 1979; West et al, 1979).

Fibronectin interacts with a variety of macromolecules including itself (Table 11.1). Specific regions of the fibronectin molecule have been shown to be involved in the interactions (Hahn & Yamada, 1979; Balian et al, 1979; Ruoslahti & Engvall, 1980; McDonald, 1980; Yamada et al, 1980; Mosher et al, 1980) in the cases of collagen, fibrinogen, heparin, hyaluronic acid, and transglutaminases. Transglutaminase can crosslink fibronectin to other fibronectin molecules, to fibrin and to collagen (Mosher et al, 1980). Each interaction could be important in vivo during wound healing or tissue growth as some patients with factor XIII (protransglutaminase) deficiency suffer from poor wound healing (Duckert, 1972). The role of the interactions of fibronectin with heparin and hyaluronic acid is less well understood but could relate to the adhesive role of this glycoprotein. Heparan sulphate, a proteoglycan whose sugar components resemble those of heparin, and hyaluronic acid are present with fibronectin (Culp et al, 1978) in the cell-substrate interface of cells. These macromolecules may act to stabilize (Ruoslahti et al, 1979) or enhance (Jilek & Hörmann, 1979; Johansson & Höök, 1980) the fibronectin-collagen interaction at adhesion sites.

Recently, the oligosaccharide portions of certain complex gangliosides have been demonstrated to bind to fibronectin (Kleinman et al, 1979). When added to fibroblasts (Kleinman et al, 1979) or red blood cells (Yamada, unpublished observations), the gangliosides inhibit the adhesion or agglutination of these cells respectively. The gangliosides do not interfere with the fibronectin-collagen interaction, suggesting that these gangliosides or glycoconjugates with similar oligosaccharides could be the cell surface receptors for fibronectin.

A recent report (Keski-Oja et al, 1979) also has described the interaction of fibronectin with actin. Since actin is an intracellular protein and fibronectin is extracellular, it is unlikely that they bind to one another in vivo. From immunofluorescent studies, however, it appears that fibronectin and actin show a partial codistribution at the cell surface (Mautner & Hynes, 1977).

In summary, fibronectin is a major glycoprotein of plasma and of the cell surface and extracellular matrices. Due to its adhesive properties and interactions with other matrix components, it is most likely involved in cell-matrix interactions in vivo.

INTERACTION OF FIBRONECTIN WITH COLLAGEN

Binding site for fibronectin on collagen

Collagen binds to fibronectin and appears to contain a specific amino acid sequence which is recognized by fibronectin (Kleinman et al, 1976; Hopper et al, 1976; Engvall & Ruoslahti, 1977; Jilek & Hörmann, 1978; Dessau et al, 1978a; Kleinman et al, 1978b; Engvall et al, 1978; Vuento & Vaheri, 1979; Gold et al, 1979). All the mammalian collagens were found capable of binding fibronectin based on both radioimmunoassays and their ability to promote cell attachment (Kleinman et al, 1978b; Jilek & Hörmann, 1978; Engvall et al, 1978; Dessau et al, 1978a). The activities of various peptides produced from types I, II, and III collagen by digestion with cyanogen bromide are summarized in Figure 11.1.

Each collagen chain contains one major active cyanogen bromide peptide all from similar regions including residues 693–795. In addition, a peptide of 35 amino acids (residues 757–791) has been isolated which binds to fibronectin. Synthetic peptides of 20 amino acids (residues 766–785) and 8 amino acids (residues 773–780) are active, while a 7 residue peptide (residues 774–780) is inactive (Kleinman, unpublished observations). Thus, a small region of as few as 8 amino acids contains the fibronectin binding site. The integrity of residues 775–776 (the collagenase cleavage site) and of residues 779–780 is necessary for activity. The binding region is unusually hydrophobic for collagen

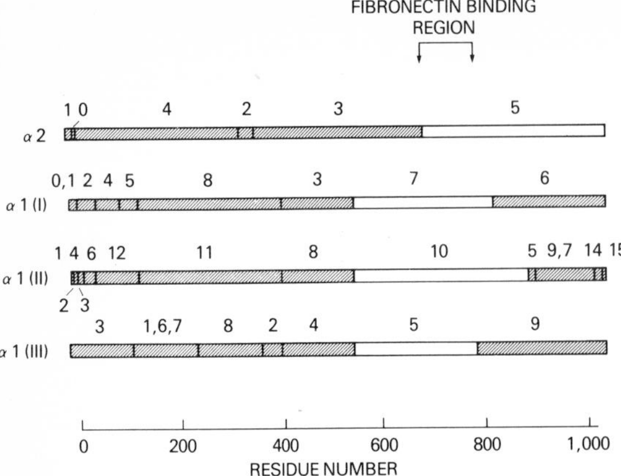

Fig. 11.1 Binding sites on collagen α chains for fibronectin. The unshaded areas designate the major active peptides in each chain. Data were obtained from Kleinman et al (1976) and Dessau et al (1978a).

sequences (Ramachandran & Reddi, 1977) and lacks hydroxyproline and proline which stabilize the helix of collagen. As a result, in this region collagen is less tightly coiled. Further, if the collagen is made more hydrophobic through chemical modification of arginine residues with 1,2-cyclohexanedione, the interaction between fibronectin and collagen is enhanced (Kleinman et al, 1978a). These studies indicate that collagen contains a unique binding site for fibronectin which lacks carbohydrate and is less helical than other segments of the molecule (Highberger et al, 1979).

Collagen can also be cross-linked to fibronectin via transglutaminase (Mosher et al, 1979; Mosher et al, 1980). The α1(I) chain and α(I)–CB7 peptide are crosslinked while *Ascaris* collagen is not. This interaction may be important in further stabilizing the extracellular matrix and in wound healing.

Interaction of fibronectin with collagens

Many of the studies exploring the interaction of fibronectin with collagen have been carried out in vitro. A variety of assays have been employed and the results vary depending upon the method, the temperature, and the length of time the molecules are allowed to interact. It is generally agreed that denatured collagens bind to fibronectin better than native collagens (Kleinman et al, 1976; Kleinman et al, 1978b; Dessau et al, 1978a; Engvall et al, 1978; Jilek & Hörmann, 1978). However, native type III collagen is nearly as effective as denatured type III while type V collagen is less active than other collagens. The collagenous portions of C1q and acetylcholinesterase also bind fibronectin while the cuticle collagen from *Ascaris* and elastin do not bind fibronectin. The relative affinity of fibronectin for collagen can be summarized as follows:

Denatured type III > denatured type I, II, IV
and native type III > denatured V > native I, II, IV

Reduced binding to native collagen may be due to internalization of the binding site within the collagen fibre. Type III collagen which forms smaller fibrils binds more fibronectin (Lapière et al, 1977).

While fibronectin binds to native collagen less well than to denatured collagen, the interaction with native collagen is substantial and probably physiologically significant. In vitro fibronectin binds to collagen as it forms fibrils (Fig. 11.2) as well as after the fibrils have formed (Kleinman,

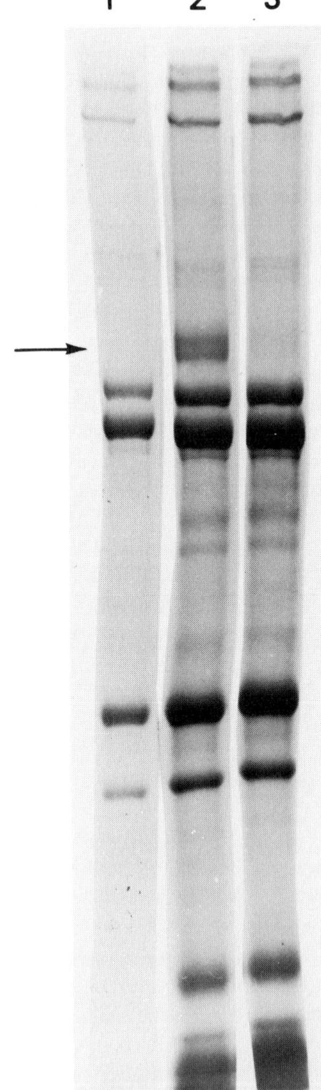

Fig. 11.2 Interaction of serum fibronectin with native collagen. Native collagen at 0.2 mg/ml in 0.02 M phosphate buffer, pH 7.4, was mixed with 0.1 ml human serum in the cold and then incubated for 1 hour at 37°. The fibrils were collected by centrifugation, washed twice, redissolved in 0.1 N acetic acid, dialyzed vs water and lyophilized. Lane 1: collagen without serum. Lane 2: collagen with serum. Lane 3: collagen with serum and 0.1 mg α1(I)–CB7. Note how the peptide, α1CB7, prevents the fibronectin (marked with an arrow) from binding to the native collagen.

Wilkes & Martin in preparation). Fibronectin binds to denatured chains in a 1:1 molar ratio while it binds at a ratio of approximately 1:13 to native collagen. Although this binding is low, it is probably significant in vivo since the two molecules are found in close association. For example, immunofluorescent staining of cultured cells demonstrates that collagen and fibronectin are codistributed (Vaheri et al, 1978). At the ultrastructural level using antibody, fibronectin appears as 'beaded strands' with a periodicity of ~ 70 nm, suggesting that fibronectin is periodically distributed along collagen fibres (Furcht et al, 1980). Fibronectin and collagen are also codistributed in such connective tissues as dermis and basement membranes (Stenman & Vaheri, 1978). Following collagenase treatment, fibronectin is released from alveolar basement membranes (Bray, 1978).

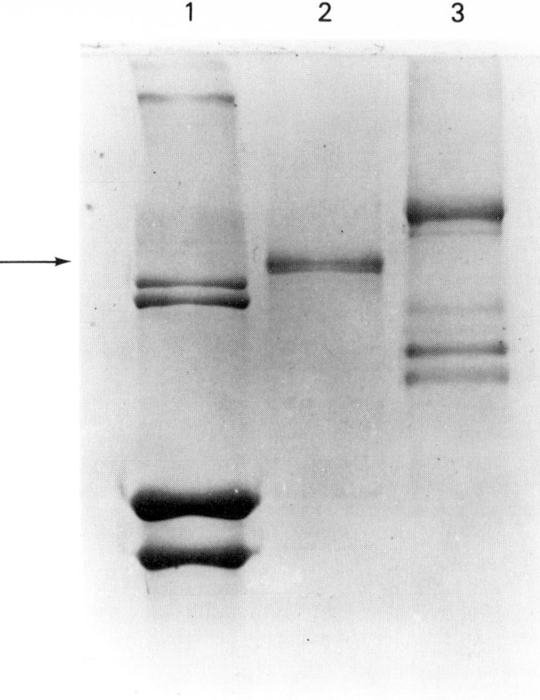

Fig. 11.3 Electrophoresis of fibronectin purified from serum by collagen-Sepharose affinity chromatography. Serum is allowed to remain on the column 1 hour at 4°. Then the unbound material is washed from the column with phosphate buffered saline and the bound material is eluted from the column with 1M KBr, 0.05 M Tris-HCl, pH 5.3, containing 0.025 M 6-aminohexanoic acid. Lane 1 is type I collagen from lathyritic rat skin. Lane 2 is the purified serum fibronectin. Lane 3 is murine type IV collagen. Arrow indicates the migration position of fibronectin.

Binding site for collagen on fibronectin

The affinity of fibronectin for collagen has been extremely useful in purifying fibronectin. Affinity columns containing covalently bound collagen specifically bind fibronectin which can then be eluted with chaotropic agents such as KBr, NaSCN, urea or arginine (Hopper et al, 1976; Engvall & Ruoslahti, 1977; Vuento & Vaheri, 1979) (Fig. 11.3). Fibronectin has a specific region which contains the binding site for collagen (Balian et al, 1979; Hahn & Yamada, 1979; Ruoslahti et al, 1979; McDonald, 198O). This has been isolated from proteolytic digests of fibronectin (Table 11.3). The collagen binding domain resists digestion and can be isolated by adsorption to collagen-Sepharose. A collagen binding fragment in fibronectin has also been prepared by protease treatment of fibronectin bound to collagen-Sepharose beads (Hahn & Yamada, 1979). The unbound, non-collagen binding fragments are removed and the bound fragment containing the collagen binding region is eluted. Using these approaches, a 30 000 dalton peptide has been isolated that binds to collagen. Those fragments of 40 000 daltons or less that bind collagen lack the cell binding site and do not promote cell adhesion. However, a 50 000 dalton peptide has been isolated from a subtilisin digest of fibronectin (Gold et al, 1979), with both activities suggesting that the collagen binding and cell binding regions are close together. This portion of the fibronectin molecule lacks carbohydrate (Fig. 11.4) and is relatively rich in glycine (14 per cent) (Ruoslahti et al, 1979; Gold et al, 1979) suggesting it may have collagen-like domains. The collagen-binding region, unlike the intact molecule, is poorly immunogenic (Ruoslahti et al, 1979) and probably is highly structured since it is very resistant to proteolysis.

Table 11.3 Fibronectin fragments known to interact with collagen

Investigators	*Fragment size* (Daltons)	*Enzyme used to generate fragments*	*Fibronectin source*
Ruoslahti et al (1979b)	30 000	Trypsin	Human plasma
Hahn & Yamada (1979)	40 000	Chymotrypsin	Chick embryo Fibroblast cell surface
Hahn & Yamada (1979)	42 000	Chymotrypsin	Human plasma
Balian et al (1979)	42 000	Cathepsin D and plasmin	Human plasma
Gold et al (1979)	50 000	Subtilisin	Human plasma
McDonald et al (1980)	39 000	Neutrophil elastase	Human plasma

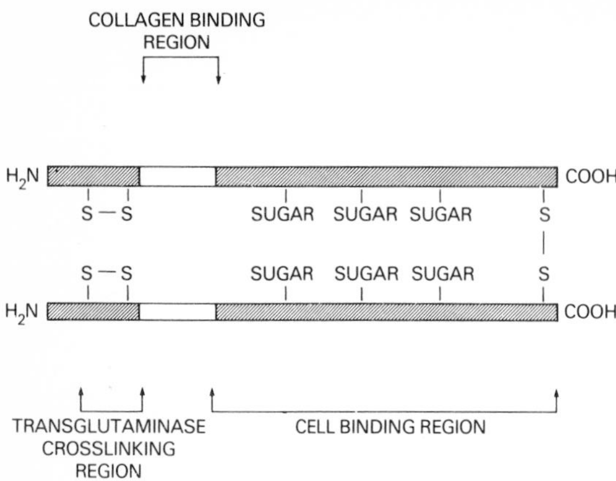

Fig. 11.4 Schematic model of the fibronectin molecule. Location of the carboxyl and amino terminal ends is tentative. Data were obtained from references Balian et al (1979), Hahn & Yamada (1979), Ruoslahti et al, (1979b) and McDonald (1980).

A specific region of the fibronectin molecule (Mosher, 1980) is utilized in crosslinking by transglutaminase. The crosslinking site is adjacent to the collagen-binding domain (Fig. 11.4).

Specific regions of collagen and fibronectin are involved in their interactions. Denatured collagen appears to bind fibronectin better than native collagen possibly due to the greater availability of the binding sites in denatured collagen and to the fact that a linear sequence of amino acids in the collagen is recognized by fibronectin.

BIOLOGICAL SIGNIFICANCE OF COLLAGEN FIBRONECTIN INTERACTIONS

Cell adhesion and differentiation

Fibronectin has been demonstrated to mediate the attachment of fibroblasts to collagen (Klebe, 1974; Pearlstein, 1976). These studies have shown that fibronectin binds to collagen and that the cells in the presence of calcium or magnesium bind to the fibronectin-collagen complex in an energy dependent process. A similar sequence may occur in vivo during embryogenesis, tissue differentiation and wound repair. Further, it has been demonstrated that both a collagen substrate and fibronectin are required for myoblast fusion in vitro (Hauschka & White, 1972; Chicquet et al, 1979).

Adult cartilage lacks fibronectin (Dessau et al, 1978b) and chondrocytes do not utilize fibronectin for cell adhesion (Hewitt et al, 1980). Instead cartilage cells utilize a different protein, termed chondronectin, which is smaller and more heat labile than fibronectin. Chondronectin is produced by chondrocytes and can be extracted from cartilage but not other tissues. It is found in fetal plasma and serum. Current data suggest that chondronectin is a cartilage-specific protein and will not function, for example in fibroblast attachment. Fibronectin, however, can influence the differentiation of the chondrocyte (Pennypacker et al, 1979; West et al, 1979). When added to chondrocytes in vitro, fibronectin causes these cells to become fibroblastic, to synthesize fibronectin and to decrease proteoglycan synthesis. This 'dedifferentiation' response of chondrocytes in vitro to fibronectin could be important in vivo. If an injury occurs, the cartilage would be exposed to serum fibronectin. The responses observed in culture would serve in vivo to promote repair of the damage. With repeated injury, the quality of the tissue could be altered to a fibrous matrix as seen, for example, in osteoarthritis.

Wound healing

Perhaps the most convincing role for the interaction of fibronectin and collagen is demonstrated directly in wound repair. At the site of injury, fibronectin and collagen may have multiple important functions. Fibronectin binds to fibrinogen (Engvall et al, 1978) and is present in the fibrin clot. Through the action of transglutaminase, it could be crosslinked to itself, to fibrin, and to collagen to stabilize the clot and link the hemostatic plug to the margins of the wound (Mosher et al, 1979). Fibronectin enhances platelet spreading and appears to be required (Santoro & Cunningham, 1979) in the reaction with collagen but probably not in the initial interaction. In the early stages of wound repair, fibronectin and collagen both promote the formation and stabilizion of the fibrin clot. In addition, both macromolecules can attract fibroblasts into the area of the wound (Postlethwaite et al, 1978; Gauss-Müller et al, 1980) since both fibronectin (Gauss-Müller et al, 1980) and collagen (Postlethwaite et al, 1978) are chemotactic for fibroblasts. These macromolecules could stimulate the cells at the margin of the wound to migrate into the lesion. The new cells would adhere well to collagen substrates in the presence of fibronectin (Klebe, 1974; Pearlstein, 1976) and both collagen and fibronectin could stimulate the further deposition of more matrix proteins for repair (Dodson & Hay, 1974; Foidart et al, 1980). Other studies have also demonstrated that fibronectin is required for maximal phagocytic activity of macrophages (Hopper et al, 1976; Saba et al, 1978). Thus, both collagen and fibronectin have key roles in many stages of the host's response to an injury.

Growth and transformation

Both fibronectin and collagen are important for normal growth and development. Most cells are maintained in tissues by their adhesion to an extracellular matrix. This, however, is not true of transformed and metastatic cells which are less adherent. The synthesis of both fibronectin and collagen are reduced after cell transformation

(Abrogast et al, 1977; Adams et al, 1977; Vaheri & Mosher, 1978). The cause of the reduction is not clear, but decreased mRNA levels (Adams et al, 1977), increased protease activity, and decreased cell surface receptors may all be involved (for discussion see Hynes et al, 1979). Transformed cells have less fibronectin on their surfaces and do not require collagen for growth in culture (Liotta et al, 1978). However, a more normal morphology is obtained when transformed cells are grown with exogenous fibronectin (Ali et al, 1977; Yamada et al, 1977b). Under these conditions the cells flatten, elongate and align in a fashion more typical of normal cells. Under these conditions the microfilaments are organized into bundles, but the ability of the cells to grow in agar, the levels of cAMP and the high rate of nutrient uptake, are not restored to normal. Thus, alterations in fibronectin and collagen appear to contribute to some of the properties of transformed and malignant cells suggesting the importance of these two matrix proteins in normal cell growth and differentiation.

SUMMARY

1. Fibronectin and collagen interact specifically and strongly. Distinct domains in each molecule have been identified as participating in the interaction.

2. Fibronectin binds to collagens I-V, C1q and acetylcholinesterase, but not to elastin or *Ascaris* cuticle collagen. It binds better to denatured than to native collagen, in part because of a greater availability of the fibronectin binding sites in the denatured collagen.

3. Transglutaminase can cross-link fibronectin to itself and to collagen and thus strengthen and stabilize connective tissues.

4. The biological importance of the interaction of fibronectin with collagen is seen in cell adhesion, cell differentiation, and in wound repair where platelet aggregation, cell migration and matrix formation are required. Alterations in fibronectin and collagen may explain some of the events in cell transformation and malignancy.

REFERENCES

Abrogast B W, Yoshimura M, Kefalides N A, Holtzer H, Kaji A 1977 Failure of cultured chick embryo fibroblasts to incorporate collagen into their extracellular matrix when transformed by Rous sarcoma virus. Journal of Biological Chemistry 252: 8863-8

Adams S L, Sobel M E, Howard B H, Olden K, Yamada K M, DeCrombrugghe B, Pastan I 1977 Levels of translatable mRNAs for cell surface protein, collagen precursors, and two membrane proteins are altered in Rous sarcoma virus-transformed chick embryo fibroblasts. Proceedings of the National Academy of Science USA 74: 3399-403

Ali I U, Mautner V M, Lanza R, Hynes R O 1977 Restoration of normal morphology, adhesion and cytoskeleton in transformation-sensitive surface protein. Cell 11: 115-26

Ali I U, Hynes R O 1978 Effect of LETS glycoprotein on cell motility. Cell 14: 439-46

Balian G, Click E M, Crouch E, Davidson J M, Bornstein P 1979 Isolation of a collagen-binding fragment from fibronectin and cold-insoluble globulin. Journal of Biological Chemistry 254: 1429-32

Bornstein P, Ash J F 1977 Cell surface-associated structural proteins in connective tissue cells. Proceedings of the National Academy of Science USA 74: 2480-4

Bray B A 1978 Cold-insoluble globulin (fibronectin) in connective tissues of adult human lung and trophoblast basement membrane. Journal of Clinical Investigation 62: 745-52

Chen L B, Maitland N, Gallimore P H, McDougall J K 1977 Detection of the large external transformation sensitive protein on some epithelial cells. Experimental Cell Research 106: 39-46

Chicquet M, Puri E C, Turner D C 1979 Fibronectin mediates attachment of chicken myoblasts to a gelatin-coated substratum. Journal of Biological Chemistry 254: 5745-82

Culp L A, Rollins B J, Buniel J, Hitri S 1978 Two functionally distinct pools of glycosaminoglycans in the substrate adhesion site of murine cells. Journal of Biological Chemistry 79: 788-801

Dessau W, Adelmann B C, Timpl R, Martin G R 1978a Identification of the sites in collagen α-chains that bind serum antigelatin factor (cold-insoluble globulin). Biochemical Journal 169: 55-9

Dessau W, Sasse J, Timpl R, Jilek F, von der Mark K 1978b Synthesis and extracellular deposition of fibronectin in chondrocyte cultures. Response to the removal of extracellular cartilage matrix. Journal of Cell Biology 79: 342-55

Dodson J W, Hay E D 1974 Secretion of collagen by corneal epithelium. Effect of the underlying substratum on secretion and polymerization of epithelial products. Journal of Experimental Zoology 189: 51-72

Duckert F 1972 Documentation of the plasma factor XIII deficiency in man. Annals of the New York Academy of Science 202: 190-9

Engvall E, Ruoslahti E 1977 Binding of soluble form of fibroblast surface protein, fibronectin, to collagen. International Journal of Cancer 20: 1-7

Engvall E, Ruoslahti E, Miller E J 1978 Affinity of fibronectin to collagens of different genetic types. Journal of Experimental Medicine 147: 1584-95

Foidart J M, Berman J J, Paglia L, Rennard S I, Abe S, Perantoni A, Martin G R 1980 Synthesis of fibronectin, laminin and several collagens by a liver-derived epithelial line. Laboratory Investigation 42: 525-32

Fukuda M, Hakomori S 1979 Carbohydrate structure of galactoprotein a, a major transformation-sensitive glycoprotein; released from human embryo fibroblasts. Journal of Biological Chemistry 254: 5451-7

Furcht L T, Mosher D F, Wendelschafer-Crabb G, Foidart J M 1979 Reversal by glucocorticoid hormones of the loss of a fibronectin and procollagen matrix around transformed human cells. Cancer Research 39: 2077-83

Furcht L T, Wendelschafer-Crabb G, Woodbridge P 1977 Cell surface changes accompanying myoblast differentiation. Journal of Supramolecular Structure 7: 307-22

Furcht L T, Wendelschafer-Crabb G, Mosher D F, Foidart J M 1980 An axial periodic fibrillar arrangement of antigenic determinants for fibronectin and procollagen on ascorbate treated human fibroblasts. Journal of Supramolecular Structure 13: 15-33

Gauss-Müller V, Schiffmann E, Martin G R, Kleinman H K 1980 Characterization of fibroblast chemotaxis. Journal of Laboratory and Clinical Medicine 96: 1071-80

Gold L I, Garcia-Pardo A, Frangione B, Franklin E C, Pearlstein E 1979 Subtilisin and cyanogen bromide cleavage products of fibronectin that retain gelatin-binding activity. Proceedings of the National Academy of Science USA 76: 4803-7

Hahn L H, Yamada K M 1979 Identification and isolation of a collagen-binding fragment of the adhesive glycoprotein fibronectin. Proceedings of the National Academy of Science USA 76: 1160-3

Hassell J R, Pennypacker J P, Kleinman H K, Pratt R M, Yamada K M 1979 Enhanced cellular fibronectin accumulation in chondrocytes treated with vitamin A. Cell 17: 821-6

Hauschka S D, White N K 1972 Studies of myogenesis in vitro. In: Banker B Q, Prybylski R J, van der Meulen J P, Victor M (eds) Research in muscle development and the muscle spindle. Excerpta Medica, p 53

Hewitt A T, Pennypacker J P, Kleinman H K, Martin G R 1980 Identification of an adhesion factor for chondrocytes. Proceedings of the National Academy of Science USA 77: 385-8

Highberger J H, Corbett C, Gross J 1979 Isolation and characterization of a peptide containing the site of cleavage of the chick skin collagen $\alpha 1$(I) chain by animal collagenases. Biochemical Biophysical Research Communications 89: 202-8

Hopper K E, Adelmann B C, Gentner G, Gay S 1977 Recognition by guinea pig peritoneal exudate cells of comformationally different states of the collagen molecule. Immunology 30: 249-59

Hynes R O, Destree A T, Perkins M E, Wagner D D 1979 Cell surface fibronectin and oncogenic transformation. Journal of Supramolecular Structure 11: 95-104

Jaffe E A, Mosher D F 1978 Synthesis of fibronectin by cultured human endothelial cells. Journal of Experimental Medicine 147: 1779-91

Jilek F, Hörmann H 1978 Cold-insoluble globulin (fibronectin) IV. Affinity to soluble collagen of various types. Hoppe-Seyler's Zeitschrift for Physiological Chemistry 359: 247-50

Jilek F, Hörmann H 1979 Fibronectin (cold-insoluble globulin) VI. Influence of heparin and hyaluronic acid on the binding of native collagen. Hoppe-Seyler's Zeitschrift for Physiological Chemistry 360: 597-603

Johansson S, Höök M 1980 Heparin enhances the rate of binding of fibronectin to collagen. Biochemical Journal 187: 521-4

Keski-Oja J, Sen A, Todaro G 1979 Soluble form of fibronectin binds to purified actin. Journal of Cell Biology 83: 49a 1975

Klebe R J 1974 Isolation of a collagen-dependent cell attachment factor. Nature 250: 248-51

Kleinman H K, Martin G R, Fishman P H 1979 Ganglioside inhibition of fibronectin mediated cell adhesion to collagen. Proceedings of the National Academy of Science USA 76: 3367-71

Kleinman H K, McGoodwin E B, Klebe R J 1976 Localization of the cell attachment region in types I and II collagen. Biochemical Biophysical Research Communications 72: 426-32

Kleinman H K, McGoodwin E B, Martin G R, Klebe R J 1978a Binding of cell attachment protein to collagen: effect of chemical modifications. Annals of the New York Academy of Science 312: 436-8

Kleinman H K, McGoodwin E B, Martin G R, Klebe R J, Fietzek P O, Woolley D E 1978b Localization of the binding site for cell attachment in the $\alpha 1$(I) chain of collagen. Journal of Biological Chemistry 253: 5642-6

Kleinman H K, Murray J C, McGoodwin E B, Martin G R 1978c Connective tissue structure: cell binding to collagen. Journal of Investigative Dermatology 71: 9-11

Lapière C M, Nusgens B, Pierard G E 1977 Interaction between collagen type I and type III in conditioning bundle organization. Connective Tissue Research 5: 21-9

Linder E, Vaheri A, Ruoslahti E, Wartiovaara J 1975 Distribution of fibroblast surface antigen in the developing chick embryo. Journal of Experimental Medicine 142: 41-9

Liotta L A, Vembu D, Kleinman H K, Martin G R, Boone C 1978 Collagen required for the proliferation of cultured connective tissue cells but not their transformed counterparts. Nature 272: 622-4

Mautner V M, Hynes R O 1977 Surface distribution of LETS protein in relation to the cytoskeleton of normal and transformed fibroblasts. Journal of Cell Biology 75: 743-66

McDonald J A, Kelley D G 1980 Degradation of fibronectin by human leucocyte elastase: Production of collagen binding and cell adhesive peptides. Journal of Biological Chemistry 255: 8848-58

Morrison P R, Edsall J T, Miller S G 1948 Preparation and properties of serum and plasma proteins XIII. The separation of purified fibrinogen from fraction I of human plasma. Journal of the American Chemical Society 70: 3103-8

Mosher D F, Schad P E, Vann J M 1980 Cross-linking of collagen and fibronectin by Factor XIII_a: Localization of participating glutaminyl residues to a tryptic fragment of fibronectin. Journal of Biological Chemistry 255: 1181-8

Mosher D F, Schad P E, Kleinman H K 1979 Cross-linking of fibronectin to collagen by blood coagulation factor XIII_a. Journal of Clinical Investigation 64: 781-7

Parry G, Soo W-J, Bissell M J 1979 The uncoupled regulation of fibronectin and collagen synthesis in Rous sarcoma virus transformed avian tendon cells. Journal of Biological Chemistry 254: 11763-6

Pearlstein E 1976 Plasma membrane glycoprotein which mediates adhesion of fibroblasts to collagen. Nature 262: 497-500

Pearlstein E, Gold I I, Garcia-Pardo A 1980 Fibronectin: a review of its structure and biological activity. Molecular and Cellular Biochemistry, 29: 103-28

Pennypacker J P, Hassell J R, Yamada K M, Pratt R M 1979 The influence of an adhesive cell surface protein on chondrogenic expression in vitro. Experimental Cell Research 121: 411-5

Postlethwaite A E, Seyer J M, Kang A H 1978 Chemotactic attraction of human fibroblasts to type I, II and III collagens and collagen-derived peptides. Proceedings of the National Academy of Science USA 75: 871-5

Ramachandran G N, Reddi A H (eds) 1976 Biochemistry of collagen. Plenum Press, New York

Ruoslahti E, Engvall E 1980 Complexing of fibronectin, glycosaminoglycans and collagen. Biochimica Biophysica Acta 322: 352-8

Ruoslahti E, Hayman E G, Kuusela P, Shively J E, Engvall E 1979 Isolation of a tryptic fragment containing the collagen-binding site of plasma fibronectin. Journal of Biological Chemistry 254: 6054-9

Saba T M, Blumenstock F A, Weber P, Kaplan E 1978 Physiological role of cold-insoluble globulin in host defense: impllcations of its characterization as an opsonic A_2 surface binding glycoprotein. Annals of the New York Academy of Science 312: 43-55

Santoro S A, Cunningham L W 1979 Fibronectin and the multiple interaction model for platelet-collagen adhesion. Proceedings of the National Academy of Science USA 76: 2644-8

Stenman S, Vaheri A 1978 Distribution of a major connective tissue protein, fibronectin in normal human tissues. Journal of Experimental Medicine 147: 1054-64

Vaheri A, Kurkinen M, Lehto V P, Linder E, Timpl R 1978 Codistribution of pericellular matrix proteins in cultured fibroblasts and loss in transformation: fibronectin and procollagen. Proceedings of the National Academy of Science USA 75: 4944-8

Vaheri A, Mosher D F 1978 High molecular weight cell surface glycoprotein (fibronectin) lost in malignant transformation. Archives of Biochemistry and Biophysics 185: 214-21

Vaheri A, Ruoslahti E, Westermark B, Ponten J 1976 A common cell-type specific surface antigen in cultured human glial cells and fibroblasts. Journal of Experimental Medicine 143: 64-72

Vuento M, Vaheri A 1979 Dissociation of fibronectin from gelatin-agarose by amino compounds. Biochemical Journal 175: 333-6

Yamada K M, Olden K, Hahn L E 1980 Cell surface protein and cell interactions. In: S Subtelny and N K Wessells (eds) The cell surface: mediator of developmental processes. Academic Press, New York p 43-77

Yamada K M, Kennedy D W 1979 Fibroblast cellular and plasma fibronectins are similar but not identical. Journal of Cell Biology 80: 492-7

Yamada K M, Olden K 1978 Fibronectins-adhesive glycoproteins of cell surface and blood. Nature 275: 179-84

Yamada K M, Yamada S S, Pastan I 1977a Quantitation of a transformation-sensitive adhesion, cell surface glycoprotein. Journal of Cell Biology 74: 649-54

Yamada K M, Yamada S S, Pastan I 1977b Cell surface protein partially restores morphology, adhesiveness and contact inhibition of movement to transformed fibroblasts. Proceedings of the National Academy of Science USA 73: 1211-21

West C M, Lanza R, Rosenbloom J, Lowe M, Holtzer H 1979 Fibronectin alters the phenotypic properties of cultured chick embryo chondroblasts. Cell 17: 491-501

12

Experimental modifications of collagen synthesis and degradation and their therapeutic applications

M. CHVAPIL *

INTRODUCTION

The purpose of this chapter is to briefly review and emphasize some aspects of the pharmacology of fibrosis, specifically those related to the collagenous component of fibrotic, cirrhotic or sclerotic lesions. In doing this, I shall present my views on this area of collagen research, which integrates both the basic and clinical information and needs.

Pharmacology of fibrosis is concerned with all possible methods of inhibiting the formation of the fibrotic tissue. Fibrosis is, however, a final stage of the fibroproductive inflammation which could be induced by any noxious agent of physical (temperature, radiation, incision), chemical (CCl_4, bleomycin, etc.), or biological (infection, immune reaction) nature. A noxious agent initiates a cascade of humoral-cellular reactions with microcirculatory changes in the injured tissue. The various activators and mediators of inflammation in early stages of the tissue injury affect the fibroblast. The chemical environment of an injured tissue can activate fibroblasts, to both proliferate at an increased rate and increase synthesis of structural macromolecules, glycosaminoglycans and collagen. My reason for presenting this simplified outline of fibroproliferative reaction is to indicate that the final fibrosis may be affected by various factors interfering with any feature of the inflammatory reaction. Thus, an anti-inflammatory agent inhibiting, for instance, histamine or serotonin release, prostaglandin synthesis or some cellular reactions (release of lysosomal enzymes, chemotaxis, formation of free oxygen radicals by activated granulocytes, macrophages, etc.) or preserving the structure and function of microcirculation (pO_2), etc., should ultimately modify the magnitude of the fibrotic reaction.

Specificity and selectivity

For the purpose of this review, I will call all factors acting on various inflammatory reactions before these involve fibroblast *non-specific*, while those factors affecting various metabolic aspects of collagen inside or outside of fibroblasts will be classified as *specific*.

Specific pharmacological interference with collagen metabolism is related to several rather unique features of the synthesis, secretion, maturation and degradation of this protein. For the purposes of this review, Table 12.1 summarizes the sequence of events in collagen metabolism and proposed methods of inhibition. The pivotal role of the *hydroxylation* of prolyl and lysyl residues in the synthesis of collagen molecules indicates that inhibition of this step will affect solely collagen and not noncollagenous proteins. Similarly, selective inhibition of *maturation* of collagen by inhibiting lysyl oxidase will be reflected only in the degree of polymerization of collagenous structures. In view of the recent findings of several similarities between both C1q complement component and acetylcholinesterase and the collagen molecule, the uniqueness of collagen and, thus, its specific inhibition is questionable.

I will limit, therefore, the scope of this review to the collagenous component of the fibrosis and to methods of inhibiting abnormal collagen deposition.

The chances that a certain drug will selectively inhibit collagen synthesis only in a pathological lesion are because the rate of collagen synthesis and turnover is significantly higher in diseased than in normal tissue. Biological structures with higher turnover rates are more susceptible to metabolic modifications by pharmacological or physical interference. Thus, it appears that collagen metabolism could be inhibited selectively in the injured tissue. In other words, any substance affecting collagen metabolism would exert its most prominent effect in the scar where collagen turnover is higher, rather than in the surrounding tissues (Berlin & Schimke, 1965; Goldstein et al, 1974). The principle of specificity and selectivity is illustrated in Figure 12.1.

Although in this chapter I will review much basic information on the modifications of collagen structure and function derived mainly from research of isolated biological systems (fibroblast cultures, tissue slices), the ultimate aim is the therapeutic applications of these data. Thus, we will test whether many quite ingenious methods of interference with various steps of collagen metabolism, established in

*Supported in part by Grants GM25159 and AM18706-04 from National Institutes of Health.

Table 12.1 Pharmacological interferences with post-translational steps of collagen biosynthesis

Metabolic step	*Enzyme involved*	*Cofactors*	*Controlling drug*
Hydroxylation	Prolyl hydroxylase	O_2, Ascorbic acid	Depletion of Ascorbic Acid.
	Lysyl hydroxylase	α-Ketoglutarate	—
		$Fe^{2+/3+}$	Iron chelators
			α, α-dipyridyl
			o-phenanthroline
		Substrate	Proline analogs
			Lysine analogs
		$^{-}O_2$.	Free radicals inhibitors, scavengers
Glycosylation	Galactosyl transferase	Mn^{2+}	
	Glucosyl transferase		
	N-acetylglucosaminyl transferase		
	Mannosyl transferase		
Secretion	Functional microtubules	Ca^{2+}	Colchicine, vinblastin
	microfilaments		Cytochalasin B
	Procollagen N — protease(s)	Ca^{2+}, Mg^{2+}	Cu^{2+}, Zn^{2+}, EGTA
	C — protease(s)		
Polymerization	Lysyl oxidase	Cu^{2+}, O_2	Cu^{2+}-deficiency
		Pyridoxal	BAPN
			D-penicillamine
Degradation	Tissue collagenases	Ca^{2+}, Zn^{2+}	EDTA, colchicine

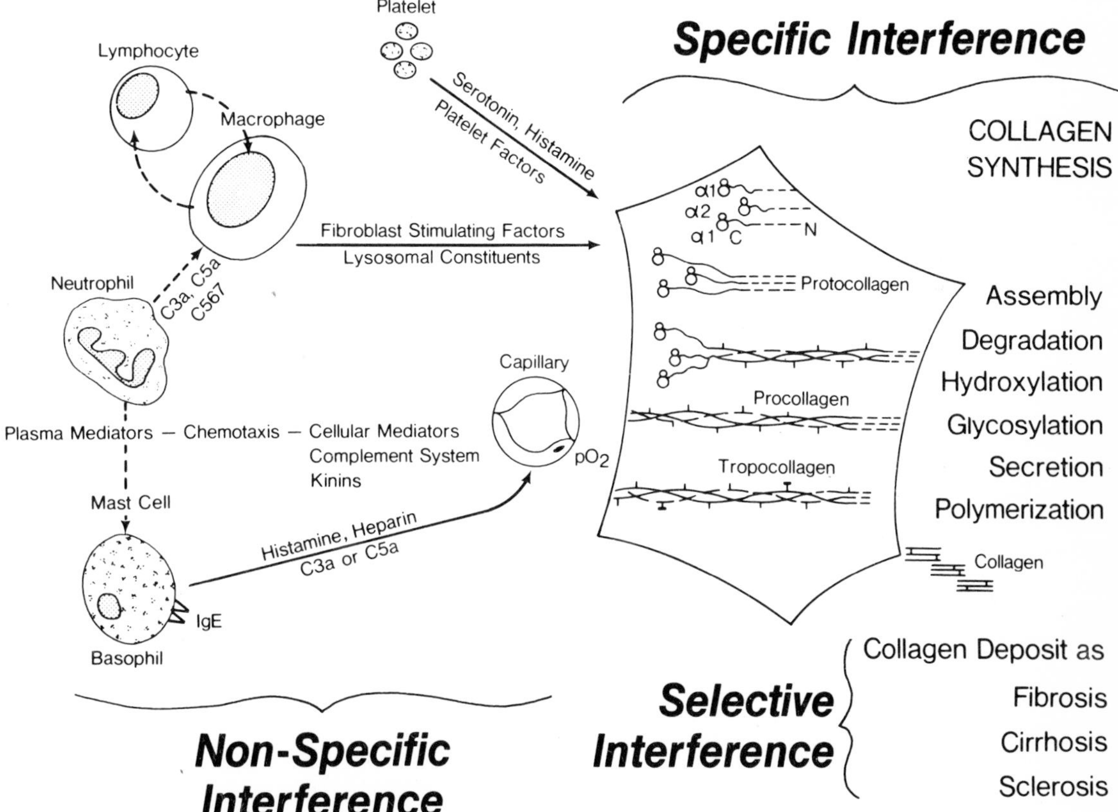

Fig. 12.1 Schematic representation of fibroproliferative inflammation. The figure indicates the nonspecific, specific and selective pharmacological modifications of the process.

isolated cellular or cell-free systems, would be applicable to collagen regulation in vivo. Dealing with the whole organism, every clinician is concerned mainly with the risk to benefit ratio, or toxic versus desired therapeutic effects of a certain treatment. In laboratory animals, the most obvious indication of general toxicity is change in body growth, loss of body weight and reduced food intake. These parameters will be carefully analyzed with regard to each method of specific and selective interference with the collagen molecule. I would like to stress that loss of body mass itself affects almost every aspect of collagen metabolism. Lysyl oxidase activity is also reduced by loss of body weight (Madia et al, 1979).

Finally, one should keep in mind that evaluating the effectiveness of anticollagenous medication, that only a substantial inhibition of collagenous structures is clinically meaningful. Thus, statistical significance may not be the same as therapeutic significance.

SELECTIVE INHIBITION OF COLLAGEN

The characteristic steps involved in collagen biosynthesis are shown in Table 12.1. Each step is controlled by specific enzymes, several classified as metalloenzymes or metal dependent. The requirement for metal offers an opportunity for interference by complexing or chelating agents. This aspect will be discussed in detail in the analysis of individual post-translational modifications. The rather poor specificity of most chelating agents to bind particular metals makes this approach a matter of challenge for the future.

METHODS CONTROLLING THE HYDROXYLATION STEP

Hydroxylation of some proline residues is important for the structural stability of the final collagen molecule. Underhydroxylated collagen is more susceptible to heat denaturation and to bacterial collagenase degradation (see review by Prockop et al, 1980). Several recent data indicate that the hydroxyl group of hydroxyproline plays a critical role in stabilizing the triplehelical conformation of collagen. In fact, it was shown that fibrogenic cells incubated in the presence of Cis-Hyp or any other proline analogs prevent the collagen polypeptide chains from becoming triplehelical (Inouye et al, 1976). Nonhelical procollagen containing the analogue is retained within the RER of the fibroblast in tissue culture system (Uitto et al, 1975). By this mechanism, the secretions of the 'product' and its deposition in the extracellular space is inhibited. Hydroxylation of lysine residues is a prerequisite for the following glycosylation step and further secretion of collagen out of the cell.

Hydroxylation of some Pro or Lys residues in the collagenous polypeptide is catalysed by two different hydroxylases having similar cofactors or cosubstrates: Fe^{2+}, O_2, ascorbic acid and α-ketoglutarate. Interference with any of these factors results in the modification of the activity of prolyl or lysyl hydroxylase and to the above structural consequences in the collagen molecule.

Ascorbic acid deficiency

Although several modes of action of ascorbic acid on connective tissue structure and synthesis of its macromolecular components were postulated (for review, see Barnes, 1975), we will consider its effect on collagen hydroxylation only. It has been proven that in isolated systems, and to a lesser degree in vivo this cofactor of prolyl and lysyl hydroxylase affects the degree of collagen hydroxylation and, therefore, the secretion of the collagen molecule. A controversy exists as to the role of ascorbic acid in the activation of an inactive form of prolyl hydroxylase.

Considering the difficulties of decreasing the content of Vitamin C in tissues of adult animals under in vivo conditions, ascorbic acid deficiency has been shown to be a very effective method of inhibiting collagen accumulation in various animal models of fibrotic tissues. Ascorbic acid deficiency has no effect on already deposited collagen as there is no evidence of increased collagen degradation (Barnes, 1975). Newly synthesized collagen in ascorbate deficient guinea pigs is partially hydroxylated and this form is degraded at a faster rate (Barnes et al, 1970). Inherited human collagen lysyl hydroxylase deficiency responding to ascorbic acid supplementation produces congenital hypotonia, lax joints, friable skin, haemorrhagic scars, and high-arched palate (Elsas et al, 1978). Only primates, guinea pigs and shrimps do not synthesize ascorbate and so develop scorbutic symptoms by reducing its supply (Magarelli et al, 1979). The predictability of inducing a controlled ascorbate deficiency for therapeutic purposes in primates, mainly in man, is rather doubtful. Enormous individual variability in the susceptibility to Vitamin C deficiency in man is reported and would make this method of controlling collagenous fibrosis for human pathology quite impractical.

Furthermore, it is documented that, following an operation, ascorbic acid deficiency is a common and significant factor in the pathogenesis of wound complications not directly related to collagen deposition (Irvin et al, 1978).

Chelation of iron

Since the first report that divalent iron chelators, such as α,α'-dipyridyl or o-phenanthroline in isolated systems of tissue slices on fibrogenic cells inhibit the hydroxylation of collagen by interference with Fe^{2+} of prolyl and lysyl hydroxylase, this approach was successfully used to elucidate several basic problems of collagen biosynthesis (see review by Prockop et al, 1979). Trivalent iron chelators (Desferrioxamine-β, EDTA, Tiron) were also effective only when they permeated the cell membrane (Hurych and Chvapil, unpublished results).

Administration of either α,α'-dipyridyl or o-phenanthroline, to animals resulted in a decrease of collagen deposition in liver injury induced by i.v. instillation of silica particles (Chvapil & Hurych, 1968; Chvapil et al, 1967, 1969, 1974) or ethionine treatment (Brada et al, 1972a, b). Inhibition of collagen deposition in colostomy wounds (Bora et al, 1972) or in skin wounds (Whitson & Peacock, 1967) by divalent iron chelators were also reported. It was assumed that the inhibitory effect was related to chelation of Fe^{2+} of the appropriate hydroxylases. Direct measurement of prolyl hydroxylase activity in various tissues of animals treated systemically or locally with *o*-phenanthroline or α,α'-dipyridyl or desferrioxamine failed, however, to demonstrate inhibition of the enzyme. On the contrary, an enhancement of prolyl hydroxylase activity was shown (Chvapil et al, 1974). Stimulation of the activity of prolyl hydroxylase by *o*-phenanthroline was also shown in cultures of 3T3 fibroblasts at lower concentrations of the chelating agent than commonly used (Chvapil, 1977). Recently, Takeda et al (1979) suggested that stimulation of prolyl hydroxylase activity by chelating agents may be related to the activation of oxygen by the complex of chelating agent — $Fe^{2+/3+}$.

Taking into consideration the toxicity-effectiveness ratio of in vivo administered chelating agents, their nonspecificity in binding various metals and even some other effects not related to chelation (such as supply of SH groups by diethyldithiocarbonates and D-penicillamine or induction of hepatic mixed function oxidases by phenanthrolines (Chvapil & Ryan, 1971), the actual mechanism of the previously reported inhibitory effect of some Fe^{2+} chelating agents on collagen synthesis in various models of fibrosis may not be related to the inhibition of prolyl hydroxylase or to specific interference with collagen metabolism. Even the nonchelating analogue of *o*-phenanthroline, m-phenanthroline, reduces the liver injury and collagen deposition induced by ethionine (Brada & Chvapil, 1972; Brada et al, 1972).

Proline analogues

The ingenious idea of using proline or lysine analogues to interfere with the hydroxylation of some Pro or Lys residues in the collagen polypeptide resulted in an avalanche of studies elucidating many essential features of collagen metabolism (for review, see Grant & Prockop, 1976; Prockop et al, 1979). Besides the usual proline analogues tested (Table 12.2), new analogues as potential inhibitors of collagen biosynthesis were synthesized (Shirota et al, 1977).

While the in vitro studies are impeccable, and clearly demonstrate inhibition of various features of collagen metabolism, the use of analogues in whole animals resulted in conflicting results which could be classified into two groups:

1. Inhibition of collagen accumulation without toxic side effects.
2. No effect on collagen or inhibition of collagen accumulation only at toxic dosages of the drug.

In the first group belong the studies of Bora et al (1972) and Lane et al (1972) who found a significant decrease of the breaking strength of peritendinous adhesions in rats treated with D,L-3,4-dehydroxyproline (3,4 DHP) or cis-hydroxyproline. Daly et al (1973) reported a decrease in the bursting strength of colostomy wounds in rats treated with cis-hydroxyproline. 3,4 DHP significantly reduced collagen accumulation in the in vivo system of estradiol-stimulated rat uterus (Salvador et al, 1976). At least two studies report on effective inhibition of liver fibrosis induced by carbon tetrachloride in rats treated with either L-azetidine-2-carboxylic acid (Rojkind et al, 1973) or by 3,4-DHP (Kewar et al, 1977). There are few reports on the use of proline analogues in patients with tendon injury and in the treatment of patients with keloids (Lane et al, 1975).

Recently, Riley et al (1980) prevented the deposition of collagen in the lungs of rats exposed to a high oxygen atmosphere by simultaneous treatment with cis-4-hydroxy-L-proline. They observed that the mean body weight of the O_2-exposed and proline analogue treated group was significantly less than the controls. Nevertheless, the authors found no gross toxic effect of the cis-hydroxyproline, and they believe that the striking inhibition of collagen deposition in the injured lung is due to a specific effect of this analogue on collagen synthesis.

The second group (inhibition of collagen synthesis only at toxic dosages) is illustrated by the study of Madden et al (1973). They found that, in mice, 3,4-DHP is 15 times more toxic than L-proline. With chronic administration they observed no effect on collagen synthesis and accumulation in normal or repairing tissues. After a single injection of 3,4-DHP several signs of cytotoxicity of this analogue were noted in liver hepatocytes and fibroblasts of reactive granuloma capsule. Studies by Chvapil et al (1974), Cohen & Diegelman (1978), and Ohuchi et al (1979) showed that cis-hydroxyproline or N-acetyl-cis-4-hydroxyproline has no effect on the collagen synthesis

Table 12.2 Proline structural analogues interfering with collagen synthesis

l-acetidine-2-carboxylic acid
3,4-dehydroxy-L-proline
cis-4-fluoro-L-proline
trans-4-cis-hydroxy-L-proline
trans-4-fluoro-L-proline
thiazolidine-4-carboxylic acid
4,4-difluoro-L-proline
4,4-dimethyl-DL-proline

or deposition in skin wounds. The breaking strength of the incision wound is not affected. In fact, Cohen & Diegelman (1978) found enhancement of the synthesis of both collagenous and noncollagenous proteins in skin wounds of rats treated chemically with N-acetyl-cis-4-hydroxyproline (50 mg to 200 mg/kg body weight). Madden et al (1973) also showed an increased breaking strength of skin incision wounds of animals treated with 3,4-DHP. Ohuchi et al (1979) found little or no effect of three various proline analogues in suppressing radiation fibrosis in the skin of guinea pigs.

The discrepancies between the high efficacy of proline analogues in in vitro situations and toxic problems with in vivo administration are not typical for this category of drugs, but are quite common with several other medications suggested for the treatment of fibrotic lesions. There are several possible reasons for such a differing activity:

The efficiency of proline analogues in inhibiting collagen hydroxylation depends on the size of the pool of the analogue, which determines the amount of incorporation into collagenous polypeptides. Assuming that both proline and its analogue are incorporated randomly into a protein, the ratio of analogue to free proline should determine the relative incorporation rates. Decreasing the size of the free proline pool, therefore, should amplify the effect of any specific analogue dose. Madden et al (1973) showed, however, that elminating dietary proline has no effect on free proline pool size. The endogenous production of proline from glutamate, ornithine, and arginine seems sufficient to replace the exogenous source (Adams, 1970). Dilution by free proline, therefore, will significantly reduce the efficiency of any proline analogue. The dilution effect may be even more pronounced as most injured tissues have an elevated pool of free proline due to increased protein catabolism (Chvapil & Ryan, 1973; Roberts & Simonsen, 1962; Kershenobich et al, 1970).

In order to overcome the dilution of an analogue by the proline pool, the efficiency could be increased by administering larger amounts of the analogue. The general toxicity of protein analogues, mainly of 3,4-DHP, however, poses a serious problem to a therapist.

The toxicity of analogues may be related to the nonspecific incorporation of this drug into biologically active noncollagenous proteins. It is suggested that the reduced activity of prolyl hydroxylase synthesized under the effect of 3,4-DHP may reflect an aberrant form of the enzyme (Uslau et al, 1978). It would be of interest to know whether the structure and function of liver mixed function oxidases are affected by the administration of analogues — which would explain their protective effect on CCl_4 hepatotoxicity.

The assumption of random incorporation of proline or its analogues into protein may not be valid. Rosenbloom (1971) demonstrated that cis-hydroxyproline, which is incorporated into collagen and behaves as a proline analogue, is incorporated into protein at a rate approximately 10 times slower than L-proline. Rosenbloom & Prockop (1970) also showed that 3,4-DHP is incorporated into cartilage protein at a rate five times slower than that of L-proline. A reduced rate of incorporation, as well as the dilution related to free proline pool, may explain the difficulty in demonstrating the presence of 3,4-DHP in either collagen or noncollagenous protein after in vivo chronic administration (Madden et al, 1973). Using a closed system of embryonal chickens injected with 0.5 mg azetidine-2-carboxylic acid daily between days 8 and 12, Lane et al (1971) found 4 residues of this analogue per 1000 residues of amino acid in acid-soluble collagen. This represents only 2 per cent incorporation when the content of proline and hydroxyproline is considered as 100 per cent.

Regulation by oxygen concentrating

A low oxygen or increased nitrogen atmosphere in in vitro experiments results in inhibition of prolyl hydroxylase activity. The magnitude of K_m for O_2 indicates that it is almost impossible to achieve such a low pO_2 in tissues of living organisms without generalized tissue damage. Some studies indicate, however, that oxygen used by the enzymes in the hydroxylation reactions exists in the activated form, possibly as superoxide anion $\cdot O_2^-$ (Cardinale & Udenfriend, 1974; Bhatnagar, 1977). Nitroblue tetrazolium as a superoxide scavenger inhibits both hydroxylases (Tuderman et al, 1977; Liu & Bhatnagar, 1973). For unknown reasons, the superoxide dismutase (SOD) was found ineffective (Cardinale & Udenfriend, 1974; Liu & Bhatnagar, 1973). Only in the presence of ascorbate and ferrous ions in the culture medium with WI-38 fibroblast did SOD reduce the stimulatory effect of both cofactors on the formation of C^{14} collagenous hydroxyproline. Recently Myllylä et al (1979) presented evidence strongly supporting the view that $\cdot O_2^-$ is involved in the hydroxylase reactions as dismutation of the superoxide by SOD and four low molecular active copper chelates inhibited both prolyl and lysyl hydroxylases. These findings suggest various speculations about the importance of controlling the free radicals or other active oxygen forms in injured tissues in relation to the synthesis of the complete collagen molecule.

INTERFERENCE WITH COLLAGEN SECRETION

Several prerequisites are essential for the collagen molecule to be secreted by the cell. It has to be glycosylated; thus, interference with hydroxylation of lysine residues or direct effect on glycosylating transferases could be the target for interference. Secretion is related to the activity of cell microskeletons. Thus, interference with microfilaments or microtubules will affect the transport of collagen molecule within and out of the cell. Cytochalasin B is known to interfere with microfilaments; colchicine and vinblastin are representatives of drugs that reversibly disaggregate microtubules. These substances were demonstrated to inhibit collagen synthesis and conversion of procollagen to collagen in closed systems of organ or cell cultures by a mechanism related to modification of the microskeleton and not to inhibition of either procollagen peptidase or the hydroxylation step.

Colchicine

Several reports indicate the beneficial effect of in vivo colchicine administration on liver cirrhosis (Rojkind et al, 1973; Rojkind & Kershenobich, 1975), scleroderma (Alaceon-Segovia et al, 1974) and in sarcoid arthritis (Harris & Millis, 1971). Other reports, dealing mainly with the effectiveness of this drug in the treatment of scleroderma patients, produced negative findings (Harris et al, 1975; Guttadauria et al, 1977).

Colchicine has been used for centuries for the treatment of acute gout, but it is generally ineffective in other inflammatory disorders (Wellau et al, 1967). Still, colchicine given as an oral dose of 6.0 mg/kg suppresses the development of carrageenan-induced oedema in rats. This effect may be mediated by suppressing some functions of polymorphonuclear leucocytes (Chang, 1975), or may relate to the inhibition of induction of lysosomal enzymes by interference with microtubules, involved in pinocytosis and phagocytosis of inflammatory cells (Pesanti & Axline, 1975). Colchicine was tried in the treatment of CCl_4-liver cirrhosis of rats (Rojkind et al, 1973; Rojkind & Kershenobich, 1975). Young rats receiving 10 μg colchicine/day by the gastric route continued to grow at a normal rate (Rojkind & Kershenobich, 1975). When the drug was administered simultaneously with CCl_4, collagen synthesis and deposition in the liver were inhibited and the liver function remained normal. When the drug was administered after 30 days of CCl_4 administration which was then discontinued, the loss of collagen from the injured liver was enhanced by colchicine.

Several studies tested colchicine in patients with scleroderma. While Aleceon-Segovia et al (1974) noted clinical and laboratory improvements, most of the reports and personal experience found colchicine of no value in the treatment of scleroderma (Guttadauria et al, 1977). Harris et al (1975) studying the effect of the drug on the excretion of urinary hydroxyproline in scleroderma concluded that 'administration of colchicine in doses tolerated in man do not either inhibit synthesis of new collagen or increase degradation of mature collagen to be of use in treatment of fibrotic states.'

The rationale for using colchicine in the inhibition of fibrosing processes relates to the established effects of this drug on depolymerization of the microtubules of fibroblasts, thus inhibiting the secretion of synthesized collagen molecules. Another interesting effect of colchicine was reported by Harris & Krane (1971) who found that in cultures of rheumatoid synovial cells colchicine stimulates de novo synthesis of collagenase. This aspect will be discussed in the section on collagen degradation. Finally, direct effect of colchicine on the synthesis of collagen and noncollagenous protein, at least in the liver tissue, was reported (Rojkind & Kershenobich, 1975). The in vivo effect of colchicine on the synthesis of both types of proteins, at least in granuloma tissue, was just the opposite (Chvapil et al, 1980). Personally, I have come to the conclusion that the therapeutic dose of colchicine is too close to the toxic dose. This may be related, at least in the liver, to the effect of this drug on the secretion of both collagen as well as noncollagenous proteins (Redman & Banerjee, 1975).

Local anaesthetics

Local anaesthetics such as procaine and lidocaine were shown to inhibit the synthesis of proteins, DNA and RNA by a wide range of bacteria and fungi, suggesting a possible explanation for their antimicrobial activity (Schmidt & Rosenkranz, 1970). In mammalian skeletal-muscle cells, protein synthesis is inhibited by bupivacaine at concentrations which do not affect DNA or RNA synthesis (Johnson & Jones, 1978). It is also reported that local anaesthetics inhibit secretion of plasma proteins in rat liver slices and reduce histamine release from mast cells (Bannerjee & Redman, 1977). Eichhorn & Peterkofsky (1979) showed in fibroblast culture inhibition of collagen secretion by local anaesthetics, possibly by influencing the microtubular system through an effect on the cell membrane. Recently, Chvapil et al (1980) showed inhibition of collagen synthesis and prolyl hydroxylase activity in granuloma tissue of rats after local administration of lidocaine or bupivacaine.

Several molecular mechanisms have been proposed for the effects of local anaesthetics. It is possible that local anaesthetics affect the stability and fluidity of cell membranes, sodium conductance and cell-calcium movement. Interference of local anaesthetics with cell microtubules and microfilaments is demonstrated by several studies, some suggesting the displacement of Ca^{++} as a possible microtubule depolymerizing mechanism (Seeman, 1972; Nicolson et al, 1976).

Other substances

Tunicamycin (Housley et al, 1980) and monensin (M. Tanzer, personal communication) have been studied for an effect on collagen biosynthesis and may interfere with the intracellular transport and secretion of the molecule by blocking either glycosylation step or microskeleton integrity. So far, these drugs have been studied in isolated systems of cells in culture only. It seems, however, that these drugs inhibit the secretion of various glycoproteins by the cell. For this reason, specific interference with collagen synthesis is doubtful.

METHODS CONTROLLING THE MATURATION (POLYMERIZATION) OF COLLAGEN

Inhibition of maturation of collagen has so far been the most successful and powerful method of interfering with the physical properties of scar contractures and fibrotic structures (for review, see Perez-Tamayo et al, 1974). Apparently, it is not the total volume of collagenous structures within a certain tissue, but rather the physical properties of the collagenous matrix which represent the real danger to the function of the tissue or organ. When collagen is cross-linked, possibly by stable covalent cross-links involving the function of lysyl oxidase, it is less degradable by mammalian collagenase and forms a compact rigid scar.

Lysyl oxidase oxidatively deaminates specific ϵ-amino-groups of peptidyl lysine and hydroxylysine residues contained within the structural proteins collagen and elastin. The aldehyde product then forms, nonenzymatically, either Schiff base adducts with other specific ϵ-amino peptidyl lysine or hydroxylysine residues or forms aldol condensates with other preformed aldehydic components. These cross-linking reactions lend structural integrity to collagenous and elastinous connective tissue.

Two substances, possibly directly involved in the enzyme activity, i.e. copper and pyridoxal, have been shown to regulate enzyme function in vivo. Induction of copper or pyridoxal deficiency are, however, very impractical as a clinical-therapeutic method of controlling the maturation of collagen (Harris, 1976; Murray & Levine, 1977; Murray et al, 1978; Levine, 1978).

Sudden loss of body weight does result in significantly reduced activity of lysyl oxidase (Chvapil, unpublished results; Madia et al, 1979). Among other factors implicated in the control of the enzyme activity, are hypophysectomy (Everitt, 1959) and body temperature. Without going into the analysis of possible mechanisms of the effects of these factors, it is becoming clear that using BAPN to control lysyl oxidase is the most promising.

One important feature of lysyl oxidase should be mentioned: it is documented that after irreversible inhibition of the enzyme by BAPN, its activity in the tissue recovers very quickly, usually 6 to 12 hours depending on the metabolic turnover rate of the tissue (Arem et al, 1979). This recovery as well as the rapid metabolism of BAPN led to the conclusion that BAPN should be administered either at short time intervals (6 hours apart) or preferably continuously by a drug delivery system.

In principle, we may interfere directly with the function of lysyl oxidase by various lathyrogenic agents, of which BAPN is the most effective. Inhibition of lysyl oxidase by BAPN is irreversible. Another possibility is blocking the formed aldehydes, as with D-penicillamine, preventing condensation of aldehydes or formation of Schiff bases as shown in Figure 12.2. Since BAPN and D-penicillamine affect two different sites in the formation of covalent cross-links, when used together their effect is cumulative (Haney et al, 1973).

The lathyritic properties of penicillamine derive from its ability to interact with aldehydes formed by the action of lysyl oxidase on the ϵ-amino group of lysine in tropocollagen. This results in subsequent reduction of collagen aldol groups in animal models of fibrotic lesions. Direct inhibition of lysyl oxidase by D-penicillamine has been reported (Nimni, 1970). Finally, as will be shown below, chelation of Cu^{++} after topical continuous administration could be assumed.

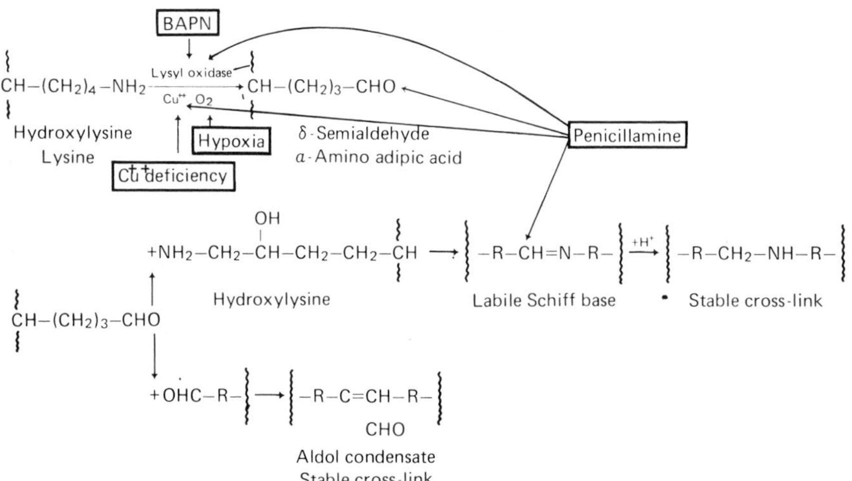

Fig. 12.2 Method of formation of covalent cross-links in the collagen structure. The scheme shows a few factors (in brackets) interfering with collagen polymerization.

BAPN

BAPN has undergone extensive evaluation and testing in our division, and we have successfully used it to reverse several conditions of pathological scarring in experimental animal models. I would like to summarize here some of these results in place of reviewing a rather extensive literature on this topic. Peacock & Madden (1966) employed BAPN in studies of basic wound biology and demonstrated cessation of gain in wound strength and an increase in soluble collagen extraction in incised and sutured rat dermal wounds during BAPN administration. Craver, Madden & Peacock (1968) employed BAPN to prevent tendon incarceration in injured chicken flexor tendons. Furlow & Peacock (1965) used BAPN to prevent joint stiffness in immobilized rat joints by altering the physical properties of collagen deposited around joints in immobilized limbs. Davis, Madden & Peacock (1972) employed BAPN in dogs, first to prevent oesophageal stricture in experimental lye burns and subsequently to reverse established strictures. In summary, we have found, in agreement with studies of several other authors, that BAPN is an effective and specific drug interfering with collagen structural stability in the animal models studied. Signs of systemic toxicity were, however, recognized. Our most recent studies (Chvapil, unpublished) indicated that.the 'lathyrogenic' effectiveness of BAPN is always associated with inhibition of the growth of body weight. There was almost no difference in the breaking strength of skin wounds between the BAPN group and pair-fed control group. In fact, if BAPN was administered to young rats at the dose which did not affect their body growth rate, no 'lathyrogenic' effect was manifest. Simple reduction of body weight by 10 to 15 per cent of control animals resulted in lower lysyl oxidase activity in the granuloma tissue.

Because of success in animal studies, Keiser & Sjoerdsma (1967) studied the effect of BAPN in patients with scleroderma. In short-term treatment with a dose of 2 g/day, no toxic side effects were noted; longer courses of treatment were, however, associated with prohibitive reactions, such as allergic skin rash and heamolytic anaemia. Peacock & Madden (1969) employed BAPN in clinical trials with humans undergoing flexor tendon surgery. Although a significant number of the patients exhibited hypersensitivity to the agent, decreased covalent bonding of human collagen with significant clinical benefit was demonstrated.

The systemic toxicity of BAPN has been the major obstacle in using this drug in large scale in human pathology. There is no doubt that at lathyrogenic dosages of BAPN, the animals stop growing, lose body weight and lower their food intake. Also, the animals' behaviour is changed — they do not clean their fur and are irritated if they are touched. All this indicates a general toxicity. One way to reduce the systemic toxicity of BAPN without interfering with its lathyrogenic activity is to inhibit the metabolism of this drug. If degradation of BAPN is blocked by pargyline, a monoamine oxidase (MAO) inhibitor, prolonged lysyl oxidase inhibition potentiates wound strength diminution without accompanying toxicity. Isoniazid (INH), both a weak lysyl oxidase and MAO inhibitor, also potentiates the lathyritic effects of BAPN. We found that the addition of isoniazid or pargyline to an otherwise effective dose of BAPN profoundly inhibited lysyl oxidase and depressed wound burst strength. All animals gained weight throughout the experiment (Arem et al, 1979).

Another method of overcoming the general toxicity of BAPN would be the topical delivery of the drug to the site of the injury either by injecting or implanting BAPN-polymer complex, where the polymer serves either as a vehicle for sustained release of the drug or reduces the release by controlling the diffusion of BAPN from the site of administration. Preliminary results with BAPN-delivery systems are reported (Speer et al, 1975). It was found that many carriers for BAPN tested (glycolmethacrylate, polyglutamic acid and polyacrylic acid) induced nonacceptable tissue reactions. Other topical delivery systems are under investigation.

D-penicillamine

The theoretical reasons for combining the BAPN with D-penicillamine were indicated above. Nimni (1970, 1972, 1977) contributed most to our understanding of the mechanism of the effect of D-penicillamine on collagen cross-linking. It seems that a lower dose affects interaction with lysine derived aldehydes (Nimni, 1977; Siegel, 1977) while at larger doses the chelation of various metals is of primary significance (Albergoin et al, 1975). Two other effects of D-penicillamine on collagen structural stability are postulated: depolymerization of nonreduced Schiff base cross-links resulting in increased extractability of collagen into neutral salts (Nimni, 1977) and a direct inhibition of lysyl oxidase shown by Nimni (1977) and recently by Misiorowski et al (1978)' The latter study indicates that the inhibition of the enzyme by D-penicillamine may not be related to chelation of the metal but to direct interaction with other functional groups of the enzyme molecule. The overall effectiveness of D-penicillamine in decreasing the structural stability of collagen has been well-documented (see review by Nimni, 1977). The long-term experience with this drug was well summarized by Sternlieb & Scheinberg (1967). All of the clinical studies related to D-penicillamine have indicated a high incidence of acute hypersensitivity reactions. These symptoms are suppressed by systemic steroids; thus a combination of D-penicillamine and prednisone should minimize toxic side effects.

The fact that D-penicillamine affects the structural stability of collagen at different sites than BAPN indicates the advantage of combining both drugs to eventually achieve an additive effect at a lower dosage than that of either drug alone. I personally feel that the potential therapeutic effectiveness of this method is very promising. More controlled clinical trials are needed to establish the value of this medication in the treatment of fibrotic lesions.

DEGRADATION OF COLLAGEN

It is obvious that the equilibrium between the rates of the synthesis and degradation of collagen determines the net deposition of this protein: Thus, controlled stimulation of the activity of mammalian collagenase or elastase could be of importance in the final outcome of collagenous fibrosis (for review see Peréz-Tamayo, 1978).

Colchicine

Harris et al (1971) found that colchicine stimulates de novo synthesis of collagenase in cultures of synovial membrane cells. Chvapil et al (1980) also found enhanced collagenase activity in reactive granuloma tissue with less deposited collagen in rats treated with rather high doses of colchicine. Unfortunately, the general body weight loss made it difficult to determine the actual reasons for the above effects. Beneficial effects of colchicine in scleroderma patients (Rojkind et al, 1973) and liver cirrhosis in $CC1_4$ treated rats (Rojkind & Kershenobich, 1975) were reported. It seems, however, that in vivo colchicine does not affect collagen degradation, at least in scleroderma patients, who did not show any increase in urinary hydroxyproline excretion during colchicine treatment (Harris et al, 1975).

EDTA

Aronson & Rogerson (1975) demonstrated marked increase in urinary Hyp excretion of rats treated with EDTA. This effect was paralleled with labilization of lysosomes. We assume that the possible mechanism of this labilization of lysosomes is related to sequestration of zinc ions from the tissues. Zinc ions were shown to stabilize various biomembranes, mainly of lysosomes (Ludwig et al, 1980). Indeed, the i.v. infusion of EDTA to sheep or goats resulted in a striking increase of first zinc excretion followed by Hyp excretion (Fig. 12.3). Chronic administration of EDTA to rats with skin wounds failed, however, to change the mechanical properties of skin wounds in spite of a marked increase in urinary excretion of Hyp (Tobin et al, 1974).

Macrophages

The presence of tissue inhibitors of collagenase would interfere not only with active enzyme but also with inactive enzyme-inhibitor complex. Deporter (1979) proposes phagocytosis and intracellular degradation of collagen by macrophages as the most probable mechanism of collagen

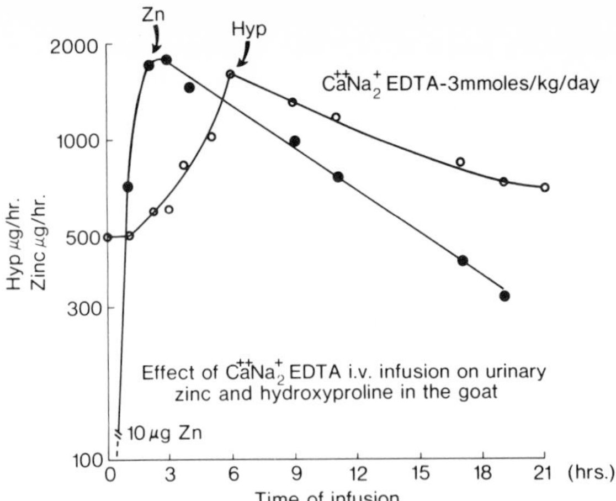

Fig. 12.3 The effect of Ca^{++},Na^+ EDTA i.v. infusion to goats on urinary excretion of zinc and hydroxyproline. The drug was infused at the rate of 3 mmol/kg body weight/24 hours (Aronson, A and Chvapil, M, unpublished results).

degradation. Increasing the invasion of activated macrophages into the fibrotic lesion should increase collagen degradation but, at the same time the activated macrophages produce factor(s) which are known to stimulate the proliferation and activity of fibroblasts. It is difficult to predict which aspect of macrophage activity in its effect on synthesis and degradation of collagen will prevail. The role of the macrophage or granulocyte in collagen resorption in chronic inflammatory disorders was recently reviewed by Deporter (1979). Several studies demonstrate enhanced activity of collagenase by cells such as macrophage, granalocyte or fibroblast when activated by plasminogen, lymphokines, endotoxin or by any stimulus enhancing phagocytosis. Nonstimulated macrophages did not produce collagenase (Wahl et al, 1974; Oronsky et al, 1973; Bienkowski et al, 1978; Horwitz et al, 1976; Werb & Aggeler, 1978). Deporter (1979) argues, however, that in the presence of at least two serum inhibitors of collagenase, α_2-macroglobulin and β_1-anticollagenase, both present also in injured tissues, 'it seems likely, that any enzymes secreted by macrophages would be inactivated or inhibited to the point where they could not produce significant destruction of extracellular collagen fibres.'

Topical collagenase

Bacterial collagenase has been used in topical debridement of dermal ulcers and decubiti. The reasons for its use are given by the study of Howes et al (1959) who showed that necrotic tissue may be anchored to wound granulation tissue by native collagen. Cleavage of the collagen is important to remove the excess debris and granulation tissue which can interfere with reepithelization and skin grafts.

Other modifications

In the introduction, we defined the specific pharmacological interference as that involving intracellular fibroblast-linked collagen synthetic steps as well as extracellular events, such as polymerization and degradation of collagen. In the light of recent findings on the role of free radicals, active forms of oxygen, and the role of the immune system and lysosomal enzymes in the activity of fibroblasts, such a definition seems rather artificial. It is becoming obvious that fibroproliferative inflammation is a highly integrated dynamic flow of events, in which every single reaction contributes to the magnitude of the final outcome, the fibrotic lesion. Thus, the reader of this chapter should complete the view of pharmacology of fibrosis by consulting several excellent reviews on steroidal and nonsteroidal anti-inflammatory drugs, which have been shown to ammeliorate the fibrotic collagenous lesion.

Our attempt to control the volume of fibroblasts in a fibrotic lesion by antifibroblast serum (Steinbronn et al, 1974) using either whole fibroblast or fibroblast membrane surface antigen failed because of great cross-reactivity and lack of specificity of the antiserum. This is now quite understandable in view of the rather large distribution of fibronectin among various cell membranes. Another interesting approach is to selectively lyse particular cells such as fibroblasts as indicated by Youle et al (1979) who are constructing highly toxic cell-type specific reagents by coupling the proper receptor-binding moiety to a native toxin (vicin). By this method, the toxin enters the cell where it is directed to specific cellular compartments to exert its effect.

SUMMARY

Among various post-translational modifications of the collagen molecule which showed a striking effect on collagen synthesis and metabolism in closed systems, only a few are promising when tested in vivo. At the present time, interference with collagen polymerization by systemic or topical administration of BAPN or D-penicillamine or a combination of both drugs seems the most effective method and is associated with less toxic side effects than the other procedures.

REFERENCES

Adams E 1970 Metabolism of proline and of hydroproline. In: Hall D A, Jackson D S (eds) International Review of Connective Tissue Research, Vol 5. Academic Press, New York. p 2

Alarcón-Segovia D, Ibánez G, Kershenobich D, Rojkind M 1974 Treatment of Scleroderma. The Lancet 1: 1054-5

Albergoni V, Cassini A, Favero N, Rocco G P 1975 Effect of penicillamine on some metals and metalloproteins in the rat. Biochemical Pharmacology 24: 1131-3

Arem A J, Misiorowski R, Chvapil M 1979 Effects of low-dose BAPN on wound healing. Journal of Surgical Research 27: 228-32

Aronson A L, Rogerson K M 1972 Effect of calcium and chromium chelates of ethylenediaminetetraacetate on intestinal permeability and collagen metabolism in the rat. Toxicology and Applied Pharmacology 21: 440-53

Banerjee D, Redman C M 1977 Effect of local anesthetics on plasma protein secretion by rat hepatocytes. Biochimica et Biophysica Acta 500: 49

Barnes M J 1975 Function of ascorbic acid in collagen metabolism. Annals of the New York Academy of Sciences 258: 264-77

Barnes M J, Constable B J, Morton L F, Kodicek E 1970 Studies in vivo on the biosynthesis of collagen and elastin in ascorbic acid-deficient guinea pigs. Biochemical Journal 119: 575-85

Barrow M V, Simpson C F, Miller E J 1974 Lathyrism: A Review. In: The Quarterly Review of Biology 49: 101-28

Berlin C M, Schimke R T 1965 Influence of turnover rates on the response of enzymes to cortisone. Molecular Pharmacology 1: 149-56

Bhatnagar R S 1977 The role of superoxide in oxidant-induced pulmonary fibrosis. In: Lee S D (ed) Biochemical effects of environmental pollutants. Ann Arbor Science Publishers, Ann Arbor, Michigan. Ch 5, p 47

Bhatnagar R S, Liu T Z 1972 Evidence for free radical involvement in the hydroxylation of proline: inhibition by nitro blue tetrazolium. FEBS Letters 26: 32

Bienkowski R S, Baum B J, Crystal R G 1978 Fibroblasts degrade newly synthesized collagen within the cell before secretion. Nature 276: 413-6

Bora F W, Lane J M, Prockop D M 1972 Inhibitors of collagen biosynthesis as a means of controlling scar formation in tendon injury. Journal of Bone and Joint Surgery 54A: 1501-8

Boxer A M, Gottesman N, Bernstein H, Mandl E 1969 Debridement of dermal ulcers and decubiti with collagenase. Geriatrics 24: 75-86

Brada Z, Bulba S, Chen M S 1972 Influence on some nitrogen derivatives of phenanthrene on chronic and acute effect of ethionine. Federation Proceedings 31: 842

Brada Z, Chvapil M, Bulba S 1972 Influence of 1,10-phenanthroline on pathologic changes in liver of ethionine fed rats. Life Sciences 11: 2277

Cardinale G J, Udenfriend S 1974 Prolyl hydroxylase. Advanced Enzymology 41: 245

Cardinale G J, Stassen F L H, Kuttan R, Udenfriend S 1975 Activation of prolyl hydroxylase in fibroblasts by ascorbic acid. Annals of the New York Academy of Science 258: 278-87

Chang Y H 1975 Mechanism of action of colchicine. I. Effects of colchicine and its analogs on the reversed passive arthus reaction and the carrageenan-induced hindpaw edema in the rat. Journal of Pharmacology and Experimental Therapeutics 194: 154-8

Chang Y H 1975 Mechanism of action of colchicine. II. Effects of colchicine and its analogs on phagocytosis and chemotaxis in vitro. The Journal of Pharmacology and Experimental Therapeutics 194: 159-64

Chang Y H 1975 Mechanism of action of colchicine. III. Anti-inflammatory effects of colchicine compared with phenylbutazone and indomethacin. Arthritis and Rheumatism 18: 493-6

Christner P, Agamemnon C, Harsch M, Rosenbloom J 1975 Inhibition of the assembly and secretion of procollagen by incorporation of a threonine analogue, hydroxynorvaline. The Journal of Biological Chemistry 250: 7623-30

Chvapil M 1974a Pharmacology of fibrosis and tissue injury. Environmental Health Perspectives 9: 283-94

Chvapil M 1974b Pharmacology of fibrosis: definitions, limits and perspectives. Life Sciences 16: 1345-62

Chvapil M, Hurych J 1968 Control of collagen biosynthesis. In: Hall D A (ed) International review of connective tissue research. Vol 4, Academic Press, New York. p 67

Chvapil M, Hurych J 1969 Factors controlling exclusively the synthesis of collagen proteins in fibrotic lesion. Bibliotheca Nutritio et Dieta 13: 111-9

Chvapil M, Ryan J N 1973 The pool of free proline in acute and chronic liver injury and its effect on the synthesis of collagen and globular proteins. Agents and Actions 3: 38-44

Chvapil M, Hurych J, Ehrlichova E, Tichy M 1967 Mechanism of the action of chelating agents on proline hydroxylation and its incorporation into collagenous and non-collagenous proteins. European Journal of Biochemistry 2: 229-35

Chvapil M, Hameroff S R, O'Dea K, Peacock E E Jr 1979 Local anesthetics and wound healing. Journal of Surgical Research 27: 367-71

Chvapil M, McCarthy D, Madden J W, Peacock E E Jr 1974 Effect of 1,10-Phenanthroline and desferrioxamine in vivo on prolyl hydroxylase and hydroxylation of collagen in various tissues of rats. Biochemical Pharmacology 23: 2165-73

Chvapil M, Misiorowski R, Tillema L, Herring C 1977 Stimulation of the activity of prolyl hydroxylase in 3T3 fibroblasts by 1,10-phenanthroline. Biochimica et Biophysica Acta 497: 488-98

Cohen I K, Diegelmann R F 1978 Effect of N-acetyl-cis-4-hydroxyproline on collagen synthesis. Experimental and Molecular Pathology 28: 58-64

Craver J M, Madden J W, Peacock E E Jr 1968 Biological control of physical properties of tendon adhesions: effect of beta-aminopropionitrile in chickens. Annals of Surgery 167: 697-704

Daly J M, Steiger E, Prockop D J, Dudrick S J 1973 Inhibition of collagen synthesis by the proline analogue cis-4-hydroxyproline. Journal of Surgical Research 14: 551-5

Davis W M, Madden J W, Peacock E E Jr 1972 A new approach to the control of esophageal stenosis. Annals of Surgery 176: 469-76

Deporter D A 1979 The role of the macrophage in collagen resorption during chronic inflammation. A New Look at an Old Hypothesis. Agents and Actions 9: 168-71

Eichhorn J H, Peterkofsky B 1979 Local anesthetic-induced inhibition of collagen secretion in cultured cells under conditions where microtubules are not depolymerized by these agents. The Journal of Cell Biology 81: 26-42

Elsas L J II, Miller R L, Pinnell S R 1978 Inherited human collagen lysyl hydroxylase deficiency: ascorbic acid response. The Journal of Pediatrics 92: 378-84

Everitt A V, Delbridge L 1972 Two phases of collagen ageing in the tail tendon of hypophysectomized rats. Experimental Gerontology 7: 45

Fujii K, Kajiwara T, Kurosu H 1979 Effect of vitamin B6 deficiency on the crosslink formation of collagen. FEBS Letters 97: 193-5

Furlow L T Jr, Peacock E E Jr 1965 Effect of beta-aminopropionitrile on the prevention and treatment of joint stiffness in rats. Surgical Forum XVI: 457-8

Goldstein A, Aronow L, Kalman S (eds) 1974 Principles of drug action 2nd edn. John Wiley & Sons. pp 329-332

Grant M E, Prockop D J 1972 The Biosynthesis of Collagen. New England Journal of Medicine 286: 194-199

Guttadauria M, Diamond H, Kaplan D 1977 Colchicine in the treatment of scleroderma. Journal of Rheumatology 4: 272-6

Haney A F, Peacock E E Jr, Madden J W 1973 The effect of multiple lathyrogenic agents upon wound healing in rats. Proceedings of the Society for Experimental Biology and Medicine 142: 289-92

Harris E D 1976 Copper-induced activation of aortic lysyl oxidase in vivo. Proceedings of the National Academy of Science 73: 371-4

Harris E D Jr, Krane S M 1971 Effects of colchicine on collagenase in cultures of rheumatoid synovium. Arthritis and Rheumatism 14: 669-84

Harris E D, Millis M 1971 Treatment with colchicine of the periarticular inflammation associated with sarcoidosis. Arthritis and Rheumatism 14: 130

Harris E D Jr, Hoffman G S, McGuire J L, Strosberg J M 1975 Colchicine: effects upon urinary hydroxyproline excretion in patients with scleroderma. Metabolism 24: 529-35

Horwitz A L, Kelman J A, Crystal R G 1976 Activation of alveolar macrophage collagenase by a neutral protease secreted by the same cell. Nature 264: 772-4

Housley T J, Rowland F N, Ledger P W, Kaplan J, Tanzer M L 1980 Effects of tunicamycin on the biosynthesis of procollagen by human fibroblasts. The Journal of Biological Chemistry 255: 121-8

Inouye K, Sakakibara S, Prockop D J 1976 Effects of the stereoconfiguration of the hydroxyl group in 4-hydroxyproline on the triple-helical structures formed by homogeneous peptides resembling collagen. Biochimica et Biophysica Acta 420: 133-41

Irvin T T, Chattopadhyay D K, Smythe A 1978 Ascorbic acid requirements in postoperative patients. Surgery, Gynecology and Obstetrics 147: 49-54

Johnson M E, Jones G H 1978 Effects of marcaine, a myotoxic drug, on macromolecular synthesis in muscle. Medical Pharmacology 27: 1753

Kao W W-Y, Prockop D J 1977 Proline analogue removes fibroblasts from cultured mixed cell populations. Nature 266: 63-4

Keiser H R, Sjoerdsma A 1967 Studies on beta-aminopropionitrile in patients with scleroderma. Clinical Pharmacology and Therapeutics 8: 593-602

Kershenobich D, Fierro F J, Rojkind M 1970 The relationship between the free pool of proline and collagen content in human liver cirrhosis. Journal of Clinical Investigation 49: 2246

Kerwar S S, Marcel R J M, Salvador R A 1976 Studies on the effect of L-3,4-dehydroproline on collagen synthesis by chick embryo polysomes. Archives of Biochemistry and Biophysics 172: 685-8

Lane J M, Bora F W, Prockop D J, Heppenstall R B, Black J 1972 Inhibition of scar formation by the proline analog cis-hydroxyproline. Journal of Surgical Research 3: 135-7

Lane J M, Parkes L J, Prockop D J 1971 Effect of the proline analogue azetidine-2-carboxylic acid on collagen synthesis in vivo. II. Morphological and physical properties of collagen containing the analogue. Biochimica et Biophysica Acta 236: 528-41

Levene C I 1978 Diseases of the collagen molecule. In: The Royal College of Pathologists, diseases of connective tissue. Symposium Supplement, British Medical Association, London. p 82

Madden J W, Chvapil M, Carlson E C, Ryan J N 1973 Toxicity and metabolic effects of 3,4-dehyroproline in mice. Toxicology and Applied Pharmacology 26: 426-37

Madia A M, Rozovski S J, Kagan H M 1979 Changes in lung lysyl oxidase activity in streptozotocin-diabetes and in starvation. Biochimica et Biophysica Acta 585: 481-7

Magarelli P C Jr, Hunter B, Lightner D V, Colvin L B 1979 Black death: an ascorbic acid deficiency disease in penaeid shrimp. Comparative Biochemistry and Physiology 63A: 103-8

Murray J C, Levene C I 1977 Evidence for the role of vitamin B-6 as a cofactor of lysyl oxidase. Biochemistry Journal 167: 463-7

Murray J C, Fraser D R, Levene C I 1978 The effect of pyridoxine deficiency on lysyl oxidase activity in the chick. Experimental and Molecular Pathology 28: 301-8

Myllylä R, Schubotz L M, Weser U, Kivirikko K I 1979 Involvement of superoxide in the prolyl and lysyl hydroxylase reactions. Biochemical and Biophysical Research Communications 89: 98-102

Nicolson G, Smith J R, Poste G 1976 Effects of local anesthetics on cell morphology and membrane-associated cytoskeletal organization in Balb/3T3 cells. Journal of Cell Biology 68: 395

Nimni M E 1970 Mechanism of inhibition of collagen crosslinking by penicillamine. Proceedings of the Royal Society of Medicine 70: 65-72

Nolan J C, Ridge S, Oronsky A L, Kerwar S S 1978 Studies on the mechanism of reduction of prolyl hydroxylase activity by D,L-3,4 dehyroproline. Archives of Biochemistry and Biophysics 189: 448-53

Ohuchi K, Chang L F, Tabachnick J 1979 Radiation fibrosis of guinea pig skin after β irradiation and an attempt at its suppression with proline analogs. Radiation Research 79: 273-88

Oronsky A L, Perper R J, Schroder H C 1973 Phagocytic release and activation of human leukocyte procollagenase. Nature 246: 417-9

Peacock E E Jr 1973 Biologic frontiers in the control of healing. The American Journal of Surgery 126: 708-13

Peacock E E Jr, Madden J W 1966 Some studies on the effect of β-amino-propionitrile on collagen in healing wounds. Surgery 60: 7-12

Peacock E E Jr, Madden J W 1969 Some studies on the effects of β-aminopropionitrile in patients with injured flexor tendons. Surgery 66: 215-23

Pérez-Tamayo R, 1978 Pathology of collagen degradation. American Journal of Pathology 92: 509-66

Pesanti E L, Axline S G 1975 Colchicine effects on lysosomal enzyme induction and intracellular degradation in the cultivated macrophage. The Journal of Experimental Medicine 141: 1030-46

Prockop D J, Kivirikko K I, Tuderman L, Guzman N A 1979 The biosynthesis of collagen and its disorders. New England Journal of Medicine 301: 13-23 & 77-85

Riley D J, Berg R A, Edelman N H, Prockop D J 1980 Prevention of collagen deposition following pulmonary oxygen toxicity in the rat by cis-4-hydroxy-L-proline. Journal of Clinical Investigation 65: 643-51

Roberts E, Simonsen D G 1962. In: Holden J T (ed) Amino acid pools. Elsevier Publishing Company, Amsterdam. p 284

Rojkind M 1973 Inhibition of liver fibrosis by L-azetidine-2-carboxylic acid in rats treated with carbon tetrachloride. The Journal of Clinical Investigation 52: 2451-6

Rojkind M, Kershenobich D 1975 Effect of colchicine on collagen, albumin and transferrin synthesis by cirrhotic rat liver slices. Biochimica et Biophysica Acta 378: 415-23

Rojkind M, Uribe M, Kershenobich D 1973 Colchicine and the treatment of liver cirrhosis. Lancet 1: 38

Rokosova B, Chvapil M 1974 Relationship between the dose of ascorbic acid and its structural analogs and proline hydroxylation in various biological systems. Connective Tissue Research 2: 215-21

Rosenbloom J 1971 Trans-hydroxyproline is not incorporated into collagen. Archives of Biochemistry and Biophysics 142: 718-9

Rosenbloom J, Prockop D J 1970 Incorporation of 3,4-dehydroproline into protocollagen and collagen. Journal of Biological Chemistry 245: 3361-8

Schmidt R M, Rosenkranz H S 1970 Antimicrobial activity of local anesthetics: Lidocaine and procaine. Journal of Infectious Diseases 121: 597

Seeman P 1972 The membrane actions of anesthetics and tranquilizers. Pharmacological Review 24: 583

Shirota F N, Nagasawa H T, Elberling J A 1977 Potential inhibitors of collagen biosynthesis. 4,4-Difluoro-L-proline and 4,4-dimethyl-DL-proline and their activation by prolyl-tRNA ligase' Journal of Medicinal Chemistry 20: 1176-81

Siegel R C 1977 Collagen cross-linking. The Journal of Biological Chemistry 252: 254-9

Speer D P, Peacock E E Jr, Chvapil M 1975 The use of large molecular weight compounds to produce local lathyrism in healing wounds. Journal of Surgical Research 19: 169-73

Steinbronn D, Carlson E, Chvapil M 1974 Antifibroblast serum: a new method of controlling collagen synthesis. Surgical Forum 25: 47-9

Takeda K, Katoh F, Kawai S, Konno K 1979 Stimulation of prolyl hydroxylase activity by chelating agents. Archives of Biochemistry and Biophysics 197: 273-6

Tobin G, Aronson A, Chvapil M 1974 Effect of CaEDTA administration on urinary hydroxyproline excretion and skin wound healing in the rat. Journal of Surgical Research 17: 346-51

Uitto J, Prockop D J 1977 Incorporation of proline analogs into procollagen. Assay for replacement of imino acids by cis-4-hydroxy-L-proline and cis-4-fluoro-L-proline. Archives of Biochemistry and Biophysics 181: 293-9

Uitto J, Hoffmann H-P, Prockop D J 1975 Retention of nonhelical procollagen containing cis-hydroxyproline in rough endoplasmic reticulum. Science 190: 1202-4

Wahl L M, Wahl S M, Mergenhagen S E, Martin G R 1974 Collagenase production by endotoxin-activated macrophages. Proceedings of the National Academy of Science USA 71: 3598-601

Wallace S L, Bernstein D, Diamond H 1967 Diagnostic value of the colchicine therapeutic trial. Journal of the American Medical Association 199: 525

Werb Z, Aggeler J 1978 Proteases induce secretion of collagenase and plasminogen activator by fibroblasts. Proceedings of the National Academy of Science USA 75: 1839-43

Whitson T C, Peacock E E Jr 1969 Effect of alpha alpha dipyridyl on collagen synthesis in healing wounds. Surgery, Gynecology and Obstetrics 128: 1061-4

Youle R J, Murray G J, Neville D M 1979 Ricin linked to monophosphopentamannose binds to fibroblast lysosomal hydrolase receptors, resulting in a cell-type-specific toxin. Proceedings of the National Academy of Science USA 76: 5559-62

13

The effect of collagen on cell division, cellular differentiation and embryonic development

E. D. ADAMSON

In most of the work to be considered, it is difficult to assess the effect of collagen per se since it is only one of the components of the extracellular matrix interacting with cells. We now know that many of the identified components of matrices interact strongly with each other and it is quite possible that single components, i.e. collagens, cannot be considered in terms of their activity towards cells because of the fact that they are so closely tuned to, and by, their interactions with other matrix components. It is necessary therefore to describe some of the effects of other components such as the glycoproteins, fibronectin (reviewed by Ruoslahti et al, 1979) and laminin (Timpl et al, 1979), proteoglycans (reviewed by Manasek, 1975) and the glycosminoglycans (GAGs) which make up 80 per cent of the mass of proteoglycans.

The role of collagen in the processes of growth and differentiation will be assessed by considering the evidence which has accumulated in four different fields:

1. Extracellular matrix components in embryos: a summary of our present knowledge of extracellular matrix components and collagen types in developing embryos to ascertain when collagens are synthesized and where they contact cells. This will be a necessary framework to establish possible functions in the new structures where growth and differentiation are both occurring in a marvellously orchestrated fashion.

2. Matrix interactions in development: the analysis of parts of the whole embryo to study matrix interactions in structures such as developing salivary and mammary glands, in somite chondrogenesis and in muscle, kidney and corneal development.

3. Effects of matrix on cell behaviour: in vitro studies using cell cultures to ask questions about the attachment, spreading, cell division, differentiation and phenotypic expression and their dependence on collagen or other extracellular matrix materials.

4. Teratocarcinomas as a model of development and differentiation: the teratocarcinoma cell system will be considered in terms of the synthesis and accumulation of extracellular matrix components since new matrix will then provide a new microenvironment which could have interactive effects on future daughter cells.

COLLAGEN AND EXTRACELLULAR MATRIX (ECM) IN THE DEVELOPING EMBRYO

Collagen has been detected in sea urchin, frog and chick embryos at relatively early stages, long before the time at which connective tissue cells are observed (Reddi, 1976). More recent studies on mammalian embryos have stressed the importance of collagen type and this is a direction which holds exciting prospects for analyses of development. A developing embryo rapidly achieves a complex state of structured tissues and organs, all of which, contain collagen (Harkness, 1961). For excellent reviews of collagen types in tissues see Miller (1976), Gay & Miller (1978) and Wartiovaara et al (1980).

With the realization that collagen exists in at least five main types came the belief that since each type has a set of unique properties, then each should also have specific functions. However, valuable studies were made before the characterization of the distinct collagen types and have much to tell us about the general importance of the cellular environment, and these are still as relevant to our understanding of the events of differentiation, morphogenesis and development. It is clear that the materials which make up the extracellular environment must be considered as interacting components and only when their distribution and proportions in all tissues are fully documented can we attempt to formulate hypotheses which link their location with their properties and to assign a function to each.

The location of collagen types in the mammalian embryo

Matrix components have a characteristic developmental sequence in their appearance in the mouse embryo (Fig. 13.1 and Table 13.1). The earliest detected materials are collagens type IV (C chain see Ch. 17) and V (B chain see Ch. 1) at the 4-cell stage (Sherman et al, 1980); these increase in quantity as development proceeds. These collagen chains are almost entirely restricted to basement membranes in adult tissues, but in embryos they appear long before any basement membranes. Sherman et al also detected type III collagen very early in development,

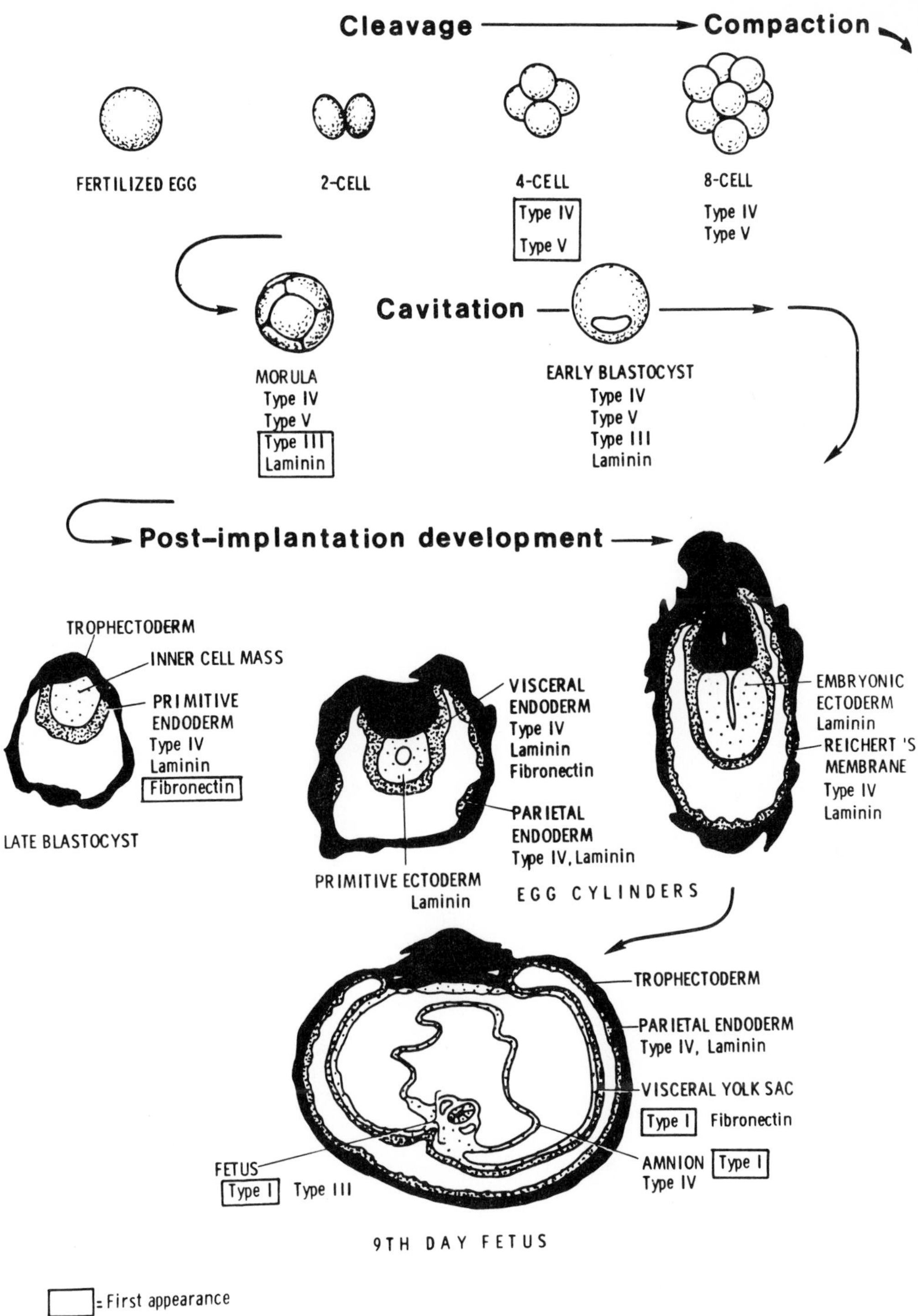

Fig. 13.1 The appearance of extracellular components during the development of the mouse.

Table 13.1 ECM components in the mouse embryo and teratocarcinoma cells.

Stage of embryo and location	I	II	III/Pro III	*Collagen types* IV (or C)	V (or AB)	*Fibronectin*	*Laminin*	*Method of detection*
2-Cell	–	–	–	± to +?	± to +?	–	–	11F
4–8-Cell	–	–	± to +	+	+	–	–	11F
Morula	–	–	– and +	+	+	–	+	11F
Mid to late blastocyst	–	–	++	++	+	+	+	11F and 11P
Unhatched blastocyst			+					11F
Delayed blastocyst (floating)			± to +	+		+	+	11F
Delayed blastocyst (attached)			++					11F
Isolated ICM	–	–	+ and –	+		+	+	11F and 11P
7–8th day egg cylinder:								
ectoderm	–	–	–	–		–	+	11F and 11P
parietal								
endoderm	–	–	–	+		+	+	11F and 11P
visceral								
endoderm	–	–	–	+		+	+	11F, 11P and synthesis
mesoderm	–	–	–	+		+	+	11F and 11P
								8th day differentiating
mesoderm	+	–	+	+		+	+	11F
trophoblast	–	–	–	patches		+	+	11F
EC cells	–		–	+ and ±		(+)	+	11F
Embryoid body endoderm	–		–	+		+	+	11F and 11P
END cells: OC15 END	+			±		+	–	synthesis
PC13 END	+			+		+	–	synthesis
F9 END				+		+	+	synthesis
PYS-2	–		–	+++		+	++	synthesis
PSASE	+			+		±	±	synthesis

11F, indirect immunofluorescence; 11P, indirect immunoperoxidase; synthesis, internal labelling, extraction and analysis.
±, trace; + staining; ++ heavy staining; +++ very intense staining or reaction. (+) does not accumulate.

perhaps as early as the 16-cell stage but here depicted as first appearing at the early blastocyst stage in Figure 13.1 as a compromise with Wartiovaara et al (1980) who detect it only later. Thus, by the time that compaction occurs in the 8-cell embryo, probably 2 or 3 types of collagen are present. Compaction entails the loss of the spherical shape of the blastomeres as greater cell contact is achieved (Graham & Lehtonen, 1979). Junctional complexes form between the plasma membranes of adjacent cells and these are probably important to the establishment of future 'inside' cells. Other changes in the biochemistry and commitment of cells at this and subsequent stages are reviewed by Adamson & Gardner (1979). At the late morula stage, cellular developmental fate is realized with the formation of 'inside' cells. Inside cells, in contrast to outside cells are enclosed by matrix and are destined to become the future inner cell mass (ICM) of the blastocyst (Fig. 13.1).

Figure 13.2 shows immunofluorescent staining of some preimplantation stages of mouse embryos. The accumulation of the glycoprotein laminin is seen in late morulae both in the cytoplasm and lining intercellular contours. Fibronectin can first be detected in the early blastocyst where it becomes concentrated between the ICM cells and the layer of primitive endoderm cells which now appear lining the blastocyst cavity. It is at this stage that a further cell compaction occurs and the first basement membrane appears.

As parietal endoderm cells multiply from the primitive endoderm and move around the trophectoderm, they synthesize and secrete a continually thickening basement membrane called Reichert's membrane. Studies on rat embryos by Minor et al (1976) have shown that the sparse overlying layer of parietal endoderm cells is responsible for the synthesis of type IV collagen which is the largest component of Reichert's membrane. The synthesis of type IV collagen by parietal endoderm cells and its location in Reichert's membrane has been confirmed in mouse embryos (Adamson & Ayers, 1979). Reichert's membrane at this stage also contains laminin (Leivo et al, 1980) and fibronectin; the latter declines as development proceeds (Wartiovaara et al, 1979). The trophoblast layer on the outer aspect of the parietal yolk sac contains large deposits of fibronectin and laminin but at later stages nothing remains of the traces of type IV collagen which were seen there at the blastocyst stage. Intracellular type IV collagen can be detected by immunoperoxidase staining in the primitive endoderm and in parietal endoderm cells. Otherwise this type of collagen is restricted to accumulations in sheets which form basement membranes underlying and separating layers of cells. Figure 13.3 shows the following basement membranes (stained for type IV collagen) on the 8th day of development: the amnion, chorion, visceral yolk sac, between the endoderm and mesoderm and between mesoderm and ectoderm, in the allantois as well as in Reichert's membrane. Fibronectin and laminin follow a similar distribution to type IV collagen in basement membrane, but they are also seen between primitive ectoderm cells, and in and around mesoderm cells. Fibronectin is known to form an integral part of the extracellular matrix of many kinds of cells as

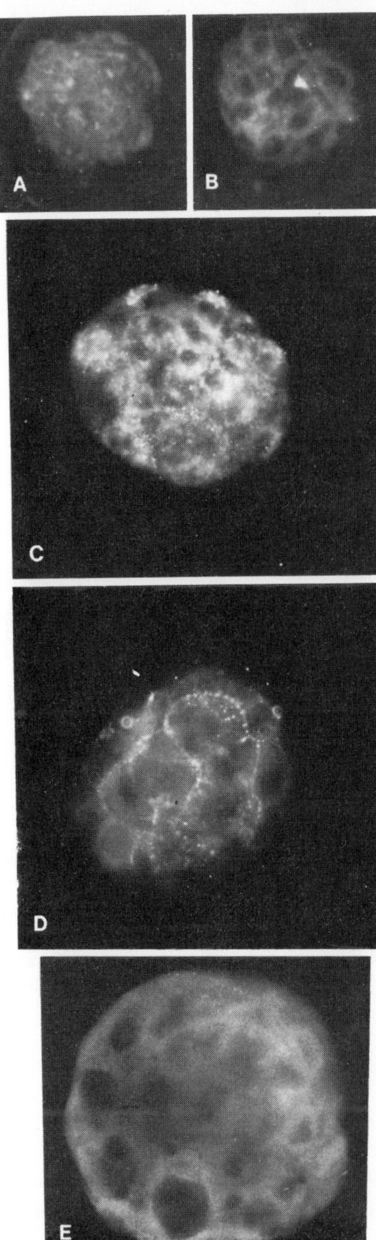

Fig. 13.2 The association of extracellular components with preimplantation mouse embryos. Immunofluorescent staining of: A, morula with anti-type V collagen (B chain); B, blastocyst with anti-type IV collagen (C chain); C and D, 16–32 cell morulae with anti-laminin, B intracellular, C, cell surface; E blastocyst with anti-type III collagen. A, B and E are published with the permission of Sherman et al (1980). C and D are published with the permission of Leivo et al (1980).

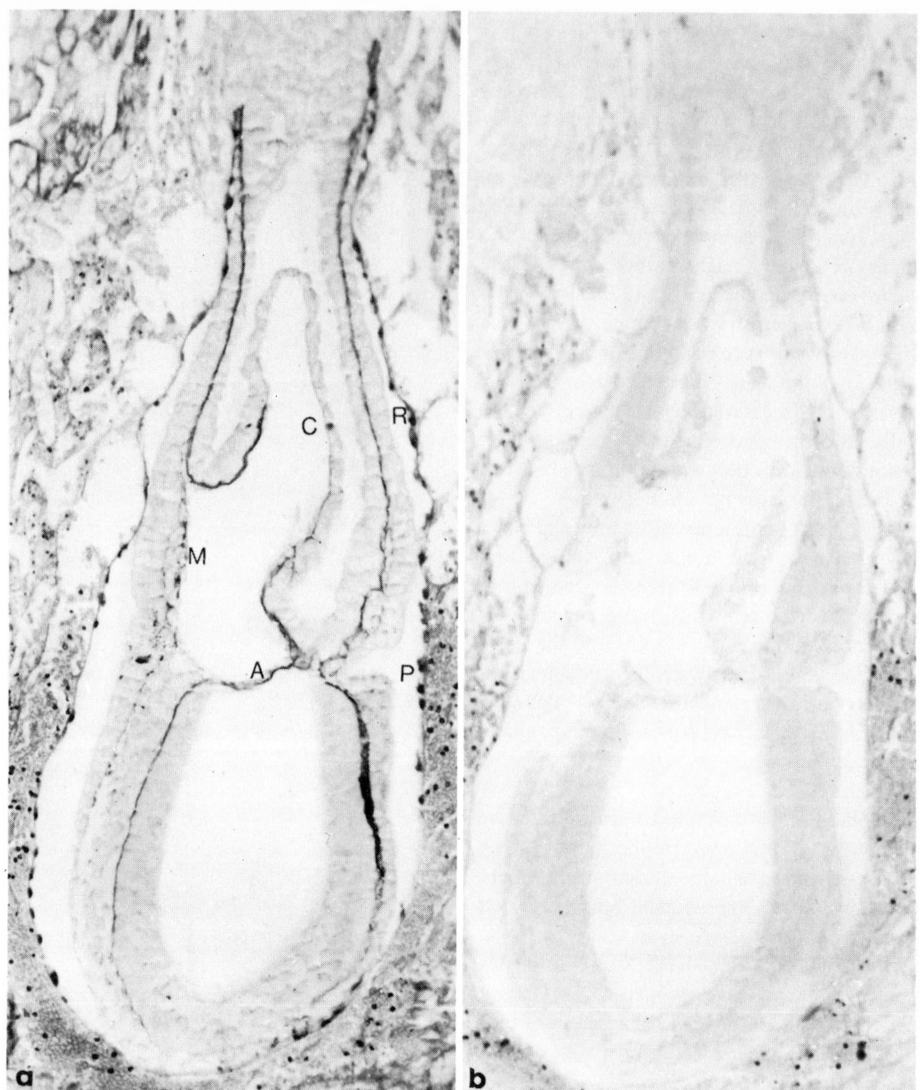

Fig. 13.3 Indirect immunoperoxidase reaction of anti-type IV collagen with sections of an 8th day embryo. a, Reaction. b, Control. Key: R, Reichert's membrane; A, amnion; M, mesoderm; P, parietal endoderm; C, chorion. (Reproduced with permission from Adamson & Ayers, 1979.)

well as being present in soluble form in serum and body fluids.

Interstitial collagens, types I and III are largely associated with mesodermal differentiation in the postimplantation embryo, though type III makes an early appearance in the late morula. Both types I and III appear in the mesenchymal stroma of head, heart and somites on the 8th day of gestation (Wartiovaara et al, 1980; Leivo et al, 1980). The dermis underlying the epidermis of the skin forms from the biosynthetic products of the mesenchymal fibroblasts. It consists of a predominance of type III collagen over type I (about 60 per cent) as massed striated fibres in fetal skin. As development proceeds, type III declines until the adult proportion of about 25 per cent is reached (Epstein, 1974). Dermis fibroblasts do not synthesize laminin or type IV collagen although both are seen in the epidermal basement membrane of mouse skin (Timpl et al, 1979). Cultured cells of ectodermal origin do not seem to synthesize fibronectin, for example, keratinocytes, cervix epithelial cells and several types of carcinoma cell lines.

Type I (and possibly type III) collagen is synthesized by the endoderm as well as the mesoderm portion of the visceral yolk sac of the 14th day mouse embryo. This represents a switch in type synthesized from type IV known to be produced by its ancestor, the primitive endoderm of the blastocyst, to type I as the major species detected in the biosynthetic products of the visceral yolk sac endoderm

(Adamson & Ayers, 1979). Whether this switch is important to the phenotypic expression of the two cell type remains to be seen, but the divergence of the characteristic macromolecular products of the two extraembryonic endoderm layers, namely visceral and parietal, is strongly marked by the 14th day. Not only differences in collagen type but the synthesis of laminin is also low in visceral endoderm while it remains high in parietal endoderm (Hogan, 1980; Hogan et al, 1980) although both cell layers are located on basement membranes containing type IV collagen. It seems essential to find out if the biosynthetic switches and relocation of matrix components are a consequence or a cause of the production of new cell types.

Basement membranes (see also Ch. 17)
Basement membrane serves not only as supporting architecture for sheets of epithelial cells through which epithelial cells cannot normally penetrate (Schor et al, 1979) but also as a filtration barrier in the kidney glomerulus and perhaps embryonic yolk sac, as a promoter of epithelial cell differentiation and metabolism (see pp. 224–234), as a support for guidance of migrating cells of the mesenchyme, and as a stimulator of underlying mesenchyme, for example, in feather formation and by maintaining the asymmetry and the organization of the cytoskeletal support of the epithelial cell.

Collagen types in cartilage and bone differentiation
Studies on human fetuses by Gay & Miller (1978) show that fibrillar collagen can be observed as extracellular matrix between the mesenchyme cells at the end of the 8th week of gestation. In all vertebrates, presumptive chondrogenic mesenchyme cells migrate to specific regions and make a model of the skeletal system surrounded by matrix containing type III (reticulin) and type I collagen fibres.

Cartilage accumulates and is characterized by the appearance of type II collagen in the matrix. Cells at the periphery of the compacted mesenchyme still make type I until they differentiate to chondroblasts which then proliferate and make type II collagen. In endochondral ossification, bone matrix then replaces the preformed cartilaginous structure by resorption and new synthesis of bone matrix is characterized by type I collagen.

The osteoprogenitor cells embedded in the fibrous network of type I and type II collagen forming the perichondrium (now called periosteum) form osteoblasts which lay down bone from the outside. Capillaries sprout from the bone marrow region (containing type III and B chain of type V collagen) and lead to ossification from the inside. Further details of collagen in these tissues are presented in later chapters of this book by R. Burgeson (Ch. 18) and S. Sakamoto (Ch. 19).

Collagen types in muscle differentiation (see also Ch. 25)
Immunochemical localization has shown that the 'polymorphic' forms of collagen have a specific distribution (Duance et al, 1977; Bailey & Sims, 1977). Type I is located mainly in the epimysium and perimysium) and type III in the perimysium (with less in the epimysium and endomysium) and type V mainly in the endomysium.

In addition, subtle roles in muscle development are suggested by Bailey et al (1979) for collagen types I, III and V (A and B chains) because they are synthesized at particular times during the differentiative process. Type V appears in the culture medium of myoblasts (note that these were not cloned, however) on the first day of culture after isolation from 13-day embryo thigh muscles. This is 3 to 4 days before fusion; type III appears next closely followed by type I around the time of fusion. Type V collagen may have a special function in muscle development, since it makes an early appearance, so much so that it has also been termed a marker of presumptive muscle cells in chicks (v. der Mark & v. der Mark, 1979).

The early appearance of type V (type IV was not determined) is consistent with the observation of patchy basement membrane in electron microscope studies of in vivo development. The work of Lipton (1977) however, suggests that myofibres cannot accumulate a basement membrane on their own although they secrete a collagenous material. Apparently such cells need the interacting presence of mesenchyme fibroblasts before a substratum can be proliferated.

Collagen types in the nervous system
As stated earlier, the central nervous system is particularly low in collagen; whereas 23 to 25 per cent of bone and cartilage, 1 to 2 per cent of muscle, only 0.2 to 0.4 per cent of the central nervous system is collagen and this is largely confined to blood vessel walls (reviewed by Harkness, 1961). However, cells of neuroectodermal origin can synthesize collagen, for example, a clonal line of Schwann cells (Church et al, 1973) and also peripheral neurinomas contain collagen. Interaction between matrix and nerve fibres was summarized on page 000. Shellswell et al (1979) have identified the distribution of collagen polypeptides in the central and peripheral nervous system of steers by extraction and analysis and by immunofluorescence. They find that extracts of sciatic nerve contain type I, IV and V collagens. Type I collagen is located in the epi-, peri- and endoneurium, while type III is mainly in the peri- and endoneurium. Both type I and III collagens form an extracellular matrix which fills the space between nerve fibres and the whole is bounded by a basement membrane on the external face. Both type IV and V collagens are present in the endoneurial basement membrane as sharply delineated rings around single nerve fibres and as laminae in the perineurium. The spinal cord neural compartment

proper does not contain collagen except for small blood vessels and fine capillaries which stain for type IV and V only. The pia mater contains large amounts of type I and III and also stains for type IV and V.

ACTIONS OF COLLAGEN IN TISSUE DIFFERENTIATION AND MORPHOGENESIS

Now we examine whether developing cells can alter their immediate environment to create new conditions that could serve as a kind of feedback of information to the same kind or to different kinds of cells. Morphogenesis in developing organs of the fetus, in many cases is accomplished by interaction of epithelia on mesenchyme (for example, notochord on somite chondrogenesis and in kidney development), by mesenchyme on the epithelia (for example lung, kidney, pancreas and salivary glands), or epithelia (for example lens on cornea). Some of these interactions have been shown to require direct contact between cell surfaces (for example kidney) and others to be mediated by extracellular matrix components, in some cases collagen: in other cases GAGs proved to be the 'inducing' materials (Slavkin & Greulich, 1975; Wessells, 1977).

Chondrogenesis (see also Ch. 18)

Somites

Somite chondrogenesis in the chick is stimulated in vitro by the epithelial mesenchymal interaction of the notochord or by the addition of exogenous matrix components to the medium. Various combinations of collagens, proteoglycans and GAGs will stimulate chondrogenesis and type II collagen is most effective of the collagens (the same type of collagen that is synthesized by the notochord). Kosher & Savage (1979) suggest that collagen acts by lowering the cyclic AMP level of embryonic somites and that this is the trigger for chondrogenesis. Induction can be followed by the secretion of type II collagen and the proteoglycans which characterize cartilage (Church & Kosher, 1975; Lash & Vasan, 1978). Since type II collagen and proteoglycans (Kosher & Lash, 1975) are all that are needed to stimulate chondrogenesis in somites, it is possible to ask if these factors have other stimulatory properties. Embryonic mouse tooth mesenchyme can also be stimulated to produce cartilage by culture with avian limb and bud epithelium. In this case, type II collagen is produced from mesenchymal tissue which normally never chondrifies and which normally synthesizes only type I and type I trimer collagen polypeptides (Hata & Slavkin, 1978). Retinal pigmented epithelium also induces scleral cartilage in embryonic chick neural crest cells. However in this case, as in mouse tooth mesenchyme, the inducing material has not been identified. Pigmented epithelial cells deposit copious collagen-containing ECM in vitro and this material after lysis of the epithelial cells is extremely potent in the stimulation of chondrogenesis. Substrata of purified type I and II collagens, however, are not effective stimulators, therefore some other component of the matrix is necessary. In addition, direct cell contact must be made (Newsome, 1976).

Limb chondrogenesis

Presumptive chondrocytes (mesenchyme) of the chick limb synthesize only type I collagen, but during chondrogenesis type II synthesis takes over (v. der Mark et al, 1976; v. der Mark & v. der Mark, 1977). The stability of phenotypic expression is rather easily disturbed by too sparse seeding, by the addition of chick embryo extract to the medium, or by senescence (Mayne et al, 1975 and 1976). Collagen type, GAG type and glycoprotein synthesis are all altered during loss of phenotypic expression. Chondrogenic development seems to occur best when mesenchymal cells are allowed to stay in contact with each other and thus build up their own matrix and condition their own environment. Miller et al (1977) and Benya & Nimni (1979) confirm this with organ cultures of rabbit articular cartilage which continue to accumulate matrix even while DNA synthesis is stimulated 30-fold.

Free hyaluronate can depress proteoglycan synthesis whereas hyaluronate in a proteoglycan complex does not. Exogenous hyaluronate added to cultured chick embryo limb chondrocytes has two distinct effects: rapid displacement of newly-synthesized proteoglycans into the medium, and a slower-acting depression of proteoglycan synthesis (Solursh et al, 1980).

Fibronectin added to embryonic chick chondrocytes stimulates a loss of phenotype to a fibroblastic morphology and depression of GAG and type II collagen synthesis. At the same time, the chondrocytes change to synthesis of type I collagen and fibronectin, a process which is accelerated on a type I collagen substrate. Removal of fibronectin from the culture medium allows chondrogenic expression on a collagen substrate. Therefore control of fibronectin synthesis or accumulation may be an important mechanism for regulating chondrogenesis (Pennypacker et al, 1979a). Antifibronectin antibodies block the effects of added fibronectin, embryo extract, 5-bromo-2-deoxyuridine and vitamin A which all cause loss of differentiated expression in chondrocyte cultures (Pennypacker et al, 1979b). These materials may inhibit the process of chondrogenesis via increased fibronectin synthesis or accumulation. Both mouse limb bud mesenchyme cells (Lewis et al, 1978) and chick sternal chondrocytes (Hassell et al, 1979) treated with vitamin A synthesize and accumulate fibronectin on the cell surface and this may be the signal to reverse the process of chondrocytic expression. It is important to note that fibronectin is not found in differentiated cartilage. On the other hand, a different cell adhesion protein (chondronectin) has been described which selectively causes chondrocytes to attach to collagen substrates, especially type II collagen although the other types have moderate activity also (Hewitt et al, 1980).

Chondrogenesis induced by demineralized bone

Demineralized bone was first shown by Urist (1965) to be a powerful inducer of cartilage, bone and bone-marrow differentiation. When transplanted as a coarse powder to subcutaneous locations (Reddi et al, 1977) a succession of collagen types (type I with 10 per cent type III) is noted as dermal tissue fibroblasts accumulate on the matrix on day 3. Abundant type III collagen fibres are seen around the fibroblasts and type I collagen accumulates later. Chondrocytes synthesizing type II collagen are detected on day 6 and these persist until the early stages of bone formation. Vascular invasion of the implant is accompanied by osteogenesis (and type I collagen) on day 10. On day 9, type IV collagen and laminin are localized in the invading vascular endothelial cells which accumulate these materials in a basement membrane (Foidart & Reddi, 1980). Decalcified bone matrix also has inductive effects in vitro when cultured up to 14 days with rat muscle (Anderson & Griner, 1977).

Rath & Reddi (1979) suggest that decalcified bone matrix is a mitogen for the connective tissue cells which invade it. Tritiated thymidine incorporation is increased in parallel with the induction of ornithine decarboxylase activity which is an early marker of cell proliferation. The inducing molecule is thought to be an insoluble bone matrix specific component. It is not clear if the mitogenic activity is the same as the bone-inducing activity. 'Bone morphogenetic protein' is destroyed by heating at 80°C for 1 hour and is trypsin sensitive but bacterial collagenase resistant (Anderson & Griner, 1977).

Induction of corneal differentiation (reviewed by Hay, 1977; see also Ch. 21)

Corneal epithelial cells rest on a basal lamina rich in chondroitin sulphate and heparin sulphate. The proteoglycan particles of the inner layer of the lamina are attached to the basal plasmalemma of the epithelial cells and collagen fibres are also attached. Intracellular cytoskeletal elements are closely associated with ECM-rich sites on the exterior. The embryonic corneal epithelium synthesizes most, if not all, of the collagen and GAG comprising the primary corneal stroma of the chick embryo. Corneal epithelium can be isolated (with enzymatic digestion) and grown on Millipore filters, plastic, or other substrata. In 24 h it will produce a new stroma consisting of orthogonally arranged type I and II collagen fibrils and GAGs. A small amount of new basement membrane is formed, but if the corneal epithelium is cultured on a collagen substratum, a much larger amount is produced. No specific type of collagen is needed, all are equally effective, but noncollagenous surfaces are not. The synthesis of collagens and GAGs is stimulated by collagen substrata or by collagens added to the medium while the synthesis of GAGs only (chondroitin sulphate and heparin sulphate) is stimulated further by the addition of the same kind of GAGs. Hyaluronate has no detectable effect. Actual contact of the epithelial cell with the collagenous surface is a necessary part of the stimulatory process. This is a clear example of the stimulatory effect of a collagen substratum on the cells which are producing collagen, that is, a positive feed-back mechanism. Further consideration of the factors affecting growth and expression of corneal epithelial cells are discussed on page 231.

Mesenchymal-epithelial inductions

Kidney development (see also Ch. 22)

Kidney development is characterized by reciprocal interactions. The ureteric bud branches in response to the nephrogenic mesenchyme and the latter forms tubules in response to the ureteric bud. Other ectodermal tissues as well as the ureteric bud of the developing kidney, can induce the differentiation of the mesenchymal metanephric tubule in vitro. In transfilter experiments mesenchyme induction is dependent on physical contacts with tissues such as the spinal cord or notochord for about 24 h, after which time the inducing tissue may be removed. By 72 h differentiation characterized by the aggregation of mesenchymal elements and organization of tubules has occurred. The 24 h induction period is sensitive to drugs which inhibit GAG and glycoprotein synthesis (6-diazo-5-oxo-norleucine, DON, a glutamine-analogue) and to tunicamycin (an inhibitor of protein glycosylation). In the presence of these drugs, morphogenesis does not occur although cell growth through the filter is normal. The separate pretreatment of the spinal cord with DON does not prevent its inducing capacity. Therefore substances produced by the induced tissue are thought to be involved. Before morphogenesis, the mesenchymal cells stain for type I and III collagens; these gradually disappear during the period of 'induction' and new matrix materials take their place. These materials include laminin and type IV collagen. These materials appear in the mesenchyme during the period 12 h after the start of culture when no overt differentiation can be observed. Tunicamycin prevents differentiation and the appearance of laminin if applied during the induction period but not if applied at 24 to 72 h when differentiation also occurs normally (Ekblom et al, 1979a and b, 1980a and b). The changes in collagen types in the cellular environment of the developing kidney tissue in the early stages of differentiation are suggestive that they may be influencing the process of differentiation itself although the evidence is still indirect.

Lung morphogenesis and salivary gland morphogenesis (see also Ch. 24)

Lung, salivary gland and mammary epithelia develop into branching structures by the formation of buds and clefts. Acidic GAGs are deposited at the tips of the buds in the interface between the epithelium and its mesenchyme. Older and deeper clefts are characterized by collagen fibres. The hypothesis proposed by Bernfield (1973) is that hydrolytic enzymes produced by the mesenchyme cause rapid turnover of the GAGs which are part of the basement membrane. The basement membrane is thought to be the stabilizing influence on the shape of the developing branches. Calcium ions may be bound by GAGs thus trapping the possible activating factor for contractile microfilaments and microtubules which alter cell shape. Earlier studies had implicated collagen as the inducing material but this was an experimental artefact.

Mammary gland development and differentiation

Embryonic mammary epithelium cultured with its own mesenchyme tissue develops into narrow tubular structures. Interestingly, this pattern can be altered to something remarkably like salivary gland morphogenesis if salivary mesenchyme replaces the homologous tissue (Kratchowil, 1972). This strongly suggests that the mesenchyme supports a specific pattern of organization to shape the overlying epithelium and it may do so by means of strategically placed GAGs in the basal lamina. The deposition of GAGs is probably a permissive influence in shaping the epithelium and the accumulation of GAGs can be increased by presence of collagen. Such an effect is obtained in secondary cultures of mouse postnatal mammary epithelial cells grown on collagen substrata (David & Bernfield, 1977). Cultures grown on collagen accumulate more GAGs in part because of reduced degradation and therefore it is possible that the basal lamina in vivo is influenced by collagen in the environment. The presence of GAGs in basement membranes may be characteristic of mammary epithelia which are undergoing morphogenesis, since they are also present in mid-pregnancy mouse mammary glands which are also undergoing folding and budding (Gordon & Bernfield, 1980).

Mammary tissue has been the focus of much attention in studies which examine the influence of the microenvironment on normal and malignant cells. Real progress is being made towards understanding the complexity of a specialized gland, the synthetic products and their cellular origins in vitro and in vivo. Drugs may be applied which inhibit the synthesis of identified components and cause the loss of specific properties and hence the influence of each component is assessed. In 1977 Emerman and Pitelka showed that dissociated normal tissue from prelactating mice could be cultured as a differentiated tissue for 1 month when grown on floating collagen membranes in media containing hormones. The cells form three-dimensional alveolar structures of epithelial cells with a basement membrane which separates them from stromal cells. The epithelial cells show polarization with microvilli and tight junctions at the luminal interface. Such cells grown on plastic, glass or collagen substrata rapidly lose the capacity to secrete the products which characterize mammary epithelium (prolactin receptor, casein and alpha-lactalbumin). If they are transferred to floating collagen gels, protein synthesis increases sharply, DNA synthesis is reduced and re-differentiation occurs. Mammary tumour epithelial cells can also be cultured successfully on such gels (Yang et al, 1979). These observations indicate the importance of a three-dimensional framework of contacts and communication to support biological activity of cells.

The ultimate aim is to use cloned cells and defined media to examine the control of growth and differentiated expression of mammary epithelial cells but so far the best results have been obtained from preparations of 'organoids' or ductal fragments and alveoli consisting of epithelial and myoepithelial cells attached to a partially intact basement membrane (Kidwell et al, 1980a). Both normal and tumourous mammary gland cultures have been prepared; they form two cell layers on dishes. The lower one is a large flattened fibroblast-like cell and the upper layer consists of cuboidal epithelial cells. The lower cells were shown to contain and secrete type IV collagen, thus showing their non-fibroblastic origin since fibroblasts synthesize only type I and III collagen. When dividing cells are identified by labelling with tritiated thymidine, epithelial cells in two positions were labelled: those at the colony periphery in the neighbourhood of the large flat cells and those in contact with the remnants of the basement membrane. The large flat cells are likely to be myoepithelial cells and seem to support the epithelial cell population not only physically by the formation of a basement membrane, but also to maintain cell division. The rate of attachment of epithelial cells to collagen substrata of various types is greatest (three times higher) to type IV collagen compared to type I, II and III. The specific dependence of attachment and cell division on type IV collagen is illustrated by adding the inhibitor cis-hydroxyproline to cultures to stop the synthesis and secretion of collagen. Cell attachment to type I collagen is almost eliminated and if cis-hydroxyproline is added after attachment, cell division is stopped and the cells die. On type IV collagen substrates, however, cell attachment is not affected and the growth rate is reduced by only 50 per cent (Wicha et al, 1979a). Kidwell et al (1980a) emphasize a key role for myoepithelial cells in the production of type IV collagen plus an unidentified collagen-dependent survival factor. Myoepithelial cells, therefore, promote the physical and biochemical environment necessary for mammary gland proliferation and function.

Hormones in the culture medium have several functions, one of which involves an endogenous inactive collagenase. When hormones are removed, the collagenase is activated, the basement membrane is degraded and the epithelial cells degenerate. Such a process is very similar to normal mammary gland involution and to that involution induced in mammary tumours by the administration of cis-hydroxyproline. Although it is clear that the maintenance of mammary epithelium is highly dependent on the presence of a basement membrane, the exact nature of the interaction is obscure.

The in vitro culture system has been further defined by omitting serum and including epidermal growth factor (EGF), insulin and dexamethasone, transferrin and fetuin. Table 13.2 shows that if growth factors are withdrawn from the medium, the resulting inhibition of cell growth is moderated if the cells are attached to a type IV substratum. EGF stimulates the cells to attach and grow on type I collagen (but no stimulation is observed on type IV collagen) and it is suggested that EGF may stimulate the production of ECM, particularly a basement membrane. The mitogenic activity of EGF is enhanced by the presence of ascorbic acid in the medium (Lembach, 1976) and this potentiation may be ascribed to increased collagen production which in turn favours cell survival.

Mammary tumour epithelial cells and their normal counterparts synthesize similar amounts of type IV collagen but the tumour cells are different in their lack of preference for attachment to type IV collagen. Although their growth is inhibited by cis-hydroxyproline, the tumour cells' sensitivity to this drug is not diminished by plating them on type IV (or type I) collagen. They have therefore overcome the marked dependence on collagen which attends normal mammary cells. Nevertheless, their growth in vivo is susceptible to inhibitors of collagen synthesis, partly because of the inhibition of basement membrane formation and partly because the collagen seems to be necessary for the production of the survival factor.

Primary cultures of mammary tumour epithelial cells stain poorly with periodic acid-Schiff's reagent, while normal cell cultures are heavily stained. This could be caused by differences in glycoprotein deposition in the matrix. Fibronectin does not seem to be present in either normal or neoplastic mouse or human mammary epithelial cells in culture (Yang et al, 1980). The absence of this glycoprotein component of the ECM is therefore not a marker of malignancy as has been suggested (Chen et al, 1979). However, there seems to be a species difference since fibronectin is found in rat dimethylbenanthracene-induced mammary tumours. In addition there is a difference between normal and malignant cell types in that laminin is not present in rat tumour cell cultures while it is present in large amounts in normal cell cultures (Kidwell et al, 1980b). This could have important implications for cell attachment to substrata and therefore to morphogenesis and metastatic invasion.

Nervous tissue development

Collagen is known to be synthesized by Schwann cells (Church et al, 1973) and to be secreted as soluble collagen polypeptides which may be responsible for the ensheathment of peripheral nerves. Nerve cells cultured alone lack a sheath, a basement membrane and extracellular fibrils, but if cultured in the presence of Schwann cells, these components are formed (Bunge et al, 1980). Collagen-coated dishes are necessary to establish these cultures but the part played by collagen has not been identified. The fibrils produced are of small diameter, collagenase sensitive, trypsin resistant and have a repeat banding pattern. The types of collagen made include type I, III and V (AB), and these become part of the endoneurium. The perineurium and the larger diameter fibres of the endoneurium seem to be formed by the interaction of connective tissue fibroblasts with Schwann cells.

Skin

Actively dividing basal epidermal cells can be cultured in vitro if their shape and orientation is maintained by a collagen substratum or if embryo extract is present in the medium (Wessells, 1964). In vivo, the mesenchyme provides both a substratum and a factor essential to the survival of epidermal cells. A factor which is known to promote the proliferation of epidermal and other cells is epidermal growth factor (EGF) (reviewed by Carpenter and Cohen, 1979). Although EGF is known to accumulate in large amounts in the ductal cells of the submandibular salivary gland of adult male mice and rats, it seems that many fetal tissues in the goat (K. Brown, personal communication) and mouse (Nexo et al, 1980) also contain this activity. It is likely that some of the supportive effect

Table 13.2 The effect of removal of growth factor from the culture medium of mammary epithelium. (Data from Kidwell et al, 1980)

Factor omitted	*Plastic* (A)	*Type I collagen* (B)	*Type IV collagen* (C)	*A/C*	*B/C*
EGF	56	45	14	3.9	3.2
Insulin	38	31	32	1.2	1.0
Fetuin	100	100	95	1.1	1.1
Dexamethasone	58	45	13	4.4	3.5
Transferrin	24	35	15	1.6	3.5

that mesoderm and chick embryo juice have on the maintenance of epidermal cells is due to an EGF-like factor. On the other hand, Eisinger et al (1979) have concluded that human epidermal cells will grow and differentiate in the absence of any dermal elements or collagen substrata, if the pH of the medium is kept at 5.6 to 5.8. Furthermore, the geometry of cell cultures affects the results since epidermal cells grow and differentiate well on floating collagen rafts and less well if attached to submerged collagen substrates (Lillie et al, 1980). These experiments raise the question that collagen per se may not be required.

The mesodermal fibroblast grown in culture is capable of secreting and accumulating several ECM components including hyaluronic acid and heparan sulphate as the major GAGs (GAGs form 55 per cent of the solid substratum material which accumulates under the cells in vitro), fibronectin (11 per cent) and procollagens type I and III (Hedman et al, 1979). The materials synthesized in vivo could be similar, but distributed in three dimensions in the dermis. They are separated from the epidermal cells by a basement membrane which contains collagen types IV and V, laminin and (in the embryo) fibronectin. Basement membrane is likely to have arisen at least in part from the epidermal cells since dermal fibroblasts do not synthesize type IV collagen. The integrity of basement membrane is disturbed in the skin disease psoriasis, in which the epidermal basal layer proliferates abnormally. There is no direct evidence for a causal nature of one abnormality on the other but when carcinogens are applied to the skin there is a disturbance of the attachment of epidermal cells to the basement membrane. One hypothesis (Mazzucco, 1972) is that loss of contact inhibition of the germinative epidermal cells leads to the increased appearance of collagenase as well as to increased proliferation.

Tendons (see also Ch. 30)

Avian tendon cells in primary culture seem to remain capable of full expression of their differentiated function only when in the correct orientation. When maintained at high density in a medium containing ascorbate, they synthesize 25 to 30 per cent of their total protein as collagen and this quickly drops unless they are grown on a collagen matrix where they achieve a morphology similar to that in vivo. The proportion of collagen synthesized can then be modulated by changes in the serum and ascorbate content of the medium (Schwarz & Bissell, 1977).

Muscle differentiation in vitro (see also p. 223 and Ch. 25)

Premuscle cells (mononucleated myoblasts) prepared from chick embryo thigh muscles cultured on glass or plastic tissue culture dishes proliferate poorly and fuse infrequently to form very low proportions of multinucleate myotubes. Konigsberg & Hauschka (1965) show conclusively that collagen is a component in 'conditioned' medium which is necessary for the promotion of fusion of myoblasts when present for a relatively short time at the start of the culture (about 24 h). Type I collagen can replace conditioned medium when applied as a substratum to dishes used for myoblast cultures. Since fibroblasts can be used to make 'conditioned' medium, presumably the fibroblasts surrounding the myoblasts in vivo are responsible for a kind of 'mesenchymal induction'. Later work (Ketley et al, 1976) has shown that the type of collagen used to promote fusion is immaterial since type I, II, III and IV are equally capable. A variety of synthetic polypeptides and noncollagenous proteins do not support the differentiation of myoblasts, however, and it is the protein and not the carbohydrate moiety which gives the effective stimulus.

Monolayer cultures of myoblasts require serum components and it is clear that fibronectin is one of them. Chiquet et al (1979) show that fibronectin is essential for cell attachment and that dishes precoated with purified fibronectin allow myoblasts to attach firmly, to spread, and to orient along fibrils without the need for exogenous collagen. Collagen is synthesized by these cells, however, and so endogenous collagen may promote the process of differentiation which follows attachment and proliferation. Differentiation precedes fusion and is marked by the production of actomyosin and other muscle proteins. The differentiation process must involve multiple steps, any of which could be stimulated by collagen.

Puri et al (1979) have studied myoblast behaviour in serum-free suspension cultures which do not contain fibronectin. The cells do not need or synthesize fibronectin, but nevertheless, proliferate and fuse into myotubes. The implication seems to be that collagen may also be unnecessary, since Puri et al conclude that perhaps fibronectin is only needed for myoblasts to attach to substrata (especially collagen substrata) and to migrate and hence to fuse, in monolayer cultures. Although suspension cultures do not need fibronectin, it is not clear if collagen is needed for myoblast differentiation. The medium utilizes a high molecular weight fraction from chick embryo juice and this could contain collagen. In addition, it is not known if suspended myoblasts synthesize collagen which may stimulate their own differentiation. It is important to determine this since three-dimensionsl suspension cultures may well be a better model of in vivo muscle development than monolayer cultures.

Other workers have used established myoblast cell lines such as rat L6 cells to study the effect of matrix components. Fibronectin is needed to maintain the cells during pre-fusion, but when added at fusion, is inhibitory. Addition of antifibronectin antibodies leads to increased fusion or onset of myogenesis (Podleski et al, 1979). Established cell lines may not give data which is relevant to the process of differentiation in embryonic myoblasts, however.

Glycosaminoglycans may also be involved in myoblast differentiation but the data are conflicting. Chick embryonic muscle cells synthesize three kinds of GAGs; hyaluronic acid, heparan sulphate and chondroitin sulphates, and the proportions change after differentiation to myotubes (Pacifici & Molinaro, 1980). It seems from this study and that of Elson (1978) that exogenous hyaluronate but not chondroitin sulphate inhibits the onset of morphological and functional differentiation. Indeed, hyaluronate synthesis is decreasing and its degradation is increasing before the time of fusion while heparan sulphate (Pacifici & Molinaro, 1980) starts to increase in synthesis and accumulation as myotubes differentiate. Ceri et al (1979) suggests that GAGs are also involved in the fusion process since both hyaluronate and dermatan sulphate are released into the medium soon after fusion. GAGs can form strong associations with cell surface receptors or endogenous lectins which seem to be under developmental regulation. Two endogenous lectins change in amounts in parallel with the GAGs present in the differentiating myoblast cultures and together they could form an agglutinating system for fusion.

The effect of hormones and growth factors on ECM development

Glucocorticoids

The ECM is a major target of glucocorticoid action. Prolonged topical treatment with glucocorticoids often leads to atrophy of the skin; both epidermal cells and dermal fibroblasts are affected. When administered to developing rats and mice, a decrease in collagen synthesis by dermal fibroblasts results in reduced gain in skin and body weight. The incorporation of radiolabelled proline into collagenous polypeptides is inhibited selectively because the activity of the enzyme prolyl hydroxylase is decreased after repeated injections of glucocorticoids into newborn rats (Newman & Cutroneo, 1978). Since underhydroxylated collagen is not accumulated, the effect is to stop the synthesis of collagen. DNA synthesis is also decreased in these treated cells. Corticosteroids do not affect the growth rate nor the synthesis of collagen by cells from keloid tissue (Russell et al, 1978) and in the case of epidermal cells enhance proliferation. Glucocorticoids stimulate the accumulation of collagen and fibronectin in human fibroblasts transformed with SV40 (Furcht et al, 1979). The hypothesis is that malignant and transformed cells are arrested at a very early stage in differentiation when glucocorticoids stimulate fibroblasts to synthesize collagen. Later in development, when fibroblasts have accumulated a matrix, glucocorticoids are inhibitory. Anabolic steroids such as nandrolone also inhibit collagen synthesis and fibroblast proliferation but if added together with corticosteroids, abolish the inhibitory effect of glucocorticoids on cell proliferation while not affecting the inhibition of collagen synthesis. It is possible that steroid hormones produce their effect via changes in the extracellular environment of target cells and this may explain why they may act synergistically with other hormones and growth factors.

Glucocorticoids in conjunction with other factors such as EGF, control the growth, elevation and fusion of the palate. They may operate through the level of cyclic AMP which is known to rise briefly before fusion. Early embryonic palatal shelves are stimulated by physiological doses of glucocorticoids, to grow and produce proteoglycans prior to and during shelf elevation; later collagen accumulates. Shelf elevation can be prevented by pharmacological doses of glucocorticoids and by drugs which prevent ECM accumulation. Delayed elevation leads to cleft palate. Exogenous EGF can also prevent fusion by preventing the epithelial cell degeneration which is necessary for fusion and this effect is counteracted by dibutyryl cyclic AMP (Salmon & Pratt, 1979).

Epidermal growth factor (EGF)

EGF has already been mentioned as a likely product of perhaps several embryonic tissues. It affects the proliferation and differentiation of epidermal cells, fibroblasts and many other types of cells. EGF stimulates the expression of fibronectin matrices in 3T3 cells (Chen et al, 1977). Its proliferative effect is enhanced by ascorbic acid (Carpenter & Cohen, 1976; Lembach, 1976) although this vitamin alone has no stimulatory activity. The addition of ascorbic acid to culture media almost wholly replaces the requirement for serum to achieve a proliferative response of human fibroblasts to EGF. Ascorbate stimulates the activity of proline hydroxylase and hence the production of collagen. Both GAG and collagen synthesis are stimulated by the action of EGF on human fibroblasts. The incorporation of tritiated glucosamine into both cellular and extracellular glycoproteins and GAGs is stimulated greatly within 4 hours. Collagen and GAGs may then form part of the extracellular environment which allows the cells to maintain cellular function and viability.

Fibroblast growth factor (FGF)

FGF is essential for the maintenance of cultures of several types of cells (Vlodavsky et al, 1979). For corneal epithelium, corneal endothelium and vascular endothelial cells, cell shape and orientation are particularly important in the response to growth factors. Cell shape and orientation can be regulated by the ECM and these will be discussed on page 231.

Insulin and nerve growth factor (NGF)

Both stimulate cell-substratum adhesion in PC12 cells (a clonal line of sympathetic ganglion-like cells) and adhesion promotes neurite outgrowth. Insulin (which has some common sequences with NGF) also stimulates the adhesion of other cell types to substrata (Schubert, 1979). Increased adhesiveness is a regularly observed characteristic for cell divivion of cells grown in monolayers (see p. 231).

THE EFFECTS OF COLLAGEN ON CELL BEHAVIOUR

On page 225 gross changes in the morphology and orientation of sheets or aggregates of cells were discussed and the influence of other cells or their secreted products on the development of tissues and organs was described. Morphogenesis in epithelia usually does not include changes in orientations of cells but individual cells may change in shape as they differentiate and take their place in the fully-formed tissue. For instance, individual epithelial cells elongate away from the basement membrane and become narrow at the apical end. The cells maintain lateral stability by complex junctions. Extracellular matrix deposition is observed and seems to act as a physical substratum for cell movements, cell attachment and hence tissue shaping. Next, we shall consider some effects of collagen on cells in culture to determine if in addition to permissive influences, there may be instructive or inductive effects on cell division or differentiation.

Cell division

Early work by Huzella and associates (1932) demonstrated greatly improved growth of cells on reconstituted fibrous collagen (type I). Ehrmann & Gey (1956) showed that several types of cells (normal and embryonic fibroblasts and carcinoma cells) grown on transparent gels of collagen have dramatically improved proliferation and outgrowth. They concluded that cells on collagen have a tendency to elongate and migrate along lines of stress in the gel. Fresh explants of keratinocytes from human skin will attach to collagen coated dishes with greater than 70 per cent efficiency and will form confluent stratified cultures whose proliferation can be stimulated by dexamethasone (Liu & Karasek, 1978).

Bovine brain capillary endothelial cells attach faster to plastic than to collagen substrata and start to divide earlier and at a faster rate. However, the final cell numbers of cultures on plastic and on collagen are similar and it is thought that the different response of the cells according to the substratum results from a difference in basic cell physiology (Schor et al, 1979). For example, these cells respond to whole platelets by proliferating at an increased rate only if they are grown on collagen. Aggregation of platelets and release of their growth factor contents can be induced by collagen and a number of other macromolecules. A collagen substratum is necessary for the synergistic effect of tumour angiogenesis factor with platelet factors on the proliferation of these cells. Several components form a complex system of inter-relationships which affect the growth of the cells. A small molecular weight tumour angiogenesis factor (about 200 daltons) isolated from tumour and other cells, is bound tightly by native but not by denatured collagen and this step seems to be crucial to its eventual mitogenic action on capillary endothelial cells (Schor et al, 1980). The nature of tumour angiogenesis factors and how they act through collagen is not yet known. The data raise the possibility that prior adsorption of some growth factors to collagen may be a general occurrence and may account for the improved proliferation and differentiation of many kinds of cells on a collagen substratum.

Cell asymmetry

Perhaps the growth of cells on a collagen substratum would be better considered in terms of the restriction in plasma membrane fluidity conferred by anchorage to a substratum or basement membrane. The strength of attachment conferred by increased extracellular matrix restricts the mobility of cell surface glycoproteins and this effect can be observed directly using a fluorescently-labelled lectin, concanavalin A. Transformed cells and cells grown on bacteriological dishes are less adhesive, have increased mobility of concanavalin A receptors, have fewer actin microfilaments and poor cytoskeletal organization (Wright & Karnovsky, 1979). Perhaps, a mechanism which increases the adhesion of cells to a matrix alters the organization of internal structure in parallel with the restriction of plasma membrane mobility and may thus alter the response of the cell to stimuli.

The blastomeres of a newly-formed eight-cell mouse embryo are spherical and have limited intercellular contacts, but the process of compaction which occurs during the late eight-cell stage is thought by Johnson et al (1980) to produce signals which lead to asymmetric distribution of plasma membrane components and hence cytoplasmic compartmentalization. The changes which are most apparent are the accumulation of ECM components, increased cell-cell contacts as the cells flatten on each other, abundant microvilli on the outer aspects, membrane bound alkaline phosphatase activity in membranes of the inner contacting cell surface (Izquierdo, 1977), and specialized junctions between the cells. Johnson et al (1980) argue that the appearance of membrane asymmetry in the embryo may be all that is needed for maintaining the differential syntheses of macromolecules which characterize the eventual formation of inner cell mass cells and outer trophectoderm cells. In other words, the response to the *position* of each of the cells of the morula (on the inside or the outside) is not the crucial design for differentiation of inner cell mass cells versus trophoblast as has been the current understanding since 1967 (Tarkowski & Wroblewska, 1967). One might speculate further that the contacting surfaces may be anchored, membrane fluidity may be altered and cytoskeletal elements rearranged by the presence of extracellular matrix components which are already present (Sherman et al, 1980; Leivo et al, 1980).

The implications of this theory could be applied equally well to other situations than the early blastomeres of the developing embryo and the mechanisms for the production of two kinds of cell from a multipotent one. The formation of sheets of epithelial cells whose bases are anchored in basement membrane, whose apical surfaces develop totally different properties, whose ability to respond to factors in the environment change, in other words, the differentiation of adult epithelial tissues could be brought about by the increasing asymmetry of the cell. The latter in turn could be organized and stabilized by the ECM and/or basement membrane. There is as yet no definite evidence that components of the ECM play a part in the production of differentiated cell types in the early embryo. There are several studies which demonstrate that certain cells growing on a basement membrane increasingly achieve physical asymmetry which precedes the expression of their differentiated phenotype in culture. Notable examples are vascular and corneal endothelial cells (Gospodarowicz et al, 1978; Vlodavsky et al, 1979). In vivo, they are monolayers of highly flattened cells which are exposed on one side to blood or aqueous humour and on the other side to basement membrane and underlying stroma. Vascular endothelial cells have functional as well as morphological polarity; the exposed surface is non-thrombogenic and the inner surface is thrombogenic and accumulates the secreted products which form the basement membrane. Only in this polarized form can these cells maintain a selective barrier capable of active transport from the blood stream as they do in vivo. Such strictly contact-inhibited sheets of cells are resistant to the uptake of externally applied low density lipoprotein (LDL) which carries cholesterol. Since their in vivo orientation is two-dimensional, it is readily simulated by culture in vitro with a substratum and fibroblast growth factor in the medium. The cells synthesize their own basement membrane coated with fibronectin which is similar in composition to that seen in vivo. A contact-inhibited and flattened cuboidal cell layer adhering to a basement membrane develops and is accompanied by all the polarities described above. At confluence there is a loss of fibronectin production associated with the synthesis of a new cell surface protein (CSP–60) which may be important in the maintenance of monolayer morphology. Whether CSP–60 occurs in vivo is not known.

Cell shape

The culture of corneal epithelial cells also illustrates the importance of the orientation of cells in culture and the complex relationships which are observed between the shape of cells, their growth characteristics, their response to growth factors and their extent of differentiation. Corneal epithelial cells in monolayer cultures respond to FGF but not EGF and this seems odd since organ cultures of the same cells show a marked proliferative response to EGF (reviewed by Gospodarowicz et al, 1979) but only small response to FGF. The difference lies in the substrate on which the cells rest. The epithelial cells proliferate on plastic as individual cells with no orientation to each other and with flattened morphology. The basal cells in organ culture maintain a columnar shape because they are attached to a basement membrane and the upper cells become wing-shaped and then flattened as they move to upper layers. In vivo the basal cell layer of the corneal epithelium rests on Bowman's membrane which is a basement membrane composed of collagen and proteoglycans. This is turn rests on the corneal stroma consisting of highly organized collagen fibres, GAGs and a few keratinocytes. In common with the epidermal cells of the skin, these cells will proliferate and differentiate in response to EGF when they are grown on collagen-coated dishes or on layers of fibroblasts. The cells remain rounded instead of flattened, they proliferate actively and eventually form a monolayer of packed, tall, columnar cells. They form multiple layers in the second week of culture and the complete array of differentiated cell types is produced.

A scheme depicting hypothetical positions of components which are known to be involved in cell attachment to a collagenous matrix has been described by Kleinman et al (1980; Fig. 6). The way in which matrix and cell surface proteins influence the shape of the cell may lie in the organization and response of the cytoskeleton. In vascular endothelial cells which are flattened, microfibrils run parallel to the surface of the dish. In epithelial cells the columnar shape is maintained by a star-shaped microfibrillar arrangement and bundles perpendicular to the plasma membrane originate from the desmosomes. There is electron microscopic evidence for a close relationship between microfibrils (actin) of the cytoskeleton and fibronectin in the extracellular matrix (Singer, 1979). In fact, soluble forms of fibronectin bind to purified actin with great avidity (Keski-Oja et al, 1979). However, there is still no direct evidence that fibronectin is attached to the cell membrane.

The requirement for cell attachment to substrata

It is generally accepted that most normal cells growing in vitro have a requirement for attachment to the substratum. Normal diploid cells except haematopoietic cells, chondrocytes and myoblasts, will not grow in suspension cultures although they may incorporate tritiated thymidine and may go through one division. Most cells require attachment before the addition of serum can stimulate mitosis. This can be by culture on glass or plastic dishes or on glass fibrils or beads over a certain size (reviewed by Folkman & Greenspan, 1975). Similarly collagen fibrils or Sephadex beads even in suspension will form a suitable substrate for cells to attach, spread and stretch out on, a phenomenon termed 'anchorage dependence' by Stoker et al (1968). In other words, a flat shape appears to be needed for cell proliferation, but how the cells become committed to cell division after attaining a flat shape is obscure. The onset of division could be regulated by plasma membrane surface area per unit volume, by the exposure or re-orientation of receptors in the cell surface, increased permeability or by increased nutrient exchange. The stimulus to proliferate given by anchorage to a surface is so great that non-tumourigenic cells (such as BALB 3T3) attached to glass beads will produce tumours (Boone, 1975). Furthermore smooth surfaces as fibres or sheets (but not powders) introduced into mice and rats will stimulate the growth of endogenous cells to form a tumour. Once cells have become 'transformed' however, they are no longer subject to the same kinds of restrictions to growth control and will now grow in agar or suspension cultures and at the same time such cells may assume a more rounded appearance.

An interesting exception to the rule that normal cells require attachment for growth is the calf aortal endothelial cell which will grow in semi-solid media (Laug et al, 1980). These cells secrete high levels of plasminogen activator and have a migratory potential, that is, some properties like those of transformed cells. Other properties show them to be normal; they are non-tumourigenic, have a limited lifespan and are karyotypically normal.

Attachment to a substratum may occur with or without the mediation of fibronectin, or may occur through other adhesion factors.

Fibronectin (See also Ch. 11)

Cells in suspension cultures are usually rounded and have very little fibronectin, for example myoblasts (Puri et al, 1979). Chondrocytes in vivo are suspended in lacunae within the cartilage matrix and there is no fibronectin in the matrix although the cells can synthesize fibronectin in culture. Cells growing in a monolayer attached to a solid substratum accumulate much fibronectin by synthesis and/or by adsorption from the culture medium. Fibronectin binding to collagen fibrils is further stabilized by cross-links, by GAGs and possibly by cell surface gangliosides (Kleinman et al, 1979; Ruoslahti et al, 1979). Fibronectin is readily detected in substrata attached material (SAM) or 'footpads' (Abercrombie et al, 1971; reviewed by Culp et al, 1978) and in pericellular fibrillar matrix. The addition of extra fibronectin has no effect on growth as such in monolayers or agar. It does not affect cyclic AMP levels or rates of nutrient transport.

The synthesis of fibronectin is reduced in transformed cells. Further, there is faster turnover of fibronectin as well as decreased binding to the cell surface. If fibronectin is added to such transformed cells, they increase their adherence to the substratum and become flattened and elongated. They align in patterns characteristic of normal cells. The cell surface and cytoskeleton change to a near normal appearance. The primary effect is increased adhesion; the other phenotypic changes including contact inhibition follow. The dissociation of cytoskeletal microfibrils with cytochalasin B leads to the release of fibronectin from the cell surface consistent with a link between the internal framework and the pericellular matrix which establishes cell attachment and shape. Fibronectin seems to be involved in the migration of cells but seemingly contradictory, there is good correlation between lack of fibronectin and the metastatic activity of tumour cells (Chen et al, 1979).

Cell attachment not mediated by fibronectin

Collagen is present in the small amounts in the SAM of cells attached to plastic dishes (Schwartz et al, 1978); fibronectin is present in much larger amounts and has been shown to account for cell attachment to collagen substrates (especially denatured collagen). Attachment of cells via fibronectin involves two stages, the attachment of fibronectin to collagen and the attachment of cells to the complex. Attachment to native collagen gels may occur by a different mechanism which is serum and fibronectin independent. Schor (1979) and Schor & Court (1979) find that HeLa and polyoma-transformed BHK cells are attached to native collagen gels in a manner that is serum-independent, relatively trypsin insensitive and not inhibited by cytochalasin B, all of which argue against fibronectin mediated attachment.

In studies using collagen substrates, type I collagen is most often used since it is readily prepared in large quantities from rat-tail tendons or bovine skin. Such substrata are similar to the in vivo environment of connective tissue cells but not at all similar to the environment of those cells which normally reside on basement membrane. Epidermal cells adhere preferentially in the absence of fibronectin to type IV collagen but this occurs with a time lag which suggests that these cells may be synthesizing an adhesion factor first (Kleinman et al, 1979). Metastatic cells cultured from T241 fibrosarcoma tumours adhere rapidly and preferentially to type IV collagen in the absence of fibronectin and do not synthesize significant amounts of either fibronectin or collagen (Murray et al, 1980). Similarly, monocytes will attach to most surfaces in the absence of fibronectin. Other specific adhesion factors may exist for each cell type. For example, such a factor has been described (chondronectin) for chondrocytes (Hewitt et al, 1980). Chondronectin is synthesized by chondrocytes and can be extracted from cartilage and will mediate their preferential attachment to type II collagen.

It makes sense that preferential attachment to type IV (or V) collagen should be a property of epithelial cells such as mammary cells. Fibronectin has no effect on this process and high concentrations of serum inhibit the attachment (Murray et al, 1979). Collagen type IV has a dramatic effect on the viability of cultured mammary cells compared to types I, II and III and this may be associated with their preferred attachment to type IV collagen (see Section II, 4 and Wicha et al, 1979). Cells plated on type I collagen do not divide for 24 to 48 hours until they have synthesized some type IV. It is concluded that primary mammary epithelial cells synthesize and require type IV collagen for sustained growth and differentiation.

Cell motility

Attachment mechanisms for tissues appear very early in development. Basement membrane arises as early as the fifth day in the gestation of mouse when there are approximately 100 cells. Obviously, a coherent sheet of collagenous material forms a firm elastic base for epithelial cells which are undergoing rapid division and morphogenesis, but apparently the scaffold need not always be quite so structured; it can be in the form of a network of fibrils which link the spaces between cells. Mesenchymal cells are quite loosely packed and they are linked to each other and to basement membranes of the overlying epithelia by matrix fibrils, largely collagenous, and also are coated by these materials. Intercellular spaces may be filled with bulky materials like hyaluronic acid to which mesenchymal cells do not attach or spread. However, these cells can spread extensively on basal lamina and take on a migratory morphology. Therefore type IV collagen may be the important surface for the migration of mesenchyme cells in vivo (Fisher & Solursh, 1979).

Neural crest cells are notable for the large migratory distances which they travel to reach specific locations and to differentiate into specific tissues (reviewed by Morriss & Thorogood, 1978). The mechanism does not seem to involve chemotaxis but it could involve either 'contact guidance' or a series of adhesions and withdrawals. Contact guidance by cells migrating along oriented fibres has been described by Wessells (1977) and Elsdale & Bard (1972) Löfberg et al (1980) also describe a complex network of collagen-like fibrils on the neural tube in axolotls just ahead of advancing crest cells. At the same time, the cells change from a round shape to an irregular and arborized or motile shape when in contact with ECM fibrils. If those fibrils are necessary for the migration of cells, then collagen must be predominantly involved. Certainly collagen promotes the rapid outgrowth of cells from chick neural tube explants (Davis, 1980).

In general oriented fibrils cannot be discerned along the migration pathways of mammalian neural crest cells and it seems more likely that migration occurs by successive cell-substrate adhesions. Neural crest cells are known to synthesize fibronectin and GAGs also accumulate around them. These materials may be involved by modulating cell attachment to the matrix along the pathway of migration. Cell surface glycoproteins may play a role in the directionality of migration. Pouyssegur & Pastan (1979) have used a mutant variant (AD6) of BALB 3T3 cells as a model of 'directionality'. AD6 has the same rate of migration as the parent cell line but has reduced directionality associated with deficient membrane glycoproteins, together with reduced adhesiveness and lower fibronectin levels. Directionality is restored to normal if fibronectin is added. The addition of N-acetyl glucosamine to the medium also restores the normal pattern of glycoproteins and glycolipids, together with adhesiveness, directionality of movement and intracellular microfilament bundles. Pouyssegur & Pastan (1979) suggest that cell substrate adhesiveness is necessary to stabilize the leading edge and promote the organization of microfilaments and axial actin cables for directing motion.

Peridontal ligament fibroblasts actively migrate in vivo and are known to secrete collagen as they do so. Intracellular accumulations can be seen polarized in the distal part of these cells as they migrate. All the intracellular organelles are polarized and cytofilaments extend from the anterior pole. Since colchicine blocks polarity and cell elongation as well as collagen secretion, Garant & Cho (1979) suggest that secretion of new collagen fibrils may be linked to active cell migration.

Couchman & Rees (1979) find that fibroblast migration from chick heart explants occurs rapidly at first and that at this phase there are no focal contacts and the cells lack adhesion, fibronectin and actin-containing bundles. Growth rate is low in the first 48 hours and only later when focal contacts, adhesion, acto-myosin bundles and fibronectin increase, does growth occur. They suggest that anchorage dependence for growth depends on the degree of cell spreading and this is specified by the cell genotype. Selden & Schwartz (1979) used cytochalasin B to inhibit bovine endothelial cell proliferation at 'wound edges' in vitro. Only the replication of the migrating cells at the edge of the wound was inhibited and this may also indicate that some form of movement may be required for initiation of wound-associated replication.

The migration of cells within three-dimensional collagen matrices is clearly dependent on cell type since no epithelial cell type will enter such matrices (Schor, 1979). These include HeLa, rat liver parenchymal, rat hepatoma, normal kidney, renal, mammary and bronchial carcinoma and normal epidermal cells. Fibroblastic cells do enter: they include BHK, 3T3, PyBHK, SV3T3, CHO, RPMI3460, melanoma, fibrosarcoma cells and mouse peritoneal macrophages. These cells enter without lysis of the collagen and there is no change in the rate of cell division whether the cells are on top or inside the collagen lattice. If fibronectin is added there is no change in the rate proliferation but there is a marked increase in the proportion of cells which migrate in.

Epithelial cell motility is likely to be independent of fibronectin and also of interstitial collagens like type I because these cells are normally found attached to basement membrane. Outgrowing mouse skin epidermal cells contain type V (AB) collagen and type IV is found in the basement membrane below them when explants are cultured to stimulate outgrowth. They require the continual production of a proline-rich macromolecule for cell motility (Stenn & Madri, 1978; Stenn et al, 1979), and if collagen synthesis is inhibited by the proline analogue, L-acetidine-2-carboxylic acid (LACA) cell motility is inhibited. However, the interpretation of this result is difficult because collagen substrates of types I, III, IV or V added to the medium cannot prevent this inhibition.

Collagen synthesis by transformed cells

There is much evidence that once fibroblasts which have been transformed by viruses (Kamine & Rubin, 1977; Moro & Smith 1977; Vaheri et al, 1978), chemicals (Hata & Peterkovsky, 1977), tumour promoters (Declos & Blumberg, 1979) or spontaneously (Vembu et al, 1979) both collagen and fibronectin deposits in the pericellular matrix are greatly reduced. Chondrocytes transformed by Rous sarcoma virus stop synthesizing their specific sulphated proteoglycans (Pacifici et al, 1977). After transformation, the cells lose adherence to substrata, become more rounded and assume the ability to grow in semi-solid media amongst other changes in growth properties. In most cases transformed cells synthesize collagen at about 20 per cent of the normal cells' rate, but this is reversible when tumour promoters have been used. It may also be reversible if transformation is brought about by temperature-sensitive mutant viruses. For example, Rous sarcoma virus transformed chick embryo fibroblasts at the non-permissive temperature, 41°C, have a normal phenotype and normal matrix deposition. At the permissive temperature, 35°C, the cells have a transformed phenotype and matrix is lost (Vaheri et al, 1978). However, BHK cells transformed by a temperature-sensitive mutant, lose the ability to synthesize collagen at both temperatures (Smith et al, 1979).

Recent studies suggest that fibronectin and collagen syntheses are controlled by different mechanisms. In chick primary tendon cells, the early effects of transformation are seen within one day as reduced rates of procollagen synthesis, but fibronectin synthesis is not altered. With long term labelling, reduction in fibronectin synthesis is also observed. In addition, the rate of fibronectin degradation and/or its release into the medium is increased (Parry et al, 1979). It is known that for collagen, depressed synthesis is caused by a reduced level of mRNA (Adams et al, 1977; Rowe et al, 1978) and that the proportions and types of collagen synthesized by transformed cells are altered, with $\alpha 1(I)$ trimer appearing in detectable quantities (Hata & Peterkovsky, 1977; Moro & Smith, 1977; Arbogast et al, 1977; Sundaraj & Church, 1978).

Reduced levels of collagen synthesis and morphology can be restored by adding dibutyryl cAMP to cultures of Kirsten virus transformed BALB 3T3 cells, whereas there is no effect on the untransformed parental lines (Peterkovsky & Prather, 1974). In addition, the transformed cells are stimulated by cAMP to increase their production of collagen but in an ascorbate-dependent fashion which is not altered by the cyclic nucleotide (Evans & Peterkovsky, 1976).

In most cases, it is established that transformed cells have normal levels of prolyl hydroxylase and the affected step in the process is not known. It could be that the failure to produce a matrix by the transformed cells largely accounts for the phenotypic characteristics of transformed fibroblasts. Certainly such cells seem to be less dependent on a matrix. We have seen above that malignant mammary cell lines are much less sensitive to growth inhibition by cis-hydroxyproline which acts by blocking the accumulation and hence the synthesis of collagen. The analogue inhibits the attachment, spreading and proliferation of normal connective tissue cells and this situation is reversed if the cells are grown in collagen-coated dishes but not on fibrin-coated dishes (Liotta et al, 1978). Different malignant lines have been analyzed for sensitivity to cis-hydroxyproline by Vembu et al (1979). All the tumourigenic lines are less sensitive to cis-hydroxyproline than their normal non-tumourigenic counterparts and the latter accumulate much higher levels of collagen in culture. The rates of collagen accumulation without cis-hydroxyproline and the growth inhibition by cis-hydroxyproline are directly related, thus supporting the hypothesis that normal cells but not tumourigenic cells require the synthesis of a collagenous extracellular substrate to support spreading and growth.

TERATOCARCINOMAS AS MODELS OF DEVELOPMENT

Origin

Teratocarcinomas arise spontaneously in the testes and ovaries of man and in many strains of mice. They are tumours which derive from germ cells or early embryonic cells and they continue to proliferate to produce growths which contain many kinds of differentiated tissues (teratomas). If the growths contain multipotent stem cells as well, they are transplantable and termed teratocarcinomas. Experimentally-derived tumours can also be produced by implanting a mouse embryo at the 3rd to the 8th day of gestation, under the kidney capsule or in the testes of a syngeneic host animal. Within a month teratocarcinomas grow in a large percentage of cases (see Solter & Sherman, 1977). The stem cells of such tumours are called embryonal carcinoma (EC) cells and they have many properties in common with multipotent early embryonic ectoderm cells (reviewed by Martin, 1977; Graham, 1977; Martin, 1978; Solter & Damjanov, 1979). EC cells will differentiate into teratomas after injection into an adult host. They will take part in normal development and colonize many tissues after incorporation into an embryonic host; either by microinjection into blastocysts (Papaioannou et al, 1975; Mintz & Illmensee, 1975) or after aggregation with morulae stage embryos (Stewart, 1980). EC cells have been cloned and can be cultured in vitro as undifferentiated EC cells or, by changing the conditions, they will differentiate into many kinds of tissues.

Biochemical studies have shown that EC cells produce differentiated cells which have biochemical properties corresponding to their morphologies, for example, skeletal muscle is formed in which striated actomyosin fibrils are present in fused myotubes in large amounts. At the same time, the cultures acquire the skeletal forms of several isoenzymes such as creatine phosphokinase (Adamson, 1977) and enolase (Fletcher et al, 1978). The earliest 'embryo equivalent' which can be recognized when EC cells differentiate in vitro is an epithelioid cell which could be a type of endoderm cell. This has been verified by the identification of newly-synthesized endoderm-specific products such as alphafetoprotein and transferrin (Adamson et al, 1977; Adamson, (in press) Developmental Biology, 1982: 91) as well as several components of the extracellular matrix (Adamson et al, 1979; Hogan, 1980; Hogan et al, 1980).

We know from page 218 that components of the ECM are synthesized very early in embryonic development and that they appear at different times (though the exact times are controversial) and that tissues may change their synthetic capacities as they develop. At the very least, we shall be able to establish the closeness of the relationships between different teratocarcinoma cell lines and true embryonic cell types by taking advantage of our growing knowledge of the appearance of specific macromolecules during development. It is also clear that we have to keep some reservations in mind when drawing such parallels since from page 225, it is evident that tissue interactions strongly influence the proliferation and character of embryonic cells. The precisely-laid geometry of developing and interacting tissues in an embryo is exactly what is missing from teratocarcinoma cell cultures and it is probably a major cause of the production of disorganized tissues in vivo as well as the generally incomplete state of differentiation that is achieved by EC cells in vitro. It will be fortunate if teratocarcinoma cells can be used as models for individual steps of the process of development and if they can, then the effect of ECM components will be an immediately accessible approach. Since teratocarcinoma cells can be both malignant and normal in different environments, they provide us with a means of testing the influence of ECM on processes which lead to malignancy or to growth control. Toward this goal, some teratocarcinoma cell lines have been analyzed for the synthesis of matrix components both as EC cells and as differentiated endoderm-like cell products.

Synthesis of matrix materials by teratocarcinoma-derived cells

PYS cells

Teratocarcinoma cells which accumulate a mass of ECM and which appear triangular and epithelioid in culture were first derived by Lehman et al (1974). At least two sublines of PYS cells exist; they were isolated as colonies from the original tumour. PYS-2 retains the tumourigenicity of the original line. PYS-2 appears to be both differentiated and malignant and is therefore thought to be transformed. The periodic acid-Schiff's staining material which they accumulate in a pericellular matrix is known to contain large amounts of type IV collagen and laminin, but very little fibronectin or other collagen types (Wolfe et al, 1979; Hogan 1980; Adamson, unpublished). They are therefore very similar to the parietal yolk sac endoderm cells after which they were named since these cells synthesize and secrete a very similar profile of macromolecules in vitro (Adamson & Ayers, 1979; Hogan et al, 1980). In Table 13.3, some macromolecular products of embryonic parietal endoderm cells (column 1) and PYS teratocarcinoma-derived cells (column 2) are compared.

PSA5E and 'END' cells

PSA5E is a teratocarcinoma-derived endoderm-like cell line (Adamson et al, 1977). It is comparable in several secretory

Table 13.3 Comparison of embryonic and teratocarcinoma-derived endoderm.

Component	*Parietal endoderm*	*PYS-1 PYS-2*	*VYS endoderm*	*PSA5E*	*PC13 END + OC15 END*
Type IV: l	+ +	+ +	+		+
s	+ +	+ +	±	±	±
Type I: l	−	−	+		
s	−	−	+ +	+	+ +
Laminin: l	+ +	+ +	+		
s	+ +	+ +	±	±	±
Fibronectin: l	+ and −	±	+ +	+ +	+ +
s	±	±	+	+	+

±, trace; +, fair amounts; + +, large amounts
l = location; s = synthesis

products to the endoderm of the visceral yolk sac (VYS, Table 13.3). PSA5E was isolated as a colony of endoderm-like cells growing in cultures of a cloned EC cell line, PSA5, and has retained its tumourigenicity (Adamson unpublished) and therefore may have spontaneously transformed. Several cloned lines of EC cell which were thought to be unable to differentiate, for example, PC13S1 in vitro, F9, nulliSCC1, can be stimulated to differentiate in vitro over a period of 4 to 7 days after exposure to 10^{-7} M to 6×10^{-6} retinoic acid (Strickland & Mahdavi, 1978) or by low density plating in reduced serum (Burke et al, 1978; Adamson & Graham, 1980). The EC cells change from small closely-packed cells with a large nuclear-cytoplasmic ratio to large flat separated epithelioid cells called 'END'. This morphological change is accompanied by the loss of some EC cell characteristics and the appearance of an entirely new set which may be either visceral endoderm-like (OC15S1 and PC13S1) or parietal endoderm-like (F9, PCC4aza1R). The expression of these characteristics is not as great as embryonic endoderm, partly because a mixture of cell types is present. Table 13.4 compares the syntheses of collagens and glycoproteins in the two kinds of cells. Refer to Table 13.3 for a comparison of END cells with the products of the embryonic endoderm which have been identified so far.

Primitive embryonic endoderm

The first endoderm cells to be differentiated from the inner cell mass (ICM) of the 5th day embryo form a layer of morphologically distinguishable cells on the surface facing the fluid-filled cavity of the blastocyst. In drawing comparisons with teratocarcinoma cells, the primitive ectoderm cells of the ICM (or slightly later ectoderm cells) are seen to be similar to EC cells. Even greater likenesses are observed when the ICM is isolated from the blastocyst (either by immunosurgery, Solter & Knowles, 1975, or by microsurgery) and incubated in suspension culture. A spherical body of inner ectoderm cells covered by an external layer of endodermal cells forms in 24 hours. It is this body which has a very similar structure to that of 'embryoid bodies' formed by EC cells cultured in suspension (reviewed by Martin, 1978). At first the outer endoderm of both structures stains intracellularly for type IV collagen by immunoperoxidase tests. Later, the stain is seen largely in a layer of basement membrane material under the endoderm (Adamson et al, 1979). It is likely that the first endoderm is a primitive type while the latter types include both parietal and visceral types (the latter characterized by the production of alphafetoprotein and transferrin (Dziadek, 1979; Adamson, 1982). The data so far are summarized in Table 13.5 in order to show the similarities between early embryonic ectoderm and EC cells and between embryonic endoderm and teratocarcinoma embryoid body endoderm.

Changes in synthetic patterns of ECM components with differentiation

In the formation of visceral yolk sac (VYS) endoderm

The VYS endoderm of the mouse is derived from the embryonic endoderm of the egg cylinder and is a product of the primitive endoderm of the ICM (Gardner, 1978). In the latter, the primitive endoderm is known to contain type IV collagen and probably synthesizes it. The endoderm of the 8th day egg cylinder also synthesizes type IV collagen (Adamson unpublished) and up to this time in

Table 13.4 Switches in synthesis of ECM components as EC cells differentiate into endoderm.

	Cell line	*Collagen Type IV*	*Collagen Type I-like*	*Fibronectin*	*Laminin*
OC15	ECC	+ +	+	+	+
	Endoderm	±	+ + °	+ +	– *
PC13	ECC	+	+		
	Endoderm	+	+ + °		
F9	ECC	+	±	+	
	Endoderm			+	
PCC4 azal	ECC	– *		+	– *
	PCC4 D	– *		+ +	– *
Nulli SCC1	ECC			+	
	Nulli D1	– *		+ +	– *
C145	ECC	±	+ +		
	END	–	+ +		
PSA1	ECC	+ +	+	+	
	Endoderm†	+ +		+	

* Conjecture since it is negative to anti-basement membrane antibody (Jetten et al, 1979)
° Excess a1 over a2, slow-migrating a1.
† Endoderm of embryoid bodies.
± trace; + fair amount; + + large amount; – none detected.
PCC4 D and Nulli D1 are endoderm lines derived from EC cell lines.

development, no type I is detected. On the 10th day of development, the VYS endoderm stains for both type I and type IV collagen (Adamson & Ayers, 1979). By the 14th to the 18th day VYS endoderm is synthesizing much type I collagen and little if any type IV. Therefore, there is a switch in collagen type during development, from type IV to type I. On the other hand, the parietal endoderm portion of the PYS continues to synthesize only type IV collagen; this endoderm also derives from primitive embryonic endoderm of the late blastocyst.

The differentiation of EC cells

Teratocarcinoma EC cells synthesize and secrete a very small proportion of collagen and this can be detected because the product of 10^8 cells or so can be readily collected and analyzed. EC cells synthesize largely type IV collagen as well as fibronectin and laminin, but these products are either lacking or sparsely deposited in a matrix (Adamson et al, 1979; Wartiovaara et al, 1980). It is likely that embryonic ectoderm can also synthesize ECM components though the difficulty of detection is great with so few cells. However, laminin, fibronectin and type IV collagen have been detected by immunofluorescence reactions. As ectoderm develops it seems to lose all deposits of fibronectin and type IV while some laminin can be detected. When teratocarcinoma EC cell lines PC13S1 and OC15S1 differentiate into END cells, they produce a larger percentage of collagen in the secreted products, and the proportions change. There is a switch to the production of a type I-like polypeptide which has slower mobility than the normal $\alpha 1(I)$ but has similar cyanogen bromide peptides. It is probably largely an $\alpha 1$ trimer since the proportion of $\alpha 2$ chains is low (usually one-sixth of $\alpha 1$). At the same time, fibronectin is incorporated into an ECM, while laminin remains undetectable or low. Similar changes occur during the formation of the VYS endoderm in the embryo.

Although similar changes accompany both the development of embryonic endoderm and the differentiation of teratocarcinoma cells into endoderm, there is nothing to suggest that collagen synthesis is in any way concerned with the mechanism of differentiation. In view of the known influence that collagen and other ECM materials have on the motility, proliferation, morphology, differentiation, stability and on auto-stimulation of synthesized products of cells and tissues described on pages 225 and 230, it would not be inappropriate to suggest some causative role in endoderm formation by the components which form the extracellular milieu. The evidence clearly points to supportive roles for collagen in some cases, and permissive roles in others, but so far there is no good data which demonstrates specific inductive stimuli during development by collagen or other matrix components.

CONCLUSIONS AND SPECULATIONS

Most of the cells of a developing embryo are loosely packed into three-dimensional space amongst a rather open framework of ECM fibrils. They therefore proliferate and differentiate neither as a 'suspension culture' nor as a 'monolayer' but something in between. This architecture is probably ideal for the plasticity (for example migration, regulation after losses of cells, epithelial morphogenesis) and rapid cell divisions which characterize development. In contrast, adult tissues are stabilized by close packing of cells and matrix and this is achieved by tight associations. Differentiating tissues may attain stability of differentiated function by interaction with their particular environment. The data so far divide into at least four types of associations of cells with their matrix: (1) Mesodermal cells such as fibroblasts which attach and stretch onto type I and type III collagen fibrils with the aid of fibronectin; (2) epithelial cells which lie on a basement membrane and whose attachment to type IV collagen may be mediated by a glycoprotein other than fibronectin, for example, laminin; (3) mesodermal cells like chondrocytes which become isolated in lacunae and may associate with type II collagen by yet a third adhesion factor, chondronectin; (4) suspended cells like blood cells and (transformed cells) which seem to be largely independent of matrix.

Table 13.5 Comparison of embryonic and teratocarcinoma cells.

Component	*Early embryonic ectoderm*	*ECC*	*Primitive embryonic endoderm*	*Isolated ICM endoderm*	*Embryoid body endoderm*
Type IV: l	–	–	+	+	+
s		+	+*	+*	+*
Type I: l	–	–	–	–	–
s		±			
Laminin: l	+	±	+		+
s		+			
Fibronectin: l	–	–	+	+	+
s		+			+

* Conjecture because of intracellular staining with all other cell types negative
± trace; + moderate amounts; – not detected. l = location; s = synthesis.

The stability of the function and the binding of each category of cell to its extracellular matrix can be modulated during development by such components as GAGs or proteoglycans: for example, heparin and heparan sulphate increase the tightness of binding between fibronectin and collagen; GAGs accumulate at specific locations of the basement membrane of mammary gland buds during morphogenesis; hyaluronic acid can inhibit chondrogenic expression while proteoglycans are stimulatory.

Experimental approaches for investigating the nature of the influence that the extracellular matrix exerts on cells have naturally followed from three-fold pathways: from analyses of the components of the matrix; from monitoring changes in the matrix brought about (either by the test cell or interacting cells) during growth, migration, morphogenesis or differentiation; and by perturbations to each component to analyze their role in the system. Perturbations have included drugs to inhibit the synthesis of components, antibodies to 'neutralize' the functions of components, and mutants which have a defective component.

The rather inconclusive studies which are described in this chapter have been best developed in the following systems.

1. Mammary epithelial cultures from normal glands and from tumours. In summary (a) collagen (type I) is important in maintaining the GAGs which are associated with the basement membrane and which are concerned with morphogenesis, (b) three-dimensional collagen substrata serve best for the maintenance of differentiated function, (c) type IV collagen is preferred for a substratum and this collagen is synthesized by the myoepithelial cell which underlies the secretory alveolar cell, (d) myoepithelial cells are essential to the system for providing type IV collagen for attachment and for maintenance of cell division as well as providing a survival factor. When they are inhibited from synthesizing collagen, only a type IV substratum will maintain the culture (e) mammary tumour cells do not prefer or depend on type IV for survival (f) laminin is lacking in tumour epithelial cell cultures and may be important to maintain normal cell adhesion and stability.

2. Myoblast cells have been particularly interesting because they can be grown in suspension cultures and can pass through the complex steps of muscle differentiation and fusion into myotubes either in suspension or as attached monolayers. Fibronectin is not involved in suspension cultures, but is necessary for monolayers to attach to collagen. Collagens (all types) stimulate myogenesis in monolayers, therefore they may play as yet unknown roles in the process of differentiation.

3. Studies with vascular endothelial cells have shown the importance of the establishment of cell symmetry for the attainment of proper function. Asymmetry is achieved by growth on a collagen substratum and by FGF in the culture medium. The two surfaces of a confluent culture in vitro have totally different properties which are consistent with their in vivo functions.

4. The importance of cell shape is elegantly demonstrated by studies on corneal epithelium. Monolayer cultures of flattened cells on plastic, respond to the mitogenic stimulus of FGF and not EGF, while cells become columnar in shape on a collagen substratum and respond to EGF but not FGF. A collagen substratum is required for these cells to proliferate into a multilayered differentiated epithelium.

The shape of a cell is not the trivial character that it might seem to be. It is most obviously important to the function of cells like corneal epithelial cells. In a more mundane way the different types of cells can be categorized on the basis of shape, such as epithelioid and fibroblastic. In this chapter, I have tried to show that the extracellular matrix can affect the behaviour of cells but how it does so has not become at all clear. I believe that ECM may affect behaviour through the shape of a cell, or more precisely, through the cytoskeleton since the latter is likely to be the way that cell shape is formed. The flattened shape of a fibroblast is established by its numerous attachments (via fibronectin) to collagen fibrils. The columnar shape of an epithelial cell is maintained by 'attachment' to type IV collagen in a basement membrane as well as by lateral junctional complexes. A system of internal cytoskeletal elements which connect directly or indirectly to the external matrix where the two make contact on the plasmalemma must be postulated. Much indirect evidence supports this. Moreover, the hypothesis stipulates that changes in the matrix can change the cytoskeletal framework in such a way that cellular function or behaviour is modulated. The most important corroborative evidence will be to find a plasma membrane component which is connected to the cytoskeleton and which will bind extracellular matrix components,and for this role perhaps, a ganglioside is the best contender.

SUMMARY

1. Extracellular matrix components appear very early in development, collagen types V and III and laminin being the earliest. Analyses of the components of the extracellular environment of the developing cells and tissues of the embryo are incomplete. Immunological methods have proved extremely useful.

2. Classical studies on the morphogenesis of organs and tissues have shown that collagen is an important component. In most cases however, in the light of more recent data, it must be concluded that there is no evidence for the specific inductive influence of collagen in morphogenesis or differentiation. Interestingly, and equally importantly, there are no critical experiments which rule such an effect out.

3. In vitro studies using simplified model systems have described the influence of collagen on cell adherence, cell motility, cell shape, tissue geometry, and cell differentiation. Its effect on cell proliferation is presumed to be permissive rather than instructive.

4. Teratocarcinoma cells mimic embryonic cells in several respects: they synthesize similar types of matrix macromolecules; they change these synthetic capabilities as they differentiate to cells thought to be equivalent to those in the embryo; they differentiate in vitro to several types of cells of which the earliest is to endoderm-like cells. This differentiation can be brought about by changes in the culture conditions. Thus a model system for an approach to the analysis of the influence of the matrix on growth and differentiation is possible.

ACKNOWLEDGEMENTS

I am grateful to J. McLachlan and E. Crutch for critical reading of the manuscript and to D. A. Mercola for invaluable discussions and constructive criticism. I am indebted to M. Hollenberg, W. Kidwell, H. K. Kleinman and D. C. Turner for personal communications and to R. Gay and I. Leivo for Figure 13.2.

REFERENCES

Abercrombie M, Heaysman J E M, Pegrum S M 1971 The locomotion of fibroblasts in culture. IV Electron microscopy of the leading lamella. Experimental Cell Research 67: 359

Adams S L, Sobel M E, Howard B H, Olden K, Yamada K M, de Crombrugghe B, Pastan I 1977 Levels of translatable RNAs for cell surface proteins, collagen precursors and two membrane proteins are altered in Rous sarcoma virus-transformed chick embryo fibroblasts. Cell 14: 3399

Adamson E D 1976 Isozyme transitions of creatinephosphokinase, aldolase and phosphoglycerate mutase in differentiating mouse cells. Journal of Embryology and Experimental Morphology 35: 355

Adamson E D, Evans M J, Magrane G G 1977 Biochemical markers of the progress of differentiation in cloned teratocarcinoma cell lines. European Journal of Biochemistry 79: 607

Adamson E D, Gardner R L 1979 Control of early development. British Medical Bulletin 35: 113

Adamson E D, Ayers S E 1979 The localization and synthesis of some collagen types in developing mouse embryos. Cell 16: 953

Adamson E D, Gaunt S J, Graham C F 1979 The differentiation of teratocarcinoma stem cells is marked by the types of collagen which are synthesized. Cell 17: 469

Adamson E D, Graham C F 1980 Loss of tumorigenicity and gain of differentiated function by embryonal carcinoma cells. In: R McKinnell (ed) Third International Conference on Differentiation, Minnesota 1978. Results and problems in cell differentiation. Springer-Verlag, Berlin Vol II p 288

Anderson H C, Griner S A 1977 Cartilage induction in vitro. Ultrastructure studies. Developmental Biology 60: 351

Arbogast B W, Yoshimura M, Kefalides N, Holtzer H, Kaji A 1977 Failure of cultured chick embryo fibroblasts to incorporate collagen into their extracellular matrix when transformed by Rous sarcoma virus. Journal of Biological Chemistry 252: 8863

Bailey A J, Sims T J 1977 Meat tenderness: distribution of molecular species of collagen in bovine muscle. Journal of Science, Food and Agriculture 28: 565

Bailey A J, Shellswell G B, Duance V C 1979 Identification and change of collagen types in differentiating myoblasts and developing chick muscle. Nature 278: 67

Benya P D, Nimni M E 1979 The stability of the collagen phenotype during stimulated collagen, gycosaminoglycan and DNA synthesis by articular cartilage organ culture. Archives of Biochemistry and Biophysics 192: 327

Bernfield M R, Cohn R H, Bannerjee S D 1973 Glycosaminoglycans and epithelial organ formation. American Zoologist 13: 1067

Boone C W 1975 Malignant hemangioendotheliomas produced by subcutaneous inoculation of Balb/3T3 cells attached to glass beads. Science 188: 68

Bunge M B, Williams A K, Wood P M, Vitto J, Jeffrey J J 1980 Comparison of nerve cell and nerve cell plus Schwann cell cultures with particular emphasis on basal lamina and collagen formation. Journal of Cell Biology 84: 184

Burke D C, Graham C F, Lehman J M 1978 Appearance of interferon inducibility and sensitivity during differentiation of murine teratocarcinoma cells in vitro. Cell 13: 243

Carpenter G, Cohen S 1976 Human epidermal growth factor and the proliferation of human fibroblasts. Journal of Cellular Physiology 88: 227

Carpenter G, Cohen S 1979 Epidermal growth factor. Annual Reviews of Biochemistry 48: 193

Ceri H, Shadle P J, Kobiler D, Barondes S H 1979 Extracellular lectin and its GAG inhibitor in chick muscle ult. Journal of Supramolecular Structure 11: 61

Chen L B, Gudor R C, Sun T T, Chen A B, Mosesson M W 1977 Control of a cell surface major glycoprotein by epidermal growth factor. Science 197: 776

Chen L B, Summerhayes J, Hsieh P, Gallimore P H 1979 Possible role of fibronectin in malignancy. Journal of Supramolecular Structure 12: 139

Chicquet M, Puri E C, Turner D C 1979 Fibronectin mediates attachment of chicken myoblasts to a gelatin-coated substratum. Journal of Biological Chemistry 254: 5475

Church R L, Kosher R A 1975 Stimulation of in vitro somite chondrogenesis by procollagen and collagen. Nature 258: 327

Church R L, Tanzer M L, Pheiffer S E 1973 Collagen and procollagen production by a clonal line of Schwann cells. Proceedings of the National Academy of Science USA 70: 1943

Couchman J R, Rees D A 1979 The behaviour of fibroblasts migrating from chick heart explants: changes in adhesion, locomotion and growth, and in the distribution of actomyosin and fibronectin. Journal of Cell Science 39: 149

Culp L A, Rollins B J, Buniel S, Hitri S 1978 Two functionally distinct pools of gycosaminoglycan in the substrate adhesion sites of murine cells. Journal of Cell Biology 79: 788

David G, Bernfield M 1977 Inhibition of mammary epithelial glycosaminoglycans degradation by collagen. Journal of Cell Biology 75: 161

Davis E M 1980 Translocation of neural crest cells within a hydrated collagen lattice. Journal of Embryology and Experimental Morphology 55: 17

Delclos K B, Blumberg P M 1979 Decrease in collagen production in normal and Rous Sarcoma virus-transformed chick embryo fibroblasts induced by phorbol myristate acetate. Cancer Research 39: 167

Duance V C, Restall D J, Beard H, Bourne F J, Bailey A J 1977 The location of three collagen types in skeletal muscle. FEBS Letters 79: 248

Dziadek M 1979 Cell differentiation in isolated inner cell masses of mouse blastocysts in vitro: onset of specific gene expression. Journal of Embryology and Experimental Morphology 53: 367

Ehrmann R L, Gey G O 1956 Growth of cells on a transparent gel of reconstituted rat tail collagen. Journal of the National Cancer Institute 16: 1375

Eisinger M, Lee J S, Hefton J M, Darzynkiewicz Z, Chiao J W, de Harven E 1979 Human epidermal cell cultures: growth and differentiation in the absence of dermal components or medium supplements. Proceedings of the National Academy of Science USA 76: 5340

Ekblom P, Lash J W, Lehtonen E, Nordling S, Saxen L 1979a Inhibition of morphogenetic cell interactions by 6-diazo-5-oxo-norleucine (DON). Experimental Cell Research 121: 121

Ekblom P, Nordling S, Saxen L, Rasilo M-L, Renkonen O 1979b Cell interactions leading to kidney tubule determination are tunicamycin sensitive. Cell Differentiation 8: 347

Ekblom P, Alitalo K, Vaheri A, Timpl R, Saxen L 1980a Induction of a basement membrane glycoprotein in embryonic kidney: possible role of laminin in morphogenesis. Proceedings of the National Academy of Sciences USA 77: 485

Ekblom P, Miettinen A, Saxen L 1980b Induction of brush border antigens of the proximal tubule in the developing kidney. Developmental Biology 74: 263

Elsdale T, Bard J 1972 Collagen substrata for studies on cell behaviour. Journal of Cell Biology 54: 626

Elson H F 1978 Regulation of differentiating muscle cell cultures by the extracellular matrix. Journal of Cell Biology 79: 156

Emerman J T, Pitelka D R 1977 Maintenance and induction of morphological differentiation in dissociated mammary epithelium on floating collagen membranes. In vitro 13: 316

Epstein E H 1974 $[\alpha 1(III)]_3$ Human skin collagen. Release by pepsin digestion and preponderance in fetal life. Journal of Biological Chemistry 249: 3225

Evans C A, Peterkofsky B 1976 Ascorbate-independent proline hydroxylation resulting from viral transformation of Balb 3T3 cells and unaffected by dibutyryl cAMP treatment. Journal of Cellular Physiology 89: 355

Fisher M, Solursh M 1979 The influence of the substratum on mesenchyme spreading in vitro. Experimental Cell Research 123: 1

Fletcher L, Rider C C, Taylor C B, Adamson E D, Luke B M, Graham C F 1978 Enolase isoenzymes as markers of differentiation in teratocarcinoma cells and normal tissues of mouse. Developmental Biology 65: 462

Foidart J-M, Reddi A H 1980 Immunofluorescent localisation of type IV collagen and laminin during endochondral bone differentiation and regulation by pituitary growth hormone. Developmental Biology 75: 130

Folkman J, Greenspan H P 1975 Influence of geometry on control of cell growth. Biochimica Biophysica Acta 417: 211

Furcht L T, Mosher D F, Wendschafer-Crabb G, Woodbridge P A, Foidart J M 1979 Dexamethasone-induced accumulation of a fibronectin and collagen extracellular matrix in transformed human cells. Nature 277: 393

Garant P R, Cho M J 1979 Cytoplasmic polarization of peridontal ligament fibroblasts: implications for cell migration and collagen secretion. Journal of Periodontal Research 14: 95

Gardner R L 1978 The relationship between cell lineage and differentiation in the early mouse embryo. In: Gehring W J (ed) Results and Problems in Cell Differentiation, vol 9. Springer-Verlag, Berlin, p 205

Gay S, Miller E J 1978 Collagen in the Physiology and Pathology of Connective Tissue. Gustav Fischer, Stuttgart

Gordon J R, Bernfield M R 1980 The basal lamina of the post-natal mammary gland epithelium contains glycosaminoglycans in a precise ultrastructural organization. Developmental Biology 74: 118

Gospodarowicz D, Greenberg G, Birdwell C R 1978 Determination of cellular shape by the extracellular matrix and its correlation with the control of cellular growth. Cancer Research 38: 4155

Gospodarowicz D, Vlodavsky I, Greenberg G, Johnson L K 1979 Cellular shape is determined by the extracellular matrix and is responsible for the control of cellular growth and function. Cold Spring Harbor Conference on Cell Proliferation: 6B Hormones and cell culture, p 561

Graham C F 1977 Teratocarcinoma cells and normal mouse embryogenesis. In: Sherman M I (ed) Concepts in mammalian embryogenesis. M I T Press, Camb., USA, ch 7

Graham C F, Lehtonen E 1979 Formation and consequences of cell patterns in preimplantation mouse development. Journal of Embryology and Experimental Morphology 49: 277

Harkness R D 1971 Biological functions of collagen. Biological Review (Cambridge) 36: 399

Hassell J R, Pennypacker J P, Kleinman H K, Pratt R M, Yamada K M 1979 Enhanced cellular fibronectin accumulation in chondrocytes treated with vitamin A. Cell 17: 821

Hata R I, Peterkovsky B 1977 Specific changes in the collagen phenotype of BALB 3T3 cells as a result of transformation by Sarcoma viruses or a chemical carcinogen. Proceedings of the National Academy of Science USA 74: 2933

Hata R I, Slavkin H C 1978 De novo induction of a gene product during heterologous epithelial-mesenchymal interaction in vitro. Proceedings of the National Academy of Science USA 75: 2790

Hay E D 1977 Interaction between the cell surface and extracellular matrix in corneal development. Society of General Physiologists Series 32: 115

Hedman K, Kurkinen M, Alitalo K, Vaheri A, Johansson S, Hook M 1979 Isolation of the pericellular matrix of human fibroblast cultures. Journal of Cell Biology 81: 83

Hewitt A T, Kleinman H K, Pennypacker J P, Martin G R 1980 Identification of an adhesion factor for chondrocytes. Proceedings of the National Academy of Science USA 77: 385

Hogan B L M 1980 High molecular weight extracellular proteins synthesized by endoderm cells derived from mouse teratocarcinoma cells and normal extraembryonic membranes. Developmental Biology 75: 330

Hogan B L M, Cooper A R, Kurkinen M 1980 Incorporation into Reichert's membrane of laminin-like extracellular proteins synthesized by parietal endoderm cells of the mouse embryo. Developmental Biology (in press)

Huzella T, Lengyel I 1932 Orientation de la croissance des cultures de tissus sur la trame fibrillaire artificielle coagulée de la solution de 'collagene A' (Nageotte) par les forces de la cristallisation. Compte Rendus de Seances Societé Biologie 109: 515

Izquierdo L 1977 Cleavage and differentiation. In: Johnson M H (ed) Development in mammals, vol 2. North-Holland, Amsterdam, p 99

Jetten A M, Jetten M E R, Sherman M I 1979 Stimulation of differentiation of several murine embryonal carcinoma cell lines by retinoic acid. Experimental Cell Research 124: 381

Johnson M H, Pratt H P M, Handyside A H 1980 The generation and recognition of positional information in the preimplantation mouse embryo. In: Glasser S R, Bullock D W (eds) Cellular and molecular aspects of implantation. Plenum Press, New York

Kamine J, Rubin H 1977 Coordinate control of collagen synthesis and cell growth in chick embryo fibroblasts and the effect of viral transformation on collagen synthesis. Journal of Cellular Physiology 92: 1

Keski-Oja J, Sen A, Todaro G J 1979 Soluble forms of fibronectin bind to purified actin molecules in vitro. Journal of Cell Biology 83: 49

Ketley J N, Orkin R W, Martin G R 1976 Collagen in developing chick muscle in vivo and in vitro. Experimental Cell Research 99: 261

Kidwell W R, Wicha M S, Salomon D, Liotta L A 1980a Hormonal controls of collagen substratum formation by cultured mammary cells: implications for growth and differentiation. In: de Asua J, Levi-Montalcini R, Shields R, Iacobelli S (eds) Control mechanisms in animal cells. Raven Press, New York p 333

Kidwell W R, Wicha M S, Salomon D, Liotta L A 1980b Differential recognition of basement membrane collagen by normal and neoplastic mammary cells. In: McGrath C, Nandi S (eds) Systematics of mammary cell transformation. Academic Press, New York p 17

Kleinman H K, Hewitt A T, Murray J C, Liotta L A, Rennard S I, Pennypacker J P, McGoodwin E B, Martin G R, Fishman P H 1979 Cellular and metabolic specificity in the interaction of adhesion proteins with collagen and with cells. Journal of Supramolecular Structure 11: 69

Kleinman H K, Klebe R J, Martin G R 1980 Role of collagenous matrices in the adhesion and growth of cells. Journal of Cell Biology 88: 473

Konigsberg I R, Hauschka S D 1965 Cell and tissue interactions in the reproduction of cell type. In: Locke M (ed) Reproduction: molecular, subcellular and cellular. Academic Press, New York. p 243

Kosher R A, Lash J W 1975 Notochordal stimulation of in vitro somite chondrogenesis before and after enzymatic removal of perinotochordal materials. Developmental Biology 42: 362

Kosher R A, Savage M P 1979 The effect of collagen on the cyclic AMP content of embryonic somites. Journal of Experimental Zoology 208: 35

Kratchowil K 1972 Tissue interactions during embryonic development: general properties. In: Tarin D (ed) Inductive tissue interactions and carcinogenesis. Academic Press, New York. p 1

Lash J W, Vasan N S 1978 Somite chondrogenesis in vitro. Stimulation by exogenous extracellular matrix components. Developmental Biology 66: 151

Laug W E, Tokes Z A, Benedict W F, Sorgente N 1980 Anchorage-independent growth and plasminogen activator production by bovine endothelial cells. Journal of Cell Biology 84: 281

Lehman J M, Speers W C, Swartzendruber D E, Pierce G B 1974 Neoplastic differentiation: characteristics of cell lines derived from a murine teratocarcinoma. Journal of Cellular Physiology 84: 13

Leivo I, Vaheri A, Timpl R, Wartiovaara J 1980 Appearance and distribution of collagens and laminin in the early mouse embryo. Developmental Biology 76: 100

Lembach K J 1976 Induction of human fibroblast proliferation by epidermal growth factor (EGF): Enhancement by an EGF-binding arginine esterase and by ascorbate. Proceedings of the National Academy of Science, USA 73: 183

Lewis L A, Pratt R M, Pennypacker J P, Hassell J R 1978 Inhibitions of limb chondrogenesis in vitro by Vitamin A: alterations in cell surface characteristics. Developmental Biology 64: 31

Lillie J H, MacCallum D K, Jepson A 1980 Fine structure of subcultured stratified squamous epithelium grown on collagen rafts. Experimental Cell Research 125: 153

Liotta L A, Vembu D, Kleinman H K, Martin G R, Boone C 1978 Collagen is required for proliferation of cultural connective tissue cells but not their transformed counterparts. Nature 272: 622

Lipton B 1977 Collagen synthesis by normal and bromedoxyuridine-modulated cells in myogenic culture. Developmental Biology 61: 153

Liu S-C, Karosek M 1978 Isolation and growth of adult human epidermal keratinocytes in cell culture. Journal of Investigative Dermatology 71: 157

Löfberg J, Ahlfors K, Fällström C 1980 Neural crest cell migration in relation to extracellular matrix organization in the embryonic axolotl trunk. Developmental Biology 75: 148

Manasek F J 1975 The extracellular matrix: a dynamic component of the developing embryo. Current topics in Developmental Biology 10: 35

Martin G R 1977 The differentiation of teratocarcinoma cells in vitro: parallels to normal embryogenesis. In: Karhinen-Jaaskelainen M, Saxen L, Weiss L (eds) Cell Interactions in Differentiation. Academic Press, New York

Martin G R 1978 Advantages and limitations of teratocarcinoma stem cells as models of development. In: Johnson M H (ed) Development in mammals, vol III. North-Holland

Mayer B W, Hay E D, Hynes R O 1979 Relation of fibronectin to extracellular matrix and migrating cells in embryonic avian cornea, neural crest and area vasculosa. Journal of Cell Biology 83: 468

Mayne R, Strah S K R 1974 Collagen synthesis by cultures of chick myotubes depleted of mononucleated cells. Journal of Cell Biology 63: 212

Mayne R, Vail M S, Miller E J 1975 Analysis of changes in collagen biosynthesis that occur when chick chondrocytes are grown in 5 Br 2′ deoxyuridine. Proceedings of the National Academy of Science USA 72: 4511

Mayne R, Vail M S, Mayne P M, Miller E J 1976 Changes in type of collagen synthesized as clones of chick chondrocytes grow and eventually lose division capacity. Proceedings of the National Academy of Science USA 73: 1674

Mazzucco K 1972 The role of collagen in tissue interactions during carcinogenesis in mouse skin. In: Tarin D (ed) Tissue interactions in carcinogenesis. Academic Press, London. p 377

Miller E J 1976 Biochemical characteristics and biological significance of the genetically-distinct collagens. Molecular and Cellular Biochemistry 13: 165

Miller E J 1977 The collagens of the extracellular matrix. In: Lash J W, Burger M M (eds) Cell and tissue interactions. Society of General Physiologists Series, 32: 71. Raven Press, New York

Minor R R, Strausse E L, Koszalka T R, Brent R L, Kefalides N A 1976 Organ cultures of the embryonic rat parietal yolk sac. II Synthesis, accumulation and turnover of collagen and non-collagen basement membrane glycoproteins. Developmental Biology 48: 365

Mintz B, Illmensee K 1975 Normal genetically mosaic mice produced from malignant teratocarcinoma cells. Proceedings of the National Academy of Science USA 72: 3585

Moro L, Smith B D 1977 Identification of collagen $\alpha 1(I)$ trimer and normal type I collagen in a polyoma virus-induced mouse tumour. Archives of Biochemistry and Biophysics 182: 33

Morriss G, Thorogood P 1978 An approach to cranial neural crest cell migration and differentiation in mammalian embryos. In: Johnson M H (ed) Development in mammals, vol 3. North-Holland, Amsterdam, p 363

Murray J A, Stingl G, Kleinman H K, Martin G R, Katz S I 1979 Epidermal cells adhere preferentially to type IV basement membrane collagen. Journal of Cell Biology 80: 197

Murray J C, Liotta L, Rennard S I, Martin G R 1980 Adhesion characteristics of murine metastatic and non-metastatic tumor cells in vitro. Cancer Research 40: 347

Newman R A, Cutroneo K R 1978 Glucocorticoids selectively decrease the synthesis of hydroxylated collagen peptides. Molecular Pharmacology 14: 185

Newsome D A 1976 Stimulation of cartilage in embryonic chick neural crest cells by products of retinal pigmented epithelium. Developmental Biology 49: 496

Nexo E, Hollenberg M D, Figueroa A, Pratt R M 1980 Detection of epidermal growth factor-urogastrone and its receptor during fetal mouse development. Proceedings of the National Academy of Science USA 77: 2782

Pacifici M, Boettiger D, Roby K, Holtzer H 1977 Transformation of chondroblasts by Rous Sarcoma virus and synthesis of sulfated proteoglycan matrix. Cell 11: 891

Pacifici M, Molinaro M 1980 Developmental changes in glycosaminoglycans during skeletal muscle cell differentiation in culture. Experimental Cell Research 126: 143

Papaioannou V E, McBurney M W, Gardner R L, Evans M J 1975 Fate of teratocarcinoma cells injected into early mouse embryos. Nature 258: 70

Parry G, Soo W-J, Bissell J 1979 The uncoupled regulation of fibronectin and collagen synthesis in Rous Sarcoma virus-transformed avian tendon cells. Journal of Biological Chemistry 254: 11763

Pastan I, Pratt R M 1978 Decreased binding of epidermal growth factor to BALB/c 3T3 mutant cells defective in glycoprotein synthesis. Nature 272: 68

Pennypacker J P, Hassell J R, Yamada K M, Pratt R M 1979a The influence of fibronectin on chondrogenic expression in vitro. Journal of Cell Biology 79: 149

Pennypacker J P, Hassell J R, Yamada K M, Pratt R M 1979b The influence of an adhesive cell surface protein on chondrogenic expression in vitro. Experimental Cell Research 121: 411

Peterkovsky B, Prather W B 1974 Increased collagen synthesis in Kirsten Sarcoma virus-transformed BALB 3T3 cells grown in the presence of dibutyryl cyclic AMP. Cell 3: 291

Podleski T R, Greenberg I, Schlessinger J, Yamada K M 1979 Fibronectin delays the first fusion of L6 myoblasts. Experimental Cell Research 122: 317

Pouysesegur J, Pastan I 1979 The directionality of locomotion of mouse fibroblasts. Experimental Cell Research 121: 373

Puri E C, Chiquet M, Turner D C 1979 Fibronectin-independent myoblast fusion in suspension cultures. Biochemical Biophysical Research Communications 90: 883

Rath N C, Reddi A H 1979 Collagenous bone matrix is a local mitogen. Nature 278: 855

Reddi A H 1976 Collagen and cell differentiation. In: Ramachandran G N, Reddi A H (eds) Biochemistry of collagen. Plenum Press, New York, p 449

Reddi A H, Gay R, Gay S, Miller E J 1977 Transitions in collagen types during matrix-induced cartilage, bone and bone-marrow formation. Proceedings of the National Academy of Science USA 74: 5589

Rollins B J, Culp L A 1979 Glycosaminoglycans in the substrate adhesion sites of normal and transformed murine cells. Biochemistry 18: 141

Rowe D W, Moen R G, Davidson J M, Byers P H, Bornstein P, Palmiter R D 1978 Correlation of procollagen mRNA level in normal and transformed chick embryo fibroblasts with different rates of procollagen synthesis. Biochemistry 17: 1581

Ruoslahti E, Hayman E G, Engvall E 1979 Fibronectin. In: Sell S (ed) Cancer markers: developmental and diagnostic significance. The Humana Press Inc, Crescent Manor, Clifton New Jersey, ch. 18

Russell J D, Russell S B, Trupin K M 1978 Differential effects of hydrocortisone on both growth and collagen metabolism of human fibroblasts from normal and keloid tissue. Journal of Cellular Physiology 97: 221

Salomon D S, Pratt R M 1979 The involvement of glucocorticoids in the development of the secondary palate. Differentiation 13: 141

Schor S L 1979 The effects of EGTA and trypsin on the serum requirements for cell attachment to collagen. Journal of Cell Science 40: 271

Schor S L, Court J 1979 Different mechanisms in the attachment of cells to native and denatured collagen. Journal of Cell Science 38: 267

Schor A M, Schor S L, Kumar S 1979 Importance of a collagen substratum for stimulation of capillary endothelial cell proliferation by tumour angiogenesis factor. International Journal of Cancer 24: 225

Schor A M, Schor S L, Weiss J B, Brown R A, Kumar S, Phillips P 1980 The stimulatory effect of a low molecular weight angiogenic factor on capillary endothelial cells in culture Br. J. cancer 41: 790

Schubert D 1979 Insulin-induced cell-substratum adhesion. Experimental Cell Research 124: 446

Schwartz C E, Hellerqvist C G, Cunningham L W 1978 A collagenous component of the microexudate carpet secreted by attaching human fibroblasts. Annals of the New York Academy of Science 312: 450

Schwartz R I, Bissell M J 1977 Dependance of the differentiated state on the cellular environment: modulation of collagen synthesis in tendon cells. Proceedings of the National Academy of Science USA 74: 4453

Selden S C, Schwartz S M 1979 Cytochalasin B inhibition of endothelial proliferation at wound edges in vitro. Journal of Cell Biology 81: 348

Shellswell G B, Restall D J, Duance V C, Bailey A J 1979 Identification and differential distribution of collagen types in the central and peripheral nervous systems. FEBS Letters 106: 305

Sherman M I, Solter D (eds) 1977 Teratomas and Differentiation. Academic Press, New York

Sherman M I, Gay R, Gay S, Miller E J 1980 Association of collagen with preimplantation and peri-implantation mouse embryos. Developmental Biology 74: 470

Singer I I 1979 The fibronexus: a trans-membrane association of fibronectin-containing fibers and bundles of 5 nm microfilaments in hamster and human fibroblasts. Cell 16: 675

Slavkin H C, Greulich R C (eds) 1975 Extracellular matrix influence on gene expression. Academic Press, New York.

Smith B D, Biles D, Gonnerman W, Faris B, Levine A, Caparell N, Modten F, Franzblau C 1979 Collagen synthesis in normal BHK cells and temperature-sensitive chemically transformed BHK cells. In Vitro 15: 455

Smith B D, Biles D, Gonnerman W, Faris B, Levine A, Caparell N, Modten F, Franzblau C 1979 Collagen synthesis in normal BHK cells and temperature-sensitive chemically transformed BHK cells. In Vitro 15: 455

Solter D, Knowles B 1975 Immunosurgery of the mouse blastocyst. Proceedings of the National Academy of Science USA 72: 5099

Solter D, Damjanov I 1979 Teratocarcinoma and the expression of oncodevelopmental genes. Methods in Cancer Research 8: 277

Solursh M, Hardingham T E, Hascall V C, Kimura J H 1980 Separate effects of exogenous hyaluronic acid on proteoglycan synthesis and deposition in pericellular matrix by cultured chick embryo limb chondrocytes. Developmental Biology 75: 121

Stenn K S, Madri J A, Roll F J 1979 Migrating epidermis produces AB_2 collagen and requires continual collagen synthesis for movement. Nature 277: 229

Stewart C L 1980 Aggregation between teratocarcinoma cells and preimplantation embryos. Journal of Embryology and Experimental Morphology 58: 289

Stoker M, O'Neill C, Berryman S, Waxman V 1968 Anchorage and growth regulation in normal and virus-transformed cells. International Journal of Cancer 3: 683

Strickland S, Mahdavi V 1978 The induction of differentiation in teratocarcinoma stem cells by retinoic acid. Cell 15: 393

Sunderraj N, Church R L 1978 Alterations of post-translational modification of procollagen by SV40 transformed human fibroblasts. FEBS Letters 85: 47

Tarkowski A K, Wroblewska J 1967 Development of blastomeres of mouse eggs isolated at the 4- and 8-cell stage. Journal of Embryology and Experimental Morphology 18: 155

Timpl R, Rohde H, Gehron-Robey P, Rennard S L, Foidart J M, Martin G R 1979 Laminin — a glycoprotein from basement membranes. Journal of Biological Chemistry 254: 9933

Urist M R 1965 Bone: Formation by autoinduction. Science 150: 893

Vaheri A, Kurkinen M, Lehto V P, Linder E, Timpl R 1978 Codistribution of pericellular matrix proteins in cultured fibroblasts and loss in transformation: fibronectin and collagen. Proceedings of the National Academy of Sciences USA 75: 4944

Vembu D, Liotta L A, Paranjpe M, Boone C W 1979 Correlation of tumorigenicity with resistance to growth inhibition by cis-hydroxyproline. Experimental Cell Research 124: 247

Voldavsky L, Johnson L K, Greenburg G, Gospodarowicz D 1979 Vascular endothelial cells maintained by the absence of fibroblast growth factor undergo structural and functional alterations that are incompatible with their in vivo differentiated properties. Journal of Cell Biology 83: 468

von der Mark K, von der Mark H, Gay S 1976 Study of differential collagen synthesis during development of the chick embryo by immunofluorescence. II Localization of type I and type II collagen during long-bone formation. Developmental Biology 53: 153

von der Mark K, von der Mark H 1977 Immunological and biochemical studies of collagen type transition during in vitro chondrogenesis of chick limb mesodermal cells. Journal of Cell Biology 73: 736

von der Mark H, von der Mark K 1979 Isolation and characterization of collagen A and B chains from chick embryos. FEBS Letters 99: 101

Wartiovaara J, Leivo I, Vaheri A 1979 Expression of the cell-surface associated glycoprotein, fibronectin in the early mouse embryo. Developmental Biology 69: 247

Wartiovaara J, Leivo I, Vaheri A 1980 Matrix glycoproteins in early mouse development and in differentiation of teratocarcinoma cells. In: Subtelny S, Wessells N K (ed) The cell surface: mediator of developmental processes, the 38th Annual Symposium of the Society for Developmental Biology. Academic Press, pp 305-13

Wessells N K 1964 Substrate and nutrient effects upon epidermal basal cell orientation and proliferation. Proceedings of the National Academy of Science USA 52: 252

Wessells N K 1977 Tissue interactions and development. W.A. Benjamin, USA

Wicha M S, Liotta L A, Garbisa S, Kidwell W R 1979a Basement membrane collagen requirements for attachment and growth of mammary epithelium. Experimental Cell Research 124: 11

Wolfe J, Mautner V, Hogan B, Tilly R 1979 Synthesis and retention of fibronectin (LETS protein) by mouse teratocarcinoma cells. Experimental Cell Research 118: 63

Wright T C, Karnovsky M J 1979 Relationships between cell substratum interactions and the distribution of concanavalin A receptors of mouse embryo fibroblasts. Experimental Cell Research 123: 377

Yang J, Richards J, Bowman P, Guzman R 1979 Sustained growth and three-dimensional organization of primary mammary tumor epithelial cells embedded in collagen gels. Proceedings of the National Academy of Science USA 76: 3401

Yang N-S, Kirkland W, Jorgensen T, Furmanski P 1980 Absence of fibronectin and presence of plasminogen activator on both normal and malignant human mammary epithelial cells in culture. Journal of Cell Biology 84: 120

14

Immunology of purified collagens and their use in localization of collagen types in tissues

T. F. LINSENMAYER

INTRODUCTION

Early work on the immunology of collagen is rather difficult to interpret, chiefly due to the fact that collagen is a relatively poor immunogen when compared to most other proteins. Thus, in many cases, it is uncertain whether the antibodies produced were against collagen, since even purified preparations could have been contaminated with other proteins now known to be associated with collagen, such as fibronectin, laminin and acidic structural proteins. In addition, proteins such as serum albumin, if present even in small amounts, can elicit a strong immunological response. Also, it was not known that the collagens constitute a large class of different genetic types of molecules with common structural properties.

During the past decade, however, much work has been done which unequivocally demonstrates the immunogenicity of the collagens. Indeed, it is now known that a collagen molecule has at least three different molecular domains, each of which contains numerous determinants capable of eliciting an immunological response.

In addition, we now know about some of the immunological properties of procollagens, the precursor forms of the collagens, which contain additional immunologically active domains. We even know that each of the different genetic types of collagens, and at least some of the different procollagen forms, can be uniquely antigenic so that antibodies can be produced and isolated which are specific for each type.

Specific antibodies to the different types of collagens and procollagens offer a number of potential uses for cell, molecular and developmental biologists interested in the synthesis and assembly of extracellular matrices. These include the identification of the biosynthetic products of in vivo and in vitro collagen synthesizing systems, and the precise localization by immunocytochemistry at the light and electron microscopic levels of collagens and procollagens in cell culture, and in tissue sections of developing embryos and pathological tissues. Indeed, with the improved techniques for antibody purification, and the recently devised technique of producing monoclonal antibodies via cell hybridization, it may be possible, when combined with proper electron microscopic procedures, to dissect the substructure of individual collagen molecules and fibrils. It may also be possible to more precisely localize within individual cells where the various biosynthetic steps in collagen synthesis occur; for example, triple helix formation and secretion.

The uses and potential uses of collagen antibodies for tissue localizations by immunocytochemical staining will constitute a major portion of the present article. However, even with the improved technology for producing and purifying the required anticollagen antibodies, the results obtained using such antibodies should, I feel, be interpreted with some portion of restraint. We should be acutely aware of the possibility that even in the most highly purified collagen antibody preparations, there may exist a minor population of high affinity, contaminating antibodies which could preferentially bind to cells and tissue sections, thus giving erroneous results. In addition, the heterogeneity of the different genetic types of collagen is much greater than was once expected. Indeed, the discovery of new collagen types has been occurring with disturbing frequency. Thus, even affinity purified antibody preparations, which have been shown to have a major interaction with only one of the known types of collagen, may very well cross react with other collagens which have not yet been identified. This caveat holds true even for monoclonal antibodies, which should have the highest degree of specificity. Thus, a positive staining reaction need not mean the presence of the major collagen type to which the antibody was produced. In fact, it may not reflect the presence of collagen at all. Conversely, a lack of staining need not mean the absence of the collagen type to which the antibody was produced, but instead may be due to masking of the antigenic sites in situ. It is already known that within hyaline cartilage, most of the antigenic sites on the collagen are masked by the presence of proteoglycan. Likewise, in bone, most of the sites are masked by the presence of hydroxyapatite. What other types of masking might occur is still a matter of conjecture. Masking could occur through binding of a molecule known to strongly interact with collagen, such as fibronectin and laminin, or it could occur by means as subtle as the placement of a collagen molecule within a fibril so that the antigenic site is not exposed on the surface. It is possible that the more specific an antibody preparation becomes, the greater the chance its binding site will be masked in situ.

Indeed, with the potential problems associated with immunohistochemical localization of collagen types, I would go as far as to say that at present the most convincing studies are still those for which there is also biochemical evidence for the presence of the specific collagen type. Therefore, whenever possible I will try to correlate known biochemical data with the immunohistochemical studies. It is obvious however that the use of immunohistochemical antibody techniques can provide information that is unobtainable through conventional biochemical methods alone.

In the present article, in addition to those studies strictly involving immunohistochemical localization of collagen and procollagen types, we will also briefly cover the structure of collagen and procollagen as it relates to the immunology of collagen. Then we will investigate what is known about the antigenicity of collagens and procollagens, and how antibodies can be purified and tested for specificity so that they can be used for immunohistochemical studies with reasonable success. Lastly, we will cover what is known about monoclonal antibody production using the recently devised hybridoma technology, and how these approaches have been applied to producing antibodies against collagens.

THE COLLAGEN MOLECULE

The structure of collagen and procollagen molecules plus descriptions of the different genetic types of collagens are covered in other chapters of this volume. Therefore I will only briefly mention these topics to the extent which is necessary for understanding the immunogenicity of these molecules.

Collagen

All of the known collagen molecules are rod-like structures, and with a few possible exceptions are 3000 Å long and 15 Å in diameter. The shape and most of the properties of native collagen molecules are determined by the triple helical domain which composes more than 95% of the molecule. This domain consists of three chains (α-chains), each containing approximately 1000 amino acids, wrapped around one another in a rope-like fashion to produce a tight, triple-helical structure. This conformation is stabilized by interchain hydrogen bonds which can be disrupted by thermal denaturation resulting in unfolding of the molecule into its constituent α-chains. The triple helical conformation is wound in such a way that the peptide bonds linking adjacent amino acids are buried within the interior of the molecule. Thus, in native molecules the triple helical region is largely resistant to attack by strong, general proteases such as pepsin. If the molecule is denatured, however, the liberated α-chains are highly susceptible to proteolysis and can be reduced to small peptides.

In addition to the triple helical region, collagen molecules as found in extracellular matrices also have short (~20 amino acids), non-triple helical extension peptides (originally called telopeptides) at the NH_2 and COOH terminal ends of each component α-chain. These are susceptible to proteolytic degradation and removal under conditions in which the triple-helical body of the molecule is left intact.

Procollagen

Cells producing collagen in culture and animals with certain genetic defects secrete collagen molecules with much higher molecular weights than the corresponding molecules extracted from extracellular matrices. These higher molecular weight forms are now known to represent the 'procollagen' or precursor forms of the molecules found in the extracellular matrix. In procollagen molecules, each chain has large additional sequences, termed propeptide extensions, at both NH_2 and COOH-terminal ends. In the normal processing to collagen, the propeptide extensions are proteolytically removed. Skin from dermatosparactic animals, a genetic mutation found in cattle and sheep, contains partially processed procollagen molecules which have only the NH_2-terminal propeptide intact. Such molecules are termed P_N-procollagen to signify that they have a NH_2-terminal extension but no COOH-terminal one.

Genetic types of collagen

The most ubiquitous type of collagen isolated from many adult connective tissues such as skin, bone, tendon, and cornea is known as type I collagen. Each type I molecule is composed of two $\alpha 1(I)$ chains and one $\alpha 2$ chain, the complete molecule being abbreviated $[\alpha 1(I)]_2\alpha 2$. When type I collagen is thermally denatured the $\alpha 1(I)$ and $\alpha 2$ chains can be separated from one another either by ion exchange chromatography on carboxymethylcellulose (CM-cellulose) columns or by polyacrylamide gel electrophoresis.

With the discovery that cartilage contains a collagen molecule quite different from type I, it became apparent that collagen constitutes a class of closely related, yet genetically distinct molecules. The new molecule was termed type II collagen. When compared to type I collagen, the most striking feature of this molecule is that it contains only a single type of α-chain called $\alpha 1(II)$. The molecule is composed of three of these chains and is abbreviated $[\alpha 1(II)]_3$. Type II was thought to occur only in embryonic and adult cartilage. More recently, however, it has been found as a major collagen type in embryonic notochord and its adult derivative, the nucleus pulposus, in the vitreous body of the eyes of both embryos and adults, and in the primary corneal stroma of early chick embryos.

Type III collagen molecules also contain a single type of chain termed α1(III), the native molecule being abbreviated $[\alpha 1(III)]_3$. Unlike type I and type II collagens, the component chains are connected by interchain disulfide crosslinks which occur in the triple helical domain of the molecule. Type III collagen has a tissue distribution similar to type I, except for bone and adult cornea in which it is either absent or present in very small amounts. Loose connective tissues such as blood vessel walls, dermis and placenta are exceptionally rich sources of type III collagen and, as will be shown, it is thought to be the collagenous component of reticular fibres.

Another major class of collagen molecules is the basement membrane collagens. Many of the studies that have been done on the biochemistry of basement membrane collagen molecules, or molecules thought to be of basement membrane origin, have come to rather diverse results (see Ch. 17). Thus no clear cut definition exists for what constitutes a basement membrane collagen molecule. Two tissues which morphologically have large amounts of basement membrane material are the lens capsule of the eye and the kidney glomerulus. These were the two sources most used for initial studies. Limited pepsin digestion resulted in a single type of collagen molecule which was composed of three α-chains that classically have been termed type IV chains. More recently, studies using pepsin extraction of these same tissues have obtained several additional collagenous components, some with molecular weights ranging from 50 000 to 140 000 instead of the 100 000 of a normal α-chain. Other rich sources of basement membrane collagens are the human placenta and a mouse tumour, the EHS sarcoma. Moreover, the highly vascular human placenta also contains a number of additional collagenous molecules — two of which are the A and B chain molecules. Originally it was observed that these chains occurred in a ratio of two A chains to one B chain, suggesting that they may occur in a triple helical molecule with the conformation A_2B. Recently it has been reported that they may occur in molecules with other conformations such as $[B]_3$. It appears that the collagens containing A and B chains are clearly different from the classical basement membrane type IV collagen. They are therefore designated as type V collagens.

MAJOR ANTIGENIC DETERMINANTS OF COLLAGENS AND PROCOLLAGENS

Antigenic determinants related to protein structure can be divided into two general classes — sequential and conformational (Sela et al, 1967). For their specificity sequential determinants depend solely upon the linear arrangement of amino acids constituting the primary sequence of a protein, or a small segment of a protein. They are completely accessible for antibody binding when the protein is in the denatured state, and may also be accessible when the protein is native. In native proteins, however, sequential antigenic determinants may be inaccessible by being buried within the protein structure, or they may be modified by conformational changes so as to prevent antibody binding. Conformational determinants, on the other hand, require a certain tertiary or quarternary structure for generation of the antigenetic determinant. So not only is the correct primary sequence of amino acids required, but they must occur in a specific three dimensional arrangement. This type of antigenic site can be generated either by the folding of a single polypeptide chain so that different parts of the chain are brought into juxtaposition to form the determinant, or it can be generated from parts of separate polypeptide chains if they are also brought close to one another during formation of the native molecules. In the various antigenic domains of collagen and procollagen, one can find examples of sequential determinants, conformational determinants involving a single polypeptide chain, and conformational determinants involving more than one polypeptide chain.

Within a collagen molecule, Beil et al (1973) were able to demonstrate the presence of three major groups of antigenic determinants (Fig. 14.1) (see also Timpl, 1976, and Furthmayer & Timpl, 1976). These were: (1) sites in the native, triple-helical domain of the molecule termed 'helical sites'; (2) sites in the NH_2 and COOH-terminal, non-triple helical extension of peptides of the molecule, called 'terminal sites'; and (3) sites located along the length of denatured α-chains in the region derived from the triple-helical portion of the molecule, termed 'central determinants'. Procollagen molecules contain additional groups of determinants in both the NH_2 and COOH-propeptide extensions (Fig. 14.1).

Helical sites

In native collagen molecules, numerous antigenic sites occur along the triple-helical portion of the molecules. These are not removed by limited digestion with non-collagenase proteases such as pepsin and pronase which are known to remove the non-helical extension peptides of the molecules. The determinants tend to be conformational dependent, since antibody-binding to them is destroyed by gentle thermal denaturation of the collagen molecules, as assayed by passive haemagglutination or haemagglutination inhibition assays. Antibodies specific for these sites can be selectively enriched from a mixed population of antibodies using immunoabsorbants of native collagen, but not of denatured collagen or isolated chains or cyanogen bromide peptides (Beil et al, 1973).

Upon renaturation of collagen molecules, full antigenic activity is returned, but only if molecules with the correct

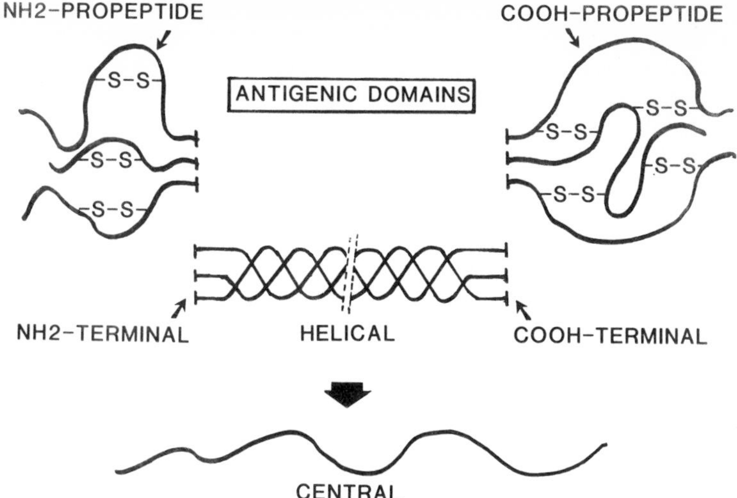

Fig. 14.1 Antigenic domains of procollagens and collagens. The individual domains specific for procollagen are the amino (NH_2-propeptide) and carboxyl (COOH-propeptide) extensions found only in the procollagen form. Native collagen molecules have determinants in the helical region as well as both the amino (NH_2-terminal) and carboxyl (COOH-terminal) non-helical extensions. Central determinants are found in the chains after denaturation of the molecules. (Modified from Beil et al, 1973.)

chain composition are made. Antibodies to helical determinants in type I collagen, $[\alpha1(I)]_2\alpha2$, react only slightly if at all with synthetic, renatured $[\alpha1(I)]_3$ or $(\alpha2)_3$ molecules but will react with renatured $[1(I)]_2\ \alpha2$ molecules (Hahn & Timpl, 1973). Conversely, antibodies made to helical determinants in synthetically renatured $[\alpha1(I)]_3$ molecules will not react with $[\alpha1(I)]_2\alpha2$ (Hahn et al, 1974). Therefore, these antibodies require the proper conformational juxtaposition of amino acids from different chains to generate an active site. That sites occur in different regions along the molecule is suggested since portions of the antibody binding activity can be retained in different triple helical fragments derived from bacterial collagenase digests of molecules.

Although most antibodies produced against the helical portion of native molecules tend to be conformational dependent, this is not always the case. Rabbits immunized with pepsin extracted, native type II collagen molecules will produce antibodies to sites within the helical portion of the molecule. Some of these antibodies react with both native and denatured molecules (Hahn et al, 1975a). Thus, both conformational and sequential antibodies can be produced.

In general, antibodies to helical sites within the molecule have a greater specificity for both collagen type and species than do antibodies made against denatured molecules or isolated α-chains. In many cases, however, they do cross species.

Terminal sites

In native molecules, the short, non-triple helical extension peptides at both the NH_2 and COOH-terminal ends of the component α-chains are antigenic. Certain animals, such as rabbits, preferentially make antibodies to these helical sites (Michaeli et al, 1979; Furthmayer et al, 1971; Timpl et al, 1972), and the antibodies produced have entirely different properties than those produced to helical sites. These determinants tend to be sequential ones occurring with equal frequency in native molecules, denatured molecules, and purified α-chains. In native molecules, determinants in terminal sites tend to be removed by limited proteolytic treatment with pepsin or pronase. All terminal sites, however, are not equally susceptible to proteolytic treatments, and some can be quite resistant (Beil et al, 1973). An additional, more definitive demonstration for the presence of antibodies to terminal sites is their ability to bind with those CNBr peptides which include the terminal peptide extension in their sequence (Michaeli et al, 1969; Timpl et al, 1970, 1972). CNBr peptides can be isolated, especially from the NH_2-terminal ends of chains which include the whole extension peptide sequence and extend only a short distance into the helical sequence. The ability of these peptides to react with antibody in passive haemagglutination or radioimmunoassay is considered good evidence that the antibodies are against determinants in terminal sites.

In general, for type I collagen, each of the COOH and NH_2-terminal extensions of the $\alpha1(I)$ and $\alpha2$ chains seem to be independently antigenic (see Timpl, 1976). That each extension contains unique determinants is consistent with what has been found concerning the uniqueness of the amino acid sequences for each extension. In some cases, the antigenic site seems to require the involvement of a single amino acid, such as pyrrolidone carboxylic acid at the NH_2-terminal end (discussed by Timpl et al, 1977). These antibodies react with collagen but not with procollagen, suggesting that the conversion of procollagen to collagen, which results in the creation of NH_2-terminal pyrrolidone carboxylic acid, creates this new antigenic site. It is thus feasible to produce antibodies specific for collagen that do not react with procollagen.

This result raised the possibility that antibodies might be produced to artificial terminal sites which do not normally occur in molecules but instead represent the products of abnormal proteolytic degradations created during collagen isolation. This indeed has been shown to occur. Antibodies produced against the COOH-terminal ends of the $\alpha 1(I)$ chain of neutral salt extracted collagen did not react with $\alpha 1(I)$ chains extracted under denaturing conditions using guanidine hydrochloride (Becker et al, 1972; Stoltz et al, 1973). Upon further analysis, the most obvious explanation for this result was that the neutral salt extracted α-chains contained a truncated COOH-terminal end, the presence of which created an artificial antigenic determinant not present in native molecules. Antibodies to such artificial sites would be useless for immunohistochemical procedures since they could not react with the native processed molecules in tissues.

Central determinants

Immunization with denatured collagen or isolated α-chains creates a whole new set of antibodies to determinants which are partially masked in native molecules. These antigenic sites, which are unmasked by denaturation of collagen molecules and tend to be of the sequential type, are termed 'central determinants' (Beil et al, 1973). When certain animals such as the chicken are immunized with native collagen, antibodies are produced against both helical and central determinants, whereas immunization with denatured collagen produces antibodies only of the central type (Beil et al, 1972, 1973). In the former case, the helical and central antibodies in the sera can largely be separated from one another by immunoabsorption on affinity columns of native and denatured collagen respectively.

Sites of central determinants occur along the length of chains. This can be demonstrated by immunizing animals with purified individual CNBr peptides derived from the central portion of the molecule (Michaeli et al, 1971; Timpl et al, 1971; Furthmayer et al, 1972). Alternatively, individual peptides can be used as inhibitors to antisera produced against whole molecules or α-chains. The results suggest that each CNBr peptide contains at least one, but probably more central determinants.

Antibodies to central determinants tend to have strong interspecies cross reactivity, probably reflecting the conservativeness of the amino acid sequence along portions of collagen α-chains. These antibodies even show some cross reactivity with denatured collagen or α-chains isolated from the same species in which the antibody was produced. Interspecies crossreactivity is found to be less pronounced in antibodies to helical determinants.

Antigenic sites of procollagen

Procollagens, which contain intact NH_2 and COOH-terminal propeptide extensions, are available mostly from cell culture. Even from this source the material is present in extremely small amounts due to its susceptibility to both specific and non-specific proteolytic cleavage. Thus, only limited information is available on the immunogenicity of the intact molecule. P_N-procollagen of type I collagen, the partially processed form of procollagen containing only the NH_2-terminal propeptide extension, is more readily available from sheep and cattle with the genetic disease dermatosparaxis, so most of the work that has been done on the immunogenicity of procollagen has been done with this material. That procollagen contains antigenic determinants independent of those in collagen molecules was initially demonstrated by Timpl et al (1973) who injected rabbits with P_N-procollagen from dermatosparactic calves. When the antisera produced were tested by passive haemagglutination against either P_N-procollagen or calf collagen, it was found that the major response was against the procollagen extension, but some antibodies were also produced against the collagenous portion. These two classes of antibodies could largely be separated from one another by affinity chromatography on columns using native collagen and P_N-procollagen as immunoabsorbants. The procollagen antibodies were further characterized. They reacted with the isolated $P_N\alpha 1(I)$ and $P_N\alpha 2$ chains from P_N-procollagen, and each chain seemed to have independent determinants. The antibody activity was not affected by thermal denaturation, nor collagenase digestion of the P_N-procollagen molecules, but most binding was destroyed by reduction and alkylation of the chains. Thus, the antigenic sites recognized by the procollagen antibodies do not depend on the conformation of the helical portion of the molecule or, in fact, on the presence of any sequences within the helical portion at all. The sites are largely conformational dependent, however, since they are destroyed by alkylation and reduction. These general properties of procollagen antibodies have been confirmed in most subsequent studies dealing with the antigenicity of type I procollagen. Using a smaller dose of procollagen from immunization, Park et al (1975) have reported eliciting an antibody response specific only for determinants in the procollagen domains with no response against the collagenous region.

A more complete study on the characteristics and localization of the antigenic determinants within the NH_2-terminal propeptide of type I P_N-procollagen and the response to the globular and triple helical domains within this region was performed by Rohde et al (1976, a, b). They demonstrated that in addition to using whole P_N-procollagen as an immunogen, similar procollagen antibodies could be produced when the immunogen was either the intact P_N-propeptide piece isolated by collagenase digestion of P_N-procollagen, or the intact $P_N\alpha 1(I)$ chain, or the globular portion isolated by collagenase digestion of the $P_N\alpha 1(I)$ chain. When the specificity of these antibodies was tested in radioimmune assays it was determined that the antigenic sites within the P_N-propeptide region are located in the main globular domain of the $P_N\alpha 1(I)$ chain. The small triple helical region within the propeptide piece is either non-antigenic or only weakly antigenic, as is the short non-helical piece which connects the triple helical region to the non-helical extension peptide of the collagen molecule. In these studies no determinants could be detected in the $P_N\alpha 2$ chain even when $P_N\alpha 2$ was used as an immunogen. The determinants in the $P_N\alpha 1(I)$ chain did not react with $P_N\alpha 2$ chains nor with the same region from type III procollagen, which appears to be uniquely antigenic (Nowack et al, 1976b). As previously established, most of the procollagen antibodies were dependent on the conformation of the globular propeptide piece since the antigenic activity was largely destroyed by reduction and carboxymethylation. Slight antibody activity still remained, however, suggesting the presence of some sequential determinants. If unreduced chains were used for immunization, the antisera produced contained antibodies to both conformational and sequential determinants, but immunization with reduced and alkylated chains resulted in antibodies only to sequential determinants.

The COOH-terminal end of intact type I procollagen is also known to be independently antigenic as suggested by the early work of Sherr & Goldberg (1973), Sherr et al (1973), Dehm et al (1974), and Nist et al (1975). This work was done before the actual discovery of the existence of the COOH-terminal propeptide. More recently Park et al (1975), Murphy et al (1975), and Olsen et al (1977), have extended this work. Park et al (1975) immunized rabbits with procollagen derived from cell cultures of dermatosparactic calf collagen, which, unlike the molecules isolated from dermatosparactic skin, have the propeptide extensions intact at both ends. As assayed by immunodiffusion, an assay which does not detect nonprecipitating antibodies, the antisera did not react with calf collagen but did react with dermatosparactic collagen isolated from skin, suggesting the presence of antibodies to the NH_2-terminal propeptide extension. An additional antigenic site in the COOH-terminal end was suggested by digesting the procollagen molecules with animal collagenase to produce two fragments, $T_C^{3/4}$ procollagen which contains the NH_2-terminal propeptide and $T_C^{1/4}$ procollagen which contains the COOH-terminal one. The antisera against intact procollagen reacted with both pieces suggesting antigenic determinants at both ends. Olsen et al (1977) injected rabbits with the purified, disulphide cross-linked COOH-terminal propeptide of type I procollagen isolated from medium of matrix-free chick tendon cell cultures. By radioimmune assay they showed that the antisera contained activity against whole procollagen and also against the disulphide-crosslinked peptide used for immunization, but not against pepsin treated procollagen. Then, the antisera were tested against the animal collagenase derived fragments, procollagen $T_C^{3/4}$ and procollagen $T_C^{1/4}$, which had been separated from one another. The only activity was against the $T_C^{1/4}$ fragment. Clearly, the antibodies were against determinants in the COOH-propeptide extension and these did not cross react with any determinants in the NH_2-terminal extension.

CELLULAR BASIS FOR THE IMMUNOGENICITY OF COLLAGEN AND PROCOLLAGEN IN MICE

The production of a humoral antibody response to protein antigens is thought usually to require the involvement of helper T-lymphocytes in addition to B-lymphocytes. The B-cells recognize the 'haptenic' determinants to which antibody is produced and the T-cells recognize 'carrier' determinants within the antigen. Recently, it has been demonstrated in mice that both collagen and procollagen are T-cell dependent antigens.

In mice, Nowack et al (1975) showed that by far the predominant antibody response to native calf type I and II collagens is to helical determinants and that this response is under genetic control. These antibodies were largely specific for the type of collagen used for immunization and did not cross react with artificial molecules with the chain composition $[\alpha 1(I)]_3$ or $[\alpha 2]_3$. The determinants were not destroyed by limited pepsinization of the collagen but were destroyed by thermal denaturation. They appeared not to be against a repeating structural component within the helical domain, since a bacterial collagenase derived, triple helical fragment, C78, which comprises about a quarter of the length of the triple-helical portion of type I, had only limited antigenic activity. Different genetic strains of mice responded with dramatically different titres to collagen types I and II. That this response is T-cell dependent was demonstrated by testing the antigenic response of athymic nude mice to native collagen (Nowack et al, 1976a). Homozygous nude mice (nu/nu) produced no detectable antibody to calf skin collagen. However, when injected with T-lymphocytes and then subsequently injected with collagen, the antibody titres elicited were nearly as high as for heterozygous nu/+ controls. Likewise, thymectomized, irradiated mice of a strain known to be a strong antibody producer against calf skin collagen, did not produce antibody when injected only with normal B-cells before immunization with collagen. When treated with both B and T-cells, however, a strong antigenic response could be detected which was proportional to the number of T-cells injected. Fuchs et al (1974), however, obtained conflicting results which suggested the antibody response to rat collagen was T-cell independent. The difference in these results is still unexplained except that they may constitute a species difference.

Support for the T-cell dependence of collagen antibody production was also obtained by immunogenetic studies. Hahn et al (1975a), using inbred strains of mice, were able to demonstrate that the immune response to native calf collagen is genetically controlled by an autosomal dominant gene which is linked to H–2, the major histocompatibility locus. Some of the strains which were low responders, when injected with procollagen, became high responders, producing antibodies to helical sites as well as to sites in the procollagen extensions. Since a genetic immune response is thought, in general, to be a T-cell dependent function, these data were interpreted to further suggest T-cell functional requirements for the production of collagen antibodies. The results with procollagen were interpreted as suggesting that the procollagen extension peptides provide additional carrier determinants which are recognized by helper T-cells. T and B-cell cooperation then would result in a higher antibody response by B-cells to haptenic determinants within the helical portion of the molecule.

Using nude mice, the production of procollagen specific antibodies to dermatosparactic collagen has also recently been shown to be T-cell dependent (Rohde et al, 1978). In this case, both carrier and haptenic determinants are located in the NH_2-terminal propeptide extension (Rohde et al, 1978). They used two strains of mice which showed an equally strong antigenic response to immunization with P_N-procollagen or complete $P_N\alpha 1(I)$ chain, but not to the collagenase derived globular propeptide piece from the NH_2-terminal end. So the small helical portion within the propeptide was necessary for eliciting antibody production. The antibody produced in response to the procollagen injections, however, was entirely against haptenic sites within the globular propeptide piece and not the helical portion. Reduction of the disulphide bonds in the globular propeptide piece destroyed its immunogenicity, showing that the haptenic determinants are conformational dependent. The helper effect exerted by the propeptide helical portion, however, was independent of whether this portion was in a trimeric molecule, and thus in the triple helical conformation, or in a monomeric, denatured peptide. Thus, the haptenic determinants, to which antibody is produced, are contained within the major globular portion of the propeptide extension and are conformational dependent. Carrier information is provided by the short triple helical portions of the propeptide piece and this is non-conformational dependent.

GENERAL METHODS USED FOR THE PREPARATION OF ANTIBODIES SUITABLE FOR IMMUNOCYTOCHEMICAL LOCALIZATIONS

The class of antigenic determinant to which a collagen antibody is produced is largely a function of the animal used for immunization. The rabbit, the animal most used for antibody production, when immunized with type I collagen, preferentially makes antibodies against the non-helical extension peptides (Michaeli et al, 1969; Furthmayer et al, 1971; Timpl et al, 1970–72). Some artifactual determinants can be created in these regions by proteolytic cleavage during isolation and purification, so a portion of the antibodies produced may be against these and thus may not be effective for immunofluorescence staining of collagen in situ. That the rabbit can also make antibodies against helical and central determinants was shown for type II collagen by Hahn et al (1975). Rabbits are also very effective for producing antibodies that are specific for the procollagen extension peptides (Timpl et al, 1973; Nowack et al, 1976b; Rohde et al, 1976b). On the other hand, rats (Beil et al, 1973; Hahn & Timpl, 1973; Hahn et al, 1974) and mice (Nowack et al, 1975), when injected with native collagens, produce antibodies almost exclusively against helical determinants. In general, these tend to be quite specific for the type of collagen used for immunization with only small amounts cross reacting with determinants in the other collagen types. The monoclonal antibodies that have been produced from mouse lymphocytes also have these latter characteristics (discussed later).

Even from very early work it became obvious that collagen preparations could still contain small amounts of noncollagenous, yet highly antigenic proteins, such as serum components (Steffen et al, 1967) or acidic proteins, which could remain tightly bound to collagen and were removable only by CM-cellulose chromatography (LeRoy, 1968, 1969). These could be present in exceedingly small amounts and yet, due to their relatively high antigenicity compared to collagen, could elicit a strong antibody response. The possibility that antibodies to such contaminants could potentially produce artifactual results in immunocytochemical studies was demonstrated by Wick et al (1975). They produced antibodies in rabbits against native rat skin collagen, and subsequently purified the antibodies by affinity chromatography on collagen immunoabsorbants. Then the unpurified sera and the fractionated antibodies were tested for their staining pattern on kidney sections in a double-antibody, indirect immunofluorescence procedure. The antibody fraction which bound to the collagen immunoabsorbant stained only the peritubular connective tissue septae and Bowman's capsule. The unfractionated serum stained these structures and in addition the glomerular basement membrane. The antibody fraction responsible for staining the basement membrane could be recovered in the antisera that did not bind to the collagen immunoabsorbant, and thus most probably represents antibodies against small amounts of noncollagenous contaminants present in the original immunogen preparation. In addition, even the population of antibodies that are produced to the collagen type used for immunization will contain some antibodies directed against determinants present on other genetic types of collagen (Wick et al, 1976). In this case, even if an absolutely pure preparation of collagen is used for immunization, undesirable antibodies will be produced which cross-react with other collagen types.

These results, among others, have given rise to the well-founded thesis that, when dealing with antibodies to the different genetic types of collagens, it is impossible to obtain the desired results by sufficiently purifying the antigen. One must instead purify the resulting antibodies. The usual means for effecting the desired purification is through the use of affinity column chromatography using immunoabsorbants of purified collagens coupled to solid phase supports. Although for various experimental purposes. these procedures have been done using various forms of collagenous proteins such as α-chains and CNBr peptides, for immunofluorescence localizations, the antibodies have usually been purified using either native molecules of specific types of collagens and procollagens or isolated propeptide extension pieces. The solid phase supports which have been used are diazotized p-aminobenzyl cellulose (Timpl et al, 1967) and CNBr activated sepharose 4B (Cuatrecasas, 1970; as described for collagens in Nowack et al, 1975b and von der Mark, 1976).

A purification scheme for the production of type I collagen antibodies is shown in Figure 14.2. The basic scheme (adapted from Timpl et al, 1977) first involves the removal of cross-reacting anticollagen antibodies by chromatography on columns of the known heterologous types of collagen such as types II and III. Subsequently, the antibodies are purified by direct chromatography on columns of the homologous collagen to which the antibody was produced. On the columns with the heterologous collagens, the unwanted cross reactive collagen antibodies bind and the desired antibodies wash through. The need for cross absorption on all the different known types of heterologous collagens and not just one type was demonstrated by Wick et al (1976). They observed that for either rat or rabbit antibodies against bovine type I collagen, extensive cross absorption against type II collagen eliminated any detectable cross-reaction for that type of collagen. However, there was still considerable cross reactivity to type III. Thus, the function of cross absorption is not just to eliminate the general anticollagen antibodies which would be present in all collagens, but in some cases at least, it is to remove more specific antibodies which may bind to determinants shared by two collagens but not a third. In this same study it was also demonstrated that in some cases a single crossabsorption is sufficient. When antibodies to type II collagen were cross absorbed against type I collagen but not type III, no detectable activity was found for either types I or III.

On the homologous type collagen, the desired specific antibodies bind to the column, while any antibodies to minor, noncollagenous contaminants wash through. The specific antibodies can then be eluted with low pH (Beil et al, 1973) or chaotropic agents such as 3M KSCN. The latter eluant gives a considerably higher yield of immunoglobulin (von der Mark et al, 1976). Although KSCN is a denaturing agent, von der Mark et al (1976) found that immunoabsorbents of native collagen coupled to

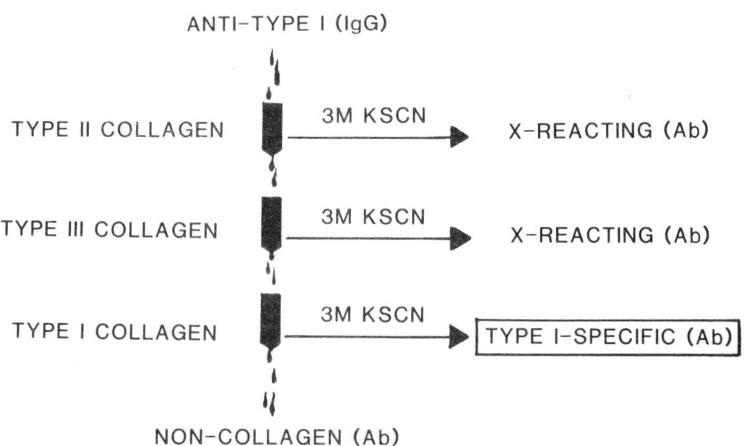

Fig. 14.2 Methods for purifying type I-specific collagen antibodies. The IgG is isolated from an animal immunized with type I collagen, and is absorbed on columns of type II and type III collagens, which remove the crossreacting, anticollagen antibodies. Lastly, the antiserum is directly absorbed on a column of type I collagen. The non-collagen antibodies wash through the column, while the type I-specific antibodies bind and can be subsequently eluted with 3M KSCN. Ab = antibody; 3M KSCN = 3 molar potassium thiocyanate. (Modified from Timpl et al, 1977.)

sepharose 4B did not lose their capacity to bind antibodies to native collagen, even after repeated use. The eluted antibodies are then rapidly dialyzed into a buffer such as 0.15M NaCl, 0.05M Tris HCl, pH 7.5, concentrated and tested for specificity.

As will be described later, an alternate method for producing specific antibodies to collagens is through the recently devised technique for producing monoclonal antibodies by lymphocyte-myeloma cell hybrids (Linsenmayer et al, 1979; Linsenmayer & Hendrix, 1980, 1981).

The specificity and titres of purified antibodies have been assayed by passive haemagglutination or inhibition of passive haemagglutination (Beil et al, 1972, 73), and numerous radioimmune assays (for example Adelman et al, 1973; Menzel, 1977; Roll et al, 1979). All of these techniques can be used with native collagens and procollagens as well as the various chains and peptides derived from them. In passive haemagglutination, collagen is covalently coupled to glutaraldehyde treated erythrocytes (Beil et al, 1972, 1973). The coated cells are then added to wells of microtitre plates containing two-fold serial dilutions of antibody, and after overnight incubation at 4°C the wells are visually scored for agglutination. Since in this case we are dealing with two-fold dilutions, the titres are usually expressed as ($-\log_2$). This assay is quick, easily done, and gives quite reproducible results. Its major limitation is quantitation which due to the two-fold dilution step is probably no better than 50 per cent. In a modification of this assay, haemagglutination inhibition, a known amount of inhibitor collagen is added to each of the antibody dilutions and preincubated for several hours to allow antibody binding to occur. Then, the collagen coated erythrocytes are added, and after an overnight incubation at 4°C, the wells are scored for haemagglutination. If significant antibody binding to the inhibitor collagen has occurred, fewer of the serial dilutions will be positive when compared to an identical series of wells in which no inhibitor collagen has been added, or to which a noninhibitor form has been added.

Radioimmune assays (RIA) offer an advantage if more quantitative data is required. In this assay, isotopically labelled collagen of a rather high specific activity is required. This can be accomplished by post synthetically labelling collagen preparations with ^{125}I (Adelmann et al, 1973; Roll et al, 1979), or with ^{14}C using ^{14}C-labelled acetic anhydride (Menzel, 1977). Alternatively, radio-labelled collagen can be obtained from cell or organ cultures which have been grown in the presence of ^{14}C or ^{3}H-proline or glycine (von der Mark et al, 1973; Dehm et al, 1974) plus β-aminopropionitrile to prevent crosslinking. The in vitro labelling removes any possibility of structural damage to antigenic determinants within the collagen molecule which theoretically could occur during ^{125}I labelling. Aliquots of the labelled collagen are then allowed to incubate with different quantities of antibody, and then the antibody-antigen complex is precipitated by the addition of a second antibody produced in a different animal species and directed against the immunoglobulin of the species in which the primary anticollagen antibody was produced. Alternatively, heat killed Staphylococcus aureus, which has IgG binding protein A on its surface, can be used as a solid phase precipitant instead of second antibody (Kessler, 1975). Inhibition type RIA's can be performed by preincubating unlabelled collagens as inhibitors before the addition of the labelled collagen.

The most recently devised assay is the ELISA or enzyme-linked immunoabsorbant assay (Rennard et al, 1980; Gosslau & Barrach, 1979), which is a colourimetric assay for the presence of antibody activity. This assay takes advantage of the observation that proteins will tightly adsorb to plastic surfaces, and thus the wells of microtitre plates can be coated with dilute solutions such as collagens. Subsequently, antibody is added to the wells and, if reactive with determinants on the coating collagen, they will also become part of the solid phase complex. Then a second antibody is added which is covalently coupled with an enzyme such as alkaline phosphatase or horseradish peroxidase and is directed against immunoglobulin of the species used to produce the primary anticollagen antibody. Lastly, a solution containing the substrate for the enzyme is added to each well and then is incubated to allow colour development. This assay is very sensitive due to amplification afforded by the enzymatic reaction, and also alleviates the need of using radioactivity. Thus, it will probably receive much future use.

AFFINITY PURIFIED ANTIBODIES THAT HAVE BEEN PREPARED TO COLLAGENS AND PROCOLLAGENS

Over the past several years, affinity purified antibodies suitable for immunohistochemical localizations have been produced against a number of different collagens and procollagens. These include collagen types I, II, and III, several different collagens thought to be of basement membrane origin, and procollagen types I and III. In this section we will examine the properties of these specific antibodies and describe some of the studies in which they have been utilized for immunocytochemical localizations at the light and electron microscopic levels.

Type I collagen and procollagen

Wick et al (1975) used affinity purified antibodies to type I collagen for immunohistochemical staining. They raised antisera to rat or calf skin type I collagen, both in rabbits, which produce antibodies predominantly to terminal sites, and in chickens, which produce antibodies to terminal sites, helical sites, and central sites. The antibodies were isolated and purified by direct affinity chromatography on collagen immunoabsorbants. Some of the antibodies were further selected for binding to determinants in the three different classes of sites by affinity chromatography on columns of native and denatured collagens. The purified antibody fractions were examined for their staining patterns on sections of skin and kidney using a double antibody immunofluorescent technique. In this type of technique, which is used in most studies with collagen antibodies, the tissue section is first reacted with the collagen antibody and washed to remove any of this primary antibody which is unbound. The section is then reacted with a rhodamine or fluorescein conjugated second antibody directed against the immunoglobulin of the animal species in which the primary antibody was produced. After washing to remove any of the unreacted second antibody, the section is viewed in a fluorescence microscope. When the collagen antibodies were used to stain skin and kidney sections, specific fluorescence was observed throughout the dermis of the skin and the interstitial connective tissue of the kidney. When the affinity purified anticollagen antibodies were subsequently fractionated for enrichment to different types of determinants within the collagen molecule, it was established that the antibodies to terminal and helical determinants gave equally good fluorescence, whereas those against central determinants gave a weaker response. Also, the antibodies made to the calf type I collagen reacted equally well with human type I collagen.

Subsequently, it was demonstrated that rabbit antibodies against native bovine type I collagen or $\alpha 1(I)$ chains could be rendered free of type II and III crossreactivity by absorption with these collagen types (Nowack et al, 1976b). When immunofluorescence staining with these type I antibodies was compared to that obtained with similarly purified antibodies specific for type III collagen, entirely different staining patterns were noted. For example, in tendon (Becker et al, 1976) the antibody to type I collagen stained the large collagen bundles whereas the antibody to type III collagen stained the tendon sheaths. Other antibodies specific for type I collagen have been produced against chick type I collagen using rabbits, rats, and guinea pigs (see, for example: von der Mark et al, 1976).

Antibodies against type I P_N-procollagen were first produced in rabbits using native dermatosparactic calf collagen as an immunogen (Timpl et al, 1973). These were rendered specific for the procollagen form by crossabsorption against native and denatured type I collagen molecules followed by direct absorption on dermatosparactic collagen. The purified antibodies were shown to react with determinants in the NH_2-terminal procollagen extension peptide. In immunofluorescence staining, the antibodies reacted with determinants present in normal calf skin and also with human tissues. In subsequent studies, it was demonstrated that antibodies specific for type I procollagen could also be produced by immunization with the NH_2-terminal propeptide extension piece derived from dermatosparactic procollagen (Nowack et al, 1976b; Rohde et al, 1976a, b). Specificity for type I P_N-procollagen was obtained by cross absorption against type III P_N-procollagen, as well as type I collagen. When these antibodies were used for immunocytochemical staining of adult skin, they reacted with determinants present only in the stratum papillare, the area of dermis directly beneath the epidermis. Antibodies against type I collagen, as shown previously, stained the whole dermis (Gay et al, 1976c).

Antibodies specific for the COOH terminal propeptide extension of type I procollagen were first produced by Dehm et al (1974), who immunized rabbits with native procollagen isolated from matrix-free chick tendon cell cultures. The antibodies were purified by direct immunoabsorption on a disulphide crosslinked trimer propeptide derived by collagenase digestion of tendon procollagen. Subsequently, Olsen et al (1977) produced an affinity purified antibody directed against the COOH-terminal propeptide extension piece isolated from the same type of tendon cultures. Other affinity purified type I procollagen antibodies have been produced against chick calvaria and tendon procollagens (von der Mark et al, 1973; Nist et al, 1975; and Murphy et al, 1975).

Type II collagen

Hahn et al (1974, 1975a), Gay et al (1976b), and Wick et al (1976) were the first to produce antibodies specific for type II collagen, thus demonstrating the feasibility of using antibodies against the different genetic types of collagens as immunological reagents. They immunized rabbits and rats with native type II collagen extracted by limited pepsin digestion of chicken and bovine cartilage, and crossabsorbed the antisera on type I collagen. There was no detectable titre against either types I or III as assayed by passive haemagglutination and haemagglutination inhibition, nor was there activity against artificially renatured molecules with the chain compositions $[\alpha 1(I)]_3$ and $[\alpha 2]_3$. In this case, then, crossabsorption against one type of collagen was sufficient to remove reactivity against the other known collagen types. The antibodies produced in the rat reacted only with helical determinants; however, those produced in the rabbit reacted with both helical and central determinants, and probably also with some terminal ones. A major determinant could be located in the CNBr peptide CB–11; however, others appeared to be located throughout the molecule. When used for fluorescence immunocytochemistry of sectioned material, positive results with the type II antibody were obtained only with hyaline cartilage and nucleus pulposus, two tissues known to contain type II collagen. The antibodies against the bovine and chick type II collagens reacted equally well with collagens from the opposite species, and the bovine antibodies also reacted with human collagen. Von der Mark et al (1976) observed that far superior staining of hyaline cartilage is obtained with antibody to type II when the chondroitin-sulphate proteoglycan is removed from the sections by hyaluronidase digestion before reaction with the antibody.

Type III collagen and procollagen

Antibodies have been produced in rabbits against native type III collagen molecules from calf skin (Gay et al, 1975; Nowack et al, 1976b) and against a 13 000 mol wt cross-link fragment of type III collagen, termed TIX (Becker et al, 1976). TIX was derived from trypsin digestion of insoluble calf skin collagen. By itself, TIX was found to be poorly immunogenic, but its immunogenicity could be increased by covalent crosslinking to bovine serum albumen with glutaraldehyde. Cross absorption against denatured type I collagen followed by direct absorption on denatured type III produced an antibody with no cross reactivity against type I collagen. In a radioimmune assay the antibody reacted well with native type III collagen and denatured $\alpha 1$(III) chains, as well as with the peptide TIX. Collagenase digestion of TIX did not destroy its ability to bind with antibody, showing that the determinants are not in the short portion of the peptide that extends into the helical region. Antibodies produced against native type III molecules can also be rendered specific by cross absorption against collagen types I and II and direct absorption on type III (Nowack et al, 1976b). The antibodies to the cross-link peptide and to the native type III molecule produce identical staining patterns on a variety of tissues. They stain the stratum papillare layer of the skin, the sheaths of tendon bundles, and the reticular fibre of spleen and liver.

Type III P_N-procollagen with intact NH_2-terminal propeptide ends can be extracted directly from calf skin (Timpl et al, 1975; Lenaers & Lapiere, 1975) and thus can serve as an immunogen. Using this source of antigen, Nowack et al (1976b & c) produced antibodies which could be made specific for the type III P_N-procollagen form by crossabsorption against type I collagen, type I procollagen, and native and denatured type III collagen. Such purified antibodies, as assayed by haemagglutination inhibition and radioimmune assay, reacted equally well with native type III procollagen, with a bacterial collagenase derived NH_2-terminal propeptide p$\alpha 1$(III) col 1–3, or with a CNBr derived propeptide from the same region p$\alpha 1$(III)–CB3A. Reduction of the disulphide bonds destroyed binding activity.

Type IV and Type V molecules

Antibodies have been produced against type IV collagen extracted from such classic sources as lens capsule. They have been demonstraled to have specificity so that they do not react with other collagen types (Gunson & Kefalides, 1976). Generally, however, they have not been purified by affinity chromatography, and only infrequently have they been used for immunofluorescence staining (Howard et al, 1976).

Recently, a mouse tumour, the EHS sarcoma, has been identified as a rich source of basement membrane materials (Orkin et al, 1977), including several different species of triple helical collagenous molecules (Timpl et al, 1978; Timpl, 1979). When animals innoculated with the tumour are made lathrytic by including β-aminopropionitrile in their diets, much of the tumour collagen is acid extractable, thus circumventing the need for extraction by proteolytic enzymes. Antibodies have been made in rabbits against these tumour basement membrane collagen(s) and purified by direct immunoabsorption (Timpl et al, 1978). When the antibodies were used for immunofluorescence staining, they reacted with the matrix of the EHS tumour and in addition with basement membrane structures in normal mouse tissues. They react with the kidney basement membrane, and in skin they react with the basement membranes at the epidermal-dermal junction, around hair follicles, in blood vessels, and around muscle bundles (Yaoita et al, 1978). They also have determinants in common with structures in human placenta (cited in Timpl et al, 1979) and the basement membranes of the avian cornea (Hay et al, 1979). Gay et al (1979) have produced an antibody against human basement membrane collagen which reacts with epithelial and endothelial basement membranes of human skin.

Several recent studies have reported the production of affinity purified antibodies directed against molecules containing A and B chains. Duance et al (1977) and Bailey et al (1978) have reported that rabbit antibodies made against AB collagen from human placenta preferentially stain the endomysium of bovine skeletal muscle. Stenn et al (1979) have reported that AB antibodies preferentially stain the epidermal layer of mouse skin. Recent data demonstrated that it is possible to produce specific antibodies to B-chain containing molecules (Gay et al, 1980a). These react with the exocytoskeleton of smooth muscle cells (Gay & Miller, 1978) as well as the pericellular matrix of chondrocytes (Gay et al, 1981).

STUDIES INVOLVING DEVELOPMENTAL SYSTEMS AND OTHER IMMUNOCYTOCHEMICAL LOCALIZATIONS USING FLUORESCENT AND FERRITIN-CONJUGATED ANTIBODIES

Skeletogenesis — mesenchyme, cartilage and bone

For developmental studies involving extracellular matrix molecules, the most frequently used systems involve the synthesis of collagen types I and II during chondrogenesis and osteogenesis. Excellent agreement has been obtained with experiments involving both biochemical analyses and immunocytochemical localizations.

In the developing chick limb (for review, see Toole and

Linsenmayer, 1977), until stage 22 (day 3 1/2 of incubation), the limb bud or mesoblast consists of a uniform population of mesenchymally-derived cells surrounded by ectoderm. At stage 22 a 'condensation' occurs in the core of the limb bud delineating the presumptive cartilage from soft tissue areas. However, histological characteristics of cartilage do not appear until stage 24 to 25 (day 4). Bone formation begins around day 7 to 8 in the perichondrium at the centre of the future shaft and gives rise to a sleeve surrounding the cartilage primordium. This is followed by calcification of the central part of the anlage, blood vessel invasion into the calcified cartilage, and division into two endochondral zones of ossification, in addition to the periosteum.

The collagens synthesized by developing limbs was one of the initial systems biochemically investigated (Linsenmayer et al, 1973a; Linsenmayer, 1974). When precartilagenous mesoblasts were labelled with ^{3}H-proline, and the collagens analyzed, type I collagen was the only type detected. At the stage when the first metachromatic matrix becomes visible in the core region of the limb (stages 25 to 26), the labelled collagen synthesized by the whole limb now showed synthesis of some type II collagen. It was demonstrated that the synthesis of type II molecules was begun preferentially in the core region, whereas the outer, soft tissue region maintained the synthesis of type I. The proportion of type II collagen synthesized in the cartilagenous core increased until it was the only molecule detected by day 7 to 8. Later, in the diaphysial region of the long bone rudiments, another transition in collagen type is signified by reappearance of detectable $\alpha 2$ chains and thus the renewed or greatly enhanced synthesis of the type I collagen characteristic of bone.

Subsequently, von der Mark et al (1976a, b), and von der Mark and von der Mark (1977), using antibodies to collagen types I and II, both confirmed and extended this pattern of synthesis. In the prechondrogenic mesoblast, the type I collagen is not distributed uniformly throughout the limb, but is localized under the epidermis where the dermis will form and in the core of the limb which will go on to become cartilage (Fig. 14.3A).

Type II staining appears in the cartilagenous region at about the same time it is detected biochemically (Fig. 14.3B), and goes on to become the only detectable collagen type in the mature embryonic cartilage. For its efficient detection, however, the tissue sections require predigestion with hyaluronidase to remove masking proteoglycan. By day 6 to 7 the fibrous perichondrial region stains intensely with antibody to type I collagen and this staining extends for several cell layers down into the type II collagen of the cartilage, probably reflecting the formation of chondrocytes from perichondrial cells via appositional growth (see the staining pattern obtained with monoclonal antibodies in Fig. 14.12). Once cartilage erosion has progressed sufficiently, the onset of endochondral ossification is signified by the deposition of type I collagen on the surface of eroded cartilage (Fig. 14.4A & B). On these surfaces, the type I collagen diffuses down into the cartilage matrix, producing again a hybrid type I-type II matrix. When these sections were analyzed by staining for calcium deposition,

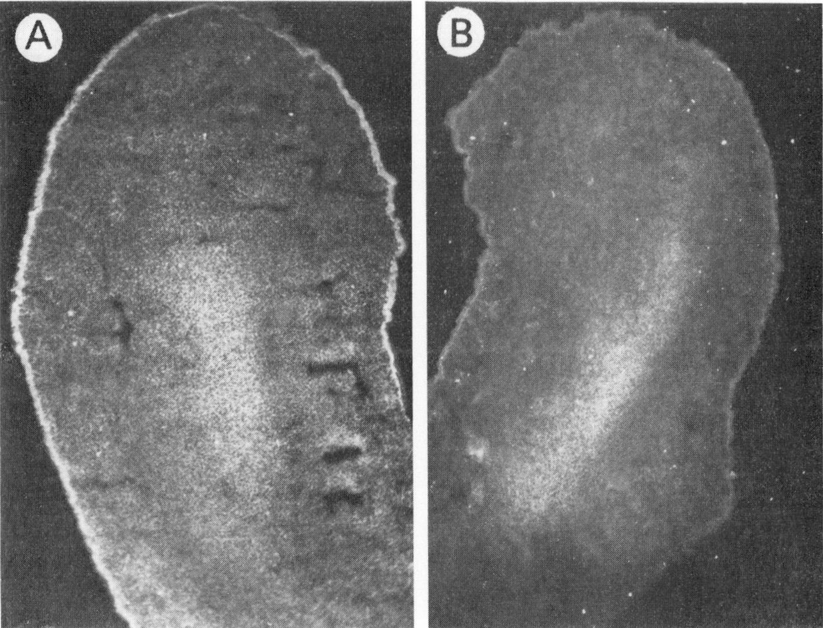

Fig. 14.3 Chick limb buds, stage 24–25, stained with guinea pig antibodies made against chick collagen. A, Type I, and B, Type II (×90). (Courtesy of W. Dessau and K. von der Mark, unpublished results.)

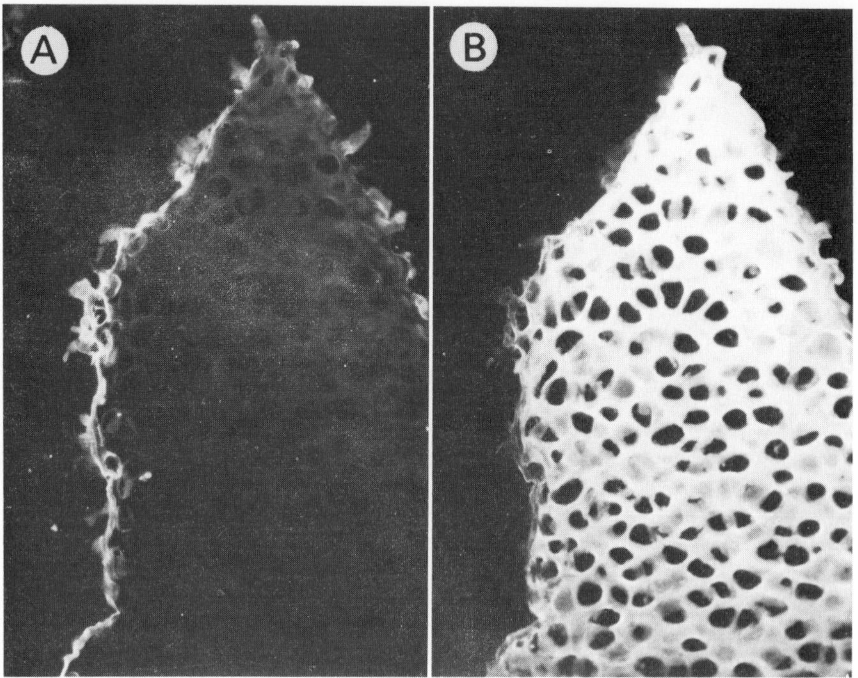

Fig. 14.4 Cartilagenous rudiment of 17 day embryonic chick tibia stained with (A) rabbit antibodies against chick type I collagen, and (B) guinea pig antibodies against chick type II collagen (×160). (K. von der Mark & H. von der Mark, 1977; courtesy of E. S. Livingstone.)

this hybrid matrix appeared to be one of the sites conducive to apatite formation. Endochondral bone containg type I collagen could be found covering both calcified and uncalcified cartilage which stained for type II. On the other hand the surface of type II staining, calcified cartilage was not necessarily covered by type I-containing osteoid. This indicated that the calcification of the matrices of endochondral bone and the underlying cartilage can occur independently. Type I-type II hybrid matrix is continuously found in the walls of the lacunae of the hypertrophied chondrocytes that are formed in the epiphysial growth plate. In this case the type I collagen is completely surrounded by type II matrix suggesting that the chondrocytes, once they begin to hypertrophy, switch to the synthesis of type I collagen.

This result confirmed the earlier observation of Gay et al (1976b) that the hypertrophic chondrocytes of human epiphysial growth plates contain both type I and type II collagen in the walls of their lacunae.

Another developing skeletal system in the chick that has been examined both biochemically and immunocytochemically for the synthesis of collagen types I and II is the embryonic notochord and the surrounding vertebral cartilages which are derived from somatic mesoderm. By biochemical analysis of radiolabelled collagens synthesized in vitro, it was demonstrated that the very early embryonic chick notochord ($2\frac{1}{2}$ days of incubation) synthesized predominantly type II collagen plus a small amount of type I (Linsenmayer et al, 1973b). Subsequently, the somatic mesoderm which comes to surround the notochord begins to undergo chondrogenesis and initiates the synthesis of type II collagen (Linsenmayer et al, 1973c). Von der Mark et al (1976) observed that the $2\frac{1}{2}$ day embryonic notochordal sheath stained strongly with antibody to type II collagen and more weakly with type I (Fig. 14.5A). Once the somatic mesoderm surrounded the notochord and began to produce metachromatic matrix, type II collagen staining also appeared in the shape of the vertebral bodies which were forming (Fig. 14.5B). The type II collagen staining present in the notochord persists into older organisms in the form of the notochordally derived nucleus pulposus of the intervertebral disc. Wick et al (1976) observed that the nucleus pulposus of the calf reacts strongly with antibodies to both types I and II whereas the annulus fibrosus stains only for type I. In human embryos and newborns they observed a similar pattern. In the adult, however, much of the type II reactivity had disappeared, possibly due to masking of sites. Eyre & Muir (1974) have biochemically demonstrated essentially the same pattern of collagen distribution within the disc.

Avian cornea and vitreous development

Several lines of evidence suggest that type II collagen, or a type II-like molecule, is involved in the early development of the chick cornea and vitreous.

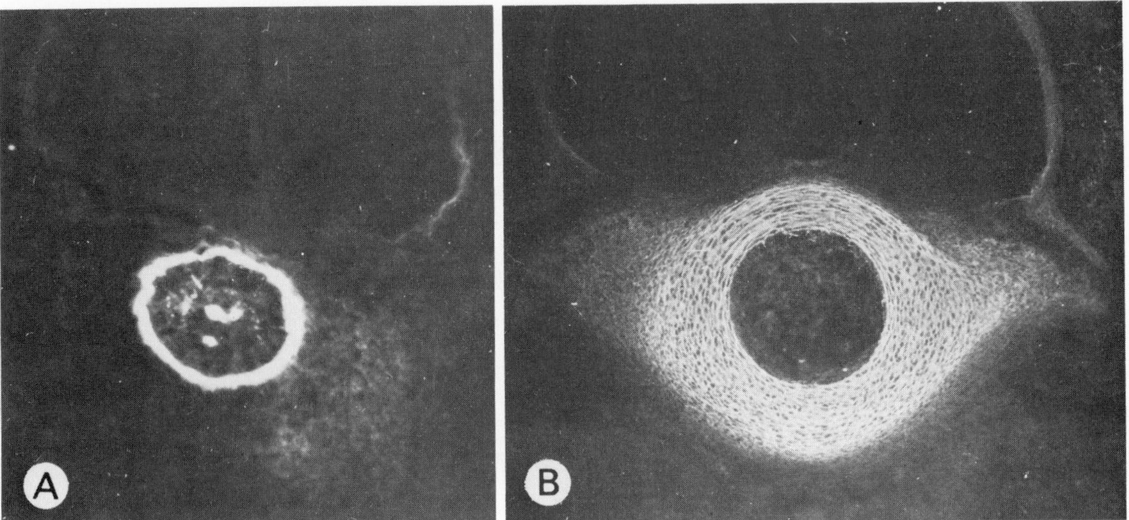

Fig. 14.5 A, Embryonic chick notochord, stage 22, and B, vertebral body, stage 30 stained with antibodies against type II collagen made in (A) rabbits and (B) guinea pigs (×360). (Courtesy K. von der Mark, unpublished results.)

The morphogenesis of the chick corneal stroma proceeds in two distinct phases (for reviews see Hay & Revel, 1969; and Hay et al, 1979). In the first phase the cornea consists of only two cell layers, an outer epithelium and an inner endothelium. Between these two layers is found an accellular matrix, the primary corneal stroma, which is composed of collagen and glycosaminoglycans. The collagen is arranged in a highly ordered array of layers or plies, each composed of numerous striated fibrils, which in alternate layers are arranged essentially orthogonal to one another. During the second phase this acellular stroma becomes populated with invading mesenchymal cells which become corneal fibroblasts and synthesize large amounts of collagen. Thus, the stroma thickens and becomes the secondary stroma which persists as the adult cornea. Studies, both in vivo and in vitro, have shown that the collagen of the primary stroma is produced largely, if not solely, by the corneal epithelium, whereas that of the secondary stroma is probably produced to a great extent by the mesenchymal cells once they are present. From a number of biochemical criteria of radiolabelled material, the collagen synthesized by the 5–6 day corneal epithelium consists of about 30–40 per cent type II, with the majority of the rest being type I (Linsenmayer et al, 1977).

In similar experiments using radiolabelled collagens, Newsome et al (1976) were able to demonstrate that the collagen within the vitreous body of the developing avian embryo also has a dual origin, first being synthesized by the neural retina and later by a cell population within the vitreous itself, possibly the hyalocytes. At both stages, biochemical analyses identified this collagen as type II (Smith et al, 1976; Linsenmayer & Little, 1979).

Subsequently, various tissues within the embryonic chick eye were examined using conventional antibodies to collagen type I–IV (von der Mark et al, 1977b; Hay et al, 1979) and monoclonal antibodies against collagen types I and II (Linsenmayer & Hendrix, 1981; Hendrix, Linsenmayer, & Hay, in preparation). There is excellent agreement between the conventional antibodies and the monoclonal ones (whose preparation will be described later). As can be seen in Figure 14.6 (A and B) the 5 day, uninvaded primary stroma stains uniformly with monoclonal antibodies against collagen type I (Fig. 14.6A) and type II (Fig. 14.6B). In the 10 day embryonic cornea (Fig. 14.6C and D), which has been invaded by mesenchymal cells, the staining pattern is now distinctly different with the two antibodies. The type I monoclonal antibody (Fig. 14.6C) gives bright fluorescence throughout the stroma with the most intense reaction localized under the corneal epithelium. This staining pattern probably reflects the continued presence of type I in the uninvaded portion of the primary stroma adjacent to the epithelium, plus new type I synthesized by the corneal fibroblasts that have invaded. The type II monoclonal antibody (Fig. 14.6D) also gives the brightest staining under the epithelium, but then shows a decreasing gradient of fluorescence across about one fourth of the anterior portion of the stroma. The remaining stroma shows little if any staining for type II except for a narrow region at the extreme posterior edge, just under the corneal endothelium (not shown). This pattern probably reflects the continued presence of type II in the remaining uninvaded primary stroma directly under the anterior epithelium. The decreasing gradient in this anterior portion probably also reflects type II remaining from the primary stroma. The anterior portion is the region most recently invaded by mesenchymal cells so the type II staining is still prominent. The more posterior regions, however, have been invaded

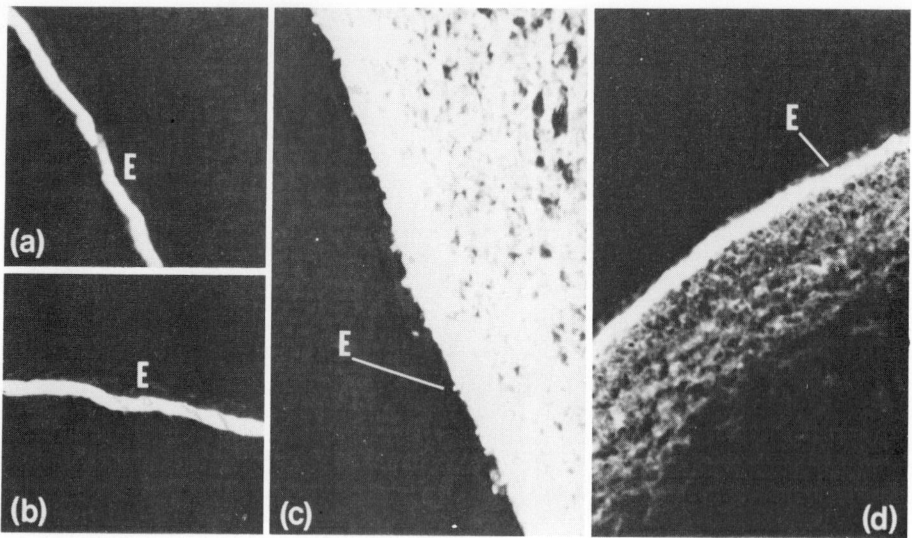

Fig. 14.6 Fluorescence micrographs of developing chick corneas from 5-day embryos (a, b) and 10-day embryos (c, d) stained with monoclonal antibody ascites fluid against type I collagen (a, c) and type II collagen (b, d) using a double layer sandwich technique. The second antibody is rhodamine-conjugated rabbit IgG directed against mouse IgG; E = epithelium. a, b = 180× c, d = 170×

by mesenchymal cells for progressively longer periods of time, so the large amount of type I synthesized by these cells has masked the type II. Alternatively, the type II may have been progressively degraded by the invading mesenchymal cells.

Additional structures that have been shown to stain for type II (von der Mark et al, 1977) are the vitreous body and the neural retina. Again, these results agree with the previously obtained biochemical data.

The two other types of collagen examined (von der Mark et al, 1977b; Hay et al, 1979), types III and IV, have a more limited distribution. Type IV is found in the basement membrane structures, including Decemet's membrane and Bowman's membranes, and type III is found only in the structures surrounding the cornea, such as the iris and eyelid. No type III was observed in either the primary or the secondary corneal stromas.

Skin

In early embryonic chick limbs, at stages before a dermis has formed, there is a slight staining with type I antibodies directly under the ectoderm (see Fig. 14.3A and von der Mark et al, 1976a). In adult skin, anti-type I collagen staining is observed in the large collagen bundles distributed throughout the dermis (Wick et al, 1975, 1976; Gay et al, 1976c; Nowack et al, 1976b). In embryonic human skin, type III collagen staining also extends through the dermis and into the subdermal connective tissue (Gay & Miller, 1978). In adult skin, however, type III antibodies stain only the fine collagen fibrils (reticulin) located largely in the part of the adventitial dermis directly under the epidermis (Becker et al, 1976; Gay et al, 1976).

A recent biochemical study on the distribution of types I and III collagen in adult human skin have obtained somewhat different results. Epstein & Munderloh (1978) used a dermatome to dissect adult human skin into layers composed of outer, middle, and inner dermis. They then digested the material with CNBr and quantitated the relative amounts of types I and III by determining the ratios of the CNBr peptides α1(I)–CB8 and αI(III)–CB8. Using this method they obtained the same ratios of types I and III throughout the whole dermis, and therefore suggest that the lack of type III immunofluorescent staining in the lower dermis may be due to masking of the sites. Another possibility, however, is that the type III collagen in the lower dermis is derived from capillaries and dermal appendages such as glands and hair follicles which do stain positive for type III (Gay & Miller, 1978; Fleischmajer et al, 1979).

When stained with antibodies to type I P_N-procollagen, embryonic calf skin stains throughout the dermis (Wick et al, 1978b). With increasing age, however, this staining becomes more restricted until, in the adult, only the area of dermis directly under the epidermis (stratum papillare) gives a positive result (Timpl et al, 1973; Wick et al, 1975, 1976, 1978b). The distribution observed when staining with type III procollagen (Nowack et al, 1976) is not unlike that found for type III collagen, thus suggesting that type III procollagen normally accumulates in skin along with type III collagen.

Recently, Wick et al (1978b) have performed electron microscopic localizations of type I P_N-procollagen in the skin of dermatosparactic calves. The antibodies were conjugated to ferritin using the glutaraldehyde method of Olsen & Prockop (1974). In dermatosparactic skin, P_N-procollagen accumulates in aberrant appearing fibrils located throughout the dermis. When these fibrils were stained with antibody, periodic localizations of ferritin were observed with a 50nm spacing (Fig. 14.7). This shows that in dermatosparactic skin, P_N-procollagen molecules with intact NH_2-terminal procollagen extensions can be arranged into fibrils with the extension peptides most probably protruding into the periodic hole zones within the fibrils.

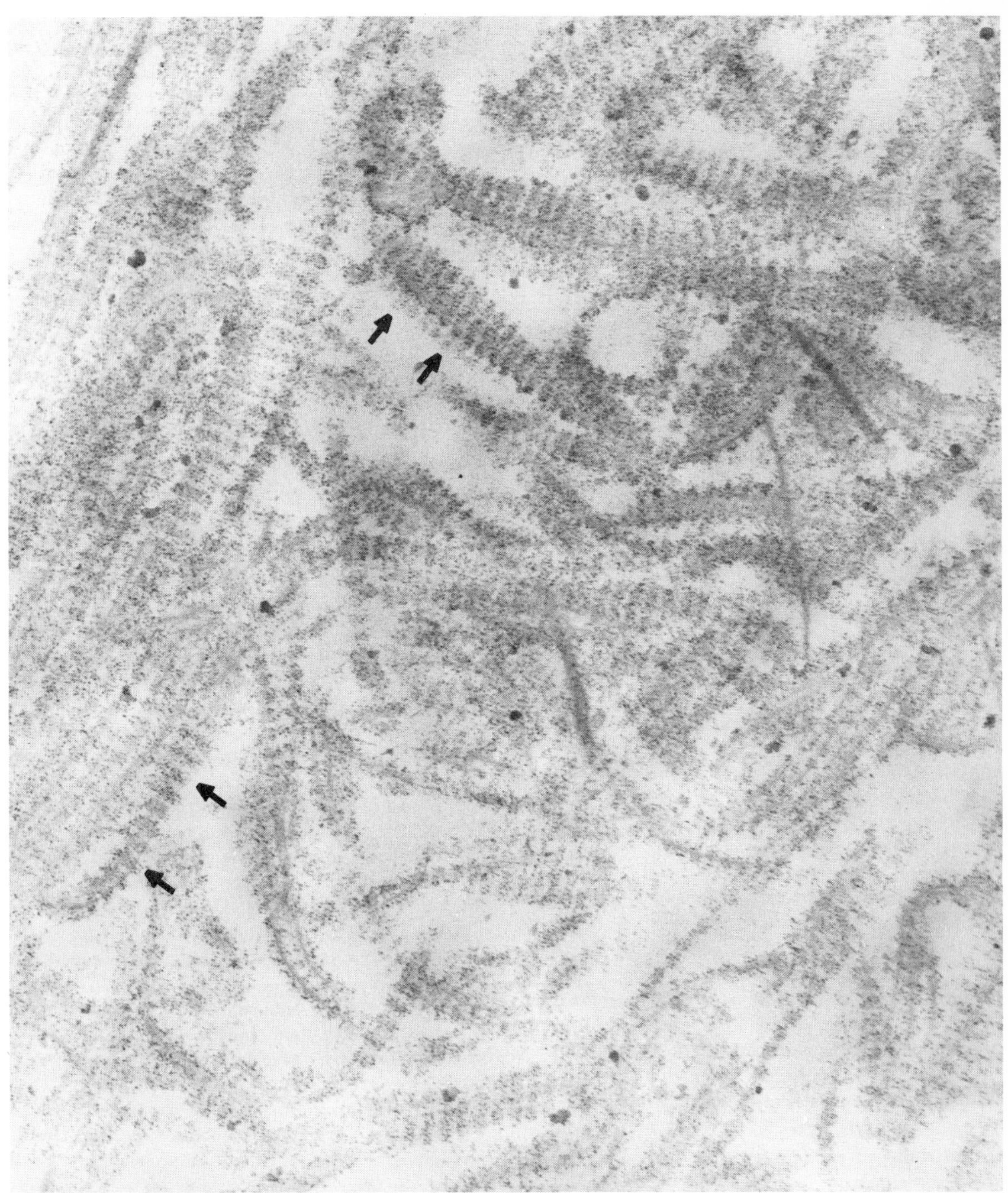

Fig. 14.7 Dermatosparactic sheep skin stained with ferritin-conjugated, anti-P_N-procollagen type I antibodies. The section was counterstained with lead citrate. Note the localization of ferritin at regular intervals along the fibrils (arrows) (×60 000). (Courtesy of B. Olsen.)

Tendons

Tendons are chiefly composed of bundles of large collagen fibres, surrounded by thin sheaths, endotendinium, containing finer collagen fibrils. The large bundles stain uniformly for type I collagen, whereas type III is present only in the endotendinium (Becker et al, 1976; Gay et al, 1976b).

Blood vessels

Elastic and muscular arteries and veins contain a complex mixture of collagen types, including I and III and A and B chain molecules (Gay et al, 1975; Gay & Miller, 1979), plus basement membrane collagen(s) (Timpl et al, 1978). The basement membranes of vessels, located at the border between the tunica intima and the tunica media, stain with antibodies to the EHS mouse tumour collagen. Type III staining is found throughout the media, but is most intense directly under the intima. Type I is also found in the media, but is mainly in the surrounding tunica adventitia. A and B chain molecules, known to be synthesized by smooth muscle cells, are found in close association with the smooth muscle of the media.

Other organs — kidney, spleen, liver

In these organs, type III collagen is frequently found in the parenchymal regions which contain fine reticular fibres. Type I is usually concentrated in the fibrous capsules surrounding these organs, the connective tissue trabeculae separating the different lobes of organs, and other regions with dense connective tissue such as the periportal tracts in the liver (Becker et al, 1976; Nowack et al, 1976b; Wick et al, 1978a; Gay & Miller, 1979; Kent et al, 1976).

Skeletal muscle

Recently, collagen types I, III and AB-molecules have been localized in sections of bovine (Duance et al, 1977) chicken (Bailey et al, 1979) and human (Duance et al, 1980) skeletal muscle. Histologically, skeletal muscle contains three divisions of connective tissue: (1) the dense, thick epimysium which surrounds the whole muscle; (2) the perimysium which separates groups of muscle fibres, and (3) the endomysium which surrounds individual muscle fibres. Type I staining was observed mostly in the epimysium and to a lesser extent in the perimysium, whereas type III staining was found predominantly in the perimysium. Type III also lightly stains the epimysium and to an even lesser extent the endomysium. AB collagen staining was found solely in the endomysium.

Localization of collagens within individual cells

One of the most interesting and promising uses of type specific collagen antibodies is for examining the possible coordinate production of different types of collagens and other matrix molecules by individual cells and for the intracellular localization of events in the synthesis, processing and assembly of collagen molecules.

Gay et al (1976a) approached the question of whether a single cell can produce more than one genetic type of collagen by examining cultured human fibroblasts for the simultaneous intracellular localization of types I and III. Cells were grown in the absence of ascorbate to increase the intracellular concentration of procollagen, and were subsequently fixed and permeabilized so that antibodies could enter. They were then treated with antibodies specific for types I or III collagens or procollagens produced in different animal species and subsequently reacted with second antibodies direct against the primary antibodies. The second antibodies had been conjugated with either fluorescein or rhodamine. Since these two dyes fluoresce at different wavelengths, the staining of each antibody could be independently visualized within the same cell. The results, shown in Figure 14.8 (A & B), clearly demonstrated that most fibroblasts from normal donors contained both types of collagens. On the other hand, fibroblasts from patients with Ehlers-Danlos IV syndrome, whose skin previously had been shown to be deficient in type III by biochemical analyses (Pope et al, 1975), stained with type I only.

Using a similar double antibody fluorescence technique, von der Mark et al (1977a) examined the synthesis of collagen types I and II during the in vitro transformation of chondrocytes into 'fibroblast-like' cells. Previous biochemical (Mayne et al, 1975, 1976) and immunocytochemical studies (Gay et al, 1976b) had demonstrated that such a transformation is accompanied by a loss of type II synthesis with the concomitant acquisition of the synthesis of a type I-like molecule and type I trimer. Von der Mark et al's (1977a) study added the additional information that this transition must be very rapid and complete, since about 99 per cent of the cells in such cultures stained either for type I or type II collagen, but not for both. The remaining 1 per cent did react positively for both types and were assumed to be in a state of transition from chondrocyte to 'fibroblast-like' cell. The cellular distribution of type-I-trimer has yet to be established.

Double antibody immunofluorescence can also be used to examine the synthesis and association of collagens with other matrix molecules. Vertel & Dorfman (1979) examined chondrocytes for the simultaneous synthesis of type II collagen and the core protein of cartilage-specific chondroitin-sulphate proteoglycan using antibodies specific for these two molecules.

After hyaluronidase treatment to remove extracellular proteoglycan, individual chondrocytes exhibited intracellular staining for both core protein and type II collagen. Sometimes specific staining for both molecules was found in the same vacuoles suggesting the possibility of their coordinate packaging.

Precise localization of intracellular events involved in

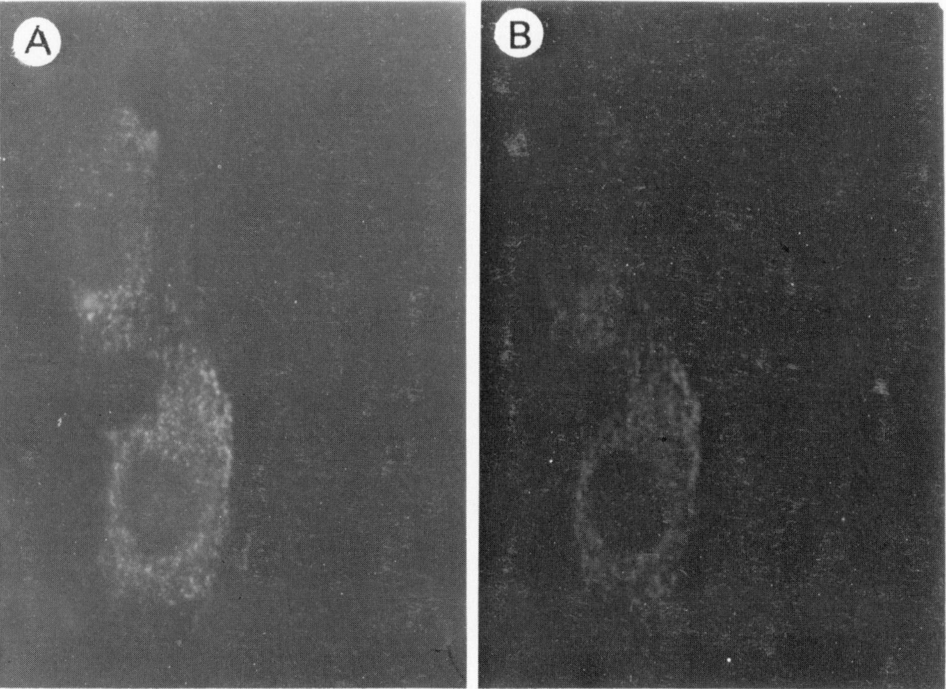

Fig. 14.8 Fetal human skin fibroblasts double stained with antibodies to type III procollagen (A. fluorescein label) and antibodies to helical determinants in type I collagen (B rhodamine). The staining pattern indicates a similar localization for these collagens in the cells suggesting that the same cell synthesized both types of collagen (×4000). (From S. Gay & E. J. Miller, 1978, courtesy of G. Fischer.)

collagen synthesis and assembly can only be accomplished through immunocytochemistry performed at the electromicroscopic level. Such studies present three major problems and numerous minor ones. The major problems are antibody specificity, which has already been discussed, antibody conjugation to an appropriate electron dense marker, and intracellular penetration of the antibody-marker complex. Penetration can be an especially difficult problem when investigating processes occurring within membrane bound intracellular organelles. Olsen and coworkers have provided adequate methods for overcoming the latter two problems. Olson & Prockop (1974) and Kishida et al (1975) have worked out conditions for using glutaraldehyde to covalently crosslink antibodies specific for procollagen and prolyl hydroxylase to the electron dense molecule ferritin. The crosslinking reaction is then followed by gel filtration chromatography to separate the desired complex from aggregated molecules and unconjugated antibody. The second problem, penetration of intracellular organelles, was adequately solved by devising a gentle homogenization procedure which ruptured the cells, but left the cellular pieces enough intact to identify to which structures the ferritin conjugated antibody was binding (Olsen et al, 1975). Using antibodies specific for the NH_2-terminal extension of procollagen, these techniques were first used on matrix-free tendon cells which had been incubated with $\alpha\alpha$-dipyridyl to produce unhydroxylated collagen (protocollagen). Such molecules are only inefficiently secreted and therefore tend to accumulate intracellularly. As shown in Figure 14.9, the cells accumulate protocollagen in the cisternae of the endoplasmic reticulum, but it is not found in the Golgi. That the normal pathway for procollagen secretion does involve passage through the Golgi was subsequently demonstrated for tendon and corneal fibroblasts (Nist et al, 1975). Using similar conditions to those just described, but without the addition of dipyridyl, several different preparations of procollagen antibodies with specificities for different parts of the molecule stained both the endoplasmic reticulum and the Golgi. The only obvious cytoplasmic staining was seen at sites where membranes had been broken which resulted in release of procollagen from the membrane bound organelles.

MONOCLONAL ANTIBODIES TO COLLAGENS

It is obvious that the production and use of antibodies to the different genetic types of collagen does present some difficult problems that we have already discussed, such as the potential lack of specificity. In addition, there are other less obvious and tangible problems such as obtaining

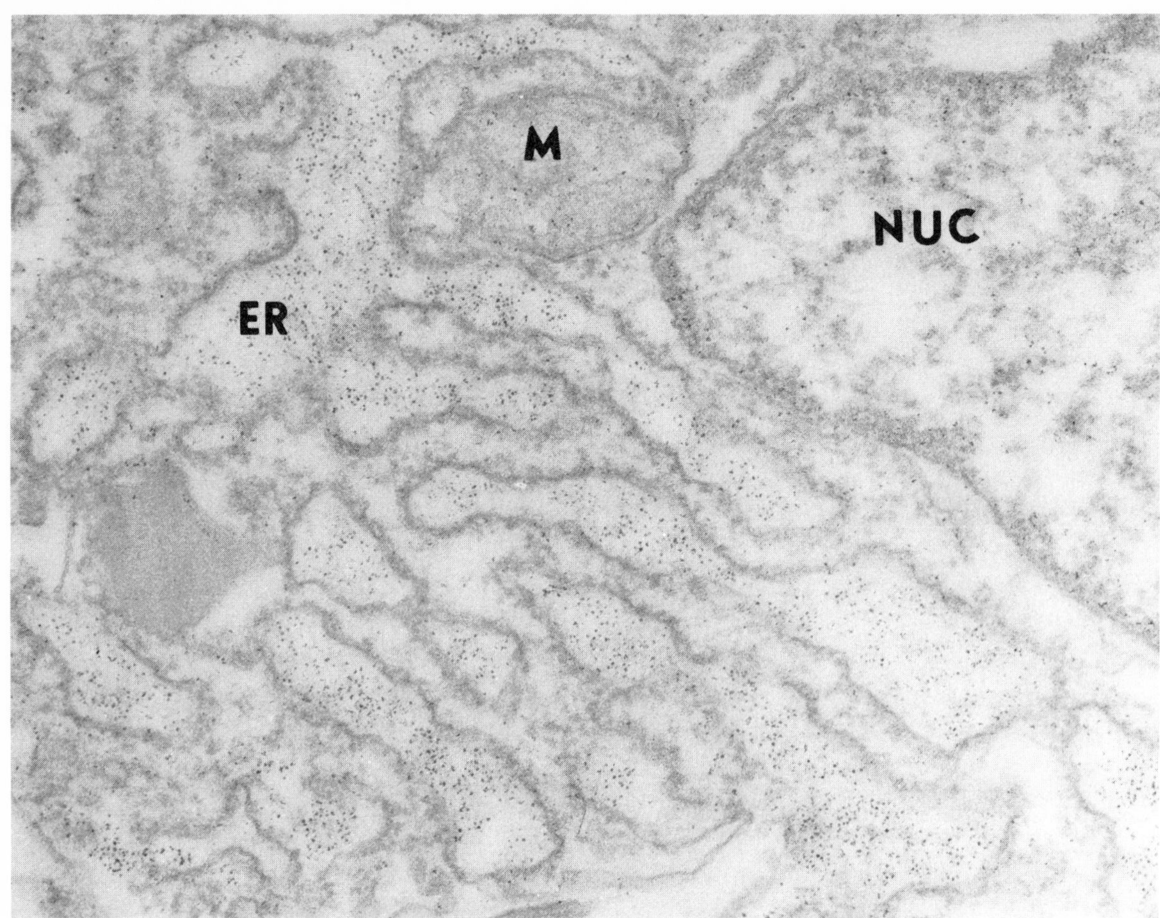

Fig. 14.9 Chick tendon fibroblasts incubated with α,α-dipyridyl to inhibit hydroxylation of procollagen. The unhydroxylated procollagen (protocollagen) is localized in the rough endoplasmic reticulum (ER) as shown by staining with ferritin-conjugated antibodies directed against determinants in the carboxyl propeptide of type I procollagen. Some background staining is observed in mitochondria (M) and the nucleus (NUC). Block staining with magnesium-uranyl-acetate (×75 000). (Courtesy of B. Olsen.)

sufficient quantities of antibodies to perform certain experiments, and the unavoidable variations in antibodies which can occur due to differences within individual animals or groups of animals. We felt that some of these difficulties, at least, could be overcome by applying the recently devised cell hybridization technology for the creation of lymphocyte-myeloma cell hybrids, 'hybridomas', capable of producing monoclonal antibodies against the different genetic types of collagen (Linsenmayer et al, 1979; Linsenmayer & Hendrix, 1980, 1981). In a hybridoma cell, the information for producing a specific antibody is supplied by the lymphocyte parent, and the ability to be propagaged indefinitely is supplied by the myeloma cell parent (Kohler & Milstein, 1975: see also Melchers & Potter, 1979; Linsenmayer & Hendrix, 1981).

In evaluating the information which will now be presented on the production and characterizations of monoclonal antibodies against purified collagens, it should be remembered that only two positive hybridoma clones have been so far isolated — one each against chicken type I and type II collagens. The data which have been obtained demonstrating the considerable advantages of this technique, plus some potential disadvantages, are from this extremely small and thus potentially unrepresentative sample. We think, however, that they can serve as a guideline for the types of results that one can expect to obtain with the use of monoclonal antibodies.

For the production of anticollagen monocloncal antibodies, we have used the parental myeloma cell line MPC 11 45.6TG1.7, which produces its own IgG composed of γ2b heavy chains and K light chains (Margulis et al, 1976). For work in progress we are using the more recently available myeloma lines which do not secrete their own antibody, but after fusion will secrete antibody specified by the lymphocyte parent. The disadvantage of using a parental myeloma cell line which makes its own nonspecific immunoglobulin molecules is that the hybridomas that are constructed produce hybrid molecules containing all combinations and permutations of heavy and light chains from both the lymphocyte and myeloma cell parents (Kohler & Milstein, 1975). Thus, while a portion of the antibodies produced by the hybridomas are completely active, many of the antigenic binding sites and even some whole antibody molecules are inactive.

The isolation of hybridoma cells requires the use of a biochemical selective technique such as HAT medium (hypoxanthine; aminopterin; thymidine) (Littlefield, 1964). To be used in the HAT medium selection procedure for hybrid cells, the myeloma parent must be deficient in the enzyme hypoxanthine phosphoribosyltransferase (HPRT) and thus be susceptible to killing by HAT selective medium. This selective mechanism, which was initially developed for use in somatic cell genetic analyses (Littlefield, 1964), depends on poisoning the metabolic pathways normally requiring folic acid by including aminopterin in the selective medium. The block to purine synthesis can be circumvented by normal cells which contain a functional HPRT enzyme and thus are able to effectively utilize hypoxanthine in the salvage pathway for purine synthesis. The HPRT $^-$ myeloma parents can not utilize the exogenously added hypoxanthanine and thus are killed by HAT selective medium — unless, that is, they have been hybridized to a normal cell such as a lymphocyte which can supply the hybrid with the information necessary to synthesize an active HPRT enzyme. Hybridomas live in HAT medium.

To produce hybridomas which will make anticollagen antibodies, the source of lymphocytes must obviously be an animal which has been immunized with the type of collagen to which antibody is desired. Since, at present, the only myeloma cell lines readily available are of mouse origin, the lymphocytes should also be of mouse origin. Unhybridized parental lymphocytes, being normal cells, are not killed in HAT medium. However, since they do not divide in vitro, they are also selectively removed with time in culture and only the hybridomas survive and divide.

An outline of the methods we have used to produce hybridomas synthesizing anticollagen monoclonal antibodies is diagrammatically shown in Figure 14.10. MPC 11 myeloma cells were fused with lymphocytes removed from ASW/SN strain mice which had previously been immunized with either type I or type II collagen from chickens. The fusion agent was 37.5 per cent polyethylene glycol 1000 used according to Gefter et al (1977), although other fusion procedures have recently proved more effective (see Linsenmayer & Hendrix, 1981). Hybridomas were selected by plating the entire cell suspension into numerous tissue culture wells containing HAT medium, and wells that showed cell growth were tested for the presence of antibody activity by passive haemagglutination (Beil et al, 1973). Cells from antibody positive wells were cloned by limiting dilution in microtitre wells. The process of cloning of the hybridomas eliminates the possibility of

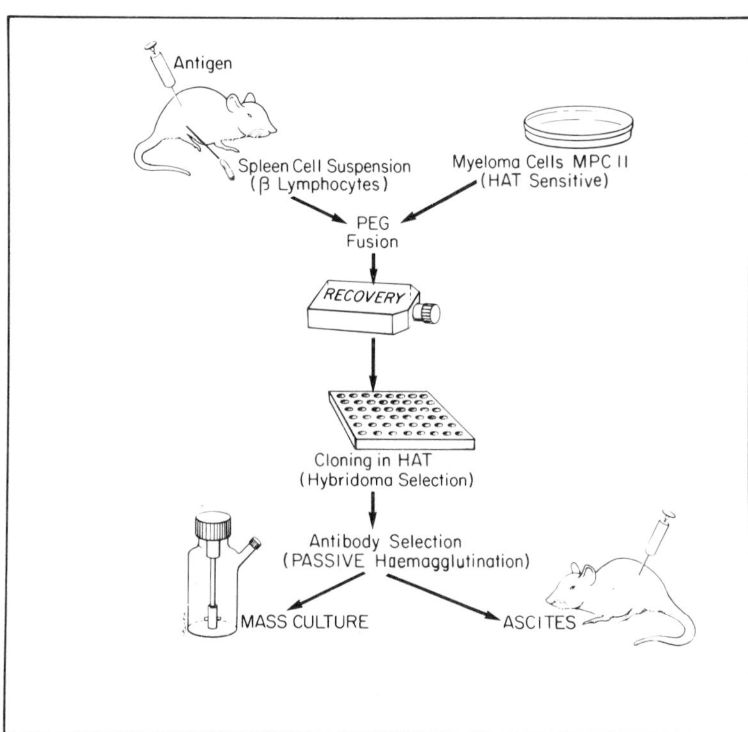

Fig. 14.10 Diagram of a method for producing monoclonal antibodies. HAT = hypoxanthine; aminopterin; thymidine. PEG = polyethylene glycol.

the production of unwanted antibodies, since each hybridoma contains the genome of a single lymphocyte parent.

The hybridomas which have already been selected for the production of monoclonal antibodies against collagen types I and II have been characterized with respect to specificity and titres obtainable, and ability to function as immunocytochemical reagents. They both belong to the IgG class of immunoglobulins.

Antibody titres were determined by passive haemagglutination (Table 14.1), and since the titres were determined by 2-fold serial dilutions, the data are expressed as ($-\log_2$). Spent culture medium from the hybridoma that had been produced from lymphocytes of a mouse immunized with type I collagen had a titre of 6–7 when tested with erythrocytes coated with type I collagen and no detectable titre when tested against type II coated cells. Culture medium from the hybridoma produced from the type II immunized mouse had a titre of 10–11 when tested against type II coated erythrocytes and no detectable titre against the type I cells. Since these media showed no crossreactivity between the collagen types, the antibody does not require affinity chromatographic purification.

Table 14.1 Monoclonal antibody titres

Monoclonal antibody	*Antibody source*	*Titres (-Log$_2$)* Chick I	Chick II
Chick type I	Culture medium	6–7	0
	Ascites fluid	15– 17	0
Chick type II	Culture medium	0	10.6 ± 0.69
	Ascites fluid	0	21.1 ± 1.95

For both antibodies, a much higher titre could be obtained by injecting the hybridoma cells into the peritoneal cavity of athymic, nude mice (nu/nu), and harvesting the ascites fluid approximately 2 weeks later. The ascites fluid from the type II hybridoma-containing nude mice had an average titre of 21 ± 1.95, which indicates a detectable average antibody response at an absolute dilution of greater than two million. The ascites fluid from the type I-containing mice had titres of 15 — 17 which gives an absolute titre of greater than a half million. Still, neither ascites fluid had any detectable activity when tested against the heterologous collagen type.

Limited pepsin digestion of either type of collagen did not affect the titres. Thus, for both antibodies the antigenic site probably resides within the helical portion of the molecule. To test whether the antigenic site in addition is conformation dependent and present only when the collagen is in the native state, we performed inhibition of haemagglutination using native and denatured collagens. The results for the type II antibody are shown in Figure 14.11 and similar results were obtainable for the type I

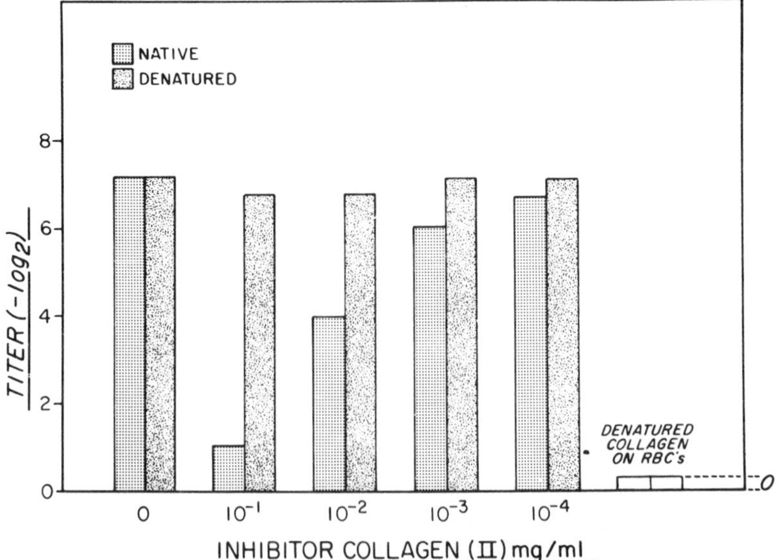

Fig. 14.11 Native and thermally denatured (50°C for 30 min.) type II collagens were examined for their ability to inhibit the haemagglutination of type II-coated RBCs by the type II monoclonal antibody. Inhibitor collagens at the concentrations shown in the figure were mixed with serial dilutions of antibody and allowed to incubate at 4°C for 1 hour. The RBCs coated with native type II were added and allowed to react overnight at 4°C. An additional experiment was to thermally denature the type II collagen on the RBCs in situ. The coated RBCs were heated to 50°C for 30 min., and after cooling were tested for agglutinability with antibody (see last two bars). (From Linsenmayer and Hendrix, 1980, courtesy Academic Press.)

antibody. When native collagen was tested using 10-fold serial dilutions, a concentration dependence was observed. Thermally denatured collagen caused no inhibition. Upon renaturation, inhibitory activity was regained. In addition, similar inhibitory activity was found for artificially renatured molecules produced from α1(II) chains which had been further purified by carboxymethylcellulose chromatography. That the antibody does not bind to denatured collagen was further demonstrated by using thermally denatured collagen on the RBC's surface. Such cells were not agglutinated by antibody (Fig. 14.11, last two bars). These results are all consistent with ones found for conventional anticollagen antibodies produced in mice.

Both the type I and type II antibodies have been shown to react well in immunocytochemical procedures. Figure 14.12 shows fluorescence micrographs of a 14-day embryonic chick tibia, including both cartilagenous and non-cartilagenous regions stained with either type I or type II monoclonal antibody using the double-antibody sandwich technique (see also sections of avian corneas in Fig. 14.7). The second antibody was rhodamine-conjugated rabbit IgG directed against mouse IgG. Sections treated with anti-type I collagen ascites fluid (Fig. 14.12a) showed the brightest fluorescence in the perichondrial region, with loose connective tissue also showing bright staining. The matrix in the cartilagenous regions, on the other hand, had at most a slight background fluorescence. Sections treated with anti-type II collagen ascites fluid (Fig. 14.12b) showed bright fluorescence over the cartilage matrix, with little, if any, over the perichondrium and surrounding connective tissue. Uniform staining of the cartilagenous matrix required pretreatment of the sections with hyaluronidase to remove proteoglycan. Both ascites-derived antibodies could be diluted many thousand fold with no detectable decrease in staining intensity.

Thus far, the only negative feature we have found about these monoclonal antibodies is that they only precipitate a fractional portion of the labelled collagen in a radioimmune assay using staphylococcal protein A or a second antibody as a precipitating agent (see Linsenmayer et al, 1979). As yet we do not know why this is the case. It could be that, due to their monoclonal nature, they recognize a subpopulation of the collagen molecules, or possibly a single antibody binding site is not strong enough to allow effective precipitation of a large rod-like molecule like collagen. Alternatively, the problem may be one of affinity. The hybridomas may have been formed with a subpopulation of lymphocytes that themselves were producing low-affinity antibodies. Possibly all anticollagen antibodies are relatively low affinity, but with conventional antibodies, due to the heterogeneity of binding sites, the low affinity is not so obvious. Alternatively, it may be that the presence of one or more inactive parental myeloma chains in the antibody may interfere with antibody binding. To discriminate among some of these possibilities we are currently trying to produce more anticollagen secreting hybridomas — this time with non-secretor and non-producer myeloma cell lines.

ACKNOWLEDGEMENTS

This is publication number 822 of the Robert W. Lovett Memorial Group for the Study of Diseases Causing Deformities. Original unpublished research and previously published work by the author was supported by NIH Research Grants EY 02261 and AM 03564, and a Research Career Development Award AM00031. I thank S. Gay for helpful criticisms of the manuscript and M. Hendrix, S. Gay, K. von der Mark and B. Olsen for contributing pictures.

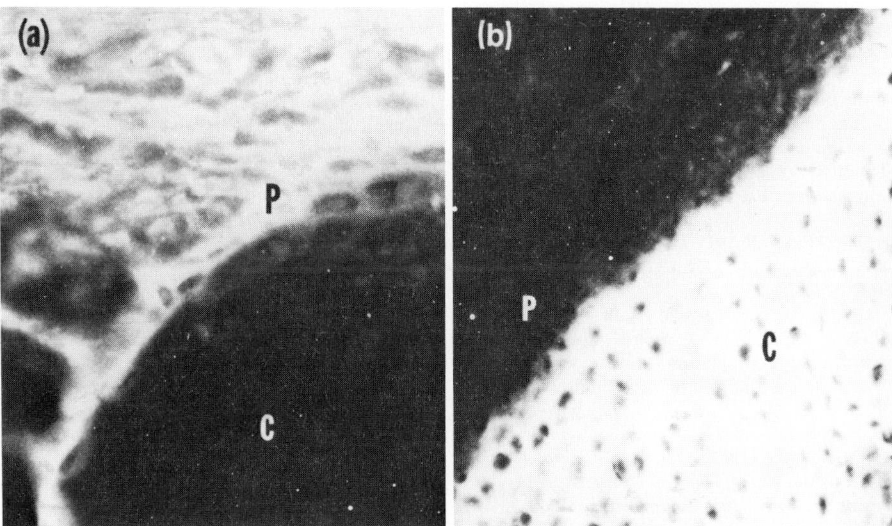

Fig. 14.12 Fluorescence micrographs of 14-day embryonic chick tibias stained with monoclonal antibody ascites fluid to (a) type I collagen and (b) type II collagen: a double-antibody sandwich technique. The second antibody is rhodamine-conjugated rabbit IgG directed against mouse IgG; C = cartilage; P = perichondrium. a = 60×; b = 540×

REFERENCES

Adelmann B C, Gentner G J, Hopper K 1973 A sensitive radioimmunoassay for collagen. Journal of Immunological Methods 3: 319

Bailey A J, Shellswell G B, Duance V C 1979 Identification and change of collagen types in differentiating myoblasts and developing chick muscle. Nature 278: 67

Becker U, Nowack H, Gay S, Timpl R 1976 Production and specificity of antibodies against the aminoterminal region in type III collagen. Immunology 31: 57

Becker U, Timpl R, Kuhn K 1972 Carboxyterminal antigenic determinants of collagen from calf skin. Localization within discrete regions of the non-helical sequence. European Journal of Biochemistry 28: 221

Beil W, Furthmayr H, Timpl R 1972 Chicken antibodies to soluble rat collagen 1. Characterization of the immune response by precipitation and agglutination methods. Immunochemistry 9: 779

Beil W, Timpl R, Furthmayr H 1973 Conformation dependence of antigenic determinants on the collagen molecule. Immunology 24: 13

Cuatrecasas P 1970 Protein purification by affinity chromatography. Journal of Biological Chemistry 245: 3059

Dehm P, Olsen B R. Prockop D J 1974 Antibodies to chick-tendon procollagen: Affinity purification with the isolated disulphide-linked NH_2-terminal extensions and reactivity with a component in embryonic serum. European Journal of Biochemistry 46: 107

Duance V C, Restall D J, Beard H, Bourne F J, Bailey A J 1977 The location of three collagen types in skeletal muscle. FEBS Letters 79: 248

Duance V C, Stephens H R, Dunn M, Bailey A J, Dubowitz V 1980 A role for collagen in the pathogenesis of muscular dystrophy. Nature 284: 470

Epstein E H, Munderloh N 1978 Human skin collagen: Presence of type I and type III at all levels of the dermis. Journal of Biological Chemistry 253: 1336

Eyre D, Muir H 1974 Collagen polymorphism: Two molecular species in pig intervertebral disk. FEBS Letters 42: 192

Fleischmajer R, Gay S, Meigel W N, Perlish J S 1978 Collagen in the cellular and fibrotic stages of scleroderma. Arthritis and Rheumatism 21: 418

Fuchs S, Mozes E, Maoz A, Sela M 1974 Thymus independence of a collagen-like synthetic polypeptide and of collagen, and the need for thymus and bone marrow-cell cooperation in the immune response to gelatin. Journal of Experimental Medicine 139: 148

Furthmayr H, Timpl R 1976 Immunochemistry of collagens and procollagens. International Review of Connective Tissue Research 7: 61

Furthmayr H, Beil W, Timpl R 1971 Different antigenic determinants in the polypeptide chains of human collagen. FEBS Letters 12: 341

Furthmayr H, Stoltz M, Becker U, Beil W, Timpl R 1972 Chicken antibodies to soluble rat collagen II. Specificity of the reactions with individual polypeptide chains and cyanogen bromide peptides of collagen. Immunochemistry 9: 789

Gay R E, Buckingham R B, Prince R K, Gay S, Rodnan G P, Miller E J 1980a Collagen types synthesized in dermal fibroblast cultures from patients with early progressive systemic sclerosis. Arthritis and Rheumatism 23: 190

Gay S, Kresina T F, Gay R, Miller E J, Montes L F 1979 Immunohistochemical demonstration of basement membrane collagen in normal human skin and in psoriasis. Journal of Cutaneous Pathology 6: 91

Gay S, Miller E J 1978 Collagen in the physiology and pathology of connective tissue. Gustav Fischer Verlag, New York

Gay S, Balleisen L, Remberger K, Fietzek P P, Adelemann B C, Kuhn K 1975 Immunohistochemical evidence for the presence of collagen type III in human arterial walls, arterial thrombi and in leucocytes incubated with collagen in vitro. Klinische Wochenschrift 53: 899

Gay S, Martin G R, Muller P K, Timpl R, Kuhn K 1976a Simultaneous synthesis of types I and III collagen by fibroblasts in culture. Proceedings of the National Academy of Science USA 73: 4037

Gay S, Muller P K, Lemmen C, Remberger K, Matzen K, Kuhn K 1976b Immunohistological study on collagen in cartilage-bone metamorphosis and degenerative osteoarthrosis. Klinische Wochenschrift 54: 969

Gay S, Muller P K, Meigel W N, Kuhn K 1976c Polymorphie des kollagens. Neue aspekte fur struktur and funktion des bindesgewebes. Hautarzt 27: 196

Gay S, Rhodes R K, Gay R, Miller E J 1981 Collagen molecules comprised of $\alpha 1(V)$-chains (B chains): An apparent localization in the exocytoskeleton. Collagen and Related Research 1: 53

Gefter M L, Margulies D H, Scharff M D 1977 A simple method for polyethylene glycol promoted hybridization of mouse myeloma cells. Somatic Cell Genetics 3: 231

Gosslau B, Barrach H J 1979 Enzyme-linked immunoabsorbent microassay for quantification of specific antibodies to collagen types I, II, III. Journal of Immunological Methods 29: 71

Gunson D E, Kefalides N A 1976 The use of radioimmunoassay in the characterization of antibodies to basement membrane collagen. Immunology 31: 563

Gunson D E, Arbogast B, Kefalides N A 1976 Rat parietal yolk sac basement membrane. An investigation of the antigenic determinants using a radio-immunoassay. Immunology 31: 577

Hahn E, Timpl R 1973 Involvement of more than a single polypeptide chain in the helical antigenic determinants of collagen. European Journal of Immunology 3: 442

Hahn E, Timpl R, Miller E J 1974 The production of specific antibodies to native collagens with the chain compositions, $(\alpha 1(I))_3$, $(\alpha 1(II))_3$ and $(\alpha(I))_2\alpha 2$. Journal of Immunology 113: 421

Hahn E, Timpl R, Miller E J 1975 Demonstration of a unique antigenic specificity for the collagen alpha 1 (II) chain from cartilagenous tissue. Immunology 28: 561

Hahn E, Nowack H, Gotze D, Timpl R 1975 H–2 linked genetic control of antibody response to soluble calf skin collagen in mice. European Journal of Immunology 5: 288

Hay E D, Revel J P 1969 Fine structure of the developing avian cornea. In: Wolsky A, Chen P S (eds) Monographs in developmental biology, vol 1. Karger, Basel

Hay E, Linsenmayer T F, Trelstad R L, von der Mark K 1979 Origin and distribution of collagens in the develping avian cornea. In: Zadunaisky, Davson (eds) Current topics in eye research, vol 1. Academic Press, New York. ch 1, p 1

Howard B V, Macarak E J, Gunson D, Kefalides N A 1976 Characterization of the collagen synthesized by endothelial cells in culture. Proceedings of the National Academy of Science USA 73: 2361

Kent G, Gay S, Inouye T, Bahu R, Minki O T, Popper H 1976 Vitamin A-containing lipocytes and formation of type III collagen in liver injury. Proceedings of the National Academy of Science USA 73: 3719

Kessler S W 1975 Rapid isolation of antigens from cells with a staphylococcal protein A-antibody adsorbent: parameters of the interaction of antibody-antigen complexes with protein A. Journal of Immunology 115: 1617

Kishida Y, Olsen B R, Berg R A, Prockop D J 1975 Two improved methods for preparing ferritin-protein conjugates for electron microscopy. Journal of Cell Biology 64: 331

Kohler G, Milstein C 1976 Derivation of specific antibody-producing tissue culture and tumour lines by cell fusion. European Journal of Immunology 6: 511

Lenaers A, Lapiere C M 1975 Type III procollagen and collagen in skin. Biochimica et Biophysica Acta 400: 121

LeRoy C E 1968 Precipitating and complement-fixing antibodies to collagen with species and collagen subunit specificity. Proceedings Society for Experimental Biology Medicine 128: 341

LeRoy C E 1969 Some characteristics of the antigenic moiety of calf skin collagen. Journal of Immunology 102: 219

Lindsley H B, Mannik M, Bornstein P 1969 Immunogenicity of rat and human collagen polypeptide chains. Arthritis and Rheumatism 12: 676

Linsenmayer T F 1974 Temporal and spatial transitions in collagen types during embyronic chick limb development. II Comparison of the embryonic cartilage collagen molecule with that from adult cartilage. Developmental Biology 40: 372

Linsenmayer T F, Hendrix M J C 1980 Monoclonal antibodies to connective tissue macromolecules: Type II collagen. Biochemical and Biophysical Research Communications 92: 440

Linsenmayer T F, Hendrix M J C 1981 Production of monoclonal antibodies to collagen and their immunofluorescence localization in embryonic cornea and cartilage. In: Furthmayr H (ed) Immunochemistry of the extracellular matrix, vol. 1. CRC Press, Boca Raton, (in press)

Linsenmayer T F, Little C D 1978 Embryonic neural retina collagen: In vitro synthesis of high molecular weight forms of type II plus a new genetic type. Proceedings of the National Academy of Sciences USA 75: 3235

Linsenmayer T F, Toole B P, Trelstad R L 1973a Temporal and spatial transitions in collagen types during embryonic chick limb development. Developmental Biology 35: 232

Linsenmayer T F, Trelstad R L, Gross J 1973b The collagen of chick embryonic notochord. Biochemical and Biophysical Research Communications 53: 39

Linsenmayer T F, Trelstad R L, Toole B P, Gross J 1973c The collagen of osteogenic cartilage in the embryonic chick. Biochemical and Biophysical Research Communications 52: 870

Linsenmayer T F, Smith G N, Hay E 1977 Synthesis of two collagen types by embryonic chick corneal epithelium in vitro. Proceedings of the National Academy of Science USA 74: 39

Linsenmayer T F, Little C D, Hendrix M J C 1979 Production and characterization of a monoclonal antibody against chicken type I collagen. Proceedings of the National Academy of Science USA 76: 3703

Littlefield J W 1964 Selection of hybrids from matings of fibroblasts in vitro and their presumed recombinants. Science 145: 709

Margulies D H, Kuehl W M, Scharff M D 1976 Somatic cell hybridization of mouse myeloma cells. Cell 8: 405

Mayne R, Vail M, Mayne P, Miller E J 1976 Changes in type of collagen synthesized as clones of chick chondrocytes grow and eventually lose division capacity. Proceedings of the National Academy of Science USA 73: 1674

Mayne R, Vail M, Miller E J 1975 Analysis of changes in collagen biosynthesis that occur when chick chondrocytes are grown in 5-bromo-2′-deoxyuridine. Proceedings of the National Academy of Science USA 72: 4511

Melchers F, Potter M, Warner N 1978 Lymphocyte hybridomas. Springer, New York

Menzel J 1977 Radioimmunoassay for anticollagen — antibodies using ^{14}C-labelled collagen. Journal of Immunological Methods 15: 77

Michaeli D, Martin G R, Kettman J, Benjamini F. Leung D Y K, Blatt B A 1969 Localization of antigenic determinants in the polypeptide chains of collagen. Science 166: 1522

Michaeli D, Benjamini E, Leung D Y K, Martin G R 1971 Immunochemical studies on collagen II. Antigenic differences between guinea pig skin collagen and gelatin. Immunochemistry 8:1

Murphy W H, von der Mark K, McEneany L S G, Bornstein P 1975 Characterization of procollagen-derived peptides unique to the precursor molecule. Biochemistry 14: 3243

Newsome D A, Linsenmayer T F, Trelstad R L 1976 Vitreous body collagen: Evidence for a dual origin from the neural retina and hyalocytes. The Journal of Cell Biology 71: 59

Nist C, von der Mark K, Hay E D, Olsen B R, Bornstein P, Ross R, Dehm P 1975 Location of procollagen in chick corneal and tendon fibroblasts with ferritin conjugated antibodies. Journal of Cell Biology 65: 75

Nowack H, Hahn E, David C S, Timpl R, Gotze D 1975a Immune response control to calf collagen type I in mice: A combined control of Ir–IA and non H–2 linked genes. Immunogenetics 2: 331

Nowack H, Hahn E, Timpl R 1975b Specificity of the antibody response in inbred mice to bovine type I and type II collagen. Immunology 29: 621

Nowack H, Hahn E, Timpl R 1976a Requirement for T cells in the antibody response of mice to calf skin collagen. Immunology 30: 29

Nowack H, Gay S, Wick G, Becker U, Timpl R 1976b Preparation and use in immunohistology of antibodies specific for type I and type III collagen and procollagen. Journal of Immunological Methods 12: 117

Nowack H, Olsen B R, Timpl R 1976c Characterization of the amino-terminal segment in type III procollagen. European Journal of Biochemistry 70: 205

Olsen B R, Prockop D J 1974 Ferritin-conjugated antibodies used for labelling or organelles involved in the cellular synthesis and transport of procollagen. Proceedings of the National Academy of Science 71: 2033

Olsen B R, Berg R A, Kishica Y, Prockop D J 1975 Further characterization of embryonic tendon fibroblasts and the use of immunoferritin techniques to study collagen biosynthesis. Journal of Cell Biology 64: 340

Olsen B R, Guzman N A, Engel J, Condit C, Aase S 1977 Purification and characterization of a peptide from the carboxy-terminal region of chick tendon procollagen type I. Biochemistry 16: 3030

Orkin R W, Gehron P, McGoodwin E B, Martin G R, Valentine T, Swarm R 1977 A murine tumour producing a matrix of basement membrane. The Journal of Experimental Medicine 145: 204

Park E, Church R L, Tanzer M L 1975 Immunological properties of procollagens obtained from the culture medium of dermatosparactic cells. Immunology 28: 781

Pope F M, Martin G R, Lichtenstein J R, Penttinen R, Gerson B, Rowe D W, McKusick V A 1975 Patients with Ehlers-Danlos syndrome type IV lack type III collagen. Proceedings of the National Academy of Science USA 72: 1314

Rennard S I, Berg R, Martin G R, Robey P G 1980 Enzyme-linked Immunoassay (ELISA) for connective tissue components. Analytical Biochemistry 104: 205

Rohde H, Becker U, Nowack H, Timpl R 1976a Antigenic structure of the aminoterminal region in type I procollagen. Immunochemistry 13: 967

Rohde H, Nowack H, Becker U, Timpl R 1976b Radioimmunoassay for the aminoterminal peptide of procollagen pα1(I)-chain. Journal Immunological Methods 11: 135

Rohde H, Nowack H, Timpl R 1978 Localization of antigenic activity and immunogenic capacity in different conformational domains of procollagen peptide. European Journal of Immunology 8: 141

Roll F J, Madri A, Furthmayr H 1979 A new method of iodinating collagens for use in radioimmunoassay. Analytical Biochemistry 96: 489

Sela M, Schechter B, Schechter M, Borck F 1967 Antibodies to sequential and conformational antigenic determinants. Cold Spring Harbor Symposium on Quantatative Biology 32: 537

Sherr C J, Goldberg B 1973 Antibodies to a precursor of human collagen. Science 180: 1190

Sherr C J, Taubman M B, Goldberg B 1973 Isolation of a disulphide-stabilized three-chain polypeptide fragment unique to the precursor of human collagen. The Journal of Biological Chemistry 248: 7035

Smith G N Jr, Linsenmayer T F, Newsome D A 1976 Synthesis of type II collagen in vitro by embryonic chick neural retina tissue. Proceedings of the National Academy of Science USA 73: 4420

Steffen C, Timpl R, Wolff I 1967 Immunogenitat und spezifitat von kollagen IV. Untersuchungen zur kollagen-spezifitat der antiserren. Zeitschrift fur Immunitatsforschung 134: 205

Steffen C, Dichtl M, Knapp W, Brunner H 1971 Immunogenicity and specificity of collagen. XII Demonstration by immunofluorescence and haemagglutination of antibodies with different specificity in human collagen. Immunology 21: 649

Stenn K S, Madri J A, Roll F J 1979 Migrating epidermis produces AB_2 collagen and requires continual collagen synthesis for movement. Nature 277: 229

Stoltz M, Timpl R, Furthmayr H, Kuhn K 1973 Structural and immunogenic properties of a major antigenic determinant in neutral salt-extracted rat skin collagen. European Journal of Biochemistry 37: 287

Timpl R, Furthmayr H, Steffen C, Doleschel W 1967 Isolation of pure anticollagen antibodies using a specific immunoadsorbent technique. Zeitschrift fur Immunitatsforschung 134: 391

Timpl R, Fietzek P P, Furthmayr H, Meigel W, Kuhn K 1970a Evidence for two antigenic determinants in the C-terminal region of rat skin collagen. FEBS Letters 9: 11

Timpl R, Fietzek P P, Furthmayr H, Meigel W, Pontz B 1971 Characterization of conformation independent antigenic determinants in the triple-helical part of calf and rat collagen. Immunology 21: 1017

Timpl R, Furthmayr H, Beil W 1972 Maturation of the immune response to soluble rat collagen: Late appearance of antibodies to N-terminal sites of the α2-chain. Immunology 108: 119

Timpl R, Wick G, Furthmayr H. Lapiere C M, Kuhn K 1973 Immunochemical properties of procollagen from dermatosparactic calves. European Journal of Biochemistry 32: 584

Timpl R, Glanville R W, Nowack H, Wiedemann H, Fietzek P P, Kuhn K 1975 Isolation, chemical and electron microscopial characterization of neutral-salt soluble type III collagen and procollagen from fetal bovine skin. Hoppe-Seyler's Zeitschrift fur Physiologische Chemie 356: 1783

Timpl R, Wick G, Gay S 1977 Antibodies to distinct types of collagens and procollagens and their application in immunohistology. Journal of Immunological Methods 18: 165

Timpl R, Martin G R, Bruckner P, Wick G, Wiedemann H 1978 Nature of the collagenous protein in a tumour basement membrane. European Journal of Biochemistry 84: 43

Timpl R, Bruckner P, Fietzek P P 1979 Characterization of pepsin fragments of basement membrane collagen obtained from a mouse tumour. European Journal of Biochemistry 95: 255

Timpl R 1976 Immunological studies on collagen. In: Ramachandran G N, Reddi A H (eds) Biochemistry of collagen. Plenum, New York. pp 319, 326

Toole B P, Linsenmayer T F 1977 Newer knowledge of skeletogenesis: macromolecular transitions in the extracellular matrix. Clinical Orthopaedics and Related Research 129: 259

Vertel B M, Dorfman A 1979 Simultaneous localization of type II collagen and core protein of chondroitin sulphate proteoglycan in individual chondrocytes. Proceedings of the National Academy of Science USA 76: 1261

von der Mark K, von der Mark H 1977 The role of three genetically distinct collagen types in endochondral ossification and calcification of cartilage. The Journal of Bone and Joint Surgery 59B: 458

von der Mark K, Click E M, Bornstein P 1973 The immunology of procollagen 1. Development of antibodies to determinants unique to the proα1 chain. Archives of Biochemistry and Biophysics 156: 356

von der Mark H, von der Mark K, Gay S 1976a Study of differential collagen synthesis during development of the chick embryo by immunofluorescence: 1. Preparation of collagen Type I and Type II specific antibodies and their application to early stages of the chick embryo. Developmental Biology 48: 237

von der Mark K, von der Mark H, Gay S 1976b Study of differential collagen synthesis during development of the chick embryo by immunofluorescence: II. Localization of Type I and Type II collagen during long bone development. Developmental Biology 53: 153

von der Mark K, Gauss V, von der Mark H, Muller P 1977a Relationship between cell shape and type collagen synthesized as chondrocytes lose their cartilage phenotype in culture. Nature 267: 531

von der Mark K, von der Mark H, Timpl R. Trelstad R L 1977b Immunofluorescent localization of collagen types I, II, and III in the embryonic chick eye. Developmental Biology 59: 75

Wick G, Furthmayr H, Timpl R 1975 Purified antibodies to collagen: An immunofluoresce study of their reaction with tissue collagen. International Archives of Allergy and Applied Immunology 48: 664

Wick G, Nowack H, Hahn E, Timpl R, Miller E J 1976 Visualization of type I and II collagens in tissue sections by immunohistologic techniques. Immunology 117: 298

Wick G, Brunner H, Penner E, Timpl R 1978a The diagnostic application of specific antiprocollagen sera II. Analysis of liver biopsies. International Archives of Allergy and Applied Immunology 56: 316

Wick G, Olsen B R, Timpl R 1978b Immunohistological analysis of fetal and dermatosparactic calf and sheep skin with antisera to procollagen and collagen type I. Laboratory Investigation 39: 151

Yaoita H, Foidart J M, Katz S 1978 Localization of the collagenous component in skin basement membrane. Journal of Investigative Dermatology 70: 191

15

Immunological disorders of collagen

S. GAY and T. F. KRESINA

INTRODUCTION

The diseases involving immunological mechanisms affecting the different collagenous proteins of connective tissue can be divided into two categories (Fig. 15.1). First there are the various acquired maladies in which collagen may induce an immune response. In the past it had been believed that collagen was a relatively weak immunogen in comparison to other macromolecular proteins. In recent years, however, numerous studies have shown that native and denatured collagen molecules, as well as certain collagen or procollagen peptides, are capable of inducing both humoral and cellular immune responses. Second are the disorders which cause similar lesions in the collagenous structures of connective tissue by certain immunopathological mechanisms that may not directly involve collagen (Table 15.1). Most of the latter conditions were originally designated as 'collagen diseases' (Klemperer, 1950; Bywaters, 1976). At the moment, however, there is still some doubt as to the direct involvement of collagen in a variety of pathophysiological changes of connective tissue. Recently, sufficient data have been accumulated to correlate certain alterations of collagen metabolism to certain aetiological entities. Initially, the term 'collagen disease' was used to describe a number of acute and chronic disorders which include: rheumatoid arthritis, systemic lupus erythematosus, progressive systemic sclerosis, polymyositis, dermatomyositis, Sjögren's syndrome, amyloidosis, certain inflammatory vascular disorders, rheumatic fever, ankylosing spondylitis and relapsing polychondritis. The term was useful in one way. Namely, it emphasized that that these disorders do not occur in a single organ, but are disseminated throughout the connective tissue which in the past was known as 'the collagen'. Presently, the genetically different collagens comprising the interstitial fibres, and the basement membranes or basement membrane-like structural elements are now recognized as distinct structural entities which exist within the various connective tissues along with other noncollagenous components. Therefore, it is now necessary to be specific about the morphological and biochemical description of the cellular and structural sites of the pathological changes in connective tissue lesions (Table 15.2). For example, pathophysiological alterations in the involved connective tissue described by light microscopy

Table 15.1 Disorders affecting connective tissue and some of the frequently occurring lesions

Disease	*Arthritis*	*Vasculitis*	*Nephritis*
Rheumatoid arthritis	↑↑	↑	↑
Syst. lupus eryth.	↑	↑	↑↑
Progr. syst. sclerosis	(↑)	↑↑	↑
Polymyositis	↑	↑↑	(↑)
Dermatomyositis	↑	↑↑	(↑)
Polyarteritis nodosa	↑	↑↑	↑
Rheumatic fever	↑	↑	↑↑

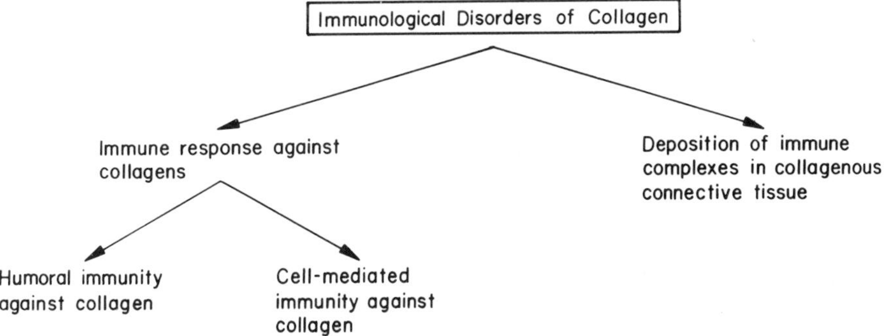

Fig. 15.1 Immunological events resulting in alteration of collagenous connective tissue.

Table 15.2 Potential cellular sites and collagenous structures affected by immunopathological alterations

Collagens		*Potential immune binding sites*	
Interstitial collagens			
Type I	$[\alpha 1(I)]_2\alpha 2(I)$	Fibroblasts	Large fibrils of dense connective tissue
Type II	$[\alpha 1(II)]_3$	Chondroblasts	Small fibrils of hyaline cartilage
Type III	$[\alpha 1(III)]_3$	Fibroblasts, Reticulum cells	Fine fibrillar reticular network
Basement membrane collagens			
Type IV*	$[\alpha 1(IV)]_3$ $[\alpha 2(IV)]_3$	Epithel- and Endothel-cells	Morphologically distinct basement membranes
Pericellular collagens			
Type V**	$[\alpha 1(V)]_2\alpha 2(V)$ $\alpha 1(V)\alpha 2(V)\alpha 3(V)$ $[\alpha 1(V)]_3$	Smooth muscle cells myofibroblasts, etc.	Basement membrane-like exocytoskeleton

*$\alpha 1(IV)$ = C-chain; $\alpha 2(IV)$ = D-chain.
**$\alpha 1(V)$ = B-chain; $\alpha 2(V)$ = A-chain; $\alpha 3(V)$ = αC-chain

such as 'fibrinoid degeneration' have failed to establish any molecular defect in collagen structure. Thus, there is currently no justification for using the term 'collagen disease' to encompass this heterogenous group of diseases.

It appears much more appropriate for organizational purposes that the disorders of connective tissue affecting collagen be grouped into general categories (Gay & Miller, 1978). Thus, the heritable disorders are those involving defects or deficiencies in the formation of the physiologically appropriate collagen, and the acquired diseases reveal either increased collagen deposition or accelarated collagen breakdown within previously normal connective tissue (Table 15.3). In this classification, then, there are the acquired diseases in which immunopathological alterations of collagen are the primary causal agent in the pathological conditions, and there are the acquired diseases in which the collagenous connective tissues are altered as a sequela to other pathological conditions not initiated within the collagenous components of the tissue.

Table 15.3 Pathology of collagen

Interstitial collagens
Inherited diseases
(e.g. Osteogenesis imperfecta, Ehlers-Danlos syndrome)
Fibroproliferative disorders
(e.g. Liver cirrhosis, Scleroderma)
Fibrodegenerative disorders
(e.g. Aging, Osteoarthrosis)
Basement membrane collagens
Excessive membrane deposition
(e.g. Diabetic angiopathy, Glomerular sclerosis)
Membrane breakdown
(e.g. Psoriasis)
Pericellular collagens
Cell accumulation
(e.g. Atherosclerotic smooth muscle plaques)

The immunological events leading to an immune response against collagen or causing a lesion in connective tissues involve several different cell types. All of these cells are thought to be derived from a single type of progenitor haematopoietic stem cell which subsequently differentiates into different types of specific effector cells responsible for the immune response. The macrophage is the primary phagocytic cell in the body and has the main function of engulfing and removing tissue debris 'foreign' materials, and antigens. This activity of the macrophage is nonspecific but can be facilitated by coating foreign, antigenic material with newly synthesized specific antibody. In this process called opsonization, cytophylic antibody enhances the macrophage's ability to recognize and endocytose the antigen. Other functions of the macrophage are the processing and presentation of antigen to other cells of the immune response. Further, it has been postulated that an important early immunological event is the transformation of antigen by macrophages into a form recognized by a particular subclass of lymphocytes. Upon incubation of antigen with macrophages in vitro a portion of the antigen becomes tightly bound to the macrophage cell surface and this remnant of the antigen becomes a potent immunogen.

The other prominent cell types known to be involved in the immune response are the two subpopulations of lymphocytes, the T- and B-cells. The T-cells, which themselves can be divided into various subpopulations, are functionally dependent on the integrity of the thymus gland. T-cells have been shown to be the primary cell types responsible for the cell-mediated immune response. In addition they can act as cytotoxic or killer cells, immunosuppressors, enhancers, inducers, or 'helpers' of the immune response. On stimulation with either free antigen, mitogen, or macrophage-processed antigen, T-cells undergo morphological changes to blast cells which subsequently undergo mitosis. After mitosis, the biological roles of T-cells are observed, e.g. activated T-cells can elaborate lymphokines in the cell-mediated immune response, or function as helper or suppressor cells in B-cell–T-cell interactions.

The B-cell lymphocytes, on the other hand, are derived from the bone marrow, fetal liver, or yolk sac. These lymphocytes are the progenitors of the antibody producing cells, the plasma cells. On stimulation by either free antigen, processed antigen, or helper T-cells, the small B-cell lymphocytes transform into active blast cells. These blast cells subsequently divide into plasma cells which can actively produce immunoglobulin or be retained as a memory cell.

The immunoglobulin molecule produced by B-lymphocytes consists of two types of disulphide-bonded chains, designated the heavy chain (H) and the light chain (L) (for reviews see Kochwa & Kunkel, 1971). At least five major classes of immunoglobulins have been described as humoral antibodies. The immunoglobulin classes vary in concentration in the sera from the abundant IgG class (1 g per 100 ml) to the exiguous IgE (0.03 mg per 100 ml). In addition to the immunoglobulins, some serum polypeptides are related to the immune response. These are a complex set of interacting proteins, called complement which are responsible in part for cytolysis of 'foreign' bacteria and cells. The complement system, although activated mainly by antigen-antibody complexes, can also be activated by numerous biological substances participating in certain tissue-damaging reactions (for review see Müller-Eberhard, 1975).

Another major area which will be discussed is that of autoimmunity. Specifically, in light of the presence of human antibodies and cellular immunity against different collagen types, the general immunological mechanisms leading to autoimmunity should be considered. Autoimmunity to collagen refers to an immune response to an individual's own connective tissue collagen. In general, the human organism develops a natural tolerance to his own tissue components (antigens) during the fetal development. The loss of this tolerance leads to autoimmunization. Further autoimmunity may be induced by the following mechanisms (Talal et al, 1976):

1. Infection by viruses, which contain cross-reacting antigens or alter host antigens, rendering them autoimmunogenic;
2. Binding of foreign haptens, such as certain drugs, to host tissues;
3. Nonspecific stimulation of helper T-cell activity;
4. Exposure to cross-reacting foreign antigens; and
5. Loss of suppressor T-cell activity.

Autoimmunity, characterized by self-destruction, plays a significant role in a variety of pathological conditions such as certain viral infections, organ specific alterations like thyroiditis, or generalized diseases, like systemic lupus erythematosus. In such conditions, the physiological regulation of the immune response appears to be altered by an abnormal or excessive activity of immune effector cells. Pathologically, this can result in the production of autoantibodies by B-lymphocytes and abnormal tissue reactions by T-lymphocytes and macrophages. Autoimmunity then is a state of immunologic imbalance in which B-lymphocyte activity is increased and suppressor T-lymphocyte activity is decreased. This imbalance may be caused by genetic factors as outlined later (p. 279), as well as viral and environmental mechanisms.

The pathophysiological events whereby the immune response may cause connective tissue damage have been subdivided into four general reactions (Fig. 15.2). Some disorders appear to be related to only one of these reactions of immune injury, whereas others may result from a combination of different immune processes. In this regard, we will discuss a variety of different types of diseases leading to a humoral and/or cellular immune response against certain antigenic determinants of the various collagen types, as well as conditions involving immunopathological mechanisms in altering collagen metabolism.

HUMORAL ANTIBODY RESPONSE TO COLLAGEN

The first evidence for the immunogenicity of collagen was provided by Watson et al (1954). Since this initial observation, the immunology of collagen has become a topic of intense investigation which has been extensively reviewed by Beard et al (1977), Furthmayr & Timpl (1976), Mestecky et al (1979), Michaeli (1977), and Timpl (1976). The discovery of unique antigenic determinants on the procollagen and collagen molecules has led to the experimental production of specific antibodies for use in immunohistochemical assays as discussed in Chapter 14 by Linsenmayer. Likewise, a number of immunoserological assays have been developed to demonstrate collagen autoantibodies in human fluids and tissues (see below).

Specificity of anticollagen antibodies

Mauer (1954) first described gelatin to be antigenic in man because of the presence of a serum factor, designed as antigelatin factor (AGF), which reacted with denatured collagen. In these studies, the 'antigelatin factor' observed in normal human sera was believed to be a serum

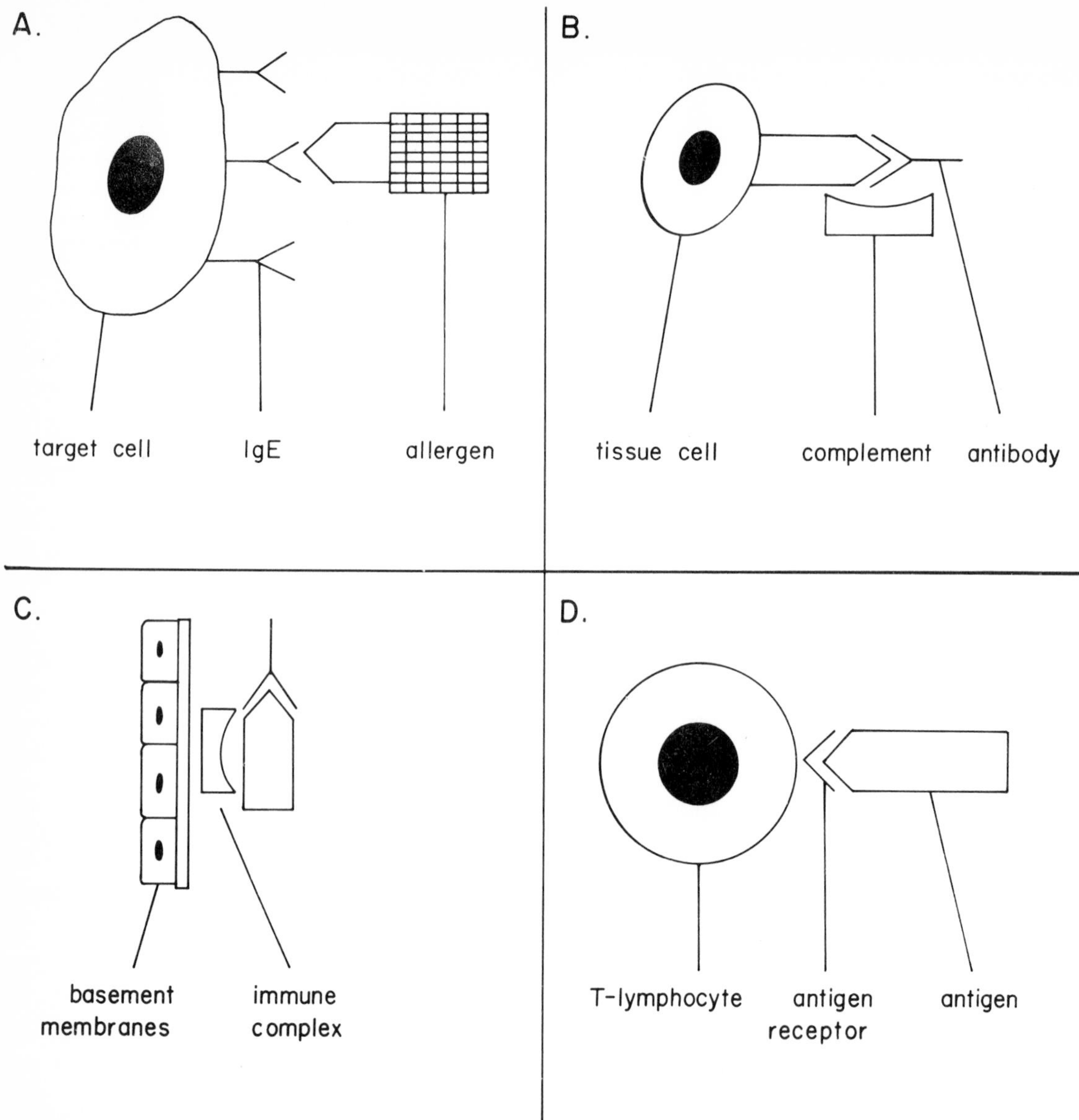

Fig. 15.2 Schematic representation of the four types of immunological reactions which may produce connective tissue damage. A, Type I — anaphylaxis. Interaction of antigen (allergen) with its specific preformed IgE antibody fixed to target cell results in an allergic reaction such as vasodilatation and oedema. B, Type II — cytotoxicity. Interaction of antibody with antigen on cell surface leads to cellular damage. C, Type III — immune complex toxicity. Antigen reaction with antibody forms complement fixing immune complexes which are deposited on connective tissue structures such as basement membranes and lead to tissue injury. D, Upon interaction with antigen, T-lymphocytes are transformed and release mediators with localize macrophages releasing tissue damaging enzymes.

autoantibody against denatured collagen. At that time, the possibility was discussed that normal individuals may produce antibodies against the gelatin present in most diets or that antibody could be made to the naturally occurring collagen in the connective tissue. Later Wolff et al (1967) described binding of human serum components with denatured acid-soluble collagen (gelatin) and indicated that human serum could contain antigelatin factor activity in two macromolecular components — one which was heat-labile macroglobulin agglutinator and a second which was a heat-stabile macroglobulin activator. The agglutinating antigelatin factor appeared to be related to the factor initially described by Maurer (1954), because of its ability to bind different kinds of gelatin (Wolff & Timpl, 1968). Recently, studies by Dessau et al (1978b) have proven that this antigelatin factor is not an antibody, but instead is similar to cold-insoluble globulin (CIG) as judged by its electrophoretic mobility, amino acid composition, identity on immunodiffusion, and capacity to mediate uptake of denatured collagen by guinea pig peritoneal exudate cells. Moreover, antigelatin factor reacted with ^{125}I-labelled denatured collagen, and the reaction could be inhibited by preincubation with unlabelled collagenous proteins such as native and denatured type I, II, III, and IV collagens from various species (Dessau et al, 1978a). It now appears conclusive that antigelatin factor resembles cold-insoluble globulin, fibronectin, and other cell-surface associated glycoproteins, and binds with varying degrees to all presently known collagen types and their denatured chains (Dessau et al, 1978a; Engvall & Ruoslahti, 1977; Engvall et al, 1978; Jilek & Hörmann, 1978; Kleinman et al, 1979; Ruoslahti et al, 1978; Yamada & Olden, 1978). Moreover, Adelmann et al (1973), Nowack et al (1975b), and Hopper et al (1976) have demonstrated that the reaction of denatured collagen with antigelatin factor in normal sera of guinea pigs and mice can be detected by radioassay.

Based on the above results, some of the conflicting data concerning collagen autoantibodies obtained using certain serological assays may be explained by interference caused by protein-binding serum glycoproteins. Nevertheless, Beard et al (1977) have summarized methods used for the detection of anticollagen antibodies in sera which include: (1) anaphylaxis (Rothbard & Watson, 1956); (2) complement fixation (Davidson et al, 1967; Schmitt et al, 1964); (3) cytotoxicity (Duksin et al, 1975; Lustig, 1970); (4) qualitative immunofluorescence (Engel & Catchpole, 1972; Lustig, 1971; Lustig et al, 1969; Mancini et al, 1965; Rothbard & Watson, 1961; Steffen et al, 1971); (5) quantitative immunofluorescence (Knapp et al, 1974); (6) quantitative immunoprecipitation in liquid media (Michaeli et al, 1968); (7) antiglobulin consumption test (Steffen, 1954; 1970); (8) passive haemagglutination with tanned human red cells (Steffen et al, 1967); (9) passive haemagglutination with glutaraldehyde-treated human erythrocytes (Beil et al, 1972); (10) double diffusion in agar and immunoelectrophoresis (Beil et al, 1972; Furthmayr et al, 1972); and (11) latex agglutination (Bray et al, 1967). However, it must be stressed that the proof of specificity for collagen and not some contaminating protein is definitely required, especially in view of significant antibody titres to impurities other than collagen which may exist (demonstrated in certain animal sera by Wick et al, 1975). This is particularly true when whole sera are used for such assays as cytotoxicity, gel-precipitation, and immunofluorescence. The development of optimal purification procedures for collagen and of more sensitive serological assays has led to the more recent use of haemagglutination/haemagglutination-inhibition assays (Beil et al, 1973), radioimmunoassay (Adelmann et al, 1973; Clague et al, 1979; Lindsley et al, 1971; Menzel, 1977; Nowack et al, 1976; Rhode et al, 1976; Roll et al, 1979), and enzyme-linked immunosorbent microassay (ELISA) (Gosslau & Barrach, 1979), which should help overcome past problems.

Antibodies to collagen in disease

The greatest volume of immunochemical work on autoantibodies to collagen in human diseases concerns the rheumatic diseases in which collagen has been implicated as playing a major role in the pathogenesis (Glynn, 1969; Waksman & Mason, 1949). In this regard, Steffen (1970; 1978) considered the pathogenesis of rheumatoid arthritis as collagen autoimmune disease. A number of immunoserological studies have been performed to demonstrate the existence of antibodies against collagen in sera and joint fluids of patients with rheumatoid arthritis (reviewed recently by Mestecky et al, 1979). In initial studies, homogenates of joint capsule tissue appeared to elicit antibodies as suggested by consumption tests (Steffen, 1954). In subsequent studies, the antigens used involved insoluble, impure, Type I collagen from calf and rat skin, as well as human dura mater and its hydroxylamine cleavage products. Consumption tests suggested that autoantibodies had been produced to collagen (for review see Steffen, 1978). These latter studies showed that about 40 per cent of sera and 70 per cent of synovial fluids from patients with rheumatoid arthritis reacted with human collagen, whereas only 10 per cent of sera and synovial fluids of patients with nonrheumatic joint disease tested positive. Although no correlation could be observed between the stages of disease and the appearance of antibodies, a correlation was apparent between the activity of the disease and the demonstration of antibodies (Steffen et al, 1973). Related studies by Michaeli & Fudenberg (1974) have shown an incidence of antibodies against denatured human Type I collagen of about 60 per cent in rheumatoid arthritis sera and about 9 per cent in age- and sex-matched control sera. The titres, using haemagglutination assays, ranged form 1:8 to 1:512 in the rheumatoid sera, compared to 1:4 in the controls. The anticollagen antibodies were shown to be independent of rheumatoid factor, were primarily of the IgG class, and were able to recognize both the $\alpha1$ and $\alpha2$ chains of Type I collagen. Assays of five sera showed that the major antigenic determinants were located in the cyanogen bromide fragments $\alpha1$(I)CBO, 1 and $\alpha2$(I)CB3, although some antigenic activity was also found in other peptides. Later studies by Cracchiolo et al (1975) demonstrated that antibodies to native and denatured Type I collagen could be found in the vast majority of rheumatoid and traumatic synovial fluids. In contrast, these antibodies were present in the sera of less than half of the rheumatoid patients and were rarely found in sera of patients with traumatic synovitis. In selected cases, antibodies to collagen Type I could be eluted from rheumatoid synovial membranes.

The discovery of the genetically-distinct collagens

influenced Andriopoulos et al (1976b) to use a passive haemagglutination assay to detect antibodies to native human collagens Type I, II, and III as well as to denatured chains in the sera of 110 rheumatoid patients and 75 normals. The incidence of antibodies in rheumatoid sera was as follows: Type I, 77 per cent; $\alpha 1(I)+\alpha 2(I)$, 88 per cent; Type II, 71 per cent; $\alpha 1(II)$, 62 per cent; and Type III, 62 per cent. No correlation was found between the stage of disease, or titres of rheumatoid factor or antinuclear antibodies (ANA), and the incidence and/or titres of antibody to any given type of collagen. Subsequent studies by the same group (Andriopoulos et al, 1976a) indicated that the greatest incidence and highest titres of antibodies to Types I and II collagens occurred in rheumatic joint fluids. The titres for all three types of collagens were lower in corresponding sera than in joint fluids. A similar pattern was observed when denatured chains from the respective collagens were used as the test antigen. Moreover, in each case titres for denatured chains were higher than those for the native collagens. Synovial fluids, but not sera, from three osteoarthritic patients contained antibodies to collagen chains. Patients with other non-rheumatic diseases possessed no anticollagen antibodies. Trentham et al (1978c) have obtained similar results by investigating the sera of 50 patients with rheumatoid arthritis. Immunochemical studies on the autoantibodies to collagen in rheumatoid arthritis have shown the latter to be specific with regard to the collagen type and the collagen chain (Andriopoulos et al, 1978c). Absorption of both sera and synovial fluids with a given type of native collagen abolished the antibody activity directed against that collagen, but did not remove antibody activity directed against the other collagen types, nor the component chains. A similar specificity of antibodies for certain collagen chains was also demonstrated. Furthermore, it was indicated in these studies that the antibodies under investigation belonged to both IgG and IgM classes.

In contrast, Menzel et al (1978) have performed a radioimmunoassay with ^{14}C-labelled collagen, in which the radioactive label appears evenly distributed along the α chains. In this investigation on rheumatoid synovial fluid, they reported that antibodies to denatured type I collagen cross-reacted with native type I and also that antibodies to $\alpha 1(III)$ chains strongly cross-reacted with type I. These results could be explained by possible contamination of the native type I collagen preparation with denatured collagen, as well as an incomplete separation of type I and III collagen molecules during the purification process.

The origin of the antibodies against collagen appears to be the plasma cells of the immunopathologically-affected synovial membrane. As outlined above, the titres of antibodies to the different collagens are higher in the synovial fluids than in the corresponding sera. In addition, antibodies to type I collagen have been directly eluted from rheumatoid synovial membranes (Cracchiolo et al, 1975). In other studies, Mestecky & Miller (1975) have indicated that inflammed synovial membranes from selected rheumatoid arthritis patients revealed a distribution of rhodamine-labelled type II collagen resembling largely the tissue localization of immunoglobulins IgG and IgM. Therefore, the immunoglobulins might be, at least in part, synthesized by a local synovial immune response. They could not, however, demonstrate the binding of labelled type I collagen which might be interpreted as binding of the antibodies against type I to the collagen type I of synovial tissue; thus, they may be unavailable for binding of labelled exogenous collagen type I. On the other hand, the presence of collagen-anticollagen immune complexes in rheumatoid arthritis fluids (Menzel et al, 1976) might interfere with type I collagen binding. What is apparent is that collagen types I, II, and III (Gay & Remberger, 1976), as well as type IV and V, occur in rheumatoid synovial exudate cells, most likely released during the proteolytic disease process (Fig. 15.3). This conclusion is supported by the presence of these different collagens within the cells frequently associated with immunoglobulins and complement components (Gay et al, 1980b; Steffen et al, 1974).

It is of considerable interest that antibodies to type I collagen have also been observed in body fluids of patients with Felty's syndrome, Sjögren's syndrome, psoriatic arthritis, lupus erythematosus, and scleroderma as reviewed recently by Mestecky et al (1979). Some controversy exists about the presence of antibodies with low titres to native and denatured collagen in synovial fluids of patients with traumatic synovitis (Cracchiolo et al, 1975), which could not be found by Andriopoulos et al (1976a) and Menzel et al (1978).

More recent studies by Huffstutter et al (1979) of sera and synovial fluids from patients with a variety of joint diseases have suggested that in addition to antibodies against collagen type I, II, and III, there occurs antibodies against native collagen type IV and V as well as their component chains. The latter finding appears to be of some interest, since type V collagen occurs in the exocytoskeleton of connective tissue cells (Gay et al, 1980c). In general, the antibodies to denatured collagen were more frequent and at higher levels than antibodies to native collagen. Levels of antibodies were also higher in synovial fluid than in the serum. In this study, the $\alpha 2(I)$ chain seemed to be the most immunogenic agent, although antibodies to denatured type II collagen were found also at high levels in degenerative joint disease, gout, and other joint diseases. Based on these results, it was concluded that collagen antibodies can be correlated with the presence of inflammatory arthritis regardless of particular diagnosis.

It should be noted that the presence of antibodies to collagen is not restricted to patients with joint disease. Antibodies to native type I collagen have been detected by

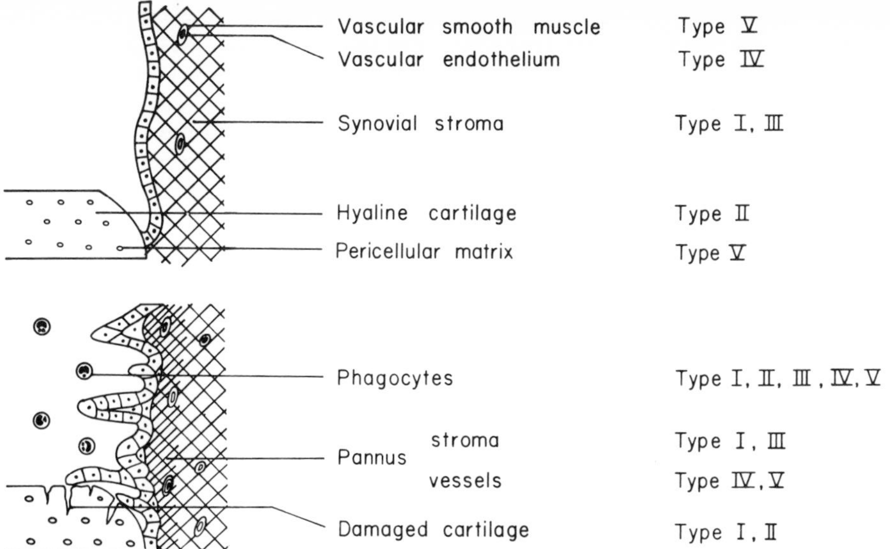

Fig. 15.3 Collagen types in normal and rheumatic joints (after Gay & Miller, 1980).

passive haemagglutination in 44 per cent of the sera of patients with selective IgA deficiency (Wells et al, 1973). In other studies, 70 per cent of the 422 patients with lung emphysema were found to have IgG antibodies to denatured type I collagen, particularly to α2(I)-CB3 (Michaeli & Fudenberg, 1974b). In this latter example, presence of antibodies could reflect the destruction of pulmonary connective tissue. In subsequent investigations by the same group antibodies to denatured type I collagen were detected in the serum of leprosy patients from two different geographical areas of Papua, New Guinea (McAdam et al, 1978). In highland patients, the prevalence of significant titres varied according to the clinical spectrum of leprosy. There was a remarkable difference from high prevalence (53 per cent) in the immunodeficient polar lepromatous patients to a low prevalence (9 per cent) at the turberculoid end of the clinical spectrum. A similar gradient was not observed in coastal patients, who had a higher overall prevalence of antibodies (53 per cent).

Foidart et al (1978) have performed an interesting study using the sera of patients with relapsing polychondritis. In the sera of 5 of 15 patients they detected antibodies directed exclusively against native type II collagen, with only little activity against α1(II) chains and none at all to cartilage proteoglycan or to other collagen types. The antibodies were found only in the acute phase of the disease. Prednisone therapy resulted in both clinical improvement and decreases in antibody titres. The occurrence of the antibodies to native type II collagen appeared almost completely restricted to relapsing polychondritis, since similar antibodies were detected in only 1 of 92 patients with other arthritic diseases. It is concluded that in the case of polychondritis, the formation of antibody to native type II collagen may be a primary event in the pathogenesis of the disease, unlike rheumatoid arthritis in which such antibody formation may represent a consequence of the initial inflammatory disease process.

The demonstration of antibodies directed against basement membrane collagen type IV, but not against type I, II, III, and V collagen, has been detected in the sera of six patients with a dominant form of epidermolysis bullosa (Gay et al, 1980d). The type IV collagen had been prepared from human placenta (Kresina & Miller, 1979) and bovine lens capsule (Gay & Miller, 1979) and had been shown to be derived from basement membrane structures (Gay et al, 1979). The presence of this antibody suggests that alterations in the basement membrane itself might be responsible for the loss of union between the basal cells of the epidermis and the underlying basement membrane which leads to the clinical manifestations of the bullous lesion. In contrast, sera of patients with bullous pemphigus, which contain antibodies against basement membranes as judged by immunofluorescence assays, do not have antibodies against type IV collagen. These data indicate that the bullous pemphigus antibody is directed against a noncollagenous basement membrane component (Gay et al, 1980d), which might also be a substantial constituent of a human skin tumour, the cylindroma (Wick et al, 1979b). This tumour may provide an optimal tissue for the isolation and identification of antigens reactive with antibodies to noncollagenous basement membrane components. The production of antibodies against noncollagenous components of basement membranes is not an isolated case. In sera from patients with Goodpasture syndrome, the use of immunohistology indicates antibodies to basement membranes of glomeruli and lung alveoli. However, it could be shown that the antibodies are not directed against basement membrane type IV collagen

(Wick et al, 1979a). Similarly, sera from patients with coeliac disease show autoantibodies to so-called reticulin by indirect immunofluorescence. These antibodies, however, fail to react with type III collagen, the major collagenous component of 'reticulin' fibres (Timpl et al, 1977). The results discussed above reinforce the fact that unless appropriate detection methods are applied, the presence of autoantibodies to different collagens might be incorrectly concluded.

Last, but not least, it is of considerable clinical interest whether collagen of collagen transplants in humans are immunologically inert (for review see Chvapil et al, 1973; Stenzel et al, 1974). At present, no significant information is available about immunopathological complications of such uses.

CELLULAR IMMUNITY AGAINST COLLAGEN

Cell-mediated immune reactions differ from the humoral immune reactions both in the nature of the immunological response and the mediator cells responsible. While the humoral response to antigenic stimulation is the production of circulating antibody by differentiated B-cell lymphocytes (bone marrow-derived), the principle mediators in cell-mediated immune reactions are specific T-cell lymphocytes (thymus-derived) (see Fudenberg et al, 1978). Upon antigenic stimulation, T-cell lymphocytes secrete soluble products called lymphokines (Table 15.4), which are responsible for the multiple effects of cellular immune reactions. The significance of cellular immunity to collagen can be related to various cell-mediated immune responses including delayed-type hypersensitivity, rejection of allographs, and autoimmune diseases.

Table 15.4 Factors (lymphokines) released from activated lymphocytes

Macrophage migration inhibition factor (MIF)
Macrophage activation factor (MAF)
Macrophage chemotactic factor
Leucocyte chemotactic factor
Leucocyte inhibition factor (LIF)
Lymphocyte mitogenic factor
Antibody production factors
Transfer factor
Lymphotoxin
Skin reactive factor
Osteoclast-activating factor (OAF)
Interferon

Delayed-type hypersensitivity

Cell-mediated immunity to native collagen molecules was initially described by Steffen (1965), who observed a positive skin reaction in guinea pigs on the sixteenth day after immunization with calf or guinea pig collagen in complete Freund's adjuvant. Subsequently, Adelmann et al (1972) showed an analogous response in guinea pigs utilizing a similar immunization regimen with native type I collagen extracted from the skins of normal calves, rats, and guinea pigs, as well as lathyritic rats. In this latter study, the animals were sensitized with 500μg of calf skin collagen or 1000 μg guinea pig skin collagen in complete Freund's adjuvant. Three weeks later the animals were challenged with either 150 μg calf or 100 μg guinea pig skin collagen in saline. A cutaneous reaction of erythema and swelling slowly appeared in the dermis of the guinea pigs sensitized and challenged with calf type I collagen. The immunological response reached maximum between 24 and 36 hours after the second injection and then gradually subsided. However, the sensitized period was shown to last at least 3 months. Skin biopsies from the reaction sites exhibited an infiltration of mononuclear cells. These data characterize the classical delayed-type hypersensitivity reaction. It is of interest to note that humoral antibody titres at the time of challenge with antigen were insignificant, indicating a low level of serum antibodies to native collagen during the delayed hypersensitivity reaction. The immunological reaction was also species specific, in that the most severe cutaneous inflammatory reaction occurred when the immunizing and challenging antigens were identical. However, guinea pigs immunized and/or challenged with guinea pig skin collagen gave no cutaneous reaction indicative of cell-mediated immunity to 'self' collagens.

Reactivity of type I collagen α chains of rat and calf skin in the cutaneous delayed-hypersensitivity reaction has also been reported by Adelmann (1972). In these experiments, immunization and challenge with denatured type I collagen or isolated collagen α chains resulted in cutaneous reactions exhibiting the typical features of cutaneous delayed hypersensitivity. This immunological reaction was shown to be both species and chain specific in that the maximum erythema and swelling occurred when the antigen utilized for immunization and challenge was identical. Qualitatively, these results were indistinguishable from the previous experiments utilizing native calf type I collagen as antigen.

Further studies by Adelmann (1973) probed the conformational specificity of the cutaneous delayed hypersensitivity reaction. These studies suggested that appropriately sensitized animals were capable of recognizing conformational alterations of the antigen. The guinea pigs hypersensitized with native collagen distinguished native molecules from constituent polypeptide α chains, as demonstrated by a higher index of skin reaction. In contrast, animals immunized with denatured collagen produced a maximum cutaneous delayed-type hypersensitivity reaction when challenged with denatured collagen. These data suggested that denatured chains of type I collagen results in both the loss of helical antigenic determinants and the exposure of new antigenic determinants.

The importance of the helical versus the nonhelical regions of the collagen molecule in the induction of cell-mediated immunity has been investigated (Adelmann & Kirrane, 1973). Utilizing both pepsin-treated and neutral salt-extracted or acid soluble type I collagen as the sensitizing and challenging antigen, no difference has been observed in the degree of inflammation or species specificity of the delayed-type hypersensitivity reaction. These data indicated that the antigenic determinants of the type I collagen molecule recognized by the reacting T-cell lymphocytes were located in the central or helical domain of the collagen molecule and not in the nonhelical regions.

Other studies (Senyk & Michaeli, 1973) have associated cutaneous cell-mediated hypersensitivity and autoimmunity. The results of these studies suggest that guinea pigs possess cells (T-cells) capable of recognizing autoantigens and that both a cell-mediated immune response and tolerance could be produced to 'self' collagen. In these studies normal guinea pigs exhibited no pre-existing cellular immunity to 'self' collagen or to related human or mouse collagens. However, when these guinea pigs were immunized with 1000 μg of human type I collagen in complete Freund's adjuvant and subsequently sensitized with the same antigen, a cellular immune reaction to human skin collagen, as well as guinea pig skin collagen could be generated. Further, when guinea pigs were immunized with their own collagen in complete Freund's adjuvant, the animals developed a cellular immune response upon challenge with the autoantigen. These data, with regard to cellular immunity to autoantigens, conflict with results of the studies by Adelmann et al (1973). A possible explanation for the discrepancy may reside in the purity of the antigenic preparations or the different genotypes of the animals used.

More recently, the studies of Gentner & Adelmann (1976a, b) have shown that animals preimmunized with native collagen in Freund's incomplete adjuvant can elicit a partially-suppressed cutaneous delayed-type hypersensitivity reaction when animals are sensitized and challenged with the appropriate antigen. The circulating humoral antibodies to collagen, induced by the preimmunization, were shown not to be the suppressive agents. The humoral antibody titres, as judged by passive haemagglutination, did not correlate with the degree of suppression, nor did passive transfer of anticollagen Type I antibodies from animals with suppressed skin reactivity affect the degree of cutaneous delayed-type hypersensitivity in animals made hypersensitive to collagen by conventional techniques. The immunologically-suppressed animals were subsequently shown to respond to skin reactive factor, a lymphokine, suggesting a specific suppression to collagen. In addition, lymphocytes from animals with induced delayed-type hypersensitivity functioned normally in animals with suppressed skin reactivity. Furthermore, the lymphoid cells from animals with suppressed delayed-hypersensitivity passively transferred the suppression to neutral recipients. It was concluded, therefore, that induction of a humoral antibody response to collagen impairs the function of T-cells activated in the cutaneous delayed-type hypersensitivity reaction.

The data presented above represent a preliminary stage in the investigation of cutaneous cell-mediated, delayed-type hypersensitivity to type I collagen (for data relating cell-mediated immunity to other collagen types, see below). Many points still remain to be elucidated, including the identification of the antigenic determinants in both native and denatured collagen, the subpopulation of T-cells activated in the immune response, the mechanisms of T-cell recognition of antigenic collagen, and the subsequent binding to the collagen molecule.

Cell-mediated immunity to collagen in diseases

Although the aetiology of many diseases involving the connective tissue components are unknown, in certain pathological cases data have been accumulated which suggest a relationship between cell-mediated immunity and collagen.

In the pathogenesis of rheumatoid arthritis a relatively large body of data has accumulated indicating cell-mediated immunity to various collagen types. Early studies of arthritic patients demonstrated the presence of an immune response to different connective tissue components which is characteristic of cell-mediated immunity. For example, lymph-node cells from patients with rheumatoid arthritis were shown to have a destructive effect on amnion cells in vitro (Braunsteiner et al, 1964). Subsequent studies with joint-fluid of arthritic patients showed the presence of mononuclear cells which were cytotoxic to fibroblasts in vitro (Hedberg, 1967). Recent studies have produced evidence which supports the concept that a cellular-mediated immune response provokes at least some of the synovial inflammation accompanying rheumatoid arthritis (for review see Panayi & Johnson, 1979). These studies have reported both the cellular infiltration of rheumatoid synovial membrane, predominantly by T-cell lymphocytes, and the production of lymphokines. These studies, however, failed to identify the antigen(s) responsible for the cellular sensitivity.

Subsequent experiments have tried to elucidate the inducers of the cellular immune response in rheumatoid arthritis. Intra-articular injections of hyaline cartilage shavings (containing impure type II collagen) produced a delayed-type hypersensitivity reaction to hyaline cartilage (Langer et al, 1972). Recent studies by Trentham et al (1977, 1978a, b) and Stuart et al (1979) have shown an induction of arthritis in rats utilizing intradermal injections of various preparations of type II collagen. Purified native type II collagen derived from autologous (rat) of heterologous (human and chicken) cartilage, emulsified in complete or incomplete Freund's adjuvant induced an experimental arthritis in approximately 40 per cent of various strains of rats. In this animal model of arthritis numerous other related molecules were found not to be arthritogenic, including native type I and type III collagen, the denatured chains from type I, II, and III collagens, as well as cartilage-derived proteoglycans. Native type II collagen without Freund's adjuvant was also ineffective in inducing arthritis. Thus, only the native type II collagen combined with adjuvant incudes arthritis indicating that the helical portion of the collagen molecule, but not the individual $\alpha 1(II)$ chains, contains the necessary antigenic determinant(s). In this regard, it should be considered that the preparation of native type II collagen may contain contaminants responsible for the arthritogenic reaction which have been removed by the isolation and purification of the single $\alpha 1(II)$ chains.

The type II collagen-induced arthritis in rats develops as early as the second week after the initial injection of antigen. Histologically, the disease is characterized by oedema, synovitis with synovial hypertrophy and infiltration by mononuclear cells as well as erosion and damage of articular hyaline cartilage. In addition, cell-mediated immunity, measured by the incorporation of radioactive thymidine into lymphocytes, was significantly elevated in arthritic rats. Moreover, the arthritis could be passively transferred to normal rats by pooled spleen and lymph node cells. In contrast, intraveneous injection of sera from arthritic donors was incapable of passively transferring the clinical and histological features of the arthritis. Also, arthritis could not be induced in animals by injecting killed cells, cells from nonimmunized rats, cells from rats immunized with type I collagen, or cells from donors injected only with complete Freund's adjuvant. Infusion of unsensitized cells along with soluble type II collagen was also not arthritogenic. The demonstration of passively transferable arthritis by injection of viable cells from rats immunized with native type II collagen, but not by application of a rat sera containing antibodies against the collagen, suggests that a cell-mediated immunity to the preparation of type II collagen may be of greater importance than the humoral immune response.

Recent studies by Courtenay et al (1980) have also used type II collagen for the induction of a similar arthritis in certain strains of mice. There are differences in the pathological characteristics of the disease between the rat and the mouse. In rats the disease is initiated earlier and can be induced with type II collagen emulsified with incomplete Freund's adjuvant. The mice responded less to the use of incomplete adjuvant and certain strains did not develop arthritis with the identical immunization schedule. The latter result might be clarified in light of the findings by Nowack et al (1975b), who demonstrated that the immune response to the helical antigenic determinants of the type II collagen molecule differs considerably among certain strains of inbred mice.

In other animal studies, cell-mediated immunity to type II collagen has been shown not to be conformationally dependent. To illustrate this point, both native and denatured type II collagen induced a cutaneous delayed-type hypersensitivity reaction in guinea pigs, previously hyperimmunized with cartilage collagen (Beard et al, 1978). In addition, cell-mediated immune responses could be elicited with type II collagen CNBr peptides, 8, 9, 10, and 12 suggesting that the antigenic sites of the type II collagen molecule are located in the central region of the collagen chain. Nevertheless, it should be noted at this point that a significant humoral antibody response to native, but not denatured type II collagen was observed in most of these animal studies. Therefore it would be inappropriate to conclude that tissue inflammation and damage was totally a result of the cell-mediated immune response to collagen.

It should be acknowledged at this point that the experimental studies on type II collagen induced arthritis in animals cannot be directly correlated with the pathogenesis of rheumatoid arthritis in humans. There is currently no available evidence that the human disease is initiated by exposure to autologous native type II collagen in a soluble form, nor is there evidence for the presence of substances which could act as adjuvants. It appears more likely that the development of cellular immunity to type II collagen in humans is a consequence of the pathophysiological alterations in cartilage which subsequently lead to an immune response and, thereby, contribute to the chronicity of the pathological process. Recently several studies have tried to determine whether a cellular immune response to the different collagens is present in patients with classically-defined rheumatoid arthritis. Trentham et al (1978c) examined patients for cellular sensitivity to human type I, II, and III collagens by utilizing in vitro assays for measuring antigen-induced lymphokines and ^{3}H-labelled thymidine incorporation by lymphocytes. Blood monocytes from individuals with rheumatoid arthritis could be induced in vitro to incorporate ^{3}H-thymidine and to synthesize lymphokines by incubation with type II and type III collagens. The data also suggested that the cellular response to both native type II and type III collagens correlated with the activity of the disease. Additional data (Endler et al, 1978) show that blood leucocytes from individuals with rheumatoid arthritis respond strongly to native type III collagen and only weakly to native type I collagen, as measured by lymphokine production. In other studies, Stuart et al (1979) have shown that peripheral blood leucocytes from patients with rheumatoid arthritis produce chemotactic activity on exposure to native and denatured collagen types I, II, and

III. Concurrently, Smolen et al (1980) have found that 58 per cent of the patients with rheumatoid arthritis who were studied, possessed blood lymphocytes that could be stimulated in vitro by denatured type I collagen. These authors suggest that type I collagen is at least as good an arthritogen as collagen types II and III.

The results of these studies, taken collectively, indicate that type I and type III collagen which comprise the synovial membrane as well as type II collagen, a constituent of cartilage, may, as a consequence of initial tissue alteration, elicit a cell-mediated immune response. This immune response warrants further investigation to assess the role of the distinct collagens in maintaining the diseased states.

Another disease in which a cell-mediated immune response to collagen has been implicated as a causal agent is pulmonary fibrosis (Kravis et al, 1976). In this condition, several histological features such as derangement of parenchymal collagen fibrils and infiltration of the involved tissue with chronic inflammatory cells have suggested a cell-mediated immune response. To test this possibility more directly, peripheral blood lymphocytes from patients exhibiting clinical features of fibrotic lung disease were exposed to human type I collagen in vitro and evaluated for their production of lymphokines. Ninety-four per cent of the cell cultures were positive for recognition of type I collagen, as assayed by the production of migration inhibition factor as well as lysis of collagen-coated sheep red blood cells. These in vitro observations suggest that T-cell lymphocytes and type I collagen may be intimately associated in the pathogenesis of human pulmonary fibrosis.

Some evidence for cell-mediated immunity to collagen in progressive systemic sclerosis has come from the work of Stuart et al (1976). Their study showed that peripheral blood leucocytes from patients demonstrating the clinical features of progressive systemic sclerosis produce a lymphokine when incubated in culture with normal human skin collagen (type I) or lathyritic chick skin collagen (type I). Other studies have shown that tissue specimens from progressive systemic sclerosis contain large infiltrates of mononuclear cells, often associated with abnormal collagen deposition and abnormal arrangement of collagen fibrils (Fleischmajer et al, 1978; Gay et al, 1980a). These data taken collectively may suggest that some cell-mediated immunity against collagen is possibly involved in the pathogenesis of scleroderma.

In summary, it can be concluded from the preceding studies with regard to cell-mediated immunity and the involvement of collagens that the various interstitial collagens distributed throughout the body may at some point participate in an immune response which may perpetuate some pathological conditions. Conclusive data, however, must still be obtained in order to firmly establish the validity of this hypothesis.

Genetic regulation of the immune response to collagen

It is now generally accepted that a large number of specific immune response genes are responsible for controlling the response of an individual to a variety of antigens (for review see Bellanti, 1978). With regard to cell-mediated immunity, the main recognizible T-cell-dependent antigenic determinants are termed lymphocyte-defined (LD). In mice these are associated with the products of the I region and in humans with the leucocyte antigen (HLA) D region of the major histocompatibility complex (MHC) (see Fig' 15.4). In mice the I region encodes for a portion of the specific antigenic receptors on T-cell lymphocytes, as well as for other specific receptors found on the surface of T- and B-cells and subpopulations of macrophages. This latter group of interacting molecules are termed the Ia or I region-associated molecules (for review see McDevitt & Landy, 1972). Utilizing antisera directed against the molecules coded by the I region, it has been shown that the I region genes regulate such functions as the genetic control of specific immune responses, graft versus host reactions, regulation of immune suppression, and regulation of the interaction between B-lymphocytes and T-lymphocytes and macrophages.

To date, the available data suggest that the immune response to type I collagen is genetically-controlled. Experiments by Hahn et al (1975), utilizing congenic strains of mice, provide evidence that the immune responsiveness to collagen as expressed by humoral antibody production, is associated with the major histocompatibility complex H-2. Immunization of inbred strains of mice with calf skin type I collagen over a broad range of antigenic concentrations resulted in the demonstration of high responder H-2 haplotypes and low responder H-2 haplotypes. Studies with off-spring of the backcross between F_1hybrids and low responder haplotypes indicated that the immune response to collagen is controlled by an autosomal dominant gene closely linked to the H-2 locus. Interestingly, this control was not demonstrated by inbred animals immunized with procollagen; since all strains which were low responders to native type I collagen molecules became high responders upon immunization with procollagen. These data can be interpreted to suggest that the procollagen extension peptides are recognized to a greater degree by T-cell lymphocytes than the helical domains of the collagen molecule. Therefore, the extension peptides can act as potent inducers of B- and T-cell interactions which lead to a high production of antibodies of plasma cells.

In further studies (Nowack et al, 1975a) demonstrated that the immune response to calf skin type I collagen in congenic strains of mice is governed by at least two genes. Apparently, one gene is not linked to the H-2 locus and probably is expressed in the immune response at the level of macrophage processing (for review see Staines, 1979).

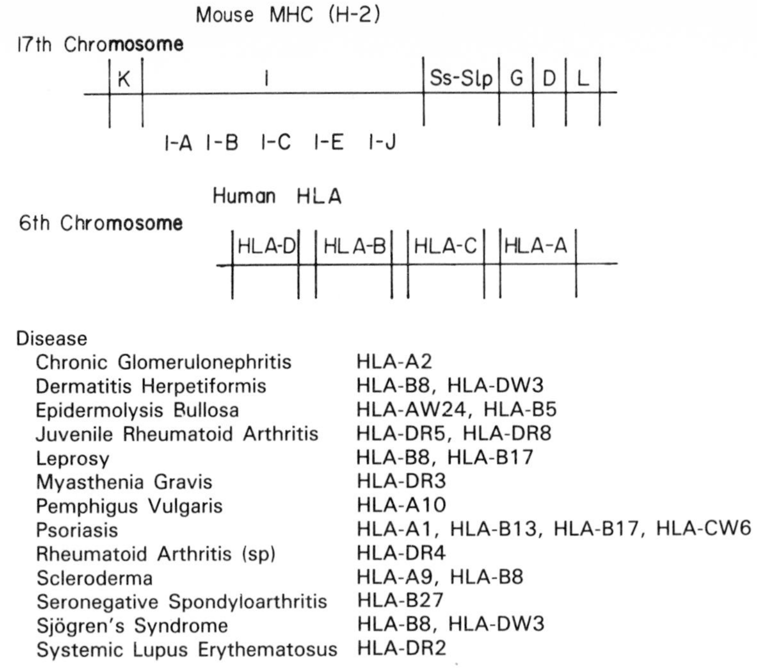

Fig. 15.4 The major histocompatibility complexes and associated diseases.

The other gene is located within the I region, in the Ia subregion, of the H-2. The data also suggest that Ia gene controls the immune response at the T-cell level, i.e. immunization with the 'carrier' procollagen transforms the haplotypes which are low responders to collagen into high responders.

Additional studies using procollagen as an immunogen in congenic, recombinant strains of mice as well as backcross populations, have shown that the immune response to this molecule is under the control of a gene located in the I region (Ia and/or Ib subregion) of the H-2 complex (Nowack et al, 1977). The immune response was also shown to be T-cell dependent since athymic mice failed to produce antibody upon immunization with procollagen.

To date virtually no data are available regarding the genetic control of the immune response to collagen types other than type I. However, data obtained by Nowack et al (1975b) indicate that there probably is also genetic control of the antigenic response to type II collagen. They found a significant difference in the immune response to type I and type II collagens in an inbred strain (DBA/IJ) of mice.

In summary, numerous studies have demonstrated specific associations between certain diseases affecting connective tissue components and specific genetic loci in the major histocompatibility complex in humans (Fig. 15.4). However, there is limited information available indicating genetic control of specific collagen types. Extensive work remains to elucidate the mode of action of the I region genes and their association with diseases affecting the collagens.

DEPOSITION OF IMMUNE COMPLEXES IN COLLAGENOUS TISSUE

During the last stages of the humoral response, antibody usually inactivates antigen through the formation of antigen-antibody complexes which are subsequently removed or destroyed by phagocytosis or complement activation. However, the deposition of such circulating immune complexes in tissues, other than the lymphoid tissues, can cause local inflammation and tissue damage.

The formation of these immune complexes in tissues per se does not induce tissue damage. The destruction results from activation of subsequent immunological events. Factors that affect the formation of circulating immune complexes include: (1) the concentration of antigen and antibody; (2) the equilibrium of immune complexes and their component parts; (3) the binding of complement to immune complexes; (4) deposition of immune complexes in situ; and (5) the phagocytosis of the complexes (for review see Barnett et al, 1979). In addition, the fate of circulating immune complexes is affected by their size and composition. The size of the antigen-antibody complex is a function of the relative concentration of antigen to antibody (Fig. 15.5). Small immune complexes, less than 19S which are usually formed in antigen excess, tend to remain in the circulatory system and do not activate the complement cascade to a high degree. Therefore, the smaller immune complexes are less pathogenic than their larger counterparts. Complexes of 19S or greater are generally formed when antibody is in excess or at the equivalence

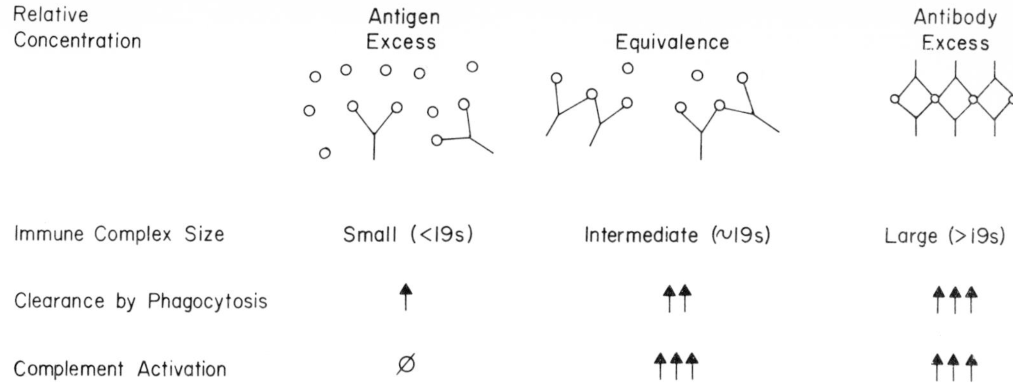

Fig. 15.5 Variables related to the formation of immune complexes by antigen (O) and antibody (Y).

point of antibody and antigen. These tend to be potent pathogens usually being entrapped in vessel walls as well as active agents in complement fixation.

Some major characteristics of immune complexes are the activation of the complement system, fixation to specific tissues, interaction with specific cell types, and release of pathogenic mediators. These molecular and cellular events have formed the basis for establishing methodologies for the detection of immune complexes (Table 15.5).

Certain mechanisms appear to be responsible for the deposition of immune complexes in rheumatoid joint tissues. Studies utilizing intra-articular injection of antigen into previously immunized animals have shown that very few preformed immune complexes are deposited in rheumatoid joint tissues. These studies suggest that the trapping of immune complexes in the joint tissue of preimmunized animals requires several events such as: (1) the presence of the antibody in the extravascular space or cartilage matrix; (2) the diffusion of antigen or soluble complexes into the extravascular space; and (3) the formation of macromolecular, insoluble immune complexes by the interaction of antigen or small immune complexes with extravascular antibody (Jasin, 1975; Teuschner & Donaldson, 1979). In addition, it has been shown that experimentally induced immune complexes can be deposited in rheumatoid-collagenous joint tissues with specific antigen and cross-reactive antibody (Teuschner & Donaldson, 1979) suggesting that structurally similar 'antigenic' proteins possibly augment the localization of immune complexes in situ.

At present, the nature of the antigenic material (altered immunoglobulin?) responsible for the presence of high concentrations of antibody and immune complexes in the synovial fluid of patients with rheumatoid arthritis has not been elucidated. The previous described studies demonstrating antibodies to the various collagens in serum and synovial fluid of arthritic patients present the possibility that at least some of the antigenic material could be collagenous in nature and participate in the formation of immune complexes. In this regard, induction of acute and chronic arthritis in rabbits can be caused by the intra-articular injection of preformed collagen-anticollagen complexes (Steffen et al, 1977; 1978).

Table 15.5 Methods utilized for the detection of immune complexes (Modified after Mannik, 1979)

Technique	*Sensitivity*
Physicochemical	
1. Analytical ultracentrifugation	Relatively insensitive, however, can be coupled with biological assays for further characterization of immune complexes
2. Sucrose gradient ultracentrifugation	
3. Gel filtration	
4. Polyethylene glycol precipitation	
Immunological	
1. Precipitation in gels with C1q or monoclonal rheumatoid factor	generally most assays are highly sensitive, however individual assays range in specificity and cost
2. Precipitation of radiolabelled C1q and immune complexes in polyethylene glycol	
3. C1q deviation test	
4. C1q or conglutinin coated polystyrene tubes	
5. Solid-phase radioimmunoassay	
A. rheumatoid factor bonded to cellulose	
B. aggregated IgG bound to agarose	
6. Platelet aggregation	
7. Raja cell assay	
8. Interaction with macrophage receptors	
9. Histamine release quantified from perfused guinea pig lung preparations	
10. Immunofluorescence	

An additional mechanism of tissue injury in rheumatoid arthritis involves the interaction of lymphocytes with immune complexes. Incubation of immune complexes and lymphocytes from patients with rheumatoid arthritis in vitro, results in the production of certain lymphokines (for review see Stastny et al, 1974). In addition, lymphokine-activated macrophages have been shown to synthesize collagenase, an enzyme important to the degradation of connective tissues (Wahl et al, 1974). Macrophages have also been reported to produce a collagenase-stimulating factor for rheumatoid synovial cells (Dayer et al, 1979; 1980) as well as a prostaglandin-stimulating factor (Dayer et al, 1979). The latter factor is noteworthy since prostaglandins appear to regulate the production of macrophage collagenase (Wahl et al, 1977). Therefore, the stimulation of lymphocytes by immune complexes in situ, resulting in the synthesis and secretion of various lymphokines, mediates numerous biological activities which can lead to tissue destruction and joint erosion.

Nevertheless, it should be noted that collagen by itself may initiate tissue injury. In this regard, type II collagen, the major component of cartilaginous tissues, has been implicated in the release of degradative enzymes from macrophages as well as activation of the alternate pathway of the complement system (Schorlemmer et al, 1979). The exact mechanism of this phenomena remains to be elucidated.

In summary, it can be concluded that two mechanisms are responsible for tissue damage in immune-complex related pathological states (Fig. 15.6). In acute inflammatory reactions, deposited macromolecular immune complexes are absorbed to the predominant cellular infiltrate, the polymorphonuclear leucocytes, through specific immunoglobulin and complement membranes receptors. Subsequently, these cells are activated to phagocytose the immune complexes with concomittant release of lysosomal enzymes (Weissmann, 1977) as well as granulocyte collagenase (see Ch. 8). These enzymes degrade the surrounding connective tissues thereby releasing tissue fragments of a noncollagenous and

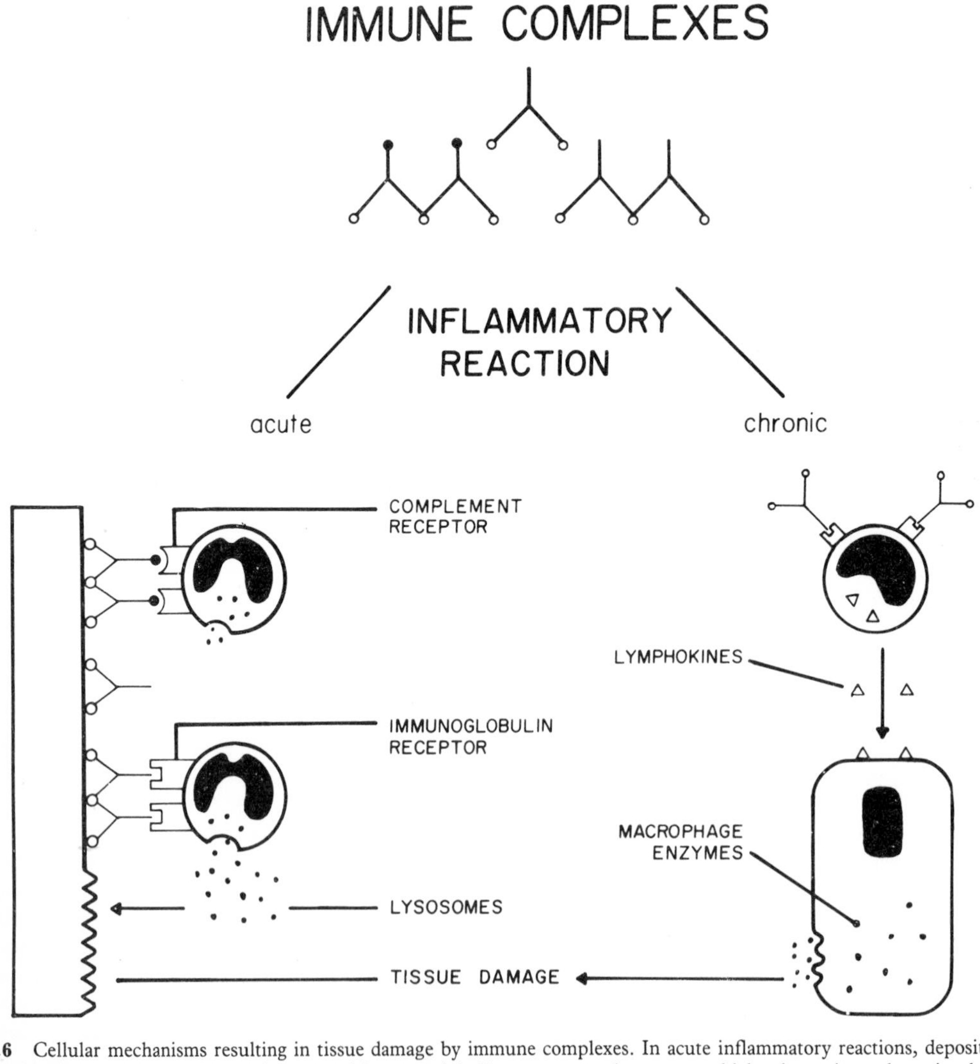

IMMUNE COMPLEXES

INFLAMMATORY REACTION

acute

chronic

COMPLEMENT RECEPTOR

IMMUNOGLOBULIN RECEPTOR

LYSOSOMES

TISSUE DAMAGE

LYMPHOKINES

MACROPHAGE ENZYMES

Fig. 15.6 Cellular mechanisms resulting in tissue damage by immune complexes. In acute inflammatory reactions, deposited immune complexes bind through complement and immunoglobulin receptors to leucocytes which release tissue damaging lysosomal enzymes. In chronic inflammatory reactions, lymphocytes sensitized by immune complexes actively secrete lymphokines, which have numerous local effects including the inhibition of macrophage migration and release of degradative enzymes.

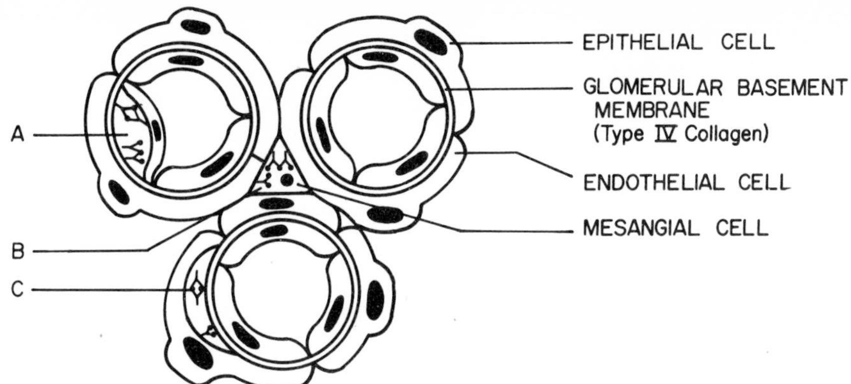

Fig. 15.7 Deposition of immune complexes in subendothelial (A), mesangial (B), and subepithelial (C) glomerular regions.

collagenous nature into the local environment. The continued release of stimulatory material into the surrounding medium results again in complement activation and increased immune complex formation. This persistent immune response transforms the acute legion into a chronic inflammatory state. The major cellular mediators of these chronic lesions, the lymphocyte and macrophage, are specifically sensitized and contribute to tissue destruction. The lymphocyte population is most likely sensitized by high concentrations of immune complexes, thereby releasing numerous lymphokines into the inflammed areas. The major results of these mediators, in general, would be increased immunoglobulin synthesis as well as increased number of macrophages. The subsequent induction of synthesis of macrophage collagenase by specific lymphokines would consequently increase the breakdown of the local collagenous tissue, adding additional antigenic material and increasing the response of the cellular constituents.

Immune complexes and specific biochemical aspects of collagen have been implicated in the pathogenesis of other chronic inflammatory diseases.

In systemic lupus erythematosus, the status of cell-mediated immunity and cellular sensitization to nuclear antigens as well as other antigens is a subject of controversy (Provost, 1979; Raveche & Steinberg, 1979). It is generally known that individuals with systemic lupus erythematosus develop antibodies directed against several autoantigens. It has also been reported that immune complexes comprised of DNA and anti-DNA antibody are the major component of the immune complexes localized in the kidney and skin (Koffler et al, 1977). Based on these data and the observation that DNA can efficiently bind to isolated glomerular basement membrane (containing type IV collagen) as well as other structures containing collagen, Izui et al (1976) have suggested that collagen-bound DNA reacts with anti-DNA antibody thereby forming immune complexes which become localized in adjacent collagenous structures. These authors suggest that the systemic manifestations of systemic lupus erythematosus are at least partially related to the widespread distribution of collagenous structures in the body.

In progressive systemic sclerosis, a disease characterized by collagen accumulation in connective tissues (Rodnan, 1979), the presence of immune complexes has been observed in the kidney. McGiven et al (1971) and McCoy et al (1976) have shown IgM and complement in scleroderma renal lesions as well as antinuclear antibody and anti-immunoglobulin activity in kidney eluates. These data, as well as the previous discussion relating a cell-mediated immune response to collagen in progressive systemic sclerosis (see p. 279), suggest an interrelationship between collagen metabolism and immune response. Recent studies utilizing normal lymphocytes and fibroblasts have supported this interrelationship. Antigen-activated T-lymphocytes have been proposed as stimulators of both collagen synthesis and of the in vitro proliferation of fibroblasts (Wahl et al, 1978). In addition, supernatants of activated lymphocyte cultures have been reported to enhance collagen accumulation by human lung fibroblasts (Johnson & Ziff, 1976). In other studies, a still uncharacterized serum factor from patients with progressive systemic sclerosis has also been shown to stimulate collagen accumulation by fibroblasts in vitro (Keyser et al, 1979). Therefore, serum factors regulating collagen biosynthesis as well as a cell-mediated immune response to collagen could probably be involved in the pathogenesis of progressive systemic sclerosis.

Two major forms of immunologically-induced glomerular diseases have been ascertained: antiglomerular basement membrane nephritis and immune complex glomerulonephritis (McCluskey, 1978). In antiglomerular basement membrane nephritis, glomerular injury is initiated by antibodies directed against an antigen localized in the basement membrane. This chemically uncharacterized antigen may be an actual constituent of the basement membrane which contains type IV collagen and other noncollagenous components. Alternatively, the antigen could be a 'foreign' substance lodged in the membrane. In either case, autoantibodies to glomerular basement membrane are generated in the host resulting in a deposition of immunoglobulin and complement along the basement membrane with subsequent tissue damage. On the other hand, immune complex glomerulonephritis is thought to be a pathological manifestation, resulting from a local deposition of immune complexes within the glomeruli (Fig. 15.7). In this case the immune complexes usually contain antigens of nonglomerular origin. The factors accounting for the localization of immune complexes on basement membranes of the kidney are not well established. However, the membrane structure, subject to a high pressure gradient during filtration, is certainly an important factor. Whether the different collagens of the basement membranes and the mesangium contribute to the trapping of immune complexes remains to be elucidated.

ACKNOWLEDGEMENTS

We are most grateful to Ms Julie Sanders for the illustrations and for typing, and Drs Donald K. Furuto, Thomas Linsenmajer, Dov Michaeli, Edward J. Miller, and R. Kent Rhodes for constructive and critical reviews.

REFERENCES

Adelmann B C 1972 The structural basis of cell-mediated immunological reactions of collagen. Reactivity of separated α chains of calf and rat collagen in cutaneous delayed hypersensitivity reactions. Immunology 23: 739

Adelmann B C 1973 The structural basis of cell-mediated immunological reactions of collagen. Recognition by the cutaneous delayed hypersensitivity reaction in guinea-pigs of conformational alterations of rat and calf skin collagen. Immunology 24: 871

Adelmann B C, Gentner G J, Hopper K 1973 A sensitive radioimmunoassay for collagen. Journal of Immunological Methods 3: 319

Adelmann B C, Kirrane J 1973 The structural basis of cell-mediated immunological reactions of collagen. The species specificity of the cutaneous delayed hypersensitivity reaction. Immunology 25: 123

Adelmann B C, Kirrane J A, Glynn L E 1972 The structural basis of cell-mediated immunological reactions of collagen. Characteristics of cutaneous delayed hypersensitivity reactions in specifically sensitized guinea-pigs. Immunology 23: 723

Andriopoulos N A, Mestecky J, Miller E J, Bennett J C 1976a Antibodies to human native and denatured collagens in synovial fluids of patients with rheumatoid arthritis. Clinical Immunology and Immunopathology 6: 209

Andriopoulos N A, Mestecky J, Miller E J, Bradley E L 1976b Antibodies to native and denatured collagens in sera of patients with rheumatoid arthritis. Arthritis and Rheumatism 19: 613

Andriopoulos N A, Mestecky J, Wright G P, Miller E J 1976c Characterization of antibodies to the native human collagens and to their component α chains in the sera and the joint fluids of patients with rheumatoid arthritis. Immunochemistry 13: 709

Barnett E V, Knutson D W, Abrass C K, Chia D S, Young L S, Liebling M R 1979 Circulating immune complexes: their immunochemistry, detection, and importance. Annals of Internal Medicine 91: 430

Beard H K, Faulk W P, Conochie L B, Glynn L E 1977 Some immunological aspects of collagen. Progress in Allergy 22: 45

Beard H K, Ueda M, Faulk W P, Glynn L E 1978 Cell-mediated and humoral immunity to chick type II collagen and its cyanogen bromide peptides in guinea-pigs. Immunology 34: 323

Beil W, Furthmayr H, Timpl R 1972 Chicken antibodies to soluble rat collagen. I. Characterization of the immune response by precipitation and agglutination methods. Immunochemistry 9: 779

Beil W, Timpl R, Furthmayr H 1973 Conformation dependence of antigenic determinants on the collagen molecule. Immunology 24: 13

Bellanti J A (ed) 1978 Immunology II. W B Saunders, Philadelphia

Braunsteiner H, Dienstle F, Eibl M 1964 Destructive effect of lymph node cells from patients with rheumatoid arthritis in tissue culture. Acta Haematologica 31: 225

Bray J P, Estess F, Bass J A 1969 Anticollagen antibodies following thermal trauma. Proceeding of the Society of Experimental Biology and Medicine 130: 394

Bywaters E G L 1976 The historical evolution of the concept of connective tissue diseases. Scandinavian Journal of Rheumatology 5: (Supplement 12) 11

Chvapil M, Kronenthal R L, van Winckle W 1973 Medical and surgical applications of collagen. International Review of Connective Tissue Research 6: 1

Clague R B, Brown R A, Weiss J B, Lennox Holt P J 1979 Solid-phase radioimmunoassay for the detection of antibodies to collagen. Journal of Immunological Methods 27: 31

Courtenay J S, Dallman M J, Dayan A D, Martin A, Mosedale B 1980 Immunisation against heterologous type II collagen induces arthritis in mice. Nature 283: 666

Cracchiolo A III, Michaeli D, Goldberg L S, Fudenberg H H 1975 The occurrence of antibodies to collagen in synovial fluids. Clinical Immunology and Immunopathology 3: 567

Davidson P F, Levine L, Drake M P, Rubin A, Bump S 1967 The serologic specificity of tropocollagen telopeptides. Journal of Experimental Medicine 126: 331

Dayer J M, Breard J, Chess L, Krane S M 1979 Participation of monocyte-macrophages and lymphocytes in the production of a factor that stimulated collagenase and prostaglandin release by rheumatoid synovial cells. Journal of Clinical Investigation 64: 1386

Dayer J M, Passwell J H, Schneeberger E E, Krane S M 1980 Interactions among rheumatoid synovial cells and monocyte-macrophages: Production of collagenase-stimulating factor by human monocytes exposed to concavalin A or immunoglobulin Fc fragments. Journal of Immunology 124: 1712

Dessau W, Adelmann B C, Timpl R, Martin G R 1978a Identification of the sites in collagen α-chains that bind serum anti-gelatin factor (cold-insoluble globulin). Biochemical Journal 169: 55

Dessau W, Adelmann B C, Hörmann H 1978b Similarity of antigelatin factor and cold insoluble globulin. Biochimica et Biophysica Acta 533: 227

Duksin D, Maoz A, Fuchs S 1975 Differential cytotoxic activity of anticollagen serum on rat osteoblasts and fibroblasts in tissue culture. Cell 5: 83

Endler A T, Zielinski C, Menzel E J, Smolen J S, Schwägerl W, Endler M, Eberl R, Frank O, Steffen C 1978 Leucocyte migration inhibition with collagen type I and collagen type III in rheumatoid arthritis and degenerative joint diseases. Zeitschrift für Rheumatologie 37: 87

Engle M B, Catchpole H R 1972 Collagen distribution in the rat demonstrated by a specific anti-collagen antiserum. American Journal of Anatomy 134: 23

Engvall E, Ruoslahti E 1977 Binding of soluble form of fibroblast surface protein, fibronectin, to collagen. International Journal of Cancer 20: 1

Engvall E, Ruoslahti E, Miller E J 1978 Affinity of fibronectin to collagens of different genetic types and to fibrinogen. Journal of Experimental Medicine 147: 1584

Fleischmajer R, Gay S, Miegel W N. Perlish J S 1978 Collagen in the cellular and fibrotic stages of scleroderma. Arthritis and Rheumatism 21: 418

Foidart J M, Abe S, Martin G R, Zizig T M, Barnett E V, Lawley T J, Katz S I 1978 Antibodies to type II collagen in relapsing polychondritis. New England Journal of Medicine 299: 1203

Fudenberg H H, Stites D P, Caldwell J L, Wells J V (eds) 1978 Basic & Clinical Immunology. Lange Medical Publications, Los Altos, California

Furthmayr H, Stoltz M, Becker U, Beil W, Timpl R 1972 Chicken antibodies to soluble rat collagen. II. Specificity of the reactions with individual polypeptide chains and cyanogen bromide peptides of collagen. Immunochemistry 9: 789

Furthmayr H, Timpl R 1976 Immunochemistry of collagens and procollagens. International Review of Connective Tissue Research 7: 61

Gay R E, Buckingham R B, Prince R K, Gay S, Rodnan G P, Miller E J 1980a Collagen types synthesized in dermal fibroblast cultures from patients with early progressive systemic sclerosis. Arthritis and Rheumatism 23: 190

Gay S, Gay R, Miller E J 1980b The collagens of the joint. Arthritis and Rheumatism 23: 937

Gay S, Kresina T F, Gay R, Miller E J, Montes L F 1979 Immunohistochemical demonstration of basement membrane collagen in normal human skin and in psoriasis. Journal of Cutaneous Pathology 6: 91

Gay S, Miller E J 1978 Collagen in the physiology and pathology of connective tissue. Gustav Fischer, Stuttgart-New York

Gay S, Miller E J 1979 Characterization of lens capsule collagen: Evidence for the presence of two unique chains in molecules derived from major basement membrane structures. Archives of Biochemistry and Biophysics 198: 370

Gay S, Remberger K 1976 Rheumatoide Arthritis: Immunohistochemische Untersuchungen mit Antikörpern gegen Kollagen Typ I, II and III. Verhandlungen der Duetschen Gesellschaft für Pathologie 60: 290

Gay S, Rhodes R K, Gay R, Miller E J 1981 Collagen molecules comprised of α1(V)-chains (B chains): An apparent localization in the exocytoskeleton. Collagen and Related Research 1: 53

Gay S, Ward W Q, Gay R, Miller E J 1980 Autoantibodies to basement membrane collagen: Epidermolysis bullosa simplex versus bullous pemphigoid. Journal of Cutaneous Pathology 7: 315

Gentner G J, Adelmann B C 1976a The relation between the cell-mediated immunological responses and the induction of circulating antibodies to collagen in guinea-pigs. Immunology 31: 95

Gentner G J, Adelmann B C 1976b Specific suppression of delayed hypersensitivity skin reactions to collagen in guinea-pigs after immunization with collagen and Freund's incomplete adjuvant. Immunology 31: 87

Glynn L E 1969 Aetiology of rheumatoid arthritis with regard to its chronicity. Annals of Rheumatic Disease 28: (Supplement) 3

Gosslau B, Barrach H J 1979 Enzyme-linked immunosorbent microassay for quantification of specific antibodies to collagen type I, II, III. Journal of Immunological Methods 29: 71

Hahn E, Nowack H, Götze D, Timpl R 1975 H-2-linked genetic control of antibody response to soluble calf skin collagen in mice. European Journal of Immunology 5: 288

Hedberg H 1967 Studies on synovial fluid in arthritis. II. Occurrence of mononuclear cells with in vitro cytoxic effect. Acta Medica Scandinavia 479: (Supplement) 79

Hopper K E, Adelmann B C, Gentner G, Gay S 1976 Recognition by guinea-pig peritoneal exudate cells of conformationally different states of the collagen molecule. Immunology 30: 249

Huffstutter J E, Stuart J M, Townes A S, Kang A H 1979 Antibodies to native and denatured collagen in various rheumatic diseases utilizing radioimmunoassay. Abstract. Sixth South-eastern Regional Meeting, American Rheumatism Section, White Sulfur Springs, West Virginia, December 7-8, 1978

Izui S, Lambert P H, Miescher P A 1976 In vitro demonstration of a particular affinity of glomerular basement membrane and collagen for DNA. A possible basis for a local formation of DNA-anti-DNA complexes in systemic lupus erythematosus. Journal of Experimental Medicine 144: 428

Jasin H E 1975 Mechanism of trapping of immune complexes in joint collagenous tissues. Clinical and Experimental Immunology 22: 473

Jilek F, Hörmann H 1978 Cold-insoluble globulin (fibronectin), IV affinity to soluble collagens in various types. Hoppe-Seyler's Zeitschrift für Physiologische Chemie 359: 247

Johnson R L, Ziff M 1976 Lymphokine stimulation of collagen accumulation. Journal of Clinical Investigation 58: 240

Keyser A J, Cooper S M, Ruoslahti E, Nimni M E, Quismimio F P 1975 Scleroderma: Enhancement of connective tissue biosynthesis by a circulating factor. Federation Proceedings 38: 1339

Kleinman H K, Hewitt A T, Murray J C, Liotta L A, Rennard S I, Pennypacker J P, McGoodwin E B, Martin G R, Fishman P H 1979 Cellular and metabolic specificity in the interaction of adhesion proteins with collagen and with cells. Journal of Supramolecular Structure 11: 69

Klemperer P 1950 Concept of collagen diseases. American Journal of Pathology 26: 505

Knapp W, Menzel J, Steffen C 1974 Microfluorometric evaluation of anti-collagen-antibodies with the defined antigen substrate spheres (DASS) system. Zeitschrift für Immunitätsforschung 148: 132

Kochwa S, Kunkel H G 1971 Immunoglobulin. Annals of the New York Academy of Science 190: 5

Koffler D, Schur P H, Kunkel H G 1967 Immunological studies concerning the nephritis of systemic lupus erythematosus. Journal of Experimental Medicine 126: 609

Kravis T C, Ahmed A, Brown T E, Fulmer J D, Crystal R G 1976 Pathogenic mechanisms in pulmonary fibrosis. Journal of Clinical Investigation 58: 1223

Kresina T F, Miller E J 1979 Isolation and characterization of basement membrane collagen from human placental tissue: Evidence for the presence of two genetically-distinct collagen chains. Biochemistry 18: 3089

Langer F, Gross A E, Greaves M F 1972 The auto-immunogenicity of articular cartilage. Clinical and Experimental Immunology 12: 31

Lindsley H, Mannik M, Bornstein P 1971 The distribution of antigenic determinants in rat skin collagen. Journal of Experimental Medicine 133: 1309

Lustig L 1970 Cytotoxic action of an antiserum to soluble collagen on tissue culture of fibroblasts. Proceeding of the Society of Experimental Biology and Medicine 133: 207

Lustig L 1971 Ultrastructural localization of a soluble collagen antigen. Journal of Histochemistry and Cytochemistry 19: 663

Lustig L, Costantini H, Mancini R E 1969 Serological and immunofluorescent study of soluble collagen in tissue culture of fibroblasts. Proceedings of the Society of Experimental Biology and Medicine 130: 283

Maini R N, Horsfall A, Roffe L 1979 Lymphokines and rheumatoid arthritis. In: Panayi G S, Johnson P M (eds) Immunopathogenesis of Rheumatoid Arthritis. Reedbooks, Chertsey, Surrey. p 37

Mancini R E, Paz M, Vilar O, Davidson O W, Barquet J 1965 Histoimmunological detection of collagen fractions. Proceedings of the Society of Experimental Biology and Medicine 118: 346

Mannik M 1979 Characteristics of immune complexes and principles of immune complex diseases. In: McCarty D J (ed) Arthritis and allied conditions, 9th end, Lea & Febiger, Philadelphia. p 256

Maurer P H 1954 I. Antigenicity of oxypolygelatin and gelatin in man. Journal of Experimental Medicine 100: 497

McAdam K P W J, Fudenberg H H, Michaeli D 1978 Antibodies to collagen in patients with leprosy. Clinical Immunology and Immunopathology 9: 16

McDevitt H O, Landy M (eds) 1972 Genetic control of immune responsiveness: Relationship to disease susceptibility. Academic Press, New York

McCluskey R T 1974 Immunologic mechanism in renal disease. In: Heptinstall R H (ed) Pathology of the kidney, 2nd edn. Little, Brown and Company, Boston. p 273

McCoy R C, Tischer C C, Pepe P F, Cleveland L A 1976 The kidney in progressive systemic sclerosis. Laboratory Investigation 35: 124

McGiven A R, Deboer W G R M, Barnett A J 1971 Renal immune deposits in scleroderma. Pathology 3: 145

Menzel J 1977 Radioimmunoassay for anticollagen-antibodies using ^{14}C-labelled collagen. Journal of Immunological Methods 15: 77

Menzel J, Steffen C, Kolarz G, Eberl R, Frank O, Thumb N 1976 Demonstration of antibodies to collagen and of collagen-anticollagen immune complexes in rheumatoid arthritis synovial fluids. Annals of the Rheumatic Disease 35: 446

Menzel J, Steffen C, Kolarz G, Kojer M, Smolen J 1978 Demonstration of anticollagen antibodies in rheumatoid arthritis synovial fluids by ^{14}C-radioimmunoassay. Arthritis and Rheumatism 21: 243

Mestecky J, Miller E J 1975 Presence of antibodies specific to cartilage-type collagen in rheumatoid synovial tissue. Clinical and Experimental Immunology 22: 453

Mestecky J, Miller E J, Gay S, Andriopoulos N A 1979 Immune response to collagen. In: Panayi G S, Johnson P M (eds) Immunopathogenesis of Rheumatoid Arthritis. Reedbooks, Chertsey, Surrey. p 63

Michaeli D 1977 Immunochemistry of collagen. In: Attassi M Z (ed) Immunochemistry of Proteins, Vol. 1. Plenum Press, New York-London. p 371

Michaeli D, Fudenberg H H 1974a The incidence and antigenic specificity of antibodies against denatured human collagen in rheumatoid arthritis. Clinical Immunology and Immunopathology 2: 153

Michaeli D, Fudenberg H H 1974b Antibodies to collagen in patients with emphysema. Clinical Immunology and Immunopathology 3: 187

Michaeli D, Kamenecka H, Benjamini E, Kettman J R, Leung D Y K, Miner R C 1968 Immunochemical studies on collagen. I. The binding and precipitation of guinea-pig skin collagen and gelatin by rabbit anti-collagen. Immunochemistry 5: 433

Nowack H, Gay S, Wick G, Becker U, Timpl R 1976 Preparation and use in immunohistology of antibodies specific for type I and type III collagen and procollagen. Journal of Immunological Methods 12: 117

Nowack H, Hahn E, David C S, Timpl R, Götze D 1975a Immune response to calf collagen type I in mice: A combined control of Ir-IA and non H-2 linked genes. Immunogenetics 2: 331

Nowack H, Hahn E, Timpl R 1975b Specificity of the antibody responses in inbred mice to bovine type I and type II collagen. Immunology 29: 621

Nowack H, Rohde H, Götze D, Timpl R 1977 Genetic control and carrier and suppressor effects in the antibody response of mice to procollagen. Immunogenetics 4: 117

Provost T 1979 The relationship between discoid lupus erythematosus and systemic lupus erythematosus. The American Journal of Dermatopathology 1: 181

Raveche E S, Steinberg A D 1979 Lymphocytes and lymphocyte functions in systemic lupus erythematosus. Seminars in Hematology 16: 344

Robbins W C, Watson R F, Pappas G D, Porter K R 1955 Some effects of anti-collagen serum on collagen formation in tissue culture: A preliminary report. Journal of Biophysical and Biochemical Cytology 1: 381

Rodnan G P 1979 Progressive systemic sclerosis (scleroderma). In: McCarty D J (ed) Arthritis and Allied Conditions. Lea & Febiger, Philadelphia, 9th edn. p 762

Rohde H, Nowack H, Becker U, Timpl R 1976 Radioimmunoassay for the aminoterminal peptide of procollagen pα1(I)-chain. Journal of Immunological Methods 11: 135

Roll F J, Madri J A, Furthmayr H 1979 A new method of iodinating collagens for use in radioimmunoassay. Analytical Biochemistry 96: 489

Rothbard S, Watson R F 1956 Antigenicity of rat collagen. Reverse anaphylaxis induced in rats by anti-rat collagen serum. Journal of Experimental Medicine 103: 57

Rothbard S, Watson R F 1961 Antigenicity of rat collagen. Demonstration of antibody to rat collagen in the renal glomeruli of rats by fluorescence microscopy. Journal of Experimental Medicine 113: 1041

Ruoslahti E, Vuento M, Engvall E 1978 Interaction of fibronectin with antibodies and collagen in radioimmunoassay. Biochimica et Biophysica Acta 534: 210

Schmitt F O, Levine L, Drake M P, Rubin A L, Pfahl D, Davison P F 1964 The antigenicity of tropocollagen. Proceedings of the National Academy of Science, U.S.A. 51: 493

Schorlemmer H U, Hanauske-Abel H, Pontz B F 1979 Cartilage specific collagen type II activates mouse peritoneal macrophages and the alternate pathway of the complement system. Immunobiology 156: 239

Senyk G, Michaeli D 1973 Induction of cell-mediated immunity and tolerance to homologous collagen in guinea pigs: Demonstration of antigen-reactive cells for a self-antigen. Journal of Immunology 111: 1381

Smolen J S, Menzel E J, Scherak O, Kojer M, Kolarz G, Steffen C, Mayr W R 1980 Lymphocyte transformation to denatured type I collagen and B lymphocyte alloantigens in rheumatoid arthritis. Arthritis and Rheumatism 23: 424

Staines N A 1979 The major histocompatibility complex and the genetic control of immune responses. In: Panayi G S, Johnson P M (eds) Immunopathogenesis of Rheumatoid Arthritis. Reedbooks, Chertsey. p 3

Stastny P, Rosenthal M, Andreis M, Cooke D, Ziff M 1974 Lymphokines in rheumatoid synovitis. Annals of the New York Academy of Sciences 256: 117

Steffen C 1954 Untersuchungen über des Vorkommen eines in Polyarthritikerseren aufscheinenden und am Bindegewebe sessil werdenden Antikörper. Wiener Zeitschrift für Innere Medizin 35: 422

Steffen C 1965 Antigenicity and autoantigenicity of collagen. Annals of the New York Academy of Sciences 124: 570

Steffen C 1970 Consideration of pathogenesis of rheumatoid arthritis as collagen autoimmunity. Zeitschrift für Immunitätsforschung 139: 219

Steffen C 1978 Grundlagenuntersuchungen über die chronische Polyarthritis als Kollagen-Autoimmunkrankheit. Zeitschrift für Rheumatologie 37: 131

Steffen C, Dichtl M, Knapp W, Brunner H 1971 Immunogenicity and specificity of collagen. XII. Demonstration by immunofluorescence and haemagglutination of antibodies with different specificity to human collagen. Immunology 21: 649

Steffen C, Kovac W, Endler T A, Menzel J, Smolen J 1977 Induction of acute and chronic arthritis by intra-articular injection of preformed collagen-anticollagen complexes. Immunology 32: 161

Steffen C, Ludwig H, Knapp W 1974 Collagen-anticollagen immune complexes in rheumatoid arthritis synovial fluid cells. Zeitschrift für Immunitätsforschung 147: 229

Steffen C, Ludwig H, Thumb N, Frank O, Eberl R, Tausch F 1973 Nachweis von Antikörpern mit verschiedener Kollagenspezifität bei progressiv chonischer Polyarthritis und Vergleich von Humankollagen und Kalbskollagen als Testantigen. Klinische Wochenschrift 51: 222

Steffen C, Timpl R, Wolff L 1967 Immunogenität und Spezifität von Kollagen. III. Die Erzeugung und Nachweis von Anti-Kollagen-Antikörpern und serologischer Vergleich von nativem und denaturiertem löslichen Kollagen. Zeitschrift für Immunitäts-Forschung 134: 91

Steffen C, Zeitlhofer J, Zielinski C, Endler A T, Menzel J 1978 Acute autoimmune collagen-induced arthritis in rabbits. Zeitschrift für Rheumatologie 37: 275

Stenzel K H, Miyata T, Rubin A L 1974 Collagen as biomaterial. Annual Review on Biophysics and Bioengineering 3: 231

Stuart J M, Cremer M A, Kang A H, Townes A S 1979 Collagen-induced arthritis in rats: Evaluations of early immunologic events. Arthritis and Rheumatism 22: 1344

Stuart J M, Postlethwaite A E, Kang A H 1976 Evidence for cell-mediated immunity to collagen in progressive systemic sclerosis. Journal of Laboratory and Clinical Medicine 88: 601

Stuart J M, Postlethwaite A E, Kang A H, Townes A S 1979 Cell-mediated immunity to collagen in rheumatoid arthritis. Arthritis and Rheumatism 22: 665

Talal N, Fye K H, Moutsopoulos H M 1976 Autoimmunity. In: Fudenberg H H, Stites D P, Caldwell J L, Well J V (eds) basic & clinical immunology. Lange Medical Publications, Los Altos. p 196

Teuscher C, Donaldson D M 1979 The deposition and formation of immune complexes in collagenous tissues. Clinical Immunology and Immunopathology 13: 56

Timpl R 1976 Immunological studies on collagen. In: Ramachandran G N, Reddi A H (eds) Biochemistry of collagen. Plenum, New York. p 319

Timpl R, Wick G, Granditsch G 1977 Reticulin autoantibodies in childhood coeliac disease not directed against type III collagen. Clinical and Experimental Immunology 28: 546

Trentham D E, Dynesius R A, David J R 1978b Passive transfer by cells of type II collagen-induced arthritis in rats. Journal of Clinical Investigation 62: 359

Trentham D E, Dynesius R A, Rocklin R E, David R J 1978c Cellular sensitivity to collagen in rheumatoid arthritis. The New England Journal of Medicine 299: 327

Trentham D E, Townes A S, King A H 1977 Autoimmunity to type II collagen: An experimental model of arthritis. Journal of Experimental Medicine 146: 857

Trentham D E, Townes A S, King A H, David J R 1978a Humoral and cellular sensitivity to collagen in type II collagen-induced arthritis in rats. Journal of Clinical Investigation 61: 89

Wahl L M, Olsen C E, Sandberg A L, Mergenhagen S E 1977 Prostaglandin regulation of macrophage collagenase production. Proceedings of the National Academy of Science U.S.A. 74: 4955

Wahl L M, Wahl S M, Mergenhagen S E, Martin G R 1974 Collagenase productive by lymphokine-activated macrophages. Science 187: 261

Wahl S M, Wahl L M, McCarthy J B 1978 Lymphocyte-mediated activation of fibroblast proliferation and collagen production. Journal of Immunology 121: 942

Waksman B H, Mason H L 1949 The antigenicity of collagen. Journal of Immunology 63: 427

Watson R F, Rothbard S, Vanamee P 1954 The antigenicity of rat collagen. Journal of Experimental Medicine 99: 535

Weissmann G 1977 Lysosomes and rheumatoid joint inflammation. Arthritis and Rheumatism 20: (Supplement No 6) 193

Wells J V, Michaeli D, Fudenberg H H 1973 Antibodies to human collagen in subjects with selective IgA deficiency. Clinical and Experimental Immunology 13: 203

Wick G, Furthmayr H, Timpl R 1975 Purified antibodies to collagen: An immunofluorescence study of their reaction with tissue collagen. International Archiv of Allergy and Applied Immunology 48: 664

Wick G, Müller P U, Timpl R, Martin G R 1979a Studies on the immunology of basement membrane collagen using antibody to a tumor basement membrane. Frontiers in Matrix Bioly 7: 120

Wick G, Munro V, Gebhart W, Timpl R 1979b Studies on the specificity of autoantibodies to basement membrane in patients with bullous pemphigoid. Immunobiology 156: 252

Wolff I, Timpl R 1968 Reaction of the human anti-gelatine factor with gelatine from different species and with collagen peptides. Vox Sanguinis 15: 459

Wolff I, Timpl R, Pecker I, Steffen C 1967 A two-component system of human serum agglutinating gelatin-coated erythrocytes. Vox Sanguinis 12: 443

Yamada K M, Olden K 1978 Fibronectins: Adhesive glycoproteins of cell surface and blood. Nature 275: 179

Note added in proof

During the printing of the chapter the following papers have been published: S. M. Hedrick and J. Watson: Genetic control of the immune response to collagen-I. Quantitative determination of response levels by multiple I-region genes. Journal of Immunogenetics 7: 271, 1980. — II. Antibody responses produced in fetal liver restored radiation chimeras and thymus reconstituted F_1 hybrid nude mice. Journal of Experimental Medicine 150: 646, 1979. — III. Coordinate restriction of cellular cooperation and antigen responsiveness by thymus-directed maturation. Journal of Immunology 125: 1782, 1980.

16

Diseases associated with collagen abnormalities *

J. UITTO and E. A. BAUER

INTRODUCTION

Collagen constitutes the most ubiquitous structural macromolecule in a variety of tissues. (For recent reviews on collagen, see Fessler & Fessler, 1978; Gay & Miller, 1978; Bauer & Uitto, 1979; Prockop et al, 1979; Bornstein & Sage, 1980.) For example, in normal human dermis collagen represents more than 70 per cent of the dry weight of the skin and about 95 per cent of the organic matrix of the bone is collagen (Miller, 1976; Uitto & Eisen, 1979). The biological function of collagen is to provide the major structural framework which is responsible for functional integrity of the tissues. The critical tensile properties necessary for structural integrity are achieved by specific interactions, not only between collagenous molecules, but also other extracellular macromolecules, such as proteoglycans and elastin.

The biochemical processes involved in the biosynthesis and degradation of collagen have been actively investigated in several laboratories (Prockop et al, 1976; Harper, 1980). Based on current knowledge of these processes, it is possible to define certain connective tissue diseases in terms of the specific biochemical aberrations which occur during synthesis and degradation (Kivirikko & Risteli, 1976; Uitto & Lichtenstein, 1976; Bornstein & Byers, 1980). In some circumstances, the defects result from a genetic abnormality in the collagen or in the enzymes involved in its biosynthesis and degradation. In other diseases, the biochemical defect is apparently acquired and represents a change in the collagen secondary to an unrelated metabolic change. In this review, we are discussing diseases which involve abnormalities in the structure and metabolism of collagen.

DISEASES WITH COLLAGEN ABNORMALITIES

Definition of 'collagen disease'

Just about a third of a century ago Klemperer and his co-workers introduced the term 'collagen disease' (Klemperer et al, 1942). In this 'classical' sense, as it is frequently used in clinical context, the term applied to a group of connective tissue diseases, including lupus erythematosus, periarteritis nodosa, dermatomyositis, and scleroderma. The basis for their suggestion was the observation that collagen in the affected tissues in these conditions appeared to be abnormally homogeneous, when examined by light microscopy. This change, known as fibrinoid degeneration, suggested to Klemperer et al that collagen in these patients was abnormal. The introduction of the term 'collagen disease' was highly useful at the time in conceptualizing these diseases, and in particular it focused attention on the fact that disease processes can be systemic, not limited to a single organ. Unfortunately, however, we do not know at the present the exact biochemical meaning of the fibrinoid degeneration, and based on the current knowledge of lupus erythematosus, periarteritis nodosa and dermatomyositis, both the structure and metabolism of collagen is largely unaltered in these conditions. Thus, these conditions, in the modern sense, are not 'collagen diseases'.

In contrast, we are now in the position to apply the term 'collagen disease' to a variety of clinical conditions which are clearly known to be associated with collagen abnormalities; these conditions could, therefore, be called 'true' collagen diseases (Uitto & Prockop, 1974) (Table 16.1). In some of these diseases, the primary defect can be identified in the structure of collagen or procollagen, or in the enzymes participating in collagen metabolism. Several inherited connective tissue disorders, as for example the Ehlers-Danlos syndrome and osteogenesis imperfecta, could serve as examples of such primary collagen diseases. On the other hand, the changes in collagen could be secondary to less specific changes in tissue metabolism and such changes could be observed both in inherited and acquired conditions. As examples of such 'secondary' collagen diseases one could mention scurvy, homocystinuria, and various fibrotic processes, such as pulmonary fibrosis and liver cirrhosis.

Mechanisms leading to manifestation of collagen diseases

Collagen is a complex macromolecule, and its synthesis and degradation involve numerous biochemical reactions (Table 16.1). Many of these reactions are catalyzed by

* This work was supported in part by US Public Health Service, National Institutes of Health Grants TO-AM 07284, AM 19357, AM 28450 and GM 28833 and by grants from the National Foundation — March of Dimes. The authors received NIH Research Career Development Awards 7-KO4-AM-00897 and 5-KO4-AM-00077.

Table 16.1 Major steps in the biogenesis and degradation of collagen fibres, their functional significance, and associated clinical or experimental conditions

Step[a]	*Functional significance*	*Associated condition*[b]
Synthesis of collagen polypeptides		
1. Gene selection	Determines the collagen type synthesized	Some forms of E–D IV[c], OI and the Marfan syndrome, osteoarthrosis
2. Transcription	Formation of mRNA templates	Some of those listed in 1 and 4
3. Translation of mRNAs	Polypeptide assembly	may have the defect in this level
4. Control of the translational rate	Determines the amount of polypeptides synthesized	Scleroderma, proliferative phase of rheumatoid arthritis, various fibrotic processes, familial cutaneous collagenoma (?), acromegaly, corticosteroid-induced changes
Intracellular Post-translational Modifications		
1. Synthesis of 4-hydroxyproline	Stabilization of triple-helix	Scurvy, tissue anoxia
2. Synthesis of 3-hydroxyproline	Unknown	None known
3. Synthesis of hydroxylysine	Stabilization of cross-links, and attachment site for glycosylation	E–D VI, alkaptonuria, scurvy, tissue anoxia, some forms of OI, vitamin D-deficiency
4. Synthesis of hydroxylysine-o-glycosides	May influence cross-link formation and determine the fiber diameter	Some forms of dominant EB simplex
5. Glycosylation of the extension peptides	Unknown	Some forms of OI
6. Removal of the signal sequence	Unknown	Incubation of cells with an arginine analogue
7. Degradation of non-helical chains	Removal of defective polypeptides and modulation of collagen production	β-Adrenergic stimulation, scurvy, anoxia, incorporation of proline analogues
8. Chain association and disulphide bonding	Facilitation of the triple-helix formation	Not known
9. Triple-helix formation	Pre-requisite for proper secretion	Incorporation of proline analogues, any condition preventing the formation of 4-hydroxyproline
Secretion	Transport of procollagen to the extracellular space	Type III collagen in some forms of E–D IV, presence of inhibitors of microtubular function
Extracellular modifications		
1. Removal of the propeptides	Necessary for fibre formation	E–D VII, dermatosparaxis in various animal species
2. Non-enzymatic glucosylation	May interfere with fibre formation	Diabetes
3. Deamination of lysine and hydroxylysine	Necessary for cross-link formation	X-linked cutis laxa, homocystinuria, Menkes syndrome, aneurysm-prone mice, lathyrism, copper deficiency, diabetes
Fibre formation		
1. Alignment of the molecules	Formation of microfibrils	Defective removal of extension peptides in dermatosparaxis
2. Formation of cross-links	Stabilization of the fibre structures	D-penicillamine-induced changes, and the same as in 3 above
3. Supramolecular assembly	Architectural organization of collagen in tissues	E–D I and II (?)
4. Interactions with other extracellular macromolecules	Determines the physiologic properties of tissues	Some forms of spondyloepiphyseal dysplasia, the Marfan syndrome (?)

Table 16.1 *(continued)*

Step[a]	*Functional significance*	*Associated condition*[b]
Extracellular degradation		
1. Cleavage by specific collagenases	Rate-limiting step	Rheumatoid arthritis, recessive dystrophic EB, Paget's disease of the bones, hyperparathyroidism, hyperthyroidism, tumor invasion, uremia, inflammatory processes involving leukocyte collagenase, postpartum involution of uterus
2. Further degradation by peptidases and enzymes metabolizing free amino acids	Removal of degradation products	Hydroxyprolinemia, hydroxylysinemia

[a] These are the major steps in a sequence most likely occurring in under physiological conditions; some of the reactions can, however, occur simultaneously and the order of some reactions can be reversed (see Prockop et al, 1979).
[b] These are conditions in which sufficient evidence allows their categorization in the present scheme; in several conditions considerable biochemical heterogeneity exists and also in some conditions more than one step is affected, thus causing the condition to be listed in more than one category.
[c] Abbreviations used: E–D, The Ehlers-Danlos syndrome; OI, osteogenesis imperfecta; EB, epidermolysis bullosa.

enzymes which are, at least to a certain extent, specific to collagen metabolism (Table 16.2). It is conceivable, therefore, that aberrations in any of these steps can occur, and such a situation might manifest as a disease. When considering the mechanisms by which aberrations in collagen can manifest at the tissue level as a clinical disease, we can visualize several possibilities. First, the biogenesis and degradation of extracellular collagen fibres have to be in a carefully controlled balance. An aberration in the control mechanisms could alter the balance between production and degradation, and thus lead to excessive or deficient deposition of structurally unaltered collagen in tissues. The excessive deposition of collagen can clearly affect the physiological properties or interfere with cellular and metabolic functions of the organs. On the other hand diminution of otherwise normal collagen in tissues could result in functional weakness and reduced tensile strength of the organ systems.

A second mechanism, which could result in a disease, involves synthesis of collagen which is structurally altered so that it is unable to form functionally competent extracellular fibres. Such alterations in collagen molecule could be in the primary sequence as a result of gene mutations or chromosomal abnormalities, or a fraction of newly-synthesized collagen polypeptides could be abnormal as a result of translational errors. An alternative possibility for the synthesis of structurally abnormal molecules arises from aberrations in the post-translational modifications. Since many of these are catalyzed by specific enzymes with stringent co-factor and co-substrate requirements, an abnormality in the synthesis or degradation of the enzyme protein itself, or in its catalytic activity, could lead to synthesis of structurally altered collagen molecules. It should be noted that all structural alterations do not necessarily manifest as a clinical abnormality at the tissue level. For example, a point mutation leading to conservative substitution of an amino acid in the α-chain may not demonstrate adverse effects at all. On the other hand, a single point mutation altering an amino acid in a critical position, for example at the cleavage site of a procollagen protease, can lead to formation of severely abnormal protein. These abnormal collagen molecules may not then form functional collagen fibres, and as a consequence severe connective tissue weakness ensues.

A third possibility for mechanisms leading to tissue alterations involves an imbalance in the relative synthesis of genetically distinct collagens. Although the exact role of various collagen types is not known, their relative ratios in various tissues appear to be characteristic and show only small variations between species. Therefore, a relative change in the deposition of genetically distinct collagens, even though the total production of collagen may be unaffected, could alter the characteristics of fibre formation and lead to abnormal physiology of the connective tissues.

Finally, a fourth possibility for manifestation of the disease involves abnormalities in the packing of collagen molecules into fibre structure or in the interactions of such fibres with other extracellular components of the connective tissue. In the latter case, no abnormality may necessarily exist in the collagen molecule, but as a consequence, the architecture of the collagen fibres is abnormal, and the overall function of the connective tissues may be defective.

Table 16.2 Characteristics of some enzymes participating in the biosynthesis and degradation of collagen

Enzyme [a]	*Product*	*Co-factors and Co-substrates*	*Inhibitors*
1. Prolyl-4-hydroxylase	4-hydroxyproline	O_2, Fe^{2+}, α-ketoglutarate, ascorbic acid	Chelators; dehydroproline-containing polypeptides; poly-(L-proline); some divalent cations
2. Prolyl-3-hydroxylase	3-hydroxyproline	O_2, Fe^{2+}, α-ketoglutarate, ascorbic acid	Chelators
3. Lysyl hydroxylase	hydroxylysine	O_2, Fe^{2+}, α-ketoglutarate, ascorbic acid	Chelators; some divalent cations
4. Collagen galactosyl transferase	gal-0-hydroxylysine	Mn^{2+}, UDP-galactose	Co^{2+}, free gal-0-hylys; UDP-gal analogs
5. Collagen glucosyl transferase	glc-gal-0-hydroxylysine	Mn^{2+}, UDP-glucose	
6. Protein disulphide isomerase[b]	S-S-bonds	Thiols	
7. Procollagen N-terminal protease	Pc-collagen or collagen[c]	Ca^{2+}	Chelators; some synthetic polypeptides
8. Procollagen C-terminal protease	Pn-collagen or collagen[c]	Ca^{2+}	Chelators
9. Lysyl oxidase	Aldehyde derivatives of lysine and hydroxylysine	Cu^{2+}, O_2	Nitriles; chelators
10. Collagenase	Cleavage products TC^A and TC^B	Ca^{2+}	Chelators; α2-macroglobulin; polypeptide inhibitors in tissues
11. Hydroxyproline oxidase	Δ'-pyrroline-3-hydroxy-5-carboxylic acid	O_2	
12. Hydroxylysine kinase	0-phosphohydroxylysine	Mg^{2+}, GTP	

[a] The action of these enzymes is somewhat limited to collagen; the complete sequences of procollagen synthesis and collagen degradation involve additional, less specific enzymes, such as those of transcription and translation, as well as extracellular proteases.

[b] It has not been established whether the formation of interchain disulphides in procollagen involves enzymatic catalysis, as occurs in some other proteins, or whether their synthesis takes place spontaneously.

[c] If intact procollagen is used as a substrate, partially modified products are formed; however, if the partially cleaved proteins serve as substrate, collagen is produced.

Inherited diseases

The Ehlers-Danlos syndrome (EDS)

This syndrome consists of a group of patients who have some of the manifestations of a generalized connective tissue weakness (Beighton, 1970; McKusick, 1972; Uitto & Lichtenstein, 1976; Hollister, 1978; Bornstein & Byers 1980). The major clinical features of EDS include hyperextensible skin, hypermobile joints, bruising tendency, atrophic scarring, and fragility of the connective tissues. The spectrum of the severity is, however, markedly variable, so that at one end of the spectrum the condition represents only a curious deviation from the normal, while in the more severe forms the disease can be life-threatening. Also, the inheritance of the disease is variable, so that autosomal dominant, autosomal recessive, and X-linked recessive patterns have been encountered. Nevertheless, in several of the patients with different forms of EDS, an apparent abnormality in the collagen biology has been detected, and it may well be that in the majority of the cases, the clinical manifestations of EDS result from different errors in the structure or metabolism of collagen.

Currently, EDS has been divided into eight separate categories, based on clinical, genetic and biochemical criteria (Table 16.3). It should be noted, however, that there are several patients reported in the literature who do not correspond to any particular type in the existing classification (see e.g. Daentl et al, 1978; Beasley & Cohen, 1979; Hernandez et al, 1979). Also, apparent genetic and biochemical heterogeneity within a given type shown in Table 16.3 suggests further heterogeneity in the classification. *EDS types I, II, and III* are the most common

Table 16.3 Clinical, genetic and biochemical heterogeneity in the Ehlers-Danlos syndrome

Type [a]	*Inheritance*	*Major manifestations*	*Biochemical defect*
I Gravis	Autosomal dominant	Marked joint hypermobility; Marked bruising, fragility, hyperextensibility of skin; Premature rupture of fetal membranes	Unknown[b]
II Mitis	Autosomal dominant	Moderate joint hypermobility; Moderately hyperextensible skin	Unknown
III Benign hypermobile	Autosomal dominant	Marked joint hypermobility; Minimal cutaneous manifestations	Unknown
IV Ecchymotic	Autosomal dominant or recessive	Hypermobility limited to digits; Marked skin fragility and bruisability; Arterial, gastrointestinal rupture	Deficiency of type III collagen in tissues
V X-linked	X-linked recessive	Minimal joint hypermobility; Marked hyperextensibility of skin with moderate bruising; Skeletal disorders	Unknown[c]
VI Ocular	Autosomal recessive	Marked joint hypermobility; Markedly hyperextensible skin with little bruising; Scleral and corneal fragility	Lysyl hydroxylase deficiency
VII Arthrocalasis multiplex congenita	Autosomal recessive or dominant[d]	Marked joint hypermobility; Moderate skin fragility, hyperexensibility and bruising; Short stature; Multiple dislocations	Defective conversion of procollagen to collagen
VIII Periodontitis	Autosomal dominant	Moderate joint hypermobility; Moderate skin fragility but minimal hyperextensibility; Advanced periodontitis	Unknown

[a] These are the major types recognized on the basis of clinical, genetic and biochemical observations; several cases observed by us or reported in the literature do not clinically, however, correspond to any of these types. Furthermore, genetic and biochemical variations in patients classifiable as type IV, V or VI suggest further heterogeneity (see text).

[b] In a report on one patient, a defective conversion of procollagen to collagen has been suggested (Shinkai et al, 1976).

[c] In one study (DiFerrante et al, 1975) lysyl oxidase deficiency has been reported; more recently (Siegel et al, 1979), however, no abnormalities in the cross-linking process have been found.

[d] Classically, type VII has been thought to be inherited in an autosomal recessive manner; demonstration of a structural mutation in one half of the collagen in an affected individual (Steinmann et al, 1980) suggests autosomal dominant inheritance.

forms of the disease. They are inherited in an autosomal dominant pattern, and they appear to represent a spectrum of severity of the clinical features (Barabas, 1967; McKusick, 1972). The patients with EDS I demonstrate the classical features of the syndrome: the skin is soft, velvety, and hyperextensible; the patients have a tendency to easy bruising as a result of the fragility of blood vessels; the bruising frequently leads to localized hyperpigmentation of the skin due to deposition of heme pigment especially on the pretibial area. The patients with EDS I also have several orthopaedic problems, such as pes planus, kyphoscoliosis, and frequent dislocations of the joints (Beighton & Horan, 1969). Cardiac manifestations include mitral valve prolapse which is frequently seen in patients with other varieties of EDS. EDS II, although genetically distinct from EDS I, shares the above clinical features. The clinical picture, however, is considerably milder and some of the features, such as prematurity and orthopaedic problems are infrequent. EDS III is characterized by striking hypermobility of the joints, while actual skin changes may be minimal. The degree of joint involvement within a family can also be somewhat variable.

The biochemical defect(s) in EDS I, II, and III is currently unknown, although a report on fibroblast cultures from a patient with EDS I has suggested defective conversion of procollagen to collagen (Shinkai et al, 1976). On the structural level, however, marked abnormalities in the organization of the collagen fibres have been demonstrated (Vogel et al, 1979; Black et al, 1980). When the skin from patients with EDS I and II was examined by scanning electron microscopy, there was a marked disorganization in the collagen architecture resulting from an apparent inability of the individual fibres to aggregate into large bundles (Black et al, 1980). This disorder was more pronounced in EDS I than in EDS II.

In the study by Black et al (1980), no abnormalities in the ultrastructure of collagen fibrils could be demonstrated by transmission electron microscopy. On the other hand, the study by Vogel et al (1979) demonstrated that the dermis in nine patients with a clinical picture consistent with EDS I was composed of collagen fibrils which have the mean diameter 13 to 40 per cent larger than in the controls. Even more strikingly, a small proportion of the fibrils had markedly larger diameter (up to 500 nm *vs.* 90nm), had a highly irregular, convoluted outline in cross-section, and were spiraled and fragmented in longitudinal view (Vogel et al, 1979). These observations clearly suggest that the collagen fibre formation is abnormal in patients with EDS I. However, the extrapolation of such observations into a specific biochemical defect in collagen is difficult for several reasons. First, several different abnormalities in the collagen molecule could produce similar disorganization on the higher level of the fibre bundle formation, and also, defects in the interaction of collagen with other extracellular components, such as proteoglycans, can affect the fibre architecture. Secondly, changes in the fibre diameter and the appearance of highly abnormal fibres with irregular border have been encountered in a variety of conditions unrelated to EDS (see e.g. Danielsen & Kobayashi, 1972; Danielsen, 1979; Scheck et al, 1979; Uitto et al, 1981). Therefore, further work is necessary to disclose the exact biochemical defects present in EDS types I, II and III.

EDS type IV. This form of EDS is considerably less common than types I–III (McKusick, 1972). Clinically, however, it is important to recognize this form of the syndrome, because it carries the most ominous prognosis, and rupture of large arteries or gastrointestinal tract frequently leads to premature demise. Patients with EDS IV typically have a thin, translucent skin, so that the underlying venous network is prominently visible. The skin is not particularly hyperextensible, and the hypermobility of the joints is mostly limited to hands and feet. The patients, however, have fragile skin and they bruise easily as a result of a minor trauma. Some of the internal organs, and the vascular and gastrointestinal tissues in particular, are very fragile, and severe complications, for example, aortic or gastrointestinal rupture and spontaneous pneumothorax, may lead to death at the second or third decade of life (Beighton, 1968a; Beighton et al, 1969; McKusick, 1972; Clark et al, 1980). There is considerable genetic heterogeneity in EDS IV, so that in some families the condition is inherited in an autosomal recessive manner while autosomal dominant inheritance is evident in others (McKusick, 1972; Pope et al, 1977, Byers et al, 1979). The underlying biochemical defect in most patients appears to involve abnormalities in the synthesis, secretion and structure of type III collagen (Pope et al, 1975; Pope et al, 1977; Byers et al, 1979; Clark et al, 1980; Uitto et al, 1982b). Initially, when tissues from patients with EDS, inherited in an autosomal recessive pattern, were examined by amino acid analysis, a marked reduction in the total content of collagen was noted. Further analyses of collagen indicated that little, if any, type III collagen was present in tissues (Pope et al, 1975). Furthermore, fibroblast cultures initiated from the skin of these patients synthesized only type I procollagen (Gay et al, 1976; Pope et al, 1977). It is possible, therefore, that these patients had a deficiency in type III collagen because of a defect in the transcriptional or translational level.

In other patients with EDS IV, only a diminution in the relative amount of type III collagen in the tissue or in the synthesis and secretion of type III procollagen by cultured fibroblasts has been noted (Byers et al, 1979; Clark et al, 1980; Jaffe et al, 1981; Uitto et al, 1982b). Examination of the skin from these patients by electron microscopy has revealed fibroblasts containing homogeneous appearing material within a highly dilated rough endoplasmic reticulum (Byers et al, 1979). Since most of the latter patients appear to have a disease inherited in an autosomal dominant pattern, it is possible that a fraction of type III collagen is not secreted properly but accumulates in the cells instead. Irrespective of the mechanism, whether decreased synthesis or an aberration in the secretory process, diminished levels of type III collagen can explain some of the clinical manifestations in tissues such as the aorta, which have been shown to be rich in type III collagen. Interestingly, in a large family with EDS IV, a correlation between the diminished type III collagen production and presence of mitral valve prolapse was demonstrated (Jaffe et al, 1981). This and similar observations (Hammer et al, 1979) suggest, therefore, that deficiency in type III collagen might be the underlying cause also in other patients with mitral valve prolapse but without other manifestations of EDS.

EDS type V is inherited in an X-linked recessive manner (Beighton, 1968b; McKusick, 1972). The clinical picture is relatively mild, resembling that of EDS II. In an earlier study, the activity of lysyl oxidase was reported to be decreased in skin fibroblast cultures from patients who supposedly had EDS V (DiFerranti et al, 1975). Thus, the connective tissue weakness in these patients could be explained on the basis of defective cross-linking of collagen. More recently the structure and cross-linking of collagen were studied in three patients with a typical clinical picture of EDS V (Siegel et al, 1979; Black et al, 1980). The pattern of reducible cross-links in dermal collagen was similar to that of normal skin (Black et al, 1980). In addition, the activity and antigenicity of lysyl oxidase in the skin of one patient were equivalent to those of normal skin (Siegel et al, 1979). However, scanning electron microscopy demonstrated a disorganization of collagen fibre structure in a manner similar but less pronounced than in EDS I (Black et al, 1980). Thus, the connective tissue abnormality in EDS V appears to involve collagen, but the mechanism for the aberration is currently unknown.

EDS type VI, the hydroxylysine deficient collagen disease, was the first form of EDS in which a specific defect in collagen could be demonstrated (Pinnell et al, 1972). Most of the patients with EDS VI have reduced levels of lysyl hydroxylase, and as a consequence, the hydroxylysine content of collagen is markedly reduced (Pinnell et al, 1972; Sussman et al, 1974; Steinmann et al, 1975; Elsas et al, 1978; Krieg et al, 1979). It should be noted that even this form of EDS is biochemically heterogeneous, in that lysyl hydroxylase levels in some patients with typical clinical presentations are normal (Judisch et al, 1976).

Clinically, EDS VI is characterized by markedly hyperextensible skin and moderately increased joint hypermobility. Easy bruising, atrophic scarring, and skeletal abnormalities, such as kyphoscoliosis and arachnodactyly, are also typical for this form of the syndrome. EDS VI is also known as the ocular type. This is due to the fact that these patients demonstrate marked ocular fragility and keratoconus, features which are usually not present in the other forms of EDS.

The markedly reduced hydroxylysine content of the collagen in patients with EDS VI is due to deficiency in the activity of lysyl hydroxylase (see above). The activity of this enzyme is reduced not only in the skin of these patients but also in fibroblasts cultures (Krane et al, 1972; Sussman et al, 1974). In some cases the mutant enzyme has been shown to have an increased Km for ascorbic acid, and in such cases it has been suggested that the hydroxylation defect could be overcome by increased levels of this cofactor (Quinn & Krane, 1976; Elsas et al, 1974). In fact, a recent study has suggested that the administration of large doses of ascorbic acid to some patients with EDS VI may increase the formation of hydroxylysine and perhaps improve the clinical situation (Elsas et al, 1978). The mechanisms by which deficient hydroxylation of lysine manifest as a connective tissue weakness are not entirely clear. It is known, however, that collagen in the skin of these patients is deficient in hydroxylysine-derived reducible cross-links (Eyre & Glimcher, 1972). It has been suggested that covalent hydroxylysine-derived cross-links are more stable than their counterparts derived from lysine residues; this stabilization has been thought to occur as a result of ketoenol tautomerism, the Amadori rearrangement (Miller & Robertson 1973). Alternatively, the carbohydrates, galactosyl and glucosylgalactosyl residues, which are attached to the hydroxylysyl residues through an O-glycosidic linkage, might stabilize the cross-links and in the absence of hydroxylysine-O-glycosides, as in EDS VI, the cross-links would be less stable. It should be noted that the hydroxylysine-deficient procollagen molecules, which lack the hydroxylysine-O-glycosides, are secreted by the fibroblasts in culture at a normal rate. This observation indicates that these sugar residues are not necessary for collagen secretion. It does not discount, however, the 'sugar-tag hypothesis' (Eylar, 1966; Winterburn and Phelps, 1972; Prockop, 1972), according to which proteins for export have to be glycosylated prior to secretion, since the extensions of procollagen also contain carbohydrate units which are not hydroxylysine-linked (Clark & Kefalides, 1976; Olsen et al, 1977).

EDS type VII, previously known as arthrocalasis multiplex congenita, is clinically characterized by bilateral hip dislocations, extreme hypermobility of the joints, and short stature (McKusick, 1972; Lichtenstein et al, 1973a). The skin is soft and velvety, but not particularly friable. The condition is classically inherited in an autosomal recessive pattern, but recent demonstration of a structural alteration in procollagen in a heterozygous, clinically affected individual is consistent with autosomal dominant inheritance (Tuderman et al, 1979). The biochemical basis in several patients with EDS VII has been shown to be a defect in the conversion of procollagen to collagen (Lichtenstein et al, 1973a, b; Tuderman et al, 1979; Steinmann, 1980). In some patients, the defective conversion appears to be due to decreased activity of the N-terminal protease, so that the N-terminal extensions are not removed and pN-collagen accumulates in the tissues.

In other cases, the conversion defect is not due to enzyme deficiency, but procollagen is structurally altered, so that removal of some of the extension peptides is not taking place. Specifically, in one case removal of the N-terminal extension peptide does not take place even in the presence of normal enzyme, perhaps as a consequence of an amino acid substitution in the cleavage site (Tuderman et al, 1979). The N-terminal sequence retained in the molecule then interferes with normal packing of the collagen molecules, and as a consequence, cross-link formation is altered (Bailey & Lapière, 1976).

A counterpart of human EDS VII is dermatosparaxis, an animal disease encountered in cattle, sheep and cats (Fjolstad & Helle, 1974; Lapière & Nusgens, 1976; Minor, 1980). This condition is marked by fragility of dermis, so that as a result of minor trauma skin tears off. In these animals the conversion of type I procollagen to collagen is defective and pN-collagen accumulates in the skin (Lenaers et al, 1971; Becker et al, 1976; Counts et al, 1980). The severity of the disease appears to correlate with the extent of the conversion defect. In sheep essentially all of the collagen is in the form of pN-collagen and the affected animals die within a few weeks of life (Becker et al, 1976). In contrast, in cattle and cats, only a relatively small portion of collagen is in the form of pN-collagen, while most of the molecules are processed normally (Lenaers et al, 1971; Counts et al, 1980); in these animals the disease is considerably milder and is reflected in the longer survival. The reason for defective conversion of pN-collagen to collagen in the case of the cattle and cat has been shown to be diminished activity of procollagen N-protease, while in sheep the basic defect is unknown. It should be mentioned that several other animal models, demonstrating connective tissue weakness in the skin and other tissues, may be counterparts of other types of human EDS (Minor, 1980). For example, dominantly inherited collagen packing defects observed in a variety of animal species, such as cats, dogs and minks, could correspond to EDS I (Hegreberg et al, 1970; Counts et al, 1977; Patterson & Minor, 1977; Minor, 1980). These animal models may, therefore, be helpful in further attempts to explore the molecular defects and the mode of genetic transmission in various forms of EDS.

EDS type VIII. This variant, the most recent addition to the current classification, is called the periodontitis type, since marked, destructive periodontitis is the hallmark of this particular subgroup of patients (Stewart et al, 1977). Other clinical features in these patients include marked fragility of skin and moderate hypermobility of joints. This condition is inherited in an autosomal dominant pattern and its aetiology is, as yet, unknown.

Osteogenesis imperfecta (OI)

This condition is one of the most common inherited connective tissue disorders (McKusick, 1972). Clinically, OI is characterized by excessively fragile bones leading to multiple fractures, thin skin, dentinogenesis imperfecta, joint hypermobility, otosclerosis, and blue sclerae. This condition is both clinically and genetically heterogeneous, however, and the severity of the disease can vary markedly between different types of OI (Table 16.4). Previously, OI has been conveniently classified according to the onset of the fractures (Seedorff, 1949). In OI congenita the fetus is born with multiple in utero fractures and the disease has a high perinatal mortality. In OI tarda, the fractures are not present at birth, but may occur any time after the birth. The clinical manifestations in these two groups are similar but less severe in OI tarda than in the congenita form.

More recently, a new classification, based on the available clinical and genetic information on OI, has been proposed (Table 16.4) (Sillence et al, 1979 a, b; Sillence, 1982). According to this classification, there are four major types of OI. It is already evident, however, that a

Table 16.4 Clinical, genetic and biochemical heterogeneity in osteogenesis imperfecta[a]

Type [c]	*Inheritance*	*Clinical features*	*Biochemical observations*
I Dominant with blue sclera	Autosomal recessive[b]	Onset of fractures variable, 10% at birth; blue sclerae; dentinogenesis imperfecta rare; hearing impairment may be present	The ratio of type I/III collagen in skin decreased
II Lethal perinatal	Autosomal recessive[b]	Multiple intrauterine fractures with growth retardation and limb abnormalities; dark blue sclerae; death before or soon after delivery	Markedly diminished synthesis of type I collagen; increased hydroxylysine content of the bone collagen
III Recessive with blue or normal sclerae	Autosomal[b] recessive	Fractures at birth, with progressive limb deformation; sclerae may be blue in childhood, with improvement in adult years; dentinogenesis imperfecta common; hearing loss rare	—
IV Dominant with normal sclerae	Autosomal dominant	Onset of fractures variable; sclerae normal; marked dentinogenesis imperfecta; hearing loss rare	Decreased stability of polymeric collagen in skin[d]

[a] The classification is according to Sillence (1982).

[b] Genetic heterogeneity may exist in these types.

[c] Further genetic heterogeneity appears likely as some families in each group have opalescent dentin while some families have normal teeth.

[d] The metabolic implications of this observation are unclear.

considerable amount of heterogeneity exists in some of these types, and further expansion of this classification is likely in the future.

OI type I is characterized by bone fractures which usually begin at early infancy, at the time when the child starts to stand upright. The frequency of fractures decreases after puberty, possibly due to changes in the hormonal status. Other frequent features include blue sclerae and marked hearing impairment, while dentinogenesis imperfecta is rare. OI I is inherited in an autosomal dominant manner and can be distinguished from type IV by blue sclerae, among other features.

OI type II, the lethal perinatal type, is the most severe form of the disease, and the majority of the patients die either in utero or shortly after birth. The affected infants are small and characteristically show shortened limbs due to multiple fractures in utero. Radiologically, the bones are lucent and can be unusually broad with evidence of multiple fractures. The cranium is soft and membranous with little evidence of calcification. OI II is probably inherited in an autosomal recessive manner, although some of the cases may represent new mutations.

OI type III, a rare autosomal recessive group, is also associated with marked perinatal fragility of bones but is distinguished radiologically from OI type II. The affected infants are usually of normal weight and height at birth although deformities of the limbs due to fractures may be present. The surviving patients develop a severe deformity of bones which is evident in early adolescence. Other features of OI III include short stature and dentinogenesis imperfecta, while sclerae are normal and hearing is not impaired.

OI type IV includes bone fragility which, as in type III, begins early in childhood and may lead to deformity. Dentinogenesis imperfecta is present in some but not all families, sclerae are normal and hearing is not impaired. The distinction from type III is partly based on family history, since type IV is inherited in an autosomal dominant pattern.

Biochemical studies on several patients with OI have revealed definite changes in bone and skin collagen. In some studies the ratio of type I/III collagen has been shown to be markedly reduced, suggesting abnormal synthesis of type I collagen (Sykes et al, 1977; Müller et al, 1977; Fujii et al, 1977). In accordance with this observation, skin fibroblasts from some patients with OI synthesize type I and type III procollagens in a markedly reduced ratio (Penttinen et al, 1975; Turakainen et al, 1980). Some studies have suggested that type I collagen synthesized by the fibroblasts is structurally altered, so that the triple-helix is unstable when tested by pepsin proteolysis (Penttinen et al, 1975). In one of these cases, however, the Tm of the newly-synthesized type I procollagen was normal, about 40°C, when examined by circular dichroism (Peltonen et al, 1980a). Instead, the procollagen showed marked tendency to aggregate, a property which could be attributed to the presence of excessive amounts of mannose at the C-terminal extension peptide of the molecule (Peltonen et al, 1980b). In several patients with OI, increased hydroxylysine content of the bone collagen has also been observed (Trelstad et al, 1977; Fujii & Tanzer, 1977). Although the explanation for this observation is not clear, it is possible that delayed triple-helix formation of defective procollagen polypeptides leads to excessive hydroxylation of lysyl residues. It might be mentioned that intracellular degradation of newly-synthesized collagen polypeptides is unaltered in OI skin fibroblasts in culture (Steinmann et al, 1979). And finally, the stability of polymeric skin collagen has been suggested to be decreased in some patients with OI (Bauze et al, 1975; Francis & Smith, 1975).

Although the implications of some of the biochemical findings in terms of bone fragility and other connective tissue manifestations of OI are unclear, it appears that OI is a disease of type I collagen. Since type I collagen is essentially the exclusive type in normal bone matrix, decreased synthesis or formation of abnormal fibres can clearly lead to decreased bone mass, interfere with the mineralization process and cause the bone fragility.

Cutis laxa

This relatively rare disorder of connective tissue is genetically heterogeneous, and autosomal dominant, autosomal recessive, X-linked recessive, and acquired forms are known (Table 16.5) (McKusick, 1972; Beighton, 1972; Goltz et al, 1965). The primary clinical features is pendulous, redundant and stretchable skin. The skin sags into the jowls and the eyelids tend to droop, giving the patient an apperance of premature ageing. In the most severe forms the infants are born with loosely fit, hanging skin. The skin in cutis laxa, although easily stretchable, is not resilient and does not re-coil, like the skin of the Ehlers-Danlos patients. Also, the skin is not friable, there is no bruising tendency, and the hypermobility of the joints is usually absent. The most severe complications arise from the systemic manifestations of the disease. Some forms of the disease are associated with pulmonary emphysema and stenosis of pulmonary artery. These changes can lead to cor pulmonale and premature demise. Other systemic manifestations include umbilical and inguinal hernias, gastrointestinal and bladder diverticula, and rectal and uterine prolapse. Ureteral redundancy is also present in the inherited forms of the disease. The acquired form of cutis laxa (generalized elastolysis) has been described with onset often precipitated by a non-specific illness, such as urticarial rash, drug reaction, erythema multiforme, and it also has been described in association with multiple myeloma.

The biochemical basis of cutis laxa is unknown in most cases. In several instances, however, histopathological examination of the skin has revealed fragmentation of the

Table 16.5 Clinical, genetic and biochemical heterogeneity of cutis laxa[a]

Type	*Clinical features*	*Connective Tissue[b] Abnormalities*
I Dominant	Loose, sagging and wrinkled skin; systemic manifestations absent; mostly cosmetic problem	Alterations in elastic fibers
II Recessive	Redundant, sagging skin with loss of elasticity; marked systemic manifestations; progressive disease	Abnormal collagen cross-linking; fragmentation of elastic fibers
III X-linked	Marked laxity of skin; association with systemic manifestations	Lysyl oxidase deficiency
IV Acquired	Variable skin changes; systemic manifestations absent; follows episodes of illness, drug reaction, etc.	Alterations in elastic fibers

[a] Adapted from Freiberger and Pinnell (1979).
[b] These abnormalities have been detected only in a limited number of patients and it is uncertain whether the connective tissue aberrations are the same in each patient in any given type.

elastic fibres (Reed et al, 1971; Hashimoto & Kanzaki, 1975). In addition, in some cases an abnormality in collagen cross-linking process has been suggested. For example, two patients with X-linked recessive cutis laxa have been reported to have deficient lysyl oxidase activity in their cultured skin fibroblasts (Byers et al, 1980). This observation, together with increased solubility of newly-synthesized collagen in 1 M NaCl or 0.5N acetic acid. suggests that defective cross-link formation in collagen would provide an explanation for the connective tissue weakness. It should be noted that these patients also had low serum copper concentrations. Since copper is a cofactor for lysyl oxidase and experimental copper deficiency produces a clinical picture similar to that seen in patients with cutis laxa (Carnes, 1971), it might be that the primary defect in these cases may reside in the metabolism of copper. It is not known whether other cases have a similar defect in lysyl oxidase, and further studies are required to disclose the underlying biochemical defects in various forms of cutis laxa.

The Marfan syndrome

This syndrome consists of skeletal, ocular, cardiovascular and dermatological abnormalities (McKusick, 1972; Pyeritz & McKusick, 1979). In the classic form, the skeletal manifestations include tall stature, dolichostenomelia, arachnodactyly, pectus excavatum or carinatum, and kyphoscoliosis. The ocular abnormalities include myopia and congenital dislocation of the lens, the displacement being usually upward. The cardiovascular abnormalities, the most severe manifestations of the disease, include aneurysms and aortic dissection. The rupture of the aorta is the most common cause of premature demise in the Marfan syndrome (Murdoch et al, 1972). The patients also have a variety of heart valve abnormalities, mitral valve prolapse and regurgitation being the most common ones. The skin lesions of the Marfan syndrome include striae distensae, and elastosis perforans serpiginosa, a process of transepidermal elimination of elastic fibres from the dermis, has been reported in some patients.

At least two clinically distinct subsets can be separated from the classic form of the disease. Although moderate loose-jointedness is part of the clinical picture in the Marfan syndrome, some of the patients with typical Marfanoid habitus have a strikingly increased hypermobility of the joints. This variety is known as the Marfanoid hypermobility syndrome (McKusick, 1972). On the other hand, another group of patients with typical features of the Marfan syndrome have exceptionally tight joints with contractures of the hands and fingers (Beals & Hecht, 1971). This particular group of patients, known as contractural arachnodactyly, has less frequent association of cardiovascular problems.

Because of the similarity of the clinical findings of the Marfan syndrome to experimental lathyrism, a cross-linking defect has been postulated in these patients. In fact, some investigations have suggested that cross-linking of collagen in the Marfan syndrome may be abnormal. Specifically, the collagen in skin or in skin fibroblast cultures is more extractable in aqueous or denaturing solvents than collagen in the controls (Macek et al, 1966; Laitinen et al, 1968; Priest et al, 1973). However, lysyl oxidase activity has been reported to be normal in cultured skin fibroblasts from these patients (Layman et al, 1972). On the other hand, a recent in vitro study of aorta collagen in one patient with the Marfan syndrome has suggested that an insufficient synthesis of type I collagen, rather than a cross-linking defect, may be the underlying cause of the connective tissue weakness (Krieg & Müller, 1977). In another study, a qualitative and quantitative defect in α2-chain production of type I collagen was noted in one patient with the Marfan syndrome (Scheck et al, 1979).

Examination of aorta extract by SDS-polyacrylamide electrophoresis revealed two separate bands in the $\alpha2$ region, and an increase in the $\alpha1(I)/\alpha2$ ratio was noted. These changes were accompanied by increased solubility of skin collagen in 1 M NaCl or 0.5 M acetic acid. The investigators suggested, therefore, that decreased synthesis of $\alpha2$ chains leads to decreased cross-linking of collagen, which subsequently causes the weakness of connective tissues. It should be mentioned that in this study abnormal $\alpha2$-chain synthesis was noted only in one patient while type I collagen appeared to be normal in several additional patients examined.

Although the observations mentioned above suggest abnormalities in collagen, the major pathological feature of the aorta in patients with the Marfan syndrome is degeneration of the elastic structures (McKusick, 1972). In addition, abnormalities have been observed in the synthesis of proteoglycans (Lamberg & Dorfman, 1973; Appel et al, 1979). For example, the skin fibroblasts, which also stain metachromatically, synthesize about five times more hyaluronic acid than the control cells. These observations may suggest multiple possibilities for the aetiology of the Marfan syndrome. Alternatively, some of the observed changes are secondary to a primary defect which still remains to be disclosed.

Homocystinuria

This inherited condition has features resembling the Marfan syndrome, such as skeletal manifestations (kyphoscoliosis and pectus excavatum or carinatum) and ocular findings (ectopia lentis) (McKusick, 1972). However, these two conditions can be clearly distinguished on clinical basis by associated cardiovascular, neurologic and skin findings (Table 16.6). Also the mode of inheritance is different in that homocystinuria is inherited in an autosomal recessive manner while the Marfan syndrome is an autosomal dominant disease.

The basic defect in homocystinuria is reduced activity of cystathionine synthetase, an enzyme which converts homocysteine and serine to cystathionine; with defective enzymatic activity, homocysteine, homocystine, serine and methionine accumulate in tissues.

The mechanisms of connective tissue involvement in homocystinuria are not clear. It has been demonstrated, however, that skin collagen in patients with homocystinuria is more soluble than in the controls (Harris & Sjoerdsma, 1966). This observation, together with the clinical similarity to lathyrism, have suggested that the formation or stability of collagen cross-links may be altered by the accumulation of one of the metabolites mentioned above. Because of the similarity of the structures of homocysteine and penicillamine, it was initially suggested the homocysteine might bind to lysine-derived aldehydes and thus prevent the cross-linking (Kang & Trelstad, 1973). The problem with this suggestion is that the concentrations required to prevent the formation of aldehyde-derived cross-links in vitro are about 10 times higher than those found in the serum of patients with homocystinuria. Furthermore, it has been demonstrated that in the presence of homocysteine in the concentrations found in these patients there is actually an accumulation of the aldehyde-derived collagen cross-link, dehydrohydroxylysinonorleucine (Siegel, 1975). This suggests that homocysteine may prevent the stabilization of the newly-synthesized cross-links, and as a consequence, the collagen fibres do not acquire the normal tensile strength.

Menkes kinky hair syndrome

This syndrome is inherited in an X-linked recessive pattern. The major clinical manifestations include connective tissue disorders, together with neurological and pigmentary abnormalities (Menkes et al, 1962; McKusick, 1972; Uitto & Lichtenstein, 1976). Clinically, the patients have pallid skin, and lacklustre, hypopigmented hair which is tangled and brittle. The infants are often born prematurely, and hypothermia, peripheral circulatory

Table 16.6 Comparison of clinical features in the Marfan syndrome and homocystinuria

Feature	*The Marfan syndrome*	*Homocystinuria*
Inheritance	Autosomal dominant	Autosomal recessive
Skin	Striae distensae; elastosis perforans serpiginosa	Malar flush; livedo reticularis; thin skin
Eyes	Congenital ectopia lentis, displacement upward	Acquired ectopia lentis, displacement downward
Skeletal	Marked arachnodactyly; pectus excavatum or carinatum; kyphoscoliosis; no osteoporosis; loose joints	Occasional arachnodactyly; pectus excavatum or carinatum; mild kyphoscoliosis; osteoporosis; stiff joints with contractions
Cardiovascular	Aortic dilatation and dissection; heart valve abnormalities	Thrombosis of the blood vessels causing myocardial infarcts and cardiovascular accidents
Neurologic	Normal intelligence	Frequent mental retardation

problems, deterioration of the central nervous system, and infections complicate the neonatal period, making the disease lethal in infancy. The connective tissue manifestations include luminal irregularities and generalized tortuosity of the cerebral arteries, and wormian bones and metaphyseal spurs of the long bones, when examined by radiographic techniques. Histopathology of the arteries reveals fragmentation and reduplication of the internal elastic lamina.

The primary defect in the patients with Menkes kinky hair syndrome is in copper metabolism (Danks et al, 1972 a, b). The serum levels of copper are extremely low while the intracellular copper concentrations appear to be high. It has been also demonstrated that skin fibroblasts from patients with Menkes kinky hair syndrome concentrate copper intracellularly (Danks & Cartwright, 1973). These observations suggest that the primary defect in this disease may be in a protein involved in copper binding or transport across the membranes (Goka et al, 1976).

The multiplicity of the clinical manifestations can probably be explained by deficient activities of copper-requiring enzymes in various tissues. These include ascorbic acid oxidase, tyrosinase, sulphydryl oxidase and dopamine hydroxylase, which are involved in ascorbic acid transport, melanin formation, keratinization and catecholamine formation, respectively (Freiberger & Pinnell, 1979). Deficiencies in these functions could then explain some of the changes in connective tissues, pigmentation, hair and central nervous system. In terms of connective tissue involvment, most of the abnormalities could be explained by a deficiency in lysyl oxidase activity. Since this enzyme is responsible for initiation of the cross-linking process not only for collagen but elastin, as well (see Uitto, 1979), it is clear that decreased lysyl oxidase activity could explain the connective tissue changes, such as degeneration of the arterial tissues.

Alkaptonuria with ochronosis

Another inherited disease in which the underlying defect is clearly unrelated to connective tissue but secondarily affects the collagen is alkaptonuria. The basic defect is absence of homogentisic acid oxidase, an enzyme metabolizing homogentisic acid to malethylacetoacetic acid. Thus, in homocystinuria, an autosomal recessive condition, homogentisic acid accumulates in tissues (McKusick, 1972). Clinically, the patients display dark urine, abnormal pigmentation of cartilages, degeneration of the joints, and vascular abnormalities (Lichtenstein & Kaplan, 1954). The pigmentary changes can be explained by oxidation of homogentisic acid into benzoquinone acetic acid which can polymerize into a melanin-like pigment; this pigmented compound then irreversibly binds to connective tissues (Milch, 1962).

It has been recently demonstrated that homogentisic acid inhibits lysyl hydroxylase activity in vitro (Murray et al, 1977). The inhibition was competitive with respect to ascorbic acid, and lysyl hydroxylase could be protected by the addition of reducing agents, such as ascorbic acid or dithiothreitol. On the basis of these observations it is possible that homogentisic acid in vivo prevents lysyl hydroxylation, and the collagen in affected patients is deficient in hydroxylysine. As a consequence, the cross-linking of collagen would be defective, and this would then lead to degenerative changes of the joints and vascular tissues.

Familial cutaneous collagenoma

In 1968, three brothers with asymptomatic cutaneous nodules on the back and arms were reported by Henderson et al (1968). Histologically, the nodules showed marked thickening of the skin due to excessive deposition of collagen in dermis. Based on the clinical and histological presentations of the lesions, the authors suggested the name familial cutaneous collagenoma. Subsequently, a female patient with somewhat similar cutaneous nodules was reported, but in this case there was no family history of similar dermal lesions (Hegedus & Schorr, 1972).

Recently, six patients, representing a kindred of 53, with a clinical picture similar to those described by Henderson was reported by us (Uitto et al, 1979a). These patients had multiple dermal nodules symmetrically distributed on the trunk and upper arms. Histologically, the dermal lesions were characterized by an excessive accumulation of thick, coarse collagen fibres in the dermis. Analysis of hydroxyproline in a skin biopsy including the full-thickness dermis indicated that the collagen content of the skin in a lesion was increased 8- to 10- fold over the normal-looking skin in the same patient. The skin lesions in these patients are, therefore, connective tissue nevi of the collagen type (Uitto et al, 1980a).

Because of the relatively large number of patients affected and the presence of the lesions in individuals representing three different generations, we were able to establish an autosomal dominant mode of inheritance in familial cutaneous collagenoma (Uitto et al, 1979a). An interesting observation was the fact that the lesions in all patients had an onset at the age of 15–19 years, and the total number of lesions increased during each pregnancy. It appears, therefore, that familial cutaneous collagenoma is an inherited condition whose expression is under a hormonal control. Thus, changes which occur during puberty and pregnancy may accelerate the phenotypic expression of the lesions.

The reasons for excessive accumulation of collagen in the skin are unknown at present. Preliminary studies with fibroblasts derived from the skin lesions of familial cutaneous collagenoma have indicated that, under standard tissue culture conditions in vitro, these cells synthesize procollagens of type I and type III at the same rate and in a same ratio as control cultures (Uitto et al, unpublished observations). Also, production of immunologically reacting and enzymatically active collagenase was unaltered in culture. Furthermore, the growth kinetics of the cells, in terms of mean population doubling time and final saturation density, were the same both in control and affected fibroblast cultures. Finally, serum from patients with familial cutaneous collagenoma failed to stimulate procollagen synthesis by control or affected fibroblasts more than sera from normal control subjects (Tan et al, 1980). It appears, therefore, that a local tissue factor, which is yet to be identified, is responsible for collagen accumulation in vivo. Alternatively, the cultured fibroblasts, either through selection of the cell population or under the experimental conditions, do not express the genetic abnormality in vitro.

It should be mentioned that connective tissue naevi of the collagen type can be found in tuberous sclerosis, another inherited complex of developmental anomalies. Furthermore, collagenomas have been reported in isolated cases without family history, and also as multiple dermal lesions in eruptive collagenoma syndrome. The skin lesions in all these conditions demonstrate, histologically, an excessive accumulation of collagen in tissues (Uitto et al, 1980a).

The reasons for collagen accumulation in these lesions are for the most part unclear but biochemical studies employing cultured fibroblasts have been helpful in delineating the aberrations in collagen metabolism in some of these conditions. For example, fibroblast cultures were recently used to study collagen metabolism in large cerebriform connective tissue naevi covering the plantar surfaces of both feet (Uitto et al, 1982a). Histologically, the lesions consisted of thick collagen fibres and the content of collagen, assayed as hydroxyproline content, per surface area of skin was increased about 8-fold. Thus, these lesions were connective tissue naevi of the collagen type (Uitto et al, 1982a). The fibroblast cultures established from the affected lesions were shown to produce significantly less enzymatically active and immunologically detectable collagenase than that by similar cell cultures derived from the unaffacted areas of skin. The fibroblasts derived from the lesion also displayed slightly shortened mean population doubling time as compared to control cells from the normal skin of the same patient or cells derived from unrelated control individuals. However, cell cultures derived from the lesion and from control skin synthesized procollagen at the same rate and in a normal type I/type III procollagen ratio. These results suggested that, in this particular case, the excessive deposition of collagen in the skin lesion may have resulted from decreased local degradation of collagen, while enhanced proliferative capacity of the regional fibroblasts could have contributed to the accumulation of collagen as well. It was postulated that the fibroblasts of the lesion represented a clonal population of cells; in these cells there may have been an aberration at the transcriptional or translational level of the synthesis of collagenase protein. Alternatively, an abnormality at the post-translational level of protein synthesis, such as increased intracellular degradation of enzyme protein, could provide an explanation for diminished accumulation of collagenase in the affected cultures (Uitto et al, 1982a).

Focal dermal hypoplasia

This syndrome is characterized by widespread anomalies of cutaneous, osseus, ocular and dental structures (Goltz et al, 1962, 1970). This syndrome is predominantly seen in females, a fact probably explained by an X-linked dominant inheritance, so that the heterozygous females live to demonstrate the congenital abnormalities. In hemizygous males, however, it has been postulated that the disease is so severe that intrauterine death occurs.

The syndrome, as defined by Goltz (1962), consists of a congenital decrease in the dermal connective tissue in association with other defects involving tissues of ectodermal and mesodermal origin. Histopathologically, the skin lesions are characterized by absence of dermal collagen and other connective tissues, so that mature fat cells, usually located in the subcutaneous tissue, occupy large areas of the upper dermis (Lever & Schaumburg-Lever, 1975).

Recent study of a patient with focal dermal hypoplasia demonstrated that fibroblasts derived from the affected skin were characterized by a markedly compromised growth potential, with a mean population doubling time twice that of the controls and a final saturation density of one-fifth that of control cultures (Uitto et al, 1980b). Phase contrast microscopy revealed that fibroblasts from the skin lesions were strikingly abnormal and characterized by large granular cytoplasm with cytoplasmic vacuoles. In spite of these findings, the rate of collagen production per cell was normal, and procollagens type I and III were synthesized in a normal ratio. These findings suggest that an abnormality in cell kinetics may have relevance to the absence of collagen and other connective tissue components of the dermis in focal dermal hypoplasia. The abnormalities observed in the growth kinetics and morphology of the fibroblasts might reflect an inherent cellular defect in a structure essential for normal cell proliferation; such defect might, for example, reside in the membrane structures of these cells. It should be mentioned that only the fibroblasts in lesions, but not in normal-appearing skin, demonstrated the cellular abnormalities (Uitto et al, 1980b).

Thus, the fibroblasts in the lesions of focal dermal hypoplasia appear to represent a distinct population, and the patchy distribution of the lesions in the skin of affected females may reflect mosaicism as a consequence of random inactivation of the X-chromosome.

Recessive dystrophic epidermolysis bullosa

In order to maintain the necessary tensile properties of the skin, specific mechanisms for controlled degradation of collagen must exist. Collagenases, enzymes capable of degrading native collagen, are now known to exist in a number of human and animal tissues, and studies indicate that this group of enzymes occupy a crucial position in both the normal and pathological remodelling of collagen in vivo (Eisen, Bauer & Jeffrey, 1970). In this section, we shall describe certain properties and control of human skin collagenase, focusing only on those areas which may be pertinent to the regulation of this enzyme in pathological states in the skin.

The aetiologies of the various forms of epidermolysis bullosa are unknown. However, electron microscopic observations of recessive dystrophic epidermolysis bullosa have disclosed collagen degeneration and phagocytosis of collagen fibrils by macrophages in the area of blister formation (Pearson, 1962), suggesting that mechanisms involved in collagen breakdown might be important in the pathogenesis of blister formation. Indeed, the collagenase activity of skin from friction blisters produced in patients with recessive dystrophic epidermolysis bullosa was approximately 6-fold greater than that found in the normal skin (Eisen, 1969; Lazarus, 1972). In addition, in one study, enzyme activity in nonbullous skin of these patients was also elevated (Eisen, 1969). Despite the data which suggested that the blistering in recessive dystrophic epidermolysis bullosa was at least in part due to excessive collagenase activity, it remained unclear whether the in vitro observation of increased enzyme reflected the primary cause of the disease or represented a nonspecific or secondary (wound healing) response limited to the blistered skin (Eisen, 1969). If the genetic abnormality were to result in a fundamental biochemical change characterized by an excess of collagenase, this should be reflected in the unaffected skin as well.

A major difficulty in determining the significance of collagenase in the in vivo degradation of collagen has been the inability to detect active enzyme readily in vivo. Thus, to evaluate further in vivo role of collagenase in epidermolysis bullosa, we developed a specific radioimmunoassay for quantitating collagenase in biological material (Bauer, Eisen & Jeffrey, 1972).

Utilizing this assay, human skin collagenase was quantitated by radioimmunoassay in 40 patients with various forms of epidermolysis bullosa to compare levels of the enzyme in blistered and clinically unaffected skin (Bauer, Gedde-Dahl & Eisen, 1977). Immunoreactive human skin collagenase was significantly elevated in blistered skin both in patients with the recessive and with the dominant form of epidermolysis bullosa. Of greater importance, however, was the fact that patients with recessive dystrophic epidermolysis bullosa manifested a mean 4-fold increase in collagenase protein in their normal-appearing skin and in some patients immunoreactive collagenase was as high as 12-fold greater. In contrast, patients with dominantly inherited dystrophic epidermolysis bullosa failed to display a significant increase in immunoreactive collagenase in their nonblistered skin. The finding of elevated collagenase in normal-appearing skin of patients with recessive dystrophic epidermolysis bullosa suggested that the enzyme could, in part, provide an explanation at the molecular level for the formation of the blistering in this disease (Bauer, Gedde-Dahl & Eisen, 1977).

Such a hypothesis would imply a fundamental aberration in the regulation of synthesis, degradation and/or activity of enzyme. Since previous studies established fibroblasts as the primary source of human skin collagenase under physiological conditions, if an aberration in collagenase were basic to the aetiology of recessive dystrophic epidermolysis bullosa, it might be expected that it would be expressed in fibroblast cultures. This possibility was explored using cell cultures from patients with the severe form of recessive dystrophic epidermolysis bullosa to examine the properties of the collagenase produced by the mutant cell lines (Bauer, 1977).

Purified procollagenase preparations from the cell cultures of these two patients were shown to be significantly more thermolabile than control enzyme preparations at low Ca^{2+} concentration (Fig. 16.1). Furthermore, they showed a decreased affinity for Ca^{2+}, a cofactor required both for enzyme activity and thermal stability (Table 16.7). In addition, the collagenase from each mutant cell line displayed diminished catalytic efficiency (activity per unit immunoreactive protein), a finding which subsequent studies have suggested can be attributed to the marked lability of the recessive dystrophic epidermolysis bullosa collagenase. The data support the postulate that the increased synthesis of the altered collagenase may be the result of a structural gene mutation, a defect in a post-translational modification of the enzyme or a mutation in a gene regulating the synthesis of collagenase.

Table 16.7 Apparent Km for Ca^{2+} of fibroblast collagenases from patients with epidermolysis bullosa (EB)

Collagenase source	*Apparent Km (mM)*
Normal controls	1.14 ± 0.09[a]
Recessive dystrophic EB	3.98 ± 0.67[b]
Dominant EB simplex	1.06
Recessive EB letalis	1.07

[a] Expressed as mean ± SE.
[b] $p < 0.001$ compared to controls or other EB collagenases.

The expression of an altered form of the enzyme in fibroblast cultures of patients with recessive dystrophic epidermolysis bullosa suggested that a detailed study

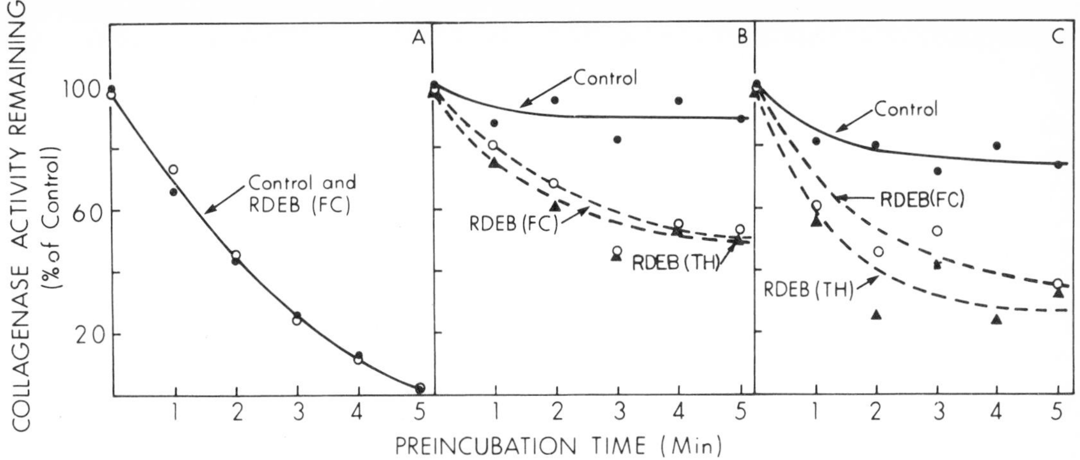

Fig. 16.1 Thermal inactivation of control and recessive dystrophic epidermolysis bullosa collagenases. Portions of purified procollagenase preparations were heated at 60°C for 0–5 min after which residual collagenase activity was measured. A, Thermal stability in the complete absence of Ca^{2+}. B, Thermal stability in 10 mM Ca^{2+}. C, Thermal stability in 2 mM Ca^{2+} for the control and in 2 mM and 4 mM Ca^{+} for collagenases from RDEB(TH) and RDEB(FC) respectively. ●——● control procollagenase; O——O, RDEB(FC) procollagenase; ▲——▲, RDEB(TH) procollagenase. (Adapted from Bauer, 1977.)

should be undertaken to determine if overproduction of an altered form of collagenase were an in vitro characteristic of this disorder. Examining fibroblast cultures from 10 patients with recessive dystrophic epidermolysis bullosa, we found the cells from 8 patients to have an increased capacity to synthesize and secrete collagenase (Fig. 16.2) (Bauer & Eisen, 1978). Furthermore, the finding of increased collagenase appeared to be a specific manifestation of these cells in that prototypic lysosomal and cytoplasmic enzymes were present in approximately normal concentrations. The elevated concentrations of immunoreactive collagenase in fibroblast cultures in patients with recessive dystrophic epidermolysis bullosa were, in certain circumstances, accompanied by increased enzyme activity and reflected those previously observed in explant cultures (Eisen, 1969).

More recent studies examining detailed biosynthetic mechanisms in recessive dystrophic epidermolysis bullosa fibroblast cultures strongly suggest the existence of a defect in the regulation of synthesis of collagenase in this disease (Valle and Bauer, 1980). These findings lend strong support to the concept of some pathogenetic role for the enzyme in the blistering phenomenon.

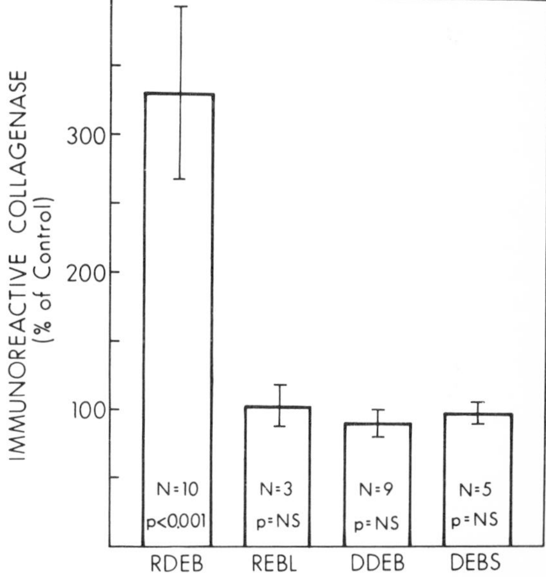

Fig. 16.2 Immunoreactive collagenase concentration in epidermolysis bullosa fibroblast cultures. Human skin collagenase was quantitated in the culture medium after a 24-hr serum-free period by radioimmunoassay (Bauer, Eisen & Jeffrey, 1972) using cells from 10 patients with recessive dystrophic epidermolysis bullosa (RDEB), 3 patients with recessive epidermolysis bullosa letalis (REBL), 9 patients with dominant dystrophic epidermolysis bullosa, and 5 patients with dominant epidermolysis bullosa simplex (DEBS). The values are presented as mean ± SE per cent of control, so that comparisons can be made between experiments. (Adapted from Bauer & Eisen, 1978.)

Acquired diseases

In several acquired diseases, the metabolism or structure of collagen has been shown to be abnormal, usually as a consequence of a non-specific pathological process. Although the collagen abnormality, such as excessive deposition of collagen in various fibrotic processes, is not the primary event in these conditions, the collagen aberrations can have serious consequences and may be responsible for most of the clinical symptoms (Kivirikko & Risteli, 1976; Prockop et al, 1979, Bailey & Duance, 1980).

Since most of the localized processes are discussed in this text in the context of specific tissue collagens, here we are concentrating on two acquired diseases which have multisystem involvement of collagen; scleroderma and diabetes, and localized processes associated with cutaneous neoplasms.

Scleroderma

One of the acquired conditions, which has received considerable attention among the collagen chemists, is scleroderma. This disease consists of a group of related conditions characterized by excessive deposition of collagen in the skin and subcutaneous tissue (Table 16.8) (Eisen et al, 1979). In the generalized form of scleroderma, progressive systemic sclerosis, several internal organs, such as kidneys, lungs and the gastrointestinal tract are affected (Rodnan, 1965; Winkelmann, 1976). A subset of generalized scleroderma, the CREST-syndrome, which has a more favourable prognosis, consists of Calcinosis cutis, Raynaud's phenomenon, Esophageal dysmobility, Sclerodactyly and Teleangiectasia (Velayos et al, 1979). In the localized form, the tissue involvement is exclusively limited to the skin, either in the form of isolated lesions as in localized morphea or with extensive cutaneous involvement as in generalized morphea (Fleischmajer & Nedwich, 1972; Uitto et al, 1980c). Finally, scleroderma-like skin changes can be observed as an associated feature in a variety of metabolic or immunologic disorders (Jablonska, 1975); LeRoy et al, 1980). Some of them are mentioned in Table 16.8.

Table 16.8 Various forms of scleroderma in the skin

Generalized:
1. Progressive systemis sclerosis
2. CREST-syndrome

Localized:
1. Isolated lesions of morphea
2. Linear morphea
3. Generalized morphea

Associated feature in:
1. Mixed connective tissue disease
2. Overlap syndromes with lupus erythematosus and dermatomyositis
3. Eosinophilic fasciitis
4. Chronic graft-vs-host reaction
5. Porphyria cutanea tarda
6. Phenylketonuria

Most of our knowledge of various aspects of collagen metabolism in scleroderma has been gained through studies on progressive systemic sclerosis. The early evidence clearly pointed to the conclusion that increased synthesis, rather than deficient removal, is responsible for excessive deposition of collagen in tissues (Uitto, 1972). This conclusion was based on the observations that the activity of prolylhydroxylase, incorporation of radioactive proline into collagen, and the synthesis of radioactive hydroxyproline in vitro were increased in skin biopsy specimens taken from patients with active scleroderma. This conclusion was further supported by cross-link analyses: skin collagen in active scleroderma contained newly formed labile cross-links, a finding consistent with increased collagen synthesis (Herbert et al, 1974).

In addition to these studies on collagen biosynthesis, one report has suggested that the activity of collagenase is decreased in scleroderma skin (Brady, 1975). Furthermore, immunofluorescence studies have demonstrated that lower dermis in affected skin in scleroderma contains increased amounts of fibronectin which may act as an inhibitor of tissue collagenase (Cooper et al, 1979). On the basis of the latter results, the accumulation of collagen in skin and other tissues could be explained by decreased removal rather than increased production of collagen fibres.

These questions have also been addressed by studies employing skin fibroblasts in culture. Several studies have shown that fibroblast cell lines derived from patients with active scleroderma synthesize procollagen at an increased rate (LeRoy, 1972, 1974; Jimenez & Bashey, 1977; Buckingham et al, 1978, 1980; Uitto et al, 1979b). On the other hand, production of collagenase, measured as immunologically reacting or enzymatically active enzyme, has been shown to be normal in eight lines of scleroderma fibroblast cultures, five of which demonstrated increased procollagen synthesis (Uitto et al, 1979b). More recently, examination of fibroblast cultures, which have been separately established either from the upper or lower portion of the dermis, has suggested that the most active cell population, in terms of procollagen production, is located in the lower reticular dermis (Fleichmajer et al, 1981). It is possible, therefore, that in scleroderma, there is a population of fibroblasts which excessively produce procollagen, and the deposition of collagen in the skin and other organs is responsible for the clinical manifestations of the disease.

Another aspect of collagen metabolism examined in scleroderma is the synthesis of genetically distinct types of collagen in the skin. Assay of the two major types of procollagen, types I and III, synthesized in fibroblast cultures revealed that these procollagens were produced in an unaltered ratio in spite of up to 4-fold increased total procollagen production (Uitto et al, 1979b).

This observation is supported by chemical analyses of type I and type III collagens in the affected skin in scleroderma: no marked changes in the relative distribution of these genetically distinct collagens have been noted (Lovell et al, 1979). It has been demonstrated, however, that in early stages of the disease process type III collagen is deposited in the lower dermis and subcutaneous tissue, as detected by immunofluorescence (Fleischmajer et al, 1978, 1980). Later on, the dermis mostly consists of type I collagen. In addition to types I and III, the synthesis of A–B collagen has been detected in dermal fibroblast cultures (Gay et al, 1980). In progressive systemic sclerosis, cultures derived from lower dermis accummulated significantly more A–B collagen, detected by antibody staining techniques, than cells derived from upper or lower portion of the control skin.

The mechanisms which might be responsible for increased collagen production by scleroderma fibroblasts are largely unknown at present. One of the theories suggest that the initial event in scleroderma is a vascular insult, which through events like reduced blood flow, local ischaemia and proliferative vascular response, might lead to clinical fibrosis of the skin (Campbell & LeRoy, 1975). In support of the vascular hypothesis it has been demonstrated that sera from a majority of patients with scleroderma or Raynaud's syndrome contain a factor which is cytotoxic to endothelial cells in culture (Kahaleh et al, 1979). It is postulated then that the endothelial injury leads to proliferation and influx of cells characteristically being active in collagen production. This attractive hypothesis certainly merits further testing in experimental models of vascular injury.

In addition to the vascular hypothesis, it has been suggested that scleroderma fibroblasts in culture synthesize more procollagen in response to fetal calf serum or that scleroderma cells have more stringent requirements for ascorbic acid than control cells (Bashey & Jimenez, 1977; Jimenez & Bashey, 1977). It has also been suggested that scleroderma patients' sera contain factor(s) which stimulate procollagen production by normal fibroblasts more than sera from healthy controls (Keyser et al, 1979, 1980). Although such factors may be present in sera of some patients, this observation is not a constant feature in all patients with scleroderma, and the observed increases are relatively small, about 1.5-fold at best (Tan et al, 1981).

An interesting observation related to the pathogenesis of scleroderma is the occurrence of scleroderma-like skin lesions in patients with chronic graft-vs-host reaction. (Shulman et al, 1978). This finding suggests that immunological aberrations might modulate the collagen production in vivo, and that scleroderma may have an underlying immunological cause. Indeed, it has been demonstrated that lymphokines, which are capable of causing fibroblast proliferation, chemotactic attraction and increased collagen production, can be synthesized by stimulated lymphocyte cultures (Kondo et al, 1976; Johnson & Ziff, 1976; Postlethwaite et al, 1976; Wahl et al, 1978).

Diabetes mellitus

Diabetes is clearly accompanied by changes in the metabolism and properties of connective tissues, and collagen in particular. The clinical manifestations of such changes include, for example, poor wound healing, atrophy of the skin, and thickening of the basement membranes (Freinkel & Freinkel, 1979). The precise nature of the collagen changes in the tissues of patients with diabetes is largely unknown, and some of the reported observations are contradictory. For example, Beisswenger & Spiro (1973) suggested that the thickening of the glomerular basement membrane in diabetes is a result of synthesis of abnormal basement membrane collagen rich in hydroxylysine and glucosylgalactosyl-O-hydroxylysine. In support of this suggestion it was also noted that the activity of collagen glucosyltransferase was increased in diabetic kidneys (Spiro & Spiro, 1971). The observation on abnormal basement membrane collagen in diabetes was, however, disputed by other workers (Westberg & Michael, 1973; Kefalides, 1974). Their results showed that the α-chains isolated from normal and diabetic basement membranes had similar amino acid and carbohydrate compositions (Kefalides, 1974).

Several subsequent studies, employing experimental animal models of diabetes, have explored the chemical and metabolic changes occurring in collagen. These studies suggest that the basement membrane changes occurring in diabetes induced by streptozotocin are similar to those observed in human disease, and, therefore, the streptozotocin-diabetes is an appropriate model for studies relating to the pathogenesis of diabetic complications (Fox et al, 1977; Cohen & Klein, 1979). Studies with diabetic rats also indicated that the synthesis of glomerular basement membrane collagen is markedly increased (Grant et al, 1976; Cohen & Khalifa, 1977a; Brownlee & Spiro, 1979). Concomitant with the increased basement membrane collagen synthesis, the activities of prolyl and lysyl hydroxylases as well as of glycosyltransferases involved in the biosynthesis of collagen are significantly increased in the kidneys of drug-induced diabetic rats (Khalifa & Cohen, 1975; Cohen & Khalifa, 1977b; Grant et al, 1976; Risteli et al, 1976; Haft & Reddi, 1979). Taken together, these results are consistent with accelerated production of collagen in diabetes, thus suggesting an explanation for thickening of the basement membranes.

Another interesting observation made in the streptozotocin-induced diabetes relates to the solubility of collagen in various animal tissues. For example, collagen in the tail-tendon of diabetic rats is markedly less soluble in 0.5 M acetic acid than collagen of the control animals (Golub et al, 1978). Also, the collagen synthesized in a tissue implant inserted in the subcutis of a diabetic rat is markedly less soluble than collagen synthesized in control rats (Chang et al, 1980). The decreased solubility of collagen is probably due to accelerated formation of lysine- and hydroxylysine-derived cross-links, since in animals treated with β-aminopropionitrile or D-penicillamine, the solubility of collagen from diabetics is equal to that of controls (Chang et al, 1980). This postulate is also consistent with the observation that lysyl oxidase activity is markedly increased in lungs of rats with streptozotocin-induced diabetes (Madia et al, 1979).

Of further interest is the observation that collagen can be glucosylated non-enzymatically in a similar manner as has been demonstrated in case of several other proteins, including haemoglobin A, serum albumin, other serum proteins, and erythrocyte membrane proteins (see Bailey et al, 1976; Spicer et al, 1979; McFarland et al, 1979). The addition of glucose moeity occurs through a ketoamine linkage, and the sugar residues are attached either to the α-amino group of the N-terminal amino acid or to the ϵ-amino group of internal lysyl residues in the protein (Bookchin & Gallop, 1968). In experimental diabetes, the glucose content of collagen isolated from the thoracic aorta has been shown to be increased (Rosenberg et al, 1979). Also, preliminary studies on glomerular basement membrane collagen, isolated from kidneys of patients who died from diabetic complications, have indicated that the non-enzymatic glucosylation is increased 2- to 3-fold over the corresponding controls (Uitto et al, 1980d).

On the basis of observations made in diabetic patients, as well as in the animal models of diabetes, one could conclude that over-glycosylated collagen, which is extensively cross-linked, is synthesized perhaps at an accelerated rate in diabetes. Two lines of evidence suggest that this abnormal collagen is not removed from the basement membranes at a control rate, but an accumulation of collagen occurs instead. First, it has been demonstrated that cross-linked collagen is less susceptible to degradation by specific collagenases (Vater et al, 1979). Secondly, genetically distinct collagens with high carbohydrate content are characteristically more resistant to collagenases of tissue origin, and specific collagenolytic enzymes are required for degradation of collagens, as for example type IV (Liotta et al, 1979; Uitto V-J et al, 1980). It appears, therefore, that the removal of basement membrane collagen is impaired, and the accumulation of collagen then contributes to the development of vascular complications in diabetes (Williamson & Kilo, 1977).

Cutaneous neoplasms

Since the invasive properties of a variety of malignant tumours may depend in part upon proteases, as suggested by the correlation of increased proteolytic activity with both in vivo and in vitro markers of malignancy, a variety of experimental methods have been utilized to assess the potential role of collagenase in cutaneous tumours. Initial studies (Dresden, Heilman & Schmidt, 1972) utilized tissue specimens cultured for a short period of time in serum-free medium or on reconstituted native collagen gels. Utilizing this in vitro technique, a variety of cutaneous neoplasms, most noteworthy, basal cell carcinoma and squamous cell carcinoma, were found to contain increased amounts of collagenase activity. In certain circumstances, these enzymes were partially characterized (Dresden, Heilman & Schmidt, 1972) and found to resemble the collagenase derived from short-term serum-free cultures of normal human skin (Eisen, Jeffrey & Gross, 1968). It was, thus, unclear whether the increase in collagenase was in fact derived from the tumour tissue itself or was present as part of a normal tissue response to the tumours.

Employing a somewhat different approach, Hashimoto and his associates (Yamanishi, Dabbous & Hashimoto, 1972; Hashimoto, Yamanishi & Dabbous, 1972; Yamanishi et al, 1973; Hashimoto et al, 1973) examined tissue extracts from basal cell carcinomas, malignant melanomas, and squamous cell carcinomas of the skin. In each of these cases, increased collagenase activity was reported in the crude tissue extracts of the tumours. However, the overall levels of activity described were low, and it seems possible that the existence of proenzyme species and the presence of a variety of inhibitors of collagenase may have partially compromised complete recovery of the enzyme.

Since basal cell carcinomas are tumours of epithelial origin which typically produce local invasion but rarely metastasize, they should be an ideal prototypic tumour in which to examine the mechanisms by which tumours produce local destruction and invasion. The use of immunological techniques to measure collagenase in extracts of normal and diseased tissues has permitted us to assess the potential role of collagenase in tumour invasion without depending upon collagenase activity, which can be influenced by the factors noted above (Bauer et al, 1977). Human skin collagenase was quantitated by radio-immunoassay in 21 basal cell carcinomas and found to be approximately 2-fold greater in extracts of these tumours than in normal skin. These findings suggested that the enzyme may be important in the pathogenesis of soft tissue destruction in vivo.

To define further the role of collagenase in such destruction, immunofluorescence staining with antiserum to human skin collagenase was used to localize the enzyme in the tumours (Fig. 16.3). The enzyme was found only in the stromal elements surrounding the tumour islands (Bauer et al, 1977). No staining of the epithelial components of the basal cell carcinomas was found. Although it is possible that the collagenase could have been produced by the tumour cells and rapidly bound to the surrounding collagenous matrix, the findings suggest that the normal connective tissue elements may have been stimulated to produce increased amounts of collagenase. It is of interest that electron microscopic studies of basal cell carcinoma demonstrate the loss of collagen adjacent to the tumour (Hashimoto et al, 1972; McNutt, 1976), a morphological finding that would seem to correlate well with the immunofluorescent localization of collagenase. It is, thus, possible that the tumours may be producing an as yet unidentified diffusable factor capable of stimulating collagenase production by adjacent fibroblasts.

In this regard, it is of interest that fibroblast cultures derived from human basal cell carcinomas demonstrated an increased capacity to synthesize and secrete collagenase (Bauer et al, 1979). The levels of collagenase were up to 8-fold greater than those of normal control cell lines.

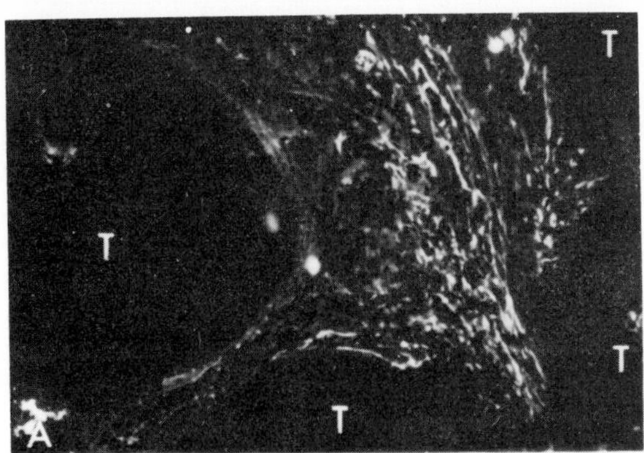

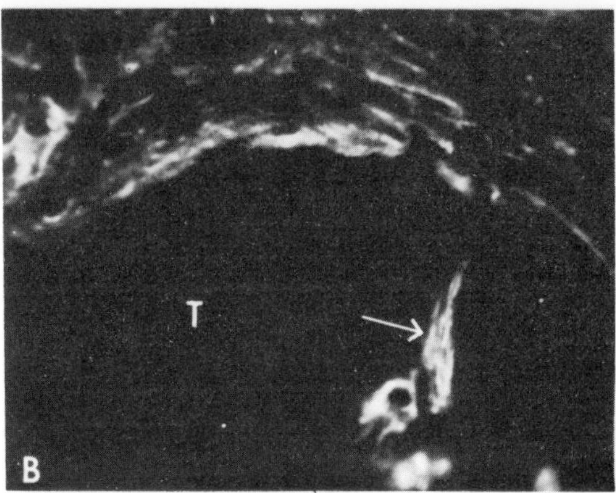

Fig. 16.3 Immunofluorescent localization of human skin collagenase in basal cell carcinoma. Sections were stained with rabbit anti-collagenase serum followed by fluorescein isothiocyanate-labeled goat anti-rabbit IgG as the second antibody. Note the intense staining of the stromal elements adjacent to the tumour islands (T) of basal cell carcinoma. A, 163 ×. B = 312 ×; the arrow denotes an area of stroma in the midst of a tumour island (T). (Adapted from Bauer, Gordon, Reddick & Eisen, 1977.)

However, this phenotypic trait was not permanent and was expressed only for a few passages following primary explantation of the tumour fragments. The basal cell carcinoma fibroblast collagenase was secreted as a proenzyme and the kinetics of activation and the catalytic efficiency of the basal cell carcinoma fibroblast enzyme were equal to control collagenase, indicating that increased activity was due to increased synthesis of enzyme protein. Increased synthesis of collagenase was not due either to altered cell growth or to an overall increase in protein synthesis. Furthermore, synthesis of another major protein, collagen, was not enhanced. Thus, the data suggest that the tumours may have stimulated adjacent fibroblasts to produce more collagenase, which is of importance in tumour invasion.

REFERENCES

Appel A, Horwitz A L, Dorfman A 1979 Cell-free synthesis of hyaluronic acid in Marfan syndrome. Journal of Biological Chemistry 254: 12199

Bailey A J, Lapière C M 1973 Effect of an additional peptide extension of the N-terminus of collagen from dermatosparactic calves on the cross-linking of collagen. European Journal of Biochemistry 34: 91

Bailey A J, Robins S P, Tanner M J A 1976 Reducible components in the proteins of human erythrocyte membranes. Biochimica et Biophysica Acta 434: 51

Bailey A J, Duance V C 1980 Collagen in acquired connective tissue diseases: an active or passive role? European Journal of Clinical Investigation 10: 1

Barabas A P 1967 Heterogeneity of the Ehlers-Danlos syndrome; description of three clinical types and a hypothesis to explain the basic defect(s). British Medical Journal 2: 612

Bashey R I, Jimenez S A 1977 Increased sensitivity of scleroderma fibroblasts in culture to stimulation of protein and collagen synthesis by serum. Biochemical and Biophysical Research Communications 76: 1214

Bauer E A, Uitto J 1979 Collagen in cutaneous diseases. International Journal of Dermatology 18: 251

Bauer E A, Eisen A Z, Jeffrey J J 1972 Radioimmunoassay of human collagenase. Specificity of the assay and quantitative determination of in vivo and in vitro human skin collagenase. Journal of Biological Chemistry 247: 6679

Bauer E A 1977 Recessive dystrophic epidermolysis bullosa: evidence for an altered collagenase in fibroblast cultures. Proceedings of the National Academy of Sciences USA 74: 4646

Bauer E A, Gedde-Dahl T, Eisen A Z 1977 The role of human skin collagenase in epidermolysis bullosa. Journal of Investigative Dermatology 68: 119

Bauer E A, Eisen A Z 1978 Recessive dystrophic epidermolysis bullosa: evidence for increased collagenase as a genetic characteristic in cell culture. Journal of Experimental Medicine 148: 1378

Bauer E A, Gordon J M, Reddick M E, Eisen A Z 1977 Quantitation and immunocytochemical localization of human skin collagenase in basal cell carcinoma. Journal of Investigative Dermatology 69: 363

Bauer E A, Uitto J, Walters R C, Eisen A Z 1979 Enhanced collagenase production by fibroblasts derived from human basal cell carcinoma. Cancer Research 39: 4594

Bauze R J, Smith R, Francis M J O 1975 A new look at osteogenesis imperfecta. A clinical, radiological and biochemical study of fourty-two patients. Journal of Bone and Joint Surgery 578A: 2

Beals R K, Hecht F 1971 Contractural arachnodactyly, a heritable disorder of connective tissue. Journal of Bone and Joint Surgery 53A: 987

Beasley R R, Cohen M M 1979 A new presumably autosomal recessive form of the Ehlers-Danlos syndrome. Clinical Genetics 16: 19

Becker U, Timpl R, Helle O, Prockop D J 1976 NH_2-terminal eftensions on skin collagen from sheep with a genetic defect in conversion of procollagen into collagen. Biochemistry 15: 2853

Beighton P 1968a lethal complications of the Ehlers-Danlos syndrome. British Medical Journal 3: 656

Beighton P 1968b X-linked recessive inheritance in the Ehlers-Danlos syndrome. British Medical Journal 2: 9

Beighton P 1970 The Ehlers-Danlos Syndrome. William Heinemann Medical Books Ltd, London

Beighton P 1972 The dominant and recessive forms of cutis laxa. Journal of Medical Genetics 9: 216

Beighton P, Horan F 1969 Orthopaedic aspects of the Ehlers-Danlos syndrome. Journal of Bone and Joint Surgery 51B: 444

Beighton P, Murdoch J L, Votteler T 1969 Gastrointestinal complications of the Ehlers-Danlos syndrome. Gut 10: 1004

Beisswenger P J, Spiro R G 1973 Studies on the human glomerular basement membrane. Composition, nature of the carbohydrate units and chemical changes in diabetes mellitus. Diabetes 22: 180

Black C M, Gathercole L J, Bailey A J, Beighton P 1980 The Ehlers-Danlos syndrome: an analysis of the structure of the collagen fibres of the skin. British Journal of Dermatology 102: 85

Bookchin R M, Gallop P M 1968 Structure of haemoglobin A_{1c}: nature of N-terminal β-chain blocking group. Biochemical and Biophysical Research Communications 32: 86

Bornstein P, Byers P H 1980 Collagen Metabolism. The Upjohn Company, Kalamazoo

Bornstein P, Sage H 1980 Structurally distinct collagen types. Annual Review of Biochemistry 49: 957

Brady A H 1975 Collagenase in scleroderma. Journal of Clinical Investigation 56: 1175

Brownlee M, Spiro R G 1979 Glomerular basement membrane metabolism in the diabetic rat. In vivo studies. Diabetes 28: 121

Buckingham R, Prince R K, Rodnan G P, Taylor F 1978 Increased collagen accumulation in dermal fibroblast cultures from patients with progressive systemic sclerosis (scleroderma). Journal of Laboratory and Clinical Medicine 92: 5

Buckingham R B, Prince R K, Rodnan G P, Barnes E L 1980 Collagen accumulation by dermal fibroblast cultures of patients with linear scleroderma. Journal of Rheumatology 7: 30

Byers P H, Holbrook K A, McGillvray B, MacLeod P M, Lowry R B 1979 Clinical and ultrastructural heterogeneity of type IV Ehlers-Danlos syndrome. Human Genetics 47: 141

Byers P H, Siegel R C, Holbrook K A, Narayanan A S, Bornstein P, Hall J G 1980 X-linked cutis laxa. Defective cross-link formation in collagen due to decreased lysyl oxidase activity. New England Journal of Medicine 303: 61

Campbell P M, LeRoy E C 1975 Pathogenesis of systemic sclerosis: a vascular hypothesis. Seminars in Arthritis and Rheumatism 4: 351

Carnes W H 1971 Role of copper in connective tissue metabolism. Federation Proceedings 30: 995

Chang K, Uitto J, Ronnald E A, Grant G A, Kilo C, Williamson J R 1980 Decreased collagen extractability in diabetes; Reversal by β aminopropionitrile (βAPN) and D-penicillamine. Diabetes, 29: 778

Clark C C, Kefalides N A 1976 Carbohydrate moieties of procollagen: incorporation of isotopically labeled mannose and glucosamine in propeptides of procollagen secreted by matrix-free chick embryo tendon cells. Proceedings of the National Academy of Sciences USA 73: 34

Clark J G, Kuhn C, Uitto J 1980 Lung collagen in type IV Ehlers-Danlos syndrome: Ultrastructural and biochemical studies. American Review of Respiratory Disease 122: 971

Cohen M P, Khalifa A 1977a Renal glomerular collagen synthesis in streptozotocin diabetes. Reversal of increased basement membrane synthesis with insulin therapy. Biochimica et Biophysica Acta 500: 395

Cohen M P, Khalifa A 1977b Effect of diabetes and insulin on rat renal glomerular protocollagen hydroxylase activities. Biochimica et Biophysica Acta 496: 88

Cohen M P, Klein C V 1979 Glomerulopathy in rats with streptozotocin diabetes. Accumulation of glomerular basement membrane analogous to human diabetic nephropathy. Journal of Experimental Medicine 149: 623

Cooper S M, Keyser A J, Beaulieu A D, Ruoslahti E, Nimni M E, Quismorio F P 1979 Increase in fibronectin in the deep dermis of involved skin in progressive systemic sclerosis. Arthritis and Rheumatism 22: 983

Counts D F, Knighten P, Hegreberg G 1977 Biochemical changes in the skin of mink with Ehlers-Danlos syndrome: Increased collagen biosynthesis in the dermis of affected mink. Journal of Investigative Dermatology 69: 521

Counts D F, Byers P H, Holbrook K A, Hegreberg G A 1980 Dermatosparaxis in a Himalayan cat: I. Biochemical studies of dermal collagen. Journal of Investigative Dermatology 74: 96

Daentl D L, Scheck M, Siegel R C, Goodman J R, Brasch R C, Larsen L J 1978 A probable new variant of Ehlers-Danlos syndrome: Clinical, structural and biochemical studies. Birth Defects: Original Article Series 14(6B): 368

Danielsen L 1979 Morphological changes in pseudoxanthoma elasticum and senile skin. Acta Dermato-venereologica 59 (supplement 83): 1

Danielsen L, Kobayashi T 1972 Degeneration of dermal elastic fibres in relation to age and light exposure. Preliminary report on electron microscopic studies. Acta Dermato-venereologica 52: 1

Danks D M, Campbell P E, Walker-Smith J, Stevens B J, Gillespie J M, Blomfield J, Turner B 1972 Menkes kinky hair syndrome. Lancet 1: 1100

Danks D M, Campbell P E, Stevens B J, Mayne V, Cartwright E 1972 Menkes's kinky hair syndrome: an inherited defect in copper absorption with widespread effects. Pediatrics 50: 180

Danks D M, Cartwright E 1973 Menkes' kinky hair disease: further definition of the defect in copper transport. Science 179: 1140

Dresden M H, Heilman S A, Schmidt J D 1972 Collagenolytic enzymes in human neoplasms. Cancer Research 32: 993

DiFerrante N, Leachman R D, Angelini P, Donnelly P V, Francis G, Almazon A 1975 Lysyl oxidase deficience in Ehlers-Danlos syndrome type V. Connective Tissue Research 3: 49

Eisen A Z, Uitto J, Bauer E A 1979 Scleroderma. In: Fitzpatrick T B, Eisen A Z, Freedberg I M, Austen K F, Wolff K (eds) Dermatology in general medicine, 2nd edn. McGraw-Hill, New York, pp 1305-13

Eisen A Z, Jeffrey J J, Gross J 1968 Human skin collagenase: isolation and mechanism of attack on the collagen molecule. Biochimica et Biophysica Acta 151: 637

Eisen A Z 1969 Human skin collagenase: relationship to the pathogenesis of epidermolysis bullosa dystrophica. Journal of Investigative Dermatology 52: 449

Eisen A Z, Bauer E A, Jeffrey J J 1970 Animal and human collagenases. Journal of Investigative Dermatology 55: 359

Elsas L J, Hollins B, Pinnell S R 1974 Hydroxylysine-deficient collagen disease: effect of ascorbic acid. American Journal of Human Genetics 26: 28A

Elsas L J, Miller R L, Pinnell S R 1978 Inherited human collagen lysyl hydroxylase deficiency: ascorbic acid response. Journal of Pediatrics 92: 378

Eylar E H 1966 On the biological role of glycoproteins. Journal of Theoretical Biology 10: 89

Eyre D R, Glimcher M J 1972 Reducible cross-links in hydroxylysine-deficient collagens of a heritable disorder of connective tissue. Proceedings of the National Academy of Sciences USA 69: 2594

Fessler J H, Fessler L I 1978 Biosynthesis of procollagen. Annual Review of Biochemistry 47: 129

Fjolstad M, Helle O 1974 A hereditary dysplasia of collagen tissues in sheep. Journal of Pathology 112: 183

Fleishmajer R, Nedwich A 1972 Generalized morphea. I. Histology of the dermis and subcutaneous tissue. Archives of Dermatology 106: 509-514

Fleischmajer R, Gay S, Meigel W N, Perlish J S 1978 Collagen in the cellular and fibrotic stages of scleroderma. Arthritis and Rheumatism 21: 418-428

Fleischmajer R, Gay S, Perlish J S, Cesarini J—P 1980 Immunoelectron microscopy of type III collagen in normal and scleroderma skin. Journal of Investigative Dermatology 75: 189

Fleischmajer R, Perlish J S, Krieg T, Timpl R 1981 Variability in collagen and fibronectin synthesis by scleroderma fibroblasts in primary culture. Journal of Investigative Dermatology 76: 400

Fox C J, Darby S C, Ireland J T, Sonksen P H 1977 Blood glucose control and glomerular capillary basement membrane thickening in experimental diabetes. British Medical Journal 2: 605

Francis M J O, Smith R 1975 Polymeric collagen of skin in osteogenesis imperfecta, homocystinuria and Ehlers-Danlos and Marfan syndromes. Birth defects: Original Article Series XI (6): 15

Freiberger H F, Pinnell S R 1979 Heritable disorders of connective tissue. Moschella S L, Dermatology Update, Elsevier, New York, p 221

Freinkel R K, Freinkel N 1979 Dermatologic manifestations of endocrine disorder. In: Fitzpatrick T B, Eisen A Z, Wolff K, Freedberg I M, Austen K F (eds) Dermatology in general medicine, 2nd edn. McGraw-Hill, New York, p 1247

Fujii K, Tanzer M L 1977 Osteogenesis imperfecta. Biochemical studies of bone collagen. Clinical Orthopedics 124: 291

Fujii K, Kajiwara T, Kurosu H, Tanzer M L 1977 Osteogenesis imperfecta: Altered content of type III collagen and proportion of the cross-links in skin. FEBS Letters 82: 251

Gay R E, Buckingham R B, Prince P K, Gay S, Rodnan G P, Miller E J 1980 Collagen types synthesized in dermal fibroblast cultures from patients with early progressive systemic sclerosis. Arthritis and Rheumatism 23: 190

Gay S, Miller E J 1978 Collagen in the physiology and pathology of connective tissue. Gustav Fischer Verlag, Stuttgart

Gay S, Martin G R, Müller P K, Timpl R, Kühn K 1976 Simultaneous synthesis of types I and III collagen by fibroblasts in culture. Proceedings of the National Academy of Sciences USA 73: 4037

Goka T J, Stevenson R E, Hefferson P M, Howell R R 1976 Menkes disease: A biochemical abnormality in cultured human fibroblasts. Proceedings of the National Academy of Sciences U.S.A. 73: 604

Goltz R W, Peterson W C, Gorlin R J, Ravits H G 1962 Focal dermal hypoplasia. Archives of Dermatology 86: 708

Goltz R W, Hult A-M, Goldfarb M, Gorlin R J 1965 Cutis laxa: a manifestation of generalized elastolysis. Archives of Dermatology 92: 373

Goltz R W, Henderson R R, Hitch J M, Ott J E 1970 Focal dermal hypoplasia syndrome: A review of the literature and report of two cases. Archives of Dermatology 101: 1

Golub L M, Greenwald R A, Zebrowski E J, Ramamurthy H S 1978 The effect of experimental diabetes on the molecular characteristics of soluble rat-tail tendon collagen. Biochimica et Biophysica Acta 534: 73

Grant M E, Harwood R, Williams I F 1976 Increased synthesis of glomerular basement membrane collagen in streptozotocin diabetes. Journal of Physiology 257: 56

Haft D E, Reddi A S 1979 Glucosyltransferase activity in kidney fractions of normal and streptozotocin-diabetic rats Biochimica et Biophysica Acta 584: 1

Hammer D, Leier C V, Baba N, Vasco J S, Wooley C F, Pinnell S R 1979 Altered collagen composition in a prolapsing mitral valve with ruptured chordae tendineae. American Journal of Medicine 67: 863

Harper E J 1980 Collagenases. Annual Review of Biochemistry 49: 1063

Harris E D Jr, Sjoerdsma A 1966 Collagen profile in various clinical conditions. Lancet 2: 707

Hashimoto K, Yamanishi Y, Dabbous M K 1972 Electron microscopic observations of collagenolytic activity of basal cell epithelioma of the skin in vivo and in vitro. Cancer Research 32: 2561

Hashimoto K, Yamanishi Y, Maeyens E, Dabbous M K 1973 Collagenolytic activities of squamous cell carcinoma of the skin. Cancer Research 33: 2790

Hashimoto K, Kanzaki T 1975 Cutis laxa: Ultrastructural and biochemical studies. Archives of Dermatology 111: 861

Hegedus S I, Schorr W F 1972 Familial cutaneous collagenoma. Cutis 10: 283

Hegreberg G A, Padgett G A, Ott R L, Henson J B 1970 A heritable connective tissue disease of dogs and mink resembling Ehlers-Danlos syndrome of man: I. Skin tensile strength and properties. Journal of Investigative Dermatology S4: 377

Henderson R R, Wheeler C E, Abele D C 1968 Familial cutaneous collagenoma. Report of cases. Archives of Dermatology 98: 23

Herbert C M, Lindberg K, Jayson M I V, Bailey A J 1974 Biosynthesis and maturation of skin collagen in scleroderma and effect of D-penicillamine. Lancet I: 187-192

Hernández A, Aguirre-Negrete M G, Ramírez-Soltero S, González-Mendoza A, Martínez y Martínez R, Velazquez-Cabrera A, Cantú J M 1979 A distinct variant of the Ehlers-Danlos syndrome. Clinical Genetics 16: 335

Hollister D W 1978 Heritable disorders of connective tissue: Ehlers-Danlos syndrome. Pediatric Clinics of North America 25: 575

Jablonska S 1975 Scleroderma and pseudoscleroderma, 2nd edn. Polish Medical Publishers, Warsaw. pp 1-579

Jaffe A S, Geltman E M, Rodey G E, Uitto J 1981 Mitral valve prolapse. A consistent manifestation of type IV Ehlers-Danlos syndrome. The pathogenetic role of abnormal type III collagen synthesis. Circulation 64: 121

Jimenez S A, Bashey R I 1977 Collagen synthesis by scleroderma fibroblasts in culture. Arthritis and Rheumatism 20: 902

Johnson R L, Ziff M 1976 Lymphokine stimulation of collagen accumulation. Journal of Clinical Investigation 48: 20

Judisch G F, Waziri M, Krachmer J H 1976 Ocular Ehlers-Danlos syndrome with normal lysyl hydroxylase activity. Archives of Ophtalmology 94: 1489

Kahaleh M B, Sherer G K, LeRoy E C 1979 Endothelial injury in scleroderma. Journal of Experimental Medicine 149: 1325

Kang A H, Trelstad R L 1973 A collagen defect in homocystinuria. Journal of Clinical Investigation 52: 2571

Kefalides N A 1974 Biochemical properties of human glomerular basement membrane in normal and diabetic kidneys. Journal of Clinical Investigation 53: 403

Keyser A J, Cooper S M, Ruoslahti E, Nimni M E, Quismorio F P 1979 Scleroderma: Enhancement of connective tissue biosynthesis by a circulating factor. Federation Proceedings 38: 1339 (abstract)

Keyser A J, Cooper S M, Nimni M E 1980 The role of a circulating factor in the pathogenesis of scleroderma. Federation Proceedings 39: 874

Khalifa A, Cohen M P 1975 Glomerular protocollagen lysylhydroxylase activity in streptozotocin diabetes. Biochimica et Biophysica Acta 386: 332

Kivirikko K I, Risteli L 1976 Biosynthesis of collagen and its alterations in pathological states. Medical Biology 54: 159

Klemperer P, Pollack A D, Baehr G 1942 Diffuse collagen disease. Acute disseminated lupus erythematosus and diffuse scleroderma. Journal of the American Medical Association 119: 331

Kondo H, Rabin B S, Rodnan G P 1976 Cutaneous antigen-stimulating lymphokine production by lymphocytes of patients of progressive systemic sclerosis (scleroderma). The Journal of Clinical Investigation 59: 1388

Krane S M, Pinnell S R, Erbe R W 1972 Lysyl-protocollagen hydroxylase deficiency in fibroblasts from siblings with hydroxylysine-deficient collagen. Proceedings of the National Academy of Sciences USA 69: 2899

Krieg T, Müller P K 1977 The Marfan's syndrome. In vitro study of collagen metabolism in tissue specimens of the aorta. Experimental Cell Biology 45: 207

Krieg T, Feldmann U, Kessler W, Müller P K 1979 Biochemical characteristics of Ehlers-Danlos syndrome type VI in a family with one affected infant. Human Genetics 46: 41

Laitinen O, Uitto J, Iivanainen M, Hannuksela M, Kivirikko K I 1968 Collagen metabolism in the skin in Marfan's syndrome. Clinica Chimica Acta 21: 321

Lamberg S, Dorfman A 1973 Synthesis and degradation of hyaluronic acid in the cultured fibroblasts of Marfan's disease. Journal of Clinical Investigation 52: 2428

Layman D L, Narayanan A S, Martin G R 1972 The production of lysyl oxidase by human fibroblasts in culture. Archives of Biochemistry and Biophysics 149: 97

Lazarus G S 1972 Collagenase and connective tissue metabolism in epidermolysis bullosa. Journal of Investigative Dermatology 58: 242

Lenaers A, Ansay M, Nusgens B V, Lapière C M 1971 Collagen made of extended α-chains, procollagen, in genetically-defective dermatosparaxic calves. European Journal of Biochemistry 23: 533

LeRoy E C 1974 Increased collagen synthesis by scleroderma skin fibroblasts in vitro. A possible defect in the regulation or activation of the scleroderma fibroblast. Journal of Clinical Investigation 54: 880

LeRoy E C 1972 Connective tissue synthesis by scleroderma skin fibroblasts in culture. Journal of Experimental Medicine 135: 1351

LeRoy E C, Maricq H R, Kahaleh M B 1980 Undifferentiated connective tissue syndromes. Arthritis and Rheumatism 23: 341

Lever W F, Schaumburg-Lever 1975 Histopathology of the skin, 5th edn. Lippincott, Philadelphia, pp 67-8

Lichtenstein J R, Kohn L, Byers P, Martin G R, McKusick V A 1973a Procollagen peptidase deficiency in a form of the Ehlers-Danlos syndrome. Transactions of the American Association of Physicians 86: 333

Lichtenstein J R, Martin G R, Kohn L D, Byers P H, McKusick V A 1973b Defect in conversion of procollagen to collagen in a form of Ehlers-Danlos syndrome. Science 182: 298

Lichtenstein L, Kaplan L 1954 Hereditary ochronosis. Pathological changes observed in two necropsied cases. American Journal of Pathology 30: 99

Liotta L, Abe S, Robey P, Martin G 1979 Preferential digestion of basement collagen by an enzyme derived from a metastatic murine tumour. Proceedings of the National Academy of Sciences USA 76: 2268

Lovell C R, Nicholls A C, Duance V C, Bailey A J 1979 Characterizations of dermal collagen in systemic sclerosis. British Journal of Dermatology 100: 359

Macek M, Hurych J, Chvapil M, Kaddlecova V 1966 Study of fibroblasts in Marfan syndrome. Humangenetik 3: 87

Madia A M, Rozovski S J, Kagan H M 1979 Changes in lung lysyl oxidase activity in streptozotocin-diabetes and in starvation. Biochimica et Biophysica Acta 585: 481

McNutt N S 1976 Ulstrastructural comparison of the interface between epithelium and stroma in basal cell carcinoma and control human skin. Laboratory Investigation 35: 132

McFarland K F, Catalano E W, Day J F, Thorpe S R, Baynes J W 1979 Nonenzymatic glucosylation of serum proteins in diabetes mellitus. Diabetes 28: 1011

McKusick V A 1972 Heritable Disorders of Connective Tissue 4th edition. Mosby, St. Louis

Menkes J H, Alter M, Steigleder G K, Weakley D R, Sung J H 1962 A sex-linked recessive disorder with retardation of growth, peculiar hair and focal cerebral and cerebellar degeneration. Pediatrics 29: 764

Milch R A 1962 Biochemical studies on the pathogenesis of collagen tissue changes in alkaptonuria. Clinical Orthopaedics 24: 213

Miller E J 1976 Biochemical characteristics and biological significance of the genetically distinct collagens. Molecular and Cellular Biochemistry 13: 165

Miller E J, Robertson P B 1973 The stability of collagen cross-links when derived from hydroxylysyl residues. Biochemical and Biophysical Research Communications 54, 432

Minor R R 1980 Collagen metabolism. A comparison of diseases of collagen and diseases affecting collagen. American Journal of Pathology 98: 227

Müller P K, Raisch K, Matzen K, Gay S 1977 Presence of type III collagen in bone from a patient with osteogenesis imperfecta. European Journal of Pediatrics 125: 29

Murdock J L, Walker B A, Halpern B L, Kusman J W, McKusick V A 1972 Life expectancy and causes of death in the Marfan syndrome. New England Journal of Medicine 286: 804

Murray J C, Lindberg K A, Pinnell S R 1977 In vitro inhibition of chick embryo lysyl hydroxylase by homogentisic acid: a proposed connective tissue defect in alkaptoptonuria. Journal of Clinical Investigation 59: 107

Olsen B R, Guzman N, Engel J, Condit C, Aase S 1977 Purification and characterization of a peptide from the carboxy terminal region of chick tendon procollagen type I. Biochemistry 16: 3030

Patterson D F, Minor R R 1977 Hereditary fragility and hyperextensibility of the skin of cats: A defects in collagen fibrillogenesis. Laboratory Investigation 37: 170

Pearson R W 1962 Studies on the pathogenesis of epidermolysis bullosa. Journal of Investigative Dermatology 30: 551

Peltonen L, Palotie A, Hayashi T, Prockop D J 1980a Thermal stability of type I and type III procollagens from a patient with osteogenesis imperfecta. Proceedings of the National Academy of Sciences, U.S.A. 77: 162

Peltonen L, Palotie A, Prockop D J 1980b A defect in the structure of type I procollagen in a patient with osteogenesis imperfecta. Excess mannose in the C-terminal propeptide. Proceedings of the National Academy of Sciences, U.S.A. 77: 6179

Penttinen R P, Lichtenstein J R, Martin G R, McKusick V A 1975 Abnormal collagen metabolism in cultured cells in osteogenesis imperfecta. Proceedings of the National Academy of Sciences, U.S.A. 72: 588

Pinnell S R, Krane S M, Kenzora J E, Glimcher M J 1972 A heritable disorder of connective tissue. Hydroxylysine-deficient collagen disease. New England Journal of Medicine 286: 1013

Pope F M, Martin G R, Lichtenstein J R, Penttinen R P, Gerson B, Rowe D W, McKusick V A 1975 Patients with Ehlers-Danlos syndrome type IV lack type III collagen. Proceedings of the National Academy of Sciences, USA 72: 1314

Pope F M, Martin G R, McKusick V A 1977 Inheritance of Ehlers-Danlos type IV syndrome. Journal of Medical Genetics 14: 200

Postlethwaite A E, Snyderman, Kang A H 1976 The chemotactic attraction of human fibroblasts to a lymphocyte-derived factor. Journal of Experimental Medicine 144: 1188

Priest R E, Moiuddin J F, Priest J H 1973 Collagen of Marfan's syndrome is abnormally soluble. Nature 245: 264

Prockop D J 1972 A subtle disease and a dilemma: Can cells secrete collagen that does not contain a sugar-tag? New England Journal of Medicine 286: 1055

Prockop D J, Berg R A, Kivirikko K I, Uitto J 1976 Intracellular steps in the biosynthesis of collagen. Ramachandran G N, Reddi A H: Biochemistry of Collagen, Plenum, p 163

Prockop D J, Kivirikko K I, Tuderman L, Guzman N A 1979 Biocynthesis of collagen and its disorders. New England Journal of Medicine 301: 13 & 17

Pyeritz R E, McKusick V A 1979 The Marfan syndrome: diagnosis and management. New England Journal of Medicine 300: 772

Quinn R S, Krane S M 1976 Abnormal properties of collagen lysyl hydroxylase from skin fibroblasts of siblings with hydroxylysine-deficient collagen. Journal of Clinical Investigation 57: 83

Reed W B, Horowitz R E, Beighton P 1971 Acquired cutis laxa: primary generalized elastolysis. Archives of Dermatology 103: 661

Risteli L, Koivisto V A, Akerblom H K, Kivirikko K I 1976 Intracellular enzymes of collagen biosynthesis in rat kidneys in streptozotocin diabetes. Diabetes 25: 1066

Rodnan G P 1965 Progressive systemic sclerosis (diffuse scleroderma). In: Samter M (ed) Immunological diseases. Edited by M Samter. Little-Brown, Boston, pp 769-783

Rosenberg H, Modrak J B, Hassing J M, Al-Turk W A, Stohs S J 1979 Glycosylated collagen. Biochemical and Biophysical Research Communications 91: 498

Scheck M, Siegel R C, Parker J, Chan Y-H, Fu J C C 1979 Aortic aneurysm in Marfan's syndrome: Changes in the ultrastructure and composition of collagen. Journal of Anatomy 129: 645

Seedorff K S 1949 Osteogenesis imperfecta. A study of clinical features and heredity based on 55 Danish families comprising 180 affected members. Universitetsforlaget, Copenhagen

Shinkai H, Hirabayashi O, Tamaki A, Matsubayashi S, Sano S 1976 Connective tissue metabolism in altered fibroblasts of a patient with Ehlers-Danlos syndrome type I. Archives of Dermatological Research 257: 113

Shulman H M, Sale G E, Lerner K G, Barker E A, Welden P L, Sullivan K, Galluchi B, Thomas E D, Storb R 1978 Chronic cutaneous graft-versus-host disease in man. American Journal of Pathology 91: 545

Siegel R C, Black C M, Bailey A J 1979 Cross-linking of collagen in the X-linked Ehlers-Danlos type V. Biochemical and Biophysical Research Communications 88: 281

Siegel R C 1975 The connective tissue defect in homocystinuria (HS). Clinical Research 23: 263A (abstract)

Sillence D O 1982 Osteogenesis imperfecta: Clinical variability and classification. Glimcher M, Bornstein P, Heritable Disorders of Connective Tissue. C. V. Mosby, St. Louis

Sillence D O, Senn A, Danks D M 1979a Genetic heterogeneity in osteogenesis imperfecta. Journal of Medical Genetics 16: 10

Sillence D O, Rimoin D L, Danks D M 1979b Clinical variability in osteogenesis imperfecta-Variable expressivity or genetic heterogeneity. Birth Defects: Original Article Series XV(5B): 113

Spicer K M, Allen R C, Hallett D, Buse M G 1979 Synthesis of hemoglobin A_{1c} and related minor hemoglobins by erythrocytes. In vitro study of regulation. Journal of Clinical Investigation 64: 40

Spiro R G, Spiro M J 1971 Effect of diabetes on biosynthesis of the renal glomerular basement membrane. Studies on the glucosyltransferase. Diabetes 20: 641

Steinmann B, Gitzelmann R, Vogel A, Grant M E, Harwood R, Sear C H J 1975 Ehlers-Danlos syndrome in two siblings with deficient lysyl hydroxylase activity in cultured skin fibroblasts but only mild hydroxylysine deficit in skin. Helvetica Pediatrica Acta 30: 255

Steinmann B U, Martin G R, Baum B I, Grystal R G 1979 Synthesis and degradation of collagen by skin fibroblasts from controls and from patients with osteogenesis imperfecta. FEBS Letters 101: 269

Steinmann B, Tuderman L, Peltonen L, Martin G, McKusick V A, Prockop D J 1980 Evidence for a structural mutation of procollagen type I in a patient with the Ehlers-Danlos syndrome type VII. Journal of Biological Chemistry 255: 8887

Stewart R E, Hollister D W, Rimoin D L 1977 A new variant of Ehlers-Danlos syndrome: An autosomal dominant disorder of fragile skin, abnormal scarring and generalized periodontitis. Birth Defects: Original Artical Series 13: 85

Sussman M D, Lichtenstein J R, Nigra T P, Martin G R, McKusick V A 1974 Hydroxylysine deficient skin collagen in a patient with a form of Ehlers-Danlos syndrome. Journal of Bone and Joint Surgery 56A: 1228

Sykes B, Francis M J O, Smith R 1977 Altered relation of two collagen types in osteogenesis imperfecta. New England Journal of Medicine 296: 1200

Tan EML, Uitto J, Bauer E A, Eisen A Z 1981 Human skin fibroblasts in culture: Stimulation of procollagen synthesis by sera from normal human subjects and from patients with dermal fibroses. Journal of Investigative Dermatology 76: 462

Trelstad R L, Rubin D, Gross J 1977 Osteogenesis imperfecta congenita: evidence for a generalized molecular disorder of collagen. Laboratory Investigation 36: 507

Tuderman L, Steinmann B, Peltonen L, Martin G, Prockop D J 1979 Evidence for a structural mutation in the procollagen synthesized by a patient with Ehlers-Danlos syndrome type VII. Federation Proceedings 38: 1407

Turakainen H, Larjava H, Saarni H, Penttinen R 1980 Synthesis of hyaluronic acid and collagen in skin fibroblasts cultured from patients with osteogenesis imperfecta. Biochimica et Biophysica Acta 628: 388

Uitto J 1972 Collagen biosynthesis in human skin. A review with emphasis on scleroderma. Annals of Clinical Research 3: 250

Uitto J 1979 Biochemistry of the elastic fibres in normal connective tissues and its alterations in diseases. Journal of Investigative Dermatology 72: 1

Uitto J, Prockop D J 1974 In: Good R A, Day S B, Yunis J J (eds) Molecular defects in collagen and the definition of 'collagen disease'. The Molecular Pathology. Thomas, Springfield, p 670

Uitto J, Lichtenstein J R 1976 Defects in the biochemistry of collagen in diseases of connective tissue. Journal of Investigative Dermatology 66: 59

Uitto J, Eisen A Z 1979 Collagen. In: Fitzpatrick T B, Eisen A Z, Wolff K, Freedberg I M, Austen K F (eds) Dermatology in general medicine, 2nd edn. McGraw-Hill, New York, p 164

Uitto J, Santa-Cruz D J, Eisen A Z 1979a Familial cutaneous collagenoma: genetic studies on a family. British Journal of Dermatology 101: 185

Uitto J, Bauer E A, Eisen A Z 1979b Scleroderma. Increased biosynthesis of triple-helical type I and type III procollagen associated with unaltered expression of collagenase by skin fibroblasts in culture. Journal of Clinical Investigation 64: 921

Uitto J, Santa-Cruz D J, Eizen A Z 1980a Connective tissue nevi of the skin: Clinical, genetic and histopathologic classification of hamartomas of the collagen, elastin, and proteoglycan type. Journal of the American Academy of Dermatology 3: 441

Uitto J, Bauer E A, Santa-Cruz D J, Loewinger R J, Eisen A Z 1980b Focal dermal hypoplasia: Abnormal growth characteristics of skin fibroblasts in culture. Journal of Investigative Dermatology, 75: 170

Uitto J, Santa Cruz D J, Bauer E A, Eisen A Z 1980c Morphea and lichen sclerous et atrophicus. Clinical and histopathologic studies in patients with combined features. Journal of American Academy of Dermatology 3: 271

Uitto J, Grant G A, Perejda A J, Rowold E, Williamson J R 1980d Glycosylation of human glomerular basement membrane collagen (GBMC): Increased non-enzymatic glucosylation in diabetes. Federation Proceedings 39: 1792

Uitto J, Santa Cruz D J, Starcher B C, Whyte M P, Murphy W A 1981 Biochemical and ultrastructural demonstration of elastin accumulation in the skin lesions of the Buschke-Ollendorff syndrome. Journal of Investigative Dermatology 76: 284

Uitto J, Bauer E A, Santa Cruz D J, Holtmann B, Eisen A Z 1982a Connective tissue nevi of the skin consisting of collagen. Decreased production of collagenase by regional fibroblasts in culture. Journal of Investigative Dermatology 78: 136

Uitto J, Jaffe A S, Geltman E M, Rodey G E 1982b The Ehlers-Danlos syndrome type IV: Clinical and biochemical studies in a family. Glimcher M, Bornstein P, Heritable Disorders of Connective Tissue. C. V. Mosby, St. Louis

Uitto V-J, Schwartz D, Veis A 1980 Degradation of basement membrane collagen by a neutral protease from human leukocytes. European Journal of Biochemistry 105: 409

Valle K J, Bauer E A 1980 Enhanced biosynthesis of human skin collagenase in fibroblast cultures from recessive dystrophic epidermolysis bullosa. Journal of Clinical Investigation 66: 176

Vater C A, Harris E D, Siegel R C 1979 Native cross-links in collagen fibrils induce resistance to human synovial collagenase. Biochemical Journal 181: 639

Velayos E E, Masi A T, Stevens M B, Shulman L E 1979 The CREST syndrome, comparison with systemic sclerosis (scleroderma). Archives of Internal Medicine 139: 1240

Vogel A, Holbrook K A, Steinmann B U, Gitzelmann R, Byers P H 1979 Abnormal collagen fibril structure in the gravis form (type I) of Ehlers-Danlos syndrome. Laboratory Investigation 40: 201

Wahl S M, Wahl L M, McCarthy J B 1978 Lymphocyte-mediated activation of fibroblast proliferation and collagen production. Journal of Immunology 121: 942

Westberg N G, Michael A F 1973 Human glomerular basement membrane: Chemical composition in diabetes mellitus. Acta Medica Scandinavica 194: 39

Williamson J R, Kilo C 1977 Current status of capillary basement membrane disease in diabetes mellitus. Diabetes 26: 65

Winkelmann R K 1976 Pathogenesis and staging of scleroderma. Acta Dermato-venereologica 56: 83

Winterburn P J, Phelps C F 1972 The significance of glycosylated proteins. Nature 236: 147

Yamanishi Y, Dabbous M K, Hashimoto K 1972 Effect of collagenolytic activity in basal cell epithelioma of the skin on reconstituted collagen and physical properties and kinetics of the crude enzymes. Cancer Research 32: 2551

Yamanishi Y, Maeyens E, Dabbous M K, Ohyama H, Hashimoto K 1973 Collagenolytic activity in malignant melanoma: physicochemical studies. Cancer Research 33: 2507

17

Basement membrane collagen

N. A. KEFALIDES

INTRODUCTION

A renewed interest in basement membranes became noticeable in recent years as new knowledge concerning the nature of their components, especially of the collagen component, began to accumulate through novel biological and biochemical approaches (Kefalides et al, 1979).

In this chapter, I propose to discuss the structural chemistry of isolated, intact basement membranes with emphasis on basement membrane collagen and procollagen. The physicochemical, immunochemical and biosynthetic properties of basement membrane collagen and procollagen will be discussed, an attempt will be made to relate the structure of the collagenous component to the overall structure and function of basement membranes, and a discussion of changes in disease will be made.

STRUCTURAL CHEMISTRY OF BASEMENT MEMBRANES

Any discussion on the biochemical structure of a tissue component requires that criteria first be established for the appropriate identification of that component. In the case of basement membranes, this should require the isolation of the basement membrane being studied, its identification using morphologic criteria and, finally, some definition of what will be considered a basement membrane component and what will not. For example, one of the functions of a basement membrane is that of a filter. Should molecules of serum proteins which are trapped in transit at the time the basement membrane is isolated be considered to be a basement membrane component? In this particular instance, I have taken the position that such molecules are not basement membrane components nor should molecules which are adsorbed onto the surface of basement membranes, e.g., antibodies, be considered as basement membrane components. A more difficult situation arises when, during the isolation of the basement membrane, substances such as lipids or glycoproteins are lost. Here, it cannot be stated so definitively that these are not basement membrane components for their presence or absence may depend solely upon the method of isolation. Several studies have claimed that proteoglycans constitute an integral component of basement membranes. In the developing embryo such substances are synthesized by the same cell which makes basement membrane and they can be detected in ultrastructural studies as they traverse the basement membrane on their way to the adjacent connective tissue. In the mature animal heparan sulphate has been detected in isolated glomerular basement membrane but its content is quite low, not exceeding 0.1 to 0.2 per cent by weight (Kanwar & Farquhar, 1979). An issue not yet satisfactorily resolved is the degree of cell membrane contamination which may contribute to the small amount of glycosaminoglycan isolated from glomerular basement membrane.

In this discussion I have chosen to consider as basement membrane components only those proteins which constitute the major components of a given preparation and which are not easily removed by mild non-degradative procedures.

Solubility properties of basement membranes

The solubility properties of basement membranes were established in the earlier literature and have been included in a number of comprehensive reviews (Kefalides, 1971a, 1973; Kefalides et al, 1979). Briefly, basement membranes are highly insoluble in buffers at neutral pH. They can be solubilized with alkali but this is undoubtedly the result of degradation. A small amount of material can be brought into solution with acidic buffers. Treatment with chaotropes or strong denaturants can solubilize a small percentage of basement membrane material but it is still not clear whether the extracted materials are components of the basement membrane or contaminants which are trapped in or adsorbed onto it. Reduction of disulphide bonds is only partially successful in bringing basement membranes into solution unless the reduction is performed in the presence of strong denaturants such as guanidine HCl, urea or sodium dodecyl sulphate (SDS). This has been the most successful approach to solubilizing basement membranes and, depending upon the source, will bring from 60 to 100 per cent of the material into solution.

However, upon removal of the denaturants, the solutions often become very unstable and reprecipitation is encountered. On the basis of these properties, it appears that the components of basement membranes are held together by hydrogen bonding forces, disulphide crosslinkages and, perhaps, other types of covalent crosslinkages.

Amino acid and carbohydrate composition

Although the amino acid compositions of various basement membranes have been extensively reviewed, it is pertinent to this discussion to present a table (Table 17.1) showing the amino acid compositions of representative basement membrane preparations. Newer procedures have facilitated the isolation of basement membranes from tissues which previously had been considered too complex for the isolation of uncontaminated preparations.

Examination of the amino acid compositions in Table 17.1 reveals a number of salient features common to all basement membranes. First is the presence in large amounts of 4-hydroxyproline and hydroxylysine, indicative of the presence of collagenous components within the basement membrane. Second is the presence of considerable amounts of 3-hydroxyproline resulting in an unusually high ratio of 3-hydroxyproline to 4-hydroxyproline. This appears to be a major characteristic of basement membranes. A third feature is the presence of large amounts of half-cystine.

Examination of the carbohydrate composition of the various basement membranes reveals the presence of large amounts of sugars indicative of the glycoprotein nature of basement membranes. Present in particularly large amounts are glucose and galactose. All of the glucose and most of the galactose have been shown to be covalently

Table 17.1 Amino acid and carbohydrate compositions of various basement membranes

	Human glomerular basement membrane [a]	*Canine anterior lens capsule* [b]	*Ovine Descemet's membrane* [c]	*Bovine renal tubular basement membrane* [d]	*Rat Reichert's membrane (Day 14.5)* [e]	*Mouse sarcoma* [f]
Amino acid residues/1000 residues						
Hydroxylysine	24.5	32.0	20.0	28	18.4	38
Lysine	26.0	11.0	24.0	18	33.0	11
Histidine	18.7	12.0	11.6	16	19.9	11
Arginine	48.3	38.3	39.5	38	45.0	30
3-Hydroxyproline	7.0	18.0	6.8	20	6.0	5
4-Hydroxyproline	66.0	80.0	77.0	83	46.2	99
Aspartic	65.0	57.8	58.0	60	84.0	52
Threonine	40.0	31.0	36.4	40	48.0	34
Serine	60.0	48.0	42.1	57	67.0	60
Glutamic	103.0	95.0	94.0	96	107.0	103
Proline	62.0	66.0	95.0	55	61.5	66
Glycine	227.0	228.0	230.0	218	179.0	280
Alanine	58.0	46.1	53.0	54	62.0	45
Half-cystine	23.0	18.0	11.0	11	18.8	7
Valine	36.0	35.0	45.0	39	44	30
Methionine	7.0	6.2	8.2	12	13.3	12
Isoleucine	28.0	30.0	28.5	30	30	25
Leucine	66.0	56.5	75.2	58	70	54
Tyrosine	14.5	11.0	21.0	19	18.4	9
Phenylalanine	28.0	29.0	25.0	28	31	31
Sugar (g/100 g)						
Glucose	2.5	5.0	3.5	3.6	2.2	n.d.
Galactose	2.6	5.1	3.7	3.8	3.0	n.d.
Mannose	1.7	0.4	2.0	1.1	1.8	n.d.
Fucose	0.7	0.6	0.6	0.2	0.4	n.d.
Glucosamine	1.7	0.85	1.2	0.9	4.6	n.d.
Galactosamine	0.3	0.15	0.3	tr	0.4	n.d.
Sialic acid	1.5	0.4	0.7	0.2	1.7	n.d.

[a] Kefalides (1970)
[b] Kefalides (1969b)
[c] Kefalides & Denduchis (1969)
[d] Ferwerda et al (1974b)
[e] Clark et al (1975a)
[f] Timpl et al (1978)

associated with hydroxylysine residues and thus are associated with the collagenous portion of the membrane (Kefalides & Winzler, 1966; Kefalides, 1969; Spiro, 1967). Subsequent studies have shown that about 80 per cent of the hydroxylysine residues are glycosylated and that about 90 per cent of the substituted hydroxylysine exists as glucosyl-α(1 → 2)-galactosyl-β-O → hydroxylysine. This appears to be one of the most characteristic chemical properties of basement membrane collagen since the hydroxylysine residues of other collagens are substituted to a far lesser degree (Kefalides, 1973; Kefalides et al, 1979).

In addition to the glucose and galactose, glucosamine and, to a lesser extent, galactosamine, mannose, fucose and sialic acid are present indicating that in addition to the characteristic collagen-derived carbohydrates, typical glycoprotein heteropolysaccharide units are also present.

The most notable differences between the various basement membranes appear to reside in the proportion of the membrane taken up by the collagen component. This appears to be lowest in Reichert's membrane and highest in the lens capsule and retinal basement membranes. Interestingly, the nonvertebrate basement membrane from *Ascaris suum* apparently contains no 3-hydroxyproline although it, too, is collagenous.

Based upon these gross observations, it appears that both collagenous and noncollagenous proteins are present in basement membranes, and this appears to be true for basement membranes from nonvertebrate animals as well as from vertebrates.

The question next arises as to whether the collagenous protein in basement membranes represents a distinct collagen type such as is found for types I, II and III collagens and whether there are more than one collagen molecule.

The collagen component of basement membranes

In almost all basement membranes examined so far, it has been impossible to isolate the collagenous component without resorting to some form of mild proteolytic digestion. Two notable exceptions stand out: the isolation of procollagen-like molecules from lens capsule, using weak acid extraction (Denduchis et al, 1970; Olsen et al, 1973), and from a sarcoma tumour (Timpl et al, 1978).

When native undenatured collagens are exposed to proteases such as pepsin, it is found that the triple helical portions of the molecule are resistant to proteolytic attack whereas nonhelical portions are digested. This approach has been applied to the isolation and characterization of the basement membrane collagen component (Kefalides, 1968; Kefalides & Denduchis, 1969; Dehm & Kefalides, 1978; Dixit & Kang, 1979).

Upon treatment of basement membranes with pepsin under acidic conditions in the cold, the basement membranes are brought into solution. The collagen fraction is then isolated by salt precipitation and further purified.

Studies of the physical properties of collagen preparations isolated from lens capsule and glomerular basement membrane revealed the high intrinsic viscosities and highly negative specific optical rotations characteristic of collagens. Circular dichroism spectroscopy revealed a melting temperature (Tm) of about 40°C of the triple-helical basement membrane collagen (Kefalides, 1968, Denduchis et al, 1970; Gelman et al, 1976). Wide angle X-ray diffraction studies of glomerular basement membrane revealed a powder diagram and reflections similar to those seen with tendon collagen (Kefalides & Winzler, 1966). A strong meridional reflection with an axial repeat of 2.85 Å, an equatorial reflection with a spacing of about 11 Å and another equatorial intense halo with a repeat of 4.23 Å were the characteristic measurements (Table 17.2).

Table 17.2 X-Ray diffraction measurements of basement membrane and interstitial collagen[a]

Collagen fibre d (Å)		*Heat-denatured collagen d (Å)*		*Dog basement Membrane d (Å)*	
Arc	11.32	Halo	11.62	Intense Halo	10.27
Arc	7.25	Line	7.62		
Arc	5.71	Line	6.02		
Broad halo	4.28	Broad halo	4.18	Intense halo	4.23
Broad halo	2.19	Line	2.86	Line	2.85

[a] Kefalides & Winzler, 1966

These studies are consistent with the view that the collagen in GBM exhibits a triple-helical structure and that the collagen molecules are randomly oriented in the tissue. Roveri et al (1979) performed wide and low angle diffraction studies on bovine anterior lens capsule basement membrane and concluded that the collagen molecules have a triple-helical structure with the characteristic axial periodicity of 2.9 Å of tendon collagen. They further suggest that in the relaxed tissue the collagen molecules form a network of randomly oriented collagen molecules. The lack of a well defined fibrillar structure in basement membranes is responsible for the failure to observe typical periodic striations by electron microscopy. Since the collagen molecules in basement membranes retain their terminal propeptide extensions (Olsen et al, 1973; Minor et al, 1976), the persistence of such procollagen-like molecules may explain the lack of a well defined fibrillar structure.

The amino acid compositions of basement membrane collagens from several sources are shown in Table 17.3. The analyses show an amino acid composition typical of a collagen, i.e., approximately one third of all of the residues is glycine and a significant amount is contributed by 4-hydroxyproline and hydroxylysine. There are, however,

Table 17.3 Amino acid and carbohydrate composition of collagen components isolated from various basement membranes

	Human GBM [a]	*Anterior Lens Capsule* ovine [a]	bovine [b]	*Descemet's membrane* [a]	*Mouse sarcoma* [c]
Residues/1000 residues					
Hydroxylysine	44.6	57.0	53	43.0	46
Lysine	10.0	10.0	10	15.2	5
Histidine	10.4	8.0	6	7.8	8
Arginine	33.0	27.0	23	30.0	29
3-Hydroxyproline	11.0	12.0	8	8.0	7
4-Hydroxyproline	130.0	120.0	137	156.0	127
Aspartic	51.0	50.0	50	30.0	50
Threonine	23.0	20.0	19	18.0	27
Serine	37.0	38.0	37	25.0	53
Glutamic	84.0	92.0	80	78.0	93
Proline	61.0	67.0	62	90.0	61
Glycine	310.0	330.0	335	320.0	319
Alanine	33.0	32.0	33	32.0	30
Half-cystine	8.0	8.0	—	8.0	6
Valine	29.0	26.0	27	25.0	28
Methionine	10.0	10.0	13	9.5	11
Isoleucine	30.0	20.0	26	24.0	22
Leucine	54.0	43.0	50	52.0	45
Tyrosine	6.0	2.0	2	3.0	5
Phenylalanine	27.0	30.0	28	22.0	29
Sugars (g/100 g)					
Glucose	5.5	6.0	5.5	5.0	n.d.
Galactose	6.0	6.3	5.7	5.2	n.d.
Mannose	tr	tr	tr	—	n.d.
Fucose	—	—	—	—	n.d.
Hexosamines	tr	tr	—	—	n.d.
Sialic Acid	—	—	—	—	n.d.

[a] Kefalides (1971b)
[b] Material obtained after pepsin digestion using the three-step procedure of Dehm & Kefalides (1978)
[c] Timpl et al (1978)

some distinctive features which are characteristic of basement membranes. First is the extremely high ratio of hydroxylysine to lysine, by far the highest for any collagen previously isolated. Second is the unusually high content of 3-hydroxyproline and 4-hydroxyproline. The proportion of 3-hydroxyproline to total hydroxyproline (i.e. 3-hydroxyproline plus 4-hydroxyproline) can be as high as 12 per cent. As will be seen in the section on biosynthesis, this has provided a valuable criterion for the demonstration of basement membrane collagen biosynthesis. Additional features include an unusually low content of alanine and arginine, as compared with other collagens, and a low content of tyrosine. In material isolated after a single pepsin treatment up to eight residues of half-cystine have been reported.

Carbohydrate analyses reveal a content of total neutral sugar of about 10 per cent composed of nearly equimolar amounts of galactose and glucose with traces of mannose and hexosamine. This indicated that most of the sugars were attached to hydroxylysine and, in fact, the proportion of glycosylated hydroxylysine observed for intact basement membranes is preserved in the collagen fraction.

Upon fractionation of the collagen fraction on CM-cellulose, Kefalides (1971a) found a single peak eluting in the region of type I collagen α chains. Gel filtration of the denatured collagen yielded a significant peak eluting with a molecular weight of about 108 000. These data suggest first that because of its resistance to pepsin digestion the basement membrane collagen was present to a significant extent as a triple-helix composed of three identical α chains, and second, that the α chain was somewhat larger than that from other collagen types. On the basis of this information it was suggested that the collagen component of basement membranes is a true collagen and it is now referred to as 'type IV collagen'.

Daniels & Chu (1975) performed a similar set of studies on pepsin-digested bovine glomerular basement membrane (GBM). They utilized a unique homogenization procedure in the preparation of very large amounts of renal glomeruli and GBM although they did not characterize their GBM preparation morphologically or chemically. After an exhaustive pepsinization of the GBM, followed by gel filtration on agarose gels, they were able to isolate a series of collagen polypeptides ranging in size from over 300 000 daltons to very small peptides. One of the polypeptide fractions, which accounted for about 10 per cent of the pepsin digest eluted in a position corresponding to α chains from type I collagen (95 000 daltons) and this was resolved into two components on CM cellulose one of which was retained on CM cellulose and one which was not. After reduction and alkylation of another of the higher molecular weight fractions, a polypeptide fraction with a gel filtration elution position corresponding to about 140 000 daltons was obtained and this too was resolved into two components on CM cellulose. They hypothesized the presence of two different α chain types in GBM on the basis of differences in amino acid composition and also suggested that each of the lower molecular weight fractions were derivatives of a higher molecular weight fraction, arising presumably from more extensive proteolysis. Their data also suggested that these different α chains were linked by disulphide bonds.

A closer examination of these studies reveals that the basis for inferring the presence of two distinct collagen chains may not be a good one. The differences observed in the amino acid compositions were based upon arginine. If the authors had chosen cysteine or aspartic acid for their comparison they might have drawn an opposite conclusion. Their results may have been due to an extensive overpepsinization of the GBM and to the fact that protease inhibitors were not utilized during preparation and purification of the GBM. Most workers using pepsinization procedure incubate no longer than 24 hours whereas in this study, the GMB was pepsinized for 8 days using a tremendous excess of pepsin. The conclusions of Daniels and Chu are, therefore, difficult to accept.

Nevertheless, the possibility that there is more than one collagen chain in basement membranes surfaced again when Dixit (1979) and Gay & Miller (1979) reported on the isolation of two collagenous polypeptide chains from whole glomeruli and anterior lens capsule, respectively. Dixit (1979) digested lyophilized human glomeruli with pepsin at an enzyme substrate ratio of 1:10 for 62 hours at 4°C. The solubilized collagenous protein was purified by salt fractionation. Following molecular sieve filtration, the fraction eluting in the region of α-chains of tendon collagen was chromatographed on a CM-cellulose and the two main fractions, C and D, which emerged were examined by SDS-gel electrophoresis and amino acid analysis. The molecular weight of the C-chain corresponded to 95 000 and that of the D-chain, after reduction of disulphide bonds, to 75 000. On amino acid analysis, both the C and D fractions had features characteristic of basement membrane collagen; however, the D-chain had a lower content of hydroxylysine. Gay & Miller (1979) isolated similar collagenous chains from bovine anterior lens capsules (ALC). Unlike Dixit, they treated the lens capsules with a solution of 5M urea containing 10mM 2-mercaptoethanol before digesting with pepsin. Gay & Miller used excessive amounts of pepsin ranging from 1:1 to 1:10 enzyme:substrate ratio. The claim that the C and D fractions are distinct collagen chains or that they arise from separate molecules must be viewed with caution since in both instances excessive amounts of pepsin were used which could have given rise to artefactual cleavage of regions of basement membrane where the procollagen molecules are highly crosslinked by nondisulphide covalent linkages. The latter interpretation is supported by the following series of observations. Dehm & Kefalides (1978a) used mild conditions of pepsin digestion (enzyme:substrate ratio 1:100) to isolate the collagenous peptide from bovine ALC. After an initial mild pepsin digestion the mixture was reduced and alkylated under nondenaturing conditions. The material was pepsinized a second time and then subjected to agarose gel filtration. This three-step procedure resulted in the recovery of about 70 per cent of the hydroxyproline in a single peak with a molecular weight of 95 000. This fraction was devoid of cystine and had an amino acid composition typical of basement membrane collagen (Tables 17.3 and 17.4). Only about 5 to 10 per cent of the collagenous component eluted as a fraction corresponding to the 70 000 m.wt. (D-chain). In the Dixit (1979) and Gay & Miller (1979) studies the D-chain represented between 40 and 50 per cent of the recovered collagen. When ALC was treated once with pepsin under mild conditions and the material reduced and alkylated under non-denaturing conditions as described by Dehm & Kefalides (1978a) two large molecular weight species were obtained after CM-cellulose chromatography. The apparent molecular weight of these fractions was 125 000 and 115 000 and their amino acid composition resembled that of the C and D chains, respectively (Table 17.4). This suggested that the above fractions were precursors of the smaller 95 000 (C) and 70 000 (D)-chains, respectively. What was unique, however, about the 115 0O0 and 70 000 m.wt. D-chains was the persistence of significant amounts of sugars found on the propeptide noncollagen extensions, namely mannose, glucosamine and galactosamine (Table 17.5). Similarly, the glucose and galactose content was lower than in the 95 000 m.wt C-chain, suggesting the persistence of non-collagen peptides. Another consistent feature of the D-chain was the persistence of half-cystine.

Dehm & Kefalides (1978a) further demonstrated that if fresh lens capsules containing viable cells were incubated in the presence of ^{14}C-proline and then subjected to the three-step procedure, a hydroxy[^{14}C]proline containing fraction was obtained which on gel filtration and CM-cellulose chromatography coeluted with the 95 000 m.wt. peptide. Similar results were obtained with GBM (Dehm & Kefalides, 1978b). It was concluded from these studies that basement membranes contain at least one triple helical collagen polypeptide composed of identical chains.

The data further suggested that the D-chains may be truncated forms of the same precursor procollagen molecule from which the 95 000 α chain (C-chain) arises

Table 17.4 Amino acid composition[a] of lens capsule collagen chains

	Single pepsin[b] + Red-Alk 'C'-125K	Method of Gay & Miller (1979) 'C'-95K	Method of Dehm & Kefalides (1978a) 'C'-95K	Single pepsin[b] + Red-Alk 'D'-115K	Method of Gay & Miller (1979) 'D'-70K
Hydroxylysine	54	55	49	42	42
Lysine	8	7	8.6	6	4
Histidine	6	7	6.3	6	7
Arginine	20	19	26	43	43
3-Hydroxyproline	6	6	6.9	8	8
4-Hydroxyproline	145	137	133	132	129
Aspartic acid	46	41	51	48	42
Threonine	19	19	20	23	23
Serine	39	54	37	46	48
Glutamic acid	90	85	79	80	74
Proline	62	56	65	54	49
Glycine	344	348	328	322	342
Alanine	33	35	37	45	41
1/2 Cysteine	1–3	0	0[c]	0–1	2
Valine	19	23	28	23	20
Methionine	13	14	13	12	15
Isoleucine	16	19	29	23	25
Leucine	49	48	52	55	58
Tyrosine	2	5	2.3	5	4
Phenylalanine	25	28	29	32	28

[a] Expressed as residues/1000 residues
[b] Anterior lens capsules were digested once with pepsin according to the method of Dehm & Kefalides (1978a) and were reduced and alkylated under non-denaturing conditions. The solubilized material was subjected to gel filtration and the peak eluting at about 110–130 000 m.wt. was chromatographed on CM-cellulose. Two fractions with apparent m.wt. of 125 000 and 115 000 were obtained.
[c] Sum of cysteic acid, cysteine and S-carboxymethylcycsteine

Table 17.5 Carbohydrate content of lens capsule collagen chains

Compound	*Single Pepsin*[a] *+ Red-Alk 'C'-125K*		*Method of Gay & Miller (1979) 'C'-95K*		*Method of Dehm & Kefalides (1978a) 'C'-95K*		*Single Pepsin*[a] *+ Red-Alk 'D'-115K*		*Method of Gay & Miller (1979) 'D'-70K*	
	moles/100 g	% w/w	moles/100 g	% w/w	moles/100 g	% w/w	moles/100 g	% w/w	moles/100 g	% w/w
Galactose	28	5.1	23	4.2	30	5.4	22	4.0	21	3.8
Glucose	2	5.8	23	4.2	32	5.8	27	4.8	21	3.8
Mannose	0.8	0.15	Trace	—	0	0	3.0	0.54	2.3	0.41
Glucosamine	0.42	0.09	0.48	0.1	0	0	2.31	0.5	3.35	0.74
Galactosamine	0.46	0.1	0.45	0.1	0	0	0.45	0.1	0.51	0.11

[a] Anterior lens capsules were digested once with pepsin according to the method of Dehm & Kefalides (1978a) and were reduced and alkylated under non-denaturing conditions. The solublized material was subjected to gel filtration and the peak eluting at about 110–130 000 m.wt. was chromatographed on CM-cellulose. Two fractions with apparent m.wt. of 125 000 and 115 000 were obtained.

and that they may be aggregates of shorter peptides, held together by non-disulphided covalent cross-links which still retain portions of the propeptide terminal extensions (Fig. 17.1).

Confirmatory evidence has recently been presented by Schwartz & Veis (1978) who were able to prepare segment-long-spacing (SLS) aggregates of lens capsule collagen isolated by the three-step procedure. In another study, the above authors (1980) provided evidence for the existence of large N-terminal and C-terminal extensions in collagen extracted from bovine ALC under minimally degradative conditions (1:200, enzyme:substrate ratio). Using the same conditions Schwartz et al (1980) carried the pepsin digestion for as little as 24 hours and as long as 16 days.

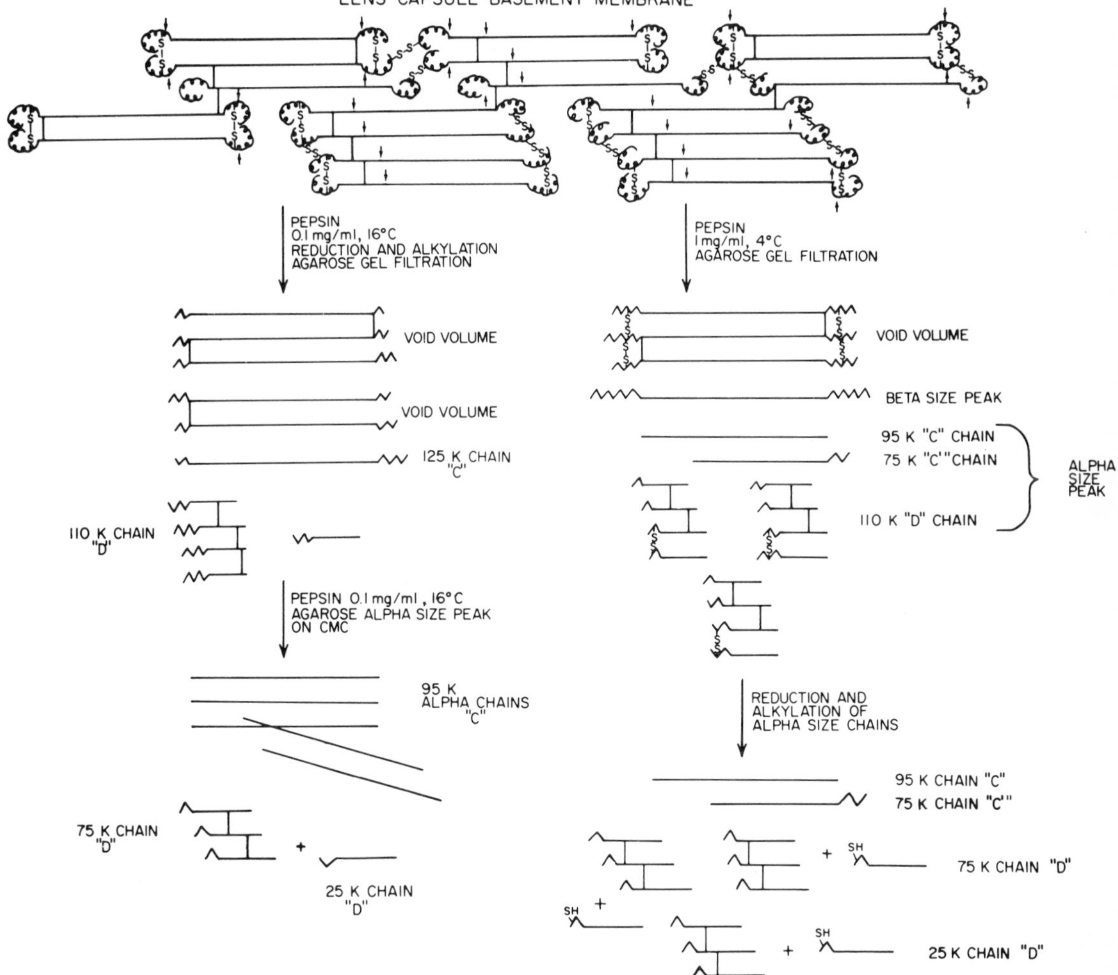

Fig. 17.1 Effects of low and high concentrations of pepsin on the degradation of lens capsule basement membranes. Procollagen molecules are held together by disulphide bonds (–S–S–) and lysyl derived covalent crosslinks (solid lines). Using mild pepsin digestion (0.1 mg/ml, enzyme:substrate ratio 1:100) followed by reduction and alkylation and then a second mild pepsin digestion leads to the formation of predominantly 95 000 m.wt. α-chains of collagen (C-chain) (Dehm & Kefalides, 1978). A small proportion of the 75 000 component (D-chain) is also formed. Use of larger amounts of pepsin (1 mg/ml, enzyme:substrate ratio 1:10, Gay & Miller, 1978) yields a larger proportion of the 75 000 m.wt. (D-chain) component. In either case, the 95 000 and the 75 000 m.wt. chains could arise from the same precursor procollagen molecules or from separate molecules.

Studies from other laboratories (Dixit, 1978; Gay & Miller, 1979; Kresina & Miller, 1979) suggest that the two polypeptide chains (C and D) may be synthesized as two genetically distinct products and have been designated as $\alpha 1$(IV) and $\alpha 2$(IV). Other investigators (Gehron, Robey & Martin, 1981) have suggested that the two chains form distinct collagen molecules and have given them the designation $\alpha 1(IV)_3$ and $\alpha 2(IV)_3$. Biosynthetic studies with rat parietal yolk sac (Clark & Kefalides, unpublished observations) give rise to a doublet which migrates on SDS-gel electrophoresis in the region of basement membrane procollagen. The ratio of the two components is not constant but varies between 3:1 and 5:1. Peptide mapping after digestion with submaxillary protease of the large molecular weight C (125 000) and D (115 00 chains shows similarities as well as differences between the two (Kefalides, unpublished observations).

Amino acid analysis of the collagen extracted on days 1, 2, 7, 11 and 16 showed no evidence of release of D-like chain based on the arginine content although the half-cystine content increased to 16 residues per 1000 on day 16 compared to 5 residues per 1000 on days 1 and 11. This finding, along with the decrease in glycine and 4-hydroxyproline content would suggest the release of pepsin resistant collagenous fragments which still retained portions of disulphide-linked terminal extensions. Unfortunately, the authors did not provide us with a carbohydrate analysis.

It would appear then that the 95 000 m.wt. α chain, whether obtained by the three-step procedure of Dehm & Kefalides (1978a,b) or the more vigorous pepsin digestion of Dixit (1979) or of Gay & Miller (1979), is a product of proteolysis of a triple-helical collagen whose α chain must have a molecular weight greater than 95 000 analogous to pro-α-chains. The ends of this collagen molecule are composed of cystine-containing sequences which apparently hold the molecules together through disulphide bridges and render the termini resistant to mild pepsin digestion. It was only after mild reduction of these disulphide bridges as shown by Dehm & Kefalides (1978a,b) that these terminal sequences were digested by the pepsin. It appears then that there is a collagen type which is characteristic for basement membranes and which is composed of α-like chains.

The basement membrane collagen α-chains were further characterized by analyzing the peptides obtained after cyanogen bromide digestion.

Preliminary studies on CNBr peptides have been reported (Kefalides, 1972a). CNBr peptides were prepared from pepsin-treated (single step) ALC. CM cellulose chromatography revealed a peptide pattern which was different from those of the other collagen types. The data from the CNBr studies demonstrated that of the 12 peptide fractions isolated, glycine accounted for one third of amino acids, 4-hydroxyproline was present in all, hydroxylysine in 9, and 3-hydroxyproline in 7. These analyses revealed a relatively even distribution of 3- and 4-hydroxyproline and hydroxylysine along the α-chain. Only one peptide contained cystine as well as glucosamine and mannose (Table 17.6).

Dixit & Kang (1979) repeated the studies of Kefalides (1972a) on the 95 000 m.wt. α-chain which they refer to as the C-chain and also obtained 12 peptides. The amino acid composition and molecular weights of the CNBr peptides of the C-chain are in substantial agreement with the results reported earlier by Kefalides (1972a).

Although no amino acid sequence data are yet available

Table 17.6 Amino acid composition of CNBr peptides of the $\alpha 1$ chains of bovine lens capsule collagen[a]

Amino acid	1	2	3	4	5	6	7	8	9	10	11	12	Total CNBr peptides
Hydroxylysine[b]	0	0	1	1	0	4	7	7	9	8.5	13	8	58.5
			(0.7)			(3.9)	(6.8)	(6.6)			(13.4)	(8.3)	
Lysine[b]	0	0	1	1	2	0	1	1	3	1	3	2	15
			(0.5)				(1.2)	(1.4)		(1.3)	(2.6)	(1.7)	
Histidine	0	0	1	0	1	0	1	2	2	1	1	1	10
Arginine	0	0	0	0	0	0	1	1	2	5	5	5	19
3-Hydroxyproline[b]	0	0	0	0	0	1	1	1	1	1.5	2	2	9.5
			(0.2)			(0.8)	(1.1)	(0.5)	(0.5)			(1.7)	
4-Hydroxyproline[b]	1	1	1	3	2	8	13	10	14	27	31	21	132
	(0.7)	(0.6)	(1.2)			(7.7)	(12.9)	(9.5)	(13.5)			(21.3)	
Aspartic	0	0	1	2	5	2	5	4	5	8	9	9	50
Threonine	0	0	0	1	3	2	2	2	2	2	3	5	22
Serine	1	1	0	1	3	2	3	3	8	7	8	5	42
Glutamic	1	1	0	2	4	6	8	6	7	12	16	15	78
Proline[b]	0	0	1	1	4	4	7	5	7	12	14	13	68
	(0.3)	(0.4)	(0.6)				(6.9)			(12.4)			
Glycine	2	3	3	9	31	20	33	26	37	58	72	54	348
Alanine	0	0	0	1	4	2	3	4	4	7	8	6	39
Valine	0	1	1	1	3	1	3	2	2	5	5	5	29
Half-cystine	0	0	0	0	0	0	0	0	0	0	0	4	4
Isoleucine	0	0	0	1	2	2	2	2	3	6	7	4	29
Leucine	0	0	0	2	4	4	6	3	6	9	11	9	54
Tyrosine	0	0	0	0	1	0	0	0	0	0	0	2	3
Phenylalanine	0	0	0	1	1	1	3	1	3	5	6	5	26
Homoserine	1	1	1	1	0	1	1	1	1	1	1	1	11
Total	6	8	11	28	70	60	100	81	116	176	215	176	1047
Molecular weight	593	749	1153	2704	6022	5718	9648	7817	11 217	16 906	19 728	17 196	100 033

[a] Residues per peptide, rounded off to the nearest whole number (from Kefalides, 1972a).
[b] Actual values for lysine, hydroxylysine, proline, and hydroxyproline are given in parentheses because of the possibility of partial hydroxylation giving rise to nonintegral values.

for basement membrane collagen, Gryder et al (1975) did sequence a 3-hydroxyproline containing tripeptide from a collagenase digest of swine renal cortex and detected 3-hydroxyproline in only one sequence, gly-3-hypro-4-hypro. Their data also suggested that the 4-hydroxyproline occurred predominantly, if not exclusively, in the Y position of the gly-X-Y triplet sequence.

Recently, two collagen fractions termed αA and αB have been isolated from pepsin digests of human skin (Chung et al, 1976) and placenta (Burgeson et al, 1976). While the amino acid composition of these fractions had some similarity to that of basement membrane collagens, the chromatographic properties differ from those reported for collagen fractions of ALC or GBM. Glanville, et al (1979) isolated type IV (basement membrane) collagen from placenta and demonstrated that it was structurally and immunologically distinct from αA and αB-chains isolated from the same tissue. They suggested that the αA and αB fractions may be representative of yet another collagen type which they called type V. It should be pointed out that at no time were αA and αB-chains isolated from isolated authentic basement membranes.

In addition to the αA and αB chains, Chung et al (1976) isolated a 55 000 dalton fraction from human aortic intima having an amino acid composition similar to that of a basement membrane collagen although it lacked 3-hydroxyproline. It was suggested that this fraction originated in endothelial cell associated basement membranes whereas the αA and αB-chains are derived from epithelial and smooth muscle basement membranes. However, Schwartz & Veis (1978) demonstrated that pepsin digested ALC resulted in the production of small amounts of a 55 000 dalton peptide which appeared to be a cleavage product of the 95 000 MW peptide.

Trelstad & Lawley (1977) found that they could remove interstitial collagens from pepsin digests of kidney, lung and spleen by thermal gelation of the native collagens. Analysis of the supernate of the gels revealed that basement membrane-like collagen did not form gels and could be isolated in this manner from the supernate. Chromatographic and electrophoretic separation of the basement membrane-like collagen supernate revealed a group of molecules of similar composition but with different molecular sizes.

From these studies it might appear that basement membranes contain a heterogeneous class of collagens. However, this should be taken with caution. In each case, the collagen fractions were minor components isolated from a pepsin digest of whole tissue. The conclusion that these fractions are of basement membrane origin are based, for the main part, upon their apparent similarity in amino acid composition to collagens isolated from purified basement membranes. Unless it can be shown that the collagen chains can be isolated in reasonable yield from a *purified* basement membrane preparation, it cannot be assumed solely from its amino acid composition that it was derived from a basement membrane. It is just as probable that they were derived from different collagen types, unrelated to basement membranes. It is possible, however, that basement membranes from different sources contain genetically distinct collagens and this is presently an area of active interest.

In summary, it appears that basement membranes contain unique collagen-like molecules, that these molecules are triple-helical in nature and exist as procollagen, that collagenous peptides equivalent in size to α-chains can be isolated from digests of basement membranes and that the triple helix appears to consist of identical α-chains. It is not yet clear whether homologous basement membranes contain genetically identical collagen components.

The noncollagen components

Several lines of evidence have indicated that in addition to the collagen component basement membranes also contain noncollagen protein material. The proportions of this noncollagen material vary from basement membrane to basement membrane with the highest amounts found in Reichert's membrane of the fetal parietal yolk sac and the lowest in anterior lens capsule and retinal basement membranes. It is conceivable that the major differences between basement membranes reside in the quantity and nature of the noncollagen components (Kefalides et al, 1979).

It has been difficult to isolate a noncollagen protein from basement membranes without resorting to proteolysis of some sort. Kefalides (1966) extracted GBM with 8M urea and isolated a high molecular weight fraction which was poor in hydroxyproline and hydroxylysine and was rich in half-cystine, sialic acid, galactose and mannose.

Upon digestion of GBM with bacterial collagenase, Kefalides (1972b) reported the formation of an insoluble 'residue' which could be solubilized by reduction and alkylation and was further purified by gel filtration. This glycoprotein fraction contained only traces of collagen-derived amino acids and had a carbohydrate composition consistent with that of a noncollagen glycoprotein containing heteropolysaccharide units. The collagenase solubilized material gave rise to a number of glycopeptides of low molecular weight also containing only trace amounts of collagen-derived amino acids. When a rabbit antiserum against reduced and alkylated GBM was reacted with the immunogen by double diffusion, two precipitin lines were formed. It was found that the 'residue' fraction formed a line of identity with one of these precipitin lines, and that the collagenase solubilized peptides formed lines of identity with the other precipitin line. The data suggested the presence of at least two immunologically distinct noncollagen glycoprotein components in GBM, one of high molecular weight and one of low molecular weight.

When Hudson & Spiro (1972) attempted to fractionate reduced and alkylated GBM by gel filtration, they found a large number of polypeptide fractions ranging in size from 30 000 to greater than 700 000 daltons. The amino acid compositions of these polypeptides were very heterogeneous, some having large amounts of collagen derived amino acids and others having much smaller amounts. In no instance was a fraction isolated which was devoid of collagen-derived amino acids. They also found that the heteropolysaccharide units tended to be associated with the larger molecules. It is possible that the low molecular weight collagenase-solubilized glycopeptides isolated by Kefalides (1972b) may have been derived from collagenase-resistant glycopeptide portions of larger molecules containing both collagenous and non-collagenous regions, analogous to procollagen. There is evidence from biosynthetic studies that such peptides can be isolated from collagenase-resistant newly synthesized basement membrane procollagen (Clark & Kefalides, 1978).

These studies suggested the presence of noncollagen subunits in basement membranes. However, the association of small but significant amounts of collagen-derived amino acids in these fractions raises questions as to the origin of these proteins. It is now well known that collagen is secreted from cells as the precursor, procollagen. It is conceivable that the noncollagen glycoprotein fractions described above represent fragments of a procollagen-like molecule which may have been produced from proteolytic cleavages either in vivo or during the isolation of the GBM.

It is important to recognize that basement membranes are generally isolated as insoluble residues after extraction and sonication. If contaminating proteins remain adsorbed onto the basement membranes, they would behave as noncollagen components. Thus, Mohos & Skoza (1970) reported that epithelial foot processes, which remained associated with the GBM, were responsible for much of the sialic acid in the GBM and could have been the source of nephritogenic components. Of equal importance is the possibility that proteins are trapped in the GBM during renal filtration and these could be extracted using chaotropes or denaturants as has been reported by Marquardt et al (1973). In making comparisons of GBM, such proteins would tend to maximize differences and minimize similarities.

Recently, a non collagen glycoprotein was isolated from a mouse sarcoma by Timpl et al (1979a) and characterized immunologically by Rohde et al (1979). This protein, called laminin has been extracted from the extracellular matrix of the tumour which among other things contained type IV (basement membrane) collagen. It consists of at least three disulphide-bonded polypeptide subunits, two having m.wts. of 220 000 and one of 440 000. Immunofluorescent as well as immunoelectron microscopy have demonstrated localization of antibodies of laminin in the lamina lucida of epidermis and the lamina rara interna and externa of renal glomerulus. Laminin has been localized in the basement membrane matrix usually referred to as lamina densa. This and the earlier report by Kefalides (1966) are the only reported instances where a noncollagen glycoprotein has been isolated from a tissue by a non-degradative method.

THE ROLE OF COLLAGEN AND NONCOLLAGEN PROTEINS IN THE SUPRAMOLECULAR ORGANIZATION OF BASEMENT MEMBRANES

From the preceding discussion, it should be obvious that basement membranes are composed of two types or proteins, collagen and noncollagen. Several questions regarding the origins of these proteins and the nature of their association require consideration.

To answer these questions, it is necessary to consider evidence not only from chemical studies but also from morphological, immunological and biosynthetic studies. In this section, I will attempt to examine the nature of the bonds holding basement membranes together and ultimately derive a model for their supramolecular organization.

Hydrogen bonds

The major forces which stabilize the collagen triple helix are those due to hydrogen bonding. It is now recognized that the large amount of 4-hydroxyproline in collagens is of prime importance in this process (Prockop et al, 1979). If the hydroxylation of collagen is prevented, the triple helix will denature at a temperature of about 25°C as compared with the 37°C needed for the denaturation of fully hydroxylated collagen. In the case of basement membranes, it has been found that the 'melting' temperature (Tm) of its collagen component is even higher than that of type I collagen (Kefalides et al, 1979). This is probably due to the significantly higher content of 4-hydroxyproline in basement membrane collagen. The resistance of basement membrane collagen (and other collagens as well) to the action of proteases is indirectly attributable to the hydrogen bonding forces holding the triple-helix together.

There is one observed difference in the behaviour of basement membrane collagen as compared to most other collagens with regards to the susceptibility of pepsin. Under certain conditions, basement membrane collagen can be degraded to molecules smaller than α-chains. This may be particularly true for newly synthesized basement membranes. It is not clear if this is due to a pepsin susceptible amino acid sequence within the α chains, to a partial denaturation of the collagen during isolation, or to the removal of peptides which mask the site of action of the protease.

Disulphide crosslinkages

It appears that cystinyl disulphide bonds are of major importance in maintaining the supramolecular organization of basement membranes. In the presence of strong denaturing agents, reduction and alkylation will result in the nearly total solubilization of most basement membranes, whereas basement membranes are only sparingly soluble without prior reduction. Studies by Hudson & Spiro (1972) have shown that all of the cysteine in basement membranes is tied up in disulphide bond formation. Most of the cystine in basement membranes is found in the noncollagen portions, and some cystine may be located near terminal regions of the collagenous domain in the procollagen molecule (Alper & Kefalides, 1978).

It is probable that disulphide bonds are present within a single procollagen α-chain, between proα-chains and noncollagen proteins and between noncollagen proteins; this serves to organize the basement membrane into an insoluble matrix. Dehm & Kefalides (1978) were able to isolate a 95 000 dalton collagen fraction from a pepsin digest of bovine anterior lens capsule only after reduction and alkylation was interposed between two pepsin digestions in their three-step procedure. The product contained no half-cystine (or at most a trace) indicating the removal by pepsin of short, peptide sequences which apparently contained interchain disulphide crosslinkages. This is consistent with the observation of Olsen et al (1973) who isolated a citrate soluble fraction from bovine lens capsule and showed that it consisted of a globular protein portion at the ends of a filamentous collagen portion. Upon reduction some of the globular components were removed, suggesting that disulphide bonds linked collagen and noncollagen components of the lens capsule and again, that the location of cystine residues in the collagen portion may be near the ends of the α-chain. Alper & Kefalides (1978) isolated a very high molecular weight fraction from a hydroxylamine digest of bovine anterior lens capsule. This fraction contained small but significant amounts of hydroxyproline, hydroxylysine and half-cystine. Upon reduction and alkylation of this product, they found that most of the half-cystine and all of the collagen-derived amino acids were lost but that the fraction remained macromolecular. Upon treatment with bacterial collagenase, all of the collagen-derived amino acids were removed but the half-cystine remained with the macromolecular fraction. This suggested that there were noncollagenous peptide extensions at the ends of the collagen molecules and that these were linked through disulphide bonds to a highly crosslinked noncollagen protein fraction. In addition, the collagenous peptides apparently were joined together through disulphide bonds. (This would explain the loss of cystine after reduction but not after collagenase digestion.) It appears then that terminal portions of the collagen component of lens capsule bear some resemblance to those of procollagen molecules. It is interesting to note that the entire complement of amino acids of the lens capsule and GBM could be accounted for, if the assumption were made that it consisted entirely of disulphide crosslinked basement membrane procollagen. This can be calculated by assuming a content of 134 residues per thousand of 4-hydroxyproline, and molecular weights of 95 000 and 160 000 for the collagen portion and the procollagen α-chain, respectively.

Other covalent crosslinkages

Tanzer & Kefalides (1973) demonstrated the presence of borohydride reducible covalent crosslinkages, which arise from lysine and hydroxylysine, in lens capsule and GBM collagen preparations similar to those found in interstitial collagens. This provides one explanation for the heterogeneity of reduced basement membrane fractions. The high molecular weight fractions might represent crosslinked polymers of the collagen component.

A procedure which selectively cleaves cystinyl residues led to the isolation of highly crosslinked noncollagen fraction from ALC. This fraction contained small amounts hydroxylysine and little, if any, hydroxyproline and radioactivity from sodium ^{3}H borohydride was incorporated in it. This study suggested the existence of covalent, noncollagen, nondisulphide crosslinkages within noncollagen portions of the lens capsule. This is consistent with the observation of a similar fraction from a hydroxylamine digest of ALC (Alper & Kefalides, 1978). Thus, another source of heterogeneity can be postulated, that of differing degrees of covalent attachment of noncollagen proteins to either collagen or to other noncollagen components.

THE SUBUNIT COMPOSITION OF BASEMENT MEMBRANES

The observations that basement membranes contain collagenous and noncollagenous components and that these appear to be held together, at least in part, by disulphide crosslinkages have led to the concept that basement membranes are composed of a series of subunits, which are associated with each other in a regular fashion through the different kinds of crosslinkages. A number of models for the supramolecular organization of basement membranes have been presented (Kefalides, 1971a, 1973; Kefalides et al, 1979). A major problem encountered by investigators in attempting to unravel this subunit structure is the marked heterogeneity of the solubilized materials obtained after reduction of disulphide bonds.

When one examines biosynthetic systems, a much less complex situation is observed. Here it has been shown for a number of systems (Kefalides et al, 1979) that basement membrane collagen is secreted as a procollagen molecule and that little or no cleavage of the procollagen extension peptides takes place. Thus, basement membrane procollagen appears to be a major building block of basement membranes and may constitute the major 'subunit.' Whether there is more than one type of basement membrane procollagen has yet to be demonstrated. It is possible that at least some of the noncollagen components are derived from the procollagen extension peptides and that other proteins are synthesized independently and eventually are transported and organized into the matrix through some mechanism of crosslinking. It has been suggested that further modifications of the matrix occur, such as cleavage of peptide bonds within the collagen and non-collagen portions of the matrix, although there is no evidence to distinguish this from processes of turnover. Upon examination of the final product as isolated from tissues, the system would appear to be much more complex than it really is.

Some very important questions remain concerning the structure of basement membranes. Among these are: (1) Do homologous basement membranes contain different collagen chains?; (2) What is the nature of the noncollagen components?; are they all derived from procollagen or are genetically distinct noncollagen proteins synthesized, secreted and organized into the matrix by the cells making the basement membranes?; (3) What controls the composition of basement membranes from different tissues? A proposed structure of the subunit composition of basement membranes appears in Figure 17.2.

BIOSYNTHESIS OF BASEMENT MEMBRANE

Biosynthetic studies of basement membranes have been used as an additional approach to understanding the

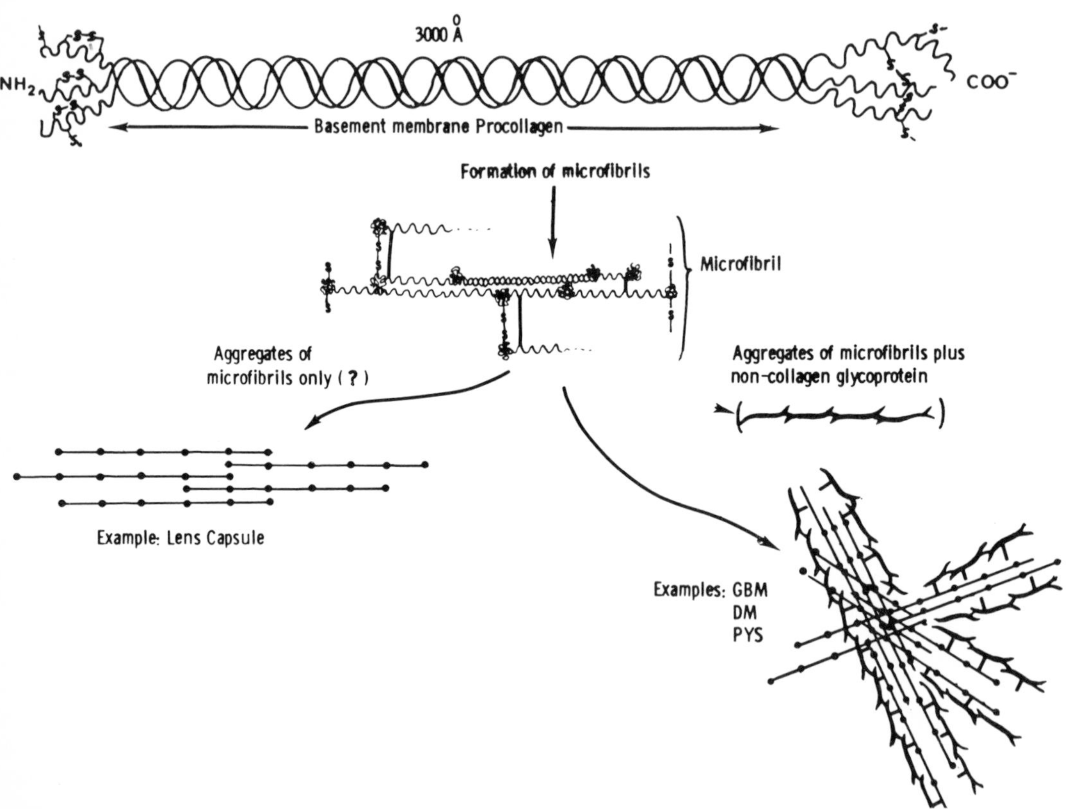

Fig. 17.2 Diagram of a hypothetical model of the supramolecular organization of basement membranes. The newly synthesized and secreted procollagen molecule is composed of 3 identical α-chains having noncollagen extensions at both the NH_2 and COO-termini. There are interchain disulphide crosslinks at the COO-terminus and intrachain disulphide crosslinks at the NH_2 terminus. Procollagen molecules are thought to form microfibrils which are stabilized by intermolecular disulphide crosslinks (–S–S–) and covalent crosslinks involving lysine and/or hydroxylysine (solid line). The microfibrils polymerize to form a larger matrix as is the case in lens capsule. The presence of a distinct noncollagenous glycoprotein within the basement membrane matrix has been postulated for certain tissues. This glycoprotein would be linked to procollagen molecules via disulphide bonds and, possibly, through other types of covalent crosslinkages. It is suggested that the proportion of the noncollagenous glycoprotein varies among basement membranes including glomerular basement membrane (GBM), Descemet's membrane (DM) and rat embryo parietal yolk sac (PYS). (From Kefalides et al, 1979.)

structure and function of these connective tissue matrices. In this section, the emphasis will be on the intracellular events necessary for completion and ultimate secretion of the collagenous component. A discussion of the extracellular maturation of this component will be provided and an attempt to suggest a structure of basement membrane procollagen will be made.

It is now accepted that the cells which rest upon a basement membrane are responsible for its synthesis. In a number of laboratories, basement membrane biosynthesis has been studied using either in vivo or in vitro systems. Although the observations from a variety of biosynthetic systems have contributed to our knowledge and understanding of basement membranes, a majority of the results have been obtained using isolated kidney glomeruli, corneal endothelium, vascular endothelium, embryonic lens capsule and embryonic rodent parietal yolk sac (Kefalides et al, 1979).

Based primarily on structural and immunochemical studies, it has been proposed that intact basement membrane is composed of a collagenous component and one or more noncollagenous glycoprotein components. Because of the relative ease and specificity in detecting collagen synthesis, the collagenous component of newly-synthesized basement membranes is relatively well-characterized compared to the noncollagenous component(s).

Characterization of the collagenous component

Most of our knowledge of the structure and biosynthesis of collagen (or procollagen) has come from systems that synthesize interstitial collagens. Since the processes involved in the synthesis of basement membrane procollagen are most likely analogous to those elucidated for other types of procollagen, the emphasis in this section will be on those features of biosynthesis which appear to be unique for basement membranes. Where possible, comparisons will be made between basement membrane procollagen and other types of procollagen, primarily type I procollagen.

Hydroxylation of peptidyl proline

Compositional studies have shown that basement membrane collagen differs from other collagen types in 3- and 4-hydroxyproline content. Similar results to these have been obtained in vitro by incubating tissues rich in basement membrane in the presence of labelled proline, and measuring the production of labelled hydroxyproline. Table 17.7 summarizes the results for several basement membrane synthesizing systems. Since basement membrane collagen is reported to have at least 60 per cent of its total amino acid as 4-hydroxyproline, it can be seen that from 5 per cent (100 × 3/60) to 43 per cent (100 × 26/60) of the total incorporated ^{14}C is in newly synthesized basement membrane procollagen in these systems. It is alsc possible to estimate from the above ratios the percentage of the newly synthesized protein represented by basement membrane collagen (Clark et al, 1975). From such calculation, values range from a low of about 1 per cent in several tissues to a high of 6 to 12 per cent in the rat embryo parietal yolk sac.

Studies on other types of collagen have shown that only about 45 per cent of the total amino acid is 4-hydroxyproline (Table 17.8). In two systems widely used for studying the synthesis of type I (matrix-free chick embryo tendon cells) and type II (matrix-free chick embryo sternal cells) procollagens, the ratio of 4-hydroxy[^{14}C]-proline to total ^{14}C averaged about 0.30. Thus, in these systems about two-thirds (100 × 30/45) of the total incorporated ^{14}C is in newly synthesized procollagen.

One characteristic of basement membrane collagen which

Table 17.7 Comparison of radioactive amounts of 3- and 4-hydroxyproline and glycosylated hydroxylysine in various tissues synthesizing basement membrane[a]

Tissue	$\frac{\text{4-Hypro}}{\text{Total Pro}} \times 100$	$\frac{\text{3-Hypro}}{\text{Total Hypro}} \times 100$	$\frac{\text{Glycosylated Hylys}}{\text{Total Hylys}} \times 100$
Chick embryo			
Lens cells	5	11–15	92
Rat			
Glomerulus	8.5	14–16	91
Lens capsule	3–6	5	n.d.[c]
Rabbit			
Corneal endothelium	11–14	14–16	94
Rat embryo			
Parietal yolk sac	10–18 20–26[b]	9–11	94–97
Bovine			
Aortic endothelium	3	10–13	91

[a] From Kefalides et al (1979)
[b] Trophoblast was removed prior to incubation
[c] n.d. = not determined

Table 17.8 Summary of differences between newly-synthesized interstitial and basement membrane procollagens

Procollagen type	3-Hyp / total Hyp × 100	4-Hyp / total Pro × 100	Glyco-Hyl / total Hyl × 100	*S–S bonding and helix formation*	*Secretion time*	*M.W. of α-chain after pepsin*
I	1–3%	44%	21%	5–10 min	20 min	95 000
II	1–3%	44%	67%	5–15 min	35 min	95 000
III	1–2%	50%	?	?	?	95 000
IV	10–15%	60%	95%	45 min	60 min	115 000 (95 000)[a]
V	3%	50%	64%	?	?	110 000

[a] M.Wt. in parenthesis after three-step procedure involving pepsin digestion followed by reduction and alkylation under non-denaturing conditions and then a second pepsin digestion, all three-steps at 16°C.

distinguishes it from other types of collagen is its content of 3-hydroxyproline. In most of those biosynthetic systems tested, the content of 3-hydroxy[^{14}C]proline ranged between 10 and 15 per cent of the total hydroxy[^{14}C]proline (Table 17.7) — a value consistent with amino acid analysis (Table 17.3). The corresponding value for other types of collagen is about 1 per cent (Table 17.8).

Hydroxylation of peptidyl lysine and glycosylation of hydroxylysine

Another characteristic of basement membrane collagen is its content of hydroxylysine and glycosylated hydroxylysine (Table17.3 and 17.7). In all of the in vitro systems studied by labelling with [^{14}C]lysine, greater than 80 per cent of the hydroxy[^{14}C]lysine was glycosylated and greater than 90 per cent of the glycosylated hydroxy-[^{14}C]lysine was glucosyl-galactosyl-hydroxy[^{14}C]lysine (Kefalides et al, 1979). These values are consistent with quantitative hydroxylysine glycoside analyses of intact basement membranes. The corresponding values for the hydroxy[^{14}C]lysine glycosylation of type I is 21 per cent and for type II is 67 per cent (Table 17.8).

Disulphide bonding, triple helix formation and secretion

An important step in the intracellular processing of procollagen that precedes triple-helix formation is the formation of disulphide bonds (Prockop et al, 1979). The presence of disulphide bonds in basement membrane collagen has been demonstrated in several biosynthetic systems (Kefalides et al, 1979). Compared with the formation of disulphide bonds in systems synthesizing either type I or type II procollagen, the formation of disulphide bonds in basement membrane procollagen appears to occur relatively late in the intracellular processing. Since disulphide formation is closely related to triple-helix formation these observations are consistent with the finding that intracellular basement membrane procollagen is predominantly nontriple-helical as measured by susceptibility to limited protease digestion (Grant et al, 1973). In turn, these findings may help explain why basement membrane procollagen requires about 60 min to be secreted (Kefalides et al, 1979), while type II and type I procollagens are secreted in 35 min and 20 min, respectively. Table 8 briefly summarizes some differences between newly synthesized interstitial and basement membrane procollagens.

There is adequate evidence to suggest that interstitial procollagens and probably basement membrane procollagen proceed from the rough endoplasmic reticulum, to the smooth endoplasmic reticulum, to the Golgi, and then to the extracellular space (Prockop et al, 1979).

Extracellular processing of procollagen

Initial studies on the extracellular processing of basement membrane procollagen suggested that there was a time-dependent conversion of newly-synthesized basement membrane procollagen to collagen, analogous to that found for other types of procollagen. More recent studies, however, indicate that there is no such conversion and that it is intact procollagen which is incorporated into the basement membrane matrix (Kefalides et al, 1979; Minor et al, 1976).

After incorporation of procollagen into the basement membrane matrix, it is likely that at least two types of intermolecular covalent bonds are formed — dusulphide and lysyl-derived crosslinks. Pulse chase experiments using rat embryo parietal yolk sacs in the presence or absence of β-aminopropionitrile (an inhibitor of lysyl-derived crosslinks) and extraction in the presence or absence of reducing agents suggest that the integrity of the basement membrane is initially stabilized by disulphide bonds, and is further reinforced by a time-dependent formation of lysyl-derived crosslinks. These conclusions are in accord with structural studies on basement membranes (Kefalides et al, 1979).

Structure of procollagen

The structure of the newly-synthesized extracellular collagenous component of basement membrane has been studied primarily by SDS-polyacrylamide gel electrophoresis, SDS-agarose gel filtration and sucrose density gradient rate zonal ultracentrifugation both before and after treatment with disulphide bond reducing agents. In the absence of reducing agents, the procollagen molecule elutes in the void volume of an SDS-agarose column (m.wt. 300 000) (Clark & Kefalides, 1978). Upon disulphide bond reduction, the molecular weight of the basement membrane pro-α-chains which are liberated appears to be greater than that of the pro-α-chains from the interstitial procollagens. Based on SDS-gel filtration, the molecular weight values for the former have ranged from 140 000 to 180 000 (Kefalides et al, 1979). Similar molecular weight values have been obtained by SDS-polyacrylamide gel electrophoresis. These values are significantly higher than the values of 135 000–145 000 reported for types I or II procollagen which were obtained by the same procedures. In addition, it has been shown by sucrose density gradient rate zonal ultracentrifugation that basement membrane pro-γ-(I) and pro-α(I), respectively (Clark & Kefalides, 1978).

Specific proteolytic digestion of basement membrane procollagen and analysis of the denatured products on SDS-agarose in the absence of reducing agents, shows that a disulphide-bonded aggregate persists. Upon disulphide bond reduction and denaturation, the released basement membrane polypeptides have a molecular weight similar to intact interstitial pro-α-chains (i.e. about 135 000). It has recently been reported, however, that when bovine lens capsule procollagen is treated with pepsin as above and the disulphide bonds are subsequently reduced after non-denaturing conditions, further pepsin digestion followed by denaturation will generate polypeptides with molecular weights comparable to the α-chains of interstitial collagen (Dehm & Kefalides, 1978). One implication of these results is that the collagenous domain (protease-resistant) of basement membrane procollagen is comparable to that found in interstitial procollagens, and thus the apparent larger molecular weight of the former may be due solely to the noncollagenous propeptide domain(s) (protease-susceptible). More evidence is needed to confirm this hypothesis.

Digestion of procollagens with bacterial collagenase and characterization of the resultant propeptide domain has proven to be a useful tool in the elucidation of interstitial procollagen structure. Preliminary results of similar experiments using basement membrane procollagen are somewhat more complex, but one interpretation of the results suggests that in contrast to type I and II procollagens, basement membrane procollagen contains a disulphide bond(s) in a hydroxyproline-containing, collagenase-resistant peptide (Clark & Kefalides, 1978).

Basement membrane collagen heterogeneity

Compared to knowledge of the different genetic collagen types present in the interstitium, little is known about the possible types of collagenous components in basement membranes. The majority of the biosynthetic evidence accumulated thus far strongly suggests that there is no collagen heterogeneity within a single basement membrane. However, there are recent reports which indicate two types of heterogeneity in newly synthesized basement membrane procollagen. Sage et al (1979) analyzed cell associated and medium fractions of cultured bovine aortic endothelial cells. They found type IV (basement membrane) to be the predominant species in the cell associate fraction, whereas type III procollagen was the major species in the medium fraction. The synthesis of type III procollagen has not been previously reported for endothelial cells in culture. One possible explanation for these results may be found in the fact that the endothelial cells were isolated from a mixture of smooth muscle and endothelial cells after exposure to large quantities of tritiated thymidine. The possibility of induction of type III procollagen synthesis by endothelial cells as a result of exposure to tritiated thymidine should be kept in mind.

In another report, Tryggvason et al (1980), reported the synthesis of two collagenous polypeptide chains in systems known to synthesize only basement membrane collagen, namely the mouse sarcoma tumour (Timpl et al, 1978), and the mouse parietal yolk sac (Clark et al, 1975). The two collagenous components were identified by SDS-gel electrophoresis and found to have apparent molecular weights of 185 000 and 170 000, respectively. Pulse-chase experiments showed no conversion of the 185 000 m.wt. component to the 170 000 one.

Contrary to these findings, Killen & Striker (1979) found that cultures of human glomerular epithelial cells synthesize basement membrane collagen and that the protein precipitated from the medium with specific antibody yielded a single collagenase labile component with an apparent m.wt. of 168 000. Analysis of hydroxylproline isomers yielded a ratio of 3-hydroxyproline to total hydroxyproline in both the medium and cell layer of 17 per cent.

It would appear, therefore, that the question of collagen heterogeneity remains unsettled; if it occurs it must do so in only specific types of basement membranes.

Regulation of basement membrane collagen synthesis

The mechanisms which regulate both the genetic types of collagen synthesized and the quantity of a given pro-α chain are not clearly understood. Environmental factors seem to influence the mechanisms for gene selection of collagen. This is exemplified by the switching from type II collagen to type I collagen synthesis in cultured chrondrocytes under a variety of conditions including growing the cells in monolayer, growing the cells until they become senescent and growing them in the presence of bromodeoxyuridine or calcium. Viral transformation of cultured fibroblasts decreases the rate of collagen synthesis which is accompanied by a decrease in procollagen mRNA in the transformed cells (Prockop et al, 1979).

Very little is known about the mechanisms which control basement membrane collagen synthesis. A limited number of studies indicate that conditions which specifically inhibit hydroxylation of proline and lysine interfere with secretion of procollagen, a situation comparable to that with interstitial procollagen. Newly synthesized unhydroxylated basement membrane procollagen fails to deposit on parietal yolk sac basement membrane (Kefalides et al, 1979).

In recent studies, attempts were made to map the chromosome which controls basement membrane collagen synthesis. Using the approach of somatic cell hybridization between the thymidine kinase deficient hamster or mouse fibroblasts and normal human vascular endothelial cells, Kefalides (1979) demonstrated concordance between positive immunofluorescence with antibody specific for basement membrane collagen and the presence of human chromosome 17. When such positive clones were grown in the presence of bromodeoxy uridine and chromosome 17 was eliminated by back selection, the selected clones lost their ability to react with the antibody to basement membrane collagen and also failed to synthesize thymidine kinase and galactose kinase. The genes for these enzymes are closely linked and are located on the long arm of human chromosome 17. These data suggest that the gene regulating the synthesis of human basement membrane collagen may be located on chromosome 17.

Turnover and degradation of basement membrane collagen

Studies on the turnover of basement membrane and its components are few. It has been suggested that glomerular basement membrane turns over very slowly requiring almost 1 year for complete replacement.

The turnover of the collagenous component in GBM appears to require more than 100 days, whereas the non-collagenous proteins turn over at a much faster rate. Similar findings were reported for Reichert's membrane of the rat embryo parietal yolk sac which is disrupted and resorbed by day 18 of gestation (Kefalides et al, 1979).

The collagenases which have been isolated from vertebrate tissues and shown to cleave interstitial collagens do not act on basement membrane collagen or procollagen. In recent studies Liotta et al (1979) reported the isolation of a collagenase from a metastatic murine tumour capable of degrading basement membrane (type IV) collagen but not collagen types I, II, III and V. The fragments produced indicated a single cleavage point within the triple-helical domain of the molecule.

Enzymes with similar activities have been isolated from human leucocytes by Uitto et al (1980) and Mainardi et al (1980). The enzymes were distinct from the leucocyte collagenase active against interstitial collagens I, II and III.

IMMUNOCHEMISTRY OF BASEMENT MEMBRANE COLLAGEN

The antigenic nature and the immunologic cross-reaction between homologous and heterologous basement membranes has been adequately documented (Kefalides 1972b; 1973). The cross-reactions observed are due primarily to two general types of antigenic components — a collagenous glycoprotein and one or more noncollagenous glycoproteins.

In this section I shall discuss recent studies on the immunochemistry of the collagenous components isolated from basement membranes and the use of antibodies against these components to study the immunochemistry of newly synthesized basement membrane procollagen. It should be emphasized here that depending on the method used for the preparation of the collagenous component, the immunogen may contain either collagenous sequences alone or both collagenous and noncollagenous sequences, the latter arising from persisting terminal extensions of the procollagen-like molecule. Single, mild pepsin digestion of isolated basement membranes tends to produce collagen molecules which still retain noncollagenous terminal sequences.

The specificity of antibodies against the collagen component of bovine anterior lens capsule, isolated after a single limited digestion with pepsin, was investigated by Gunson & Kefalides (1976). Using a radioimmunoassay, they demonstrated that the above antibodies were type specific for basement membrane collagen (type IV) and did not cross-react with interstitial collagen types I, II or III. Using the same approach, Gunson et al (1976) demonstrated that basement membrane procollagen synthesized by a variety of cell systems including rat parietal yolk sac endoderm, rabbit Descemet's membrane endothelium or vascular endothelium, could be precipitated with the above antiserum. Antigenic cross-reaction between bovine anterior lens capsule collagen and the procollagen synthesized by bovine aorta endothelial cells in culture was demonstrated by Howard et al (1976). These studies indicate that there is tissue and species non-specificity of antibodies to basement membrane collagen. Arbogast et al (1976) showed, in addition, that the antigenicity of the basement membrane procollagen (type IV) depended on the hydroxylation of proline as well as on the integrity of disulphide bonds. Subsequent studies by Wick et al (1979) and Timpl et al (1979) using antibodies to basement membrane collagens isolated from a mouse sarcoma tumour and from human placenta essentially confirmed the above observations of Gunson, Kefalides & Arbogast. These studies demonstrated, in addition, that antibodies to type IV collagen failed to react with αA and αB chains (type V collagen) isolated from human placenta.

It can be stated with certainty that there is immunologic cross-reaction among homologous and heterologous basement membranes and their components; that the antigenicity of basement membranes resides in glycoprotein components having the composition of collagen, procollagen and noncollagen peptides. Hydroxylation of proline as well as integrity of disulphide bonds may influence the antigenicity of the collagen and procollagen components, possibly through their conformational effects on these molecules.

In those tissues where the presence of basement membrane has been demonstrated only by electron microscopy and its isolation has not been accomplished for one reason or another, the demonstration of one or more of its protein components must depend on the use of antibodies prepared against basement membrane components isolated from other tissues. This situation holds particularly true for tissues such as skin, aorta, smooth and skeletal muscle fibres and in developing embryos where it has been almost impossible to isolate pure basement membranes.

BASEMENT MEMBRANE ALTERATIONS IN DISEASE

The morphological and functional alteration of basement membranes in a variety of diseases has been well documented. A number of mechanisms have been implicated including immunological injury, congenital and hereditary abnormalities, and mechanisms which remain largely unknown.

Any one of the structural components of the glomerular capillary wall, including the endothelium, epithelium, basement membrane or mesangium may be affected. The ultrastructural changes in GBM and in basement membranes of other tissues may be characterized by diffuse thickening, splitting and localized rarefaction, deposition of electron-dense antigen-antibody complexes, polypoid changes and wrinkling.

It has generally been assumed that the morphological and functional alterations of basement membranes in human and experimental disease must be accompanied by associated changes in the chemical composition and structure of their protein and carbohydrate moieties' This may not necessarily be the case but, even if it is, the studies with GBM in human disease and in experimentally induced disease in animals produced incomplete and contradictory data (Kefalides et al, 1979). There are serious limitations encountered in the effort to carry out these studies which include the unavailability of adequate amounts of tissue in the early stages of human disease and the difficulty in obtaining pure basement membrane from patients with advanced disease.

The pathogenesis of vascular lesions and particularly of the basement membrane thickening in diabetes mellitus is at present unknown. The relationship of the muscle capillary lesion to that seen in the glomerulus is not clear, although a common pathway may be operating to bring about the changes in both. The thickening of the peripheral capillary basement membrane and the increased amount of the mesangial matrix in the glomerulus of diabetic kidneys is thought to reflect the relative state of cell function. The thickening of basement membrane may be the result of increased synthesis by the epithelial and/or endothelial cells, it may reflect failure of normal degradation and removal by mesangial cells or it may be due to true increase in protein mass or simply oedema.

The biochemical basis for the thickening of GBM in diabetes still remains poorly understood (see Ch. 00). The claim of Beisswenger & Spiro (1973) that human diabetic GBM contained an abnormally high amount of hydroxylysine and hydroxylysine-linked glycosides without a concomitant increase in the other amino acids which characterize collagen, namely 3-, and 4-hydroxyproline and glycine, could not be substantiated subsequently by four independent studies (Westberg & Michael, 1973; Kefalides 1974; Sato et al, 1975; Westberg, 1976) (Table 17.9). The data to date are more compatible with the view that if any changes occur they must reflect an increase in the synthesis of both the collagen and noncollagen components; however knowledge of the pathogenesis of the changes in diabetes mellitus still escapes us.

Table 17.9 Partial list of the amino acid composition of human glomerular basement membrane from normal and diabetic patients (Residues/1000 residues)

Amino acid Residue	*Normal*					*Diabetic*					
HO-Lysine	24.9[a]	24.7[b]	24.5[c]	28.0[d]	25.4[e]	27[a]	29.5[b]	25.6[c]	29.0[d]	27.0[e1]	27.3[e2]
Lysine	20.4	25.4	26	23.9	20.1	22.2	20	30	21.9	—	—
3-HO-Proline	18.5	8.9	8.0	—	20.4	16.8	—	8	—	18.6	16.8
4-HO-Proline	82.5	80.6	66	84.2	83.8	88.6	87.8	71	93.4	88.6	88.1
Proline	62.5	74	70	70.9	61.7	59.5	69.7	63.2	68.6	58.4	59.5
Glycine	210.5	214	227	191.0	219.4	220.1	238.5	242	198.2	206.5	220.1
Half-cystine	26.1	20.3	23	20.1	25.2	19	19.5	18	15.6	18.9	19.6

[a] Westberg & Michael (1973)
[b] Beisswenger & Spiro (1973)
[c] Kefalides (1974)
[d] Sato et al (1975)
[e] Westberg (1976): [1] Patients with early diabetes; [2] Patients with advanced diabetes

CONCLUSIONS

Basement membranes are extracellular matrices whose ultrastructural morphology reveals the presence of fine fibrils 40 to 60 Å in diameter arranged randomly within a granular matrix. Chemical and physical studies demonstrated the presence of procollagen molecules within the matrix. X-ray diffraction studies of GBM and anterior lens capsule produced diagrams and reflections consistent with triple-helical collagen molecules which are arranged in a poorly-ordered fibrillar assembly. The procollagen molecules are held together by disulphide and lysyl derived covalent bonds. Noncollagenous glycoprotein(s) are thought to be associated with procollagen aggregates in some basement membranes. Although the major collagenous component is a molecule composed of three identical pro-α chains (type IV), the question of additional collagen molecules cannot be ruled out (See Ch. 1).

Metabolic studies indicate that basement membrane collagen is, like type I interstitial collagen, initially synthesized in a precursor form, procollagen. The molecular structure of basement membrane procollagen is consistent with a triple-helical collagen molecule having non-triple-helical precursor-specific appendages at the amino and carboxyl termini. Unlike interstitial procollagens, basement membrane procollagen does not undergo a time dependent conversion to a smaller molecular form.

Immunochemical studies have shown that there is immunological cross-reaction between homologous and heterologous basement membranes. At least three major antigenic components have been identified; one noncollagenous and one collagenous, consistent with procollagen molecules, and a third, a noncollagenous glycoprotein independent of procollagen, possibly related to laminin.

The biochemical basis of basement membrane changes in diseases such as glomerulonephritis and diabetes mellitus remains unknown. In diabetes mellitus the thickening of basement membrane may result from either increased deposition or decreased turnover. The collagenous component appears to be qualitatively unchanged.

Future studies on basement membranes should be directed at unravelling its structural organization, understanding its function in embryonic and adult tissues and elucidating the steps which control their synthesis and secretion.

ACKNOWLEDGEMENT

This work was supported by NIH Grants AM 20553, HL 15061 and HL 18827.

REFERENCES

Alper R, Kefalides N A 1978 The use of hydroxylamine cleavage as a probe of the supramolecular organization of bovine anterior lens capsule basement membrane. In: Kefalides N A (ed) Biology and chemistry of basement membranes. Academic Press, New York, p 239

Arbogast B W, Gunson D E, Kefalides N A 1976 The role of hydroxylation of proline in the antigenicity of basement membrane collagen. Journal of Immunology 117: 2181

Beisswenger P J, Spiro R G 1973 Studies on the human glomerular basement membrane. Composition, nature of the carbohydrate units and chemical changes in diabetes mellitus. Diabetes 22: 180

Burgeson R E, El Adli F A, Kaitila I I, Hollister D W 1976 Fetal membrane collagens: Identification of two new collagen alpha chains. Proceedings of the National Academy of Sciences USA 73: 2579

Chung E, Rhodes R K, Miller E J 1976 Isolation of three collagenous components of probable basement membrane origin. Biochemical and Biophysical Research Communications 71: 1167

Clark C C, Kefalides N A 1978 Comparison of newly synthesized basement membrane procollagen to interstitial Type I procollagen. In: Kefalides N A (ed) Biology and chemistry of basement membranes. Academic Press, New York, p 287

Clark C C, Tomichek E A, Koszalka T R, Minor R R, Kefalides N A 1975 The embryonic rat parietal yolk sac. The role of the parietal endoderm in the biosynthesis of basement membrane collagen and glycoprotein, *in vitro*. Journal of Biological Chemistry 250: 5259

Daniels J R, Chu G H 1975 Basement membrane collagen of renal glomerulus. Journal of Biological Chemistry 250: 3531

Dehm P, Kefalides N A 1978a The collagenous component of lens basement membrane. Journal of Biological Chemistry 253: 6680

Dehm P, Kefalides N A 1978b Comparison of α-chain size collagenous peptides isolated from bovine glomerular basement membrane and lens capsule. Federation Proceedings 37: 1527

Denduchis B, Kefalides N A 1969 Structural components of epithelial and endothelial basement membranes. Biochemistry 8: 4613

Denduchis B, Kefalides N A, Bezkorovainy A 1970 The chemistry of sheep anterior lens capsule. Archives of Biochemistry and Biophysics 138: 582

Dixit S N 1978 Isolation and characterization of two α-chain size collagenous polypeptide chains C and D from glomerular basement membrane. FEBS Letters 106: 379

Dixit S N, Kang A H 1979 Anterior lens capsule collagens: cyanogen bromide peptides of the C chain. Biochemistry 18: 5686

Gay S, Miller E J 1979 Characterization of lens capsule collagen: evidence for the presence of two unique chains in molecules derived from major basement membrane structures. Archives of Biochemistry and Biophysics 198: 370

Gehron Robey P, Martin G R 1981 Type IV collagen contains two distinct chains in separate molecules. Collagen Research 1: 27

Gelman R A, Blackwell J, Kefalides N A, Tomichek E A 1976 Thermal stability of basement membrane collagen. Biochimica et Biophysica Acta 427: 492

Glanville R W, Rauter A, Fietzek P P 1979 Isolation and characterization of a native placental basement membrane collagen and its component α chains. European Journal of Biochemistry 95: 383

Grant M E, Schofield J D, Kefalides N A, Prockop D J 1973 The biosynthesis of basement membrane collagen in embryonic chick lens. III. Intracellular formation of the triple-helix and the formation of aggregates through disulphide bonds. Journal of Biological Chemistry 248: 7432

Gryder R M, Lamon M, Adams E 1975 Sequence position of 3-hydroxyproline in basement membrane collagen. Journal of Biological Chemistry 250: 2470

Gunson D E, Kefalides N A 1976 The use of the radioimmunoassay in the characterization of antibodies to basement membrane collagen. Immunology 31: 563

Gunson D E, Arbogast B, Kefalides N A 1976 Rat parietal yolk sac basement membrane; an investigation of the antigenic determinants using a radioimmunoassay. Immunology 31: 577

Hudson B G, Spiro R G 1972 Studies on the native and reduced alkylated renal glomerular basement membrane. Journal of Biological Chemistry 247: 4229

Kanwar Y S, Farquhar M G 1979 The isolation of glycosaminoglycans (heparan sulfate) from the glomerular basement membrane. Proceedings of the National Academy of Sciences USA 76: 4493

Kefalides N A 1966 A collagen of unusual composition and a glycoprotein isolated from canine glomerular basement membrane. Biochemical and Biophysical Research Communications 22: 26

Kefalides N A 1968 Isolation and characterization of the collagen from glomerular basement membrane. Biochemistry 7: 3103

Kefalides N A 1969 Characterization of the collagen from lens capsule and glomerular basement membranes. In: Östman J (ed) Diabetes. Excerpta Medical Foundation, Amsterdam, p 307

Kefalides N A 1971a Chemical properties of basement membranes. International Review of Experimental Pathology 10: 1

Kefalides N A 1971b Isolation of a collagen from basement membranes containing three identical α-chains. Biochemical and Biophysical Research Communications 45: 226

Kefalides N A 1972a Isolation and characterization of cyanogen bromide peptides from basement membrane collagen. Biochemical and Biophysical Research Communications 47: 1151

Kefalides N A 1972b The chemistry of the antigenic components isolated from glomerular basement membrane. Connective Tissue Research 1: 3

Kefalides N A 1973 Structure and biosynthesis of basement membranes. International Review of Connective Tissue Research 6: 63

Kefalides N A 1974 Biochemical properties of human glomerular basement membrane in normal and diabetic kidneys. Journal of Clinical Investigation 53: 403

Kefalides N A 1979 Persistence of basement membrane collagen phenotype in hybrids of human vascular endothelium and rodent fibroblasts. Federation Proceedings 38: 816

Kefalides N A, Winzler R J 1966 The chemistry of glomerular basement membrane and its relation to collagen. Biochemistry 5: 702

Kefalides N A, Alper R, Clark C C 1979 Biochemistry and metabolism of basement membranes. International Review of Cytology 61: 167

Kresina T, Miller E J 1979 Isolation and characterisation of basement membrane collagen from human placental tissue — evidence for the presence of two genetically distinct chains. Biochemistry 18: 3089

Liotta L A, Abe S, Robey P G, Martin G R 1979 Preferential digestion of basement membrane collagen by an enzyme derived from a metastatic murine tumor. Proceedings of the National Academy of Sciences USA 76: 2268

Mainardi C L, Dixit S N, Kang A H 1980 Degradation of Type IV (basement membrane) collagen by a proteinase isolated from human polymorphonuclear leucocyte granules. Journal of Biological Chemistry 255: 5435

Marquardt H, Wilson C B, Dixon F J 1973 Human glomerular basement membrane. Selective solubilization with chaotropes and chemical and immunologic characterization of its components. Biochemistry 12: 3260

Minor R R, Clark C C, Strause E L, Koszalka T R, Brent R L, Kefalides N A 1976 Basement membrane procollagen is not converted to collagen in organ cultures of parietal yolk sac endoderm. Journal of Biological Chemistry 251: 1789

Mohos S C, Skoza L 1970 Variations in the sialic acid concentration of glomerular basement membrane preparations obtained by ultrasonic treatment. Journal of Cell Biology 45: 450

Olsen B R, Alper R, Kefalides N A 1973 Structural characterization of a soluble fraction from lens capsule basement membrane. European Journal of Biochemistry 38: 220

Prockop D J, Kivirikko K I, Tuderman L, Guzman N A 1979 The biosynthesis of collagen and its disorders. New England Journal of Medicine 301: 13 and 77

Rohde H, Wick G, Timpl R 1979 Immunochemical characterization of the basement membrane glycoprotein laminin. European Journal of Biochemistry 102: 195

Roveri N, Ripamonti A, Bigi A, Volpin D, Giro M G 1979 X-ray diffraction study of bovine lens capsule collagen. Biochimica et Biophysica Acta 576: 404

Sato T, Manakata H, Hoshinaga K, Yosizawa Z 1975 Comparison of the chemical composition of glomerular and tubular basement membranes obtained from human kidneys of diabetics and non-diabetics. Clinica Chimica Acta 61: 145

Schwartz D, Veis A 1978 Characterization of the basement membrane collagen of bovine anterior lens capsule via segment-long-spacing crystallites and the specific cleavage of the collagen by pepsin. FEBS Letters 85: 326

Schwartz D, Veis A 1980 Characterization of bovine anterior lens capsule basement membrane collagen. European Journal of Biochemistry 103: 29

Schwartz D, Chin-Quee T, Veis A 1980 Characterization of anterior lens capsule basement membrane collagen. European Journal of biochemistry 103: 21

Spiro R G 1967 The structure of the disaccharide unit of the renal glomerular basement membrane. Journal of Biological Chemistry 242: 4813

Timpl R, Martin G R, Bruckner P, Wick G, Wiedemann H 1978 Nature of the collagenous protein in a tumor basement membrane. European Journal of Biochemistry 84: 43

Timpl R, Rohde H, Gehron Robey P, Rennard S I, Foidart J M, Martin G R 1979a Laminin — a glycoprotein from basement membranes. Journal of Biological Chemistry 254: 9933

Timpl R, Glanville R W, Wick G, Martin G R 1979b Immunochemical study on basement membrane (Type IV) collagens. Immunology 38: 109

Trelstad R L, Lawley K R 1977 Isolation and initial characterization of human basement membrane collagens. Biochemical and Biophysical Research Communications 76: 376

Tryggvason K, Gehron Robey P, Martin G R 1980 Biosynthesis of type IV procollagens. Biochemistry 5: 3460

Uitto V-J, Schwartz D, Veis A 1980 Degradation of basement membrane collagen by neutral proteases from human leucocytes. European Journal of Biochemistry 105: 409

Westberg N G 1976 Biochemical alterations of the human glomerular basement membrane in diabetics. Diabetes 25: (Suppl 2) 920

Westberg N G, Michael A F 1973 Human glomerular basement membrane: Chemical composition in diabetes mellitus. Acta Medica Scandinavica 194: 39

Wick G, Glanville R W, Timpl R 1979 Characterization of antibodies to basement membrane (Type IV) collagen in immunohistologic studies. Immunobiology 156: 372

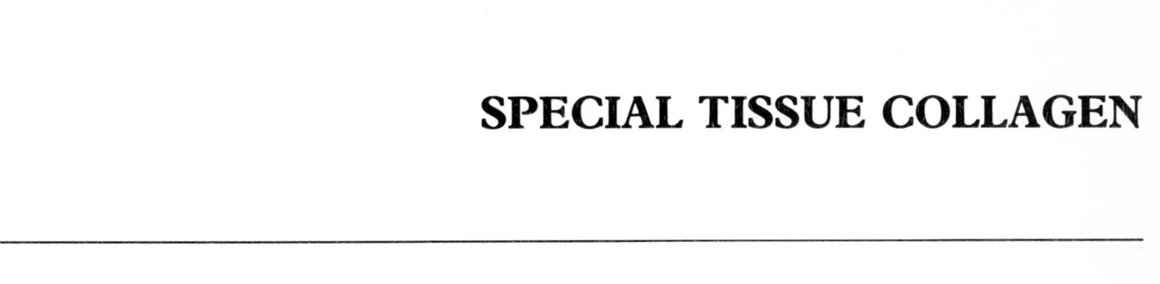

SPECIAL TISSUE COLLAGEN

18

Articular cartilage, intervertebral disc, synovia

R. BURGESON

INTRODUCTION

The term cartilage is used to describe a variety of skeletal elements which share several morphological, biophysical and functional properties. At the gross level, all cartilage appears uniformly amorphous, hypocellular relative to most nonskeletal tissues, avascular and nonenervated. By light microscopy, at least three types of cartilage, hyaline cartilage, fibro cartilage and elastic cartilage, can be distinguished morphologically by the degree and type of fibrous elements each contains. At the level of transmission electron microscopy, morphologically distinct zones may be defined within each of the cartilage types, indicating a degree of complexity which is only now beginning to be appreciated biochemically.

It is generally believed that the observed structural differences reflect functional specialization. One would expect that the mechanical properties of the elastic auricular cartilage would be substantially different from that of articular surfaces of hyaline cartilage. Likewise, the epiphyseal plate region of hyaline cartilage would be expected to function differently from the superficial zone of the articular surface. Therefore, our ability to morphologically distinguish functionally specialized areas has encouraged identification of the structural elements and attempts to understand their interactions.

The purpose of this chapter is to attempt to summarize recent advances resulting from these ongoing investigations. It includes studies of several inherited and acquired disease conditions which directly or indirectly suggest a collagen-related aetiology. This data acquisition has substantially increased our knowledge of the collagens at the molecular level. We are aware of the heterogeneity of gene products which make up the collagen family. We have an appreciation of the complex biosynthetic pathways involved in the synthesis, secretion and processing of the collagen precursors. The mechanisms involved in the control of collagen production and accumulation are under intense study. These major advances tell us a great deal about the subunits of collagen fibres, but tell us very little about the functional subunits of connective tissues, that is, the collagen fibres themselves.

The study of connective tissues has been approached from two directions. In addition to characterizing the collagenous and noncollagen components as molecular entities, each of these newly defined species is being quantitated and microlocalized within the different types of tissues. Both normal and diseasd specimens are being described as a function of age with the hope that these data will suggest testable hypotheses of the functions of these multiple elements.

These two distinct approaches are only beginning to encroach upon the missing block of knowledge so important to our understanding of connective tissue physiology. At present, we are trying to comprehend the architecture and engineering of whole buildings by studying bricks. We need to know how the bricks interact; why certain kinds of brick make up one section of the structure and other types are exclusively used in other parts. We have only the most elementary concepts of the mortar which mediate the interactions of the basic building blocks. We know essentially nothing about the articulations of walls and floors to form recognizable structures. We know that glass and steel are required components of the building, yet their function and interaction with brick and mortar continue to elude us. To answer these critical questions, we need to develop the technology to disassemble the structure without a wrecking ball. Or alternatively, we need to find the workmen responsible for subunit assembly so that we can reproduce the complex architecture which our present methodologies destroy. Lacking this ability, we continue to catalogue the disassembled components. The purpose of this chapter is to present such a current catalogue.

HYALINE CARTILAGE

The morphology of the articular surface and the growth plate of hyaline cartilage

The relevant aspects of the morphology of hyaline cartilage has been recently reviewed by Meachim & Stockwell (1979). For purposes of description, it is convenient to subdivide articular cartilage into four major zones as

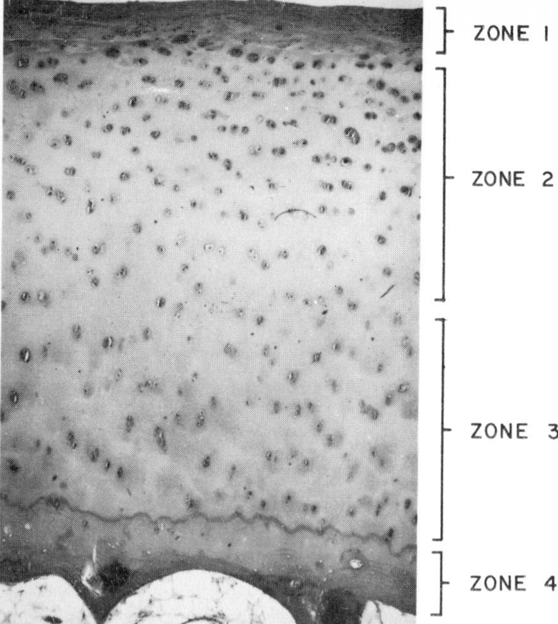

Fig. 18.1 Illustrates the morphology of human adult articular cartilage. Zone 1 defines the articular surface. Zone 4 represents the calcified cartilage immediately adjacent to the subchondral bone. The specimen is from a 21-year-old woman, and is stained with trichrome.

illustrated in Figure 18.1. Zones 1 and 4 are morphologically distinctive. Zone 1 represents the superficial zone, or articular surface. Zone 4 denotes the calcified cartilage immediately adjacent to the subchondral bone. Zones 2 and 3 are less easily defined, and represent the deep uncalcified zones of cartilage.

The major protein throughout all four zones in the articular cartilage is collagen. The distribution and orientation of collagen fibres throughout the various zones of the matrix are nonuniform. Electron microscopic assessment of the fibrous nature of the matrix indicates differences between the intercellular regions of the matrix and the areas immediately surrounding the chondrocytes (Fig. 18.2). In general, all zones of the matrix demonstrate fibres with typical banded morphology. The vast majority of the fibres seen in the intercellular space have diameters ranging from 30 to 80 nm, though occasionally in mature cartilage fibres 3 to 5 times that diameter can be seen. In contrast, the pericellular areas contain only small fibres and slender filamentous structures (Weiss et al, 1968). These distinct morphological differences may well be related to the different types of collagens which have been recently described in human cartilage, and which are discussed in detail in the next section. Between the collagen fibres of the intercellular matrix are materials traditionally described as ground substance which appear to be granular and are relatively electron-lucent. The ground substance represents a large variety of components, the most abundant of which are the glycosaminoglycans.

Zone 1, the superficial zone of articular cartilage, is made up of large numbers of collagen fibres oriented parallel to the articular surface. The fibre density in this zone is higher than the deeper zones and demonstrates greater organization. The chondrocytes embedded in this superficial layer are flattened and discoidal with their long axes parallel to the articular surface. The articular surface itself is not smooth, but rather contains large numbers of shallow depressions varying from 15 to 30 μm in diameter and 1 to 6 μm in depth (Clarke, 1971). These bowl-shaped depressions may serve to trap synovial joint fluid and aid in the lubrication of articulating surfaces. The articular surface itself is lined with an electron dense fibrous material not yet determined to be collagen. The identification of this material is clearly important to our understanding of the physiology and pathology of the articular surface.

The middle zones, 2 and 3, show fibres with a more random orientation. The fibres in zone 2 have been described as a tangled open meshwork, where those of zone 3 appear more tightly packed and are orientated radially to the articular surface (McCall, 1969). The chondrocytes in these deeper cartilage layers appear to be spherical. The zone 3 chondrocytes are often seen in clusters of three or more cells aligned perpendicularly to the articular surface.

The fourth zone of articular cartilage represents the calcified interface of the cartilage and the underlying subchondral bone. This zone is demarcated from zone 3 by a basophilic line which has become known as the 'tidemark'. This zone contains chondrocytes which are both smaller and more sparsely distributed. The calcium salts in this zone appear to be in the form of hydroxyapatite. The growth of these crystals is mediated by matrix vesicles similar to those seen in the calcified regions of the cartilage growth plate. Blood vessels originating in the subchondral bone often penetrate the deeper layers of this fourth zone.

The morphology of the growth plate of hyaline cartilage

There are four morphologically distinguishable regions of the normal growth plate as shown in Figure 18.3. The first zone, the zone nearest to the articular surface, has been defined as the resting, or reserve cartilage. This zone has an appearance similar to that of zones 2 and 3 of the articular cartilage. The chondrocytes in this zone are spherical in shape, randomly distributed and separated by large quantities of extracellular matrix. Adjacent to this is the region known as the proliferative zone in which the chondrocytes begin mitotic division. The daughter cells resulting from the division align parallel to the long bone axis. These divisions result in long columns of chondrocytes extending through the proliferative zone.

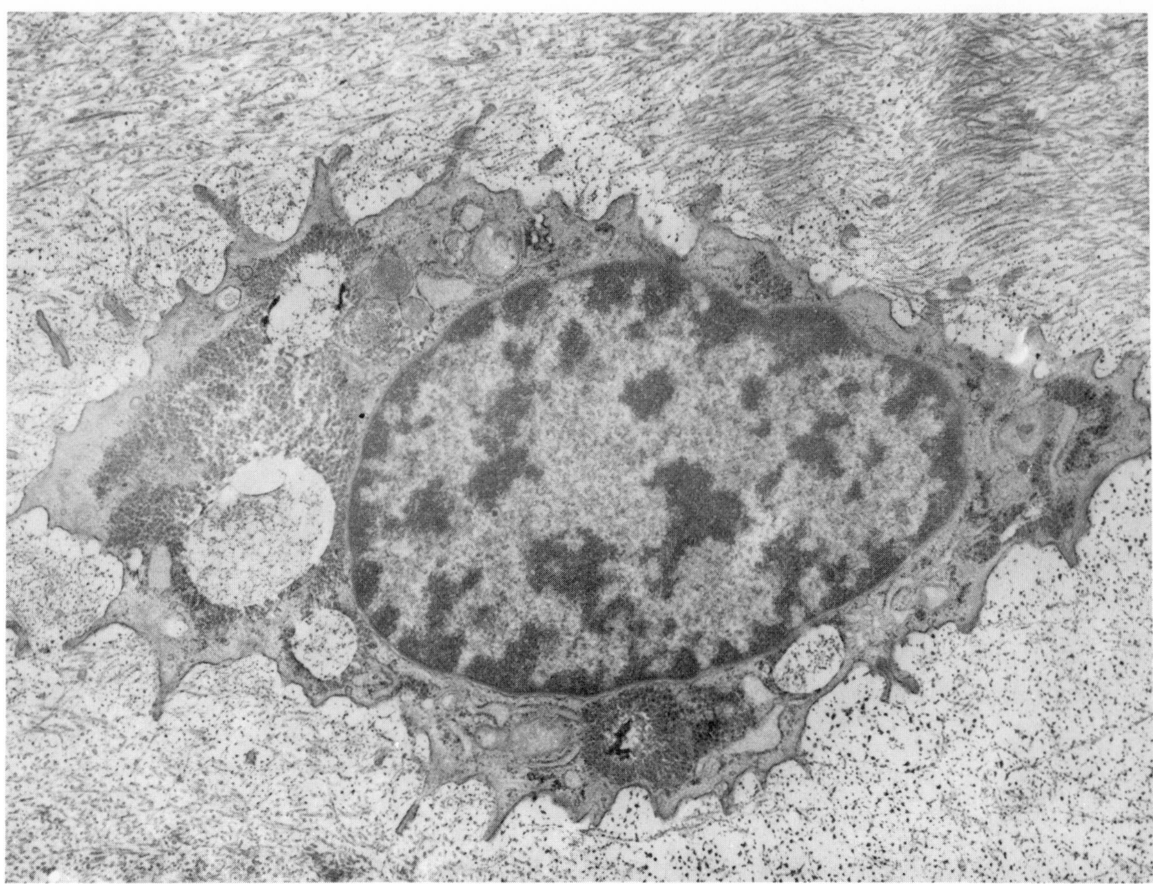

Fig. 18.2 A transmission electron micrograph of a chondrocyte from the resting zone of articular cartilage. The chondrocyte is surrounded by collagen fibres from the intercellular matrix. In the region immediately adjacent to the cell surface, the matrix has a much finer fibrous appearance. It is not known if these two fibre forms represent more than a single collagen type. The specimen was stained with uranyl acetate and lead citrate.

The chondrocytes at the base of the column hypertrophy, leaving electron-lucent and enlarged lacunae. This region of the growth plate, known as the hypertrophic zone, has a spongy appearance with spicules of cartilage remaining between the now empty cellular lacunae. The lower extremities of this zone merge with a region known as the zone of chondro-osseous transformation in which vascular elements originating from the subchondral bone invade the remaining cartilage matrix. The cartilage in this region becomes calcified, and bone collagen is deposited upon the calcified cartilage spicules.

The collagens of hyaline cartilage

The meaning of the term 'collagen' has changed drastically over the preceding 10 years due to the dramatic increase in our knowledge of this class of skeletal proteins. The term no longer applies to a single molecular entity, but rather to a class of structural elements which have the collagen triple helix as their major structural domain. This helicity is essential to the rod-like shape of the molecule, to its resistance to proteolytic degradation, and to its ability to cross-link with adjacent molecules to form an insoluble fibrous matrix. In turn, this triple helix is a consequence of the unique amino acid sequence of all collagen helical regions. Each collagen α chain contains glycine in every third position to allow close packing of the subunit α chains into the triple helical array. The helix is stabilized by hydrogen-bonding through the unusual imino acid, hydroxyproline. Therefore, every collagen must contain some minimum value of hydroxyproline residues for molecular integrity under physiological conditions. Hydroxylation of specific lysine residues is also required for the formation of cross-links between molecules. In addition, short nonhelical segments must extend from both the amino and carboxy-terminal ends of the helical domain. These short nonhelical domains provide a relatively high degree of flexibility which allows greater freedom of movement of hydroxylysine residues contained within them to cross-link with neighbouring cross-linking sites. Beyond these stringent requirements, the amino acid sequence can be varied without disruption of either the characteristic helical conformation, or the ability of the

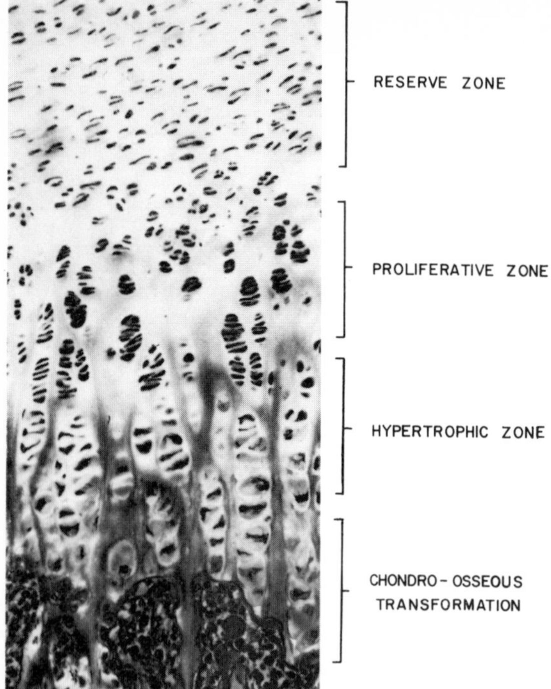

Figure 18.3 The morphology of the growth plate. The regions of the growth plate are identified. The uppermost region, the reserve zone, is the region nearest the articular surface. The zone at the bottom of the illustration, the zone of chondro-osseous transformation, is adjacent to the subchondral bone. Elongation of the bone results from mitotic division of cells in the proliferative zone. The transition from cartilage-type collagens to bone-type collagens occurs between the proliferative zone and the region of chondro-osseous transformation. This specimen is stained with trichrome.

molecules to form the stable, ordered arrays which are fundamental to biological function.

In view of the diversity of morphology and function of connective tissues as different as skin, tendon, bone or cartilage, it is not surprising that each contains a unique collagen or a mixture of different collagens. Recent evidence suggests that the maintenance of this tissue-specific collagen composition is a dynamic process. The relative content of different collagens in the same tissue varies with respect to the developmental stage of that tissue, the age of the mature tissue, as well as with the tissue's attempt to repair injury. All these data strongly support the suggestion that a direct relationship exists between the form and function of a connective tissue matrix and the type or types of collagen contained therein.

Type II collagen

Cartilage was one of the first tissues to be recognized to be composed of collagen molecules which were genetically different from the collagen which had previously been characterized (Miller & Matukas, 1969; Trelstad et al, 1970; Miller, 1971; Strawich & Nimni, 1971). We now know that this collagen species, currently referred to as type II collagen, has an extremely limited tissue distribution. It appears to be restricted to cartilage and its developmental precursors, to the cartilaginous sclera (Trelstad & Kang, 1974), and to the vitreous body of the eye (Swann et al, 1972).

Although the characterization of the different collagen types has been extensively discussed in preceding chapters, I feel it is worthwhile to review this information in specific regard to cartilage.

The major collagen in cartilage is the type II molecule. Each molecule is 300 nm in length and 1.5 nm in diameter. The flexibility of each molecule is more like that of a piece of heavy cord than a rigid rod. This molecule is a triple helical arrangement of three identical subunit chains which are denoted as α1(II) chains. The Type II α chains contain about 1020 amino acids. The amino acid compositions of α1(II) is shown in Table 18.1. Like all known collagens, one-third of its amino acids are glycine. The imino acids, proline and hydroxyproline, account for another 20 per cent. The most significant difference between the composition of type II collagen chains and those of the other major collagenous structural elements, types I and III, is the fact that nearly one-half of all the hydroxylysine residues contain covalently bound neutral hexose; either galactose or glucosylgalactose. The functional consequences of this elevated glycosylation are totally unknown. The presence of bulky sugar side chains might be expected to sterically impede the side-by-side alignment of individual molecules, and therefore, modulate the rate of fibre formation or the average fibre diameter. Since lysine and hydroxylysine are required for cross-linking of molecules within fibres, it is also possible that the addition of galactose or galactosyl-glucose to hydroxylysine affects the quantity and type of cross-links formed in cartilage.

Type II collagen may represent more than a single gene product. In the course of determining the amino acid sequence of the α1(II), chain, Butler, Finch & Miller (1977) found evidence of genetic heterogeneity in the type II collagen sequence of bovine nasal septum. At a single position, the α1(II) chain was found to contain 0.211 residues of alanine and 0.77 residues of leucine. Their data also suggest a substitution of serine for glutamine in another position. The data indicate that the type II collagen accumulated in the bovine nasal septum is the product of two genes. Since cells of higher organisms carry duplicate genes on all autosomal chromosomes due to their diploid genetic character, the finding of amino acid substitutions in the same gene on different chromosomes is not unexpected. However, the products of these allelic pairs would be predicted to be synthesized and accumulated at the same rate; therefore, the two resulting α1(II) chains would occur in cartilage in a 1:1 ratio. The finding of a 7:1 ratio of the major to minor chains suggests that they are products of

Table 18.1 Residues/1000 amino acids

	A	*B*	*1α*	*2α*	*C* [a]	*α1(I)*	*Type IV* [b]
OH-PRO	109	109	95	91	92	95	140
ASP	51	50	46	50	42	45	51
THR	26	19	17	24	19	16	20
SER	31	36	24	28	34	37	37
GLU	84	91	107	97	98	80	79
PRO	97	118	109	118	99	134	65
GLY	341	344	330	322	332	340	328
ALA	52	46	54	49	49	122	37
CYST/2	0	0	0	0	1.3	0	1
VAL	24	25	27	18	29	22	28
MET	11	8	10	9	8.1	7	13
ILEU	16	19	15	16	20	7	29
LEU	35	39	35	39	56	20	52
TYR	2	2	2	3	2.4	2	2
PHE	14	12	11	11	9.2	13	29
OH-LYS	24	35	37	40	43	4	49
LYS	18	20	18	15	15	31	9
HIS	11	8	6	11	14	2	6
ARG	50	45	42	47	42	50	26
PRO+OH-PRO	206	227	204	209	191	229	205
LYS+OH-LYS	42	55	55	55	58	35	58

[a] H Sage & P Bornstein, Biochemistry *18* (1979)
[b] Dehm & Kefalides (1978)

genes in separate loci. The proposed interpretation of these studies is that at least two, but possibly more, gene loci code for the α1(II) chain, and the accumulated matrix is the product of these several type II genes.

A second independent line of evidence supports this hypothesis. DNA sequence studies of the α2 gene of type I collagen demonstrate differences which can most easily be explained by assuming that there are multiple copies of the α2 gene. Therefore, it is reasonable that all collagen genes might be duplicated.

Thirdly, attempts to localize the α1(I) gene to a specific human chromosome have resulted in the assignment of that gene to both chromosome number 7 and number 17. Similarly, the α1(III) gene has been localized both to chromosome 17 and chromosome 4 (Raj et al, 1977; Sykes & Salomon, 1978). These data further support the hypothesis that there are multiple genes for each collagen αchain.

Finally, studies of human neonatal cartilage by Burgeson & Hollister (1979) suggest differences in the accumulated type II collagens in that tissue. Solubilization of the total collagens of the tissue was obtained by limited proteolysis with pepsin under optimal conditions. From this solution, a fraction was isolated on the basis of solubility in acidic and neutral solutions which had distinct electrophoretic mobility from the vast bulk of the type II collagen as can be seen in Figure 18.4. The material was extensively purified by chromatographic procedures, and the resulting αchain (termed 3α for purposes of identification) was compared by amino acid composition and cyanogen bromide peptide mapping to authentic α1(II) chain. The results of the amino acid analyses are shown on Table 18.1. The only significant and reproducible difference demonstrated between 3α and α1(II) was in the content of hydroxylysine. Fifty-eight per cent of the total lysine residues of the 3α chain were hydroxylated whereas the value determined for the majority of the type II chain was 39 per cent. For both chains, the total of lysine plus hydroxylysine was 36 residues. Although the major detected difference between the two chains is the result of post-translational modifications, the possibility that they represent two gene products cannot be ruled out.

The electrophoretic difference demonstrated for the 3α and α1(II) chains can also be seen between each of the major cyanogen bromide digestion products. Treatment of the isolated chains with cyanogen bromide causes cleavage of the peptide bond wherever methionine occurs in the amino acid sequence. Therefore, comparison of these peptides is an indirect comparison of the primary structure of the chains. Cyanogen bromide peptide maps of 3α and α1(II) are shown in Figure 18.5. The pattern seen for both chains is nearly identical except that the mobility of each of the 3α peptides is retarded relative to the analogous α1(II) peptide.

Similarly, when the chromatographic elution profiles of each of the materials are compared (Fig. 18.6) the patterns are only marginally different. From these studies, the authors conclude that 3α and α1(II) are nearly identical by all the criteria examined. The difference between the chains can be most easily accounted for by differences in the hydroxylation of lysine and the glycosylation of hydroxylysine. Since both of these events are post-

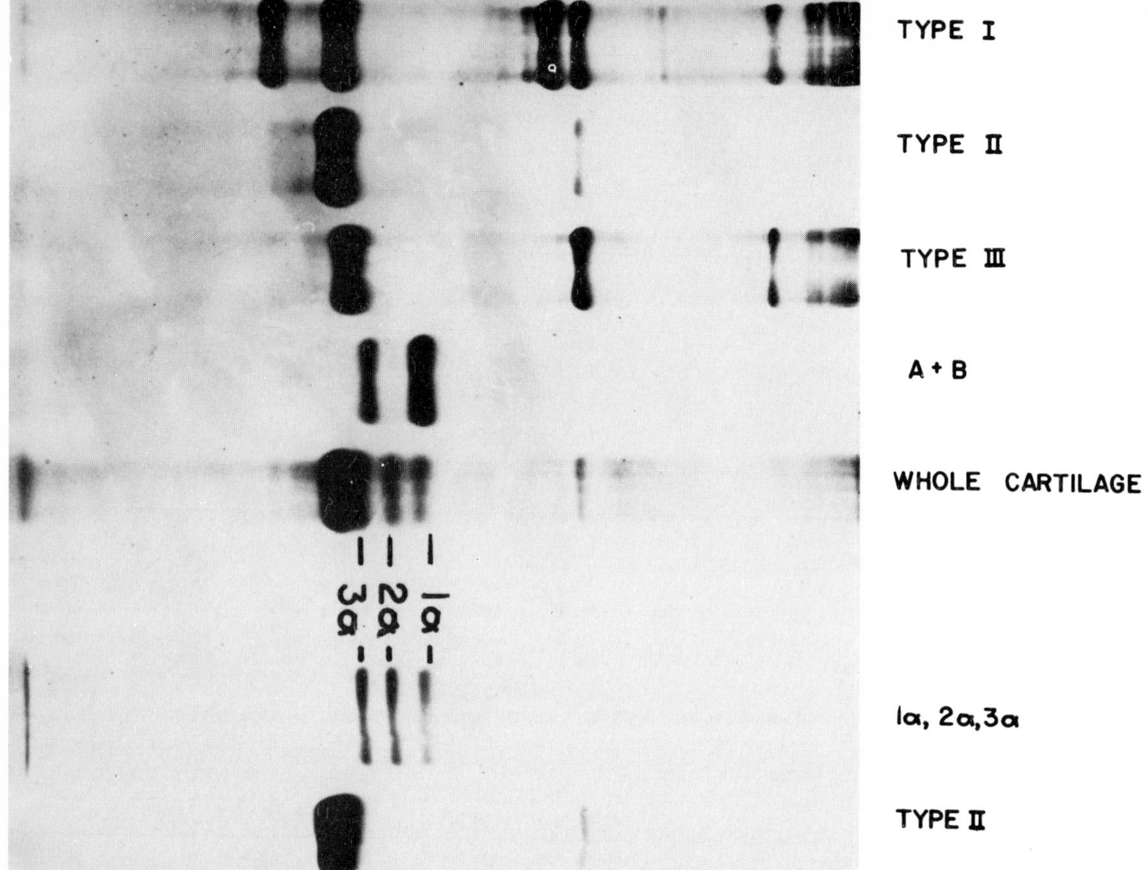

Fig. 18.4 The alpha chains of collagen can be separated by polyacrylamide gel electrophoresis in sodium dodecyl sulfate. The patterns obtained from several collagen types are illustrated here. The alpha chains isolated from normal cartilage by limited proteolytic digestion are illustrated in the channel labeled 'whole cartilage'. In addition to type II collagen, three other materials are present. These are denoted as 1α, 2α, and 3α. These three components can be separated from the type II collagen, and the isolated materials are shown in the next two channels. The relative electrophoretic mobilities of total cartilage collagen chains are compared to the mobilities of collagens type I, type III, A and B collagen chains.

translational modifications, the question of whether the 3α and α1(II) chains are products of different genes remains unanswered. However, in so far as the 3α chains represent a distinct class of α1(II)-like molecules which must be modified differently and separately from the bulk of the type II molecules, it is quite possible that 3α does represent the product of a second type II collagen gene. The relationship of the 3α chain to the minor α1(II) chain reported by Butler, Finch and Miller is not presently known.

Taken together, all these data strongly suggest that the collagen content of the cartilage matrix is derived from several different structural genes. If the physiological properties of these gene products are different, then they are clearly important to our understanding of the function of the matrix. Even if multiple genes specify products with identical function, this knowledge is critical to our understanding of rate of matrix accumulation during normal development and growth in response to tissue injury and during the pathological progress of various disease states.

Non-type II collagens of hyaline cartilage

Although there is general agreement that type II accounts for the majority of the cartilage collagen content, there have been several reports of collagens other than type II which have been found in relatively small amounts. Early reports of type I collagen uniformly present in hyaline cartilage were most likely due to perichondral contamination, and will not be discussed here. In 1974, Linsenmayer described three collagenous peptides isolated from embryonic chick limb cartilage. Each of these materials differed in amino acid composition from the chick α1(II) chain. Each was reported to have a lower content of alanine and elevated values for tyrosine, hydroxylysine, histidine, and half-cystine relative to α1(II). The three non-type II chains

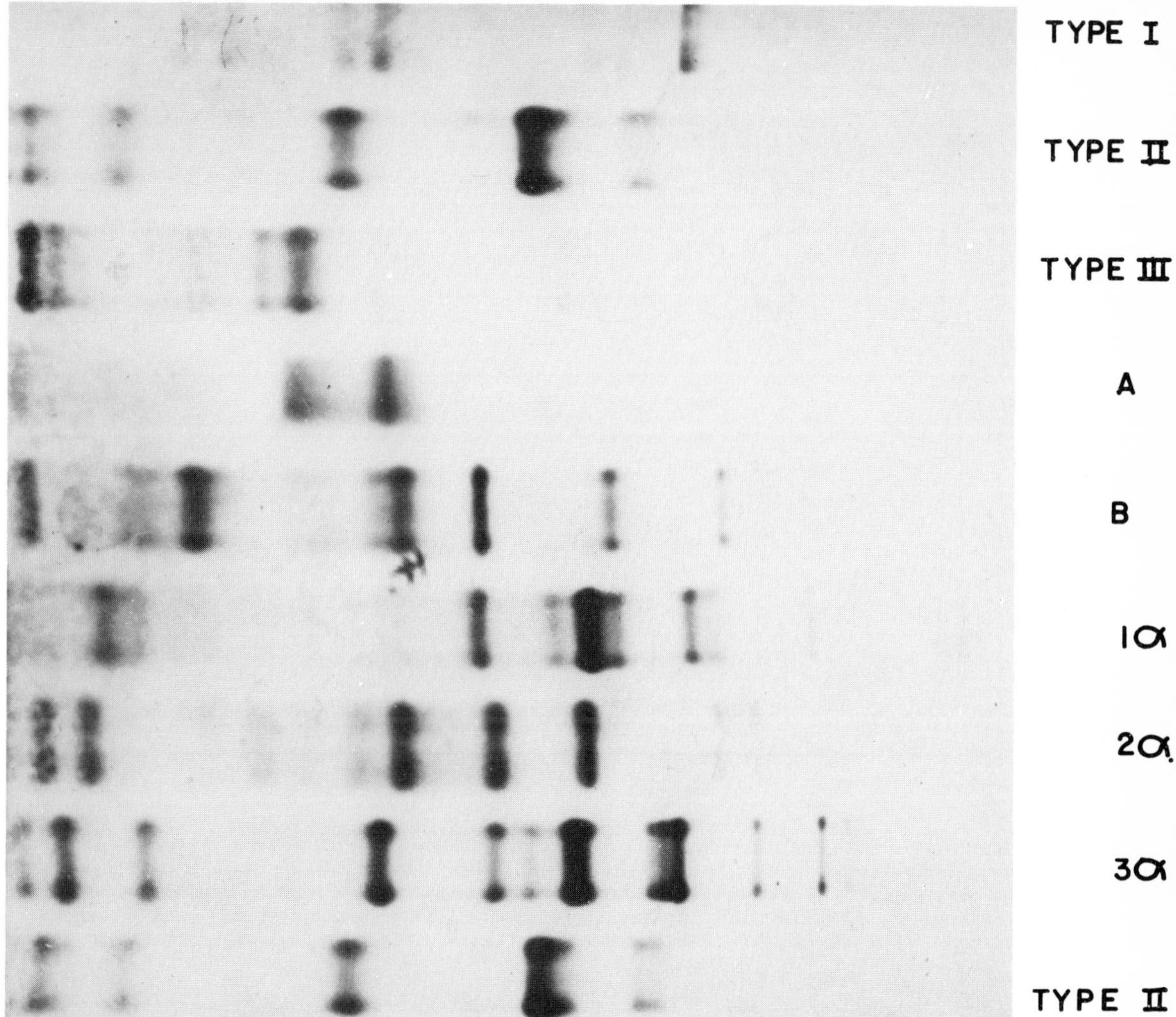

Fig. 18.5 Isolated collagen chains can be identified by mapping the peptides obtained from each chain following digestion with cyanogen bromide. This figure illustrates the separation obtained for the cyanogen bromide peptides of several collagen chains by polyacrylamide slab gel electrophoresis in sodium dodecyl sulphate. The patterns obtained for 1α and 2α can be distinguished from the A chain, B chain, and the chains of collagens types I, II and III. The two channels to the far right of this electrophoretogram compare the patterns obtained from 3α and the type II chain. Although the position of each of the peptides is different, the pattern is essentially the same. Each of the three alpha peptides has a slightly retarded mobility relative to the equivalent type II peptide.

together accounted for less than 25 per cent of the total solubilized matrix. Also in 1974, Trelstad & Kang reported finding both type II collagen and an unknown collagenous material in chick cartilaginous sclera. This new material was characterized by lower values for hydroxyproline, isoleucine, leucine and alanine, and elevated amounts of histidine, hydroxylysine and half-cystine.

Rhodes & Miller (1978) reported finding a collagen α chain in human infant epiphyseal cartilage. This collagen chain was similar in amino acid composition and chromatographic elution position to the B chain which has been reported in a large number of vertebrate tissues (Burgeson et al, 1976; Chung et al, 1976; Madri & Furthmeyr, 1978; Rojkind et al, 1979; Brown et al, 1978; Jimenez et al, 1978; Bailey et al, 1979; Stenn et al, 1979).

Investigations of the collagens of human cartilage carried on in our laboratory have supported the above-cited findings. In addition to the α1(II) chain and the closely related 3α chain, we have documented the presence of two additional collagen α chains in this complex tissue. When total collagen is solubilized from neonatal femoral head cartilage under conditions which minimize losses of any of the species due to problems of solubility, four collagenous α chain species can be detected by electrophoresis in sodium dodecyl sulphate-polyacrylamide gels as shown in Figure 18.4. As indicated in the electrophoretogram, the

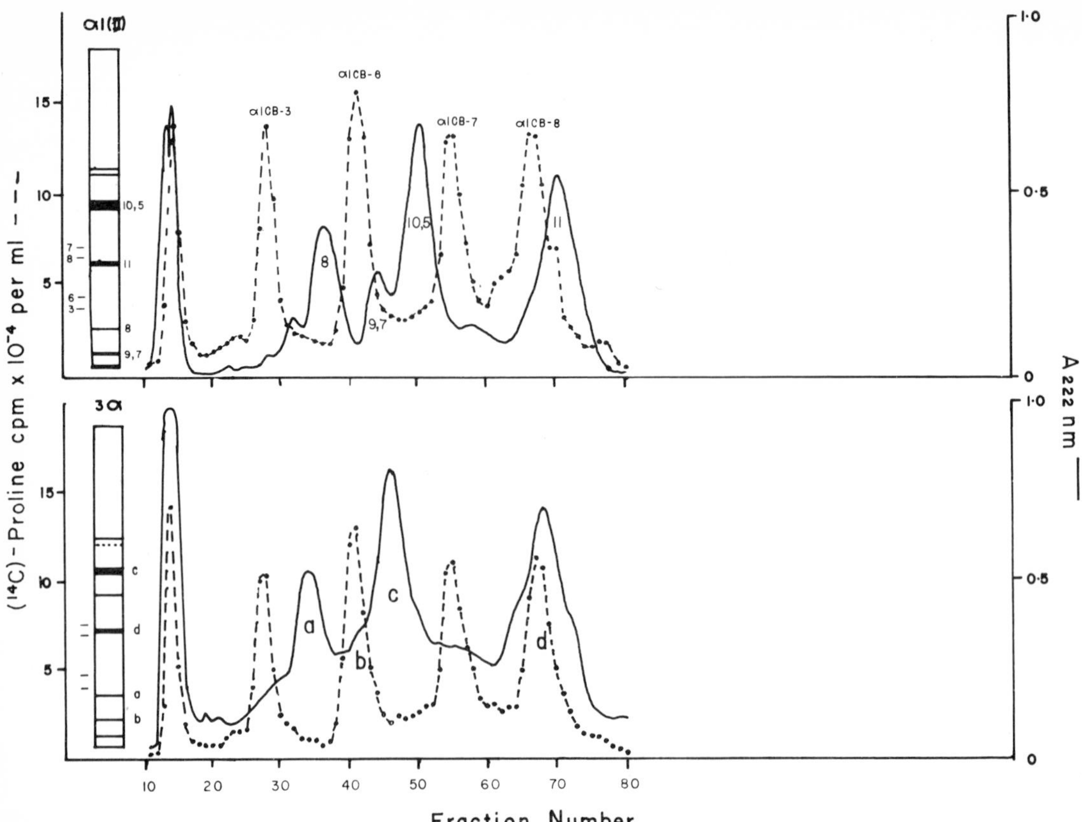

Fig. 18.6 Different collagen chains can be identified by the chromatographic elution position of their constituent cyanogen bromide peptides. The cyanogen bromide peptides of the α1 type II chain and the peptides of the 3α chain are compared in this illustration. Each of the chains was co-digested with radioactive α1 type I chain, which serves as an internal marker. The relative elution positions of the major peptides of both chains are nearly identical. To the left of the figure is shown the electrophoretic positions of the major isolated peaks. These data indicates that the 3α chain is very closely related to the α1 type II chain.

major species has the mobility of an α1(II) chain. Electrophoresing just more slowly is the 3α chain discussed earlier. Above these are two additional α chains indicated as 1α and 2α. 1α and 2α account for approximately 10 per cent of the total cartilage collagens of the neonatal femoral head. They have also been detected in human costal cartilage and in human femoral head from 24 weeks fetal gestation to 14 years postnatal. They are also present in bovine costal cartilage obtained at 18 months. Older human or bovine materials have not been examined.

1α and 2α chains have been isolated by ion-exchange chromatography, and were compared to α1(II), A and B collagen chains by amino acid composition analyses and peptide mapping following digestion with cyanogen bromide. The amino acid analyses of 1α, 2α and α1(II), A and B are shown in Table 18.1. On the basis of composition alone, 1α and 2α are unequivocally different from the α1(II) chain. 1α and 2α are prominently distinguished by their low content of alanine and enhanced contents of hydroxylysine and total lysine plus hydroxylysine. The distinctions between 1α, 2α, A and B chain are less dramatic. A chain differs from the others in its relatively low content of lysine and hydroxylysine (42 residues for A, 55 residues for 1α, 2α and B). B chain can be distinguished from A, 1α and 2α by its relatively high content of proline plus hydroxyproline (B contains 227 residues versus 204–209 for A, 1α and 2α).

The nonidentity of 1α and 2α with A and B chains is further supported by comparisons of the cyanogen bromide peptide patterns. Figures 18.7 and 18.8 compare these cleavage product patterns as obtained by ion-exchange chromatography. The electrophoretic mobility of major peaks is indicated to the left of each chromatogram. The profiles are different for each of the chains. Only in a single case (the 'a' peptide of 1α and the 'a' peptide of B chain) do peptides from different chains nearly coelute and coelectrophorese.

From these data, we conclude that the 1α and B chains and the 2α and A chains are different but closely related gene products. A and B chains have a nearly ubiquitous distribution through human tissues, though are found most often underlying various epithelia. The 1α and 2α chains

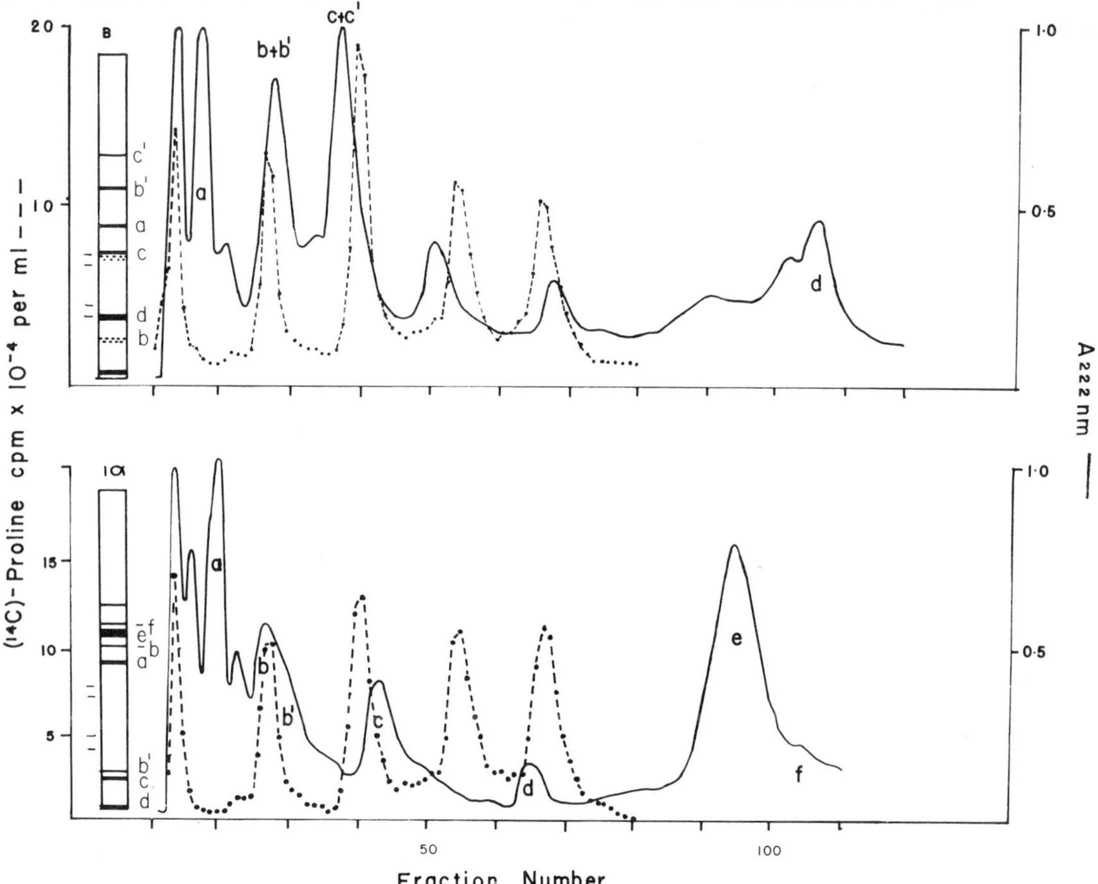

Fig. 18.7 The cyanogen bromide peptide maps of the B chain and the 1α chain are compared in this illustration. Each chain was co-digested with radioactive αI type, which serves as an internal marker. The electrophoretic position of each of the major peptides is represented at the far left of the illustration. This comparison of B chain peptides and 1α peptides indicates that the two chains contain methionine residues in different relative positions, and therefore have different amino acid sequences.

appear to be restricted to cartilaginous structures and codistribute with the α1(II) chain.

Attempts to localize these materials either to the articular surface or the epiphyseal growth plate indicate that both 1α and 2α are uniformly distributed throughout neonatal cartilage. Further investigations of their distribution will require specific fluorescent antibody probes. These studies are now in progress. On the basis of relative amount and uniform gross distribution, it might not be surprising to find these chains associated with chondrocytes or the perilacunar areas.

Recently, Ayad et al (1981) have confirmed the presence of the 1α, 2α and 3α chains in bovine nasal cartilage. In addition to these collagen chains, the authors present evidence for an additional non-type II collagen in that tissue. The triple-helical portion of the molecule obtained following limited pepsin digestion appears to be one-third the length of other collagen molecules. The authors suggest that this molecule, termed C-PS, may be a fragment of a larger native structure which has significant pepsin lability, similar to type IV-like collagens. However, compositional studies of C-PS are not reminiscent of 'type IV-like' collagens. The authors suggest that C-PS may be cartilage specific.

We have no information as to the function of these chains in cartilage at the present time. Their compositional dissimilarity not only to α1(II), but also to the α chains of types I, III and IV collagens suggests that these materials play a highly specific role in cartilage physiology. Recognition of the presence of multiple collagen types in cartilage must be an important consideration when pathological mechanisms are being hypothesized and investigated.

The synthesis of the type II collagen molecule

All collagens examined to date follow the same biosynthetic scheme. The details of this biosynthetic pathway have been extensively discussed in Chapter 7 of this book. In general, the translation product from the ribosomes is a collagenous species known as a pre-proalpha chain. This precursor

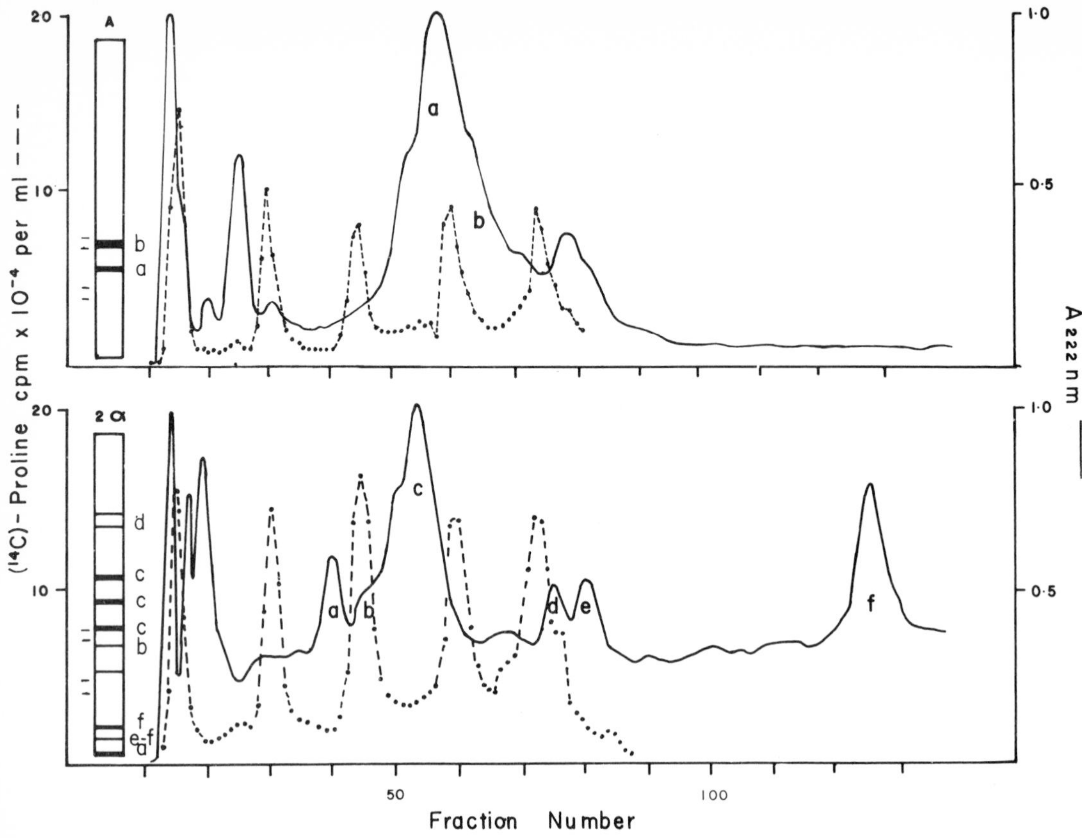

Fig. 18.8 This figure compares the elution positions of the cyanogen bromide peptides obtained from the A chain and the 2α chain. The dash line represents the pattern obtained from co-digested radioactive α1 chain, which serves as an internal positional marker. The electrophoretic positions of the major peptides are represented at the far left of the figure. This comparison indicates that the A chain and 2α chain are the products of different genes.

chain is larger than the alpha chain subunit found in the matrix associated into fibres. At the amino terminus of this precursor, there is a short tract of about 200 amino acids which has become known as the signal peptide. This short region serves to mark the protein for extracellular transport. The signal sequence is quickly excised by proteolytic action following translation. Immediately adjacent to the signal sequence is a largely nonhelical domain known as the amino terminal propeptide. The next domain in the sequence is the major helical region, consisting of approximately 1000 amino acids. Finally, the helical region is followed by a large nonhelical domain known as the carboxyterminal propeptide. Following translation and excision of the signal sequences, three proalpha chains become covalently associated through interchain disulphide bonds in the carboxyl propeptide, and the helical portions of each of these chains fold into a triple helical conformation. This triple helical array of three proalpha chains is referred to as the procollagen molecule. Procollagen is then transported from the rough endoplasmic reticulum via the golgi apparatus into the extracellular space. Following secretion, both the amino and carboxyterminal propeptides are excised by specific enzymes. The excision of the carboxy propeptide occurs simultaneously with fibre formation and is probably involved in its control and modulation.

The biosynthetic pathway for the synthesis of type II procollagen follows this general scheme. Like other collagens, the proalpha chain contains extensions at both the amino and carboxy terminus (Uitto et al, 1977). These nonhelical propeptide regions are excised from the procollagen molecule within 20 minutes following secretion (Uitto, 1977). The only reported significant difference between the processing of type II procollagen and that of type I is the order in which the procollagen extension peptides are excised. The type I collagen, amino propeptide, is removed before the carboxy propeptide. No such specific order has been reported for the removal of the propeptides from type II procollagen. What functional significance this difference may have, if any, is not immediately obvious.

Growth

Hyaline cartilage serves two major physiological processes. The first of these is to provide the resilient, self-lubricating articular surface necessary for protection of the underlying bone from abrasive erosion. The second and equally important function of hyaline cartilage is the mediating role it plays in long bone growth. This general process, known as endochondral ossification, is the only mechanism available to the developing organism for interstitial bone growth. The growth of all other bones occurs by appositional deposit of newly synthesized osseous material onto a pre-existing surface. Appositional bone growth occurs continuously throughout the life of the organism due to the ongoing processes of resorption and remodeling. In contrast, growth by endochondral ossification is limited to periods of rapid long bone growth and maturation. The careful regulation of this process is necessary for the attainment of the final correct skeletal proportions, though the mechanisms underlying this process and its control are not well understood at this time.

The general morphological and histological features of this process have been reviewed by Ham in 1950. The region most critical to this growth process has become known as the epiphyseal plate. This plate refers to a region of cartilage directly above the cartilage-bone interface and extending through the region of columnar arrays of chondrocytes into the resting cartilage. Growth occurs by an increase in length of the epiphyseal plate. This lengthening results from the division of chondrocytes in the proliferative zone and a concomitant thinning of the cartilage matrix in this region. The daughter cells resulting from chondrocyte mitoses align parallel to the direction of bone growth. As the mitoses continue, cells which become progressively lower in the growth plate show degenerative changes. At the very base of the cellular columns, this necrosis results in vacant cellular lacunae, and therefore, an increased porosity to this region of the cartilage. Vascular elements from the immediately adjacent bony region rapidly invade this region of decreased matrix density. This infiltration results in increased resorption of the cartilage matrix, and at the same time, the deposition of new osseous material on the surface of residual cartilage elements and calcification of the cartilage residue. During bony maturation, continued remodeling results in a final disappearance of all cartilage-derived elements within the mature bone.

Cartilage consists primarily of type II collagen, whereas bone results from calcification of a matrix derived from type I collagen. Much of the recent work involving collagen's role in growth has been directed toward an understanding of this conversion of collagen types between the two matrices. From compositional studies, this collagen type transition is known to occur in the epiphyseal growth plate. The exact mechanism of this changeover, both with regard to the initiation of type I synthesis and resorption of type II collagen elements, is not clearly understood. It was initially thought that the cartilage-derived cellular elements continue to synthesize type II cartilage-specific collagen. The type II to type I transition then occurred by an infiltration of type I synthesizing cells from bone which were transported into this area by the invading vascular network. The synthesis of type II collagen was then thought to cease due to the death of the chondrocytes. The matrix in this transition area then contained cartilage elements which were becoming calcified and newly synthesized bony elements derived from type I collagen production. The type II to type I transition would then be completed by the synthesis and localization of a specific collagenase capable of degrading the remaining type II collagen without affecting the newly developing type I matrix. Attempts to isolate this specific type II collagenase have been markedly nonproductive. To date all mammalian collagenases capable of degrading type II collagen also degrade type I collagen. In fact, type I collagen appears to be a somewhat better substrate for all of these enzymes in vitro. However, it is not clear that the collagen type-specific differences in rate seen between these enzymes are biologically significant. The results of Von der Mark, Von der Mark and Gay in 1976 indicate that the transition in collagen type synthesis occurs somewhat earlier than was suggested by morphological studies. Using fluorescent antibodies directed towards type I collagen, the authors observed regions of fluorescence within the lacunae of the hypertrophic chondrocytes. These results indicate that the switchover of type II to type I synthesis is initiated within the chondrocytes themselves. This change in collagen type synthesis is probably initiated by unknown control mechanisms at the time the chondrocytes first begin rapid cell division. This is consistent with results obtained in vitro by Deshmukh and Kline in 1976. Chondrocytes removed from their surrounding matrix and grown in vitro in monolayer culture initially produce type II collagen, and in subsequent passages, synthesize increasing amounts of type I collagen. If cells isolated in the same way are grown in suspension culture in the absence of calcium chloride, the cells continue to synthesize their tissue-specific type II collagen. All these results imply that the synthesis of type I collagen accompanies a rapid increase in the division rate of the chondrocytes.

This beginning of the transition from a type II collagen matrix to one consisting of type I collagen is accompanied by a loss in cartilage proteoglycan. From the edge of the degenerative zone, the matrix progressively loses its alcian blue positivity. This gradient of decreasing proteoglycan concentration is probably due to both a decreased synthesis of proteoglycan by the proliferating and degenerating chondrocytes and an increase in degradative processes in response to protease infiltrating upward from the regions of vascular invasion. The direct role, if any, of the chondrocytes in the elaboration of the proteoglycan-specific proteases is not known.

In summary, our present knowledge suggests that endochondral growth is initiated by some signal received by the chondrocytes within the resting zone of cartilage near the periphery of the epiphyseal plate. In response to that signal, the chondrocytes begin rapid cell division. Soon after cell division begins, the chondrocytes switch their synthesis from predominantly type II molecules to type I molecules and decrease their production of cartilage proteoglycans. Following a limited number of mitoses, the chondrocytes degenerate, leaving behind a mixed type I, type II collagen matrix. This mixed matrix has a spongy appearance due to the now vacant cellular lacunae and proteoglycan depletion. Invading vascular elements bring osteoprogenitor cells into this region which begin synthesis of osseous-specific type I collagen. Calcification of both the residual type II matrix and the newly synthesized type I matrix occurs simultaneously. The final conversion of this mixed collagen matrix to a type I-containing collagen matrix results from remodeling processes occurring as the bone front advances. This remodeling involves the controlled synthesis or activation of specific collagenases capable of degrading both type I and type II collagens. The collagenolytic activity is concurrent with increasing type I collagen synthesis. As a result, the remnants of type II collagen initially present in the cartilage matrix are effectively diluted out.

Maturation

As the final length and proportion of the long bone is attained, a secondary ossification centre develops in the central region of the epiphyseal hyaline cartilage. The advancing bone front eventually fuses with the metaphyseal margin of this epiphyseal centre. At maturity, only a narrow region of cartilage, the articular cartilage, remains. The chondrocytes in the articular layer decrease their rate of collagen synthesis, their mitotic rates, and the extent of production of glycosaminoglycans and other matrix elements. Thus established, the articular cartilage is functionally mature and normally remains metabolically and structurally stable for the lifetime of the adult organism. Present data would indicate that this lifetime is temporally limited and genetically determined. The apparently low metabolic rate of the avascular cartilage chondrocytes is maintained by a diffusional flow of vital nutrients and oxygen across the articular surface from the synovial fluid. The secretory activity of the chondrocytes is directed toward maintenance of the proteoglycan moieties of the matrix. The collagen network, once established, is not subject to significant turnover. The failure of the articular cartilage to renew its major structural scaffold would appear to be the major limiting factor in the preservation of the articular surface. This surface is subjected to continual assault during the life of the organism. In addition to normal use, the joints are especially sensitive to infection and injury. Developmental aberrations result in architectural irregularities of the joint which may predispose the articular surface to premature erosive damage. The tissue attempts to respond to these insults, but is limited by its inability to effect substantial reversal of the damage to the type II collagen fibre system'

Age-related changes in the cartilage matrix

Ageing of cartilage, as it will be considered here, can be defined as the changes which occur in normal matrix subsequent to growth. These changes are exclusive of injury or disease, and occur progressively with chronological age. For cartilage, many of these events will be the result of the tissue's response to mechanical forces. Constant use of a joint surface would be expected to cause progressive deterioration of the cartilage matrix if a system were not provided for the renewal of the matrix structural elements. This renewal process may exactly reconstruct the cartilage so that no compositional changes will be found, or the newly replaced tissue element may be somewhat different qualitatively or quantitatively from the pre-existing components. In addition to the phenomenon of replacement, one might expect to see specific changes in the residual accumulated structural element occurring as the result of continuing maturational processes, such as collagen cross-linking. The results of these two processes, tissue renewal and continued tissue maturation, might result in age-related changes in the ability of the cartilage matrix to resist the mechanical abuse to which it is exposed.

Changes in the biomechanical properties of articular cartilage have been documented. These processes were recently reviewed by Kempson (1979) and by Schofield & Weightman (1978). Kempson measured the ability of isolated superficial layer of human articular femoral condyl to withstand stress until fracture occurred as a function of increasing age. In these studies, the required tensile fracture stress was shown to decrease linearly by about 60 per cent from 10 to 90 years of age. Similar measurements of tensile stiffness at increasing ages indicate the same linear decrease. In related studies, Weightman, Chappell and Jenkins (Weightman et al, 1978) measured the number of repeated applications of tensile stress required to fracture isolated cartilage specimens. Data obtained in this way were expressed as 'fatigue strength,' which also decreased linearly with age. Evidence from Armstrong, Bahrani & Gardner (1977) demonstrated that while young cartilage is nearly rigid, old specimens could be compressed as much as 15 per cent.

Taken together, these studies document significant alterations in the mechanical properties of the articular surface. They imply that changes in the components or organization of the structural macromolecules also occur with increasing age. Our conception of cartilage structure to which these changes must be related was first proposed by Fessler (1960), who demonstrated that hyaluronate which is entrapped in a fibrous collagen network can produce a matrix with elastic consistency similar to that of cartilage. With increasing knowledge of the complex structure of the cartilage proteoglycans (see Muir, 1979, for review), this concept has been extended. The tensile strength and fracture resistance are thought to be a function of the fibrous collagen network made firm by covalent cross-links. However, the forces applied to cartilage are not resisted by the collagen fibres directly. It is more likely that the collagen serves as a meshwork woven around molecules of proteoglycan. These entrapped structures are extensively hydrated. Cartilage then can be thought of as a hydraulic system in which the water bound to the glycosaminoglycans must be displaced from a region of compression into adjacent areas of the cartilage if compression takes place. But glycosaminoglycans bind water avidly. The internal osmotic pressure of cartilage due to this water binding has been measured at 4 kg/cm^2 (Ogston, 1970). Compression failure will occur if the glycosaminoglycans can be displaced from theirs fixed positions within the collagen network. Although the exact mechanisms for fixation of the proteoglycans to collagen fibres is not known, rupture is most likely to occur as a function of disruption of the collagenous fibre structure.

Shear forces and the distribution of tensile stress are probably more directly mediated by the collagen matrix architecture itself. We know that intermolecular cross-links contribute to the strength of the collagen fibre skeleton, but we know almost nothing about the interactions between fibres within bundles or between fibre bundles. It is possible that interactions between the assembled fibres and proteoglycans provide some of this structural definition (Muir, 1978). Electromicroscopic evidence suggests that periodic bands of glycosaminoglycans correspond to banding patterns of underlying collagen (Serafini-Faracassini, 1974). Whatever the source of these interactions, their maintenance is critical to the structural integrity of the cartilage matrix.

Age-related changes in the composition of the cartilage matrix

Numerous age-related changes in the glycosaminoglycan content of the articular cartilage matrix have been reported (for review, see Schofield & Weightman, 1978, and Freeman & Meachim, 1979). However, most of these variations appear to be due to maturational changes occurring only in the first years of life. At later times, the amount and character of the glycosaminoglycans appear to plateau and remain relatively constant. The most thoroughly documented exception to this generalization concerns the content of keratan sulphate. Keratan sulphate, unlike condroitan-4 and controitan-6 sulphate, accumulates in large quantities only in the mature matrix. The distribution of the keratan sulphate is restricted to the pericellular areas of the deepest layers of uncalcified cartilage. It has been suggested by Mason (1971) that the nonuniform distribution of keratan sulphate results more from differences in the rate of turnover of this particular glycosaminoglycan than from a zonal specialization of the mature matrix. While the glycosaminoglycan content remains relatively stable with time, the ability of each of the proteoglycan aggregates to interact with each other, or to interact with collagen, may be diminished. Perricone, Palmoski & Brandt (1977) examined the proteoglycans of aged hip cartilage and found that they were aggregated to a much lesser degree than control. The size of the extracted proteoglycans was not affected by removal of hyaluronic acid by enzymatic digestion. In contrast, the addition of hyaluronic acid obtained from normal bovine articular cartilage caused dramatic aggregation of the proteoglycans isolated from aged cartilage. These results suggest that the proteoglycan subunits present in aged cartilage are less able to form high molecular weight aggregates with hyaluronic acid from older individuals, probably due to some defect in the hyaluronic acid itself. Similar results were obtained by Adams & Muir (1976) when they compared the extracted proteoglycans from intervertebral discs of 44-year-old versus 16-year-old individuals.

Other consistently found variations with age in articular cartilage include a slow, but measurable decrease in water content and a decreased extractability of glycosaminoglycan. Since the total glycosaminoglycan present in the articular cartilage appears to be constant, this decreased extractability must be due either to increased specific interactions between the proteoglycan and the fibrous structural elements, or increased entrapment of the proteoglycan by the collagen fibre network.

The percentage of collagen content of articular cartilage decreases substantially when measured as a percentage of dry weight. When measured as the percentage of the wet weight, this decrease is masked by the concomitant loss of water from articular cartilage with age (Venn, 1978). The observed decrease in collagen content may not be an absolute decrease in the amount of collagen protein in that tissue, however, since there is a substantial increase of noncollagen materials accumulating over the same time period. Venn (1978) has suggested that these noncollagenous materials may consist of mineral deposits as well as an increase in the protein component of proteoglycan.

The major age-related change in the collagen network probably involves covalent cross-linking. It is well documented that the collagens of cartilage become substantially less extractable with time, yet the mechanism underlying this increased insolubility is not know. The formation of covalent intermolecular cross-links in collagen has been recently reviewed (Bailey et al, 1974; Tanzer, 1976). Newly accumulated cartilage collagen is stabilized by a covalent cross-link involving the epsilon amino group of lysine or hydroxylysine residues. The first step in cross-link formation is the oxidative deamination of specific lysine or hydroxylysine residues to form the aldehyde derivatives, allysine or hydroxyallysine, respectively. This oxidative deamination is catalyzed by the specific enzyme, lysyl oxidase. The formation of these active aldehydes appears to be restricted to the nonhelical segments of the collagen molecule at the carboxy-and amino-terminal ends. The major cross-link found in cartilage is hydroxylysinohydroxynorleucine. The formation of this cross-link is thought to arise from the condensation of allysine with the epsilon amino group of hydroxylysine, or hydroxyallysine with the epsilon amino group of lysine. This resulting aldimine cross-link spontaneously undergoes a molecular rearrangement to a more stable form of a cross-link. As the collagens mature, aldehydes are more likely to occur within the helical region of the molecule (Deshmukh & Nimni, 1971; Fujii et al, 1975; Scott et al, 1976). It is likely that the cross-links which stabilize mature cartilage result from these covalent helical region interactions. The exact nature of the cross-links stabilizing mature cartilage is not yet determined.

In summary, the above discussion indicates that articular cartilage matrix is relatively stable with time. Little or no change occurs in either the amount of glycosaminoglycan present, or in the amount of collagen on an absolute basis. The major observable change is a continual and progressive insolubility of the entire matrix. This insolubility appears to result from increased collagen-collagen interactions, as well as increased interactions between collagen and the glycosaminoglycans. However, it should be emphasized that these studies reflect the state of 'normal' regions of the articular cartilage surface. Changes which occur in the cartilage matrix due to fibrillation will be considered later as a pathological process. The continual increase in collagen cross-links is not necessarily beneficial to the structural integrity of the cartilage matrix. Harkness (1971) has compared the increase in cross-linking to the artificial cross-links which result from the tanning of leather. Tanned leather becomes more rigid, but has a far lower tensile strength than untanned leather. Similarly, the tensile strengths of natural and noncrystallizing rubber have been shown first to increase with increasing degree of cross-linking, and then to gradually decrease as the degree of cross-linking increases (Bueche & Berry, 1959). Either example might be a model for the observed decrease in mechanical strength of cartilage with age without a concomitant change in the composition of the matrix.

Cartilage degenerative processes

Fibrillation

Fibrillation can be defined as that degenerative process which causes spliting and fraying of the articular surface. The incidence of fibrillation increases with age. Mild fibrillation of the superficial zone of articular cartilage can often be seen in young adults, and is characteristic of the cartilage from elderly individuals. Individuals in which mild superficial zone fibrillation is seen are usually asymptomatic for degenerative joint disease. Areas of mild fibrillation are regional in distribution. This distribution varies from individual to individual, and the extent of fibrillation can vary from joint to joint within the same individual.

The progression of fibrillation is focal in nature. That is, areas of mild fibrillation can extend concentrically over the articular surface. The occurrence of new centres of fibrillation is also commonly seen. In more severe stages of this degenerative process, the splits seen in the superficial zone in the mild cases can extend into zones 2 and 3 of the uncalcified cartilage. Separations can also be seen along the junction of the calcified and the uncalcified cartilage. The end result of severe fibrillation is the erosion of the articular surface in the fibrillated area with concomitant changes both in the structural macromolecular composition of the affected area and in the biomechanical properties of the entire articular surface. In the most severe stages of this progressive condition, the erosion of the articular cartilage is so extensive that the underlying bone is exposed to the articular surface, resulting in the classical symptoms of osteoarthritis.

As mentioned above, the occurrence of fibrillation is clearly age-related. Mild fibrillation is seen in the articular surfaces of all older individuals. The extent of fibrillation in any given individual cannot be predicted by age alone. Further, young individuals showing mild fibrillation are not necessarily disposed towards degenerative joint disease later in life.

The primary cause of these degenerative changes is totally unknown. Various mechanisms, both mechanical and biochemical, have been proposed. Fibrillation must occur and progress by a rupture of the collagen fibre network underlying the articular surface. Whether the splitting of the hyaline surface results from degenerative changes in the collagen fibre structure, or conversely, whether the fibre structure is subjected to forces greater than it can withstand, is totally unknown. The lesions produced by fibrillation are histologically and morphologically variable, suggesting that fibrillation may be a heterogeneous class of processes with multiple primary mechanisms. Also, the presence of nonprogressive fibrillar lesions in certain individuals suggests that we are dealing with a variety of disease processes. To date, we do not have enough information to adequately assess this heterogeneity. The majority of our knowledge regarding this process comes from studies of osteoarthritic cartilage. Since our present knowledge is insufficient to distinguish the mild fibrillation from the severe forms found in osteoarthritis, the data regarding biochemical and mechanical changes seen in fibrillar cartilage will be discussed in the following section.

Osteoarthritis

Osteoarthritis is a painful and crippling joint disease resulting from erosion of the articular cartilage and subsequent exposure of the underlying bone to the mechanical abrasion of joint movement. In a portion of individuals affected with this condition, the pathology is believed to be secondary to another process, such as congenital architectural abnormalities, physical trauma or sepsis. Those patients who demonstrate degenerative joint disease, but for whom no predisposing factors can be found, are considered to show primary osteoarthritis. The causal agents active in these conditions are not yet known, and are the subject of intense research.

The incidence of osteoarthritis increases with age, suggesting that even primary osteoarthritis is really secondary to the ageing process itself. As a result, much attention has been given to the changes in biophysical and biochemical properties of the articular surface in midlife individuals. Progressive increases in degree of fibrillation have been documented in both normal and affected individuals. Accompanying biochemical changes have likewise been reported.

A second hypothetical explanation for the progressive loss of the articular surface is the suggestion that this tissue is simply eroded by normal 'wear and tear' resulting from joint movement. Multiple mechanical parameters of the articular cartilage have been assessed. The results of these studies suggest that cartilage does have a use threshold which, when exceeded, subjects the tissue to progressive injury.

If the articular surface were a static tissue, metabolically inactive and incapable of repair, one might be willing to accept one or the other of these hypotheses. However, current evidence suggests that articular cartilage is capable of responding to injury, and is capable of some degree of replacement of its structural components. The disease of osteoarthritis is most likely to be the result of many interacting factors involving both age-related changes in the composition of the matrix due to continual renewal of the joint surface and to continuing abrasion of the repairing surface by normal use of the joint.

Changes in the matrix of osteoarthritic articular cartilage. The above discussion proposes that osteoarthritis has a varied aetiology. Histological evidence demonstrates that this is the case. While it is well documented that severe fibrillation results in the symptoms of arthritis, the same symptoms have been exhibited by individuals whose cartilage has eroded by a nonfibrillation-related mechanism. Thinning of the articular surface in the absence of fibrillation can occur presumably as a result of abrasive wear. Often tracks can be seen in the cartilage parallel to the direction of joint movement (Freeman & Meachim, 1979). Also, separation of cartilage from underlying tissue has been seen along the calcified and uncalcified cartilage interface. In this type of osteoarthritis, the lesion appears to spread from these deep layers of uncalcified cartilage. Very often, all three forms of lesion can be seen in the same individual. Since osteoarthritis resulting from extensive fibrillation has been the best studied, and therefore the best understood of all of these types, we will restrict our discussion to this pathological process. The histological and biochemical characteristics of severely fibrillated articular cartilage have been well studied. Areas of cartilage immediately adjacent to the split matrix show extensive cellular depletion and death. This necropathy is particularly evident in the superficial articular zone. In cases in which the fibrillation has extended into deeper layers, the chondrocytes between the deep splits appear to have responded to the injury with increased cell division. These areas are characterized by multicellular round clusters. Ultrastructural examination of the matrix in the affected areas shows a thickening of the collagen fibres (Weiss, 1973). Increases in the interfibre distance have also been noted by Meachim and Roy in 1969.

Several compositional changes in the affected areas of the matrix have been consistently noted. The most striking changes in the matrix include increased water content (Bollet & Nance, 1966; Mankin & Thrasher, 1975) and a decrease in total glycosaminoglycan content as measured by fixed charge density (Maroudas et al 1968). The decrease in the glycosaminoglycan content is reported to reflect losses primarily of keratan sulphate with a relative increase in chondroitin-4 sulphate (Mankin et al, 1970; Benham et al, 1969; Larsson et al, 1975), and Hardingham & Muir (1972) have reported a decrease in hyauronic acid. Also, mildly fibrillated articular surface demonstrates marginally greater thickness of the uncalcified cartilage matrix (Freeman & Meachim, 1980).

It should be noted that the gross changes in the osteoarthritic matrix, the decreased content of glycosaminoglycan and the increased water binding are directly opposed to the changes which occur in cartilage with age, that is, a gradually decreasing content of water and increasing proteoglycan percent composition. This indicates that the pathology of fibrillation is not simply an extension of the ageing process, but rather proceeds by an entirely different mechanism.

In a recent treatise of the pathogenesis of 'primary' osteoarthritis, Freeman & Meachim (1980) have presented the hypothesis for the pathogenesis of fibrillation based on presently accumulated data. They suggest that fragmentation of the fibre network is the initial event causing fibrillation. The splitting of the articular cartilage seen in fibrillation implies the presence of multiple ruptures in the fibre network. The decrease in mechanical strength of either fibrillated articular cartilage or cartilage obtained from aged individuals also indicates some degenerative change in the underlying fibre structure. The observed increase in the thickness of mildly fibrillated cartilage and its increased water content can only take place if the fibre network has first become abnormally distensible. Increased fibre distensibility is also observed in transmission electron microscopic studies which show abnormally wide separations and fragmentation of collagen fibres in the superficial cartilage layer. These same changes have been seen in a canine experimental model by McDevitt & Muir (1976). Freeman & Meachim (1980) speculate that the cause of the disruption of the fibrous component of the matrix is due to failure of the 'linkages' between collagen fibres rather than decreased interactions of the individual collagen molecules to form fibres. While the authors acknowledge that a loss of proteoglycan may predispose the cartilage to network fragmentation, they interpret the bulk of the evidence to suggest that the reduced proteoglycan concentration is secondary to modifications of the fibre network. They cite evidence for both altered metabolism of the glycosaminoglycan and proteoglycan leakage in support of this concept. In addition, the finding that the biomechanical properties of the cartilage can change without a concomitant loss of proteoglycan implies that network fragmentation can precede losses of the glycosaminoglycan. The degenerative changes caused by fibrillation result from the increasing rate of fibre network fragmentation due to a diminishing fatigue strength in the fibre network with age and the age-related decrease in the ability of the tissue for intrinsic repair.

This hypothesis is consistent with many of the observations made in osteoarthritis. It directs the attention of those of us interested in molecular mechanisms for disease toward some explanation for the progressive structural failure of the fibre network. As hypothesized, the cause of that failure most reasonably resides in some alteration in the interaction of collagen fibres. We presently have little or no sound knowledge of the mechanics or dynamics of those interactions. Once elaborated, the fibre network in cartilage does not appear to be extensively remodeled or turned over. Based on studies of the rate of hydroxyproline synthesis in the mature human femoral head cartilage, a turnover time of approximately 400 years has been calculated (Maroudas, 1979). That is not to say that the collagen remains entirely static. One would expect that the elaboration of cross-links, either between collagen molecules, microfibrils, fibrils, or major fibres would continue throughout the ageing process. Therefore, one would expect that the fibrous matrix would become more rigid with age, though the benefit of such increased rigidity has been questioned. It does seem unlikely, though, that increased rigidity necessarily results in increased fragility. It is entirely possible that the breaking of fibre-fibre interactions is secondary to other changes. At this time, we can only speculate as to what those parameters might be.

It may be useful to think of cartilage structure as a system in which all the forces acting upon cartilage and within cartilage are balanced, such that the sum of the forces is zero. We are used to thinking about externally applied force acting upon cartilage. But the extent to which the fibre structure is affected by such external forces may be insignificant in comparison to the stress applied to the collagen structure by internal forces such as the swelling pressure resulting from the high affinity of the glycosaminoglycan for water. While the total amount of collagen is stable with chromological age, the glycosaminoglycans are constantly turning over. The turnover time for glycosaminoglycan of approximately 3 years (Maroudas, 1980) is biologically significant. Other data, summarized above, suggest that turnover involves a net replacement of the total fixed charge, a change in distribution of individual proteoglycan subunits, and changes in the state of aggregation of the proteoglycans. This relatively rapid change in the proteoglycan domain is likely to occur with concomitant changes in the exposure of the collagen moiety to swelling pressure. If this speculation is correct, one would expect some local micro-environmental change in the total force applied to any individual collagen fibre in the normal course of ageing. This imbalanced force may cause mechanical breaks in the bonds responsible for fibre-fibre interactions. One might expect to observe a decreasing ability of the fibre structure to compensate for the microenvironmental change in the force distribution if the bonding sites can be saturated, or if the progressive disaggregation of the proteoglycans somehow interferes with inter-fibre bonding. Such phenomena would then account for the fibre separations seen ultrastructurally.

Ultimately, the mechanical failure of articular cartilage can be seen as a consequence of the inability of the contained chondrocytes to respond to damage in the fibrous network. In vivo, the chondrocytes do not appear to produce significant amounts of cartilage-specific collagen. This can be either a consequence of the failure of the chondrocytes to recognize the structural damage and to supplement their type-specific collagen synthesis, or it may be a consequence of the difficulty transporting the large newly synthesized collagen molecules through the vast intercellular matrix. The physical-chemical properties of articular cartilage are such that transport of bulky molecules with a net positive charge, such as collagen, would be difficult at best. It is not unreasonable to expect the passage of newly synthesized collagen can only occur through extended cell processes. In the absence of an elaborate system of cytoplasmic extensions throughout the cartilage matrix, it is unlikely that collagen could ever reach the site of fibre injury without previous destruction of the proteoglycan domain. Conceivably, intrinsic repair of the articular surface may be more deleterious to the structural integrity of the matrix than the cumulative effect of the injury itself.

It is quite possible that the non-type II collagen present in cartilage may also play a direct role in the pathological processes occurring in osteoarthritis. To date, we have no information regarding their function, or even their microlocalization. One would like to think that these materials provide some sort of link between the major collagen fibres, or perhaps provide the fine scaffolding for the attachment of the proteoglycans. Obviously, a large number of hypotheses for their function might be proposed, but until more facts are known regarding their structural characterization and their involvement in tissue organization, such as exercise would be sheer speculation.

Collagen-related growth failure

Skeleton growth failure can result from defects in either cartilage or bone. A large number of these conditions have been defined which result in disproportionate short stature, that is, bony structures resulting from appositional bone growth appear to be relatively normal, whereas structures which elongate via endochondral ossification show markedly delayed growth. From these observations, it has been hypothesized that defects in the structure or metabolism of cartilage collagens, or the transition of cartilage to bone collagens, account for many of these growth-deficient states. These defects have been recently classified as osteochondrodysplasias (Rimoin, 1975). A number of these abnormalities are defined as bony defects, such as the osteogenesis imperfecta syndromes, and will not be dealt with here. The remaining diseases, the chondrodystrophies, are a heterogeneous group of disorders now encompassing more than 50 clinically, radiographically, or morphologically separable syndromes. Although the underlying molecular defect has not been determined for any of these syndromes, recent morphological and ultrastructural studies reveal abnormalities suggestive of collagen defects. The details of these studies have been summarized recently by Rimoin (1975). It is clearly outside the scope of this chapter to review the vast amount of work in this area; however, it is worthwhile to summarize the conclusions of several investigators who have implicated collagen to be relevant to the matrix pathology.

A lethal disorder known as achondrogenesis (Langer-Saldino type) demonstrates morphologically ballooned chondrocytes with little intervening matrix, suggesting a defect in the synthesis or secretion of one or more matrix components (Sillence et al, 1979). The metaphyseal dysplasias are associated with ball-like clusters of chondrocytes surrounded by dense fibrous tissue, suggesting a defect in type II collagen, or proteolytic destruction of the matrix (Sillence et al, 1979). In dysosteosclerosis, an autosomal recessive trait characterized by massive hyperostosis of bone in the skull and long bones, there appears a specific defect in the transformation of calcified cartilage spicules to bone with failure of resorption of calcified cartilage (Kaitila & Rimoin, 1976). The chondrocytes of a number of these chondrodystrophic matrices show extensive dilatation of the endoplasmic reticulum, suggesting specific or nonspecific storage of material synthesized for secretion. These include psuedoachondroplasia (Cooper et al, 1973; Cranley, 1975), spondyloepiphyseal dysplasia (Williams & Cranley, 1974), Kniest dysplasia (Siggers et al, 1974), spondylometaphyseal dysplasia (Stanescu et al, 1977), autosomal recessive multiple epiphyseal dysplasias (Stanescu et al, 1977) and various other rare skeletal dysplasias. Although there is no clear demonstration that the stored component is a collagen precursor, defective products of post-translational modification of procollagen might be expected to be accumulated intracellularly and result in the observed histopathology.

A number of the skeletal dysplasias demonstrate collagen fibres up to 500 nm in diameter, that is, 5 to 10 times larger than any of the usual species of collagen in cartilage. A distinct corona of large collagen fibres has been seen around the chondrocytes of cartilage from diastrophic dysplasia (Sillence et al, 1978; Sillence et al, 1979; Horton et al, 1979). Fibrous long spacing collagen crystallites (see Ch. 3) and parallel side-by-side aggregates of collagen molecules have been reported in one case of Kniest dysplasia (Sillence et al, 1979). Giant fibres have also been observed in one case of metaphyseal dysplasia (Sillence, 1979), a rare disorder characterized by hyperostosis and defective remodeling at the ends of the long bone. The finding of giant collagen fibres in the cartilage matrix are similar to those observed with ageing, or osteoarthritis, which are thought to occur due to proteoglycan depletion of the matrix. It is likely, then, that the large collagen fibre aggregates seen in the chondrodystrophies represent defects in proteoglycan synthesis or secretion, structural defects in the proteoglycan rendering it incapable of properly interacting with collagen, or structural defects in the collagen resulting in failure to immobilize cartilage proteoglycans.

THE SYNOVIUM

Anatomy and histology of the joint capsule

The joint capsule is intimately associated with the articular surface of the diarthritic joint. It provides both structural and metabolic support for the articular cartilage. Although it is not a cartilaginous structure, it is appropriate that it can be considered here because the destruction of the articular surface in rheumatoid arthritis, primary gout, and occasionally in relapsing polychondritis have their origins in the noncartilaginous structures of this joint.

The collagens of the joint capsule have been described by Eyre & Muir (1975) and Lovell et al, (1978). The epiphyses of the diarthroses are contained within a dense fibrous capsule composed primarily of type I collagen. The capsule is continuous with the metaphyseal periosteum and defines the hollow space surrounding the articular surfaces of the joint. The inner surface of the capsule is lined by a synovial membrane. The region of synovial membrane immediately adjacent to the joint cavity is composed of a cell layer 0-3 cells thick overlying a vascular network. This superficial cell layer is not a true epithelium in that it is not separated from deeper layers of the synovial membrane by a basement membrane. The cells of this lining are of two types, designated A and B cells. The A and B cells are polar with multiple processes extending into the synovial cavity. The A cells have ultrastructural features of macrophages and interchange of materials from the synovial cavity into these cells has been demonstrated. The B cells have the ultrastructural morphology of secretory cells. Their highly developed rough endoplasmic reticulum and golgi apparatus suggest that they are very metabolically active. Explants of these cells grown in vitro have been demonstrated to secrete large amounts of hyaluronic acid, one of the major components of synovial fluid. Unlike the deeper layers of the synovial membrane, the superficial layer is markedly devoid of morphologically identifiable collagen fibres. Within the deeper layers of the membrane, the density of fibrous components increases and becomes continuous with the very dense fibre network of the capsule. The primary structural elements of the synovial membrane are composed of type I collagen. Type III and basement membrane collagens have also been found in this membrane, though the largest amount of these materials may be derived from the vascular structures.

The joint space is filled with a viscous fluid having a composition expected for a transudate of serum. Only the very largest of the serum components, such as fibrinogen and alpha 2-macroglobulin, are excluded from the synovial fluid. Substantial exchange with capillary blood is expected since the deeper layers of the synovial membrane containing the capillary network are often contiguous to the synovial space due to discontinuities in the superficial layer of lining cells. This efficient nutrient transfer from the serum to the synovial fluid is critical, as the avascular articular cartilage derives its nutrients from the synovial fluid bathing it. In addition to serum-derived components, the synovial fluid contains several specific products of the B cells in the synovial lining. The most abundant of these is hyaluronic acid, an unbranched long polysaccharide chain which gives synovial fluid its characteristic viscosity and 'string sign.' Presumably, the hyaluronate found in the synovial fluid is identical to that found in the glycosaminoglycans of the hyaline cartilage, but the cartilage polysaccharide is a product of the chondrocytes and is not derived from the synovial fluid. The synovial membrane also synthesizes and secretes prostaglandins, the fatty acid hormones involved in the modulation of vascular permeability. In addition, the synovial membrane infuses the fluid with a variety of proteolytic enzymes. These include plasminogen activator, collagenase and a variety of proteases capable of degrading the proteoglycans of the articular cartilage. The synovial collagenase is secreted in an inactive form, either as a zymogen or a proenzyme. Its activity, and those of the other neutral proteases secreted into the synovial fluid, is probably limited to the remodelling and turnover of the synovial membrane in normal joints, though it may play a role in the turnover of the proteoglycans of the articular surface. The fluid also contains white blood cells, 7 per cent of which are polymorphonuclear leucocytes.

Rheumatoid arthritis

Rheumatoid arthritis is a chronic disease of diarthritic joints involving the synovial membrane, the enclosed fluid, and in severe cases, the articular cartilage. Rheumatoid arthritis is clinically separated from other forms of polyarthritis by the presence in serum of antibodies directed against the patient's own immunoglobulin G molecules known as rheumatoid factors. The earliest manifestation of the disease is an inflammation of the synovial lining. This inflammation progresses to the production of a painful and invasive pannus. Cells included in this pannus produce a large spectrum of proteolytic enzymes which are secreting into the synovial fluid and cause increased degradation of the proteoglycans in the articular cartilage. As the pannus grows, it eventually reaches the interface of the synovial membrane and the articular cartilage. Cells at the growing edge of the pannus secrete proteolytic enzymes, including collagenase, into the adjacent articular cartilage which is partially depleted of proteoglycan. Complete destruction of the articular cartilage occurs very rapidly, resulting in exposure of the subchondral bone. Joint tension provided by the capsule becomes progressively more lax due to degradative changes within the connective tissue elements of the capsule and due to disappearance of the articular cartilage.

Pathogenesis of rheumatoid arthritis

The diverse literature dealing with the pathophysiology of rheumatoid arthritis has been recently reviewed (Harris, 1974; Harris, 1979; Harris, 1979b; Barland, 1979; Cohen & Skinner, 1979; & Maini, 1977). The causative agent of the initiating inflammation is unknown. Streptococcal infection, mycoplasma and viruses have all been implicated. Whatever the infective agent, the first pathological change seen in the synovium is a proliferation of the synovial membrane cells. Included in this growing cell mass are serum-derived cell populations including lymphocytes and monocytes. Samples of synovial fluid indicate the occurrence of an acute inflammatory response. The production of synovial fluid increases with progression of the lesion. Large numbers of polymorphonuclear leucocytes invade the synovial membrane and fluid in response to chemotatic factors. The synovial fluid becomes markedly enriched in polymorphs, lymphocytes and other mononuclear cells of synovial membrane origin and their secretory products, including lymphokines, kinins, complement, proteolytic enzymes, immunoglobulins and cellular debris resulting from the rapid infiltration and death of the polymorphonuclear leucocytes. The sum of these materials, in addition to the presumed infective agents, help to sustain the chronic inflammatory character of this disease.

It has been suggested that collagen plays a direct role in the immunopathological process. Antibodies directed specifically against collagen have been found both in the serum and in the synovial fluid of rheumatoid patients (see Ch. 15). Recently, it has been found that intradermal immunization with either homologous or heterologous type II collagen induces proliferative synovitis in rats (Trentham et al, 1973; Trentham et al, 1978) and in mice (Courtney et al, 1980). The response is specific to type II collagen, as when type I or type III collagens were used as immunogens no disease resulted. It has also been shown that the disease can be induced in rats by intravenous injection of pooled spleen and lymph node cells from donors that had been injected intradermally with type II collagen (Trentham et al, 1978). The relevancy of these results to rheumatoid arthritis is not known. It is possible that the collagen-specific antibodies found in human disease might result from antibody production directed against the debris generated by the destruction of the articular cartilage. The presence of these antibodies would contribute to the chronic nature of the disease, but their identity as the causative agent has not been demonstrated.

While a direct role for collagen in the initiation of the disease state is unclear, progression of the disease results in major modifications of the connective tissues of the entire joint. These changes can be considered as two interrelated events. The first is the establishment and growth of the pannus. This is a proliferative process which results in massive collagen accumulation (Uitto et al, 1972), as well as increased cell number and diversification. The accumulated collagens in the synovium and the joint capsule are more easily solubilized by limited digestion with proteolytic enzymes (Steven, 1966; Weiss et al, 1975; Eyre & Muir, 1975; Lovell et al, 1978). Limited proteolysis under the conditions used by these authors degrades the very small peptides at the amino and carboxy-termini of the helical portion of the collagen molecule. Most of the covalent cross-links found in young tissues and in newly synthesized fibre systems occur between these short nonhelical areas. It is likely then that these results confirm the rapid accumulation of newly synthesized collagen, rather than imply some fundamental change in the cross-linking of the pre-existing collagen network. The majority of the evidence suggests that the newly synthesized collagens in the rheumatoid joint are the same as those found in the normal synovium. This cannot be interpreted as an indication that the increased collagen synthesis is directed towards replacement of pre-existing structures. It is more likely that the relatively high portion of type III collagen molecules which are synthesized in the rheumatoid joint are characteristic of the collagens accumulated by granulation tissue. It is only coincidental that the normal joint has a similar composition.

As indicated above, one major event in the progression of rheumatoid arthritis results in increased collagen synthesis and deposition. The second major event results in the proteolytic destruction of the articular cartilage. These apparently conflicting processes occur simultaneously within the joint capsule resulting in the net destruction of the anatomical features of the joint at the expense of the proliferation of the pannus. The irreversible destruction of the articular cartilage occurs centrifugally from the intersection of the synovial membrane and the articular surface. Prior to the invasion of the articular cartilage by the pannus, there is indication of biochemical changes occurring within the hyaline cartilage. The most consistent of these changes is the observation of a net decrease in the cartilage proteoglycan. This depletion is thought to result from the action of proteolytic enzymes, principally elastase and cathepsin D, accumulating in the synovial fluid as a result of the destructive processes occurring there. Proteoglycan depletion alone has been shown inadequate for irreversible destruction of the cartilage structure (Harris et al, 1972). In animal models, depletion of the proteoglycan by injection of the appropriate proteolytic enzymes into the joint fluid does not result in further degradative changes of the collagen matrix (Galway & Cruess, 1970; Curtis & Klein, 1963). Once the enzymatic activity is neutralized, functional cartilage is regenerated by replacement of the proteoglycan moiety by the synthetic activity of the chondrocyte. Biomechanical properties of the glycosaminoglycan-poor matrix are drastically affected, however. Without a full complement of hydrated polysaccharide, matrix becomes more compressible and more subject to damage due to abrasion resulting from joint usage. In the severe forms of human rheumatoid arthritis, proteoglycan degradation continues relentlessly, and the final destruction of the matrix by collagenolytic attack occurs from the margins.

The ultimate destruction of the collagen matrix of the articular cartilage is catalyzed by at least two specific enzymes. The first is a collagenase derived from polymorphonuclear leucocytes (Turto et al, 1977). The greatest destruction is probably catalyzed by another collagenase produced by the dendritic cells of the proliferating synovial pannus (Woolley et al, 1979; Woolley et al, 1978). This enzyme has been immunologically localized to the leading edge of the invading pannus (Woolley et al, 1977). Proteolytic activity of purified enzyme is restricted to collagen. While the enzyme accepts types I, II and III collagens as substrates, in vitro, type I collagen fibres have been shown to be six times more susceptible to synovial collagenase than are fibres of type II origin (Woolley et al, 1975). In addition, the susceptibility of type II collagen fibres has been reported to have a marked temperature sensitivity. Small increases in temperature significantly increased the susceptibility of type II collagen fibres to this collagenase (Harris & McCroskey, 1974). These differences demonstrated in vitro may have a physiological significance as well. Very often, the invading pannus degrades the subchondral bone at a more rapid rate than it destroys the articular cartilage. In a histological section, frequently one can see a region of cartilage overhanging an area of depleted subchondral osseous material. The increase in temperature accompanying joint inflammation is likely to be a large factor in the rapid destruction of the articular surface.

The activity of mammalian collagenases in vivo in the articular cartilage is likely to be modulated by a number of naturally occurring agents. Woolley & Evanson (1977) have suggested that the proteoglycans in articular cartilage may play a role in protecting the fibrous network from collagenase destruction. Even though it is now clear that proteoglycans do not directly inhibit the activity of isolated collagenase, in the cartilage matrix the proteoglycan aggregates may effectively prevent diffusion of the enzyme into the interfibre spaces. The depletion of the glycosaminoglycans found in rheumatoid cartilage would be expected to predispose the tissue to rapid collagenolysis. Serum substances have been isolated which have direct inhibitory activity upon mammalian collagenases. The major inhibitory component is $\alpha 2$-macroglobulin, though this protein is unlikely to be present in the region of cartilage destruction due to its very large size. A second inhibitory serum component has been identified as β_1-anticollagenase (Woolley et al, 1976). This 40 000 mol. wt. protein is specific for mammalian collagenase, and might be small enough to play a direct role in the regulation of the degenerative processes occurring in rheumatoid arthritis.

The pathology involved in the erosion of the articular surface in rheumatoid arthritis is markedly different from that seen in osteoarthritis. The degeneration of the osteoarthritic joint surface appears to be a self-destructive process, whereas the rheumatoid articular matrix is actively undergoing proteolytic destruction mediated by the invading pannus. The invasive characteristics of this pannus are reminiscent of a malignant neoplastic tissue. This is quite different from the attempts at extrinsic repair seen in osteoarthritis. The osteoarthritic repair tissue is probably of periosteal origin.

THE INTERVERTEBRAL DISC

The anatomy of the disc and its related structures

The anatomy of the intervertebral disc and its relationship to the vertebral bodies has been adequately described (DePalma & Rothman, 1975). The amphiarthroses of the spinal column are composed of three major elements which interact to allow partial mobility between the individual vertebral bodies. Just as in the case of the diarthrotic joint, the articulation of the bony vertebral bodies is mediated by cartilaginous end plates which have the appearance of typical hyaline cartilage. Unlike the true synovial joint, the articulation of the cartilaginous portions of the vertebral bodies is mediated by an intervening structure known as the intervertebral disc. The cartilaginous discs of the vertebral bodies do not move freely over the adjoining surface of the intervertebral disc, but rather they are affixed to the surface of the disc by a series of dense collagenous fibre originating within the disc itself and inserting into the cartilage end plates. As a result, the cartilaginous end plates are as much a part of the structure of the intervertebral disc as of the vertebral body itself.

The intervertebral disc contains a central gel-like region known as the nucleus pulposus which is surrounded by concentric rings of highly ordered dense collagen fibres known as the annulus fibrosus (Fig. 18.9). The nucleus

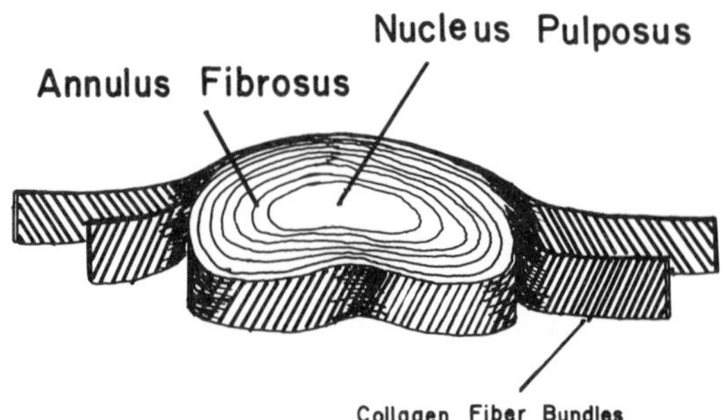

Fig. 18.9 Diagrammatic representation of the structure of the intervertebral disc.

pulposus is a highly hydrated gel of collagen fibres enveloping glycosaminoglycan molecules similar to that found in hyaline cartilage. The nucleus lacks the rigidity of hyaline cartilage and has much more the consistency of a highly viscous fluid. Presumably, the lack of rigidity results from the decreased collagen content, a less orderly fibre orientation, and diminished collagen cross-linking. The nucleus is firmly encapsulated by the surrounding fibrous structure. The fluid nature of the nucleus allows uniform distribution of the forces applied from one vertebral body to the next, irrespective of the angular relationship of the two vertebral bodies. Under maximum compression, as long as the integrity of the encapsulating annulus fibrosus is maintained, the nucleus also serves as a pivotal point for movement between adjacent vertebrae.

The annulus fibrosus is a highly complex structure. It can best be visualized as a viscous gel similar to the nucleus pulposus through which dense fibre bundles of type I collagen transit diagonally from their insertions in the end plate cartilage on either side of the intervertebral disc. The dense fibre bundles occur in concentric rings radiating from the nucleus pulposus. All the fibres of one ring are aligned in parallel creating a diagonally oriented sheath around the nucleus (Fig. 18.9). This first sheath of dense fibres is separated from the second by proteoglycan-rich connective tissue. The second concentric ring of dense fibres are also ordered diagonally through the intervertebral disc, but in the opposite direction to those of the first ring of fibres. This crisscross pattern of alternating fibre directions continues through the subsequent rings of the annulus fibrosus. This unique architecture serves to be highly resistant to lateral displacement of the nucleus pulposus under compressive pressure. In addition, it resists tortional force while allowing for lessened compressional resistance, thereby effectively relaying the compressional forces to the nucleus pulposus. Under maximal compression, the annulus opposes both the forces generated from above and below by the articulating vertebral bodies and concentric lateral forces generated by the distortion and maximal distention of the nucleus pulposus. The outermost rings of fibre bundles insert directly into the vertebral bodies themselves rather than into the cartilaginous end plates, and are known as Sharpey's fibres. The outermost anterior and posterior fibres insert into the longitudinal ligaments.

There are twice as many cells in the annulus fibrosus than are found in the nucleus pulposus. Yet, the annulus contains less than half the number of cells of the hyaline cartilage end plate which has approximately the same cellularity as other articular cartilages. The cells of the cartilage end plate are typically chondrocytic in appearance while those of the annulus and nucleus have been described either as chondrocytes or fibrocytes. It is unclear whether these represent more than a single population of cells, though the heterogeneity of the macromolecules present within the annulus or the nucleus suggests that multiple cell types may be responsible for the biosynthetic activity within these tissues.

The collagens of the intervertebral dics

The cartilaginous end plate of the intervertebral disc would be expected to have a composition very similar to hyaline cartilage. The analyses of Ludowieg, et al support this prediction (Ludowieg et al, 1973). In contrast to this hyaline cartilage, the nucleus pulposus and annulus fibrosus represent a mixed connective tissue matrix of at least two collagen types. The quantitation and identification of these collagens have been recently reviewed (Eyre, 1979).

The principal collagen type found in the nucleus pulposus is type II collagen. This collagen type represents greater than 85 per cent of the total collagen present, the remainder being type I collagen (Eyre, 1977). Analyses of the collagens of whale nucleus pulposus indicate that collagen content at the periphery of the nucleus may be higher than that in the more central regions (Hashimoto, 1968). The spatial arrangement of the type I and type II collagens in the nucleus is not presently known. The collagen fibres appear to be randomly oriented and intimately associated with proteoglycan. Extraction of the proteoglycan causes aggregation of the collagens into fibres of larger diameter (Smith & Serafini-Fracassini, 1968). Just as in the case of hyaline cartilage, the association of the proteoglycan or glycosaminoglycans with the fibrous collagen structures is not known in detail. It is currently thought that the fluid nature of the nucleus results from the association of proteoglycans with a deformable fine collagenous network. This is conceptually similar to the situation occurring in hyaline cartilage where the hydrated proteoglycan is immobilized by a nearly rigid scaffolding of the collagen network. This concept can then be extrapolated to explain the gel-like nature of the nucleus by proposing a decreased rigidity of the collagen network resulting from a reduced collagen content and a more randomized fibre orientation. The factors responsible for this apparently decreased degree of order are not known, nor is the role of type I collagen found in the nucleus understood in reference to the colloidal properties of the nucleus. The glycosaminoglycans of the nucleus are less strongly associated with the collagen network than in hyaline cartilage as demonstrated by their increased extractability (Rosenberg et al, 1967). Whether this decreased affinity results from a difference in specific collagen-proteoglycan interaction, or whether it merely reflects the decreased collagen content of the nucleus compared to hyaline cartilage is also unknown.

The structure of the annulus fibrosus is morphologically more complicated than that of the nucleus. Two distinct fibre forms can be seen ultrastructurally in the annulus. The most prominent of these are the dense parallel fibre bundles forming the concentric ringed pattern radiating from the nucleus pulposus. Surrounding these rings is an amorphous matrix which is rich in proteoglycan. The morphological suggestion of two interacting matrix types is supported by studies of the collagens of the annulus. Both type I and type II collagens are clearly present. In the human, type I collagen accounts for approximately one-half of the total collagens identified in the annulus at 5 years of age (Eyre & Muir, 1977). The amount of type II collagen increases with age and represents approximately two-thirds of the total collagens from year 16 through the lifetime of the tissue. In addition, the distribution of type I and type II collagens is not uniform from the region surrounding the nucleus to the outer extremity of the annulus. The predominant collagen of the transition zone between the nucleus and the annulus is clearly type II collagen, but the amount of type I collagen increases dramatically as one examines a radial series of samples to the outer rings of the annulus where the predominant collagen is type I. It is very tempting to correlate the morphological and biochemical findings. One would expect the dense fibre bundles to be composed of type I collagen, while the amorphous surrounding matrix would be composed primarily of type

II collagen and proteoglycan. But, as pointed out by Eyre (1979), this is probably too simplistic a view as it does not account for the very large amount of type II collagen in the annulus. The quantitative studies suggest that even the coarse fibre bundles themselves are a hybrid matrix of type I and type II collagens. Even in this morphologically distinctive matrix, the distribution of type I and type II collagens is not clearly defined. This question may be resolved in the near future by immunochemical methods applied at the ultrastructural level.

In addition to types I and II collagens, Ayad et al (1981), have recently reported the presence of 1α, 2α and a newly described collagen molecule, C-PS, in bovine annulus fibrosis and nucleus pulposis. These collagen species comprise only a small percentage of the total disc connective tissue matrix. As in hyaline cartilage, the function of these minor collagen species relative to disc physiology is unknown.

Age-related changes in the biochemistry of the intervertebral disc matrix

From age 25, the collagen content of the intervertebral disc is relatively constant. The ratio of type I to type II collagens in the human disc is also constant after maturity. In contrast. the water content of the disc substantially decreases with age. The nucleus in particular loses approximately 20 per cent of its water content from birth to the end of the 8th decade of life. The nuclear dehydration is concurrent with solidification of the nucleus due to deposition of fibrous materials. The best available evidence suggests that these changes result from a progressive loss of sulphated glycosaminoglycan and a reciprocal increase in noncollagen glycoprotein. Some of these glycoproteins may be firmly bound to collagen fibres as suggested by Anderson (1976). Just as in hyaline cartilage, the turnover rate of the proteoglycans of the intervertebral discs is biologically significant. The apparent loss of proteoglycan might be due to either a decreased cellular production of proteoglycan, production of proteoglycan incapable of aggregation or the production of proteoglycan with reduced regions of condroitin sulphate. Whatever the mechanism, the result of the decreased affinity of the nucleus for water is a progressive solidification of the nucleus. The loss of colloidal property of the nucleus impairs its ability to re-distribute forces to the surrounding annulus and predisposes the annulus to rupture or prolapse.

The nuclei pulposi of all mammals are not equally subject to solidification. The nuclei of most breeds of dog remain gelatinous throughout life. In contrast, those breeds displaying a chondrodystrophic habitus have nuclei similar to the human in that they lose their fluid behaviour at maturity. These short-limbed animals are similarly subject to premature disc degeneration. The biochemical characterization of the discs of these dogs are not yet complete enough for generalizations to be made concerning the genetic difference in their chemical makeup. Further, it is not known whether the nucleus of the disc becomes solidified due to stresses resulting from a re-distribution of force upon the disc due to the skeletal dysmorphology, or whether the underlying biochemical defect resulting in the growth deficiency of these animals directly influences all cartilaginous structures, including the disc (Ghosh et al, 1976).

Pathology of the intervertebral disc related to collagen

Degenerative changes in the disc are usually age-related, similar to the changes which occur in the articular cartilage in osteoarthritis. The early signs of degeneration probably result from excessive overloading of a disc in which the nucleus pulposus has lost its gel-like character due to dehydration and proteoglycan depletion. As a result of ageing, the disc becomes less capable of effectively buffering forces transmitted between vertebral bodies. The unequal forces thus generated can cause tearing of the surrounding annulus, or herniation of the nucleus into the annulus or into weakened regions in the hyaline end plate. The majority of the biochemical changes seen in degenerating or herniated discs probably reflects a response from the cells of the disc to repair injury rather than indicating changes predisposing the disc to further degeneration. For example, the increased collagen in the disc may result from scar formation or the infiltration of granulation tissue which would not occur prior to violent injury.

To date, no direct correlation between changes in collagen and age-related disc degeneration has been made. In most cases, disc degenerative changes are most readily related to the type and duration of occupational physical stress such as compressional overload or tortional injury. The studies of Farfan (1977) support this conclusion, though the possibility of predispositional factors cannot be excluded (Lawrence, 1977). The occurrence of Schmorl's nodes and predisposition to degeneration have been documented (Hilton et al, 1976). Schmorl's nodes are herniations of the nucleus pulposus into the cartilaginous end plate. Farfan, in 1977, proposed that these herniations are caused by compressional overload, though it's clear that herniation would be facilitated by some underlying defect in the hyaline cartilage of the end plate predisposing it to rupture. However a Schmorl's node is formed, the herniation results in a mechanically defective disc, and it is thus directly related to further degeneration (Nachemson, 1960). All of these studies support the concept that most disc degeneration results from a combination of age and excessive physical force rather than underlying defects in the collagen matrix itself.

Non-age-related biochemical changes in the intervertebral discs have been demonstrated to result from severe scoliosis. A recent study by Brickley-Parsons (1980) of thoracic and lumbar discs from adolescent idiopathic scoliotic spines indicated an abnormal distribution of type I and type II collagens in the annulus fibrosus. The scoliotic annulus concave to the curvature was found to have a significantly increased proportion of type I collagen, whereas the annulus convex to the curvature demonstrated a decreased proportion of type I collagen. Although it's not known whether these shifts in the distribution of collagen types temporally precedes the first indications of scoliosis, it is likely that the increased accumulation of type I collagen is secondary to spinal curvature. These studies also suggest that the composition of the intervertebral disc responds to changes in the relational architecture of the vertebral bodies to compensate for skeletal deformity.

While it is likely that most degenerative changes in the intervertebral disc are not directly caused by collagen abnormalities, studies of a number of conditions of inheritable defects of collagen do show pronounced effects on the vertebral column. Severe kyphoscoliosis is a prominent symptom of Ehlers-Danlos type IV syndrome. In this disorder, the hydroxylysine content of type I collagen is substantially reduced (Pinnell et al, 1972). The hydroxylation of lysine residues is required for covalent collagen cross-linking. Deficient cross-linking would be expected to result in a substantially weakened connective tissue. Similar results have been obtained from studies of animals which have been made lathyritic by treatment with beta-aminopropionitrile (Tanzer, 1965). In either of these studies, however, there is little indication that the resulting kyphoscoliosis was directly due to weakened discs. Mechanical dysfunction of tendons and muscular attachments must be at least as important a causative agent of this condition.

CONCLUDING REMARKS

The common theme running throughout this chapter is that all types of cartilage have two compositional features which make them unique among the connective tissues. The first is that the fibrous elements are derived from collagens unique to cartilage. The major cartilage collagen, type II collagen, and the minor non-type II collagens, are restricted in their tissue distribution to cartilagenous structures. The fibres formed from these collagens are relatively small in diameter, and are far more random in their orientation than fibres seen in other connective tissues primarily composed of type I collagen. Once the cartilage fibre structures are elaborated and allowed to mature, they are stable for the life-time of the organism. Their turnover times are not biologically significant. Once injured, they are not easily repaired or replaced. The static nature of these structures makes them particularly susceptible to degeneration.

The second unique compositional feature of cartilagenous structures is their high content of proteoglycans. The high affinity of these negatively charged macromolecules for water impart to the cartilage its characteristic resiliancy and impermeability. The specific interaction of the glycosaminoglycans with type II collagen are not known, though we assume that there is some primary structural difference between type II collagen fibres and type I collagen fibres, which promotes specific interactions between the glycosaminoglycans and type II collagen fibres, that do not occur with fibres derived from type I collagen. The precise nature of these type II collagen-proteoglycan interactions is a key piece of missing information in our understanding of the structure of cartilage.

The present review of the degenerative processes involving cartilage suggests a central role of the high content of glycosaminoglycan for the continued integrity of the articular surface. In every case, depletion of the glycosaminoglycan preceeds cartilage destruction. In normal growth, the matrix of the hypertrophic and degenerative zones of cartilage are depleted of glycosaminoglycans before the type II collagen is resorbed and replaced by type I containing osteoid. A strong association of type II collagen with glycosaminoglycan presents a permeability barrier to the enzymes specific for collagen degradation. Specific or non-specific destruction of the glycosaminoglycans results in the ultimate loss of the cartilage structure. We can visualize a model in which randomly oriented type II collagen fibres are surrounded by a coating of fully hydrated proteoglycans. These hydrophilic macromolecules fill the interfibre spaces. The high osmotic pressure generated by glycosaminoglycans inflate the fibre network. The maintenance of this internal pressure serves multiple functions. Its contribution to the biochemical and impermeability characteristics have already been noted. Perhaps one of the most important of these functions is to effectively separate the individual collagen fibres and prevent their aggregation. Since the amount of collagen in cartilage is relatively static, aggregation of the small diameter fibres into larger fibre aggregates decreases the collagen surface area available for proteoglycan interaction, and destroys the fine fibre network so characteristic of cartilage. Decreased collagen-glycosaminoglycan interaction would be expected to substantially change the biomechanical properties of the tissue. One would also expect that such a matrix would be more susceptible not only to increased wear by normal use, but also it would be more susceptible to enzyme catalyzed degeneration.

Presently, we are only beginning to accumulate the data necessary for our understanding of the structure of cartilage. We know that type II collagen is unique to cartilage, but we do not understand how its primary structural differences contribute to the control of cartilage collagen fibre diameters, or to its interactional specificity with glycosaminoglycans. We know that proteoglycans aggregate along a hyaluronic acid backbone through specific link proteins, yet, we do not understand what controls the degree of aggregation, or what the significance of the amount of different glycosaminoglycans within the same proteoglycan aggregate might be. Our model suggests that proteoglycans are synthesized and transported into a fine collagen network, yet it is just as likely that the glycosaminoglycans first form an aggregate, into which the collagen molecules are secreted and elaborated into a fine fibre structure. If this were the case, many of the characteristics of the fibre network which have been traditionally thought to be a consequence of the type II collagen molecules, may be modulated by the glycosaminoglycans. While collagen and glycosaminoglycans are the major structural elements found in cartilage, they are by no means the only components of the cartilage matrix. Noncollagen glycoproteins and enzymes, such as lysozyme, are also present in substantial amounts, but no specific functions have been assigned to these species. Recent studies indicate that maintenance of chondrocyte phenotype is quite fragile in vitro, but the factors responsible for that phenotype in vivo are not known.

During the next 5 years we can anticipate an increase in the definition of the components of cartilage. Recent advances in the production of specific antibodies to the various collagens of cartilage, the core proteins of the glycosaminoglycans, and the noncollagen glycoproteins will help to localize these materials within the matrix. Continuing studies of the structure of the glycosaminoglycans will aid in our understanding of these important cartilage components. One of the most promising areas of investigation of cartilage structure is the description of disease states primarily involving cartilage. In particular, the inherited diseases of cartilage are expected to provide new insights into the function of various cartilage components. Defining the defective gene products in these 'experiments of nature' should provide a great deal of new information regarding the interrelationships of cartilage macromolecules. In vitro cell culture and organ culture systems are currently being exploited in an attempt to reconstruct the initial events of cartilage neogenesis. Analyses of these systems with immunological and biochemical probes promise to substantially augment our knowledge of cartilage structure.

REFERENCES

Adams P, Eyre D, Muir H 1979 Biochemical aspects of development and aging of human lumbar intervertebral discs. Rheumatology and Rehabilitation 16: 22-9

Anderson J C 1976 Glycoproteins of the connective tissue matrix In: Hall D A, Jackson D S (eds) International review of connective tissue research 7: 251. Academic Press, New York

Armstrong C G, Bahrani A S, Gardner A L 1977 Alterations with age in compliance of human femoral head cartilage. (Letter) Lancet 1: 1103-4

Ayad S, Abedin M A, Grundy S M, Weiss J B 1981 Isolation and characterization of an unusual collagen from hyaline cartilage and intervertebral disc. FEBS Letters 1981, in press.

Bailey A J, Robins S P, Balian E 1974 Biological significance of the intermolecular cross-links of collagen. Nature (London) 251: 105-9

Bailey A J, Shellswell G D, Duance B C 1979 Identification and change of collagen types in differentiating myoblasts and developing chick muscle. Nature (London) 287: 67-9

Baluzs E A, Bloom G D, Swann D A 1966 Fine structure and glycosaminoglycan content of the surface layer of articular cartilage. Federation Proceeding 25: 1813-6

Barland P 1979 Synovial membrane. In: Cohen A S (ed) Rheumatology and Immunology. Grune and Stratton, Inc., New York. pp 37-45

Benhaman J D, Ludowieg J J, Anderson C E 1969 Glycosamine and Galactosamine distribution in human articular cartilage relationship to age and degenerative joint disease. Clinical Biochemistry 2: 461-4

Bjelle A O E, Sundstrom B K G, 1975 An ultrastructural study of the articular cartilage in calcium pyrophosphate dehydrate (CPPD) crystal deposition disease (chondrocalcinosis articularis). Calcified Tissue Research 19: 63-71

Bollet A J, Nance J L 1966 Biochemical findings in normal and osteoarthritic articular cartilage II chondroitant sulfate concentration and chain length, water and ash content. Journal of Clinical Investigation 45: 1170-7

Brickley-Parsons D 1980 A collagen defect in the intervertebral disc. Abstract, The Western Connective Tissue Society

Brown R A, Shuttleworth C A, Weiss J B 1978 Three new α-chains of collagen from a non-basement membrane source. Biophysical Biochemical Research Communication 80: 866-72

Bueche A M, Berry J P 1959 In: Auerbach J L, Felbeck D K, Hahn G T, Thomas D A The mechanism of polymer failure in fracture. Technology Press and Wiley, New York. pp 365-80

Burgeson R E, El Adli F A, Kaitila I I, Hollister D W 1976 Fetal membrane collagens: Identification of two new collagen alpha chains. Proceedings of National Acadamy of Sciences (USA) 73: 2579-83

Burgeson R E, Hollister D W 1979 Collagen heterogeneity in human cartilage: Identification of several new collagen chains. Biophysical Biochemical Research Communications 87 (4) 1124-31

Butler W T, Finch J E Jr, Miller E 1977 The covalent structure of cartilage collagen. Journal of Biological Chemistry 252: 639-43

Byers P D, Contempomi C A, Farkas T A 1970 A postmortem study of the hip joint. Annals of the Rheumatic Disease 29: 15-31

Byers P D, Maroudas A, Oztop F, Stockwell R A, Venn F 1977 Histological and biochemical studies on cartilage from osteoarthritic femoral heads with special reference to surface characteristics. Connective Tissue Research 5: 41-8

Cameron C H S, Gardner D L, Longmore R B 1976 The preparation of human articular cartilage for scanning electron microscopy. Journal of Microscopy 108: 1-12

Chung E, Rhodes R K, Miller E J 1976 Isolation of three collagenous components of probable basement membrane origin from several tissues. Biochemical and Biophysical Research Communication 71: 1167-75

Clarke I C 1971 Surface characteristics of human articular cartilage — a scanning electron microscope study. Journal of Anatomy 108: 23-38

Cohen A S, Skinner M 1979 Synovial fluid. In: Cohen A S (ed) Rheumatology and Immunology. Grune and Stratton, Inc., New York

Cohen M P, Surma M 1980 Renal glomerular basement membrane. Journal of Biological Chemistry 255: 1767-70

Cooper R R, Ponseti I V, Maynard J A 1973 Pseudoachrondoplastic dwarfism. Journal of Bone and Joint Surgery (Am.) 55: 475-84

Courtney J S, Dallman M J, Dayan A D, Martin A P, Mosedale B 1980 Immunization against heterologous type II collagen induces arthritis in mice. Nature (London) 283: 666-8

Cranley R E, Williams B R, Kopits S E, Dorst J P 1975 Pseudoachondroplastic dysplasia: Five cases representing clinical, roentgenographic, and histologic heterogeneity. Birth Defects: Original Article Series 11(6): 205-10

Curtis P H Jr, Klein L 1963 Destruction of articular cartilage in septic arthritis. Journal of Bone Joint Surgery 45A: 797-806

Dehm P, Kefalides N A 1978 The collagenous component of lens basement membrane. Journal of Biological Chemistry 253: 6680-6

DePalma A F, Rothman R H 1970 In the intervertebral disc. Saunders, Philadelphia

Deshmukh K, Kline W G 1976 Characterization of collagen and its precursors synthesized by rabbit-articular-cartilage cells in various culture systems. European Journal of Biochemistry 69: 117-23

Deshmukh K, Nimni M E 1971 Characterization of the aldehyde present on the cyanogen bromide peptides from mature rat skin collagen. Biochemistry 10: 1640-7

Eyre D R 1979 Biochemistry of the intervertebral disc. In: Hall D A, Jackson D S (eds) International Review of Connective Tissue Research volume 8: 227-91. Academic Press, New York

Eyre D R, Muir H 1975a Type III collagen: A major constituent of rheumatoid and normal human synovial membrane. Connective Tissue Research 4: 11-6

Eyre D R, Muir H 1975b The destruction of different molecular species of collagen in fiberous, elastic and hyaline cartilages of the pig. Biochemical Journal 151: 595-602

Eyre D R, Muir H 1977 Quantitative analyses of Types I and II collagens in human intervertebral discs at various ages. Biochimica Biophysica Acta 492: 29-42

Farfan H F 1977 A reorientation in the surgical approach to degenerative lumbar intervertebral joint disease. Orthopedic Clinics of North America 8: 9-21

Fessler J H 1960 A structural function of mucopolysaccharide in connective tissue. Biochemical Journal 76: 124-132

Freeman M A R 1973 Adult articular cartilage. Grune & Stratton, New York

Galway R, Cruess R L 1970 Continuing study of synovectomy upon articular cartilage. Journal of Bone and Joint Surgery 52A: 606-12

Ghosh P, Taylor P K, Braund K G, Larsen L H 1976 A comparative chemical and histochemical study of the chondrodystrophoid and nonchondrodystrophoid canine intervertebral disc. Veterinary Pathology 13: 414-27

Gregory J D 1973 Multiple aggregation factors in cartilage proteoglycans. Biochemical Journal 133: 383-6

Ham A W 1950 Histology. J B Lippincott, Philadelphia, PA

Hardingham T E, Muir H 1972 The specific interaction of hyaluronic acid with cartilage proteoglycans. Biophysica Biochemica Acta 279: 401-5

Harkness R D 1971 Mechanical properties of skin in relation to biological function and its chemical components. In: Elden H (ed) Biophysical properties of the skin. Wiley-Interscience, New York. pp 393-436

Harris E D Jr. 1974 In: Harris E D Jr (ed) Rheumatoid arthritis. Medcom Press, New York, N.Y.

Harris E D Jr 1979 Collagenases. In: Cohen A S (ed) Rheumatology and Immunology Grune and Stratton, Inc., New York, N.Y.

Harris E D Jr 1979 Rheumatoid arthritis: Epidemiology, etiology, pathogenesis and pathology. In: Cohen A S (ed) Rheumatology and Immunology. Grune and Stratton, Inc., New York.

Harris E D Jr, McCroskey P A 1974 The influence of temperature and fibril structure on degradation of cartilage collagen by rheumatoid synovial collagenase. New England Journal of Medicine 290: 1-6

Harris E D Jr, Parker H D, Rodin E L, Krane S M 1972 Effects of proteolytic enzymes on structural and mechanical properties of cartilage. Arthritis and Rheumatism 15: 497-503

Hashimoto A, Ludowieg J J 1968 The protein polysaccharides from the nucleus pulposus of whale intervertebral discs. Effects of disulfide reducing reagent. Biochemistry 7: 2469-75

Hilton R C, Ball J, Benn R T 1976 Vertebral end plate lesions (Schmorl's nodes in the dorso lumbar spine). Annals of the Rheumatic Diseases 35: 127-31

Horton W A, Rimoin D L, Hollister D W, Silberberg R 1979 Diastrophic dwarfism: A histological and ultrastructural study of the endochondral growth plate. Pediatric Research 13: 904-9

Jimenez S A, Yankowski R, Bashey R I 1978 Identification of two new collagen α-chains in extracts of lathyritic chick embryo tendon. Biochemical Biophysical Research Communication 81: 1298-306

Kaitila I, Rimoin D L 1976 Histologic heterogeneity in the hyperastotic bone dysplasias. Birth Defects: Original Article Series 12(6): 71-9

Kempson G E 1979 Mechanical properties of articular cartilage. In: Freeman Mar (ed) Adult articular cartilage Pitman Medical Publishing Co., Ltd., Kent

Larsson S D, Lemberg R K, Jones I 1975 Distribution and metabolism of glycosaminoglycans in different layers of human articular cartilage in normal adults and in initial osteoarthritis. Paper presented at 21st Annual Meeting of the Orthopedic Research Society, San Francisco, CA.

Lawrence J S 1977 Rheumatism in populations. Heinemann, London

Linsenmayer T F 1974 Temporal and special transitions in collagen types during embryonic chick limb development II. Comparison of the embryonic cartilage collagen molecule with that from adult cartilage. Developmental Biology 40: 373-7

Lovell C R, Nicholls A C, Jayson M I B, Bailey A J 1978 Changes in the collagen of synovial membrane in rheumatoid arthritis and effect of D-penicillamine. Clinical Science and Molecular Medicine 55: 31-40

Ludowieg J J, Adams J, Wang A C, Parker J, Fundenberg H H 1973 The mammalian intervertebral disc: The collagen of whole fetal nucleus pulposus. Connective Tissue Research 2: 21-9

Madri J A, Furthmayr H 1979 Isolation and tissue localization of type AB_2 collagen from normal lung parenchyma. American Journal of Pathology 94: 323-30

Maini R N 1977 Immunology of the rheumatic diseases. The Williams and Wilkins Company, Baltimore, MD.

Mankin H J, Lippiello L 1970 Biochemical and metabolic abnormalities in articular cartilage from osteo-arthritic human hips. Journal of Bone and Joint Surgery (AM) 52: 424-34

Mankin H J, Thrasher A Z 1975 Water content and binding in normal and osteo-arthritic human cartilage. Journal of Bone and Joint Surgery (AM) 57: 76-9

Maroudas A 1975 Glycosaminoglycan turnover in articular cartilage. Phil Trans R. Society, London B 271: 293-8

Maroudas A 1979 In vivo and in vitro studies of the matrix turnover in articular cartilage: A quantitative approach. In: Nuki G (ed) Models of Osteoarthritis, Pitman Medical Tunbridge Wells, in press

Maroudas A, Bullough P, Swanson A S B 1968 The permeability of articular cartilage. Journal of Bone Joint Surgery (BR) 50: 166-77

Mayne R, Vail M S, Miller E J 1978 Characterization of the collagen chains synthesized by cultured smooth muscle cells derived from rhesus monkey thoracic aorta. Biochemistry 17: 446-52

McCall J G 1969 Load-deformation studies of articular cartilage. Journal of Anatomy (London) 105: 212-9

McDevitt C A, Muir H 1976 Biochemical changes in the cartilage of the knee in experimental and natural osteoarthritis in dogs. Journal of Bone and Joint Surgery 58B: 94-101

Meachim G, Roy S 1969 Surface ultrastructure of mature adult human articular cartilage. Journal of Bone and Joint Surgery 51B: 529-32

Meachim G, Stockwell R A 1979 The matrix: In: Freeman MAR (ed) Adult articular cartilage. Pitman Medical Publishing Co., Ltd., Kent

Miller E J 1971 Isolation and characterisation of collagen from chick cartilage containing three identical chains. Biochemistry 10: 1652-9

Miller E J, Matukas V J 1969 Chick cartilage collagen: A new type of α_1 chain not present in bone or skin of the species. Proceedings of the National Academy of Science USA 65: 1264-8

Muir H 1977 Molecular approach to the understanding of osteoarthrosis. Annals of Rheumatic Disease 36: 199-208

Muir I H M 1979 Biochemistry. In: Freeman MAR (ed) Adult articular cartilage. Pittman Medical Publishing Co., Kent

Nachemson A 1960 Lumbar interdiscal pressure. Experimental studies on postmortem material. Acta Orthopaedica Scandinavica Supplement 43: 1102-10

Ogston A G 1970 Biological functions of the glycosaminoglycans. In: Balazs E A (ed) Chemistry and molecular biology of the intercellular matrix. Academic Press, New York

Parke W W 1975 Applied anatomy of the spine. In: Rothman R H, Simeone F A (ed) The spine. W B Saunders Co., Philadelphia

Pinnell S R, Krane S M, Kenzora J E, Glimcher N J 1972 A heritable disorder of collective tissue; Hydroxylysine defficient collagen disease. New England Journal of Medicine 286: 1013-20

Raj C Z, Church R L, Klobutcher L A, Ruddle F H 1977 Genetics of the connective tissue proteins: Assignment of the gene for human Type I procollagen to chromosome 17 by analysis of cell hybrids and microcell hybrids. Proceedings of the National Academy of Science, (USA) 74: 4444-8

Rhodes R R, Miller E J 1978 Physiochemical characterization and molecular organization of the collagen A and B chains. Biochemistry 17: 3442-8

Rojkind M, Giambrone M, Biempica K 1979 Collagen types in normal and cirrhotic liver. Gastroenterology 76: 710-19

Rosenberg L, Schubert M, Sandson J 1967 The protein polysaccharides of bovine nucleus pulposus. Journal of Biological Chemistry 242: 4691-701

Sage H, Bornstein P 1979 Characterization of a novel collagen chain in human placenta and its relationship to AB collagen. Biochemistry 18: 3815-22

Schofield J D, Weightman B 1978 New knowledge of connective tissue aging. Journal of Clinical Pathology 31 Suppl. (Roy. Coll. Path.) 12: 174-90

Scott P G, Veis A, Mechamic G 1976 The identity of a cyanogen bromide fragment of bovine dentin collagen containing the site of an intermolecular cross-link. Biochemistry 15: 3191-8

Siggers D C, Rimoin D L, Dorst J P, Doty S B, Williams B R, Hollister D W, Silberberg R, Cranley R E, Kaufman R L, McKusick V A 1974 The Kniest Syndrome. Birth Defects: Original Article Series 10(9): 193-08

Sillence D O 1979 Personal observation

Sillence D O, Horton W A, Rimoin D L 1979 Morphologic studies in the skeletal dysplasias. American Journal of Pathology 96: 813-70

Sillence D O, Rimoin D L, Silberberg R 1978 Ultrastructural studies of cartilage in human genetic disorders of skeletal growth. Proceedings of the 9th World Conference on Electron Microscopy 2: 668-9

Smith J W, Serafini-Fracassini A 1968 The distribution of the proteinpolysaccharide complex in the nucleus pulposus matrix in young rabbits. Cell Science 3: 33-40

Stanescu V, Stanescu R, Maroteaux P 1977 Archives Francaises de Pediatrie 34, Suppl. No. 3: 1

Stenn K S, Madri J A, Roll F J 1979 Migrating epidermis produces AB_2 collagen and requires continual collagen synthesis for movement. Nature (London) 277: 229-32

Steven F S 1966 The depolymerizing action of pepsin on collagen. Molecular weights of the component polypeptide chains. Biochimica Biophysica Acta 130: 190-5

Swann D A, Constable I J, Harper E 1972 Vitreous structure III composition of bovine vitrous collagen. Investigative Ophthalmology 11: 735-8

Sykes B, Solomon E 1978 Assignment of a type I collagen structural gene to human chromosome 7. Nature (London) 272: 548-9

Tanzer M L 1965 Experimental lathyrism. International Revue of Connective Tissue Research 3: 91-112

Tanzer M L 1975 Isolation and structure of a cross-linked tripeptide from calf bone collagen. Biochemistry 14: 4409-13

Tanzer M L 1976 In: Ramachandra G N, Reddi A H (eds) Cross-linking in biochemistry of collagen. Plenum, New York pp 137-157

Trelstad R L, Kang A H 1974 Collagen heterogeneity in the avian eye: Lens, vitreous body, cornea and sclera. Experimental Eye Research 18: 395-406

Trentham D E, Dynesius R R, David J R 1978 Passive transfer by cells of type II collagen-induced arthritis in rats. Journal of Clinical Investigation 62: 359-66

Trentham D E, Townes A S, Kang H H 1977 Autoimmunity to type II collagen: An experimental model of arthritis. Journal of Experimental Medicine 146: 857-68

Trentham D E, Townes A S, Kang A H, David J R 1978 Humoral and cellular sensitivity to collagen in type II collagen-induced arthritis in rats. Journal of Clinical Investigation 61: 89-96

Turto H, Lindy S, Uitto V, Wegelius O, Uitto J 1977 Human leukocyte collagenase: Characterization of enzyme kinetics by a new method. Annals of Biochemistry 83: 557-69

Uitto J 1977 Biosynthesis of type II collagen. Removal of amino and carboxyterminal extensions from procollagen synthesized by chick embryo cartilage cells. Biochemistry 16: 3421-9

Uitto J, Hoffmann H, Prockop D J 1977 Purification and partial characterization of type II procollagen synthesized by embryonic cartilage cells. Archives of Biochemistry, Biophysics 179: 654-62

Uitto J, Linde S, Rokkanen P, Vanio K 1970 Increased protocollagen hydroxylase activity in synovial tissue in rheumatoid arthritis. Clinica Chimica Acts 30: 741-4

Uitto J, Linde S, Turto H, Vanio K 1972 Collagen biosynthesis in rheumatoid synovial tissue. Journal of Laboratory Clinical Medicine 79: 960-71

Von der Mark H, Von der Mark K, Gay S 1976 Study of differential collagen synthesis during development of the chick embryo by immunofluorescence. Developmental Biology 48: 237-249 and 53: 153-170

Weightman B, Chappel D, Jenkins E A 1978 A secondary study of tensile fatigue properties of human articular cartilage. Annals of Rheumatic Disease 37: 58-63

Weiss C 1973 Ultrastructural characteristics of osteoarthritis. Federation Proceedings 32: 1459-66

Weiss C, Rosenberg L, Helfet A J 1968 An ultrastructural study of normal young adult human articular cartilage. Journal of Bone and Joint Surgery 50A: 663-7

Weiss J B, Shuttleworth C A, Brown R, Sedowfia K, Baildam A, Hunter J A 1975 Occurrence of type III collagen in inflamed synovial membranes: A comparison between nonrheumatoid, rheumatoid and normal synovial collagen. Biophysical Biochemical Research Communications 65: 907-12

Williams B R, Cranley R E 1974 Morphologic observations on four cases of SED congenita. Birth Defects: Original Article Series 10(9): 75-87

Woolley D E, Brinkerhoff C E, Mainardi C L, Vater C A, Evanson J M, Harris E D Jr 1979 Collagenase production by rheumatoid synovial cells: Morphological and immunohistochemical studies of the dendritic cell. Annals of Rheumatic Disease 38: 262-70

Woolley D E, Crossley N J, Evanson J M 1977 Collagenase at the site of cartilage erosion in the rheumatoid joint. Arthritis and Rheumatism 20: 1231-9

Woolley D E, Evanson J M 1977 Collagenase and its natural inhibitor in relation to the rheumatoid joint. Connective Tissue Research 5: 31-5

Woolley D E, Harris E D Jr, Mainardi C L, Brinkerhoff C E 1978 Collagenase immunolocalization in cultures of rheumatoid synovial cells. Science 200: 773-5

Woolley D E, Lindberg K A, Granville R W, Evanson J M 1975 Action of rheumatoid synovial collagenase on cartilage collagen. European Journal of Biochemistry 50: 437-44

Woolley D E, Roberts D R, Evanson J M 1976 Small molecular weight β_1 serum protein which specifically inhibits human collagenases. Nature 261: 325-7

19

Bone

S. SAKAMOTO

INTRODUCTION

Although the mineral phase provides strength and rigidity of bone, the organic matrix supports and scaffolds the structure of bone. Except for the organic matrix of dental enamel, the fibrous protein, collagen, is the major organic structural component of all the calcified tissues of the vertebrates (Miller & Martin, 1968; Herring, 1972; Glimcher, 1976). Collagen accounts for more than 90 per cent of the total organic component of bone tissue. Bone collagen largely consists of type I collagen which has the same general chemical composition, molecular structure, molecular chain composition, and macromolecular aggregation state as other type I collagens such as those of skin, tendon, and fascia (see Ch. 2). Bone collagen, however, differs markedly from the other type I collagens. It has different mechanical properties, is almost completely insoluble as the undenatured protein, has the ability to renature after thermal denaturation, and is resistant to swelling in mild acids at low ionic strength (for review, see Glimcher, 1976).

While bone collagen has the same collagen type as soft connective tissues, investigators have difficulty in isolating it in pure form to study its chemistry and biology. Insoluble and surrounded by mineral, it can only be studied in relation to bone mineral. A number of studies have been done because bone tissue collagen contributes to such unique biological occurrences as bone formation (calcification) and bone resorption (Campo & Toutellotte, 1967; Eastoe, 1968; Glimcher & Krane, 1968; Miller & Martin, 1968; Herring, 1972; Glimcher, 1976; Raisz, 1977).

The solid mineral phase has been studied for different reasons. Aside from providing scaffold, it serves as an 'ion reservoir' for the ions required for such diverse biological phenomena as neuromuscular function, membrane permeability, blood coagulation, certain enzyme reactions, and hormone action (Nichols & Wasserman, 1971). Importantly, only a very small fraction of the solid mineral phase of bone in humans (1 to 5 per cent) equilibrates with or is even available for immediate or rapid physiochemical exchange with the ions of the extracellular fluids because of the unique way in which the organic matrix and mineral phases are organized in bone (Glimcher, 1976). One can now appreciate why a number of investigators have become intrigued with the study of bone formation and bone resorption.

For detailed accounts of bone formation and bone resorption, readers may refer to a number of reviews (Vaes, 1969; Bachra, 1970; Zipkin, 1973; Glimcher, 1976; Raisz, 1976; Goldhaber et al, 1978). This chapter covers briefly the morphology of normal bone collagen, the biochemistry of collagen and its relation to bone mineral, and collagen disorders in the skeletal system viewed as defects at various stages of the molecular processing of collagen.

BONE COLLAGEN MORPHOLOGY

The details of the morphology at light and electronmicroscopic levels of bone tissue have been well presented in a number of sources (Ham, 1974; Vaughan, 1975; Cameron, 1972; Doty et al, 1976; Garant, 1978). Therefore, only points relevant to the manner in which bone collagen is organized in bone tissue will be covered here. Since bone collagen is surrounded by mineral salt, the morphology of bone collagen is limited to the sites where bone formation or resorption takes place. Mesenchymal precursor cells, called osteoprogenitor cells, differentiate into osteoblasts (Ham, 1974; Vaughan, 1975) which are morphologically characteristic secretory cells with large Golgi zones and abundant granular endoplasmic reticulum (Cameron, 1972; Doty et al, 1970). The osteoblasts synthesize collagen, glycoprotein, and proteoglycan which serve to form matrix for subsequent calcification. The matrix is laid down forming a thin layer between the osteoblasts and the calcification front. This thin layer of matrix is called osteoid, consisting by electron-microscopy of the characteristic structure of collagen bundles (Fig. 19.1). When osteoblasts are completely surrounded by the intercellular substance they secrete, and the osteoid is subsequently calcified, they are termed osteocytes. The osteocytes are not cut off from oxygen and nutrition because they are interconnected with canaliculi which

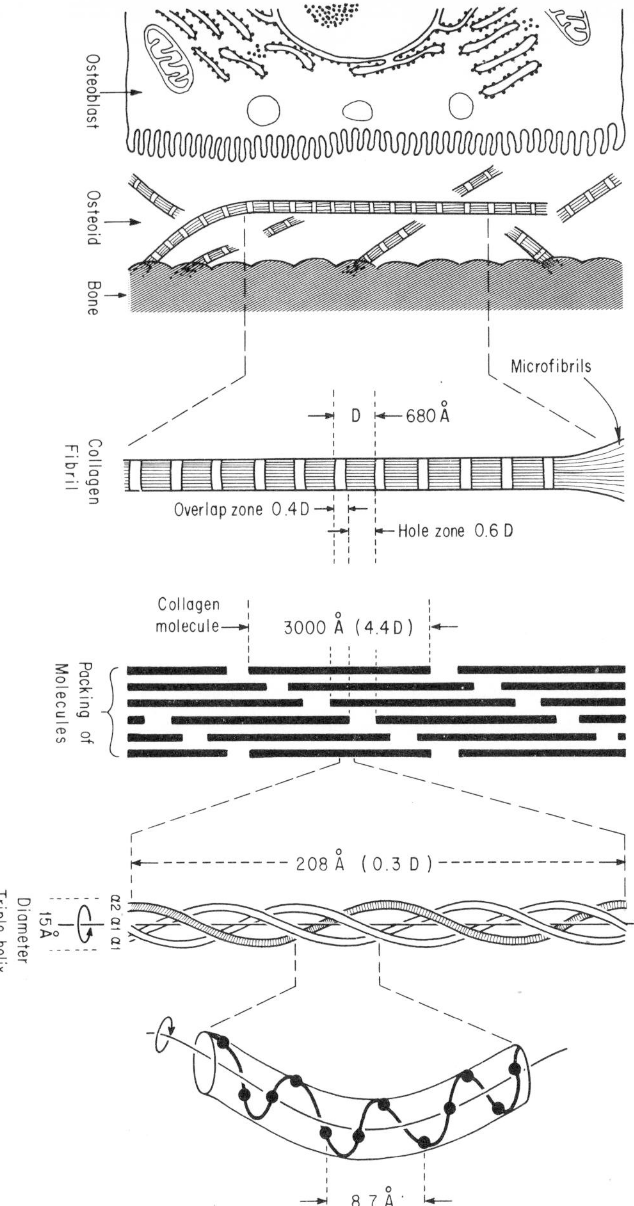

Fig. 19.1 Hierarchies of bone collagen structure from the polypeptide up to the fibril in bone tissue.

provide a means for transporting materials between surfaces and the cells buried in the calcified intercellular substance.

Although electronmicroscopic and histochemical evidence shows a decrease of cellular activity when osteocytes are finally enveloped in mature mineralized bone (Doty & Schofield, 1972), it is possible that these cells may develop a new activity and become resorbing osteocytes. The physiological importance and magnitude of osteocytic osteolysis (Belanger, 1969) has not yet been established. However, the enlargement of lacunea around osteocytes, which had been in the midst of highly mineralized bone tissue, indicates that bone tissue is highly active in the metabolism and transfer of oxygen, nutrients, salts and even proteins (Owen et al, 1977). Collagen fibrils in the osteoid, made of newly synthesized collagen by osteoblasts, can thus be observed electronmicroscopically with characteristic 680 Å striations (Fig. 19.1).

Another area to study collagen fibrils in bone tissue may be the site of bone resorption. The cell responsible for most of the resorption of bone is the osteoclast. The morphological process of bone resorption by the osteoclasts has been well documented (Gaillard, 1961; Hancox, 1972; Holtrop & King, 1977). Despite extensive studies, the function and origin of this cell are not fully understood. For light microscopic observation, bone tissue is usually demineralized. This procedure fails to demonstrate precisely the role of the osteoclasts in mineral dissolution. The osteoclasts are often found adjacent to the concave surface of bone called 'Howship's lacunae' which is believed to be the bone surface resorbed by osteoclasts (Ham, 1974). Despite extensive electronmicroscopic study of bone resorption by osteoclasts, the morphology of bone collagen degradation at the site of bone resorption is not yet established. The majority of electronmicroscopic studies, except a few reports (Hancox & Boothroyd, 1963; Cameron, 1972), fail to demonstrate collagen fibrils engulfed and degraded by the osteoclasts (Scott & Pease, 1956; Dudley & Spiro, 1961; Gonzales & Karnovsky, 1961; Bonucci, 1974). Whereas osteoclasts are often demonstrated to contain a large amount of mineral crystallite in their cytoplasm which appears to be phagocytosed and further degraded. Bone collagen, therefore, does not appear, morphologically at least, to be degraded by the osteoclasts during bone resorption.

It is conceivable that bone collagen may be degraded into small fragments which are morphologically not discernible prior to its incorporation into the osteoclasts. Heersche (1978) has postulated two separate cell systems for the removal of mineral and the degradation of organic matrix in the process of bone resorption. At present, however, neither morphological nor biochemical evidence exists to indicate that bone mineral and bone collagen are degraded independently by different kind of cells. It is generally assumed, chiefly based upon the biochemical data (Neuman & Neuman, 1953; Neuman et al, 1960; Stern et al, 1970), that the osteoclasts initiate resorption by removing mineral. However, as just described, demineralized bone collagen fibrils are rarely apparent in the spaces adjacent to the osteoclasts, in the spaces between cell processes of the ruffled border, or in the cytoplasm when undemineralized specimens are observed electronmicroscopically. Thus, it is unclear if bone mineral is removed before bone collagen or the reverse, or if both components are degraded at the same time during bone resorption. Further extensive studies are necessary.

BONE COLLAGEN BIOCHEMISTRY

General chemistry and structure of bone collagen

The details of the chemistry, structure, aggregation states, interaction properties, biosynthesis, and maturation of collagen have been well documented in a number of recent review articles (Piez & Miller, 1974; Gallop & Paz, 1975; Prockop et al, 1976; Gay & Miller, 1978; Bornstein & Traub, 1979) (see Ch. 2). Bone collagen chemistry has also been covered by several review articles (Miller & Martin, 1968; Herring, 1972; Glimcher, 1976). Therefore, this section will only cover points relevant to the characteristics of bone collagen, including information derived from the latest developments.

The study of bone collagen has encountered several problems. The main one is the presence of hard mineral which makes dissection extremely difficult and normal extraction methods almost impossible. Solubilization of bone collagen with acid brings forth a small amount of soluble collagen. Alternatively, the collagen can be obtained from bone tissue in its denatured form by extraction with hot water, and the resulting soluble gelatin can be more readily purified. Amino acid analysis of bone collagen compared with collagen or other tissues has been studied by a number of investigators. The evidence indicates that bone collagen is essentially type I collagen.

Pinnell and associates (1971) and Royce & Barnes (1977) studied the glycosylation of bone collagen. Bone collagen has less amount of diglycosylated hydroxylysine compared with skin collagen. About one-third of hydroxylysyl residues are glycosylated in both skin and bone, but the ratio of glucosylgalactosylhydroxylysine to galactosylhydroxylysine is 2.06 in skin and 0.47 in bone. Bone collagen also has less hydroxylysine than skin type I collagen; it has fewer sites for hydroxylysine glycosylation than cartilage (type II collagen).

Biosynthesis of bone collagen

During the last decade, the existence of procollagen, a biosynthetic precursor of collagen, was discovered almost simultaneously by several research groups (for review, see Bornstein & Traub, 1979). For instance, biosynthetic studies with newborn rat cranial bones indicated that this protein functioned as a precursor of the fibrous protein collagen (Bellamy & Bornstein, 1971). The procollagen is a larger molecule, differing chemically from the triple helix. These peptide extensions are considered to be involved in chain association, triple-helix formation, and extracellular polymerization. For a detailed account of the biosynthesis of procollagen, the functions of propeptides, and the removal of the propeptides by specific procollagen peptidases, readers may refer to several studies which have elucidated the various mechanisms of collagen biosynthesis. For reviews see Grant & Prockop, 1972; Schofield & Prockop, 1973; Veis, 1975; Martin et al, 1975; Prockop et al, 1976; Prockop et al, 1979; Bornstein & Traub, 1979 and Chapter 6. Among them are the formation of hydroxyproline and hydroxylysine, procollagen biosynthesis, and the removal of propeptides. Generally, they have been carried out on collagen-synthesizing tissue other than bone partly because of the difficulties of working with calcified tissues. Briefly, using the genetic information related to the functional activity of the collagen-synthesizing cell (osteoblast in the case of bone), pro-α

chain polypeptides are synthesized using the classical machinery of protein synthesis. The collagen precursor, pro-α chain has extension peptides at both amino- and carboxytermini. The sections of the collagen precursor are called the propeptides and are removed later in the processing of the molecules. The initial polypeptide produced by the ribosomes undergoes a series of covalent modifications. Most of the post-translational reactions are mediated by enzymes. Some of them occur shortly after formation of the peptide bonds. Suitably located proline residues are hydroxylated to hydroxyproline under the activity of prolylhydroxylase. Hydroxylation of lysine is mediated by lysyl-hydroxylase. Some of the hydroxylysine residues contain sugar moiety, enzymatically attached through an O-glycosidic linkage by sugar-transferase. The molecules are then transported via intracellular organelles to the cell surface and extruded into the extracellular space, where they aggregate in a highly specific way to form the collagen fibrils (Fig. 19.1). A most important post-translational change occurs extracellularly after extrusion of the molecule and after assembly of the molecules into fibrils — the formation of cross-links (maturation) (Ch. 6).

Insolubility of bone collagen: collagen cross-linking
The most distinctive feature of bone collagen is its insolubility in the usual reagents. In neutral salt solutions, less than 0.5 per cent of the total collagen is soluble and less than 1 per cent is soluble in dilute acid solution (Herring, 1972). The insolubility of bone collagen arises from its cross-linkages. Cross-links are vital for strength and for the normal functioning of collagen fibrils. Their chemistry has been reviewed by Tanzer (1976) and Bailey & Robins (1973). There is physical, structural, and chemical evidence that the number, chemical nature, distribution, and stability of the intra- and intermolecular cross-linkages in bone collagen differ from those of unmineralized soft tissues (for review, see Glimcher, 1976). For instance, rat Achilles tendon collagen is acid labile whereas there are a number of acid-stable intermolecular bonds in bone collagen.

Although various cross-links of different structure and distribution have been identified, they are mostly characterized after in vitro reduction. Whether a natural reduction of cross-link occurs is a controversial issue (Tanzer, 1976). All the genetic types of vertebrate collagen and most invertebrate collagens exhibit this cross-linking mechanism. Collagen cross-linking can be blocked in experimental animals by feeding them with β-aminopropionitrile and related compounds, which inhibit lysyloxidase and produce the condition called lathyrism (a disorder discussed later).

A new, nonreducible, fluorescent cross-linking amino acid was recently isolated by Fujimoto et al (1977) from tendon collagen without reduction. This compound was identified as a 3-hydroxypyridinium probably derived from three hydroxylysyl residues, and the name 'pyridinoline' was proposed. Eyre & Oguchi (1980) confirmed and extended this new nonreducible cross-linking amino acid showing that the same compound is especially abundant in collagen of bone and cartilage: adult articular cartilage contains about one residue per collagen molecule, with about one fifth as much in adult bone. As the dihydroxylysinonorleucine content of cartilage falls with age, the 3-hydroxypyridinium cross-link increases proportionately, suggesting a precursor-product relationship. The molar ratio of the 3-hydroxypyridinium cross-link to dihydroxylysinonorleucine reaches about 100:1 in adult cartilage. Radiochemical studies on collagen synthesized by rabbit cartilage in vivo proved that the 3-hydroxypyridinium cross-links were derived from lysine and supported their product-precursor relationship with dihydroxylysinonorleucine (Eyre, 1980).

The production of 3-dihydroxypyridinium has also been studied in experimental rickets in chicks and an increase of this cross-linking compound was demonstrated in vitamin D deficient chick bone collagen compared to vitamin D supplemented control chick bone collagen (Fujimoto et al, 1979). The bone collagen prepared from vitamin D deficient chicks, which contained an increased amount of 3-dihydroxypyridinium, has been shown to be much more resistant to pepsin and papain digestion. The vitamin D deficient chicken bone collagen has also been shown to be significantly more resistant to tissue collagenase attack as compared to control bone collagen (Sakamoto et al, unpublished results). Eyre & Oguchi (1980) proposed a mechanism for the formation of the trivalent 3-hydroxypyridinium cross-links of collagen by the interaction of two residues of hydroxylysino-5-ketonorleucine. Fujimoto (1980) has reported evidence for the natural existence of the pyridinoline cross-links in collagen in vivo. Thus, this new, nonreducible collagen cross-link within and between fibrils may account for the unique physical properties of bone and cartilage collagens (Eyre, 1980).

Bone collagen and bone formation
The role of bone collagen in the mechanism of calcification and its structural and chemical factors facilitating tissue calcification were proposed by Glimcher & Krane (1968), and Glimcher (1976). Other important research issues have been: (1) to identify the particular properties of bone collagen that permit the fibrils to become impregnanted with a solid phase of Ca-P during the calcification of bone tissue and (2) to determine why the same type I collagen in other tissues does not allow this process. Studying the extent, geometry, and distribution of the intrafibrillar space within collagen fibrils, Katz & Li (1973) found that there are significant differences between the collagen fibrils of rat tail tendon and those of bone and dentin. They point out that the average gap between collagen molecules in a bone

collagen fibril (6 Å) is twice that of a rat tail tendon collagen fibril (3 Å). This geometric property may play an important biological role by limiting and regulating the diffusion by hydrated inorganic orthophosphate ions (~4 Å) into the interstices of the collagen fibril. Organically bound phosphate, which may serve as a nucleation site, has also been found in the $\alpha2$(I) chain of collagen and it is tentatively identified as phosphoglutamic acid (Cohen-Solal et al, 1979). However, the evidence for whether bone collagen itself serves as a nucleation catalyst necessary for the initiation of normal biological mineralization is not sufficient and is still debated. In this connection, non-collagenous matrix constituents may be important. These constituents include phosphoproteins, which have long been proposed as regulators of mineral deposition (Veis et al, 1972; Butler et al, 1972), and the bone protein containing γ-carboxyglutamate which is suspected of having some regulatory role in mineral metabolism (Hauschka et al, 1975).

During the last decade, membrane-bound structures (matrix vesicles) were demonstrated intracellularly and extracellularly (Anderson, 1969; Ali et al, 1970; Anderson, 1973). The presence of increased concentrations of Ca^{2+} and Pi, and more specifically, the accumulation of solid phases of Ca-P in certain matrix vesicles has suggested their central role in tissue calcification, i.e. the site where mineral formation in the tissue begins. Thus, at present, the following issues are unresolved and require extensive studies: (1) whether collagen or noncollagenous matrix constituents serve as a nucleation catalyst, (2) whether matrix vesicles serve as performed nuclei, and (3) whether the specific interaction among them initiates tissue mineralization.

Bone collagen and metabolic regulation

There is an overwhelming amount of morphological evidence that collagen production and deposition of mineral in bone are closely coordinated activities (Ham, 1974; Vaughan, 1975). As stated earlier, in bone, the mineral is deposited within and upon recently formed collagen fibrils (osteoid). Because of the close relationship between collagen formation and mineral deposition,.there is great interest in various factors altering the rate of collagen synthesis in bone. Several studies indicate that collagen synthesis decreases in bone with age. In large part, this can be attributed to a decrease with age in the number of cells in the fully mineralized bone. Considerable interest has been evoked by the observation that parathyroid hormone, in addition to increasing the rate of resorption of bone collagen, also decreases the rate of collagen synthesis by bone (Goldhaber et al, 1968). Prostaglandin E_2 also decreases the rate of bone synthesis (Raisz & Koolemans-Beynen, 1974) and, as is well known, enhances bone resorption (Klein & Raisz 1970).

Experiments using intact bone measure the net result of the diverse cellular activities, bone formation, remodelling, and resorption. Such studies have established that certain characteristic biochemical changes occur during stimulation of bone function or resorption by various agents (Rasmussen & Bordier, 1974). In experiments in which whole bone is used, however, one cannot easily answer questions pertaining to metabolic controls which are exerted ultimately at the cellular level. Wong & Cohn (1974) recently developed an experimental system for the isolation of functionally different bone cell populations and initiated a series of studies on the premise that such an experimental system could provide more detailed insights into the biochemical basis of bone formation or resorption (Cohn & Wong, 1979). They prepared different types of bone cells by sequential digestion of mouse calvaria and yielded at least two classes of bone cell populations enriched in cells that differ from each other in morphology and surface properties and in parathormone- or calcitonin-altered metabolic activity. The cells released early in the extraction procedure (predominantly in populations 1 and 2) are denoted CT cells. They have the characteristics of osteoclasts. The cells released later in the procedure (predominantly in populations 4 and 5) and denoted PT cells. They have the characteristics of osteoblasts. Collagen prolyl hydroxylase activity of the cell types has been determined as an indication of collagen processing. Greater basal prolyl hydroxylase activity has been found in PT cells than in CT cells, and parathormone has inhibited this activity in the former populations. Calcitonin has shown no effect on this activity (Cohn & Wong, 1979). The study of bone collagen synthesis using isolated bone cells enriched in osteoblasts may obviously provide clear-cut information for bone matrix formation.

Degradation of bone collagen

It is not well established how bone collagen is degraded during bone resorption. No agreement exists as to whether bone mineral or matrix is removed first. As a detailed account of the mechanism of bone resorption is covered by many articles (Vaes, 1969; Raisz, 1976; Goldhaber et al, 1978), only a few relevant studies will be discussed here. As described in the section on morphology, some electronmicroscopic studies support the removal of bone mineral prior to matrix collagen removal and others support the opposite sequence. The two activities are normally closely coordinated and interdependent, for example, as indicated by their parallel rates of removal (Ca-mineral, hydroxyproline-collagen) in resorbing bone (Sakamoto et al, 1979). It is generally believed that bone is demineralized by acid produced by osteoclasts at the site of bone resorption (Vaes, 1969). The changes in acid production by bone explants, during bone resorption in tissue culture have been studied and a temporal relationship between the amount of citric acid released into culture medium and the extent of bone resorption has been determined (Kenny et al, 1959).

Some electronmicroscopic studies (Hancox & Boothroyd, 1963; Schenk et al, 1967) suggest that the bone surface which is in the process of being resorbed is isolated from the external environment by the surface membrane of the osteoclast on either side of its ruffled border. Vaes (1969) postulated that this isolated extracellular resorption zone is probably an essential condition for the efficiency of the resorption process; it allows the cell to create a microenvironment suitable to the lytic processes of bone mineral and bone collagen by acid and lysosomal hydrolases. However, the involvement of lysosomal hydrolases in the extracellular events of collagen degradation under physiological conditions is still debated (Gross, 1976).

Native collagen fibres are markedly resistent to attack by the normal proteolytic enzymes under physiologic temperature, pH, and ionic strength. Non-specific neutral proteinases and acid cathepsins can attack collagen only after its denaturation by an acidic milieu or by a higher temperature than its melting point. Native collagen can be extracted in dilute acid from bones of animals which have received a lathyrogen (Levene, 1973), indicating the bone collagen is not denatured by being mineralized. Thus, it is not difficult to postulate a manner in which bone collagen is degraded by specific collagenase (see Ch. 8). There is an increasing body of evidence indicating that bone collagen is degraded by specific tissue collagenase during bone resorption (Sakamoto et al, 1975, 1979; Matsumoto et al, 1979).

During the parathyroid hormone-stimulated resorption of bone in tissue culture, mineral and collagen are removed at similar rates, and hydroxyproline-containing peptides are found in the media (Goldhaber et al, 1973). In 1964, Walker and co-workers reported studies on a collagenolytic factor in rat bone promoted by parathyroid hormone extract. Fullmer & Lazarus (1967) found collagenase in the media used to culture human, goat, or rat bone. Walker and associates, as well as Fullmer & Lazarus, assayed collagenolytic activity by incubating bone fragments in vitro or collagen fibres and by measuring the release of small peptides from the collagen. The collagenolytic activity was markedly increased in bone from animals receiving parathyroid hormone (Walker et al, 1964), Shimizu and associates (1969) took the study by Fullmer & Lazarus a step further, isolated a specific collagenase from the cultures of mouse bones, and studied its mode of enzyme action. This study has been extended by Sakamoto and co-workers (1978) who have purified the enzyme and prepared an anti-mouse bone collagenase antibody.

Stern and colleagues (1963) studied in tissue culture the relationship between collagenolytic activity produced by bone explants and the extent of bone resorption. The study yielded indirect evidence that tissue collagenase is involved in the phenomenon of bone resorption in vitro. Extensive collagenolysis of radiolabelled bone matrix was observed in cultures in which rapid bone resorption was stimulated by parathyroid hormone extract whereas far less collagenolysis was detected in unstimulated control cultures. Furthermore, Kaufman et al (1965), using a similar bone culture system, demonstrated that radioactive collagen peptides were released into the culture medium from undenatured radiolabelled collagen gels attached to bone explants maintained in the presence of parathyroid hormone extract. These studies failed to establish the specific involvement of tissue collagenase in the degradation of bone matrix due to the possibility that matrix collagen was denatured and degraded by nonspecific tissue proteinases.

It has been impossible to isolate and quantify collagenase directly from culture fluids in which extensive bone resorption occurred since the serum added to the medium contains collagenase inhibitors (Gross, 1973). Using heparin-Sepharose affinity chromatography, Sakamoto et al (1975) have been able to isolate and quantify collagenase released into a serum-supplemented culture medium. Their results indicate that the amount of collagenase activity detected in culture fluids is directly correlated to the extent of bone resorption under specific conditions.

Recently, a novel pathway of degradation of newly synthesized collagen was proposed. Using bone organ culture systems, several studies (Stern et al, 1965; Golub et al, 1968; Asher et al, 1974) demonstrated that hydroxyproline in the tissue culture medium of bone, undergoing both formation and resorption, is derived from two sources. It results from the degradation of the structural bone collagen in the tissue at the time of explant, and from collagen synthesized during the period of tissue culture, but not incorporated into the tissue's structural elements (for details, see Sakamoto et al, 1979). These findings are similar to the in vivo findings of Lapière et al (1966). Studies of hydroxyproline excretion in patients with Paget's disease by Krane et al (1970) also demonstrated the presence of hydroxyproline-containing peptides. presumably derived from the breakdown of newly synthesized collagen macromolecules which were not incorporated into the tissue fabric. Independently, using tissue and cell culture systems, Bienkowski et al (1978a, 1978b) carried out a series of extensive studies. They showed that in addition to the pro-αchains, which are subjected to the multiple post-translational modifications and transported from the cell to extracellular space, 20 to 40 per cent of the pro-αchains of newly synthesized collagen is destroyed intracellularly within minutes of being synthesized and excreted from the cell as small hydroxyproline-containing peptides. Degradation of newly synthesized collagen is probably a normal process, independent of phagocytosis, by which tissues modulate the quantity or quality, or both, of collagen being secreted from the cell.

DISORDERS OF BONE COLLAGEN

The pathology of collagen at the molecular level is extensively reviewed by Lapière & Nusgens (1976) who take advantage of the rapid advancements in collagen molecular biology during the last decade. Prockop & Guzman (1977) and Prockop et al (1979) provide clinicians with an explicit account of collagen diseases and of the biosynthesis of collagen. McKusick (1972) amply discusses the clinical expression of many collagen disorders in his textbook.

Heritable disorders of the connective tissue

The 1974 Birth Defect Conference focuses upon disorders of connective tissue and compiles a number of reports of collagen disorders (Bergsma, 1975).

The discovery of apparently related connective tissue disorders has also expedited the study of the molecular biology of collagen. Osteolathyrism, for example, opened up and stimulated the rapid study of collagen cross-linking. The finding of unique disorders of connective tissue in animals and in experimental models may suggest homologus diseases in humans. Due to the multiple post-translational modification, the maturation in tissue, and the unique process of degradation, malfunction of any step required for the normal structure and function of collagen could potentially lead to defective mechanical properties. Thus, Lapière & Nusgens (1976) proposed a classification of collagen disorders based upon a relationship between a specific defect and a malfunction of one defined step responsible for synthesis, organization, maturation, or degradation of collagen. In view of the recent rapid progress in understanding the molecular biology of collagen (Bornstein & Traub, 1979), the classification of collagen disorders based upon this criterion seems most appropriate. It will facilitate understanding of the known disorders and will unveil possible relevant disorders in the future.

Since bone collagen consists entirely of type I collagen and studies of this type provide most of the information about the biosynthetic pathways involved in the production, subsequent maturation, and catabolism of the collagen molecule, the disorders of bone collagen will be reviewed here according to this classification system. The formation and fate of collagen can be divided schematically into closely related steps: (1) synthesis; (2) molecular packing and cross-linking; (3) maturation; and (4) degradation (Table 19.1). The first step is intracellular (see Ch. 7). The second step is the further modification which occurs in the extracellular space, Procollagen peptidase, a specific endopeptidase, removes the propeptides and then the remaining collagen is polymerized. The oxidation of lysyl and hydroxylysyl residues into the corresponding aldehyde is performed by oxidase(s) requiring Cu^{2+} as a cofactor. The third step is the final coherence of the fibres achieved by the function of various reducible and nonreducible covalent bonds between molecules. Tissue collagen interacts with other tissue components, such as

Table 19.1 Molecular basis of bone collagen disorders

Step	*Molecular processing*	*Biochemical event*	*Disorder* Heritable (genetic)	Acquired (environmental)
1	Synthesis	Transcription and translation	Osteogenesis imperfecta	Paget's disease of bone
		Prolyl hydroxylation	—	Scurvy
		Lysyl hydroxylation	Ehlers-Danlos VI Osteogenesis imperfecta	Rickets
		Glycosylation	—	—
2	Molecular Packing and cross-linking	Conversion of procollagen to collagen	(Dermatosparaxis) (Ehlers-Danlos VII)	—
		Lysyl oxidation	Menkes' kinky hair syndrome Aneurysm prone mice	Osteolathyrism
3	Maturation	Interaction with proteoglycans	Marfan's syndrome	—
		Interaction with glycoprotein	—	Ectopic calcification
		Regulation	—	Ageing
4	Degradation	Collagenolysis	Osteopetrosis	Invasive processes Inflammation Endocrine disturbances Heparin-osteoporosis

proteoglycans and glycoproteins through maturation. Bone collagen is featured by its subsequent mineralization and this extracellular biological event makes bone collagen different from other soft tissue collagens; i.e. it may alter the susceptibility of bone collagen especially to acquired disorders. Thus, some disorders of collagen are apparent in those of skin and other soft tissues but not in bone collagen and vice versa. The final step is the degradation of fibrous collagen in the extracellular space. The initial degradation of native collagen results from the action of collagenase (Ch. 8), and in bone collagen its degradation is accompanied by the removal of bone mineral. Again bone collagen may be resistant to some disorders because of its being calcified or in some instances may be more prone and specifically affected. Collagen disorders primarily observed in bone diseases are presented here (Table 19.1) according to a classification based upon the defect at each step of molecular processing of collagen just described.

Disorders related to synthesis

Osteogenesis imperfecta

This human heritable disorder affects most connective tissues containing type I collagen as a predominant form. The main clinical signs are bone fragility (McKusick, 1972). Several observations support the speculation about the presence of 'immature' collagen in tissue, thinner than normal fibrils. Teitelbaum et al (1974) describe the abnormal architecture of the collagen bundles and the fibres in the bones of these patients. Other observations point to the reduced thickness of cortical bone (Rily et al, 1971). The defect may be related to an abnormally persistent synthesis of type III collagen (Penttinen et al, 1975) after fetal and postnatal development although calcified connective tissues are supposed to contain little or no type III collagen even during development (Linsenmayer et al, 1973). Increased hydroxylation of lysine has been observed in osteogenesis imperfecta (Eastoe et al, 1973; Gross et al, 1975). The major defect, however, appears to be a failure to synthesize enough type I collagen (Bornstein & Traub, 1979).

Paget's disease of bone

It is possible that the metabolic disorder observed in this condition depends upon defective genetic information. The osteoclasts contain intranuclear inclusions (Rebel et al, 1974), and the condition is known to evolve sometimes into osteosarcoma. The cells participating in the process divide rapidly; they synthesize a structurally abnormal calcifying tissue and secrete collagen-derived peptides (Krane et al, 1970) (for review, Singer et al, 1978).

Scurvy

Suitably located proline residues of procollagen are hydroxylated to hydroxyproline by prolylhydroxylase. Using atmospheric oxygen and α-ketoglutarate as cosubstrates, this enzyme requires ascorbate and ferrous ions (Fe^{2+}) as cofactors. Hydroxyproline is required to stabilize at body temperature the triple helix of the crystalline part of the molecules (see Ch. 7). Hydroxylation of lysine is mediated by lysyl hydroxylase. It uses the same cosubstrates and cofactors as prolyl hydroxylase. In the absence of ascorbate, a deficient activity of hydroxylating enzyme results in the production of collagen polypeptide containing too little hydroxyproline to be stable and secreted (Barnes & Kodicek, 1972). The vascular system of bone is markedly affected (Phillips, 1971). Little is known about the defective hydroxylation of lysine in scurvy.

Ehlers-Danlos type VI

Two types (VI and VII) of Ehlers-Danlos ('rubber man') syndrome have been shown to be primary molecular defects in collagen (Prockop & Guzman, 1977). The syndrome is characterized by hyperelasticity of the skin and hypermobility of joints (McKusick, 1972). The type VI is the effect of lysyl hydroxylase. This disease is the first demonstration in human of collagen molecular pathology in a heritable disorder of the connective tissue (Pinnell et al, 1972). An extremely low level of hydroxylysine is found in skin collagen, and a reduced lysyl hydroxylation is also found in fascia and bone. This defect results from a defective enzyme, lysylhydroxylase. The patients suffer from severe scoliosis and recurrent joint dislocations. Although hydroxylation of lysine is not required for secretion and polymerization of procollagen, the lack of this hydroxylated amino acid apparently impairs subsequent cross-linking of the fibrous protein (Eyre & Glimcher, 1972). The observation of reduced activity of this enzyme in the mother of the affected children supports the heritable basis of the disease and suggests its autosomal recessive inheritance (Krane et al, 1972).

Rickets

In rickets, an acquired disorder induced by vitamin D deficiency (Mechanic et al, 1972; Toole et al, 1972; Barnes et al, 1973a; Gross et al, 1975), as well as in hypocalcemia, and in hypoparathyroidism (Barnes et al, 1973b), the hydroxylation of lysine in bone collagen is increased (Gross et al, 1975). In rickets the pattern of the cross-links is modified. The proportion of compounds derived from hydroxylysine and its aldehyde is increased (Mechanic et al, 1972). Non-reducible cross-links are increased in the bone collagen of vitamin D deficient chicks (Fujimoto et al, 1979).

Disorders related to molecular packing and cross-linking

Heritable deficiency of procollagen peptidase

Dermatosparaxis in the calf is the first heritable disorder of the connective tissue that has received a satisfactory answer at the molecular level (see Ch. 16). The defective activity of procollagen peptidase is responsible for the accumulation in the extracellular space of procollagen in the form of polymers. In the human, Ehlers-Danlos type VII (McKusick, 1974) seems to be related to the same enzyme deficiency (Lichtenstein et al, 1973). The main pathology is related to skin, tendon, and fascia, resulting in hypermobility of the joints and multiple dislocations.

Osteolathyrism

Lathyrism demonstrates the accumulation of cold extractable collagen (Levene & Gross, 1959) indicating the blockage of interchain cross-links of collagen (Martin et al, 1961) and elastin (Sykes & Partridge, 1972). The original observations on osteolathyrism were reported by Geiger et al (1933). Ponseti et al (1952, 1954) provided careful descriptions of the skeletal abnormalities, among them severe distortion of the spinal column due to osteophytosis (for review, see Gross 1973). Osteolathyrism is produced in most animal species by administration of the active principle, lathyrogen which was isolated from the sweet pea, crystallized, and identified as β amino propionitrile (βAPN; Dupuy & Lee, 1954; McKay et al, 1954; Dasler, 1954; Schilling & Strong, 1955). Pinnell & Martin (1968) and Siegel & Martin (1970) found and characterized the enzyme, lysyloxidase, responsible for converting the specific lysine residue to an aldehyde and also discovered that the lathyrogen βAPN functions by inhibiting this enzyme. The pathological changes in lathyrism occur in all tissues in which collagen or elastin is being synthesized, thus explaining the tissue specificity of the defect and its relationship to growth (Levene & Gross, 1959), development (Pratt & King, 1972), and remodelling (for reviews, see Levene, 1973; Barrow et al, 1974).

Menkes' kinky-hair syndrome

The fragility of the connective tissue including bone alteration is found in this inherited human disease. The disorder is ascribed to the genetically determined deficient copper supply due to defective intestinal absorption (Danks et al, 1972; Dekaban & Steusing, 1974; Goka et al, 1976). Lysyloxidase is inactive in the absence of cuprous ion (Pinnell & Martin, 1968). Thus, a deficient copper supply produces alterations similar to lathyrism.

Aneurysm-prone mice

These mice display inherited abnormalities that are, in many respects, similar to those found in lathyrism: aneurysms, reduced tensile strength of skin, and bone abnormalities. This pathology is related to impaired formation of the cross-links in the collagen and elastin because of a failure to generate the lysine-derived aldehyde (Rowe et al, 1974).

Disorders related to maturation

Marfan's syndrome

This is a heritable disease affecting various connective tissues including the skeletal system (excessive growth of bone) (for details, see McKusick, 1972). The increased urinary excretion of collagen breakdown products in a large proportion of the patients presenting Marfan's syndrome (Jones et al, 1964) suggests the possibility of a defective collagen framework in this disorder. However, the nature of the defect is unknown. Modifications in polysaccharides have been observed that might be either the cause or the result of the defective mechanical properties of the connective tissues (Bolande, 1963). It is conceivable that a disturbed metabolism of proteoglycan is responsible for an enhanced rate in the turnover of collagen. There is an obvious relationship between various components of the connective tissue and particularly between collagen and proteoglycans.

Ectopic calcification

Acidic glycoproteins are involved in calcification of bone (Lapière & Nusgens, 1970). Some of the peptides isolated from bone (Shuttleworth & Veis, 1972) are similar to the phosphoprotein isolated from dentin (Veis et al, 1972; Carmichael & Dodd, 1973). They might be contained in those vesicles which migrate from the cells to the calcifying front in dentin (Weinstock et al, 1972; Weinstock & Leblond, 1973). A protein of that class might act as an inducing factor, promoting ectopic osteogenesis (Urist et al, 1972). Under pathological conditions, such glycoproteins participate in calcification of soft connective tissues as in tumoral calcinosis in paraosteoarthropathy (Nusgens et al, 1972).

Ageing

All modifications of collagen framework related to ageing support a progressive reduction in the rate of turnover of its constitutive molecules. In bone, the proportion of recently synthesized noncalcified matrix also diminishes with age (Nusgens et al, 1972). The reduced metabolic activity ultimately results in modified mechanical properties of the connective tissue described by Grahame (1970) as a 'stiffening up' of the soft connective tissue.

Disorders related to degradation

Osteopetrosis

This is a systemic disorder of bone in which resorption fails to keep pace with accretion. In the mouse, it is present in three forms (variable in intensity and expression): increased bone density, lack of tooth eruption, and retardation of growth. In contrast to the failure of bone resorption in vivo in the mouse, increased collagenase activation occurs in bone in vitro (Walker, 1966). The observation of a lack of release of lysosomal enzymes under the influence of parathormone has led Marks (1974) to postulate that osteopetrosis is caused by defective activities in the release mechanism of proteases necessary for bone resorption. This thesis is supported by Walker's experiments (1973a, 1973b) showing that parabiosis and recruitment of competent osteolytic cells correct the defect in the mouse (for review, see Walker, 1978).

Invasive processes

Collagenase is needed to initiate degradation of polymeric collagen. This enzyme may occur in increased amounts in all pathological conditions in which connective tissue breakdown is required (see Ch. 8). This has been demonstrated in various invading tumours (Harris et al, 1972; Hashimoto et al, 1973a; Yamanishi et al, 1973; Matsumoto et al, 1979), cholesteatoma of the ear (Abramson, 1969), and rheumatoid nodule (Hashimoto et al, 1973b). Collagen degradation in metastatic cancers invading bone is further supported by many observations of an increased amount of urinary hydroxyproline (for review, see Kivirriko, 1970).

Inflammation

Collagen degradation in various inflammatory processes has received much attention (for review, see Gross, 1976). The large proportion of collagenase present under an inactive form suggests that some control mechanism of this enzyme in the tissue is modulated by inflammatory processes (see Ch. 8). Granulocyte collagenase and lysosomal enzyme may be involved in degrading collagen in several types of inflammation (Nigra et al, 1972). Periodontal disease featured by alveolar bone loss is associated with tissue degradation and the production of collagenase (Fullmer et al, 1972) which has been isolated from crevice fluid (Golub et al, 1974). The procollagenase is activated by products issued from the microbial plaque (Robertson et al, 1974). Its activity has also been related to a mast cell factor blocking the action of serum inhibitors (Simpson & Taylor, 1974).

Endocrine disturbances

Parathormone and calcitonin are polypeptide hormones mainly involved in the homeostasis of calcium and phosphorus. Their action in part mediated by the activity of the cells of the calcified connective tissues. Parathormone enhances the catabolism of bone in vivo (Avioli & Prockop, 1967); in bone culture it stimulates collagenase activity (Walker et al, 1964; Sakamoto et al, 1975), and the release of lysosomal enzymes (Vaes, 1969). The physiological effect of calcitonin on bone is still debated. It suppresses bone resorption induced by parathormone (Robinson et al, 1972), although its direct activity in bone cell metabolism is minimal (Marks, 1972).

Heparin-osteoporosis

Osteoporosis in humans results from the long-term use of heparin as in the treatment of thromboembolic diseases (for review, see Avioli, 1975). Goldhaber (1965) showed that the addition of small amounts of heparin to the culture media of calvarial explants enhanced the bone resorption. This effect was subsequently found to be accompanied by an increase in the collagenolytic activity released from the explants (for review, see Sakamoto & Sakamoto, 1980).

ACKNOWLEDGEMENTS

The author thanks Drs M. Sakamoto, D. R. Eyre, D. Fujimoto and P. R. Garant for their help in the preparation of the manuscript. The editorial and secretarial assistance of Pam Wolfson, Kathee Egan, Brian Ardel, Jean Thompson, Nancy White, and Kaori Sakamoto is gratefully acknowledged. Original research from the laboratory of the author was supported by NIH Grants DE 05255, K04 DE 00048, DE 02849, and AM 15671.

REFERENCES

Abramson M 1969 Collagenolytic activity in middle ear cholesteatoma. Annales of Otology, Rhinology and Laryngology 78: 112

Ali S Y, Sajdera S W, Anderson H C 1970 Isolation and characterization of calcifying matrix vesicles from epiphyseal cartilage. Proceedings of the National Academy of Sciences U S A

Anderson H C 1969 Vesicles associated with calcification in the matrix of epiphysical cartilage. Journal of Cell Biology 41: 59

Anderson H C 1973 Calcium-accumulating vesicles in the intercellular matrix of bone. In: Elliott K, Fitzsimons D W (ed) Ciba Foundation Symposium, Hard Tissue Growth, Repair and Remineralization. Elsevier, Amsterdam. p 213

Asher M A, Sledge C B, Glimcher M J 1974 The effect of inorganic orthophosphate on the rates of collagen formation and degradation in bone and cartilage in tissue culture. The Journal of Clinical Endocrinology and Metabolism 38: 376

Avioli L V, Prockop D J 1967 Collagen degradation and the response to parathyroid extract in the intact rhesus monkey. Journal of Clinical Investigations 46: 217

Avioli L V 1975 Heparin-induced osteopenia. In: Bradshaw R A, Wessler S (ed) Heparin. Advances in experimental medicine and biology 52: 375. Plenum, New York

Bachra B N 1970 Calcification of connective tissue. In: Hall D A, Jackson D S (ed) International review of connective tissue, vol 5. Academic Press, New York. p 165

Bailey A J, Robins S P 1973 Frontiers of matrix biology. Ageing of connective tissues-skin. Karger, Basel. p 130

Barnes M J, Kodicek E 1972 Biological hydroxylatons and ascorbic acid with special regard to collagen metabolism. Vitamins and Hormones 30: 1

Barnes M J, Constable B J, Morton L F, Kodicek E 1973a Bone collagen metabolism in vitamin D deficiency. Biochemical Journal 132: 113

Barnes M J, Constable B J, Morton L F, Kodicek E 1973b The influence of dietary calcium deficiency and parathyroidectomy on bone collagen structure. Biochimica et Biophysica Acta 328: 373

Barrow M V, Simpson C F, Miller E J 1974 Lathyrism: A review, Quaternal Review of Biology 49: 101

Belanger L F 1969 Osteocytic osteolysis. Calcified Tissue Research 4: 1

Bellamy G, Bornstein P 1971 Evidence for procollagen, a biosynthetic precursor of collagen. Proceedings of the National Academy of Sciences U S A 68: 1138

Bergsma D (ed) 1975 Disorders of connective tissue. Symposia Specialist Miami

Bienkowski R S, Baum B J, Crystal R G 1978a Fibroblasts degrade newly synthesized collagen within the cell before secretion. Nature 276: 413

Bienkowski R S, Cowan M J, McDonald J A, Crystal R G 1978b Degradation of newly synthesized collagen. The Journal of Biological Chemistry 253: 4356

Bolande R P 1963 The nature of the connective tissue abiotrophy in the marfan syndrome. Laboratory Investigation 12: 1087

Bonucci E 1974 The organic-inorganic relationships in bone matrix undergoing osteoclastic resorption. Calcified Tissue Research 16: 13

Bornstein P, Traub W 1979 The chemistry and biology of collagen. In: Neurath H, Hill R L (ed) The proteins, Volume IV, 3rd edn. Academic Press, New York. ch 4 p 411

Butler W T, Finch J E, DeSteno C V 1972 Chemical character of proteins in rat incisors. Biochimica et Biophysica Acta 257: 167

Cameron D A 1972 The ultrastructure of bone. In: Bourne G H (ed) The biochemistry and physiology of bone, vol 1, 2nd edn. Academic Press, New York. ch 6 p 191

Campo R D, Tourtellotte C D 1967 The composition of bovine cartilage and bone. Biochimica et Biophysica Acta 141: 614

Carmichael D J, Dodd C M 1973 An investigation of the phosphoprotein of the bovine dentin matrix. Biochimica et Biophysica Acta 317: 187

Cohen-Solal L, Cohen-Solal M, Glimcher M J 1979 Identification of γ-glutamyl phosphate in the $\alpha 2$ chains of chicken bone collagen. Proceedings of the National Academy of the Sciences U S A 76: 4327

Cohn D V, Wong G L 1979 Bone cells, cartilage cells and organ culture. In: Simmons D J, Kunin A S (ed) Skeletal research. Academic Press, New York. Part 1, p 3

Danks D M, Campbell P E, Stevens B J, Mayne V, Cartwright E 1972 Menkes' kinky hair syndrome: an inherited defect in copper absorption with widespread effects. Pediatrics 50: 188

Dasler W 1954 Isolation of toxic crystals from sweet peas (Lathyrus odoratus). Science 120: 307

Dekaban A S, Steusing J K 1974 Menkes' kinky hair disease treated with subcutaneous copper sulphate. Lancet 2: 1523

Doty S B, Schofield B H 1972 Metabolic and structural changes within osteocytes of rate bone. In: Talmage R V, Munson P L (ed) Calcium, parathyroid hormone and the calcitonins. Excerpta Medica. Amsterdam p 353

Doty S B, Robinson R A, Schofield B 1976 Morphology of bone and histochemical staining characteristics of bone cells. In: Greep R O, Astwood E B, Aurbach G D, Geiger S R (ed) Handbook of physiology, Section 7, Volume VII, American Physiological Society, Washington, D.C. ch 2, p 3

Dudley H R, Spiro D 1961 The fine structure of bone cells. The Journal of Biophysical and Biochemical Cytology 11: 627

Dupuy H P, Lee J G 1954 Isolation of material capable of producing experimental lathyrism. Journal of American Pharmacology 43: 61

Eastoe J E 1968 Chemical aspects of matrix concept in calcified tissue organization. Calcified Tissue Research 2: 1

Eastoe J E, Martens P T, Thomas N R 1973 The amino-acid composition of human hard tissue collagens in osteogenesis imperfecta and dentinogenesis imperfecta. Calcified Tissue Research 12: 91

Eyre D R, Glimcher M J 1972 Reducible cross-links in hydroxylysine deficient collagens of a heritable disorder of connective tissue. Proceedings of the National Academy of Sciences U S A 69: 2594

Eyre D R 1980 Collagen: molecular diversity in the body's protein scaffold. Science 207: 1315

Eyre D R, Oguchi H 1980 The hydroxypyridinium cross-links of skeletal collagens: their measurement, properties and a proposed pathway of formation. Biochemical and Biophysical Research Communications 92: 403

Fujimoto D, Akiba K, Nakamura N 1977 Isolation and characterization of a fluorescent material in bovine achilles tendon collagen. Biochemical and Biophysical Research Communications 76: 1124

Fujimoto D, Fujie M, Abe E, Suda T 1979 Effect of vitamin D on the content of the stable cross-link, pyridinoline, in chick bone collagen. Biochemical and Biophysical Research Communications 91: 24

Fujimoto D 1980 Evidence for natural existence of pyridinoline cross-link in collagen. Biochemical and Biophysical Research Communications 93: 948

Fullmer H M, Lazarus G 1967 Collagenase in human, goat and rat bone. Israel Journal of Medical Science 3: 761

Fullmer H M, Taylor R E, Guthrie R W 1972 Human gingival collagenase: Purification, molecular weight and inhibitor studies. Journal of Dental Research 51: 349

Gaillard P J 1961 Parathyroid and bone in tissue culture. In: Greep R O, Talmage R V (eds) The parathyroids. Thomas, Springfield p 20

Gallop P M, Paz M A 1975 Post-translational protein modifications with special attention to collagen and elastin. Physiological Reviews 55: 415

Garant P R 1978 Microanatomy of the oral mineralized tissues. In: Shaw J H, Sweeney E A, Cappuccino C C, Meller S M (ed) Textbook of oral biology. W. B. Saunders, Philadelphia. ch 5, p 181

Gay S, Miller E J 1978 Collagen in the physiology and pathology of connective tissue. Gustav Fischer Verlag, Stuttgart

Geiger B J, Steenbock J, Parsons H T 1933 Lathyrism in rats. Journal of Nutrition 6: 427

Glimcher M J 1976 Composition, structure, and organization of bone and other mineralized tissues and the mechanism of calcification. In: Greep R O, Astwood E B, Aurbach G D, Geiger S R (eds) Handbook of Physiology, Section 7, Volume VII. American Physiological Society, Washington, D.C. ch 3 p 25

Glimcher M J, Krane S M 1968 The organization and structure of bone and the mechanism of calcification. In: Ramachandran G N, Gould B S (ed) Treatise on collagen. Biology of collagen, vol 11B. Academic Press, New York. p 68

Goka T J, Stevenson R E, Hefferan P M, Howell R R 1976 Proceedings of the National Academy of the Sciences U S A 73: 604

Goldhaber P 1965 Heparin enhancement of factors stimulating bone resorption in tissue culture. Science 147: 407

Goldhaber P, Stern B D, Glimcher M J, Chao J 1968 The effect of parathyroid extract and thyrocalcitonin on bone remodelling in tissue culture. In: Talmage R V, Belanger L F (ed) Parathyroid hormone and thyrocalcitonin (calcitonin). Excerpta Medical Foundation, New York p 182

Goldhaber P, Rabadjija L, Beyer W R, Kornhauser A 1973 Bone resorption in tissue culture and its relevence to periodontal disease. Journal of American Dental Association 87: 1027

Goldhaber P, Rabadjija L, Szabo G 1978 Degradative processes of bone. In: Berlin R D, Herrmann H, Lepow I H, Tanzer L M (ed) Molecular basis of biological degradative processes. Academic Press, New York. p 313

Golub L, Glimcher M J, Goldhaber P 1968 The effect of sodium fluoride on the rates of synthesis and degradation of bone collagen in tissue culture. Proceedings of the Society for Experimental Biology and Medicine 129: 973

Golub L M, Stakiw J E, Singer D L 1974 Collagenolytic activity of human gingival crevice fluid. Journal of Dental Research 53: 1501

Gonzales F, Karnovsky M J 1961 Electron microscopy of osteoclasts in healing fractures of rat bone. Journal of Biophysical and Biochemical Cytology 9: 299

Grahame R 1970 A method for measuring human skin elasticity in vivo with observations on the effects of age, sex and pregnancy. Clinical Science 39: 223

Grant M E, Prockop D J 1972 The biosynthesis of collagen. New England Journal of Medicine 286: 194; 242; 291

Gross J 1973 Collagen biology: structure, degradation, and disease. Harvey Lect 68: 351

Gross J 1976 Aspects of the animal collagenases. In: Ramachandran G N, Reddi A H (eds) Biochemistry of collagen. Plenum, New York. ch 6 p 275

Gross J, Toole B P, Trelstad R L 1975 Bone cell biology: The emerging role of hydroxylysine. In: Slavkin H C, Greulich R C (eds) Extracellular matrix influences on gene expression. Academic Press, New York

Ham A W 1974 Histology 7th edn. Lippincott, Philadelphia

Hancox N M 1972 The osteoclast. In: Bourn G H (ed) The biochemistry and physiology of bone, vol 1, 2nd edn. Academic Press, New York. ch 3 p 45

Hancox N M, Boothroyd B 1963 Structure-function relationships in the osteoclast. In: Sognnaes R F (ed) Mechanism of hard tissue destruction. American Association for the Advancement of Sciences, Washington, D.C. ch 18 p 497

Harris E D, Faulkner C S, Wood S 1972 Collagenase in carcinoma cells. Biochemical and Biophysical Research Communications 48: 1247

Hashimoto K, Yamanishi Y, Maeyens E, Dabbous M K, Kanzaki T 1973a Collagenolytic activities of squamous cell carcinoma of the skin. Cancer Research 33: 2790

Hashimoto K, Yamanishi Y, Dabbous M K, Maeyens E 1973b Collagenase activity in rheumatoid nodules. Acta Dermatovener 53: 439

Hauschka P, Lian J, Gallop P M 1975 Direct indentification of the calcium-binding amino γcarboxyglutamate in mineralized tissue. Proceedings of the National Academy of Sciences. U S A 72: 3925

Heersche J N M 1978 The mechanism of osteoclastic bone resorption: A new hypothesis. Calcified Tissue Research 26: 81

Herring G M 1972 The biochemistry and physiology of bone, 2nd edn. Academic Press, New York. Volume 1, ch 5

Hodge A J, Petruska J A 1963a Recent studies with the electron microscope on ordered aggregates of the tropocollagen macromolecule 1963 In: Ramachandran G N (ed) Aspects of protein structure. Academic Press, New York. p 289

Holtrop M E, King G J 1977 The ultrastructure of the osteoclast and its functional implications. Clinical Orthopaedics and Related Research 123: 177

Jones C R, Bergman M W, Kittner P J, Pigman W 1964 Urinary hydroxyproline excretion in marfan's syndrome as compared with age matched controls. Proceedings of the Society for Experimental Biology and Medicine 116: 931

Katz E P, Li S T 1973 Structure and function of bone collagen fibrils. Journal of Molecular Biology 80: 1

Kaufman E J, Glimcher M J, Mechanic G L, Goldhaber P 1965 Collagenolytic activity during active bone resorption in tissue culture. Proceedings of the Society for Experimental Biology and Medicine 120: 632

Kenny A D, Draskoczy P R, Goldhaber P 1959 Citric acid production by resorbing bone in tissue culture. American Journal of Physiology 197 (2): 502

Kivirikko K I 1970 Urinary excretion of hydroxyproline in health and disease. In: Hall D A, Jackson D S (eds) International review of connective tissue, vol 5. Academic Press, New York. p 9

Klein D C, Raisz L G 1970 Prostaglandins: stimulation of bone resorption in tissue culture. Endocrinology 86: 1436

Krane S M, Munoz A J, Harris E D Jr 1970 Urinary polypeptides related to collagen synthesis. Journal of Clinical Investigation 49: 716

Krane S M, Pinnell S R, Erbe R W 1972 Lysyl-protocollagen hydroxylase deficiency in fibroblasts from siblings with hydroxylysine-deficient collagen. Proceedings of the National Academy of Sciences U S A 69: 2899

Lapière C M, Onkelinx C, Richelle L J 1966 Collagen metabolism in skin and bone. In: Comte P (ed) Biochimie et physiologie du tissu conjonctif, Societe Ormeco et Imprimerie du Sud-Est, Lyon p 505

Lapière C M, Nusgens B 1970 Maturation related changes of the protein matrix of bone. In: Balaz E A (ed) Chemistry and molecular biology of the intercellular matrix, collagen, basal laminae, elastin, Vol 1. Academic Press, New York. p 55

Lapière C M, Nusgens B 1976 Collagen pathology at the molecular level. In: Ramachandran G N, Reddi A H (ed) Biochemistry of collagen. Plenum, New York, ch 8 p 377

Levene C I, Gross J 1959 Alterations in state of molecular aggregation of collagen induced in chick embryos by β-amino-propionitrile (Lathrus factor). Journal of Experimental Medicine 110: 771

Levene C I 1973 Lathyrism. In: Perez-Tamayo R, Rojkind M (ed) Molecular pathology of connective tissues, vol 3. Marcel Dekker, New York. ch 4 p 175

Lichtenstein J R, Martin G R, Kohn L D, Byers P H, McKusick V 1973 Defect in conversion of procollagen to collagen in a form of Ehlers-Danlos syndrome. Science 182: 298

Linsenmayer T F, Toole B P, Trelstad R L 1973 Temporal and spatial transitions in collagen types during embryonic chick limb development. Developmental Biology 35: 232

Marks S C 1972 Lack of effect of thyrocalcitonin on formation of bone matrix in mice and rats. Hormone and Metabolic Research 4: 296

Marks S C 1974 A discrepancy between measurements of bone resorption in vivo and in vitro in newborn osteopetrotic rats. American Journal of Anatomy 141: 329

Martin G R, Byers P H, Piez K A 1975 Procollagen. Advances in Enzymology 42: 167

Martin G R, Gross J, Piez K A, Lewis M S 1961 On the intramolecular cross-linking of collagen in lathyritic rats. Biochimica et Biophysica Acta 53: 599

Matsumoto A, Sakamoto S, Sakamoto M 1979 Stimulation of bone collagenase synthesis by mouse fibrosarcoma in resorbing bone in-vitro culture. Archives of Oral Biology 24: 403

McKay G F, Lalich J J, Schilling E D, Strong F M 1954 A crystalleine 'Lathyrus Factor' from Lathyrus odoratus. Archives of Biochemistry and Biophysics 52: 313

McKusick V A 1972 Heritable disorders of connective tissue, 4th edn. C. V. Mosby, St. Louis

Mechanic G L, Toverud S U, Ramp W K 1972 Quantitative changes of bone collagen crosslinks and precursors in vitamin-D deficiency. Biochemical and Biophysical Research Communications 47: 760

Miller E J 1976 Biochemical characteristics and biological significance of the genetically-distinct collagens. Molecular & Cellular Biochemistry 13: 165

Miller E J, Martin G R 1968 The collagen of bone. Clinical Orthopaedics and Related Research 59: 195

Neuman W F, Neuman M W 1953 The nature of the mineral phase of bone. Chemical Reviews 53: 1

Neuman W F, Mulryan B J, Martin G R 1960 A chemical view of osteoclasts based on studies with Yttrium. Clinical Orthopaedics and Related Research 17: 124

Nigra T P, Friedland M, Martin G R 1972 Controls of connective tissue synthesis: collagen metabolism. Journal of Investigative Dermatology 59: 44

Nichols G Jr, Wasserman R H (ed) 1971 Cellular mechanisms for calcium transfer and homeostasis. Academic Press, New York

Nusgens G, Chantraine A, Lapière C M 1972 The protein in the matrix of bone. Clinical Orthopaedics and Related Research 88: 252

Owen M, Howlett C R, Triffitt J T 1977 Movement of 125–I albumin and 125–polyvinylpyrrolidone through bone tissue fluid. Calcified Tissue Research 23: 103

Penttinen R P, Lichtenstein J R, Martin G R, McKusick V A 1975 Abnormal collagen metabolism in cultured cells in osteogenesis imperfecta. Proceedings of the National Academy of Science U S A 72: 580

Phillips H J 1971 The vascularization of scorbutic bone. An experimental study in the guinea pig. Journal of Anatomy 108: 347

Piez K A, Miller A 1974 The structure of collagen fibrils. Journal of Supremolecular Structure 2: 121

Pinnell S R, Martin G R 1968 The cross linking of collagen and elastin: Enzymatic conversion of lysine in peptide linkage to α-aminoadipic-δ-semialdehyde (allysine) by an extract from bone. Proceedings of the National Academy of Sciences U S A 61: 708

Pinnell S R, Fox R, Krane S M 1971 Human collagens: Differences in glycosylated hydroxylysines in skin and bone. Biochimica et Biophysica Acta 229: 119

Pinnell S R, Krane S M, Kenzora J E, Glimcher M J 1972 A heritable disorder of connective tissue: hydroxylysine deficient collagen disease. The New England Journal of Medicine 286: 1013

Ponseti I V, Baird W A 1952 Scoliosis and dissecting aneurysm of the aorta in rats fed with Lathyrus odoratus seeds. American Journal of Pathology 28: 1059

Ponseti I V, Shepard R S 1954 Lesions of the skeleton and other mesodermal tissues in rats fed sweet-pea (Lathyrus odoratus) seeds. Journal of Bone and Joint Surgery 36A: 1031

Pratt R M, King C T G 1972 Inhibition of collagen cross-linking associated with β-aminopropionitrile-induced cleft palate in the rat. Developmental Biology 27: 332

Prockop D J, Berg R A, Kivirikko K I, Uitto J 1976 Intracellular steps in the biosynthesis of collagen. In: Ramachandran G N, Reddi A H (ed) Biochemistry of collagen. Plenum, New York. ch 5 p 163

Prockop D J, Guzman N A 1977 Collagen diseases and the biosynthesis of collagen. Hospital Practice 61

Prockop D J, Kivirikko K I, Tuderman L, Guzman N A 1979 The biosynthesis of collagen and its disorders. The New England Journal of Medicine 301: 13

Raisz L G 1976 Mechanisms of bone resorption. In: Greep R O, Astwood E B, Aurback G D, Geieger S R (ed) Handbook of physiology, Section 7, Vol VII. American Physiological Society, Washington, D.C. ch 4 p 117

Raisz L G 1977 Bone metabolism and calcium regulation. In: Avioli L V, Krane S M (eds) Metabolic bone disease, vol 1. Academic Press, New York. ch 1 p 1

Raisz L G, Koolemans-Beynen A R 1974 Inhibition of bone collagen synthesis by prostaglandin E2 in organ culture. Prostaglandins 8: 377

Rasmussen H, Bordier P 1974 The physiological and cellular basis of metabolic bone disease. Williams & Wilkins, Baltimore

Rebel A, Malkani K, Basle M 1974 Anomalies nucleaires des osteoclastes de la maladie osseuse de Paget. Nouvelle Presse Medicale 3: 1299

Robertson P B, Cobb C M, Taylor R E, Fullmer H M 1974 Activation of latent collagenase by microbial plaque. Journal of Periodontal Research 9: 81

Riley F C, Jowsey J, Brown D 1971 Connective tissue ultrastructure and bone remodelling in osteogenesis imperfecta. Journal of Bone and Joint Surgery 53A: 801

Robinson C J, Rafferty B, Parsons J A 1972 Calcium shift into bone: A calcitonin-resistant primary action of parathyroid hormone, studied in rats. Clinical Science 42: 235

Rowe D W, McGoodwin E B, Martin G R, Sussman M D, Grahn D, Farris B, Franzblau C 1974 A sex-linked defect in the cross-linking of collagen and elastin associated with the mottled locus in mice. Journal of Experimental Medicine 139: 180

Royce P M, Barnes M J 1977 Comparative studies on collagen glycosylation in chick skin and bone. Biochimica et Biophysica Acta 498: 132

Sakamoto S, Sakamoto M, Goldhaber P, Glimcher M J 1975 Collagenase and bone resorption: Isolation of collagenase from culture medium containing serum after stimulation of bone resorption by addition of parathyroid hormone extract. Biochemical and Biophysical Research Communications 63: 172

Sakamoto S, Sakamoto M, Goldhaber P, Glimcher M J 1978 Mouse bone collagenase: Purification of the enzyme by heparin-substituted sepharose 4B affinity chromatography and preparation of specific antibody to the enzyme. Archives of Biochemistry and Biophysics 188: 438

Sakamoto S, Sakamoto M, Goldhaber P, Glimcher M J 1979 Collagenase activity and morphological and chemical bone resorption induced by prostaglandin E2 in tissue culture. Proceedings of the Society for Experimental Biology and Medicine 161: 99

Sakamoto M, Sakamoto S, Brickley-Parson D, Glimcher M J 1979 Collagen synthesis and degradation in embryonic chick-bone explants. The Journal of Bone and Joint Surgery 61–A: 1042

Sakamoto S, Sakamoto M 1981 Heparin and bone metabolism. In: Brown W V, Mann K G, Robert H R, Lundblad R L (eds) The chemistry and biology of heparin. Elsevier, North Holland, Inc. New York. p 133

Scott B L, Pease D C 1956 Electron microscopy of the epiphyseal apparatus. Anatomical Record 126: 465

Schenk R K, Spiro D, Wiener J 1967 Cartilage resorption in the tibial epiphyseal plate of growing rats. The Journal of Cell Biology 34: 275

Schilling E D, Strong F M 1955 Isolation, structure and synthesis of a Lathyrus factor from L. Odoratus. Journal of the American Chemical Society 77: 2843

Schofield D, Prockop D J 1973 Procollagen: a precursor form of collagen. Clinical Orthopaedics and Related Research 97: 175

Shimizu M, Glimcher M J, Travis D, Goldhaber P 1969 Mouse bone collagenase: isolation, partial purification and mechanism of action. Proceedings of the Society for Experimental Biology and Medicine 130: 1175

Shuttleworth C A, Veis A 1972 The isolation of anionic phosphoproteins from bovine cortical bone via the periodate solubilization of bone collagen. Biochimica et Biophysica Acta 257: 414

Siegal R C, Martin G R 1970 Collagen cross-linking. Enzymatic synthesis of lysine-derived aldehydes and the production of cross-linked components. Journal of Biological Chemistry 245: 1653

Simpson J W, Taylor A C 1974 Regulation of gingival collagenase: A possible role for a mast cell factor. Proceedings for the Society of Experimental Biology and Medicine 145: 42

Singer F R, Mills B G, Terry R 1978 Bone Resorbing Cells in Paget's Disease. In: Horton J E, Tarpley T M, Davis W F (eds) Mechanisms of localized bone loss. Information Retrieval, Washington D.C. p 365

Stern B D, Mechanic G L, Glimcher M J, Goldhaber P 1963 The resorption of bone collagen in tissue culture. Biochemical and Biophysical Research Communications 13: 137

Stern B D, Glimcher M J, Mechanic G L, Goldhaber P 1965 Studies of collagen degradation during bone resorption in tissue culture. Proceedings of the Society for Experimental Biology and Medicine 119: 577

Stern B, Golub L, Goldhaber P 1970 Effects of demineralization and parathyroid hormone on the availability of bone collagen to degradation by collagenase. Journal of Periodontal Research 5: 116

Sykes B C, Partridge S M 1972 Isolation of a soluble elastin from lathyritic chicks. Biochemical Journal 130: 1171

Tanzer M L 1976 Cross-linking. In: Ramachandran G N, Reddi A H (eds) Biochemistry of collagen. Plenum, New York. ch 4, p 137

Teitelbaum S L, Kraft W J, Lang R, Avioli L V 1974 Bone collagen aggregation abnormalities in osteogenesis imperfecta. Calcified Tissue Research 17: 75

Toole B P, Kang A H, Trelstad R L, Gross J 1972 Collagen heterogeneity within different growth regions of long bones of rachitic and non-rachitic chicks. Biochemical Journal 127: 715

Urist M R, Iwata H, Strates B S 1972 Bone morphogenetic protein and proteinase in the guinea pig. Clinical Orthopaedics and Related Research 85: 275

Vaes G 1969 Lysosomes and the cellular physiology of bone resorption. In: Dingle J T, Fell H B (eds) Lysosomes in biology and pathology Volume 1. North-Holland Publishing Company, Amsterdam. ch 8, p 217

Vaughan J 1975 The physiology of bone, 2nd edn, Oxford Univ. Press, London

Veis A 1975 The biochemistry of collagen. Annals of Clinical and Laboratory Science 5: 123

Veis A, Spector A R, Zamoscianyk H 1972 The isolation of an EDTA-soluble phosphoprotein from mineralizing bovine dentin. Biochimica et Biophysica Acta 257: 404

Walker D G 1966 Elevated bone collagenolytic activity and hyperplasia of parafollicular light cells of the thyroid gland in parathormone-treated grey-lethal mice. Zeitschrift für Zellforschung and Mikroskopische Anatomie 72: 100

Walker D G 1973a Osteopetrosis cured by temporary parabiosis. Science 180: 875

Walker D G 1973b Experimental osteopetrosis. Clinical Orthopaedics and Related Research 97: 158

Walker D G 1978 Abbrogation of congenital osteopetrosis by leukocyte subpopulations. In: Horton J E, Tarpley T M, Davis W F (eds) Mechanisms of Localized Bone Loss. Information Retrieval. Washington D.C. p 383

Walker D G, Lapière C M, Gross J 1964 A collagenolytic factor in rat bone promoted by parathyroid extract. Biochemical and Biophysical Research Communications 15: 397

Weinstock A, Weinstock M, Leblond C P 1972 Autoradiographic detection of H^3-fucose incorporation in glycoprotein by odontoblasts and its deposition at the site of the calcification front in dentin. Calcified Tissue Research 8: 181

Weinstock M, Leblond C P 1973 Radioautographic visualization of the deposition of a phosphoprotein at the mineralization front in the dentin of the rat incisor. Journal of Cell Biology 56: 838

Wong G, Cohn D V 1974 Separation of parathyroid hormone and calcitonin-sensitive cells from non-responsive bone cells. Nature 252: 713

Yamanishi Y, Maeyens E, Dabbous M K, Ohyama H, Hashimoto K 1973 Collagenolytic activity in malignant melanoma: physiochemical studies. Cancer Research 33: 2507

Zipkin I (ed) 1973 Biological mineralization. Wiley A — Interscience Publication, New York

20

The blood vessel

R. K. RHODES

INTRODUCTION

The mammalian vascular system provides the network for the distribution of nutrients to and removal of metabolic wastes from all parts of the organism. To a large extent the success of this system can be attributed to the adaptation which has been achieved through the specialized extracellular matrix synthesized by the various cell types found along its course. These provide the tensile strength to withstand the pressures of the arterial system, the elasticity to accommodate the pulsatile flow of blood, and the physiological capacity to allow and possibly regulate the diffusion of substances from blood to tissue and vice versa.

Collagen accounts for a large proportion of these intercellular substances and in recent years has gained increasing attention among investigators with the discovery that the various collagen morphotypes display a very discrete distribution pattern within the vasculature (Table 20.1). Indeed, every collagen described to date with the exception of type I-trimer and type II is present at some point in the mammalian vessels. Though the role of all the various collagens has not been defined, their restricted microanatomical occurrence suggests that each has certain features which confer on a given type and only that type the physiological characteristics necessary to maintain normal function.

Table 20.1 Occurrence of collagen types in vascular tissue

Collagen type	*Anatomical location* [a]	*Fibre structure*
Type I	Adventitia, media, subendothelium	Large, well-defined fibres from 400–1800 Å in diameter
Type III	Media, subendothelium, adventitia	Small fibres from 50–400 Å in diameter or reticular meshwork
Type IV	Basement membrane	Unknown
Type V	Media, subendothelium, adventitia	Unknown
55K dalton polypeptides	Unknown	Unknown

[a] The anatomical locations are listed in decreasing order of relative abundance for the given coloagen type.

VASCULAR MORPHOLOGY

The cardiovascular system is generally subdivided into several parts for ease of discussion. These in order of occurrence proceeding from the heart are elastic arteries, muscular arteries, arterioles, capillaries, venules, and small, medium, and large veins. (For a discussion of heart collagen see Ch. 25.) However, the components are not precisely demarcated but rather gradually appear as the vascular system undergoes its continuous transition. Thus, there are shared characteristics throughout which exhibit similar morphological, biochemical, and in most instances functional characteristics.

Capillaries

The capillaries, which constitute the smallest and simplest of the blood vessels are generally divided into three categories: continuous, fenestrated, and sinusoid (Fig. 20.1). The first two can be considered true capillaries in that their luminal wall is composed of a single layer of elongated endothelial cells which rest on a continuous basement membrane. However, in the fenestrated capillary the endothelial lining is penetrated by numerous pores, or fenestrations. Sinusoids, on the other hand, are lined with cells of the reticuloendothelial system which contain numerous gaps and in the case of the liver none or only minute amounts of loosely associated basement membrane material (see Ch. 23).

Associated with the periphery of capillaries at various points are cells known as pericytes which are believed to help regulate blood flow and have origins relating them to smooth muscle cells. These cells may be partially surrounded by a basement-membrane-like structure. Within the perivascular space is a reticular meshwork of collagen fibres which serves to connect the capillaries with the surrounding tissue.

Arteries and arterioles

Morphologically all of the arterial elements are similar in that they all possess an intimal, a medial, and an adventitial layer. Differences in the size and composition of these three layers determine the classification of the artery. In addition

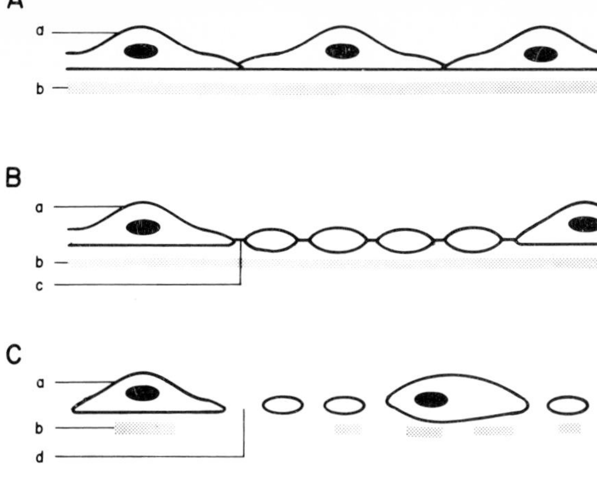

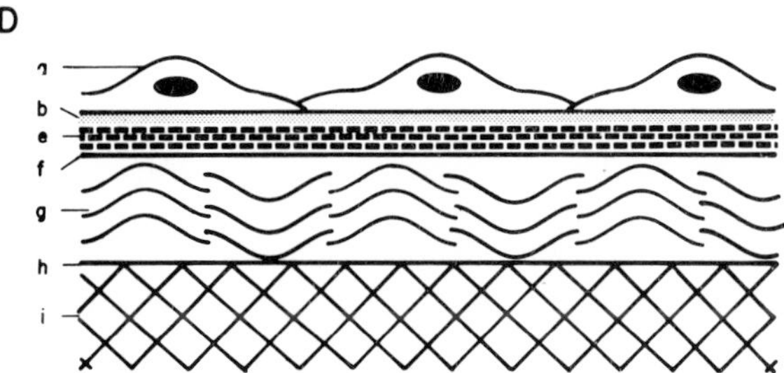

Fig. 20.1 Schematic representation of the structure of vessel walls. A, Normal capillary. B, Fenestrated capillary. C, Sinusoidal capillary. D, Medium to large artery. Key: a, endothelial cells; b, basement membrane; c, fenestration; d, gap between cells lining sinusoid; e, subendothelium; f, internal elastic lamina; g, media; h, external elastic lamina; i, adventitia.

to these layers there are two other components which may be present, the internal elastic lamina between the intima and media, and the external elastic lamina between the media and adventitia (Fig. 20.1).

Arterioles and small arteries

Arterioles and small arteries have a characteristic endothelium and basal lamina supported by a sparse subendothelial reticular network. In the larger arterioles and small arteries a continuous internal elastic lamina is present with a very discrete media ranging from a single to several layers of smooth muscle cells in thickness with interspersed collagen and elastin fibres. The adventitia, which has the same approximate thickness as the media, is composed of a loose connective tissue layer containing collagen and elastin fibres oriented parallel to the longitudinal axis of the vessel. No clearly distinguishable external elastic lamina is present.

Muscular arteries

Muscular arteries have an endothelium which is closely applied to a well-defined internal elastic lamina. Numerous processes extend from the endothelial cells through fenestrations in the elastica to make contact with the first layer of smooth muscle cells of the media. The media constitutes the largest portion of the muscular arteries and is populated almost exclusively by smooth muscle cells. Distributed throughout the media are several distinct extracellular entities, a reticular network of collagen fibres as well as some dense collagen fibre bundles, concentric layers of loosely arrayed elastic fibres, and an amorphous basement-membrane-like matrix surrounding each smooth muscle cell. The media is encircled by an easily distinguishable external elastic lamina which in turn is surrounded by a less organized adventitia containing a mixture of collagenous fibre bundles, fibroblasts and elastic fibres.

Elastic arteries

The large elastic arteries have a much thickened intima compared to the other vessels. The wall of the lumen is covered by polygonal-shaped endothelial cells resting on a discontinuous basement membrane. Subjacent to these is a somewhat extensive subendothelial layer. The subendothelium is composed of a collagen reticular network on its luminal side and contains some longitudinally-oriented smooth muscle cells with collagen and elastin fibres toward the medial aspect. The internal elastic lamina is not clearly evident but can be considered the first of the many elastic laminae which are found throughout the medial layer. Smooth muscle cells are the major cell type found in the media though some fibroblasts are also present. Extracellularly, there are large quantities of elastin, collagen, and some amorphous substances all in close juxtaposition to the smooth muscle cells. A proportionately thin adventitia covering the elastic arteries blends rather indistinguishably with the surrounding connective tissue and no clearly discernible external elastic lamina exists to separate it from the underlying media. Fibroblasts are the major cell type present though there is penetration by neural and vascular (vasa vasorum) tissues.

Veins and venules

Veins and venules, like their arterial counterparts, are considered to have a more or less pronounced intima, media, and adventitia. However, they differ substantially from arteries in that they have much larger calibers with less well developed muscular and elastic components. In addition, veins generally have a more variable morphology and layers which may not be readily distinguished.

Venules, which are formed by the anastamosis of several capillaries, have essentially the same structure as the capillary. As the venule increases in size to a small vein, smooth muscle cells begin to appear eventually forming a continuous concentric layer around the intimal endothelium and its basement membrane and increasing numbers of fibroblasts form the adventitia along with collagen and elastin fibres. The depth of the medial and adventitial layers increases as the veins enlarge with the adventitia generally becoming the predominant layer in the large veins.

In summary, we can view the vasculature as being comprised of three morphologically distinct components, the intima, media and adventitia. In all but the smallest of the vessels all three layers are present, possessing the same cell types. Indeed it is the presence of these cells throughout the cardiovascular system which seem to govern the biochemical characteristics of the extracellular matrix and thereby the collagen types present.

ENDOTHELIUM AND BASEMENT MEMBRANE

The endothelium of the entire vascular system rests on the basement membrane. Chemical studies on the collagen of purified vascular basement membrane have been limited to isolated glomerular basement membranes from kidneys. Initial studies indicated that a single α-sized collagen chain designated $\alpha 1$(IV) was present (Kefalides, 1971). Subsequent studies in several other laboratories demonstrated more than one and possibly several types of collagen chains were present in this isolated vascular basement membrane (Daniels & Chu, 1974; Trelstad & Lawley, 1977; Tryggvason & Kivirikko, 1978). Recent investigations into the nature of basement membrane collagens from tissues other than the renal glomerulus have revealed that two approximately α-chain sized molecules exist, namely the $\alpha 1$(IV) and $\alpha 2$(IV) chains (Glanville et al, 1979; Kresina & Miller, 1979; Gay & Miller, 1979; Sage et al, 1979). A retrospective examination of the data of Daniels & Chu (1974) showed that the glomerular basement membrane was likely to contain both the $\alpha 1$(IV) and $\alpha 2$(IV) chains and indeed this was recently confirmed by Dixit (1979) who isolated the two chains from human glomeruli. The organization of these chains within native collagen molecules is presently unknown though the majority of data would suggest that they exist in separate molecular species. (For a more detailed discussion of glomerular basement membrane collagens and the chemistry of basement membrane collagens in general see Ch. 22 and 17, respectively.) Corroboration of the presence of the type IV chains in the endothelial basement membrane is apparent from immunohistochemical studies. Gay et al (1979) demonstrated that antibodies to the $\alpha 1$(IV) chain intensely stained the basement membrane of skin capillaries.

The reticular network of collagen fibrils found in the capillary and venule perivascular space and in the subendothelium of the larger arteries has been examined using indirect immunofluorescent techniques. These regions have been found to contain type III and type V collagen (Gay, personal communication; Gay et al, 1975; 1976; 1976a; Timpl et al, 1977).

In order to understand the possible role of the vascular endothelium in the elaboration of a collagenous matrix, several laboratories have studied endothelial cell collagen synthesis in vitro. The results of these experiments are somewhat inconclusive since there are discrepancies in the data obtained. Howard et al (1976) described the synthesis of a collagenous protein resembling type IV collagen which was secreted into the medium of bovine aortic endothelial cell cultures. These cells were shown to stain with antibodies to type IV collagen, while no other collagens were detected. Using human endothelial cells, Jaffe et al (1976) described the synthesis of a basement-membrane-like component, but also found a collagen polypeptide whose behaviour on SDS-polyacrylamide gels indicated it to be $\alpha 1$(III). Type III collagen was also described as a product of porcine endothelial cells in culture (Barnes et al, 1978), but in addition these cells synthesized type I collagen. Two basement membrane collagen chains have been found using transformed human endothelial cells (Kay et al, 1979). It is likely that these correspond to some forms of the $\alpha 1$(IV) and $\alpha 2$(IV) chains though at present this has not been confirmed. Sage et al (1979) studying bovine aortic endothelium in vitro found that the different collagen types were selectively secreted into either the culture medium or into the matrix formed by the cell layer. Type III collagen was the predominant species synthesized and was found in the medium. Two other collagen types, types IV and V, were also synthesized and remained within the cell layer. In conclusion, it is evident that endothelial cells in vitro have the capability of synthesizing all of the collagen types found associated with them in vivo. In particular the type IV collagen of the basement membrane and the type III and type V collagens of the subendothelium have been demonstrated in cells from several species by different laboratories.

MEDIA

Smooth muscle cells are the predominant type found in the media of all arteries and veins. Studies on the collagen types found in aorta whose wall is largely composed of medial tissue revealed the presence of type III collagen as a major species in addition to type I (Chung & Miller, 1974). Localization of the type III collagen to media has subsequently been demonstrated using immunofluorescene techniques and the separated medical layer of large vessels. Gay et al (1976a) demonstrated the presence of type III in aortic media using indirect immunofluorescence. In addition, ferritin-labelled antibodies used for immunelectronmicroscopy revealed that the type III is found in the fine collagen fibrils whereas the type I is present in large collagen fibres. McCullagh & Balian (1975) using isolated media from human aortas estimated the proportion of type III to type I at 70 per cent and 30 per cent respectively.

More recent investigations have revealed the presence of a third collagen type in medial tissue, type V (Chung et al, 1976). Only two chains, α1(V) and α2(V), of the three chains described for the type V collagen family (Bentz et al, 1978; Brown et al, 1978; Burgeson et al, 1976; Chung et al, 1976; Rhodes & Miller, 1978; Sage & Bornstein, 1979; also see Ch. 2) have been found in vascular media. Immunofluorescence data indicate that type V collagen is distributed throughout the smooth muscle cell layers (Fig. 20.2) (Gay & Miller, 1978) and appears to be part of a matrix which surrounds the smooth muscle cell bundles of the media.

Chung et al (1976) reported yet another collagenous molecule with a molecular weight of approximately 55 000 daltons which could be isolated from aortic tissue. Further characterization of this component has revealed that it contains two different polypeptide chains with unusual amino acid compositions (Furuto & Miller, 1980). The cell type(s) responsible for the synthesis of these chains and their tissue distribution is presently unknown.

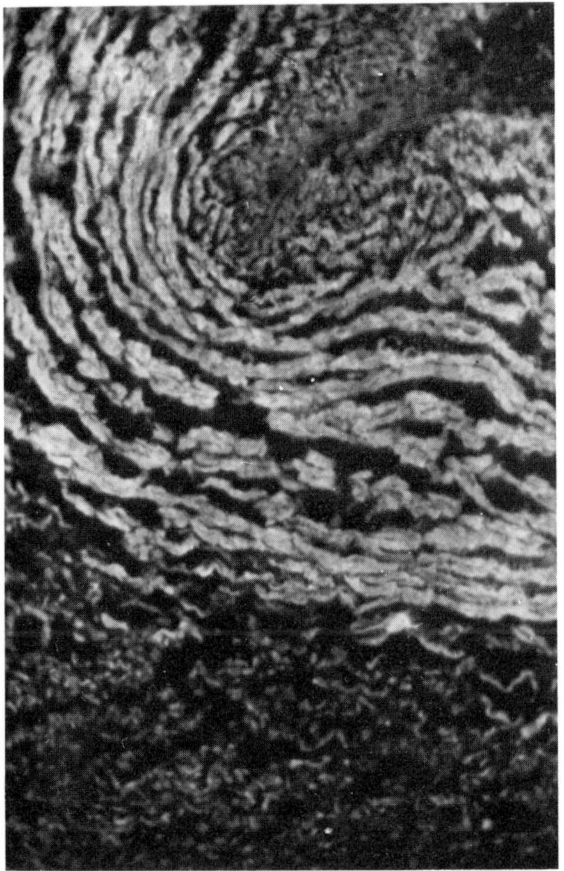

Fig. 20.2 Transverse section of human umbilical vein stained with antibodies to type V collagen (140×). Note the intense staining around the circular smooth muscle cell bundles of the media. (Photograph kindly provided by Drs Renate and Steffan Gay.)

Extensive experimentation has been performed using smooth muscle cells in culture (for review see Chamley-Campbell et al, 1979). Evidence that collagen was synthesized in vitro was apparent in early morphological studies on aortic medial explants and primary cell cultures (Boissel et al, 1976; Daoud et al, 1974; Jarmolych et al, 1968). Biosynthetic studies soon confirmed the potential for smooth muscle cells to produce collagen, when attempts were made to describe the synthesis of the different collagen types following the isolation of type III collagen from aortic tissue. Layman & Titus (1975) reported that human fetal smooth muscle cells synthesized only type I collagen. Numerous investigations by others, however, showed that cells derived from various species over a range of ages synthesized both type I and type III collagens (Barnes et al, 1976; Burke et al, 1977; Layman et al, 1977; Mayne et al, 1977; Rauterberg et al, 1977; Scott et al, 1977), though discrepancies existed in the proportions of collagens synthesized in the various systems. Layman et al (1977) and Rauterburg et al (1977) using human aortic smooth muscle cells found type I to be the predominant species, accounting for 70 to 75 per cent and type III only 25 to 30 per cent. Ratios approximating the proportions of type III to type I found in whole vascular media were documented by Burke et al (1977), Mayne et al (1977), and Scott et al (1977). Differences in the species used, the method of isolation of the collagen and the culture conditions appeared to be the reasons for discrepancies in the proportions of collagen types produced. Underestimates of the proportion of type III collagen occurred when pepsin was used to solubilize the collagens (Burke et al, 1977) and subsequent studies have demonstrated that certain serum factors and phase of cell growth markedly affect the cells' biosynthetic activity (Burke & Ross, 1977).

The synthesis of type V collagen was demonstrated in cultures of monkey aortic cells by Mayne et al (1978). A specialized function has been suggested for the type V collagen based on the immunofluorescent staining pattern observed for smooth muscle cells in culture. It has been proposed that this collagen may serve as an external cytoskeleton since the antibody staining is closely associated with the plasma membrane and it does not appear to form fibres in an extracellular matrix (Gay & Miller, 1978; Miller et al, 1978).

In addition to the biochemically characterized collagens, smooth muscle cells in culture synthesize a collagenous peptide of approximately 45 000 daltons (CP45) (Mayne et al, 1977; 1978). The significance of the protein is unclear and its presence in intact tissue has not been established. It is likely that this material is derived from a partially degraded higher molecular weight collagen. However, the behaviour of CP45 on gel filtration and carboxymethylcellulose chromatography clearly distinguish it from the 55 000-dalton peptide described by Chung et al (1976) and Furuto & Miller (1980).

The identification of collagen types I, III, and V as products of vascular smooth muscle cells has established the ability of these cells to synthesize the major collagenous components found in situ. The presence of an additional collagen-like protein (CP45) in culture (Mayne et al, 1977; 1978) indicates that more collagen species may remain to be isolated from the intact tissue. In addition, the absence of the 55 000-dalton component isolated from aortic media (Chung et al, 1976) suggests that either other cell types also contribute to the collagenous matrix of the media or that the smooth muscle cell in culture may be altered in its ability to synthesize such a protein.

From the distribution of the collagens in the vascular system we may also speculate about their adaptive function. All the collagens serve to some extent as structural proteins for maintenance of tissue integrity, while at the same time permitting other normal activity. For example, type IV collagen of the basement membrane must be integrated into the structure so as to permit or participate in the movement of substances from the vascular lumen into the vessel wall and perivascular space. In addition, the collagen types III and V of the subendothelium cannot inhibit processes of diffusion. Thus, these collagens normally do not form dense accumulations of thick fibres which if surrounding a vessel might inhibit the exchange of nutrient and waste materials. Indeed type IV and type V collagens have no readily discernible, well-defined fibrous structure and type III is found only in small fibre bundles or loosely arranged in reticular matrices (Table 20.1). This lack of large, highly organized fibres for type III and type V may also explain their location in the medial layer where in the larger arteries they must accommodate the expansions and contractions of the elastic walls. Conversely, the media is not rich in type I collagen since large quantities of type I fibres would reduce the plasticity of the vascular wall. The type I fibres which are more abundant in the adventitia provide the necessary strength to anchor the vessels in the surrounding tissue.

COLLAGEN METABOLISM

Relatively few quantitative studies are available on the deposition and accumulation of collagen in the intact vascular system. Madhavan (1977), in an examination of different anatomical regions of the aorta, found that the proportion of collagen per dry tissue weight varied only slightly. Studies in neonatal rabbits indicated that the proportions of collagen may become fixed shortly after birth (Leung et al, 1977). Within 2 weeks after birth the proportion of collagen in the ascending aorta and pulmonary artery had increased to and remained at a constant level. In addition, the pulmonary artery showed a more dramatic increase within the initial 2-week period with a final collagen concentration 1.7 times that of the ascending aorta.

Labelling studies in vivo and in vitro have been used for analyzing collagen synthesis in relatively short-term experiments. Fischer (1971; 1973) determined that the specific activity of hydroxyproline incorporated into rat aortas was constant within 3 hours of isotope administration. In vitro studies on embryonic chick aortae revealed that collagen synthesis decreased during the later stages of development (Eichner & Rosenbloom, 1979). Analysis of the percentage of radiolabelled glycine incorporated into procollagen indicated a decrease from 14 per cent on day 8 to below 10 per cent on days 14 to 18.

These studies demonstrate that collagen is not a metabolically inert protein but is continuously being synthesized and can undergo rather marked changes in its metabolism. Also evident from these few studies is the paucity of data concerning collagen synthesis, accumulation and degradation in vivo with regards to the cardiovascular system. The demonstration of collagen polymorphism in blood vessels severely restricts any interpretation of the existing data as the results do not provide any information concerning the types of collagen being synthesized nor the location within the vessel wall of the synthetic activity.

COLLAGEN AND VASCULAR DISEASE

Pathological conditions which may result in perturbations of normal collagen metabolism can be divided into two groups: (1) inherited disorders; and (2) acquired diseases (Gay & Miller, 1978). The direct involvement of collagen in the pathophysiology of the vascular system has been established in only a limited number of conditions. Examples of genetic disorders of consequence include the Ehlers-Danlos syndromes, Marfan syndrome, and homocystinurea where alterations in the collagen result in vascular dysfunction. These are discussed in detail in Chapter 16. Among the acquired diseases, two arteriopathies, hypertension and atherosclerosis, have received considerable attention with respect to collagen and will be discussed here. Many so-called 'collagen diseases' have also been described. However, this is being recognized as a misnomer because of lacking evidence for the participation of collagen in these diseases. Nonetheless, some attention will be given to the group of diseases commonly known as vasculitis.

Hypertension

Considerable data has accumulated showing clearly that collagen metabolism is affected by hypertension. Wolinsky (1972) observed that a hypertensive state led to increased accumulation of collagen and elastin in the affected vessel. Rats with either spontaneous or artificially induced hypertension were shown to have increased collagen synthesis, a greater accumulation of collagen, and higher prolyl hydroxylase activities in aortas and mesenteric arteries (Ooshima et al, 1974). Further studies provided evidence that the microvasculature was similarly affected in desoxycorticosterone acetate (DOCA)-induced hypertension (Ooshima et al, 1975). Treatment with the antihypertensive drugs reserpine or chlorothiazide reversed or inhibited the changes. The action of these drugs was found in part to be mediated through the hypothalamus (Ooshima et al, 1977), but the mechanism of action of the drugs or any mediators which they elicit on the metabolism of the vessel wall are presently unknown.

The causative factor for the increased synthesis appeared to be the increased blood pressure. Smith et al (1976) subjected veins to haemodynamic stress by performing arteriovenous anastamoses. Collagen content and salt extractable collagen increased 17 per cent and 267 per cent respectively in the affected veins. Similar conclusions were drawn from studies on collagen synthesis in the veins of hypertensive rats (Iwatsuki et al, 1977). The blood pressure in the veins of DOCA-treated rats did not increase and despite increases in collagen content and synthesis in the hypertensive arteries, the veins showed control levels for collagen synthesis and accumulation. Also, Newman & Langner (1978) reported that increased collagen synthesis in spontaneously hypertensive rats was not observed until well after the blood pressure increased, suggesting that the mechanical stress factors were important in the altered collagen synthesis.

The actual accumulation of collagen in the vascular wall may also perpetuate the condition. Iwatsuki et al (1977) observed that animals treated with DOCA and with the lathyrogen β-aminopropionitrile (βAPN) did not develop high blood pressure and even showed a reduction in arterial collagen content. Presumably the decrease in collagen accumulation caused by the lathyrogen resulted in maintenance of normotensive conditions.

The observation that βAPN would reverse an existing hypertensive condition coupled with the proposal that the accumulated collagen helped to perpetuate high blood pressure led to an investigation of collagen turnover (Nissen et al, 1978). It was found that the half-life of collagen in the vascular system of animals with DOCA-induced hypertension was selectively affected when compared with skin or tendon, being reduced from 60 to 70 days to 17 days. These data correlate with the observations of Smith et al (1976) that hypertensive vessels yielded larger quantities of low molecular weight collagenous peptides than normotensive vessels when extracted with saline. These peptides presumably resulted from increased collagenolytic activity. However, quantitation of collagenase activity was not done and the extractions were performed without inhibitors for endogenous proteases.

Collagen, though secondarily involved in hypertension, clearly plays a critical role in the sequence of events leading to chronic hypertension. Increases in both collagen accumulation and collagen degradation are potentially dangerous due to the normal fibrotic response that occurs in the presence of persistent tissue insult or injury (Gay & Miller, 1978). Though no data is currently available regarding hypertension, tissues which are undergoing repair generally show increased quantities of type I deposition which in the case of the vasculature would disrupt the normal ratios of collagen types, leading to arteriosclerosis and significant clinical sequelae.

Atherosclerosis

Atherosclerosis is the most common cardiovascular disease in man. Yet, despite its position as the leading cause of death in western societies, it remains one of the least understood diseases in terms of its aetiology. The pathophysiology, however, has been investigated extensively and is well defined.

The lesions associated with atherosclerosis are confined to the intimal layer of the arterial wall and fall into three categories: (1) the fatty streak; (2) fibrous plaque; and (3) the complicated lesion. Fatty streaks appear as slightly raised areas composed of a series of contiguous dots immediately underlying the endothelium. Histochemical staining shows the presence of large quantities of fatty material within certain cell populations which ultrastructurally appear as smooth muscle cells. The history of fatty streaks is unknown and their occurrence in all populations at an early age raise questions as to their involvement in the atherosclerotic process. Also, the streaks in humans are more prevalent in areas such as the aortic arch which do not ordinarily become populated by the true atheromatous lesions.

Fibrous plaques are recognized as the definitive feature of progressing atherosclerosis. Identifiable by the gray to whitish appearance, these lesions are well defined lumps which protrude into the lumen of the vessel. They are largely composed of smooth muscle cells which are filled with lipid and which are surrounded extracellularly by collagen, elastin, and proteoglycans. These cells with the surrounding matrix form a cap covering the deeper layers of the lesion which contains extracellular lipid, cell debris, and infiltrating macrophages.

The complicated lesion apparently results from changes to the fibrous plaque and marks the most advanced stage of atherosclerosis where the vessel may be occluded. Characteristic of this stage is the occurrence of mural thrombosis, extensive cell necrosis, and calcification. This type of lesion may of itself interfere with the flow of blood depending on its size, but more importantly may indirectly effect the cessation of circulation by producing conditions which lead to the formation of a secondary thrombosis.

Epidemiological studies have indicated that there are many contributing factors such as diet, heredity, sex, environment, work habits, etc., which may be involved in the incidence and subsequent complications of the atherosclerotic process. However, despite these indicators of probability of disease, the actual pathobiological mechanism which initiates the disease remains unknown. One hypothesis which attempts to explain the aetiology of atherosclerosis is the 'response-to-injury,' which has been proposed by Ross and coworkers (Ross, 1972; Ross & Glomset, 1973; 1976; Ross et al, 1975). The basis of this model are the results observed upon experimental desquamation of the arterial endothelium. Removal of the nonthrombogenic endothelium results in platelet aggregation at the site of the lesion which is probably induced by the type III collagen fibres of the subendothelium (see Ch. 10). The adherent platelets release their granules which contain mitogenic factors. These serve to stimulate focal smooth muscle cell proliferation which results in a thickened intima. Provided repeated injury does not occur the endothelial cells will eventually reach confluency over the injured site, re-establishing the integrity of the nonthrombogenic neointima, and the lesion will regress. However, repeated injury at the site causes a cycle of proliferation and regression wherein the intima continues to thicken and the lesion progresses to more advanced stages with lipid deposition and cell necrosis becoming prevalent. Such a situation can finally lead to the complicated lesion which will be of clinical significance.

A second hypothesis currently being investigated is the 'monoclonal' hypothesis put forward by Benditt & Benditt (1973; Benditt, 1977). In this model the lesion is viewed as being akin to a benign tumour where a single smooth muscle cell in the arterial wall becomes neoplastic as a result of mutagenesis. The transformed cell migrates to the intima where it continues to replicate causing the formation of a plaque. The basis for this hypothesis comes from the observation that atherosclerotic plaques from humans usually contain only one isozyme of the X-linked enzyme glucose-6-phosphate dehydrogenase, suggesting that all of the cells in the plaque were derived from a single parent cell.

Martin & Sprague (1973) proposed another hypothesis which would account for smooth muscle cell proliferation in plaques. In this model smooth muscle cells of the media secrete substances called 'chalones' which inhibit replication of smooth muscle stem cells. These 'chalones' also diffuse to the intima to inhibit cell division. With age, the number of stem cells decline and subsequently the smooth muscle cell population decreases. This leads to a drop in the level of 'chalones' which eventually releases the stem cells of the intima from inhibition and results in smooth muscle cell proliferation and plaque formation.

As noted above the atherosclerotic plaque contains sizeable quantities of collagen, elastin, and glycosaminoglycans. In an attempt to further understand the disease numerous biochemical studies of collagen metabolism have been undertaken. Levene & Poole (1962) found that the collagen content of intimal plaques was increased by 50 per cent when compared to uninvolved tissue in humans. Studies on prolyl hydroxylase using rabbits with thyroxine-epinephrine induced atherosclerosis revealed as much as a six-fold increase in enzyme activity in plaque regions (Fuller & Langner, 1970; Fuller et al, 1976) suggesting not only an increase in collagen content but also an increase in the rate of synthesis.

Several factors appear to affect the metabolism of collagen. The thyroxine-epinephrine induced lesions in rabbits showed increased prolyl hydroxylase within 9 days of treatment (Fuller & Langner, 1970). However rabbits maintained on a hypercholesterolaemic diet, though having pronounced atherosclerotic plaque by day 60, showed no increase in collagen content or prolyl hydroxylase activity (Langner & Modrak, 1976a). Significant increases were evident by day 90 of the experiment, when approximately a two-fold increase in prolyl hydroxylase activity was observed (Langner & Modrak, 1976b). A similar delay in the onset of stimulated collagen synthesis has been demonstrated in pigeons. St. Clair et al (1975) reported that after 8 months on a high cholesterol diet no increase could be found for collagen synthesis as measured by prolyl hydroxylase activity, whereas, animals maintained for 18 months had lesions which synthesized collagen at four times the rate of normal tissue (McCullagh & Ehrhart, 1977). These data indicate that the phenomenon of increased collagen synthesis appears to be secondary in nature in the hypercholesterolaemic model and that the method of inducing experimental atherosclerosis may markedly affect the time course and level of the increased synthetic response.

The rate of collagen synthesis and deposition in the atherosclerotic lesion appears to be a function of the location and the degree of involvement of the tissue. McCullagh & Ehrhart (1974) using various canine arteries observed that the rate of collagen synthesis is highest in arteries nearest the heart, decreasing as the distance increases. In atherosclerotic femoral arteries they found that the rate of synthesis ranged from 5-fold, for regions showing 40 per cent involvement, to 20-fold in cases of 100 per cent involvement. Moreover, the relative amount of collagen synthesized rose from 5 per cent in normal branch arteries up to 14 per cent in branch arteries with advanced lesions, thus indicating a stimulation in collagen synthesis above any increase in overall protein synthesis. Fisher et al (1980) obtained similar results in rabbits finding the highest rates of collagen synthesis in the most pulsatile arteries. However, unlike the canine model the greatest degree of involvement and most severe lesions were localized to the arteries nearest the heart and consequently these showed a greater stimulation in collagen synthesis.

Relatively little information is available on what factors may be involved in stimulating collagen synthesis in the plaque areas. Since lipid accummulation is a hallmark of the lesion and is known to infiltrate from the blood, some studies have investigated their ability to stimulate collagen production by smooth muscle cells in culture. Rabbit smooth muscle cells from aortic media when grown in homologous, hyperlipidaemic serum for 14 days accumulated lipid intracellularly but showed no changes in either collagen or total protein synthesis (Pietila & Nikkair, 1978). Hypercholesterolaemic rat serum failed to stimulate collagen synthesis in smooth muscle cell cultures or aortic organ cultures. However, liver extracts from hyperlipidaemic animals did stimulate synthesis in both systems. The significance of the response to liver extracts is to be regarded with caution as it also stimulates collagen production in fibroblasts and has not been evaluated for its affect on general protein synthesis. Recently, Chidi et al (1979) have obtained evidence that a cell to cell interaction may be necessary for increased collagen synthesis. Using balloon catheters to injure the endothelium, they found that re-endothelialization had to occur before collagen accumulation and intimal thickening proceeded.

Despite the numerous investigations of the synthesis of collagen in atherosclerosis, only recently has there been an examination of the collagen types involved. McCullagh & Balian (1975) examined normal and atherosclerotic tissue from human aortas for quantities of type I and type III collagen. Normal samples of media were estimated to contain 70 per cent type III and 30 per cent type I. On the other hand atherosclerotic intima had nearly opposite ratios with 65 per cent type I and 35 per cent type III. Examination of the cells populating the involved areas showed morphology uncharacteristic of typical smooth muscle cells. The atypical collagen ratio and the altered morphology indicated that the intimal cells were no longer phenotypically true smooth muscle cells, but had undergone a transformation.

Immunohistochemical techniques have also been used to characterize the collagens in fibrous plaques. This has provided the advantage of being able to investigate individual lesions and also facilitated the study of progressive changes in collagen with the stage of the disease. Early atherosclerotic lesions show an intense staining to type V collagen in the region of smooth muscle cell proliferation (Gay & Miller, 1978). In addition, Gay & Gay (personal communication) have found that type IV collagen is also present not only along the discontinuous basement membrane, but throughout the plaque. They suggest that in addition to smooth muscle cells some transformed endothelial cells may also participate in the collagen deposition in the lesion. Studies on advanced lesions confirm the biochemical studies with only minimal staining of tissue treated with antibodies to type III collagen and intense staining when treated with type I collagen antibodies (Gay & Miller, 1978).

In conclusion, it is evident that the commonly agreed upon feature of atherosclerosis is that intimal thickening and plaque formation is the result of smooth muscle cell proliferation with some degree of transformation occurring. These cells are by some undetermined mechanism stimulated to produce increased quantities of collagen. Though the response of collagen production is a secondary one, it is probably important in leading to further complications since the eventual replacement of the type III collagen normally present in the intima by type I leads to a loss of normal physiological function and to conditions which favour alterations such as calcification (Reddi et al, 1977). Hopefully, future studies will be designed to further detail and correlate collagen synthesis and type with the stage of the disease and investigate other mechanisms which cause the fibrotic processes to take place.

Vasculitis

Vasculitis is a pathological process characterized by the inflammation and necrosis of blood vessels which is a common feature of a broad spectrum of diseases (Fauci et al, 1978). Several well defined disorders have vasculitis as one of their clinical sequelae, but in recent years because of their distinctive clinical and pathological features are no longer considered within the domain of vasculitis per se. Examples of these diseases include systemic lupus erythematosus, rheumatoid arthritis, and progressive systemic sclerosis (scleroderma). In each of these, immunopathological mechanisms have been established and in the cases of rheumatoid arthritis and progressive systemic sclerosis autoimmunity to collagen appears to play a role (see p. 273).

However, the majority of diseases which fall under the heading of vasculitis cannot be easily categorized because of the many overlapping features and unknown aetiologies. As a result, the vasculitic disorders are generally grouped into categories which classify the disease according to its histological characteristics and anatomical location (Table 20.2). The factors which predispose a given anatomical location to any of the various vasculitides is presently unknown.

Within recent years immunological processes have been implicated in the pathology of several kinds of vasculitides. This evidence is derived from three sources: (1) the presence of vasculitis in diseases with established immunopathologies; (2) similar clinical findings between vasculitides of unknown origin and diseases having definite immunopathogenesis; and (3) animal model studies. As noted above diseases such as systemic lupus erythematosis and others have systemic vasculitis as a consequence establishing that immunological phenomena can lead to vasculitic lesions. In addition, patients with various forms of vasculitis of unknown aetiology have been found to have rheumatoid factor, cryoglobulinaemia (Conn et al, 1976) and circulating immune complexes (Cream, 1976) suggesting the involvement of immunological processes.

Animal models have provided in addition to a link

Table 20.2 Characteristics of vasculitic disorders

Classification	*Vessel involvement*	*Organ involvement*	*Histopathologic features*
Polyarteritis nodosa	Small and medium muscular arteries commonly at branches	Kidney, gastrointestinal liver urogenital, coronary artery	PMN leucocyte, plasma cell and lymphocyte infiltration; fibrinoid necrosis, elastica interna disruption, lesions at all stages present
Allergic granulomatosis	Small arteries, arterioles, capillaries, venules	Widespread with lung being most frequent	Eosinophilic and giant cells in granulomas; PMN leucocyte and lymphocyte infiltration; lesions at all stages present
Hypersensitivity angiitis	Small arteries, arterioles, postcapillary venules	Skin, kidney, lung, serosa	PMN neutrophilic leucocytes, some eosinophilia, extravasation of erythrocytes, purpura in skin, no giant cells, lesions all at same stage
Wegener's granulomatosis	Small arteries, arterioles, capillaries, venules	Upper and lower respiratory, kidney, eyes	Necrotizing granulomas, giant cells, glomerulitis with fibrin thrombi and focal necrosis of tufts, lesions at all stages present
Giant cell arteritis	Large and medium arteries	Aorta, coronary, carotid temporal and other large arteries	Giant cells, lymphocyte infiltration of the media, elastica interna disruption, fibrinoid deposition, inflammation without necrosis
Lymphomatoid granulomatosis	Small arteries, arterioles, capillaries, venules	Lung, skin, kidney, occasionally CNS; no involvement of spleen, lymph nodes or bone marrow	Infiltration by lymphoid, abnormal lymphocytoid, plasmacytoid, and reticuloendothelial-like cells giving appearance of lympho-proliferative disorder
Thromboangiitis obliterans (Buerger's disease)	Intermediate and small arteries and veins	Widespread	Thrombi at sites of inflammation; acute stages show PMN leucocyte infiltration and abscesses; sub-acute stages show mononuclear and giant cells
Mucocutaneous lymph node syndrome (limited to infants and children)	Muscular arteries	Coronary artery primarily	Intimal thickening and proliferation, mononuclear cell infiltrates,elastica disruption, aneurysm, thrombosis

between immune complex diseases and vasculitis some understanding of the mechanisms involved. (For a review see Cochrane & Dixon, 1976.) In these models either the antigen or antibody is injected locally while the other is circulating in the blood. The two agents come in contact and precipitate in the vessel wall. Complement is activated by the complex and serves as a chemotactic substance causing the infiltration of polymorphonuclear leucocytes. These release lysosomal enzymes which result in focal necrosis. In summary, when considering vasculitides of unknown aetiology, it must be emphasized that although the immune mechanisms which are apparently operative in vasculitis affect the vascular wall which is rich in collagen, there is no direct evidence that collagen is involved in the deposition of the offending immune complexes. Nonetheless, there is evidence that collagen may play a role in binding of the immune complexes found in systemic lupus erythematosis (Izui et al, 1976) which leaves the possibility the collagen could be a factor in the generalized vasculitides but simply has not been identified as such. (For a discussion of collagen and immune complex deposition, see Ch. 15.) Further investigation of vasculitis conditions will lead to the identification of the aetiological agents and either establish or refute the role which collagen may play.

ACKNOWLEDGEMENTS

The author would like to express his gratitude to Drs Donald K. Furuto and Steffan Gay for their suggestions and helpful discussions while writing this chapter. A special thanks also is extended to Drs Renate and Steffen Gay for use of the photomicrograph in Figure 20.2 and to Ms Julia Sanders for preparing the figures and typing the manuscript.

REFERENCES

Barnes M J, Morton L F, Levene C I 1976 Synthesis of collagens types I and III by pig medial smooth muscle cells in culture. Biochemical and Biophysical Research Communications 70: 339

Benditt E P 1977 The origin of atherosclerosis. Scientific American 236: 74

Benditt E P, Benditt J M 1973 Evidence for a monoclonal origin of human atherosclerotic plaques. Proceedings of the National Academy of Science, U.S.A. 70: 1753

Bentz H, Bächinger H P, Glanville R, Kühn K 1978 Physical evidence for the assembly of A and B chains of human placental collagen in a single triple helix. European Journal of Biochemistry 92: 563

Boissel J P, Bourdillon M C, Loire R, Crouzet B 1976 Histological arguments for collagen and elastin synthesis by primary cultures of rat aortic media cells. Atherosclerosis 25: 107

Brown R A, Shuttleworth C A, Weiss J B 1978 Three new α-chains of collagen from a non-basement membrane source. Biochemical and Biophysical Research Communications 80: 866

Burgeson R E, El Adli F A, Kaitila I I, Hollister D W 1976 Fetal membrane collagens: Identification of two new collagen alpha chains. Proceedings of the National Academy of Science, USA 73: 2579

Burke J M, Ross R 1977 Collagen synthesis by monkey arterial smooth muscle cells during proliferation and quiescence in culture. Experimental Cell Research 107: 387

Burke J M, Balian G, Ross R, Bornstein P 1977 Synthesis of types I and III procollagen by monkey aortic smooth muscle cells in vitro. Biochemistry 16: 3243

Chamley-Campbell J, Campbell G R, Ross R 1979 The smooth muscle cell in culture. Physiological Reviews 59: 1

Chidi C C, Klein L, De Palma R G 1979 Effect of regenerated endothelium on collagen content in the injured artery. Surgery, Gynecology and Obstetrics 148: 839

Chung E, Miller E J 1974 Collagen polymorphism: Characterization of molecules with the chain composition $[\alpha 1(III)]_3$ in human tissues. Science 183: 1200

Chung E, Rhodes R K, Miller E J 1976 Isolation of three collagenous components of probable basement membrane origin from several tissues. Biochemical and Biophysical Research Communications 71: 1167

Cochrane C G, Dixon F J 1976 Antigen-Antibody Complex Induced Disease. In: Miescher P A, Müller-Eberhard, J H (eds) Textbook of immunopathology, 2nd edn. Grune & Stratton, New York

Conn D L, McDuffie F C, Holley K E, Schrocter A L 1976 Immunologic mechanisms in systemic vasculitis. Mayo Clinic Proceedings 51: 511

Cream J J 1976 Clinical and immunological aspects of cutaneous vasculitis. Quarterly Journal of Medicine 45: 255

Daniels J R, Chu G H 1975 Basement membrane collagen of renal glomerulus. Journal of Biological Chemistry 250: 3531

Daoud A S, Fritz K E, Singh J, Augustyn J M, Jarmolych J 1974 Production of mucopolysaccharides, collagen and elastic tissue by aortic medial explants. Advances in Experimental Biology and Medicine 43: 281

Dixit S N 1979 Isolation and characterization of two α chain size collagenous polypeptide chains C and D from glomerular basement membrane. FEBS Letters 106: 379

Eichner R, Rosenbloom J 1979 Collagen and elastin synthesis in the developing chick aorta. Archives of Biochemistry and Biophysics 198: 414

Fauci A S, Haynes B F, Katz P 1978 The spectrum of vasculitis. Annals of Internal Medicine 89: 660

Fischer G M, 1971 Dynamics of collagen and elastin metabolism in rat aorta. Journal of Applied Physiology 31: 527

Fischer G M 1973 Comparison of collagen dynamics in different tissues under the influence of estradiol. Endocrinology 93: 1216

Fischer G M, Swain M L, Cherian K 1980 Increased vascular collagen and elastin synthesis in experimental atherosclerosis in the rabbit. Atherosclerosis 35: 11

Fuller G C, Langner R O 1970 Elevation of aortic proline hydroxylase: A biochemical defect in experimental arteriosclerosis. Science 168: 987

Fuller G C, Matoney A L, Fisher D O, Fausto N, Cardinale G J 1976 Increased collagen synthesis and the kinetic characteristics of prolyl hydroxylase in tissues of rabbits with experimental arteriosclerosis. Atherosclerosis 24: 483

Furuto D K, Miller E J 1980 Isolation of a unique collagenous fraction from limited pepsin digests of human placental tissue. Journal of Biological Chemistry 255: 290

Gay S, Balleisen L, Remberger K, Fietzek P P, Adelmann B C, Kühn K 1975 Immunohistochemical evidence for the presence of collagen type III in human arterial walls, arterial thrombi, and in leucocytes, incubated with collagen in vitro. Klinische Wochenschrift 53: 899

Gay S, Kresina T F, Gay R, Miller E J, Montes L F 1979 Immunohistochemical demonstration of basement membrane collagen in normal human skin and in psoriasis. Journal of Cutaneous Pathology 6: 91

Gay S, Miller E J 1978 Collagen in the Physiology and Pathology of Connective Tissue. Gustav Fischer, Stuttgart-New York

Gay S, Miller E J 1979 Characterization of lens capsule collagen: Evidence for the presence of two unique chains in molecules derived from major basement membrane structures. Archives of Biochemistry and Biophysics 198: 370

Gay S, Müller P K, Meigel W N, Kühn K 1976a Polymorphie des kollagens neue aspekte für struktur und funktion des bindegewebes. Der Hautarzt 27: 196

Gay S, Walter P, Kühn K 1976b Characterization and distribution of collagen types in arterial heterografts originating from the calf carotis. Klinische Wochenshrift 54: 889

Glanville R W, Rauter A, Fietzek P P 1979 Isolation and characterization of a native placental basement-membrane collagen and its component α chains. European Journal of Biochemistry 95: 383

Howard B V, Macarak E J, Gunson D, Kefalides N A 1976 Characterization of the collagen synthesized by endothelial cells in culture. Proceedings of the National Academy of Sciences, USA 73: 2361

Iwatsuki K, Cardinale G J, Spector S, Udenfriend S 1977a Hypertension: increase of collagen biosynthesis in arteries but not in veins. Science 198: 403

Iwatsuki K, Cardinale G J, Spector S, Udenfriend S 1977b Reduction of blood pressure and vascular collagen in hypertensive rats by β-aminopropionitrile. Proceedings of the National Academy of Science, USA 74: 360

Izui S, Lambert P H, Miescher P A 1976 In vitro demonstration of a particular affinity of glomerular basement membrane and collagen for DNA complexes in system lupus erythematosis. Journal of Experimental Medicine 144: 428

Jaffe E A, Minick C R, Adelman B, Becker C G, Nachman R 1976 Synthesis of basement-membrane collagen by cultured human endothelial cells. Journal of Experimental Medicine 144: 209

Jarmolych J, Daoud A S, Landau J, Fritz K E, McElvene E 1968 Aortic media explants: cell proliferation and production of mucopolysaccharides, collagen and elastic tissue. Experimental and Molecular Pathology 9: 171

Kay E, Fareed G C, Ruoslahti E, Fessler J H 1979 Basement-membrane collagen and glycoprotein synthesis by normal and transformed human endothelial cells. Federation Proceedings Abstracts 38: 817

Kefalides N A 1971 Isolation of a collagen from basement membranes containing three identical α-chains. Biochemical and Biophysical Research Communications 45: 226

Kresina T F, Miller E J 1979 Isolation and characterization of basement-membrane collagen from human placental tissue. Evidence for the presence of two genetically distinct collagen chains. Biochemistry 18: 3089

Langner R O, Modrak J B 1976a Hypercholesterolemia and aortic collagen synthesis in rabbit aortas. Atherosclerosis 24: 149

Langner R O, Modrak J B 1976b Collagen metabolism during the early stages of cholesterol-induced atherogenesis in rabbits. Blood Vessels 13: 257

Layman D L, Epstein E J Jr, Dodson R F, Titus J L 1977 Biosynthesis of type I and III collagens by cultured smooth muscle cells from human aorta. Proceedings of the National Academy of Science, USA 74: 671

Layman D L, Titus J L 1975 Synthesis of type I collagen by human smooth muscle cells in vitro. Laboratory Investigations 33: 103

Leung D Y M, Glagov S, Mathews M B 1977 Elastin and collagen accumulation in rabbit ascending aorta and pulmonary trunk during postnatal growth. Circulation Research 41: 316

Levene C I, Poole J C F 1962 The collagen content of the normal and atherosclerotic human aortic intima. British Journal of Experimental Pathology 43: 469

McCullagh K A, Balian G 1975 Collagen characterization and cell transformation in human atherosclerosis. Nature 258: 73

McCullagh K G, Ehrhart L A 1974 Increased arterial collagen synthesis in experimental canine atherosclerosis. Atherosclerosis 19: 13

McCullagh K G, Ehrhart L A 1977 Enhanced synthesis and accumulation of collagen in cholesterol-aggravated pigeon atherosclerosis. Atherosclerosis 26: 341

Madhavan M 1977 Glycosaminoglycans, elastin and collagen content of normal adult human aorta at different anatomical levels. Indian Journal of Experimental Biology 15: 132

Martin G M, Sprague C A 1973 Symposium on in vitro studies related to atherogenesis: Life histories of hyperplastoid cell lines from aorta and skin. Experimental and Molecular Pathology 18: 125

Mayne R, Vail M S, Miller E J 1978 Characterization of the collagen chains synthesized by cultured smooth muscle cells derived from rhesus monkey thoracic aorta. Biochemistry 17: 446

Mayne R, Vail M S, Miller E J, Blose S H, Chacko S 1977 Collagen polymorphisms in cell cultures derived from guinea pig aortic smooth muscle: Comparison with three populations of fibroblasts. Archives of Biochemistry and Biophysics 181: 462

Miller E J, Rhodes R K, Gay S, Kresina T F, Furuto D K 1979 Useful approaches in the isolation of the collagenous constituents of basement membranes. In: Robert L (ed) Frontiers in matrix biology, vol 7. Karger, Basel

Newman R A, Langner R P 1978 Age-related changes in the vascular collagen metabolism of the spontaneously hypertensive rat. Experimental Gerontology 13: 83

Nissen R, Cardinale G J, Udenfriend S 1978 Increased turnover of arterial collagen in hypertensive rats. Proceedings of the National Academy of Science, USA 75: 451

Ooshima A, Fuller G C, Cardinale G J, Spector S, Udenfriend S 1974 Increased collagen synthesis in blood vessels of hypertensive rats and its reversal by antihypertensive agents. Proceedings of the National Academy of Science, USA 71: 3019

Ooshima A, Fuller G C, Cardinale G J, Spector S, Udenfriend S 1975 Collagen biosynthesis in blood vessels of brain and other tissues of the hypertensive rat. Science 190: 898

Ooshima A, Fuller G C, Cardinale G J, Spector S, Udenfriend S 1977 Reduction of collagen biosynthesis in blood vessels and other tissues by reserpine and hypophysectomy. Proceedings of the National Academy of Science, USA 74: 777

Pietilä K, Kikkari T 1978 Effect of phase of growth and hyperlipidemic serum on the synthesis of collagen in rabbit aortic smooth muscle cells in culture. Medical Biology 50: 11

Rauterberg J, Allam S, Brehmer U, Wirth W, Hauss W H 1977 Characterization of the collagen synthesized by cultured human smooth muscle cells from fetal and adult aorta. Hoppe-Seyler's Zeitshrift für Physiologische Chemie 358: 401

Reddi A H, Gay R, Gay S, Miller E J 1977 Transition in collagen types during matrix-induced cartilage, bone, and bone marrow formation. Proceedings of the National Academy of Science, USA 74: 5587

Rhodes R K, Miller E J 1978 Physicochemical characterization and molecule organization of the collagen A and B chains. Biochemistry 17: 3442

Rönnemaa T, Dohertz N S 1977 Effect of serum and liver extracts from hypercholesterolemic rats on the synthesis of collagen by isolated aortas and cultured aortic smooth muscle cells. Atherosclerosis 26: 261

Ross R 1973 The arterial smooth muscle cell. In: Wissler R W, Geer J C (eds) The pathogenesis of atherosclerosis. Williams and Wilkins, Baltimore

Ross R, Glomset J A 1973 Atherosclerosis and the arterial smooth muscle cell. Science 180: 1332

Ross R, Glomset J A 1976 The pathogenesis of atherosclerosis. New England Journal of Medicine 295: 368 & 420

Ross R, Glomset J A, Kariya B, Harker L 1974 A platelet dependent serum factor that stimulates the proliferation of arterial smooth muscle cells in vitro. Proceedings of the National Academy of Science, USA 71: 1207

Sage H, Bornstein P 1979 Characterization of a novel collagen chain in human placenta and its relation to AB collagen. Biochemistry 18: 3815

Sage H, Crouch E, Bornstein P 1979a Collagen synthesis by bovine aortic endothelial cells in culture. Biochemistry 18: 5433

Sage H, Woodbury R G, Bornstein P 1979b Structural studies on human type IV collagen. The Journal of Biological Chemistry 254: 9893

St. Clair R W, Toma J J Jr, Lofland H B 1975 Proline hydroxylase activity and collagen content of pigeon aortas with naturally-occurring and cholesterol-aggravated atherosclerosis. Atherosclerosis 21: 155

Scott D M, Harwood R, Grant M E, Jackson D S 1977 Characterization of the major collagen species present in porcine aortae and the synthesis of their precursors by smooth muscle cells in culture. Connective Tissue Research 5: 7

Smith R A, Stehbens W E, Weber P 1976 Hemodynamically-induced increase in soluble collagen in the anastomosed veins of experimental arteriovenous fistulae. Atherosclerosis 23: 429

Timpl R, Wick G, Gay S 1977 Antibodies to distinct types of collagens and procollagens and their application in immunohistology. Journal of Immunological Methods 18: 165

Trelstad R L, Lawley K R 1977 Isolation and initial characterization of human basement membrane collagens. Biochemical and Biophysical Research Communications 76: 376

Tryggvason K, Kivirikko K I 1978 Heterogeneity of pepsin-solubilized human glomerular basement membrane collagen. Nephron 21: 230

Wolinsky H 1972 Long term effects of hypertension on the rat aortic wall and their relation to concurrent aging changes. Circulation Research 30: 301

21

The eye

I. L. FREEMAN

INTRODUCTION

The eye is essentially a highly sophisticated device for collecting and processing light energy so that information is provided to the brain in a suitable form for interpretation. To optimize this process a variety of exquisite collagen-containing tissues have been evolved. For example, the cornea and sclera form a completely closed protective tunic around the delicate light-sensitive retina (see Fig. 21.1). The multilayered cornea (vide infra) is remarkable by virtue of its transparency, and its powerful refractive properties; the sclera by its opacity and by its resistance to deformation — it enables the eyeball to be rotated through nearly 180° by quite powerful muscles without significant distortion. Inside this fibrous tunic is the visoelastic vitreous which is not only the largest concentration of extracellular material in the body but is also able to transmit up to 90 per cent of visible light through its mass. At various strategic locations, e.g. surrounding the lens, on the posterior surface of the cornea, between the retina and choroid, basement lamina structures are interposed, each playing a crucial structual role in the optimization of the light-gathering activities of the eye. The purpose of this chapter is to review the current knowledge of ocular

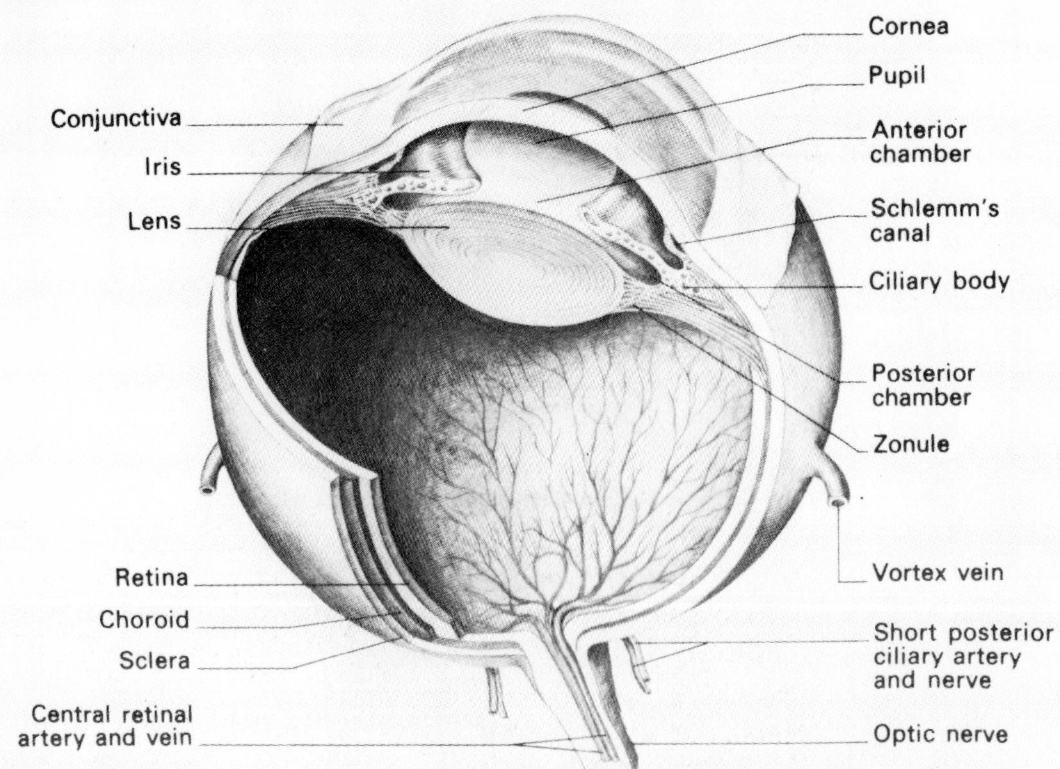

Fig. 21.1 Gross anatomy of the human eye. (From Trevor-Roper P D 1980 Lecture notes on ophthalmology. Blackwell, Oxford)

collagens so that the unique properties of the eye tissues can be better understood and comparisons with other tissues can be made. This will be followed by a discussion of the changes in structure and the resultant functional defects that are manifest in disease.

STRUCTURE AND BIOSYNTHESIS OF THE COLLAGENS

It is now well established that the collagens are a family of evolutionarily highly successful molecules, whose role is mainly structural. The total genetic potential for the collagens is not yet known, but at least 10 distinct α-chains have been described in vertebrate tissues. Each type has a unique amino acid sequence and is characterized by a distinct amino acid pattern (for review see Ch. 1). All the known collagen types have been found in the various tissues of the eye.

The physiological significance of each collagen type is yet to be determined, but some details are now emerging. Fibrous collagen is the native quaternary form of collagen type I-III. The collagen fibril is best described as a quasi-crystalloid, because it is a highly symmetrical insoluble structure, built up of identical subunits. The subunits are packed such that an asymmetric cross-striation of period 67 mm is a microscopic characteristic of the fibril. The precise number of fibrils, their diameter range and their weave vary according to the function of the particular tissue of which they are major constituents.

The other collagen types appear to be mainly basement lamina constituents or poorly characterized cell-surface components. In addition, collagenous sequences have been found elsewhere (see Ch. 2).

Like many other extracellular proteins, the collagens are synthesized as high-molecular weight precursors known as procollagens. (For further details see this volume, Ch. 5). Most of these procollagens are poorly characterized. During the assembly process, the polypeptide chains of the procollagens of the fibrous types are subject to at least six different enzyme-mediated modifications not found with other proteins. These post-translational modifications are hydroxylation of proline, hydroxylation of lysine; galactosylation of hydroxylysine; glucosylation of galactosyl-hydroxylysine, oxidative deamination of lysine and hydroxylysine and proteolytic cleavage of the extension peptides at both ends of the molecule. The resultant postsynthetic microheterogeneity probably represents the 'fine tuning' of the collagen molecules for their ultimate biological function.

The structure and biosynthetic details of the nonfibrous collagens are not as well known, but many of the assembly and post-translational processes appear to be similar to those discussed above for the fibrous collagens (see Ch. 17).

COLLAGENOUS TISSUES OF THE EYE

Cornea

The cornea is the transparent window occupying approximately one-sixth of the protective coat of the eyeball. It is the most important refractive medium of the eye. Details of the fine structure of the cornea have been reviewed (Tripathi, 1974; Marshall & Grindle, 1978) and will be briefly summarized here.

The cornea consists of five layers. The outer surface which is in intimate associate with the pre-corneal tear film, is a multilayered non-keratinized squamous epithelium of ectodermal origin. The epithelium is approximately 50 to 70 μm thick, and it rests on a thin basal lamina. Directly underneath is Bowman's 'membrane' which is not a true basal lamina, but is a thin (8 to 14 μm) modified, hyalinized anterior layer of the stroma. The corneal stroma accounts for about 90 per cent of the total corneal thickness (it is about 500 μm thick). As will be described below, it consists of highly organized, uniform diameter, collagen fibrils and associated interfibrillar matrix, together with a relatively small population of cells. Under the corneal stroma is Descemet's membrane, the basement membrane of the corneal endothelial cells. This membrane is unusual both because of its thickness (3 to 15 μm depending on age) and substructure, and because of its histological staining reactions. The corneal endothelium consists of a single layer or cuboidal cells that is 5 μm thick. These cells appear hexagonal when viewed in a flat preparation. The endothelial cells rest on Descemet's membrane and project into the anterior chamber of the eye.

Collagen accounts for about 70 per cent of the total solid content of the cornea (Maurice, 1969). Unlike other connective tissues of high collagen content, the cornea is transparent. The basis for this transparency is the precise packing order of uniform-diameter (approximately 30 μm) collagen fibrils in the corneal stroma (Maurice, 1957). Here, the corneal fibrils are organized into parallel sheets or lamellae. These lamellae are laid down with fibre axes at right angles to one another in near crystalline array giving the cornea an overall structure similar to that of plywood (Fig. 21.2).

Intensive studies over the past several years have provided considerable information on the nature of corneal collagen. It is generally agreed that the major molecular species present is a type I collagen related to the type I collagens of other tissues. This molecule species accounts for over 90 per cent of the total corneal stromal collagen (Freeman, 1978; 1981). However, there is considerable disagreement among investigators as to the nature of the minor collagen types present in the tissue. While some workers believe that the mammalian corneal stroma is exclusively type I collagen (Crabbe & Harding, 1980), others have shown the presence of type II (Harnisch, et al, 1978), type III (Schmut, 1977, 1978; Praus, et al, 1979),

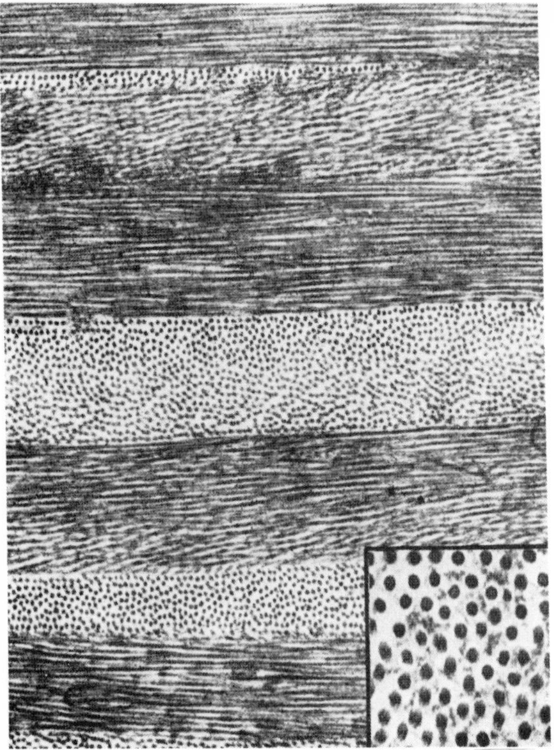

Fig. 21.2 Electron micrograph of mid-corneal stroma, showing nearby canal width of lamellae which cross each other approximately at right angles × 32 500. Inset shows fine web-like material interspersed amongst regularly spaced collagen fibrils cut transversely × 90 000. (From Tripathi R C, 1974)

type AB (Freeman, 1978; Davison, et al, 1979; Welsh, et al, 1980) and type I trimer (Freeman, 1980). In my laboratory we were unable to confirm the presence of type III collagen in any significant quantity in rabbit, bovine or human tissue, although we do not exclude the possibility of the presence of tiny amounts of this molecular species at levels detectable only by type-specific antibodies. We found type AB (Type V) collagen to represent about 7 per cent of the total corneal stromal collagen. Our results have been confirmed on rabbit and bovine cornea by other workers (Davison, et al, 1979; Welsh, et al, 1980). Type I trimer accounts for approximately 1 per cent of the total stromal collagen (Freeman, 1980).

Our studies on normal and scar tissue collagens led us to the suggestion that Type V collagen may be involved in maintenance of corneal transparency, perhaps by facilitation of interaction of the collagen with the interfibrillar matrix materials (Freeman, 1978). It should be noted that the actual position of this molecular species in the stroma is not known, although our preliminary studies have indicated it may be on the surface of the corneal fibrils or associated with corneal stromal fibroblast surface membranes.

Structural studies on corneal type I collagen show that the molecule is very similar to type I collagens from other sources (Harding et al, 1979; Freeman, 1974, 1978, 1981a). However, the level of hydroxylysine glycosylation appears to be higher than that of skin and the quantity of attached hydroxylysine glycoside is larger than that seen in any other type I collagen (Freeman, 1974, 1981a). This high glycoside level appears in some way to relate to the control of the fibril diameter seen in the tissue. Schofield et al (1971) pointed out that high glycoside levels in collagen fibrils are associated both with narrow fibril diameters and with precise control over the range of fibril diameters in the tissue. It should be noted that about 90 per cent of corneal collagen fibrils are maintained within the diameter range 25 to 35 μm.

Although there is some evidence from genetic (Church, 1981) and structural (Kao & Foreman, 1980) studies that corneal type I collagen is a different gene product from skin type I collagen, structural studies of the processed molecules obtained by limited-pepsin digestion of the tissues were only able to identify differences at the post-translational level. In particular, tissue-specific cross-links appear to be present in corneal type I collagen (Freeman, 1981a).

Although investigators agree that type I procollagen is the major collagenous product of corneal fibroblasts in culture (Stoesser et al, 1978; Yue et al, 1979; Church, 1980; Freeman, 1981b), the confusion with regard to minor collagen types extends to tissue culture studies. Yue et al (1979) reported synthesis of type V in culture, in addition to type I. Others have seen type III in culture (Newsome et al, 1980; Wollensak et al, 1980).

Church's group believe that type I collagen is the only synthetic product of human and bovine stromal fibroblasts (Stoesset et al, 1978; Church, 1980). In my laboratory, rabbit fibroblasts were found to synthesize type I and type I trimer in a ratio 70:30. No other collagen types were synthesized in significant amounts (Freeman, 1981b). Presumably these differences will be clarified as more studies emerge.

In addition to the fibrous stroma many studies have recently been reported on the limiting membranes of the cornea. Descemet's membrane is relatively easy to isolate, but despite extensive work over the past several years, characterization of the collagenous constituents is not complete (Kefalides, 1978).

Biosynthetic studies have been carried out on corneal epithelial cell explants (Hay, 1977) on endothelial-Descemet's membrane explants, and on cells in culture (Sundar-Raj et al, 1980). Corneal endothelial cells appear to be relatively easy to cultivate and study (Yue et al, 1979; Sundar-Raj et al, 1979). These studies have confirmed the ability of the cells to synthesize collagenous basement membrane-like components but detailed structural studies are still lacking.

Sclera

The sclera is the most important ocular supporting tissue. It accounts for approximately five-sixths of the outer tunic of the eye. Aside from its role in protecting the intraocular contents from injury, the sclera is rigid enough to allow the intraocular pressure to be maintained under relatively constant conditions and to allow movements of the globe without distortion of the retinal image (Watson & Hazelman, 1976).

The inherent strength, elasticity and resilience of the sclera is due largely to the interlacing collagen bundles that account for approximately 80 per cent of the dry weight of the tissue. These fibrils are similar to those of tendon and skin (Fig. 21.3). Unlike the collagen fibrils of the cornea, those of the sclera vary greatly in diameter, ranging from 30 to 300 μm, even within the same fibre bundle, the dimensions and course of the bundles differ from the superficial to the deep portions of the sclera and also from the anterior to the posterior regions; they also branch extensively and intermingle in various planes. The bundles are strengthened by elastic fibres, particularly at the equator, and at the scleral spur and are contoured away from the muscle insertions to resist the stresses imposed by the extraocular muscles. The fibre interdigitations are particularly dense around the posterior pole, presumably to ensure rigidity of this optically critical area.

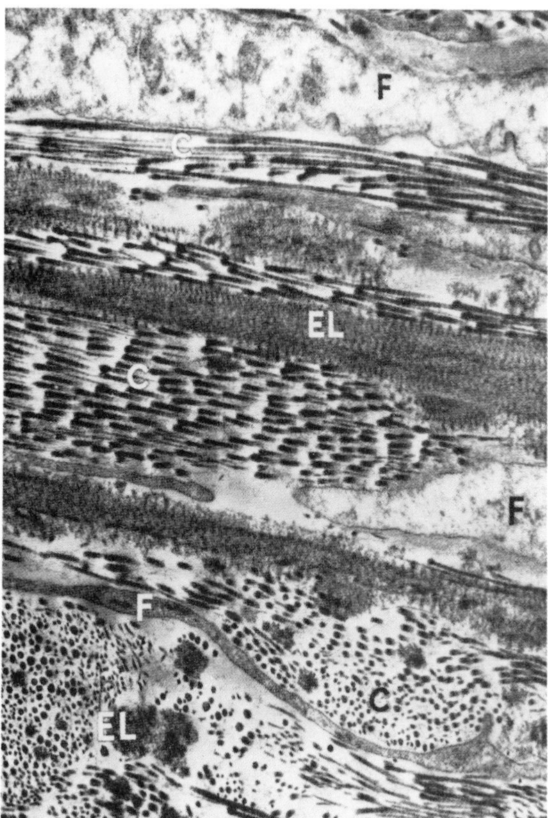

Fig. 21.3 Electron micrograph of the anterior scleral stroma, showing collagen fibrils (C), elastic fibres (EL), and fibroblasts (F). Note that the fibrils are cut in various planes, unlike the perpendicular arrangement in the cornea × 26 000. (From Tripathi T C, 1974)

Bovine sclera contains predominantly type I collagen, with type III as a minor component (Schmut, 1977; 1978). These molecular species have also been found in human sclera, with type I collagen accounting for approximately 94 per cent of the total and type III accounting for the remaining 6 per cent (Freeman 1981c). No other collagen types were found to contribute significantly to the bulk of human scleral collagen. In the avian eye a hyaline cartilagenous scleral support ring is present and type II collagen has been detected (Trelstad & Kang, 1974).

The role that these different molecular species perform in the organization and functioning of the sclera is not yet understood. Type III collagen is widely distributed throughout the tissues of the body. In vitro studies have shown that type I collagen forms thick bundles of fibres, whereas type III collagen shows thin, isolated bundles (Lapière et al, 1977). Mixtures of both type I and type III show bundles with thicknesses varying with the respective concentrations of the two types of molecule (Lapière et al, 1977; Newsome et al, 1980). Although the mechanism by which the interaction between the two types of molecule exerts its influence on the architectural organization is not yet known, it has been suggested that this is probably related to the chemical nature of the helical part of the molecules (Lapière et al, 1977). Presumably shifts in the proportion of type I and type III collagens produce simultaneous changes in mechanical properties. Type III collagen appears to be present in substantial amounts in those tissues whose physiological function requires a considerable degree of elasticity, such as skin, aorta and periodontal ligament (Epstein & Munderloh, 1975) and the presence of this molecular species in sclera may reflect the requirement for similar mechanical properties in this tissue.

An understanding of the nature of the interaction of type III collagen with type I in the sclera may provide a molecular basis for the structural changes which result in progressive myopia and some cases of low tension glaucoma.

In these cases, pathological manifestations could be due to changes in tissue distensibility produced by a shift in the rate of synthesis or degradation of one or other of the collagen types.

Changes in the proportions of collagen types may also occur during the critical phases of development. An example illustrating this possibility has been documented in the heritable disorder osteogenesis imperfecta. In one form of this disease the relative ratios of collagen type I and type III is disturbed, such that an excessive amount of type III collagen is present. Patients with this disease present with thin and supple skin and transparent scleras (Penttinen et al, 1975).

Vitreous

The vitreous body occupies about 80 per cent of the total intraocular volume. It is a formed gel which consists almost entirely (99 per cent) of water. It has evolved to serve as a transparent medium and to absorb and redistribute forces applied to the surrounding tissues (Gartner, 1975). Essentially the vitrous consists of a continuous network of fibrils embedded in a matrix consisting of highly-hydrated hyaluronic acid and soluble proteins (Reeser & Aaberg, 1979).

The collagenous nature of the vitrous fibrils has been demonstrated morphologically, biochemically and by X-ray diffraction (Reeser & Aaberg, 1979). The collagen fibrils are fine (diameters of 10 to 20 μm are usually quoted) and fairly uniform in diameter. The axial periodicity of the fibrils is indistinct. In fact, electron microscopic attempts to probe the fibrillar fine structure have led to apparently contradictory results. This confusion has been attributed to differences in tissue preparation and in staining procedures (Snowden & Swann, 1980). However, another interpretation could be that the packing arrangement of the collagen molecules is vitreous fibrils is such that the characteristic 64 μm axial periodicity is not seen in collagens from this source (Olsen, 1965; Snowden & Swann, 1980).

Recent studies by Swann and his colleagues (Swann et al, 1976, 1977; Swann & Sotman, 1980; Snowden & Swann, 1980) have established type II collagen as the major collagenous species of mammalian vitreous. Vitreous type II collagen, however, is not identical to that derived from articular cartilage. Examination of the collagen α-chains by SDS-PAGE reveals a major component that migrates at the α_1(II) position, variable amounts of a component that migrates more slowly and several low molecular weight species. After reduction alkylation and repepsinization the amount of the slower migrating (high molecular weight) material is reduced. Swann explains these findings as being due to the presence, in vitreous type II collagen, of additional terminal peptides which are resistant to pepsin attack. He suggests that pepsin-resistance indicates that these extensions are partly helical like the main body of the collagen molecule. He postulates that the presence of these extensions is necessary to promote the formation of the fine polydisperse fibrils characteristic of normal vitreous and necessary for vitreal clarity (Swann & Sotman, 1980).

Despite these differences in the extrahelical peptides many of the features of vitreous collagen are very similar to those of cartilage type II collagen, particularly with regard to the helical region of these molecules. The similarities include amino acid composition (Swann et al, 1972), the types of cyanogen bromide peptides (Swann et al, 1977), the length of the helical regions (Olsen, 1965) and the thermal stability of the molecules and distribution of polar amino acids along the helical regions (Snowden & Swann, 1980). These latter studies suggest that the organization of the collagen molecules in the collagen fibrils of these two tissues is similar.

Retina

Mechanical support for the delicate light-sensitive retina is provided by Bruch's membrane. This multi-layered structure consists of a grill-work of long thin criss-crossed elastic fibres sandwiched between two collagenous layers. The 'sandwich' is contained by the basement membrane of the pigment epithelial cells on the retinal side and by the basement membrane of the choriocapillaris endothelial cells on the choroidal side. Loosely arranged collagen fibres measuring about 60 μm in diameter and displaying the characteristic 67 μm periodicity can be found, both in the two collagenous layers and randomly passing back and forth through the elastic grill-work (Hogan et al, 1971).

Although their detailed physiological role is poorly understood, assembly and maintenance of Bruch's membrane appears to be partly the responsibility of the pigment epithelial cells. Newsome & Kenyon (1973) examined cloned colonies of chick embryo retinal pigment epithelial cells in culture. These colonies deposited basement membrane material and striated collagen fibrils intracellularly beneath the basal surfaces of the cells. The conditions chosen for tissue culture have been shown to dramatically affect pigment epithelial cell morphology characteristics (Israel et al, 1980). While the conditions chosen by Newsome and Kenyon produced colonies of cuboidal cells closely resembling their in vivo counterparts, other conditions result in rapid cell proliferation and a change to a fibroblast-like spindle morphology. This morphology change is similar to that produced in vivo by retinal pigment epithelial cells subject to insult. In the eye, these fibroblast-like cells produce opaque fibrous scar tissue bands whose traction effects may induce retinal detachment (Machemer & Laqua, 1975). Burke & Kower (1980) suggested that a substantial portion of the collagen deposited intravitreally by invading cells might be of the type I variety. Studies in my laboratory have shown that adult rabbit pigment epithelial cells grown in cell culture conditions which favour fibroblastic morphology produce type I and III collagens in a ratio of 3:1 and thus resemble skin fibroblasts in culture (Freeman, Evans & Sundar-Raj, unpublished data). This finding may be important in light of the study of Algvere & Kock (1976) who demonstrated retinal detachment after introducing collagen-producing fibroblasts into the vitreous.

In addition to the pigment epithelial cells, the neural retina itself has the capacity to synthesize collagen. The processes of the retinal Müller cells extend into the collagen layer at the vitreoretinal junction. This membranous collagen layer appears to be a product of these astrocytic glial cells (Uga & Smelser, 1973).

In tissue culture these cells secrete 90 per cent type I collagen. Most of the remaining collagen output is type V (Burke & Kower, 1980). Unlike the adult rabbit pigment epithelial cells, these glial cells did not synthesize significant quantities of type III collagen. The study by Burke & Kower (1980) also suggests that adult rabbit neural retina does not secrete vitreous type II collagen, whereas during embryogenesis the output of type II collagen is significant (Smith et al, 1976; von der Mark et al, 1977). Type II collagen synthesis appears to decline with embryonic age and the synthesis of type I collagen gradually becomes predominant (Newsome, 1976). Embryonic chick neural retina retains the capacity to synthesize type II precursors in short-term monolayer culture and also produces small amounts of other, incompletely characterized collagen species (Linsenmayer & Little, 1978).

Lens

The lens is surrounded by a prominent collagenous basal lamina. Because of its relative accessibility the nature of the collagenous components of the lens capsule have been the subject of many recent structural and biosynthetic studies. However, interpretation of experimental results has led to much controversy about the primary structure of basement membrane collagens. While pepsin-treatment has been most useful in structural studies of the fibrous collagens, the basement membrane molecules contain several centrally-located pepsin sensitive sites (Gay & Miller, 1979; Crouch et al, 1980). This chain fragility has led to difficulties in determining the exact size of the constituent molecules. However, detailed amino acid analysis of the individual components (Dixit & Kang, 1979) and bisoynthetic studies (Freeman & Sundar-Raj, 1981) have provided evidence for two procollagen sized collagen chains designated α_1(IV) and α_2(IV). A detailed discussion of the nature of the basement membrane collagens, and the heterogeneity due to current study methods are to be found elsewhere in this volume (Ch. 17).

Other eye tissues

Schmut (1978) showed that collagen accounted for approximately 41 to 49 per cent of the dry weight of the uvea (the iris, ciliary body and choroid) of the bovine eye. Studies on acid-soluble and pepsin-solubilized collagens, including differential salt precipitation, electrophoretic mobility in polyacrylamide gels and examination of CNBr-derived fragments indicated that this collagen was a mixture of type I and type III.

Although many authors still believe that the zonular fibres (suspensory apparatus of the lens) contain collagen (Gartner, 1965) the biochemical evidence is now convincing that isolated zonular fibres do *not* contain hydroxyproline and are therefore noncollagenous (Freeman, 1974; Schmut, 1978). Much of the earlier confusion appears to be due to contamination of the posterior leaf of the zonule with vitreous fibrils or with collagen from the base of the ciliary body (Freeman, 1974). It should be noted, however, that zonular fibres contain a noncollagenous protein band which migrates in the α-chain position of collagen on gel electrophoresis.

ASPECTS OF OCULAR PATHOGENESIS

Damage to the avascular cornea can result in a number of responses depending on the nature of the insult and the state of the defence mechanisms of the organism. In the cornea an initial common cellular response to injury can result in further tissue destruction by an inappropriate cellular response, which can lead to ulceration and perforation; healing with the production of an opaque vascular scar, or the invasion of the cornea with vessels, resulting in opacities due to vascular scar formation.

The cell biology of corneal ulceration

Ulceration can result from infection or chemical trauma and can exist in association with autoimmune diseases and nutritional deficiencies. Independent of the specific aetiology of the ulceration, there is a correlation between the development of the destructive process and the presence of defects in the corneal epithelium. It appears that the defective epithelial cells release plasminogen activator, which initiates several plasmin-dependent processes which result in the activation of latent degradative enzymes such as collagenase, the stimulation of de novo synthesis of destructive enzymes locally and the attraction of polymorphonuclear leucocytes (PMNs) to the site of injury (Berman, 1978). In addition, plasmin is known to cause permeability changes in blood vessels by generating kinins. Thus the damaged epithelial cells may also be partly responsible for causing an inflammatory leak into the stroma.

PMNs arrive at the site of injury by migrating directly from the perilimbal conjunctival blood vessels into the corneal stroma.

They can also arrive at the site of injury by indirect passage across the conjunctival epithelium into the tear fluid from whence they are conducted to the area of damage. Tear fluid PMNs enter the site of injury faster than stromal PMNs and are able to attach to those parts of the corneal surface denuded of epithelium. The rapid mobilization of PMNs from the vascular conjunctiva into tear fluid and thence to the site of epithelial damage is a unique transport method which has presumably evolved to circumvent the problems of corneal avascularity. Although the peak PMN response depends on the type of injury,

PMNs have been seen in the peripheral cornea within 2 to 6 hours of injury.

The activation of plasminogen in the superficial stroma by the products of the injured epithelium results in the generation of C3a from the third component of complement. This substance is chemotactic for PMNs and may be the prime attractive factor in the cornea. However, this is still a matter of controversy and one recent study has implicated arachidonic acid metabolites in the mediation of PMN chemotaxis (Srinivasan & Kulkarni, 1980). It seems likely that plasmin-dependent events are amplified both by the newly-arrived PMNs and by the activation of local corneal fibroblasts, since recent work has shown that all these cell types are capable of secreting plasminogen-activator in ulcerating corneas (Berman et al, 1980).

One of these events, the activation of latent collagenase, appears to be linked to plasminogen-activation in a dose-response manner. Although the exact details are still not clear, it has been suggested that plasminogen is the rate-limiting factor in stomal matrix degradation. The details of the mechanism of activation are currently an area of great interest and the interested reader is encouraged to turn to the chapter by Werb in this volume (Ch. 7) and to the review by Berman (1980) for further details.

The initial cellular processes of ulceration are similar to those of healing. However, it appears that the degradation processes become more established than those of repair. This suggestion seems to be borne out by the work of Pfister & Paterson (1977), and Wishard & Paterson (1980) who suggest that severe acid or alkali burns destroy the supply routes of ascorbate to the cornea. Ascorbate is a necessary cofactor in collagen biosynthesis. The tissue is therefore unable to exercise the normal reparative process. These workers showed that exogenously administered ascorbate permitted more rapid healing in the face of collagen breakdown and significantly reduced the incidence of corneal ulceration and perforation.

Although the supply of ascorbate may not be limiting in situations other than chemical burns, any factor affecting the fine balance between synthesis and degradation could compromise repair in the ulcerative situation. Compromised repair may explain the clinical observation that corticosteroids exacerbate corneal destruction, since they suppress the syntheses of matrix materials which form the bed in which the collagen fibres lie, and hence tip the balance in favour of destruction (Berman, 1978).

Corneal wound healing

An overview of the repair processes taking place in the healing cornea in health and disease has recently appeared (Baum & Silbert, 1978). The cellular response to injury has been described in the previous section. In this section, we will only consider the role of the collagens in stromal healing.

According to current theory, corneal transparency depends on restrictions in the cross-sectional diameter of collagen fibrils and the size of the interfibrillar spaces. The lack of transparency in human corneal scars has been ascribed to the increased thickness and diminished number of collagen fibrils in the tissue (Schwarz & Graf Keyserlingk, 1969).

The physical properties of corneal stromal scar have been shown to be significantly different from those of the normal cornea (Gasset & Dohlman, 1968). Scar tissue is markedly inelastic when compared to normal stroma, and it is consistently lower in mechanical strength. It is also opaque. These differences appear to be due to altered organizational patterns of the lamellae and their collagen fibrils in the scar (Jakus, 1962; Schwarz & Graf-Keyserlingk, 1969).

The differences seen in scar tissue may be the result of changes in the nature of the collagen laid down in the scar, changes in the matrix in which the fibres are laid down, or both. Cinton & Kublin (1977) showed a similarity between the glycosaminoglycans laid down in penetrating rabbit corneal wounds with those of fetal corneas, suggesting a true regenerative process. This milieu may be responsible for the remarkable similarity in collagen fibril size seen in 3-week corneal wounds and 21-day old fetal corneas (Cintron, et al, 1978).

In the healing rabbit cornea collagen accumulation is very rapid during the first 2 weeks, but becomes gradual after the second week. It is not yet known whether this reflects a decreased rate of collagen synthesis or an increased breakdown since there is evidence of a collagenolytic system playing a role in corneal wound repair (Cintron et al, 1973).

Recent studies have suggested that the collagen laid down in corneal scar is markedly different from that in normal tissue. Freeman (1980) found that like normal cornea, the scar tissue which filled a penetrating wound consisted of a type I collagen variant. However, a dramatic change in the minor collagen types present was noted. Freeman's (1980) results indicated a switchover from type V collagen to type I trimer during scar formation. Previous studies had suggested that type V collagen was an important factor in determining organization of corneal collagen, and this led to the suggestion that the opaque corneal scar could be the result of the absence of an appropriate quantity of this collagenous species in the regenerating tissue.

Sufficient information is not yet available with regard to the physical properties of type I trimer collagen or its mode of interaction with the scar components to define its structural role. It is obviously essential to determine the contribution of this collagen type to the mechanical properties of the scar, and what effect, if any, a variation of the ratio of collagen types would have on determining mechanical properties. Recent studies (Freeman, 1981) have shown that corneal fibroblasts in culture behave like those in a corneal scar with respect to their collagen production, thus providing an experimental system to test these parameters.

A changeover of collagen types in the scar correlates with the changes in a hydroxylysine glycosides (Cintron, 1974) and cross-links (Cannon & Cintron, 1975; Cintron, et al, 1978) observed by others. It should be noted, however, that the relationship of cross-links to collagen type is still not known, so that the significance of these changes in collagen cross-linking is unclear.

Further understanding of the nature of the response of the corneal fibroblast in the healing wound is very important in terms of potential pharmacological intervention. Pharmacological intervention at appropriate control points in the regenerative pathways may enable us to accelerate or slow down the healing process at will, or to induce the cells in the healing tissue to regenerate normal corneal-tissue into the wound, instead of filling the gaps with scar.

Ocular neovascularization

Neovascularization that occurs in the cornea, on the iris, from the choroid and from the retinal vessels, accounts for the greatest amount of ocular morbidity in the United States, and is a significant cause of visual loss in other countries.

Invasion of the cornea by blood vessels from the surrounding structures is a response common to a wide variety of injuries to the cornea. Although not completely understood, this process may result from the destruction of an inherent inhibitor of vascularization in the cornea, or from release of an as yet unidentified angiogenic factor. Blood vessels invade the cornea predominantly, if not exclusively, in those situations in which the acute inflammatory response is evoked.

The role of polymorphonuclear leucocytes and other leucocytes in neovascularization is not completely understood. Presumably they produce initiators or inactivate inhibitors of vascularization. Their role may be facilitatory or augmentative. Morphological studies (McCracken et al, 1979) have established that during the acute inflammatory stage, the pericorneal vessels undergo mitosis, thus demonstrating a proliferative response soon after injury. The nature and source of the initiators of corneal vascularization remains unknown, although several biogenic amines including histamines are capable of stimulating vessel growth and prostaglandin E_1 appears to be especially potent (McCracken et al, 1979). However, it appears likely that polypeptide factors related to tumour angiogenesis factor will ultimately be confirmed as the initiators of corneal new vessel formation, and the smaller molecules are probably involved in a secondary, facilitative or augmentative role.

Neovascularization in the retina is a significant complication of proliferative diabetic retinopathy. It is characterized by growth of vessels with abnormal configurotions in a plane anterior to that of the normal retinal vessels. These vessels often extend into the vitreous cavity.

Although inflammation appears to play a role in corneal neovascularization, the latest studies on the aetiology of proliferative diabetic retinopathy, retrolental fibroplasia and branch vein occlusion suggest that new vessel formation is always preceded by capillary non-perfusion (Patz, 1980). The resultant ischaemia leads to the production of 'angiogenesis (vasoproliferative) factor' which diffuses from the area of ischaemia to initiate the new vessel formation from adjacent retinal vessels (Fig. 2.4). Although much evidence for this suggestion is still lacking, the hypothesis has received circumstantial support from the success of photocoagulation in the treatment of neovascularization. Photocoagulation is often followed by regression of the new vessels. It is thought that the technique destroys or changes the ischaemic retina in such a way that the production of vasoproliferative factor is

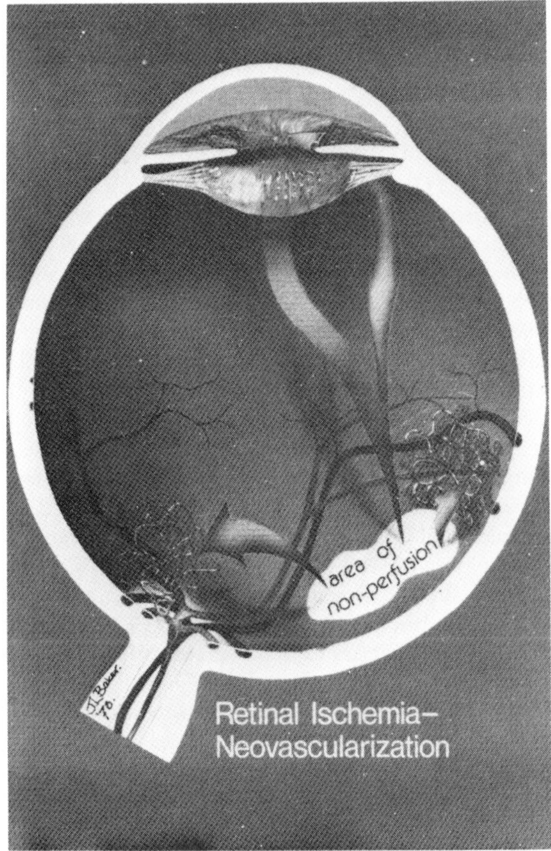

Fig. 21.4 Area of nonperfusion from retinal capillary closure. The resultant ischaemia is presumed to liberate a diffusible angiogenesis substance that stimulates neovascularization in the adjacent area, at the optic disc, or on the surface of the iris. (From Patz, 1980)

reduced or eliminated. Current work is focusing on the characterization of the angiogenic factor and on the nature and mode of action of various natural inhibitors that have been identified in relatively avascular tissues such as vitreous and cartilage. Eye tissues appear to provide a number of extremely versatile model systems for testing the role of putative inhibitors and initiators of vessel proliferation.

THE EYE AND COLLAGEN DISEASES

Osteogenesis imperfecta

This is a heterogeneous group of disorders with fragile and easily fractured bones. The ear, ligaments, tendons, dentin and the cornea and sclera are frequently involved as well. A congenital opacity in the periphery of the cornea (arcus juvenilis or embryotoxon) is a frequent finding in osteogenesis imperfecta (OI). The cornea is often thinner than normal and hypermetropia is frequently seen. Other ocular manifestations include glaucoma, ectopia lentis, keratoconus, megalocornea and maculae corneae. One of the most consistent clinical findings in OI is blue sclera (McKusick, 1972), but some patients with normal white sclera have unmistakable signs of OI. The wide variations in tissue involvements and genetic heterogeneity have been an obstacle in classification of the different types of OI, but on the basis of clinical and genetic data at least four types can currently be distinguished (Sillence et al, 1980; Bornstein & Byers, 1980). Types I and II have blue sclera.

The most common variety is probably type I (dominant with blue sclera). As the name implies, this form is inherited in an autosomal-dominant manner. Deformity is unusual and the onset of multiple fractures occurs after birth. Joint laxity is common in children and the sclera is blue. The blue scleral appearance may be due to alterations in the light scattering properties of the tissue or to a thinning such that the darkly pigmented choroid shows through.

Biochemical studies indicate that an altered ratio of collagen types is present in the skin or individuals with this disorder, due to decreased relative amounts of type I collagen in relation to type III (Sykes et al, 1977). A similar alteration may be the cause of the altered optical properties of the sclera.

OI types II and III are characterized by perinatal bone fracturing and can be diagnosed in affected infants at birth or even prenatally. In the older system of classification these forms could be 'congenital' types of OI.

Osteogenesis imperfecta type II, the lethal perinatal form, is the most severe form of OI; about 50 per cent of affected individuals are stillborn and the remainder die shortly after birth. Characteristically, the femurs have an accordion-like crumpled appearance. There is virtually no ossification of the cranial vault and the sclerae are dark blue. Trelstad et al (1977) examined pepsin-derived collagens from the cornea, sclera and other connective tissues of a deceased 4-day-old girl affected with this form of OI. They found that corneal stromal collagen was principally type I as had been found for normal corneal stroma. However, the hydroxylysine level of the collagen from the OI cornea was increased over that of a normal control by 30 to 40 per cent. A slight increase in lysyl hydroxylation was evident in the scleral collagen. These increases parallelled an increase in bone hydroxylation and confirmed the earlier findings of increased lysine hydroxylation in the connective tissues of patients with this disorder (Bleckmann et al, 1971; Eastoe et al, 1973). Examination of several tissues for covalently-linked sugars showed increased levels of hydroxylysine glycosides. This was particularly evident in bone. Although the corneal and scleral collagens were not examined, changes in the levels of glycosylation may also be part of the molecular basis of the disease. Presumably excessive or inappropriately located hydroxylysyl residues or their glycosylated derivates can have significant effects on fibril formation. Indeed, one study has reported an abnormality of collagen cross-links in bone tissue (Fuju & Tanzer, 1977). Defective fibril formation may result, for example, in the disarray of bone collagen fibrils seen in some cases (Lindenfelser et al, 1972).

However, electron microscopic examination of thin sections of fixed and embedded corneal stroma from Trelstad et al's patient showed the majority of fibrils in the normal range; with lamellar organization typical of the normal tissue. These studies were in contrast to others where the collagen fibril diameters in mid-cornea were reduced 30 per cent in comparison to controls (Blumcke et al, 1972; Riley et al, 1973). Vacuolar distentions of the rough endoplasmic reticulum in both keratocytes and scleral fibrocytes have been noted in the cornea and sclera of patients with OI, presumably reflecting the intracellular metabolic defect in protein synthesis (Blumcke, et al, 1972; Eichholtz & Müller, 1972).

Osteogenesis imperfecta type III (the progressive deforming type with normal sclerae) is also characterized by perinatal fracturing, but affected infants — in contrast to those with type II OI — are generally of normal weight and length at the time of birth. The case described by Meigel et al (1974), had normal fundi and sclerae and a hyperopia of 4 diopters. Fibroblast cultures from skin biopsies of this patient revealed the absence of collagen α_2 chains, presumably resulting in the inability to produce normal amounts of type I collagen. In another patient with this type of OI agyrophilic reticular fibres and decreased proportions of normal staining collagen were found in the skin (Follis, 1953). The agyrophilic fibres may represent type III collagen (Huang, 1977).

The fourth category, OI type IV, has dominant inheritance and normal sclera. Dentogenesis imperfecta is frequently severe and hearing loss is rare. The distinction between OI type III and OI type IV is based, in part, on the patient's family history.

Ehlers-Danlos syndrome

This syndrome has been subdivided into at least seven forms on the basis of clinical, genetic and more recently biochemical information (Bauer & Uitto, 1979; Bornstein & Byers, 1980). The common clinical features are soft, velvety, hyperextensible skin which is easily torn and often leaves gaping wounds when cut. As these gaping wounds heal, thin 'cigarette-paper' scars form. There is easy bruisability and frequently a bleeding diathesis. The joints are hypermobile and easily dislocated. Remarkably, the bones are not involved in the Ehlers-Danlos syndrome (Uitto & Lichtenstein, 1976). In general, serious ophthalmalogical problems are rare, but minor changes may include myopia, strabismus and epicanthal folds. Fuxa & Brandt (1975) compiled a literature review of alterations in the eye associated with Ehlers-Danlos syndrome.

Ehlers-Danlos syndrome type VI, the hydroxylysine deficient variant, has been called the 'ocular' form because of association with severe ocular problems. However, many of the cases currently classified as type VI variants may represent examples of 'fragilitis oculi.'

Pinnell et al (1972), reported two patients whose dermal collagen was deficient in hydroxylysine and Sussman et al (1974) made a similar finding in another patient. In both studies it has been possible to correlate the clinical observations with reduced activities of the enzyme lysyl hydroxylase (Krane et al, 1972; Sussman et al, 1974). Steinmann et al (1975) reported two cases where the deficiency of hydroxylysine in the skin was mild, but cultured fibroblasts has markedly reduced lysyl hydroxylase activity. These workers suggested that amino acid analysis of skin was therefore inadequate for diagnosis of Ehlers-Danlos type VI. A more recent report confirms its tentative diagnosis by both chemical analysis and skin fibroblast culture (Krieg et al, 1979), a two-pronged attack which may be more appropriate in the light of tissue-variability of lysine hydroxylation (Quinn & Krane, 1979).

Although fragile globes have been reported in cases with biochemically demonstrable lysyl hydroxylase deficiency, a more consistent finding associated with typical Ehlers-Danlos signs is microcorneae. It is possible that the more severe cases, including those with megalocornea, are really cases of fragilitis oculi or keratoglobus-blue sclera.

Keratoconus

Keratoconus is a non-inflammatory condition showing thinning and ectasia (dilatation) of the central cornea. It is not yet clear whether the thinning is due to a reduction in the *number* of lamellae present, or to a reduction in thickness of individual lamellae (Bron et al, 1978). The corneal ectasia appears to be due to an increased distensibility of the keratoconus cornea compared to the normal cornea (Bron et al, 1978; Foster & Yamamoto, 1978).

In the advanced stages, Bowman's membrane fragments and the superficial lamellae are replaced by an irregularly-arranged loose fibrocellular connective tissue (Patas Joyon & Roucher, 1970). Degenerative abnormalities appear in the basal epithelium and an osmophilic material accumulates between this layer and the basement membrane.

Scarring is an increasingly prominent feature of advancing keratoconus. Scarring occurs at all levels in the cornea and may present as reticular branching opacities, fine white striae, compaction of collagen at the junction of Bowman's layer and the subadjacent stroma or small focal scars which may even affect Descemet's membrane. More extensive 'Maltese cross' scarring may develop over the apex of the cone (Bron, et al, 1978).

Keratoconus may be unilateral in some patients. The disorder can occur sporadically or in association with generalized connective tissue disorders. Both recessive and dominant forms of keratoconus are encountered. Despite these variations in associated factors, the clinical morphology and natural history of the corneal changes is remarkably stereotyped. The disorder therefore appears to represent a situation where a number of different biochemical lesions can result in a similar clinical picture.

Although the changes observed could be the manifestation of a desynchronization of the relative rates of biosynthesis of collagen, proteoglycan and structural glycoprotein (Robert & Robert, 1975; Junqua et al, 1975), much of the evidence points toward an alteration in the quality of the collagen itself. The total amount of collagen is decreased in corneal tissue and this collagen has decreased levels of both hydroxylysine and glycosylated hydroxylysine. In accordance with these findings, analysis of the collagen cross-links of keratoconus corneas showed an increase in the level of lysinonorleucine, a cross-link derived from two lysyl residues (Cannon & Foster, 1978). In normal human corneas, lysinonorleucine is a minor component (0 to 5 per cent) of the total collagen cross-links; in the keratoconus samples the percentage of lysinonorleucine ranged from 9 to 67 per cent of the total collagen cross-links. As Cannon & Foster (1978) pointed out, the character of the collagen must be unusual to give rise to this high level of lysinonorleucine on reduction.

These changes could be due to alterations in the local control of post-translational modifications of the regular collagen chains or to the intrusion of other collagen types as a result of the disease process. In a cell culture study of stromal keratocytes derived from normal and keratoconus corneas, Yue et al (1979) showed that the relative proportions of type I collagen and other collagen chains was significantly altered in the keratoconus cultures. Variations in the patterns on their analytical system were interpreted as the results of heterogeneity in the disease. This appears to correlate with the clinical data, where keratoconus has been seen in a patient whose skin showed *excess* type III collagen (Ehlers-Danlos Oxford-Bron et al, 1978) and in another patient who had *decreased or absent* type III synthesis (Ehlers-Danlos IV-Kuming & Jaffe, 1977). Although collagen type III is not usually found in the cornea (vide supra), immunofluorescent studies have shown large amounts of collagen type III wrapped around the unusually spaced type I collagen in keratoconus corneas (Maumenee, 1978). These studies have to be viewed with caution, however, because they could represent secondary changes due to the repair process (Maumenee, 1978; Yue et al, 1979).

Changes in relative amounts of the genetically distinct collagen chains do not explain the observation that keratoconus has been seen in the so-called ocular form of Ehlers-Danlos syndrome (type VI) where the biochemical lesion is probably a deficiency in the enzyme lysyl hydroxylase (vide supra). Nor do they explain the fact that 50 per cent of a series of patients with Ehlers-Danlos type II — mitis type, where the biochemical disorder is unknown — had keratoconus (Robertson, 1975). It should be appreciated that in evaluating the biochemistry of this and similar heterogeneous biochemical disorders, it is important to identify the different clinical sub-groups when pooling corneal tissue for biochemical analysis or for establishing cell cultures. It is also important to exclude those tissue samples which contain excessive scar tissue since they will result in information more related to secondary changes as a result of repair.

Keratoglobus and blue sclera

Keratoglobus is a rare, bilateral globular configuration of the cornea. The cornea is transparent, but shows uniform and extreme thinning of the stroma to one-fifth of the normal thickness. It is prone to rupture following minor trauma. Although keratoglobus is considered to be a developmental anomaly, it can develop in adulthood (Biglan et al, 1977). Keratoglobus may be genetically related to keratoconus (Cavara, 1950).

A distinct heritable connective tissue disorder has been described consisting of keratoconus or keratoglobus, blue sclera and one or more of the following features: hyperextensibility of joints, abnormal teeth, reduced hearing, fractures, consanguinity and perforations of the cornea after minimal trauma (Biglan et al, 1977). Although this syndrome has some clinical features in common with the 'ocular' form of Ehlers-Danlos syndrome (type VI) and osteogenesis imperfecta, preliminary biochemical studies in my laboratory appear to confirm that keratoglobus-blue sclera is indeed a distinct entity. We could find no differences in the ratios of collagen types in skin biopsies obtained from two affected individuals and normal age and sex-matched controls. Nor could we find significant differences in the levels of lysine hydroxylation. However, both samples of skin from affected patients showed significant differences in the amount of hydroxylysine glycosides and the ratios of disaccharide to mono-saccharide-linked hydroxylysine. The skin was also more resistant to solubilization by limited pepsin digestion than the normal controls. These results may suggest that there is a primary biochemical defect at the post-translational level in the keratoglobus-blue sclera syndrome.

Fragilitis oculi

This disorder shares some clinical features in common with Ehlers-Danlos syndrome type VI, the Marfan syndrome and osteogenesis imperfecta (McKusick, 1972). There are considerable overlaps with keratoglobus-blue sclera and keratoconus is a common finding. An overlap in classification with Ehlers-Danlos syndrome has probably led to some confusion in understanding this disorder.

Fragilitis oculi is a generalized connective tissue disorder characterized by rupture of the globe, particularly the cornea, by minor trauma. Keratoglobus or keratoconus and blue sclerae are common findings. The intraocular pressure is normal. Other features include scoliosis, dolichostenomelia, hyperextensible joints, hearing defects, hernias, retinal detachment, myopia and fragilitis ossium. The disorder has autosomal recessive inheritance (Bertelgen, 1968; Stein et al, 1968; Judisch et al, 1976; Behrens-Baumann et al, 1977).

This disorder can be distinguished biochemically from Ehlers-Danlos type VI by analysis of cultured skin fibroblasts from the patients. Assays reveal normal levels of lysyl hydroxylase, the enzyme which is reduced in the Ehlers-Danlos variant (Judisch et al, 1976; Behrens-Baumann et al, 1977).

Spondyloepithelial dysplasias

The spondyloepithelial dysplasias (SEDs) are a group of inherited disorders which have in common skeletal dysplasia involving both the spine and the epipheses of the major long bones, but which differ in clinical findings, age of onset of clinically significant disability, underlying biochemical defect and mode of inheritance (Spranger & Langer, 1974).

Byers et al (1978) examined a family with a variety of this disorder characterized by punctate corneal dystrophy and markedly abnormal dermal collagen fibrils. In the electron microscope areas of atypical tissue contained collagen fibrils which were grouped adjacent to apprently normal regions, but were coiled, folded back on themselves and partly dissociated into finer component elements. Positions of some of the fibrils appeared to be 'unravelled.' The mechanism of fibril destabilization seen in this disorder is unclear, but the alterations in collagen may be secondary to changes in the control of proeoglycan deposition. It is likely that the punctate densities in the cornea are similar in organization to the abnormal areas of the dermis (Byers et al, 1978).

Marfan syndrome

This syndrome is manifested by dominant inheritance and ocular, skeletal and cardiovascular defects. The latter complications account for the decreased life span of patients with this syndrome. Like osteogenesis imperfecta, this heritable disorder may be heterogeneous biochemically (Bornstein & Byers, 1980). Careful clinical evaluation can differentiate 'contractural arachnodactyly' and 'the Marfanoid hypermobility syndrome' from the classical aesthenic variety.

The ocular complications of the Marfan syndrome are highly significant in making a diagnosis (McKusick, 1972). About 80 per cent of the patients have ectopia lentis, the manifestations of which range from frank dislocation with resultant glaucoma, myopia and retinal detachment, to mild subluxation that is evident only by careful slit-lamp examination through well-dilated pupils (Falls & Cotteman, 1943). In the slit-lamp the suspensory ligaments of the lens may appear attenuated, redundant and sometimes broken. The lens itself is most commonly displaced upward, presumably due to a weakness or to breaks in the inferior suspensory ligaments. The lens may even dislocate into the anterior chamber of the eye or dislocate backwards into the vitreous. Blue sclerae are often found in the Marfan syndrome.

The basic biochemical lesion was once thought to be a disorder of the collagen cross-linking enzymes (Neuci & Beltrami, 1968), but this is no longer thought to be the case (Bornstein & Byers, 1980). Collagen solubility is apparently increased in some cases of the Marfan syndrome (Priest et al, 1973) and there is some evidence that the collagen α_2 chain of type I collagen may be abnormal in some patients (Siegel & Chang, 1978). Another study demonstrated a reduced synthesis of type I collagen and as enhanced synthesis of type III collagen, by tissue from the aortic media and adventitia of a Marfan patient, when cultured in vitro (Kreig & Müller, 1977).

Dorfman and his colleagues showed that fibroblasts of some patients with Marfan's syndrome accummulated more hyaluronic acid than normal controls, because of increased proteoglycon synthesis (Matalon & Dorfman, 1969; Lamberg & Dorfman, 1973). Alterations in the interfibrillar matrix molecules affect the fibril formation and stability of collagen. Presumably this is the *modus operandi* in some varieties of the Marfan syndrome.

Homocystinuria

Until recently homocystinuria was not distinguished from the Marfan syndrome (Carson & Neill, 1962). However, certain clinical features, the recessive mode of inheritance and the characteristic biochemical findings, readily identify this disorder.

Although ectopia lentis and bony abnormalities are common to both homocystinuria and the Marfan syndrome, mental retardation, malar flush and increased frequency of arterial thrombosis are seen largely with homocystinuria. Various biochemical defects can result in homocystinuria. The most common is a deficiency of the enzyme cystathionine synthetase. This itself is a heterogeneous disorder, since certain persons who are treated with pyridoxal phosphate (a cofactor of cystathionine synthetase) respond with reduced plasma concentrations of homocysteine, whereas others do not (Bornstein & Byers, 1980).

The ocular hallmark of the disease is ectopia lentis. However, lens displacement tends to be downward in contrast to the upward displacement seen in the Marfan syndrome. Subluxation or dislocation of the lens is seen in 90 per cent of cases, and, unlike the Marfan syndrome, this generally does not develop before the age of 1 year (Francois, 1970). As the disorder progresses, there is usually total dislocation of the lens at age 7 years or later. Subluxation and subsequent dislocation is due to a progressive degeneration of the suspensory apparatus of the lens. The zonular fibres are deficient adjacent to the lens itself. They recoil to the ciliary body where they lie matted and retracted into a felt-work, which fuses with a greatly thickened basement membrane of the nonpigmented ciliary epithelium (Henkind & Ashton, 1965).

Other ocular features include light or blue irides in 75 per cent of cases, and depend on the albinoid appearance seen with this disorder. A high myopia is not rare in these patients and retinal detachment and optic atrophy may occur (Wollensak, 1966; Francois, 1970; Cross & Jensen, 1973).

With defective cystathionine synthetase activity, homocysteine, serine and methionine accumulate in the tissues. It was postulated that the accumulation of these metabolites interfered with the normal pattern of collagen cross-linking producing more readily extractable collagen (Harris & Sjoerdema, 1966). One postulated mechanism was by reacting with and blocking the aldehyde cross-link precursors (Kang & Trelsted, 1973). In the presence of homocysteine there is actually an accumulation of the aldehyde-derived cross-linked dehydrohydroxylysino-norleucine (Seigel, 1975). Recently an alternate theory was proposed: inhibition of the processing enzyme lysyl oxidase by the accumulated homocysteine (Lindberg et al, 1976). Either theory could account for the observed pathological changes, since changes in the cross-linking patterns of the fibrils will result in deficits in collagen tensile strength.

Alcaptonuria with ochronosis

This is an inherited disorder of amino acid metabolism in which a deficiency of the enzyme homogentisic acid oxidase causes homogentisic acid and its oxidation products to accumulate in tissues and to be excreted in the urine. The deposition in the collagen-containing tissues leads to the development of arthritis, which is the primary clinical manifestation of the disorder.

One of the first signs of the disease is deposition of pigment in the sclera at the sites of insertion of the rectus muscles. Pigmentation of the cornea, tarsal plates and eyelids may also occur. However, the ocular involvement is minor in comparison to more serious cardiovascular and rheumatological problems.

Autoimmune phenomena

The eye is often involved in systemic diseases for which an autoimmune pathology has been established (Manski et al, 1976). Criteria for establishing the extent that autoimmunity constitutes the initiating pathological mechanism as against being only a by-product of the primary disease, have been discussed with reference to the eye (Witebsky & Milgrom, 1964). However, it should be noted that much of the eye literature is restricted to studies of the autoantibody responses, since many early studies were done prior to clarification of the role of B and T-cell dependent components in the immune response, the phenomena of cellular co-operation, feedback regulation and the interplay between tolerance and immunity.

The rheumatoid group of diseases have long been known to have accompanying ocular abnormalities (Watson, 1975; Watson & Hazelman, 1976; Kearns, 1980). In children, rheumatoid arthritis (Still's disease) is associated with a triad of ocular signs — band shaped keratopathy, iridocyclitis and complicated cataract. Most often the eye signs follow the arthritic manifestations, but in rare cases they may precede the systemic disease by several years (Minton, 1957). There appears to be no relation between the severity of the systemic disease and the extent of ocular involvement. The band-shaped keratopathy develops in the interpalpebral areas of the cornea, beginning at the limbus and extending to meet axially. The keratopathy probably represents calcium deposition and scarring (Manski et al, 1976).

Ankylosing spondylitis is a rheumatic disease often accompanied by iridocyclitis. It has recently gained much attention since HLA B27 antigen is present in approximately 90 per cent of Caucasians with this disease (see Rahi, 1979; Nussenblatt, 1980).

Rheumatoid arthritis is associated with a wide variety of extraocular and intraocular complications. The most common complication is keratoconjunctivitis sicca. About 75 per cent of patients with Sjögren's disease have a rheumatoid-type of articular disease, conversely 10 per cent of patients with primary rheumatoid arthritis develop kerato conjunctivitis sicca. Other ocular manifestations of rheumatoid arthritis include episcleritis, scleritis, keratitis, scleromalacia perforans (Watson & Hazelman, 1976) and corneal ulceration (Jayson & Easty, 1977). These are all basically similar sterile inflammations involving different coats of the eye with varying severity.

They appear after pelvic or urethral infections and start with a sterile mucopurulent conjunctivitis accompanied by copious discharge. Involvement of deeper structures produces episcleritis, scleritis, iritis, optic neuritis and choroiditis. Ulcerative colitis and regional enteritis may be related in some manner to Reiter's disease. Most patients with enteritis and iritis also have inflammatory joint disturbances. Manski et al (1976), have pointed out the possibility of dissemination of the disease process from the bowel via the circulation to the eyes and joints.

Autoimmune phenomena are also thought to play a part in ocular cicatricial pemphigoid, Behcet's disease, systemic lupus erythematosus, periarteritis nodosa, Wegener's granulomatosis and Mooren's ulcer. Detailed discussion of the destructive phenomena are beyond the scope of this chapter and the reader is referred to Mondino et al (1978), Lloyd-Jones & Hemby (1978), and Watson & Hazelman (1976) for further information.

CONCLUSION

Recent advances in collagen research have added much to our understanding of the collagenous tissues of the eye. Knowledge of ocular connective tissues has been swept forward by the tide of investigation. Research has found considerable fascination with unique tissues such as the cornea and lens capsule. The eye has provided valuable models for wound healing, neovascularization, and pharmacological studies amongst others. Increased understanding of connective tissue problems have led to more sophistication in diagnosis of certain eye diseases — with the increased potential of control. Ocular connective tissue research has rapidly moved from being one of the Cinderellas of the connective tissue world to the forefront of man's attack on disease. Visual disturbances are amongst those diseases most dreaded today, and hopefully a greater understanding of the eye in health and disease will alleviate some of these problems.

REFERENCES

Algvere P, Kock E 1976 Experimental fibroplasia in the rabbit vitreous. Albrecht von Graefes, Archiv für Klinische und Experimentale Ophthalmologie 191: 215

Bauer E A, Uitto J 1979 Collagen in cutaneous diseases. International Journal of Dermatology 18: 251

Baum J L, Silbert A M 1978 Aspects of corneal wound healing in health and disease. Transactions of the Ophthalmological Society of the UK 98: 348

Behrens-Baumann W, Gebauer H J, Lagenbeck U 1977 Blaue-sklera-syndrom und keratoglobus (oculärer typ des Ehlers-Danlos syndroms). Albrecht von Graefes, Archiv for Klin und Experimentale Ophthalmologie 204: 235

Berman M 1978 Regulation of collagenase. Transactions of the Ophthalmological Societies of the United Kingdom 98: 397
Berman M 1980 Collagenase and corneal ulceration. In: Wooley D, Evanson J (eds) Collagenase in normal and pathological connective tissues. Wiley Inc, London, p 141
Berman M, Leary R, Gage J 1980 Evidence for a role of the plasminogen activator-plasmin system in corneal ulceration. Investigative Ophthalmology & Visual Science 19: 1204
Bertelsen T I 1968 Dysgenesis mesodermalis corneae et sclerae. Acta Ophthalmologica 46: 486
Biglan A W, Brown S I, Johnson B L 1977 Keratoglobus and blue sclera. American Journal of Ophthalmology 85: 225
Bleckmann H, Kresse H, Wollensak J, Buddecke E 1971 Glykosaminoglykan und kollagen analysen bei osteogenesis imperfecta. Zeitschrift für Kinderheilkund 110: 74
Blmcke S, Niedorf H R, Theil H J, Langness U 1972 Histochemical and fine structural studies on the cornea with osteogenesis imperfecta. Virchows Archives B (Zell Pathologie) 11: 124
Bornstein P, Byers P H 1980 Collagen metabolism. Current Concepts — a scope publication. The Upjohn Company
Bron A J, Tripathi R C, Harding J J, Crabbe M J C 1978 Stromal loss in keratoconus. Transactions of the Ophthalmological Society of the UK 98: 393
Burke J M, Kower H S 1980 Collagen synthesis by rabbit neural retina in vitro and in vivo. Experimental Eye Research 31: 213
Byers P H, Holbrook K A, Hall J G, Bornstein P, Chandler J W 1978 A new variety of spondyloepithelial dysplasia characterized by punctate corneal dystrophy and abnormal thermal collagen fibrils. Human Genetics 40: 157
Cannon D J, Cintron C 1975 Collagen cross-linking in corneal scar formation. Biochimica et Biophysica Acta 412: 18
Cannon D J, Foster C S 1978 Collagen cross-linking in keratoconus. Investigative Ophthalmology & Visual Science 17: 63
Cintron C, Schneider H, Kublin C L 1973 Corneal scar formation. Experimental Eye Research 17: 251
Cintron C 1974 Hydroxylysine glycosides in the collagen of normal and scarred rabbit corneas. Biochemical and Biophysical Research Communications 60: 288
Cintron C, Kublin C L 1977 Regeneration of corneal tissue. Developmental Biology 61: 346
Cintron C, Hassinger L C, Kublin C L, Cannon D J 1978 Biochemical and ultrastructural changes in collagen during corneal would healing. Journal of Ultrastructure Research 65: 13
Church R L 1980 Procollagen and collagen produced by normal bovine corneal stroma fibroblasts in cell culture. Investigative Ophthalmology & Visual Science 19: 192
Church R L 1981 Cell hybrids in ocular tissues. In: Zadunaisky J A, Davson H (eds) Current Topics in Eye Research vol III. Academic Press, New York, in press
Crabbe M J C, Harding J J 1980 Collagen cross-links in the cornea and sclera in health and disease. Proceedings of the International Society for Eye Research I, p 17 Abstract
Cross H E, Jensen A D 1973 Ocular manifestations in the Marfan syndrome and homocystinuria. American Journal of Ophthalmology 75: 405
Crouch E, Sage H, Bornstein P 1980 Structural basis for apparent heterogeneity of collagens in human basement membranes. Type V procollagen contains two distinct chains. Proceedings of the National Academy of Science 77: 745
Davison P F, Hong B S, Cannon D J 1979 Quantitative analysis of the collagens in bovine cornea. Experimental Eye Research 29: 97
Dixit S N, Kang A M 1979 Anterior lens capsule collagens: Cyanogen bromide peptides of the C-chain. Biochemistry 18: 5686
Eastoe J E, Martens P, Thomas N R 1973 The amino acid composition of human hand tissue collagens in osteogenesis imperfecta and dentinogenesis imperfecta. Calcified Tissue Research 12: 91
Eichholtz W, Müller D 1972 Electron microscopical findings of cornea and sclera in osteogenesis imperfecta. Klinische MBL Augen Heilkunde 161: 646
Epstein E H Jr, Mundeloh N H 1975 Isolation and characterization of CNBr peptides of human $[\alpha\ (III)]_3$ collagen and tissue distribution of $[\alpha\ (I)]_2\alpha_2$ and $[\alpha\ (III)]_3$ collagens. Journal of Biological Chemistry 250: 9304
Falls H F, Cotterman C W 1943 Genetic studies on ectopia lentis, a pedigree of simple ectopia of the lens. Archives of Ophthalmology 30: 610
Follis R H Jr 1953 Histodermical studies on cartilage and bone III: Osteogenesis imperfecta. Bulletin of Johns Hopkins Hospital 93: 386
Foster C S, Yamamoto G K 1978 Ocular rigidity in keratoconus. American Journal of Ophthalmology 86: 802
Francois J 1970 Homocystinuria. In: Winkleman J E & Crone R A (eds) Perspectives in ophthalmology, vol II. Excerpta Medica, Amsterdam. p 81
Freeman I L 1974 Biochemistry of some connective tissue components of the eye. PhD thesis, University of Manchester, England. p 139
Freeman I L 1978 Collagen polymorphism in mature rabbit cornea. Investigative Ophthalmology & Visual Science 17: 171
Freeman I L 1980 Collagen biosynthesis in the healing corneal wound. In: Schachar R A, Levy N S, Schachar L (eds) Keratorefraction. LAL Publishing, Denison, Texas. p 39
Freeman I L 1981a Comparative biochemistry of type I collagens from human cornea, sclera and skin. In: Hollyfield J G (ed) Proceedings of the Fourth International Symposium on the Structure of the Eye. Elsevier, Amsterdam, in press
Freeman I L 1981b Corneal collagen biosynthesis in culture: the relationship with normal and scar tissue collagens. Investigative ophthalmology and visual science, in press
Freeman I L, Sundar Raj C V 1981 Structure and biosynthesis of rabbit lens capsule collagen. Investigative ophthalmology and visual science, in press
Fujii K, Tanzer M L 1977 Osteogenesis imperfecta: biochemical analysis of bone collagen. Clinical Orthopedics and Related Research 124: 271
Fuxa G, Brant H P 1975 Beitrag zum Ehlers-Danlos-syndrome. Klinische MGL Augenheilkunde 166: 247
Gartner J 1975 Physical structure of the vitreous. Transactions of the Ophthalmological Society of the UK 95: 364
Gay S, Miller E J 1979 Characterization of lens capsule collagen: evidence for the presence of two unique chains in molecules derived from major basement membrane structures. Archives of Biochemistry and Biophysics 198: 370
Harding J J, Crabbe M J C, Panjwani N A 1979 Corneal collagen. Robert A M, Robert L (eds) Colloques Internationaux du Cnrs 287 — Biochemie des Tissus Conjonctifs Normaux et Pathologiques, Inserm, Paris
Harnisch J P, Buchen R, Sinhe P K, Barrach H J 1978 Ultrastructural identification of type I and II collagens in the cornea of the mouse by means of enzyme labelled antibodies. von Graefes Albrecht, Archiv für Klinische und Experimentale Ophthalmologie 208: 9
Harris E D Jr, Sjoerdsma A 1966 Collagen profile in various clinical conditions. Lancet 2: 707

Hay E D 1977 Interaction between cell surface and extracellular matrix in corneal development. In: Lash J W, Burger M M (eds), Society of General Physiology Series 32. Raven Press, New York. p 115

Henkind P, Ashton N 1965 Ocular pathology in homocystinuria. Transactions of the Ophthalmological Society of the UK 85: 21

Hogan M J, Alvarado J A, Weddell J E 1971 Histology of the human eye, W B Saunders Co, Philadelphia. p 328

Huang T W 1977 Chemical and histochemical studies of human alveolar collagen fibers. American Journal of Pathology 86: 81

Israel P, Masterson E, Goldman A I, Wiggert B, Chader G J 1980 Retinal pigment epithelial cell differentiation in vitro-influence of culture medium. Investigative Ophthalmology & Visual Science 19: 720

Jakus M A 1962 Further observations on the fine structure of the cornea. Investigative Ophthalmology 1: 202

Jayson M I V, Eusty D L 1977 Ulceration of the cornea in rheumatoid arthritis. Annals of rheumatic diseases 36: 428

Judisch G F, Wasiri M, Krachmer J H 1976 Ocular Ehlers-Danlos syndrome with normal lysyl hydroxylase activity. Archives of Ophthalmology 94: 1489

Junqua S, Menasche M, Brechemier D, Pouliquen Y, Robert L 1975 Study of morphogenetic disturbances of cornea by in vitro ^{14}C-L-proline incorporation. Archiv D'Ophthalmologie, Paris 35: 665

Kang A H, Trelstad R L 1973 A collagen defect in homocystinuria. Journal of Clinical Investigation 52: 2571

Kao W-W Y, Foreman C A 1980 Chick corneal collagen. European Journal of Biochemistry 106: 41

Kearns T P 1980 Collagen and rheumatic diseases: Ophthalmic aspects. In: Marsolf F A (ed) The eye and systemic disease. C V Mosby Co, St Louis. p 123

Kefalides N A 1978 Biology and chemistry of basement membranes. Academic Press, New York

Krane S M, Pinnell S R, Erbe R W 1972 Lysyl-protocollagen hydroxylase deficiency in fibroblasts from siblings with hydroxylysine deficient collagen. Proceedings of the National Academy of Sciences 69: 2899

Kreig T, Müller P K 1977 The Marfan syndrome: In vitro study of collagen metabolism in tissue specimens of the aorta. Experimental Cell Biology 45: 207

Krieg T, Feldmann U, Kessler W, Müller P K 1979 Biochemical characteristics of Ehlers-Danlos syndrome type VI in a family with one affected infant. Human Genetics 46: 41

Kuming B S, Jaffe L 1977 Ehlers-Danlos syndrome associated with keratoconus. A case report. South African Medical Journal 52: 403

Lamberg S I & Dorfman A 1973 Synthesis and degradation of hepatasonic acid in the cultured fibroblasts of Marfan's disease. Journal of Clinical Investigation 52: 2428

Lapière C M, Nusgens B, Pierard G E 1977 Interaction between collagen type I and type III in conditioning bundle organization. Connective Tissue Research 5: 21

Lindberg K A, Hassett A, Pinnell S R 1976 Inhibition of lysyl oxidase by homocysteine: A proposed connective tissue defect in homocystinuria. Clinical Research 24: 265A.

Lindenfelser R, Hasselkus W, Haubert P, Kronert W 1972 Zur osteogenesis imperfecta: Raster electron-mikroscopische untersuchungen. Virchows Archives (Zell Pathologie) 11: 80

Lindenmayer T, Little C 1978 Embryonic neural retina collagen: in vitro synthesis of high molecular weight forms of type II plus a new genetic type. Proceedings of the National Academy of Science USA 75: 3235

Lloyd-Jones D, Hemby R M 1978 Destructive corneal disease in the connective tissue disorders: Comparison with an experimental animal model. Transactions of the Ophthalmological Society of the UK 98: 383

Machemer R, Laqus H 1975 Pigment epithelium proliferation in retenal detachment (Massive perioetinal proliferation). American Journal of Ophthalmology 80: 1

Manski W, Wirostko E, Halbert S P, Hofeldt A J Auto-immune phenomena in the eye. In: Meischer P A, Müller-Ebehard H J, Grune S (eds) Textbook of Immunopathology Stratton, 1976. p 877

von der Mark K, von der Mark H, Timpl R, Trelstad R 1977 Immunofluorescent localization of collages types I, II, III in the embryonic chick eye. Developmental Biology 59: 75

Marshall J, Grindle C F J, 1978 Fine structure of the cornea and its development. Transactions of the Ophthalmological Society of the UK 98: 320

Matalon R S, Dorfman A 1969 Acid mucopolysaccharides in cultured human fibroblasts. Lancet 2: 838

Maumenee I H 1978 The cornea in connective tissue diseases. Proceedings of the American Academy of Ophthalmology & Otolarngology 85: 1014

Maurice D M 1957 The structure and transparency of the cornea. Journal of Physiology 136: 263

Maurice D M 1969 The cornea and sclera. In: Davson H (ed) The eye Vol I 2nd edn. Academic Press, New York. p 489

McCracken J S, Burger P C, Klintworth G K 1979 Morphological observations on experimental corneal vascularization in the rat. Laboratory Investigation 41: 519

McKusick V A 1972 Heritable disorders of connective tissue. St. Louis, C V Mosby Co

Meigel W N, Müller P K, Pontz B F, Sorensen N, Spranger J 1974 A constitutional disorder of connective tissue suggesting a defect in collages biosynthesis. Klinische Wochenschrift 52: 906

Minton J 1957 A clinical and pectonal survey of uveitis in childhood. Transactions of the Ophthalmological Society of the UK 77: 255

Mondino B J, Brown S I, Rabin B S 1978 Autoimmune phenomena of the external eye. Transactions of the American Academy of Ophthalmology and Otolarnyngology 85: 801

Neuci I, Beltrami C A 1968 Marfan's syndrome, a hereditary enzymopenia

Newsome D, Kenyon K 1973 Collagen production in vitro by the retinal pigmented epithelium of the chick embryo. Developmental Biology 32: 387

Newsome D, Linsenmayer T, Trelstad R 1976 Vitreous body collagen. Evidence for a dual origin from the neural retina and hyalocytes. Journal of Cell Biology 71: 59

Newsome D A, Rodrigues M M, Gross J 1980 Humas scleral collages influemes corneal collagen fibril formation. Investigative Ophthalmology and Visual Science 19: Suppl 146

Nussenblatt R B 1980 HLA and ocular disease. Proceedings Immunology of the eye: Workshop I. Steinberg G M, Gery I, Nussenblatt R B (eds) Sp Suppl Immunology Abstracts 1980, p 25

Olsen B R 1965 Electron microscope studies of collages IV. Structure of vitrosin fibrils and interaction properties of vitrosin molecules. Journal of Ultrastructure Research 13: 172

Pataa C, Joyon L, Roucher F 1970 Ultra-structure du keratocone. Archiv D'Ophthalmogie (Paris) 30: 403

Patz A 1980 I. Studies on retinal neovascularization. Investigative Ophthalmology & Visual Science 19: 1133

Pfister R R, Paterson C A 1977 Additional clinical and morphological observations on the favorable effect of ascorbate in experimental ocular alkali burns. Investigative Ophthalmology & Visual Science 16: 478

Pinnell S R, Krane S M, Kenzora J E, Glimcher M J 1972 A heritable disorder of connective tissue; hydroxylysine-deficient collagen disease. New England Journal of Medicine 286: 1013

Praus R, Brettschneider I, Adam M 1979 Heterogeneity of bovine corneal collagen. Experimental Eye Research 29: 409

Priest R E, Moinuddin J F, Priest J H 1973 Collagen of Marfan's syndrome is abnormally soluble. Nature 245: 264

Quinn R S, Krane S M 1979 Collagen synthesis by cultured skin fibroblasts from siblinge with hydroxylysine-deficient collagen. Biochimica Et Biophysica Acta 585: 589

Rahi A H S 1979 HLA and eye disease. British Journal of Ophthalmology 63: 283

Reeser F H, Aarberg T M 1979 Vitreous humor. In: Records R E (ed) Physiology of the human eye and visual system. Harper and Row, Hagerstown. p 261

Robert L, Robert B 1975 The macromolecular structure of normal cornea. Archiv D'Ophthalmologie (Paris) 35: 11

Robertson I 1975 Keratoconus and the Ehlers-Danlos syndrome. A new aspect of keratoconus. Medical Journal of Australia 1: 571

Schmut O 1977 The identification of type III collagen in calf and bovine cornea and sclera. Experimental Eye Research 25: 505

Schmut O 1978 The organization of tissues of the eye by different collagen types. Albrecht von Graefes Archiv Fur Klinische und Experimentelle Ophthalmoloqie 207: 189

Schofield S D, Freeman I L, Jackson D S 1971 The isolation and amino acid and carbohydrate composition of polymeric collagens from various human tissues. Biochemical Journal 124: 407

Seigel R C 1975 The connective tissue defect in homocystinuria. Clinical Research 23: 263A

Siegel R C, Chang Y H 1978 Defective α_2 chain synthesis in patients with sporadic Marfan syndrome. Clinical Research 26: 501A

Sillence D O, Senn A, Danks D M 1980 Genetic heterogenerty in osteogenesis imperfecta. Journal of Medical Genetics in press

Smith G Jr, Linsenmayer T, Newsome D 1976 Synthesis of type II collagen in vitro by embryonic chick neural retina tissue. Proceedings of the National Academy of Science, USA 73: 4420

Snowden J M, Swann D A 1980 Vitreous structure V. the morphology and thermal stability of vitreous collagen fibres and comparison to articular cartilage (type II) collagen. Investigative Ophthalmology and Visual Science 19: 610

Spranger J, Langer L O 1974 Spondyloepiphyseal dysplasias. Birth Defects — Original Article Series 10 9: 19

Srinivasan B D, Kulkarni P S 1980 The role of arachidonic acid metabolites in the mediation of the polymorphonuclear leucocyte response following corneal injury. Investigative Ophthalmology and Visual Science 19: 1087

Stein E, Lazar M, Adam A 1968 Brittle cornea. A familial trait associated with blue sclera. American Journal of Ophthalmology 66: 67

Steinmann B, Gitzelmann R, Vogel A, Grant M E, Harwood R, Sear C H J 1975 Ehlers-Danlos syndrome in two siblings with deficient lysyl hydroxylase activity in cultured skin fibroblasts but only mild hydroxylysine deficit in skin. Helvitica Paediatrica Acta 30: 255

Stoesser T R, Church R L, Brown S I 1978 Partial characterization of human collagen and procollagen secreted by human corneal stromal fibroblasts in cell culture. Investigative Ophthalmology and Visual Science 17: 164

Sussman M, Lichtenstein J R, Nigra T P, Martin G R, McKusick V A 1974 Hydroxylysine-deficient skin collagen in a patient with a form of Ehlers-Danlos syndrome. Journal of Bone and Joint Surgery 56A: 1228

Sundar-Raj C V, Freeman I L, Brown S I 1980 Selective growth of rabbit corneal epithelial cells in culture and basement membrane collagen synthesis. Investigative Ophthalmology & Visual Science 19: 1222

Sundar-Raj C V, Freeman I L, Church R L, Brown S I 1979 Biochemical characterization of procollagen-collagen synthesized by rabbit corneal endothehal cells in culture. Investigative Ophthalmology & Visual Science 18: 75

Swann D A, Sotman S 1980 The chemical composition of bovine vitreous-humour collagen fibres. Biochemical Journal 185: 545

Swann D A, Caulfield J B, Broadhurst J B 1976 The altered fibrous form of vitreous collagen following solubilization with pepsin. Biochimica Biophysica Acta 427: 365

Swann D A, Constable I J, Harper E 1972 Vitreous structure III. Composition of bovine vitreous collagen. Investigative Ophthalmology & Visual Science 14: 613

Swann D A, Sotman S, Snowden J 1977 Vitreous collagen — a special type II collagen. Investigative Ophthalmology & Visual Science 16, Suppl 67

Swarz W, Graf Keysenlingk D 1969 Electron microscopy of normal and opaque human cornea. In: Langham M (ed) The cornea. Johns Hopkins Press, Baltimore. p 123

Sykes B, Francis M J O, Smith R 1977 Altered relation of two collagen types in osteogenesis imperfecta. New England Journal of Medicine 296: 1200

Trelstad R L, Kang A H 1974 Collagen heterogenerty in the arian eye: lens, vitreous body, cornea and sclera. Experimental Eye Research 18: 395

Trelstad R L, Rubin D, Gross J 1977 Osteogenesis imperfecta congenita: evidence for a generalized molecular disorder of collagen. Laboratory Investigation 36: 501

Tripathi R C 1974 Fine structure of mesodemal tissues of the human eye. Transactions of the Ophthalmological Society of the UK 95: 663

Uga S, Smelsen G 1973 Electron microscopic study of the development of retinal Mullerian cells. Investigative Ophthalmology and Visual Science 12: 295

Uitto J, Lichtenstein J R 1976 Defects in the biochemistry of collagen in diseases of connective tissue. Journal of Investigative Dermatology 66: 59

Watson P G, Hazelman B L 1976 Anatomical and physiological considerations In the sclera and systemic disorders. Saunders, Philadelphia. p 183

Welsh C, Gay S, Rhodes R K, Pfister R, Miller E J 1980 Collagen heterogeneity in normal rabbit cornea. Biochimica Biophysica Acta 625: 78

Wishard P, Paterson C A 1980 The effect of ascorbic acid on experimental acid burns of the rabbit cornea. Investigative Ophthalmology and Visual Science 19: 564

Wollensak J 1966 Homocystenurie und Linsenektopie. Albrecht V Graefes Archiv für Klinische und Experimentale Ophthalmologie 169: 357

Wollensak J, Ihme A, Kneg T, Müller P K 1980 Biochemical characterization of collagen synthesized by fibroblasts derived from patients with keratoconus and controls. Proceedings of the International Society for Eye Research I: 16

Yue B Y J T, Baum J L, Smith B D 1979 Collagen synthesis by cultures of stromal cells from normal human and keratoronus corneas. Biochemical and Biophysical Research Communications 86: 465

22

Kidney

J. G. HEATHCOTE

INTRODUCTION

The amount of collagen in the kidney depends upon a number of factors: the species of animal (Neuman & Logan, 1950), its age (Schaub, 1963; Deyl et al, 1972) and the presence of disease. In general, collagen forms only a small proportion of the renal mass, e.g. 2 per cent of the dry weight of renal cortex of adult rats (Chvapil, 1967), and this may be due in part to the presence of an active collagenolytic mechanism in the kidney (Schaub, 1964). Nevertheless, the collagen is of great physiological importance as a support for the renal parenchyma and as a component of the basement membranes.

The kidney is enveloped in a capsule of connective tissue which in man is about 200 μm thick. This covers the external surface, the renal pelvis and is continuous with the connective tissue of the renal medulla (Rouiller, 1969). The collagen bundles are arranged in arcades and intertwined with elastic fibres allowing the capsule to adapt to the considerable changes in renal volume which may occur (Rouiller, 1969; Dunnill & Halley, 1973). The cortex contains little interstitial connective tissue and the collagen fibres are confined to the tunica adventitia of blood vessels and the periglomerular region (Rouiller, 1969).

Most of the interest in kidney collagen has centred on the basement membranes of the glomerulus, tubule and Bowman's capsule, together with the mesangial matrix. This reflects the involvement of these structures in a wide range of renal diseases and the significance of the glomerular basement membrane (GBM) as a filtration barrier.

THE RENAL INTERSTITIUM

The reason for the paucity of biochemical data on collagen in the renal interstitium is the difficulty in isolating sufficient pure material for analysis. Indeed almost all of the available information has come from immunohistochemical studies with antibodies prepared against collagens from other tissues. In this was type I collagen has been located in the normal human kidney in large blood vessels, the capsule and the renal pelvis (Remberger et al, 1976; Roll et al, 1980). Type III collagen and procollagen on the other hand are found in thin fibres in the interstitial space (Remberger et al, 1976; Wick et al, 1979) and also in the parietal layer of Bowman's capsule (see p. 409). Immunofluorescence studies of pathological kidneys indicate that in interstitial fibrosis of whatever aetiology the excess collagen is almost exclusively of type III (Remberger et al, 1976).

It has been suggested that increased amounts of collagen at the pelvi-ureteric junction may be involved in the development of idiopathic hydronephrosis (Notley, 1970). Gosling & Dixon (1978) reported increased numbers of collagen fibres in the dilated renal pelvis and suggested that these were synthesised by smooth muscle cells in the pelvis, although it is uncertain whether enhanced collagen biosynthesis is the primary abnormality or merely a secondary response to distension. In experimental obstructive nephropathy the number of collagen fibres in the cortex and outer medulla is elevated (Nagle & Bulger, 1978) and this has been correlated with a 100-fold increase in the quantity of interstitial collagen in the cortex (Man et al, 1978). A much smaller increase in the content of basement membrane collagen was observed and it is of interest that in a number of diseases, including experimental obstructive nephropathy (Nagle & Bulger, 1978), radiation nephritis (Churg & Madrazo, 1977) and Balkan nephropathy (Hall & Dammin, 1978), there is a close association between interstitial fibrosis and basement membrane thickening, especially in the tubule. In the isolation of tubular basement membrane (TBM) contamination with fibrillar collagen has been observed (Mahieu & Winand, 1970) and it has been suggested on morphological grounds that both interstitial cells and tubular epithelial cells contribute to the formation of the TBM (Romen & Mäder-Kruse, 1978).

THE MESANGIAL MATRIX

The glomerular mesangium was only clearly identified with the advent of the electron microscope (Tighe, 1975) and remains something of an enigma. However, the mesangial cells (Fig. 22.1) resemble smooth-muscle cells and deposit an amorphous matrix of variable density which may rarely contain collagen fibres (Yamada, 1960; Latta,

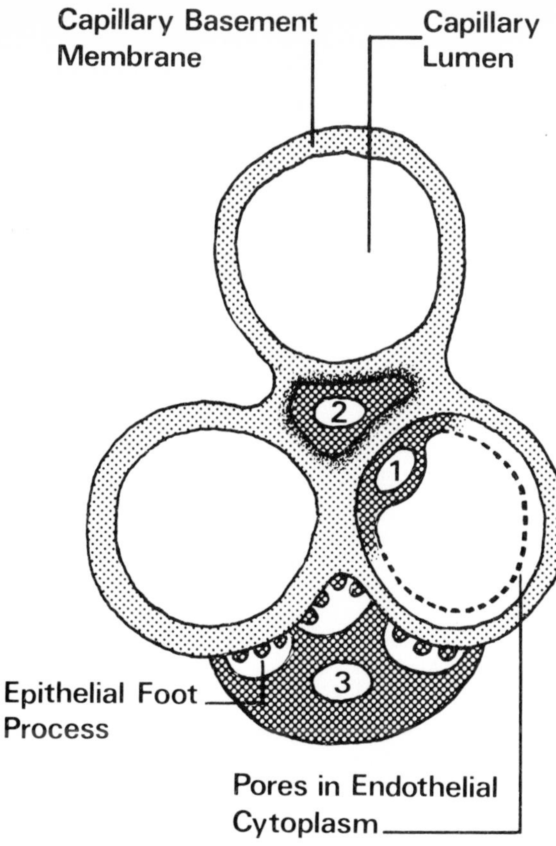

Fig. 22.1 Diagrammatic representation of a section through a glomerular capillary lobule. The cell types are indicated as follows: 1, endothelial; 2, mesangial; 3, epithelial.

1961; Tighe, 1975). These fibres are few in number, have a major period of about 60 nm and do not possess any defined relationship with the GBM (Latta, 1961). The mesangial matrix itself appears to be continuous with the lamina rara interna of the GBM but can be clearly differentiated from the epithelial component of the basement membrane (Huang, 1979).

A number of functions have been attributed to the mesangial cells but the clearance of particulate matter from the circulation is the best defined (Farquhar & Palade, 1962) and this phagocytic capacity may also be involved in the turnover of GBM (Walker, 1973; Huang, 1979). Other possible functions include mechanical support for the glomerular tuft, regulation of glomerular blood flow by virtue of their contractile properties and the synthesis and secretion of renin (Tighe, 1975). Of particular interest to the collagen biochemist is the potential of mesangial cells to synthesise part of the GBM.

The morphological similarity between the mesangial matrix and the GBM was noted by electron microscopists and when GBM is purified by detergent treatment fragments of mesangial matrix remain adherent to the basement membrane (Heathcote, 1978; Meezan et al, 1978), suggesting similarities in biochemical composition as well. Wick et al (1979) and Roll et al (1980) in immunohistochemical studies detected type IV collagen in both GBM and mesangial matrix and the latter authors also suggested that type V (AB) collagen was present in both. structures. The close association of fibronectin and collagen seen generally in connective tissues has also been observed in the mesangium (Pettersson & Colvin, 1978) although immunoelectron microscopy indicates that this glycoprotein is concentrated at the surface of the mesangial cell rather than distributed throughout the matrix (Courtoy et al, 1980; Oberley et al, 1980).

Since it is not technically possible to isolate mesangial matrix, biochemical characterization of its component macromolecules has depended upon biosynthetic experiments. When glomeruli are cultured in vitro three cell types grow out of the explants and these are thought to correspond to the epithelial, mesangial and endothelial cells (Holdsworth et al, 1978; but see Ishikawa et al, 1980). In general, the epithelial and mesangial elements predominate and these synthesise and secrete collagenous polypeptides of a similar size (Striker et al, 1978; Foidart et al, 1979a, b, 1980). However the ratios of 3-hydroxyproline: total hydroxyproline and glycosylated hydroxylysine: total hydroxylysine are less in the culture medium of the mesangial cells (Foidart et al, 1979a, 1980; Striker et al, 1980) suggesting that part of the collagen produced by these cells may be of the interstitial (I, III) or pericellular (V) types (Gay et al, 1980). Electrophoretic analysis of pepsin digests of the mesangial cell products reveals the presence of types I and III collagens together with the B chain of type V collagen (Scheinman et al, 1978; Killen & Striker, 1979a; Striker et al, 1980).

This ability of mesangial cells to synthesise non-basement membrane collagens is consistent with their smooth-muscle cell nature and with morphological observations of collagen fibres in the mesangial matrix. In a number of diseases too, e.g. diabetic glomerulosclerosis (Tisher & McCoy, 1976), Nail-Patella syndrome (Morita et al, 1973a) and chronic glomerulonephritis (Kuriyama, 1973), collagen fibrils may be laid down in the matrix and these are probably of types I and III (Remberger et al, 1976). More commonly in disease collagen fibrils are not visible and mesangial sclerosis, which ultimately may lead to obliteration of capillary lumina in the glomerulus, consists rather of cellular proliferation and increased deposition of matrix (Tighe, 1975). Such a process may occur spontaneously with age in the rat (Couser & Stilmant, 1975).

THE GLOMERULAR BASEMENT MEMBRANE

The general subject of basement membranes has been reviewed extensively both in this book (Ch. 17) and elsewhere (Heathcote & Grant, 1981) so this section will be largely restricted to a consideration of the specific features of the GBM.

The spatial relationship of the basement membrane to the three cell types in the renal glomerulus is illustrated in Figure 22.1 and morphological studies indicate that the GBM is formed by the fusion of the epithelial cell and endothelial cell basement membranes (Kurtz & McManus, 1959; Thorning & Vracko, 1977; Huang, 1979; Friis, 1980). In electron micrographs the GBM appears to consist of three layers: a central, electron-dense region (the lamina densa) flanked by two electron-lucent zones; the lamina rara interna adjacent to the endothelial cells and the lamina rara externa beneath the foot processes of the epithelial cells (Ashworth et al, 1960; Farquhar, 1978). The lamina densa is thought to be the collagenous part of the GBM (see, for example, Roll et al, 1980) and consists of a network of fine filaments no more than 4 nm in diameter (Ota et al, 1977; Farquhar, 1978). The laminae rarae may also be partly collagenous but the only components unequivocally demonstrated so far are the glycoprotein laminin (Madri et al, 1980), and a heparan sulphate proteoglycan which may contribute to the glomerular filtration barrier (Kanwar & Farquhar, 1979a, b, c; Kanwar et al, 1980). The molecular sieving properties of the GBM, which have been demonstrated in isolated preparations (Robinson & Brown, 1977; Westberg, 1979), appear to reside in the collagenous framework of the membrane. Treatment of rabbit renal basement membranes (a mixture of both GBM and TBM) with a neutral proteinase from rabbit polymorphonuclear leucocytes, resulted in the release of hydroxyproline and an alteration in the basement membranes' filtration properties (Cotter & Robinson, 1978, 1980).

One of the first indications that GBM contained a form of collagen came from immunofluorescence studies in which antibodies raised against skin collagen were deposited in the basement membrane (see, for example, Rothbard & Watson, 1969, 1972). These antibodies were not pure and it was later realized that they were reacting with noncollagenous antigenic determinants in the GBM (Wick et al, 1975). Nevertheless, by this time analysis of GBM preparations purified by sonication had shown that the membrane was rich in the amino acids and sugars characteristic of collagen (Table 22.1) (Kefalides & Winzler, 1966; Spiro, 1967; Westberg & Michael, 1970), and this has been confirmed on preparations subjected to less harsh purification procedures (Meezan et al, 1975; Ligler & Robinson, 1977). One unusual feature of the membrane is a high content of cysteine which is involved in disulphide-bonding, and this has been used as the basis of a histochemical stain for basement membrane collagen (Böck, 1978).

The isolation of a specific basement membrane collagen, type IV, from a number of tissues including GBM (Kefalides, 1971) has allowed more precise immuno-histochemical investigation of basement membranes. Immunofluorescence studies have revealed that GBM contains type IV collagen but not interstitial collagens (Remberger et al, 1976; Wick et al, 1979) and under the electron microscope ferritin-tagged antibodies to type IV collagen appeared to be concentrated over the lamina densa (Roll et al, 1980). Roll et al (1980) found that the GBM, and specifically the lamina densa, also contained type V collagen but this has not been observed by others (Gay, S, personal communication).

Kefalides' approach to the preparation of type IV collagen was to solubilise the GBM by digestion with pepsin and the use of this procedure by other workers has resulted in the isolation of a spectrum of collagenous polypeptides which are probably fragments of the native form of basement membrane collagen (Daniels & Chu, 1975; Trelstad & Lawley, 1977; Freytag et al, 1978; Spiro, 1978; Tryggvason & Kivirikko, 1978; Dixit, 1979). Daniels & Chu (1975) and Tryggvason & Kivirikko (1978) described collagenous components of molecular weight 80 000 to 100 000 and 140 000 in pepsin digests of bovine and human GBM. Subsequently Dixit (1979) isolated two α chain-sized polypeptides from human glomeruli and bulk digests of human and porcine renal cortex and these appear

Table 22.1 Composition of renal basement membranes

	GBM [a]	*TBM* [b]	*Bowman's Capsule* [c]	*Anterior Lens Capsule* [d]
residues/1000 amino acids				
Hydroxyproline	84	89	106	100
Aspartic acid	72	65	60	58
Threonine	39	37	36	31
Serine	55	55	41	48
Glutamic acid	98	97	91	95
Proline	71	69	63	66
Glycine	191	211	260	288
Alanine	54	46	51	46
Cysteine	20	16	22	18
Valine	33	38	28	35
Methionine	11	13	6	6
Isoleucine	34	35	28	30
Leucine	68	64	58	57
Tyrosine	18	19	14	11
Phenylalanine	29	29	33	29
Hydroxylysine	28	31	29	32
Lysine	24	23	23	11
Histidine	20	17	14	12
Arginine	49	41	36	38
mg/100 mg protein				
Glucose	3.23	2.87		
Galactose	3.86	2.76		
Mannose	0.76	0.47		
L-Fucose	0.19	0.13		
Hexosamine	1.48	1.02		
Sialic acid	0.87	0.46		

[a, b] Human kidney (Sato et al, 1975)
[c, d] Canine kidney and eye (Kefalides & Denduchis, 1969).

to be anologous to the C and D chains of lens capsule collagen (Gay & Miller, 1979). These chains have different amino acid compositions and cyanogen bromide-peptide patterns suggesting a distinct origin for each (Dixit, 1979) and they appear to be derived from slightly larger species, C^1 and D^1, of molecular weight 110 000 also present in the renal cortical digests (Dixit, 1980; Dixit & Kang, 1980). The C chain is believed to be identical with the α_1(IV) polypeptide of Kefalides (1971).

Spiro and his collaborators have described an even greater diversity of proteins containing collagen-like sequences in GBM (Hudson & Spiro, 1972a, b; Sato & Spiro, 1976). These were solubilised by treatment of the membrane with sodium dodecyl sulphate after reduction and alkylation and were resolved into over 50 components containing different proportions of collagenous and noncollagenous sequences (Sato & Spiro, 1976). The close proximity of such sequences has been further documented with the isolation from bovine GBM of a glycopeptide containing only 15 amino acids but both a hydroxylysinedisaccharide unit and an asparagine-linked heteropolysaccharide (Levine & Spiro, 1979). The GBM is envisaged by Spiro (1976) as a network of cross-linked polypeptides, each of different size and proportional content of collagen-like sequences, which is formed through a series of limited proteolytic cleavages of the biosynthetic precursors. Such a concept is attractive although there is no direct evidence in its favour. Certainly, the number of GBM components which can be demonstrated is probably too large to allow for individual biosynthesis and the multiple, newly synthesised hydroxylysine-containing polypeptides observed by Cohen & Klein (1978) probably resulted from degradation in vitro.

Most biosynthetic studies using isolated renal glomeruli (Grant et al, 1975; Heathcote et al, 1979; 1980b) and cultures of glomerular epithelial cells (Killen & Striker, 1979b) have confirmed the synthesis of a high-molecular-weight collagen precursor which may be composed of two distinct polypeptides (Killen & Striker, 1979b). These polypeptides have a molecular weight of 170 000 to 195 000 and are analogous to the pro-α chains of collagen types I, II and III. However, they are not converted extracellularly to α chain-sized polypeptides but are incorporated directly into the GBM matrix where they become cross-linked by lysine-derived bonds (Heathcote, 1978; Heathcote, et al, 1980b). Biosynthetic studies have demonstrated that in the lens capsule this cross-link is hydroxylysino-5-ketonorleucine (Heathcote et al, 1978; 1980a) and this may be its form in GBM also (Tanzer & Kefalides, 1973). Thus GBM collagen probably exists in situ as aggregates of a procollagen-like molecule that is stabilized by disulphide bonds and lysine-derived cross-links (for review see Heathcote & Grant, 1981; West et al, 1980).

The biosynthesis of GBM collagen by cultures of epithelial cells (Killen & Striker, 1979b) is consistent with earlier morphological observations (see, for example, Kurtz & Feldman, 1962; Romen et al, 1976). Such morphological studies on argyric rats have indicated that the turnover of GBM is slow (Kurtz & Feldman, 1962; Walker, 1973), although the interpretation of these investigations is not completely straightforward (Striker & Smuckler, 1970). Nevertheless, measurements of the loss of radioactivity from rat GBM labelled in vivo with radioactive amino acids support the contention that at least some subunits of the basement membrane are very stable (Price & Spiro, 1977; Cohen & Surma, 1980). Turnover is presumably under some form of enzymic control which has not yet been defined although α-glucosidases specific for the hydroxylysine-disaccharide have been isolated from rat renal cortical (Sternberg & Spiro, 1979) and chick embryo (Hamazaki & Hotta, 1979) homogenates.

Sternberg & Spiro (1979) found the highest levels of α-glucosidase activity in the kidneys of neonatal rats and if the enzymes concerned in the metabolism of the protein components of GBM were also most active at this period then this might help to explain the thickening of the GBM that occurs with advancing age. This thickening has been observed in a number of species including the rat (Ashworth et al, 1960; Rosenquist & Bernick, 1971; Yagihashi & Kaseda, 1978), man (Darmady et al, 1973) and the hamster (McNelly & Dittmer, 1976) and is associated with an increase in the amount of mesangial matrix (Yagihashi & Kaseda, 1978). In the case of the golden hamster the widening of the GBM is accompanied by the development of proteinuria (McNelly & Dittmer, 1976) and an increase in the proportion of type IV collagen, estimated on the basis of 3-hydroxyproline content (Man & Adams, 1975), in the renal cortex (Deyl et al, 1978). Hoyer & Spiro (1978) found an increase in the content of 3- and 4-hydroxyproline, hydroxylysine and glycine in rat GBM with age and interpreted this as evidence for a higher proportion of collagenous subunits. However, since the oldest rats examined were only 200 days old this change may not be a phenomenon of true ageing: Smalley (1980a, b) could find no firm evidence for an increased proportion of collagen in aged human GBM.

Thickening is the main response of the glomerular and other basement membranes to disease and may take the form of multiple concentric laminae (Vracko, 1974). However, other morphological changes do occur (Table 22.2; Gubler et al, 1980a, b) and there is a whole host of immune reactions which are beyond the scope of this chapter (see, for example, Wilson & Dixon, 1974; Shibata, 1978). To date, biochemical studies have contributed little to our understanding of these pathological changes although a considerable amount of research has been undertaken, especially with regard to GBM thickening in diabetes mellitus (for review see Heathcote & Grant, 1981). This thickening, which is presumably preceded by a subtle

Table 22.2 Pathological changes of glomerular basement membrane

Abnormality	*Disease*	*Associated features*	*References*
Thickening ± Lamination	Diabetes mellitus	Increased mesangial matrix (predominantly type I collagen)	Osterby (1974) Remberger et al (1976) Tisher & McCoy (1976)
	Myxoedema	TBM affected; increased mesangial matrix	DiScala et al (1967)
Electron-dense alteration	Chronic nephritis	TBM and Bowman's capsule may be affected; increased mesangial matrix	Galle & Mahieu (1975) Droz et al (1977) Churg et al (1979)
Focal splitting	Alport's syndrome	Irregular thickening of GBM	Sessa et al (1974)
Perforation	Rapidly progressive glomerulonephritis		Churg & Grishman (1975)
Separation from parenchymal cells	Haemolytic-uraemic syndrome	Widening of lamina rara interna; increased mesangial matrix	Riella et al (1976)
Excrescences	Down's syndrome		Martin & Kissane (1975)
Deposition of collagen fibres	Nail-Patella syndrome	Fibres in mesangial matrix	Morita et al (1973a)

biochemical change, might result from enhanced synthesis of the collagenous subunits of the GBM (Beisswenger & Spiro, 1970; Cohen & Vogt, 1972; Cohen & Khalifa, 1977; Canivet et al, 1979) although not all the evidence supports this (Westberg & Michael, 1973; Kefalides, 1974; Heathcote et al, 1981). Other mechanisms may operate in the pathogenesis of diabetic nephropathy, e.g. diminished basement membrane degradation (Lazarow & Speidel, 1964; Brownlee, 1976; James et al, 1980; Sato et al, 1980), trapping of serum proteins (Westberg, 1976; Michael et al, 1978) and accelerated cell death and regeneration (Vracko, 1974) but the nature of the primary biochemical defect remains obscure. It seems certain that in diffuse diabetic glomerulosclerosis there is an accumulation of collagen within the glomeruli (Klein et al, 1975) but the relative contributions of basement membrane and interstitial collagens (Remberger et al, 1976) have not been determined.

THE TUBULAR BASEMENT MEMBRANE

Purification of the TBM has been achieved by a combination of sieving and sonic vibration (Ferwerda et al, 1974; Sato et al, 1975; Krisko et al, 1977; Langeveld et al, 1978; Butkowski et al, 1979) and the product has a composition essentially similar to GBM (Table 22.1). The polypeptides present in TBM may also be similar to those of GBM since a multiplicity of components can be detected when the membrane is solubilized in sodium dodecyl sulphate (Ferwerda et al, 1974; Sato et al, 1975). Butkowski et al (1979) have suggested that this polydispersity is partly due to the existence of multimers of a collagenous polypeptide (apparent molecular weight 164 000 to 180 000) which might be equivalent to the pro-α chain(s) found in studies of GBM synthesis. Type IV collagen has been localized in the TBM by immunofluorescence (Wick et al, 1979; Roll et al, 1980) and this is demonstrated in Figure 22.2. There is still some disagreement as to the presence of type V collagen in the TBM (Roll et al, 1980; Gay S, personal communication).

Despite the apparent resemblance of TBM to GBM it is quite probable that the arrangement of subunits within the two basement membranes is different (Velican & Velican, 1970; Carlson & Kenney, 1980) especially since the TBM is as much concerned with the provision of mechanical support for the epithelial cells (Welling & Grantham, 1972; Welling & Welling, 1978) as with filtration. The tubular epithelial cells are thought to deposit the TBM, with perhaps a contribution from cells in the renal interstitium (Romen & Mäder-Kruse, 1978), and the basement membrane appears to have a meshwork sub-structure which can be demonstrated by negative staining (Makino et al, 1979). Like the GBM, it thickens with age (Ashworth et

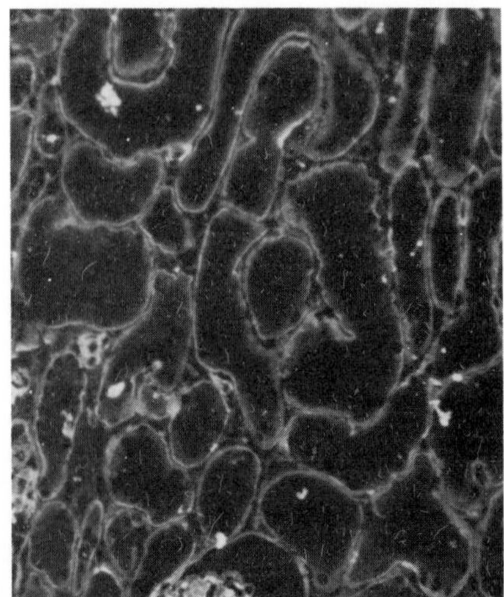

Fig. 22.2 Normal human renal tubules (× 300). The TBM is stained with antibodies to the C chain of type IV collagen as described in Gay et al (1979). (Courtesy of Dr Steffen Gay.)

al, 1960; Scott, 1964) and it displays similar morphological abnormalities in diseases, e.g. thickening in diabetes mellitus, splitting in nephropathia epidemica (Collan et al, 1978). Immunological mechanisms of renal tubular damage have been reviewed by Andres & McCluskey (1975).

BOWMAN'S CAPSULE

Bowman's capsule is a double-walled cup which surrounds the glomerular tuft of capillaries. The inner, visceral layer consists of the glomerular epithelium and is separated from the parietal layer by the urinary space. The parietal layer is composed of an epithelium and a basement membrane which is continuous with the TBM (Kurtz & McManus, 1959). Isolated Bowman's capsules have an amino acid composition similar to that of anterior lens capsule (Table 22.1) although there has been no characterization of the component polypeptides since the preparation of large amounts of tissue is extremely tedious and time-consuming (Kefalides & Denduchis, 1969). Immunofluorescence studies indicate that Bowman's capsule contains type IV collagen (Wick et al, 1979; Roll et al, 1980), but type V (Roll et al, 1980) and type III (Wick et al, 1975, 1979; Remberger et al, 1976) may also be present. In a number of forms of glomerulonephritis which are characterized by so-called 'crescent' formation the epithelial cells change shape and deposit periodic acid/Schiff-positive material that resembles basement membrane in the intercellular spaces. With time this material is replaced by fine collagen fibrils, which are probably of type I (Remberger et al, 1976), and ultimately these may replace the cells themselves (Morita et al, 1973b).

CONCLUSION

The importance of the connective tissue elements of the kidney in pathology has long been appreciated and more recently attempts have been made to define their physiological roles. Precise characterisation of the constituent macromolecules is still, however, in its early stages and will require the use of a wide range of techniques available to the biochemist and experimental pathologist. This review has concentrated on the collagenous components of the kidney although others, such as heparan sulphate proteoglycan (Kanwar & Farquhar, 1979a, b, c; Parthasarathy & Spiro, 1981) and laminin (Rohde et al, 1979), undoubtedly contribute to the architecture of the tissue. Alterations in the interaction and organization of these macromolecules will no doubt prove to be of great significance in renal diseases.

ACKNOWLEDGEMENTS

I should like to thank Drs Steffen Gay and Michael Grant for their assistance in the preparation of this chapter. Original contributions from the author and Dr Grant were supported by the British Diabetic Association and the National Kidney Research Fund and the chapter was written during the tenure of a Medical Research Council Travelling Fellowship.

REFERENCES

Andres G A, McCluskey R T 1975 Tubular and interstitial renal disease due to immunologic mechanisms. Kidney International 7: 271

Ashworth C T, Erdmann R R, Arnold N J 1960 Age changes in the renal basement membrane in rats. American Journal of Pathology 36: 165

Beisswenger P J, Spiro R G 1970 Human glomerular basement membrane: chemical alteration in diabetes mellitus. Science 168: 596

Böck P 1978 Histochemical demonstration of type IV collagen in the renal glomerulus. Histochemistry 55: 269

Brownlee M 1976 α_2-macroglobulin and reduced basement membrane degradation in diabetes. Lancet 1: 779

Butkowski R, Todd P, Grantham J J, Hudson B G 1979 Rabbit tubular basement membrane. Isolation and analysis of polypeptides. Journal of Biological Chemistry 254: 10503

Canivet J, Cruz A, Moreau-Lalande H 1979 Biochemical abnormalities of the human diabetic glomerular basement membrane. Metabolism 28: 1206

Carlson E C, Kenney M C 1980 Morphological heterogeneity of isolated renal basement membranes. Renal Physiology 3: 288

Churg J, Duffy J L, Bernstein J 1979 Identification of dense deposit disease. Archives of Pathology and Laboratory Medicine 103: 67

Churg J, Grishman E 1975 Ultrastructure of glomerular disease: A review. Kidney International 7: 254

Churg J, Madrazo A 1977 Radiation nephritis. In: Lovell Becker E (ed) Seminars in nephrology. Wiley, New York. p 83

Chvapil M 1967 Physiology of connective tissue. Butterworth, London. ch 2

Cohen M P, Khalifa A 1977 Renal glomerular collagen synthesis in streptozotocin diabetes. Reversal of increased basement membrane synthesis with insulin therapy. Biochimica et Biophysica Acta 500: 395

Cohen M P, Klein C V 1977 Evidence for heterogeneous origin of glomerular basement membrane. Biochemical and Biophysical Research Communications 77: 1326

Cohen M P, Surma M 1980 Renal glomerular basement membrane. In vivo biosynthesis and turnover in normal rats. Journal of Biological Chemistry 255: 1767

Cohen M P, Vogt C 1972 Evidence for enhanced basement membrane synthesis and lysine hydroxylation in renal glomerulus in experimental diabetes. Biochemical and Biophysical Research Communications 49: 1542

Collan Y, Lähdevirta J, Jokinen E J 1978 Electron microscopy of nephropathia epidemica. Renal tubular basement membrane. American Journal of Pathology 92: 167

Cotter T G, Robinson G B 1978 Degradation of renal basement membrane by neutral proteinases from rabbit polymorphonuclear leucocytes. Biochemical Society Transactions 6: 1359

Cotter T G, Robinson G B 1980 The effects of proteinases on the filtration properties of isolated basement membranes. International Journal of Biochemistry 12: 191

Courtoy P J, Kanwar Y S, Farquhar M G 1980 Fibronectin localization in the rat glomerulus. Federation Proceedings 39: 873

Couser W G, Stilmant M M 1975 Mesangial lesions and focal glomerular sclerosis in the ageing rat. Laboratory Investigation 33: 491

Daniels J R, Chu G H 1975 Basement membrane collagen of renal glomerulus. Journal of Biological Chemistry 250: 3531

Darmady E M, Offer J, Woodhouse M A 1973 The parameters of the ageing kidney. Journal of Pathology 109: 195

Deyl Z, Jelinek J, Rosmus J, Adam M 1972 Changes in the collagenous stroma in rat kidney in relation to age. Experimental Gerontology 7: 353

Deyl Z, Macek K, Adam M 1978a Changes in the proportion of collagen type IV with age — possible role in transport processes. Experimental Gerontology 13: 263

DiScala V A, Salomon M, Grishman E, Churg J 1967 Renal structure in myxoedema. Archives of Pathology 84: 474

Dixit S N 1979 Isolation and characterization of two α chain size collagenous polypeptide chains C and D from glomerular basement membrane. FEBS Letters 106: 379

Dixit S N 1980 Type IV collagens: Isolation and characterization of two structurally distinct collagen chains from bovine kidney cortices. European Journal of Biochemistry 106: 563

Dixit S N, Kang A 1980 Basement membrane collagens: cyanogen bromide peptides of the D chain from porcine kidney. Biochemistry 19: 2692

Droz D, Zenetti M, Noël L-H, Leibovitch J 1977 Dense deposits disease. Nephron 19: 1

Dunnill M S, Halley W 1973 Some observations on the quantitative anatomy of the kidney. Journal of Pathology 110: 113

Farquhar M G 1978 Structure and function in glomerular capillaries. Role of the basement membrane in glomerular filtration. In: Kefalides N A (ed) Biology and chemistry of basement membranes. Academic Press, New York. p 43

Farquhar M G, Palade G E 1962 Functional evidence for the existence of a third cell type in the renal glomerulus. Phagocytosis of filtration residues by a distinctive 'third' cell. Journal of Cell Biology 13: 55

Ferwerda W, Meijer J F M, van den Eijnden D H, van Dijk W 1974 Epithelial basement membrane of bovine renal tubuli. Isolation and chemical characterization. Hoppe-Seyler's Zeitschrift für Physiologische Chemie 355: 976

Foidart J B, Dechenne C A, Mahieu P R 1979a Biosynthesis of basement membrane collagen by rat glomerular epithelial and mesangial cells in culture. Frontiers of Matrix Biology 7: 60

Foidart J B, Dechenne C A, Mahieu P, Creutz C E, de Mey J 1979b Tissue culture of normal rat glomeruli. Isolation and morphological characterization of two homogeneous cell lines. Investigative and Cell Pathology 2: 15

Foidart J B, Dubois C H, Foidart J M, Dechenne C A, Mahieu P 1980 Tissue culture of normal rat glomeruli. Basement membrane biosynthesis by homogeneous epithelial and mesangial cell lines. International Journal of Biochemistry: 12: 197

Freytag J W, Dalrymple P N, Maguire M H, Strickland D K, Carraway K L, Hudson B G 1978 Glomerular basement membrane. Studies on its structure and interaction with platelets. Journal of Biological Chemistry 253: 9069

Friis C 1980 Postnatal development of the pig kidney: ultrastructure of the glomerulus and proximal tubule. Journal of Anatomy 130: 513

Galle P, Mahieu P 1975 Electron dense alteration of kidney basement membranes. American Journal of Medicine 58: 749

Gay S, Gay R, Miller E J 1980 The collagens of the joint. Arthritis and Rheumatism 23: 937

Gay S, Kresina T F, Gay R, Miller E J, Montes L F 1979 Immunohistochemical demonstration of basement membrane collagen in normal human skin and in psoriasis. Journal of Cutaneous Pathology 6: 91

Gay S, Miller E J 1979 Characterization of lens capsule collagen: evidence for the presence of two unique chains in molecules derived from major basement membrane structures. Archives of Biochemistry and Biophysics 198: 370

Gosling J A, Dixon J S 1978 Functional obstruction of the ureter and renal pelvis. A histological and electron microscopic study. British Journal of Urology 50: 145

Grant M E, Harwood R, Williams I F 1975 The biosynthesis of basement membrane collagen by isolated rat glomeruli. European Journal of Biochemistry 54: 531

Gubler M C, Levy M, Naizot C, Habib R 1980a Glomerular basement membrane changes in non-hereditary glomerular diseases. Renal Physiology 3: 395

Gubler M C, Levy M, Naizot C, Habib R 1980b Glomerular basement membrane changes in hereditary glomerular diseases. Renal Physiology 3: 405

Hall P W III, Dammin G J 1978 Balkan nephropathy. Nephron 22: 281

Hamazaki H, Hotta K 1979 Purification and characterization of an α-glucosidase specific for hydroxylysine-linked disaccharide of collagen. Journal of Biological Chemistry 254: 9682

Heathcote J G 1978 Studies on the biosynthesis of basement membrane collagen. Ph.D. Thesis, University of Manchester

Heathcote J G, Grant M E 1981 The molecular organization of basement membranes. International Reviews of Connective Tissue Research 9: 191

Heathcote J G, Sear C H J, Grant M E 1978 Studies on the assembly of the rat lens capsule. Biosynthesis and partial characterization of the collagenous components. Biochemical Journal 176: 283

Heathcote J G, Sear C H J, Grant M E 1979 Preliminary characterization of the collagenous polypeptides synthesised by lens capsules and renal glomeruli isolated from young rats. Frontiers of Matrix Biology 7: 37

Heathcote J G, Bailey A J, Grant M E 1980a Studies on the assembly of the rat lens capsule. Biosynthesis of a cross-linked component of high molecular weight. Biochemical Journal 190: 229

Heathcote J G, Muhammed S, Smith E F, Grant M E 1980b Biosynthetic studies on the collagenous components of basement membranes. Renal Physiology 3: 36

Heathcote J G, Elliott C, Smith E, Menashi S, Grant M E 1981 Influence of streptozotocin-induced diabetes on glycosyltransferase activities in plasma and renal cortex. Renal Physiology 4: 96

Holdsworth S R, Glasgow E F, Atkins R C, Thomson N M 1978 Cell characteristics of cultured glomeruli from different animal species. Nephron 22: 454

Hoyer J R, Spiro R G 1978 Studies on the rat glomerular basement membrane: age-related changes in composition. Archives of Biochemistry and Biophysics 185: 496

Huang T W 1979 Basal lamina heterogeneity in the glomerular capillary tufts of human kidneys. Journal of Experimental Medicine 149: 1450

Hudson B G, Spiro R G 1972a Studies on the native and reduced alkylated renal glomerular basement membrane. Solubility, subunit size and reaction with cyanogen bromide. Journal of Biological Chemistry 247: 4229

Hudson B G, Spiro R G 1972b Fractionation of glycoprotein components of the reduced alkylated renal glomerular basement membrane. Journal of Biological Chemistry 247: 4239

Ishikawa Y, Wada T, Sakaguchi H 1980 The possibility of three types of cells in cultured glomeruli in vitro. American Journal of Pathology 100: 779

James K, Merriman J, Gray R S, Duncan L J P, Herd R 1980 Serum α_2-macroglobulin levels in diabetes. Journal of Clinical Pathology 33: 163

Kanwar Y S, Farquhar M G 1979a Anionic sites in the glomerular basement membrane. In vivo and in vitro localization to the laminae rarae by cationic probes. Journal of Cell Biology 81: 137

Kanwar Y S, Farquhar M G 1979b Presence of heparan sulphate in the glomerular basement membrane. Proceedings of the National Academy of Sciences USA 76: 1303

Kanwar Y S, Farquhar M G 1979c Isolation of glycosaminoglycans (heparan sulphate) from glomerular basement membranes. Proceedings of the National Academy of Sciences USA 76: 4493

Kanwar Y S, Linker A, Farquhar M G 1980 Increased permeability of the glomerular basement membrane to ferritin after removal of GAG (heparan sulphate) by enzyme digestion. Journal of Cell Biology 86: 688

Kefalides N A 1971 Isolation of a collagen from basement membranes containing three identical α chains. Biochemical and Biophysical Research Communications 45: 226

Kefalides N A 1974 Biochemical properties of human glomerular basement membrane in normal and diabetic kidneys. Journal of Clinical Investigation 53: 403

Kefalides N A, Denduchis B 1969 Structural components of epithelial and endothelial basement membranes. Biochemistry 8: 4613

Kefalides N A, Winzler R J 1966 The chemistry of glomerular basement membrane and its relation to collagen. Biochemistry 5: 702

Killen P D, Striker G E 1979a Origin of the mesangial matrix. Federation Proceedings 38: 1407

Killen P D, Striker G E 1979b Human glomerular visceral epithelial cells synthesise a basal lamina collagen in vitro. Proceedings of the National Academy of Sciences USA 76: 3518

Klein L, Butcher D L, Sudilovsky O, Kikkawa R, Miller M 1975 Quantification of collagen in renal glomeruli isolated from human non-diabetic and diabetic kidneys. Diabetes 24: 1057

Krisko I, DeBernardo E, Sato C S 1977 Isolation and characterization of rat tubular basement membrane. Kidney International 12: 238

Kurtz S M, Feldman J D 1962 Experimental studies on the formation of the glomerular basement membrane. Journal of Ultrastructure Research 6: 19

Kurtz S M, McManus J F A 1959 A reconsideration of the development, structure, and disease of the human renal glomerulus. American Heart Journal 58: 357

Kuriyama T 1973 Chronic glomerulonephritis induced by prolonged immunization in the rabbit. Laboratory Investigation 28: 224

Langeveld J P M, Veerkamp J H, Monnens L A H, van Haelst U J G 1978 Chemical characterization of glomerular and tubular basement membranes of cattle of different ages. Biochimica et Biophysica Acta 514: 225

Latta H 1961 Collagen in normal rat glomeruli. Journal of Ulstrastructure Research 5: 364

Lazarow A, Speidel E 1964 The chemical composition of the glomerular basement membrane and its relationship to the production of diabetic complications. In: Siperstein M D, Colwell A R, Meyer K (eds) Small blood vessel involvement in diabetes mellitus. American Institute of Biological Sciences, Washington, D.C. p 127

Levine M J, Spiro R G 1979 Isolation from glomerular basement membrane of a glycopeptide containing both asparagine-linked and hydroxylysine-linked carbohydrate units. Journal of Biological Chemistry 254: 8121

Ligler F S, Robinson G B 1977 A new method for the isolation of renal basement membranes. Biochimica et Biophysica Acta 468: 327

McNelly N A, Dittmer J E 1976 Glomerular basement membrane width and proteinuria in the ageing hamster kidney. Experimental Gerontology 11: 49

Madri J A, Roll F J, Furthmayr H, Foidart J M 1980 Ultrastructural localization of fibronectin and laminin in the basement membranes of the murine kidney. Journal of Cell Biology 86: 682

Mahieu P, Winand R J 1970 Chemical structure of tubular and glomerular basement membranes of human kidney. Isolation, purification, carbohydrate and amino acid composition. European Journal of Biochemistry 12: 410

Makino H, Ota Z, Takaya Y, Kida K, Miyoshi A, Hiramatsu M, Takahashi K, Ofuji T 1979 Ultrastructure of rat renal tubular basement membrane. Meshwork structure demonstration by negative staining. Acta Medica Okayama 33: 133

Man M, Adams E 1975 Basement membrane and interstitial collagen of whole animals and tissues. Biochemical and Biophysical Research Communications 66: 9

Man M, Nagle R B, Adams E 1978 Chemical estimation of interstitial and basement membrane collagen in obstructive nephropathy. Experimental and Molecular Pathology 29: 144

Martin S A, Kissane J M 1975 Polypoid change of the glomerular basement membrane. Archives of Pathology 99: 249

Meezan E, Hjelle J T, Brendel K, Carlson E C 1975 A simple, versatile non-disruptive method for the isolation of morphologically and chemically pure basement membranes from several tissues. Life Sciences 17: 1721

Meezan E, Brendel K, Hjelle J T, Carlson E C 1978 A versatile method for the isolation of ultrastructurally and chemically pure basement membranes without sonication. In: Kefalides N A (ed) Biology and chemistry of basement membranes. Academic Press, New York. p 17

Michael A F, Scheinman J I, Steffes M W, Fish A J, Brown D M, Mauer S M 1978 Studies on diabetic nephropathy. In: Kefalides N A (ed) Biology and chemistry of basement membranes. Academic Press, New York. p 463

Morita T, Laughlin L O, Kawano K, Kimmelstiel P, Suzuki Y, Churg J 1973a Nail-Patella Syndrome. Light and electron microscopic studies of the kidney. Archives of Internal Medicine 131: 271

Morita T, Suzuki Y, Churg J 1973b Structure and development of the glomerular crescent. American Journal of Pathology 72: 349

Nagle R B, Bulger R E 1978 Unilaternal obstructive nephropathy in the rabbit. II Late morphological changes. Laboratory Investigation 38: 270

Neuman R E, Logan M A 1950 The determination of collagen and elastin in tissues. Journal of Biological Chemistry 186: 549

Notley R G 1970 The musculature of the human ureter. British Journal of Urology 42: 724

Oberley T D, Mosher D F, Mills M D 1979 Localization of fibronectin within the renal glomerulus and its production by cultured glomerular cells. American Journal of Pathology 96: 651

Osterby R 1974 Early phases in the development of diabetic glomerulopathy. Acta Medica Scandinavica Supplementum 574

Ota Z, Makino H, Miyoshi A, Hiramatsu M, Takahashi K, Ofuji T 1977 Electron microscopic demonstration of meshwork structure in human and bovine glomerular basement membranes. Acta Medica Okayama 31: 339

Parthasarathy N, Spiro R G 1981 Characterization of the glycosaminoglycan component of the renal glomerular basement membrane and its relation to the peptide portion. Journal of Biological Chemistry 256: 507

Pettersson E E, Colvin R B 1978 Cold-insoluble globulin (fibronectin, LETS protein) in normal and diseased human glomeruli: papain-sensitive attachment to normal glomeruli and deposition in crescents. Clinical Immunology and Immunopathology 11: 425

Price R G, Spiro R G 1977 Studies on the metabolism of the renal glomerular basement membrane. Turnover measurements in the rat with the use of radiolabelled amino acids. Journal of Biological Chemistry 252: 8597

Remberger K, Gay S, Adelman B C 1976 Immunohistochemische Charakterisierung und Lokalisation unterschiedlicher Kollagentypen bei chronischen Nierenerkrankungen. Verhandlungen der Deutschen Gesellschaft für Pathologie 60: 314

Riella M C, George C R P, Hickman R O, Striker G E, Slichter S J, Harker L, Quadracci L J 1976 Renal microangiopathy of the haemolytic-uraemic syndrome in childhood. Nephron 17: 188

Robinson G B, Brown R J 1977 A method for assessing the molecular sieving properties of renal basement membranes in vitro. FEBS Letters 78: 189

Rohde H, Wick G, Timpl R 1979 Immunochemical characterization of the basement membrane glycoprotein laminin. European Journal of Biochemistry 102: 195

Roll F J, Madri A J, Albert J, Furthmayr H 1980 Co-distribution of collagen types IV and AB_2 in basement membranes and mesangium of the kidney. An immunoferritin study of ultrathin frozen sections. Journal of Cell Biology 85: 597

Romen W, Mäder-Kruse I 1978 The basement membrane of the atrophic kidney tubule. An electron microscopic study of changes in rats. Virchows Archiv. B Cell Pathology 26: 307

Romen W, Schultze B, Hempel K 1976 Synthesis of the glomerular basement membrane in the rat kidney. Autoradiographic studies with the light and electron microscope. Virchows Archiv. B Cell Pathology 20: 125

Rosenquist T H, Bernick S 1971 Histochemistry of renal basal laminae. Adolescent compared with senescent rats. Journal of Gerontology 26: 176

Rothbard S, Watson R F 1969 Comparison of reactions of antibodies to rat collagen and to rat kidney in the basement membranes of rat renal glomeruli. Journal of Experimental Medicine 129: 1145

Rothbard S, Watson R F 1972 Demonstration of collagen in human tissues by immunofluorescence. Laboratory Investigation 27: 76

Rouiller C 1969 General anatomy and histology of the kidney. In: Rouiller C, Müller A F (eds) The kidney, vol 1. Academic Press, New York. p 61

Sato T, Spiro R G 1976 Studies on the subunit composition of the renal glomerular basement membrane. Journal of Biological Chemistry 251: 4062

Sato T, Munakata H, Yoshinaga K, Yosizawa Z 1975 Chemical compositions of glomerular and tubular basement membranes of human kidney. Tohoku Journal of Experimental Medicine 115: 299

Sato T, Saito T, Kokubun M, Ito M, Inoue M, Saito K, Yoshinaga K 1980 Urinary excretion of O-hydroxylysyl-hydroxylysylglycosides in diabetes mellitus. Tohoku Journal of Experimental Medicine 131: 97

Schaub M C 1963 Qualitative and quantitative changes of collagen in parenchymatous organs of the rat during ageing. Gerontologia 8: 114

Schaub M C 1964 Degradation of young and old collagen by extracts of various organs. Gerontologia 9: 52

Scheinman J I, Brown D M, Michael A F 1978 Collagen synthesis by human glomerular cells in culture. Biochimica et Biophysica Acta 542: 128

Scott E B 1964 Modification of the basal architecture of renal tubule cells in aged rats. Proceedings of the Society for Experimental Biology and Medicine 117: 586

Sessa A, Cioffi A, Conte F, D'Amico G 1974 Hereditary nephropathy with nerve deafness (Alport's syndrome). Electron microscopic studies on the renal glomerulus. Nephron 13: 404

Shibata S 1978 Immunologic and non-immunologic aspects of glomerulonephritis. In: Kefalides N A (ed) Biology and chemistry of basement membranes. Academic Press, New York. p 535

Smalley J W 1980a Age-related changes in the amino acid composition of human glomerular basement membrane. Experimental Gerontology 15: 43

Smalley J W 1980b Age-related changes in hydroxylysylglycosides of human glomerular basement membrane collagen. Experimental Gerontology 15: 65

Spiro R G 1967 Studies on the renal glomerular basement membrane. Preparation and chemical composition. Journal of Biological Chemistry 242: 1915

Spiro R G 1976 Search for a biochemical basis of diabetic microangiopathy. Diabetologia 12: 1

Spiro R G 1978 Nature of the glycoprotein components of basement membranes. Annals of the New York Academy of Sciences 312: 106

Sternberg M, Spiro R G 1979 Studies on the catabolism of the hydroxylysine-linked disaccharide units of basement membranes and collagens. Isolation and characterization of a rat kidney α-glucosidase of high specificity. Journal of Biological Chemistry 254: 10329

Striker G E, Smuckler E A 1970 An ultrastructural study of glomerular basement membrane synthesis. American Journal of Pathology 58: 531

Striker G E, Killen P D, Agodoa L C Y, Savin V, Quadracci L D 1978 In vitro basal lamina synthesis by human glomerular epithelial and mesangial cells, evidence for post-translational heterogeneity. In: Kefalides N A (ed) Biology and chemistry of basement membranes. Academic Press, New York. p 319

Striker G E, Killen P D, Farin F M 1980 Human glomerular cells in vitro: isolation and characterization. Transplantation Proceedings 12: Supplement 1, 88

Tanzer M L, Kefalides N A 1973 Collagen cross-links: occurrence in basement membrane collagens. Biochemical and Biophysical Research Communications 51: 775

Thorning D, Vracko R 1977 Renal glomerular basal lamina scaffold. Embryologic development, anatomy, and role in cellular reconstruction of rat glomeruli injured by freezing and thawing. Laboratory Investigation 37: 105

Tighe J R 1975 The mesangium in glomerular disease. Proceedings of the Royal Society of Medicine 68: 151

Tisher C C, McCoy R C 1976 Diabetes Mellitus and the kidney. In: Suki W N, Eknoyan G (eds) The kidney in systemic disease. Wiley, New York. p 105

Trelstad R L, Lawley K R 1977 Isolation and initial characterization of human basement membrane collagens. Biochemical and Biophysical Research Communications 76: 376

Tryggvason K, Kivirikko K I 1978 Heterogeneity of pepsin-solubilised human glomerular basement membrane collagen. Nephron 21: 230

Velican D, Velican C 1970 Structural heterogeneity of kidney basement membranes. Nature 226: 1259

Vracko R 1974 Basal lamina layering in diabetes mellitus. Evidence for accelerated rate of cell death and cell regeneration. Diabetes 23: 94

Yagihashi S, Kaseda N 1978 Age-related changes of glomerular basement membrane in normal rats. Tohoku Journal of Experimental Medicine 126: 27

Yamada E 1960 Collagen fibrils within the renal glomerulus. Journal of Biophysical and Biochemical Cytology 7: 407

Walker F 1973 The origin, turnover and removal of glomerular basement membrane. Journal of Pathology 110: 233

Welling L W, Grantham J J 1972 Physical properties of isolated perfused renal tubules and tubular basement membranes. Journal of Clinical Investigation 51: 1063

Welling L W, Welling D J 1978 Physical properties of isolated perfused basement membranes from rabbit loop of Henle. American Journal of Physiology 234: F54

West T W, Fox J W, Jodlowski M, Freytag J W, Hudson B G 1980 Bovine glomerular basement membrane. Properties of the collagenous domain. Journal of Biological Chemistry 255: 10451

Westberg N G 1976 Biochemical alterations of the human glomerular basement membrane in diabetes. Diabetes 25 (Supplement 2): 920

Westberg N G 1979 Some aspects of the physical chemistry of isolated bovine kidney glomerular basement membrane. Frontiers of Matrix Biology 7: 142

Westberg N G, Michael A F 1970 Human glomerular basement membrane. Preparation and composition. Biochemistry 9: 3837

Westberg N G, Michael A F 1973 Human glomerular basement membrane: chemical composition in diabetes mellitus. Acta Medica Scandinavica 194: 39

Wick G, Furthmayr H, Timpl R 1975 Purified antibodies to collagen: an immunofluorescence study of their reaction with tissue collagen. International Archives of Allergy and Applied Immunology 48: 664

Wick G, Glanville R W, Timpl R 1979 Characterization of antibodies to basement membrane collagen (type IV) collagen in immunohistological studies. Immunobiology 156: 372

Wilson C B, Dixon F J 1974 Immunopathology and glomerulonephritis. Annual Review of Medicine 25: 83

23

Liver

J. O'D. McGEE

The liver is the largest organ in mammals. In man it weighs about 1.5 kg. Its collagen content, in normality, is low accounting for approximately 0.5 per cent of the net weight of the organ. However, in many diseases which lead to cirrhosis — end stage liver disease — there is an enormous increase in liver collagen which completely distorts the normal macroscopic, microscopic and vascular architecture of the organ, and hence leads to a deterioration in liver function.

COLLAGEN IN NORMAL LIVER

Anatomical distribution

The liver is invested in a connective tissue capsule (Glisson's capsule), the main component of which is collagen. The large blood vessels which supply the liver (portal vein and hepatic artery) pierce this capsule at the hilum of the liver. As the vessels enter into the liver they carry with them a sheath of connective tissue from the liver

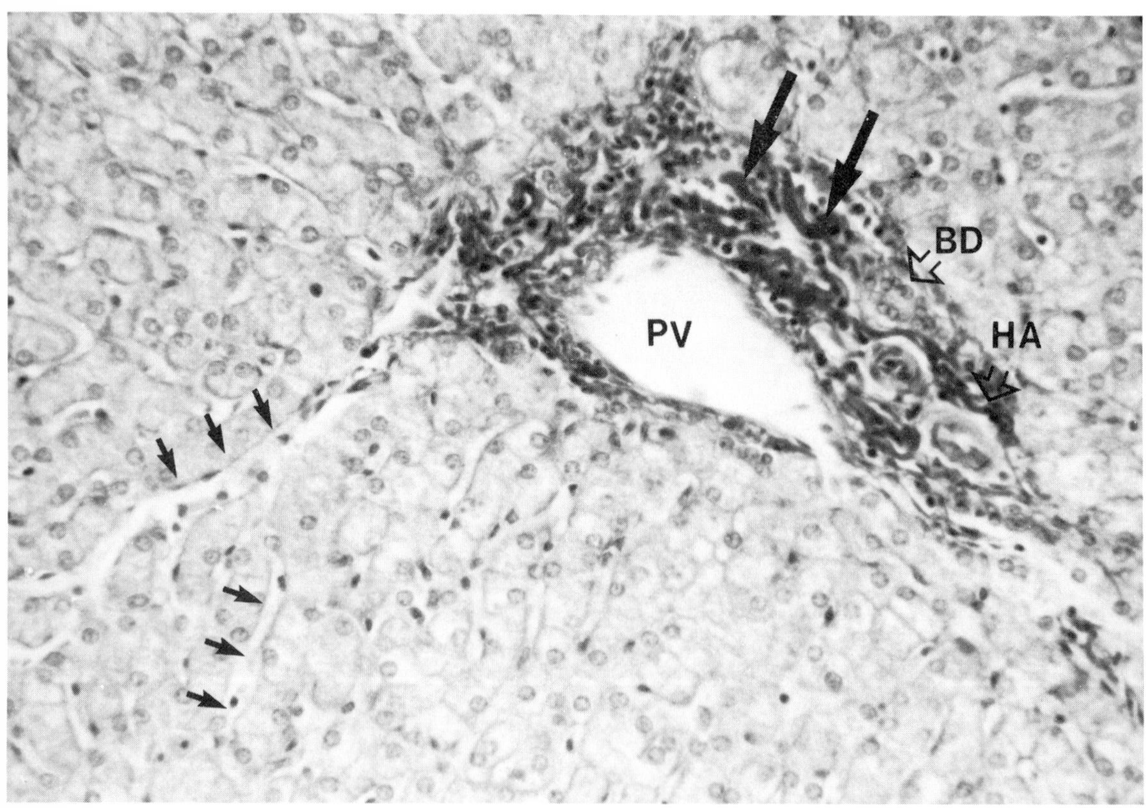

Fig. 23.1 Normal portal tract. The portal venous (PV), hepatic arterial (HA), and bile duct (BD) radicles are surrounded by thick collagen bundles (large arrows). This preparation was stained by the van Gieson technique which does not delineate the fine collagen fibrils around sinusoids (small arrows). (See Fig. 23.2.)

capsule. These vessels arborise frequently to form the microscopic blood supply of the liver which are contained in portal tracts surrounded by a small amount of connective tissue (Fig. 23.1). Hepatic arterial blood and portal venous blood flow from portal tracts into sinusoids (Figs. 23.2 and 23.3). The latter are unique vessels. They are lined by a layer of endothelial and phagocytic cells which do not make contact thus leaving distinct gaps in the cellular lining. In addition sinusoids, unlike capillaries, do not have a morphologically recognisable basement membrane or continuous connective tissue coat (Figs. 23.2 and 23.3). The consequence of this is that plasma has free access from sinusoids to the microvillous border of the hepatocyte. Sinusoids drain into larger vessels — terminal hepatic venules (also known as central veins) — which are also sheathed in connective tissue.

The connective tissue components of the liver can be demonstrated microscopically by a variety of staining techniques. Thick connective bundles in portal tracts and around central veins are delineated by van Gieson staining (Fig. 23.1) while fine fibres in portal tracts and along sinusoids are best identified by reticulin (silver impregnation) procedures. Morphologically defineable basement membranes invest bile ducts, lymphatics, blood vessels and nerves and are specifically demonstrated by periodic acid-Schiff staining; this histochemical procedure is dependant on the carbohydrate residues in basement membranes.

Electron microscopically, the interstitial collagen of portal tracts and around central veins, is composed of fibrils with a 65nM banding pattern. The fibrils are arranged in large aggregates. Basement membranes are readily identified by ultrastructural analysis around bile ducts and the other structures of portal tracts referred to above. Collagen fibrils along sinusoids are situated in the space of Disse which separates sinusoidal lining cells from hepatocytes (Fig. 23.3). Perisinusoidal fibril aggregates are smaller than those in portal tracts and each aggregate is widely separated from its neighbours. Collagen aggregates in this location lie in an amorphous electron luscent matrix, the nature of which is not completely characterised (see below).

Biochemical and immunohistochemical characterisation

The microscopic and ultrastructural heterogeneity of liver collagen is also reflected in its molecular polymorphism. As detailed in Chapter 1 at least 5 distinct collagens have been

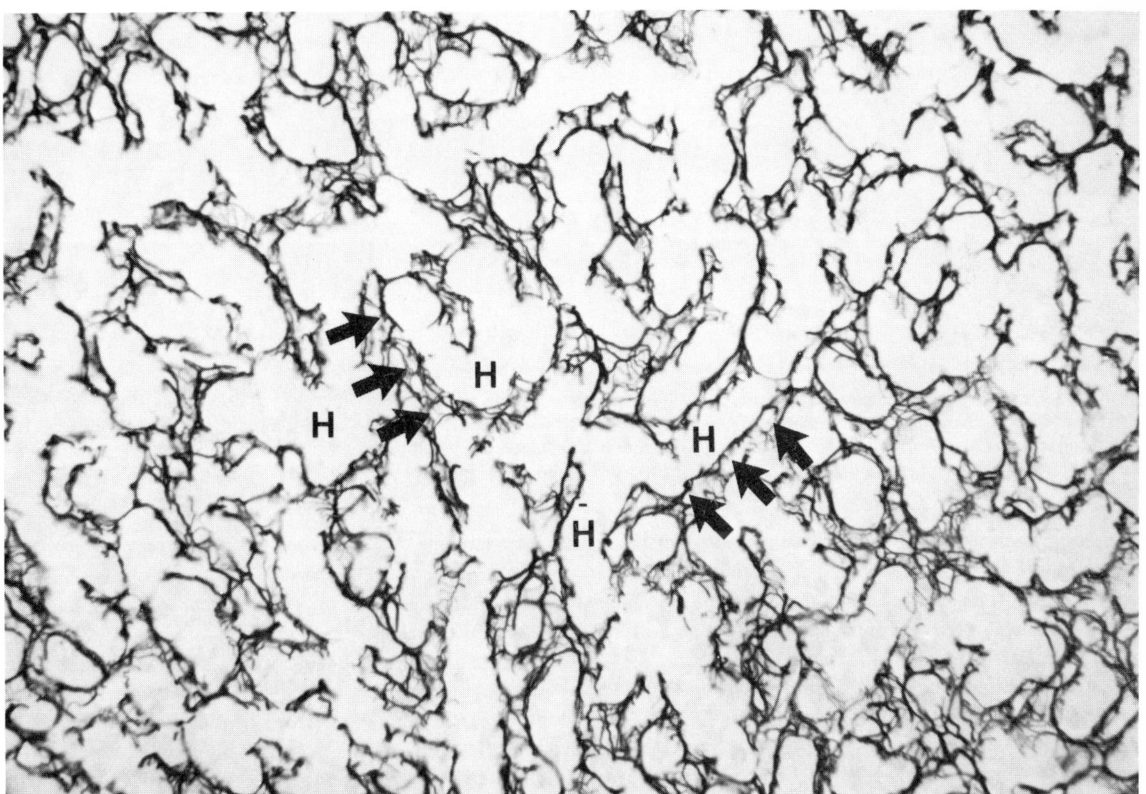

Fig. 23.2 Hepatic sinusoidal system. Portal venous and hepatic arterial blood flow from portal tracts into liver sinusoids (arrows). These lie between plates of hepatocytes (H) and are supported by a network of fine collagen fibrils which are demonstrated in this preparation by silver (reticulin) staining.

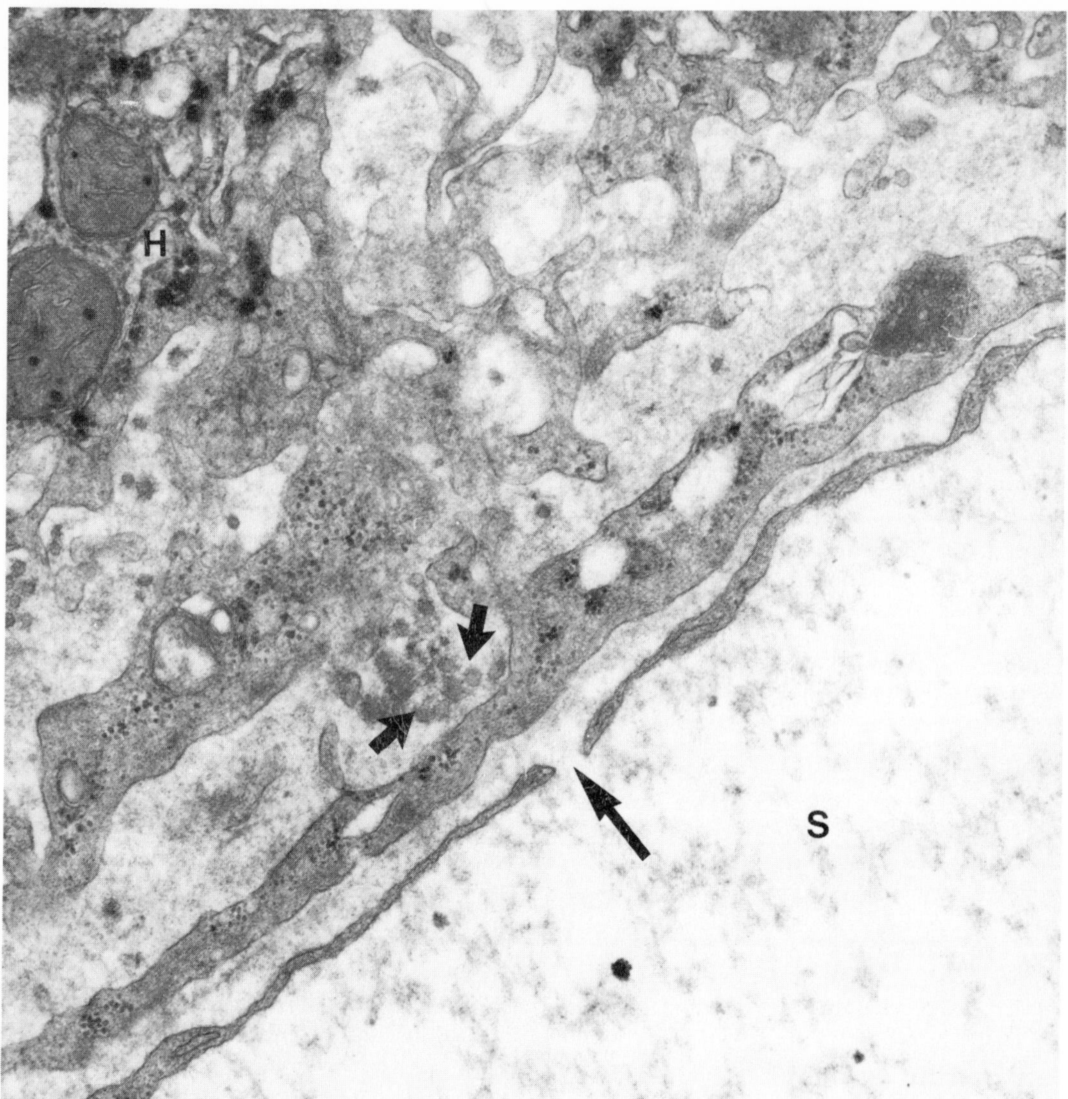

Fig. 23.3 Ultrastructure of normal hepatic sinusoid. There are physical gaps (large arrows) between the cells lining sinusoids; this allows free access of plasma to the hepatocyte. The space of Disse, which lies between the sinusoid (S) and the hepatocyte surface (H) contains electron dense flocculent material (small arrows). The latter may represent connective tissue components and/or blood plasma. Note that the sinusoidal lumen also contains electron dense plasma components. The space of Disse also contains small aggregates of collagen fibrils (small arrows).

described which have different amino acid compositions, and therefore their component polypeptide chains are products of separate genes. Although the various molecular types of collagen were first described in other organs all but one of them have now been isolated from normal liver. Repeated digestion of liver with pepsin solubilises 60 to 95 per cent of its collagen. This collagen consists of approximately equal amounts of type I, type III and basement membrane collagens (Rojkind et al, 1979). This ratio of type I/type III collagen of approximate unity has been substantiated in other experiments where collagen was isolated from liver by cyanogen bromide cleavage and characterised by identification of specific type I and III CNBr peptides (Seyer et al, 1977). Collagen type A & B, together, constitute 7 to 10 per cent of total hepatic collagen; these chains are similar to polypeptides A & B from human skin and α(A) and α(B) components of placenta (Burgeson et al, 1976). A basement membrane collagen referred to as type E, with an amino acid composition similar to a component isolated from aorta (Chung et al, 1976), has also been identified in normal liver. Another collagen resembles basement membrane collagen type IV of the renal glomerulus but this material from liver has not been fully characterised (Rojkind et al,

1979). Recently, it has been suggested that collagen containing α(A) and α(B) chains should be referred to as type V collagen (Bornstein & Sage, 1980) and the corresponding chains as α1(V) and α1(V). It is possible that further collagen types may be isolated from liver. It should be noted that the descriptions quoted above are based only on that fraction of liver collagen which is extractable with pepsin treatment. Following the latter as much as 40 per cent of hepatic collagen remains insoluble (Rojkind et al, 1979).

The anatomical location of some of the collagen types has been plotted by immunohistochemistry using polyclonal anticollagen antibodies in the indirect immunofluorescence procedure. Collagen and procollagen type I and III are present in portal tracts, around central veins and along sinusoids (Wick et al, 1978). Type IV collagen predictably is present in the basement membranes of portal tract blood vessels, lymphatics, nerves, bile ducts and central veins (Hahn et al, 1980). It is also present around smooth muscle cells of blood vessels. It does not exist in the interstitial matrix of normal portal tracts. Rather surprisingly type IV is deposited also in the space of Disse (Hahn et al, 1980), in spite of the fact that a morphological basement membrane does not occur around these blood vessels. It is possible that type IV collagen at this site does not aggregate into a visible basement membrane but rather exists free in the space of Disse complexed with other macromolecules. Ultrastructural immunohistochemistry using an immunoperoxidase procedure with polyclonal antibodies to type I, III and IV collagens has elucidated the organisation of these molecules in hepatic connective tissue (Grimand et al, 1980). Type IV collagen does indeed form a nonfibrillar network around type I and III collagen fibril aggregates in the space of Disse. Type III also exists in nonfibrillar form at this sitee. Also of interest is that fibril aggregates in this space are molecularly pure consisting either of type I or III, but not both molecules. Preliminary investigation with a mixture of antibodies has tentatively shown that type V collagen (A & B chains) is also distributed along hepatic sinusoids (Biempica et al, 1977).

Interest has also focussed recently on two other connective tissue proteins — fibronectin and laminin — which codistribute to some extent with collagen in liver. Fibronectin is a glycoprotein of molecular weight 440 000 daltons. It is composed of 2 dissimilar, disulphide bonded, subunits both of which have a molecular weight of about 200 000. The intact molecule exists in 2 forms. One is insoluble and is found in connective tissue in vivo or associated with cell surfaces in vitro. The other form is soluble and is present in human plasma, and is secreted by cells into the medium in vitro.

Fibronectin binds to collagen in vitro and the molecular domains involved in this reaction have been defined. It has been postulated that fibronectin, in the space of Disse, plays a role in the binding of hepatocytes to collagen within the liver lobule. In a cell attachment assay Klienman et al (Berman et al, 1980) have shown that isolated hepatocytes bind to collagen substrates more effectively in the presence of fibronectin. Isolated hepatocytes also agglutinate in the presence of type I collagen and form a visible precipitate (McGee, 1980). This latter reaction, is not dependant on fibronectin since it is not enhanced by the addition of fibronectin, nor is it inhibited by antibodies to fibronectin. Both of these experiments have led to opposite conclusions regarding the role of fibronectin in hepatocyte collagen interactions. The possible role of fibronectin-collagen-hepatocyte interactions at present, therefore, is not resolved. It should be noted, however, that although early experiments indicated that fibronectin mediated platelet binding to collagen, more recent experiments show that fibronectin does not facilitate collagen induced platelet aggregation but inhibits this phenomenon (McGee, 1980).

Immunohistochemistry demonstrates that fibronectin forms part of the basement membranes of portal tract structures and central veins (Hahn et al, 1980), and forms part of the electron dense amorphous matrix in the space of Disse. In addition fibronectin is associated with interstitial collagens of portal tracts (McGee, 1980).

Laminin, a more recently described glycoprotein, is a soluble component of basement membranes (Timpl et al, 1979). It has a molecular weight of 850 000 daltons and consists of several polypeptide chains of molecular weight 440 000 and 220 000; the intact molecule is dusulphide bonded. It has been isolated from a transplantable tumour which produces large amounts of morphological basement membranes. It has now been established that it also occurs in basement membranes (e.g. glomerular basement membrane) in normal animals. In liver (Hahn et al, 1980), laminin forms part of the basement membrane around bile ducts, portal tract vessels, lymphatics, nerves and the smooth muscle cells of portal veins and hepatic arterioles. It is not present along sinusoids and surprisingly it is absent from the basement membranes around central veins; ultrastructural basement membranes have been demonstrated around the latter structures.

Collagen synthesising cells

The cell types responsible for collagen and connective tissue production in liver, as in all other parenchymal organs, have not been completely established. In portal tracts it is assumed that the fibroblast is the cell of origin of interstitial collagens type I and III. The cell (or cells) which produces type IV collagen and laminin at this site is not known.

Within the hepatic parenchyma it has been postulated that perisinusoidal cells (McGee & Patrick, 1972) and or hepatocytes (Guxelian et al, 1981) produce the connective tissue which supports the major functional part of the liver. Neither of these hypotheses are proven. Electron microscopic studies show that perisinusoidal cells, which lie in the space of Disse, have all of the ultrastructural machinery necessary for the synthesis of proteins for export, viz, rough endoplasmic reticulin, and a Golgi apparatus (McGee & Patrick, 1972). The endoplasmic reticulin is filled with an electron dense material and the cell membrane is regularly associated with collagen fibril aggregates. These latter features are also found in fibroblasts. Autoradiographic investigations also support the concept that perisinusoidal cells are responsible for collagen synthesis in liver in normality and in acute liver damage (McGee & Patrick, 1972; Patrick & McGee, 1967). On the other hand, it has been postulated that hepatocytes (which produce liver specific products — albumin, fibrinogen etc) may also produce collagen (Guxelian et al, 1981). This hypothesis is based on the ability of isolated hepatocytes to form a collagenase degradeable protein and a collagen matrix in vitro. All of the preparations of freshly isolated hepatocytes which purportedly synthesise collagen have been contaminated by small number of mesenchymal cells. The latter probably derive from sinusoids or portal tracts or both. As a corollary to these findings with hepatocytes, 95 per cent pure preparations of mesenchymal cells also produce a collagen like protein as evidenced by their ability to produce a substrate which can be hydroxylated by prolyl hydroxylase, the enzyme responsible for the hydroxylation of specific prolyl residues in collagen (Shaba et al, 1973). Since isolated hepatocytes also contain prolyl hydroxylase, this observation has also been adduced in favour of the hepatocyte origin of liver collagen (Guxelian et al, 1981). However, it should be noted that virtually all cell types (including neuroblastoma cells and lymphocytes) maintained in culture contain prolyl hydroxylase and produce a collagenous protein. Since it is unlikely that specialised cells such as lymphocytes produce extracellular matrix in vivo, it would be unwise to conclude from tissue culture experiments that hepatocytes have a matrix formative function in vivo. Collagen production by hepatocytes in vitro may be necessary for cell adherence to the culture substrate and cell survival.

It has been disappointing that immunohistochemical studies with antibodies to collagen, fibronectin and laminin have entirely failed to demonstrate the collagen productive cell in the liver lobule (Hahn et al, 1980). It may well be that the net concentration of collagen protein in any cell in the liver lobule is at a concentration which is below the sensitivity of any of the immunohistochemical procedures currently available for its detection. Another possibility is, of course, that no cell within the hepatic parenchyma produces collagen but that it is produced in, and diffuses from, portal tracts into the lobule along the space of Disse. The balance of available evidence, however, suggests that the perisinusoidal cell is the connective tissue productive cell within the liver lobule, in vivo. It is probable, however, that the quantity and quality of connective tissue produced within the lobule is influenced by factors other than sinusoidal cells. It is conceivable that both sinusoidal and liver cells produce matrix components and cooperate in dictating the type of matrix in which they both exist.

The possible role of perisinusoidal cells in the production of hepatic connective tissue leaves several features of these cells unexplained. Perisinusoidal cells, like presumed fibroblasts at other sites contain prominent lipid droplets (Fig. 23.3). The lipid droplets of perisinusoidal cells contain vitamin A which can be discerned by its specific autofluorescence. It is noteworthy that a similar cell type, with large lipid droplets and abundant vitamin A also exist in the connective tissue of other parenchymal organs such as lung, kidney, adrenal and gut. It has been assumed that the latter cells have a fibroblastic function but the role of their vitamin A content in fibrogenesis has not been defined.

The rate of collagen synthesis in normal liver is low. It has been measured indirectly and directly. Prolyl hydroxylase levels in liver are higher than in most other parenchymal organs and it has been assumed that the level of this enzyme reflects the rate of collagen synthesis (Langness & Udenfriend, 1974). This assumption has been given weight by the recent observation that prolyl hydroxylase levels and collagen synthesis rates (measured as collagenase degradeable protein) show a good correlation when both were measured simultaneously in the same biopsy (McGee et al, 1974). There have been no studies of collagen type synthesis in normal liver. Fibronectin is also synthesised in normal liver. Laminin synthesis has not been quantified in liver.

COLLAGEN IN LIVER DISEASE

Almost all agents which cause acute liver disease in man and in experimental animals may be associated with the development of end-stage liver disease, viz. cirrhosis. This is a condition in which there is excessive deposition of collagen in the liver and hyperplasia of hepatocytes. This leads to complete disruption of hepatic architecture and function.

Anatomical distribution

In cirrhosis the collagen content of the liver increases up to seven times normal. Macroscopically, the liver surface and substance (which are normally smooth) become grossly nodular. Each nodule consists of regenerating liver tissue and is surrounded by thick bands of collagen. During the evolution of cirrhosis, collagen is deposited in excess in portal tracts and/or around central veins. Eventually or concomitantly, depending on the aetiological agent, collagen is also formed in increased amounts in the liver lobule which in normality has a very low content of collagen. With time the collagen in portal tracts and around central veins dissect through the liver lobules and collagen septa link these 2 structures. One result of septa formation is the creation of shunts from the portal venous to the hepatic venous system. This, together with compression of both these venous systems by excessive fibrous tissue, increases the pressure in the portal venous system (portal hypertension) which in turn results in the formation of proto-systemic shunting of blood. The latter gives rise to oesophageal varices which may bleed catastrophically, and also to hepatic encephalopathy.

The deposition of collagen in the hepatic lobule in cirrhosis may also directly compromise hepatocyte function. As mentioned earlier normal sinusoidal structure allows free access of plasma to hepatocytes through gaps in the sinusoidal cell lining which are not limited by a physically recognisable basement membrane. In cirrhosis, however, physical basement membranes appear in the space of Disse (capillarisation of sinusoids) (Schaffner & Popper, 1963) and there is also increased deposition of interstitial collagens which may ensheath large stretches of the sinusoidal system (Fig. 23.4). It is probable that the deposition of both interstitial and basement membrane collagens interfere with the free passage of plasma components to hepatocytes and vice versa. It is evident, therefore, that the formation of intrahepatic shunts and the conversion of an open to a closed sinusoidal system by collagen deposition can lead to functional liver failure in the presence of an adequate viable mass of hepatocytes.

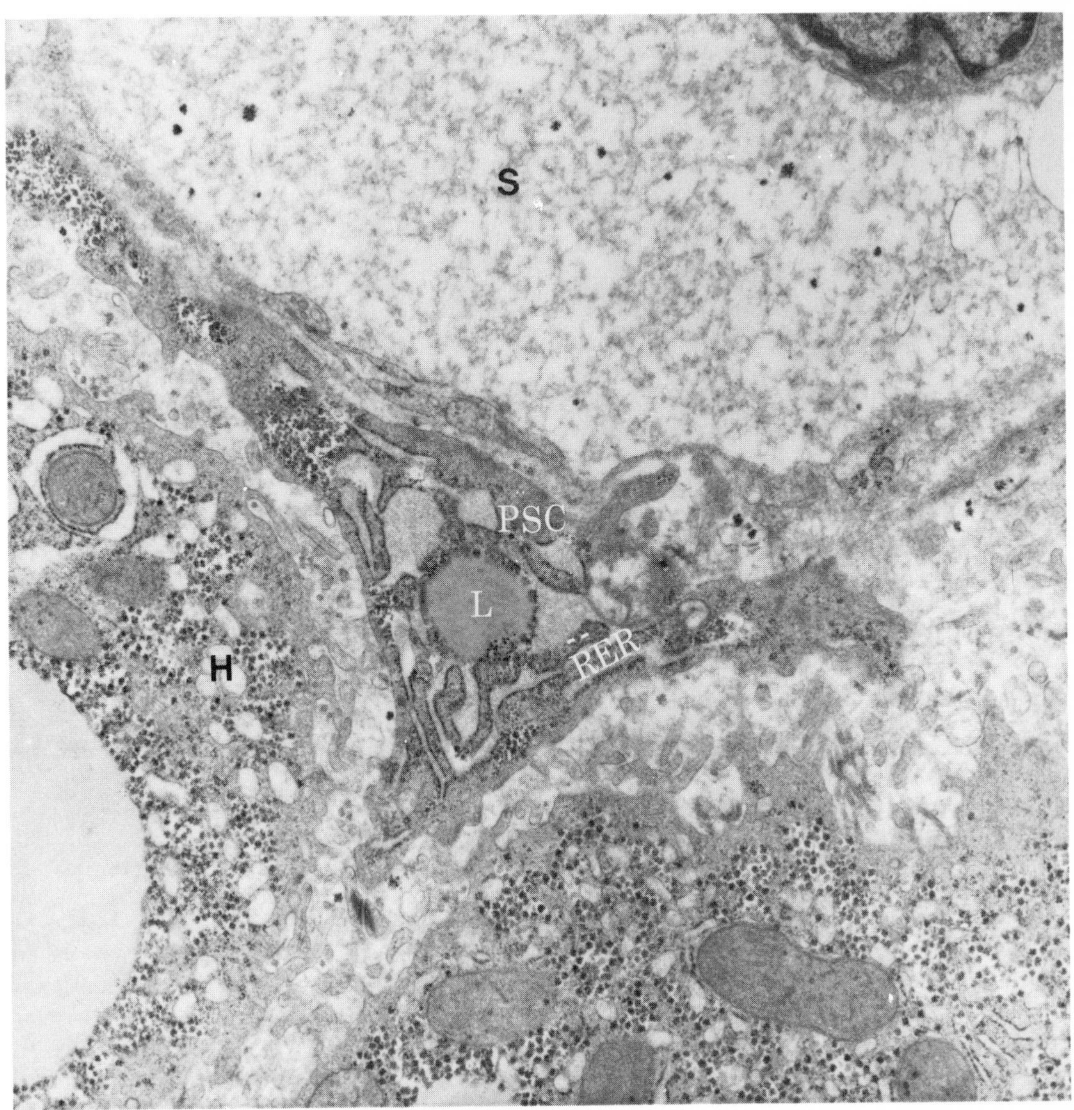

Fig. 23.4 Perisinusoidal cell (PSC). This cell lies entirely in the space of Disse between hepatocytes (H) and the sinusoidal lumen (S). It has abundant rough endoplasmic reticulum (RER) and contains a large lipid vacuole (L).

Biochemical and immunohistochemical analysis of liver collagen

The increase in liver collagen in cirrhosis has been investigated biochemically and by immunohistochemistry. The absolute quantity of type I and III collagen increases in cirrhosis whether the stimulus be alcohol abuse, haemachromatosis, or Wilsons disease (Rojkind et al, 1979). Initially it was reported that there was a preferential increase in type I collagen with a reduction in the type I to type III ratio (Seyer et al, 1977) A more recent study, however, which examined most of the known molecular types, has shown that there is a general increase in type I, III and basement membrane.collagens in cirrhosis (Rojkind et al, 1979). A preferential deposition of type I collagen was only found in cirrhotic livers where the collagen concentration was greater than 20 mg collagen/g of fresh tissue. The basement membrane collagen of cirrhotic liver comprise type IV and type V (Rojkind et al, 1979).

Type I trimer, composed of 3 $\alpha 1$ chains $(\alpha 1(I))_3$, has also been demonstrated in cirrhotic liver but not in normal liver (Rojkind et al, 1979). This trimer has been described in a number of in vitro systems but it is an unusual component of tissues in vivo.

Immunohistochemical analysis of liver tissue using antibodies to collagen types has elucidated the site of deposition of collagen in cirrhosis. Type I and III are deposited in portal tracts and along hepatic sinusoids (Wick et al, 1978). In the latter situation each collagen type coalesces to form separate fibril aggregates (Grimand et al, 1980). Type IV collagen is present in the same locations as in normal liver but rather surprisingly it also appears as part of the general matrix of collagen septa apparently unassociated with other recognised structures such as bile ducts (Hahn et al, 1980). Also of note is that type IV collagen increases around sinusoids not only in cirrhosis but also in diseases which lead to cirrhosis such as alcoholic hepatitis and chronic active hepatitis (Hahn et al, 1980). Type V collagens have not yet been localised in cirrhotic liver.

Fibronectin and laminin are also deposited in increased quantities in human cirrhotic liver (Hahn et al, 1980). Fibronectin forms part of the matrix of fibrous septa (Rudolph et al, 1979) and is increased along sinusoids and presumably codistributes with type I and III collagens (Hahn et al, 1980). Laminin, which is absent from normal sinusoids, is present around these structures in cirrhosis. Although, laminin normally codistributes with type IV collagen in normal tissues, it is not found as part of the matrix of fibrous septa as is type IV collagen (Hahn et al, 1980).

Collagen synthesising cells in liver disease

The cells responsible for increased collagen production in cirrhotic livers are controversial. It seems clear that cells with the ultrastructural features of fibroblasts populate fibrous septa and presumably synthesise type I and III collagen. However, fibroblasts do not synthesise type IV collagen which is a prominent collagen in septa. It has been postulated that myofibroblasts may be the source of type IV collagen in fibrous septa (Scheuer & Maggi, 1980). Myofibroblasts have been so named because they have many of the ultrastructural features of fibroblasts but also contain numerous cytoplasmic filaments similar to cells of smooth muscle origin. The derivation of myofibroblasts is now known. Increased collagen deposition along sinusoids may be due to the activity of perisinusoidal cells and or hepatocytes (see earlier) (McGee & Patrick, 1972; Guxelian et al, 1981). This problem has been studied in experimental models of fibrogenesis where it has been shown that after acute liver injury perisinusoidal cells proliferate and assume an ultrastructural morphology more close to that of fibroblast; (McGee & Patrick, 1972). The proliferation and change in morphology of these cells is associated spatially and temporally with collagen deposition in acute and chronic liver injury. Immunohistochemistry, has shown that in acute liver injury perisinusoidal cell activation is associated with the deposition of types I and III collagen but the other collagen types have not been studied in these models. The source of basement membrane collagens within the liver lobule in liver disease is not known. Similarly the laminin productive cells have not been identified. It seems likely that the excessive amounts of fibronectin in fibrous septa and within the hepatic parenchyma derive partially from plasma fibronectin and also from locally activated mesenchymal cells within the liver (Rudolph et al, 1979). The evidence for local production is based on in vitro incubation studies of acutely damaged liver in which it was shown that ^{3}H-leucine is incorporated into a component which has the same molecular weight as fibronectin, and like fibronectin is a disulphide bonded dimer. There is no positive immunohistochemical evidence that hepatocytes produce any of the above mentioned macromolecules in liver disease.

Regulation of the collagen productive response in liver disease

Three mechanisms have been postulated to account for the increase in collagen in cirrhotic livers: these are discussed below.

Firstly, it has been argued that the increase in collagen in liver is apparent rather than real and is due to death of liver cells which are resorbed and subsequently the stroma which normally supports these cells collapses and condenses. It is likely that this mechanism, which is based on morphological observations, operates in some liver diseases but its contribution to the massive increase in collagen found in cirrhosis is almost certainly trivial. The fact that liver collagen increases 5 to 7 fold in cirrhosis clearly demonstrates that there is a real, and not an

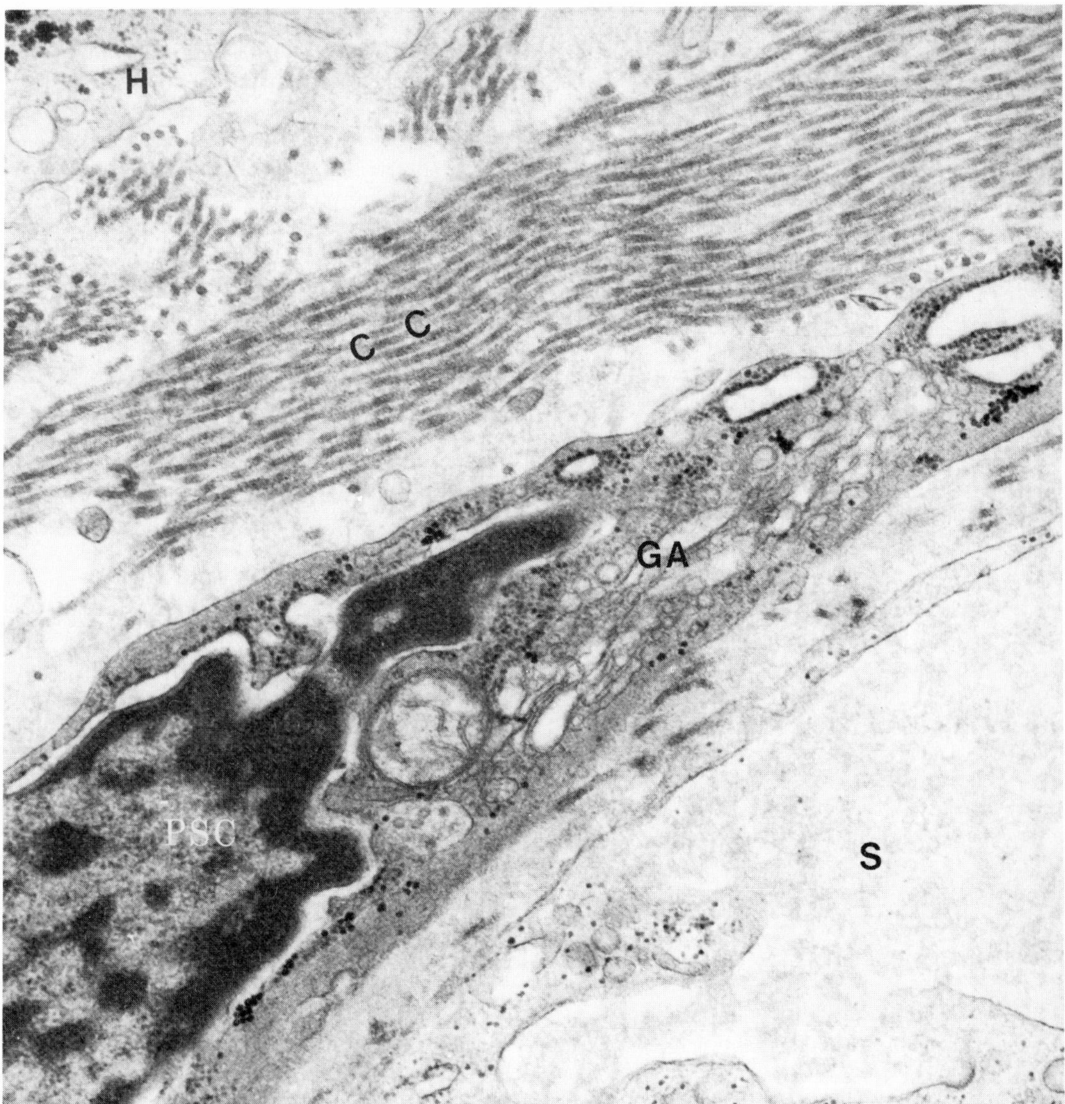

Fig. 23.5 Hepatic sinusoid in cirrhosis. The space of Disse is filled with a large aggregate of collagen fibrils (C) and part of a perisinusoidal cell (PSC) which has a prominent Golgi apparatus (GA). The sinusoidal lumen and hepatocyte surface are indicated by S & H respectively.

apparent, increase in liver collagen. Collapse of hepatic parenchyma, and subsequent collagen condensation, is found in acute hepatitis induced by viruses and other agents. Morphologically, this can be distinguished from new fibre formation by orcein staining which labels elastic tissue. In areas of collapse elastin is absent while it is present at sites of new collagen fibre formation (Scheuer & Maggi, 1980).

The second mechanism which may operate in producing excessive collagen deposition in the liver is a decrease in the rate at which collagen is degraded. Collagenase the enzyme(s) responsible for collagen degradation in man, is present in liver but accurate estimations of its activity in normality and liver disease are beset by biological difficulties. Collagenase, is inhibited by serum $\beta 2$ microglobulin and α-1-antitrypsin. Assays of collagenase activity in liver homogenates are therefore likely to be affected by both of these antiproteinases. Furthermore, there are no reliable turnover studies of collagen in cirrhosis which might also bear on this question. Although it is likely that changes in collagen degradation rates in cirrhosis influence net liver collagen, experiments to date do not allow quantitation of this mechanism.

The third mechanism, is that of increased collagen synthesis which results in a net accumulation of collagen in cirrhosis or diseases resulting in end-stage liver disease. In acute and chronic experimental liver injury associated with fibrogenesis there is abundant evidence of increased collagen synthesis. One model of acute liver damage is that induced by carbon tetrachloride. In this model hepatocyte death is evident within 6 to 24 hours of the administration of the poison. At the same time there is a burst of collagen synthesis in the damaged liver which is evident as early as 6 hours after injury and becomes maximal 2 to 3 days after the event. This is associated with activation of perisinusoidal cells and autoradiographic evidence of increased connective tissue (Patrick & McGee, 1967) and fibronectin synthesis in sinusoidal cells or mesenchymal cells which are closely associated with sinusoids (Rudolph et al, 1979). As collagen and fibronectin synthesis increase both macromolecules are extruded into the extracellular space and accumulate at the site of hepatocyte necrosis. Both glycoproteins form a sea of matrix components which after 2 days polymerise into morphologically identifiable fibres (Rudolph et al, 1979). These connective fibres persist for about 4 days after which they are resorbed, presumably by the action of specific (or nonspecific) extracellular proteases.

In human liver collagen biosynthesis in acute and chronic liver injury is also increased. The first indirect measurement of collagen synthesis in liver disease was achieved by assaying prolyl hydroxylase in fresh liver biopsies; prolyl hydroxylase is increased in a variety of physiological and pathological conditions associated with elevated collagen synthesis. The hepatic levels of this enzyme are increased in cirrhosis and conditions which lead to this condition but not in Gilbert's disease or other liver disorders which are not associated with liver fibrosis (McGee et al, 1974). More recently, it has been shown that prolyl hydroxylase and collagen synthesis in liver measured simultaneously are directly proportional, indicating that prolyl hydroxylase activity can be used to monitor hepatic collagen synthesis (McGee et al, 1974).

Theoretically, collagen production in liver disease may increase because the number of collagen synthesising cells in the liver increases and/or the rate at which each cell produces collagen increases.

Many liver diseases associated with fibrosis are characterised by lymphocytic and macrophage infiltration in the liver. This has led to the search for factors which may be released by lymphocytes and or macrophages which regulate collagen production in disease. Human peripheral lymphocytes, when stimulated by phytohaemagglutin, release a factor which increased the production of collagen by human fibroblasts in vitro; this factor(s) stimulates fibroblast growth (Wyler et al, 1977). In experimental animals, T-cells on exposure to an antigen to which they have been sensitised, also release a lymphokine which causes fibroblast proliferation and stimulates collagen production in fibroblast cultures (Chen & Leevy, 1973). Neither of these lymphokines has been investigated in human liver disease but it has been shown that the lymphokine which stimulates fibroblast growth may be active in experimental schistosomiasis, a disease in which hepatic collagen production is increased (Wahl et al, 1978).

There is one preliminary study, however, which indicates that lymphokines may modulate collagen production in human alcoholic liver disease (McGee & Fallon, 1978). Peripheral blood lymphocytes from alcoholic patients when exposed to Mallory bodies (a cytoplasmic structure present in hepatocytes damaged by alcohol) release a lymphokine which stimulates the production of collagen by fibroblasts. This action appears to be independent of an action on fibroblast proliferation.

A different group of compounds have been isolated from human and experimental liver diseases associated with fibrogenesis which have a specific effect on collagen production by fibroblasts in vitro but do not influence fibroblast proliferation. These factors, known as collagen stimulating factors, were demonstrated initially in acute liver injury induced in animals by carbon tetrachloride (Fallon & McGee, submitted). They stimulate prolyl hydroxylase activity and collagen synthesis in fibroblasts up to 10 fold. They do not influence fibroblast number, DNA synthesis or total DNA concentration in fobroblasts. Collagen stimulating factors, of which there are 4, have molecular weights below 5000 daltons. The 2 largest have apparent molecular weight of about 4500 and 1500 but the others were absorbed to the molecular sieve column which was used to measure these molecular weights. The collagen stimulating activity of all of these factors is destroyed partially or completely by trypsin indicating that they may be peptide (McGee & Fallon, 1978). More recently, similar collagen stimulating factors have been extracted from human cirrhotic liver and they appear to have the same properties as those derived from animal livers (Fallon & McGee, 1982). Not only do these factors stimulate collagen synthesis by fibroblasts but they also induce increased transport of the protein into the extracellular space. A quite different factor, from livers of normal and hyper-cholesetrolaemic rates, has also been identified as simulating collagen synthesis and it has been postulated that this may also play a role in regulating hepatic fibrogenesis (Ronnemaa et al, 1977). The source of collagen stimulating factors and those described by the Finnish group is not known. They may be released by activated macrophages, lymphocytes, or necrotic hepatocytes in liver disease. Alternatively, they may be generated in diseased liver by the action of proteases or a preformed inactive serum component in a manner analogous to the production of active kinins from an inactive serum precursor.

REFERENCES

Berman M D, Waggoner J G, Foidart J M, Kleinman H K 1980 Attachment to collagen by isolated hepatocytes from rats with induced hepatic fibrosis. Journal of Laboratory and Clinical Medicine 95: 660-70

Biempica L A, Morecki R, Wu C H, Giambrone M A, Rojkind M 1977 Isolation and immunohistochemical localisation of a component of basement membrane collagen in human liver (abstract). Gastroenterology 73: 1213

Bornstein P, Sage H 1980 Structurally distinct collagen types. Annual Review of Biochemistry 49: 957-1003

Burgeson R T, El Adli F A, Kaitila I I, Hollister D W 1976 Fetal membrane collagens: identification of two new alpha chains' Proceedings of the National Academy of Sciences of the USA 73: 2579-83

Chen T, Leevy C M 1973 Collagen biosynthesis in hepatic fibrosis (abstract). Gastroenterology 64: 178

Chung E, Rhodes R K, Miller E J 1976 Isolation of three collagenous components of probable basement membrane origin from several tissues. Biochemical and Biophysical Research Communications 17: 1167-74

Fallon A, McGee J O'D 1982 Collagen stimulating factors in hepatic fibrogenesis. Journal of Clinical Pathology (in press)

Grimand J A, Bordjevic R, Peyrol S, Chevallier M, Druguet M, Herbage D 1980 Portal fibrosis: 2 patterns of organisation of connective tissue in human liver using ultrastructural immunoperoxidase labelling of type I, III and IV collagens. (abstract). In: Rauterberg J (ed) Connective tissue of the normal and fibrotic human liver (abstracts). Munster, p 14

Guzelian P S, Qureshi G D, Diegelmann R F 1981 Collagen synthesis by the hepatocyte: Studies in primary cultures of parenchymal cells from adult rat liver. Collagen 1: 83-93

Hahn E, Wick G, Pencer D, Timpl R 1980 Distribution of basement membrane proteins in normal and fibrotic human liver: collagen type IV, Laminin and fibronectin. Gut 21: 63-71

Johnson R L, Ziff M 1976 Lymphokine stimulation of collagen accumulation. Journal of Clinical Investigation 58: 240-52

Langness U, Udenfriend S 1974 Collagen biosynthesis in non-fibroblastic cell lines. Proceedings of the National Academy of Sciences of USA 71: 50-1

McGee J O'D 1980 The healing response in liver: the role of collagen and fibronectin. In: Popper H, Bianchi L, Gudat F, Reutter W (eds) Communication of liver cells. MTP Press (England), p 39

McGee J O'D, Fallon A 1978 Hepatic cirrhosis — a collagen formative disease. Journal of Clinical Pathology (Suppl 12) 31: 150-7

McGee J O'D, Patrick R S 1972 The role of perisinusoidal cells in hepatic fibrogenesis. Laboratory Investigation 26: 429-40

McGee J O'D, O'Hare R P, Patrick R S 1973 Stimulation of the collagen biosynthetic pathway by factors isolated from experimentally injured liver. Nature. New Biology 243: 121-3

McGee J O'D, Patrick R S, Rodger M C, Luty C M 1974 Collagen prolyl hydroxylase activity and ^{35}-sulphate uptake in human liver biopsies. Gut 15: 260-7

Mann S W, Fuller G C, Rodil J V, Vidins E I 1979 Hepatic prolyl hydroxylase and collagen synthesis in patients with alcoholic liver disease. Gut 20: 825-32

Patrick R S, McGee J O'D 1967 The utilisation of proline by sinusoidal cells of mouse liver damaged by hepatotoxic agents. Journal of Pathology and Bacteriology 309-19

Rojkind M, Giamborne M A, Biempica L 1979 Collagen types in normal and cirrhotic liver. Gastroenterology 76: 710-9

Ronnemaa J, Vihersaari T, Rauta H 1977 Identification of glutamine as a hepatic factor which influences the synthesis of collagen by freshly isolated fibroblasts. Scandinavian Journal of Clinical and Laboratory Investigation 37: 351-6

Rudolph R, McClure W J, Woodward M 1979 Contractile fibroblasts in chronic alcoholic cirrhosis. Gastroenterology 76: 704-9

Ruoslahti E, Engvall E, Hayman E G 1981 Fibronectin: current concepts of its structure and functions. Collagen 1: 83-95

Schaffner F, Popper H 1963 Capillarisation of hepatic sinusoids in man. Gastroenterology 44: 239-42

Scheuer P J, Maggi G 1980 Hepatic fibrosis and collapse: histological distinction by orcein staining. Histopathology 4: 487-90

Seyer J M, Hutcheson E T, Kang A H 1977 Collagen polymorphism in normal and cirrhotic human liver. Journal of Clinical Investigation 59: 241-8

Shaba J K, Patrick R S, McGee J O'D 1973 Collagen synthesis by mesenchymal cells isolated from normal and acutely damaged mouse liver. British Journal of Experimental Pathology 54: 110-6

Sochynsky R A, Boughton B J, Burns J, Sykes B C, McGee J O'D 1980 The effect of human fibronectin on platelet collagen adhesion. Thrombosis Research 18: 521-33

Timpl R, Rhode H, Gehron-Robey P, Rennard S L, Foidart J M, Martin G R 1979 Laminin, a glycoprotein from basement membranes. Journal of Biological Chemistry 254: 9933-7

Wahl S M, Wahl L M, McCarthy J B 1978 Lymphocyte mediated activation of fibroblast proliferation and collagen production. Journal of Immunology 121: 942-6

Wick G, Brunner H, Penner E, Timpl R 1978 The diagnostic application of specific anti-procollagen antisera. II. Analysis of liver biopsies. International Archives of Allergy and Applied Immunology 56: 316-24

Wyler D J, Wahl S M, Wahl L M 1977 Hepatic fibrosis in schistosomiasis: egg granulomas secrete fibroblast stimulating factor in vitro. Science 202: 438-40

24

Lung

S. I. RENNARD and R. G. CRYSTAL

INTRODUCTION

The major function of the lung is to effect the transfer of oxygen from the atmosphere to blood and carbon dioxide from the blood to the atmosphere. To accomplish this, the lung must constantly replenish the air within the alveoli and bring blood and air into close apposition. Thus, gas exchange requires that the lung have a unique structure that both maintains the organization of its constituent parts and permits the dynamic mechanical properties of respiration.

To a large extent, these properties of the lung are defined and regulated by the extracellular connective tissue matrix. Although elastic fibres, proteoglycans, and structural glycoproteins are important in this regard, collagen is the most abundant (Hance & Crystal, 1975; Rennard et al, 1980; Crystal, 1974). By virtue of both its mechanical properties and structural organization, collagen plays a critical role in defining lung structure and function in health and disease.

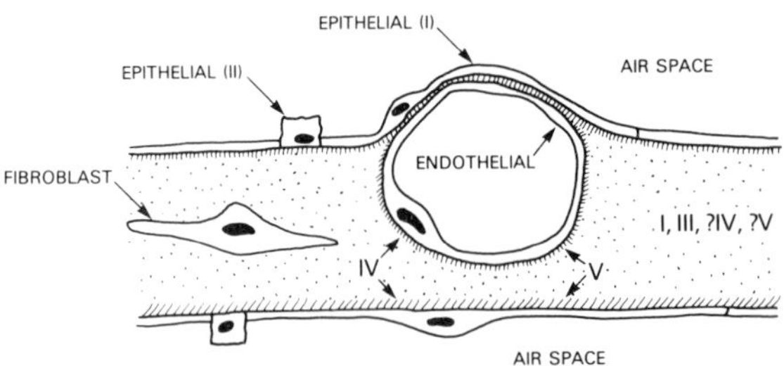

Fig. 24.1 Collagen in alveolar structures. Types I and III collagen are the major types present in the parenchyma in all species studied; these types are found in the interstitial space. Types IV and V are prominent components of alveolar and capillary basement membrane. Their presence in the interstitium has been suggested but not confirmed. Cells of the alveolar structures known to produce collagen are the fibroblast (types I, III, IV) and epithelial cells (I, III). In addition to type I, type I trimer is produced by lung epithelial cells in culture. Endothelial cells from lung parenchyma have not been studied, but endothelial cells from large vessels are known to produce I, III, IV, and V.

AMOUNT AND LOCATION OF LUNG COLLAGEN

In the adult, collagen comprises 10 to 20 per cent of the dry weight of the lung and represents 60 to 65 per cent of all lung connective tissue (Bradley et al, 1975; Pickrell & Shafer, 1971; Hoffman et al, 1972; Chvapil et al, 1973; Juricova & Deyl, 1974; Hurst et al, 1977; Collins et al, 1977; Collins & Jones, 1978; Starcher et al, 1978). There is some species variation in the relative abundance of lung collagen; for example, in the adult mouse it comprises 6 per cent of dry weight (Law et al, 1976) and in the adult human it comprises 20 per cent (Bradley et al, 1975; Hurst et al, 1977; Collins et al, 1977). On a macroscopic scale, collagen is part of a connective tissue continuum that begins at the hilar structures, courses down the bronchi, arteries and veins, branches out to the alveolar structures, and meets the connective tissue fibres coursing inward from the visceral pleura (Pierce, 1968; Low, 1978). This interconnection of lung collagen profoundly influences the mechanical behaviour of the organ throughout the respiratory cycle by providing a mechanism to distribute tensile forces within the lung and thus linking the function of the various alveolar units to the lung as a whole (Pierce, 1968; Fung et al, 1979). In addition, the mechanical properties of collagen make it ideally suited to define the shape of the component parts within the lung.

At the microscopic level, collagen is found throughout the extracellular space of the lung. In the alveolar structures, collagen is present in the alveolar interstitium as well as the endothelial and epithelial basement membranes (Fig. 24.1) (Huang et al, 1973; Madri & Furthmayr, 1979; Wick & Crystal, unpublished). In those places where the alveolar capillaries are closest to the epithelial surface, the two basement membranes join, thus bringing air and blood within 500μm of each other and allowing for efficient gas exchange (Low, 1978). In the bronchi, collagen is present in the basement membrane beneath the epithelial layer and as a sheath loosely surrounding the airway (Fig. 24.2).

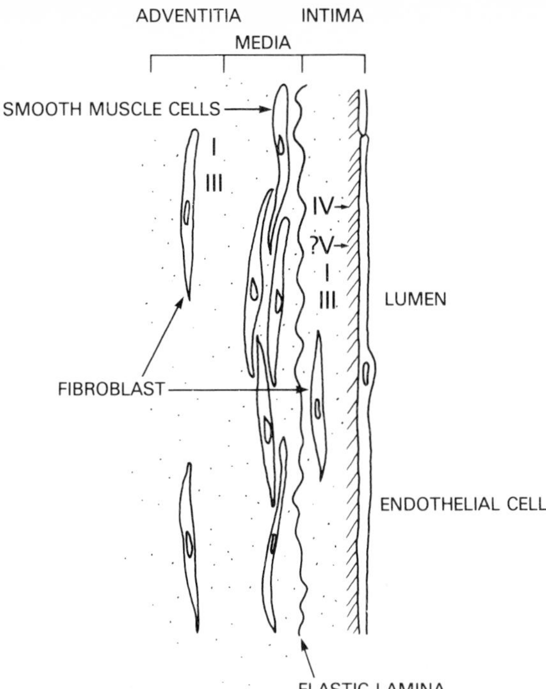

Fig. 24.2 Collagen in the pulmonary vasculature. Large blood vessels in the lung have a three-layered structure. Outermost is the serosa which is rich in type I with smaller amounts of type III; these collagens are presumably produced by serosal fibroblasts. The media is rich in smooth muscle cells and although studies have not been done with lung vascular smooth muscle cells, they probably produce most of the type III and some of the type I found in the media. The endothelium is lined with cells which, like endothelial cells from other sources, probably produce the basement membrane which certain collagen types IV and V. The relative thickness of these layers varies from arteries to veins and with the calibre of the vessel.

Collagen also comprises a large part of cartilage present in the trachea and large airways (Hurst et al, 1977; Bradley et al, 1974). In the pulmonary arteries and veins, it is present in the subendothelial basement membrane, forms a meshwork between cells of the media, and is present in the adventitial sheath loosely encasing each vessel (Fig. 24.3). Collagen is also found just beneath the mesothelial cell layer of the visceral pleura as part of a basal lamina as well as in a layer of connective tissue that connects with that of adjacent alveoli (Fig. 24.4).

Although the content of collagen (amount/dry weight) in the tracheobronchial tree and pulmonary vasculature is greater than that in the parenchyma, the total mass of the parenchyma is much larger and thus the bulk of the collagen in lung is that present in the alveolar structures. Detailed quantitative studies of the distribution of collagen among the substructures of the lung are not available from human material. In the yearling calf, collagen constitutes 40 per cent of dry weight of bronchioles, 15 per cent of dry weight of parenchyma and 5 per cent of dry weight in

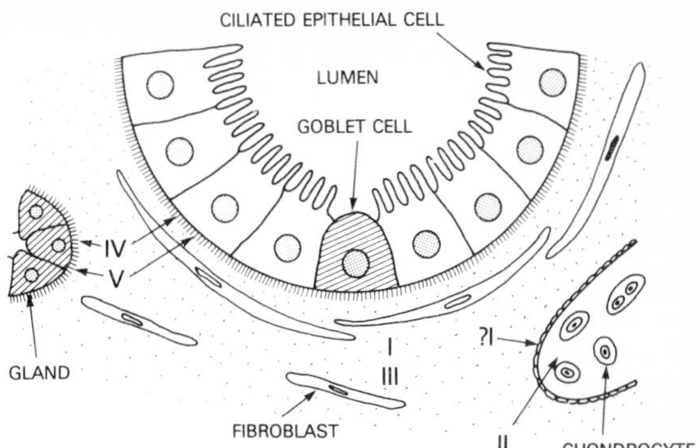

Fig. 24.3 Collagens of the tracheobronchial tree. The larger proximal airways are dominated by cartilage where chondrocytes produce the type II collagen in the matrix. The perichondrium probably has small amounts of type I collagen. Glands are prominent structures in the airways and are lined by a basement membrane containing collagen types IV and V. This basement membrane is probably produced by the glandular epithelium, but specific studies in lung have not been done. In more distal airways, cartilage and glands are less prominent. The airway epithelium is underlaid by a basement membrane containing types IV and V collagen and surrounded by smooth muscle cells. Smooth muscle cells and fibroblasts likely contribute to the types I and III found in the airways.

pleura (Seethanathan et al, 1975). In six-month-old rats, collagen comprises 25 per cent of dry weight of the trachea, bronchi and vessels, and 8 per cent of the parenchyma (Collins, personal communication). Thus, the collagen content of lung structures likely varies significantly with different species.

In general, most measurements of the quantity of

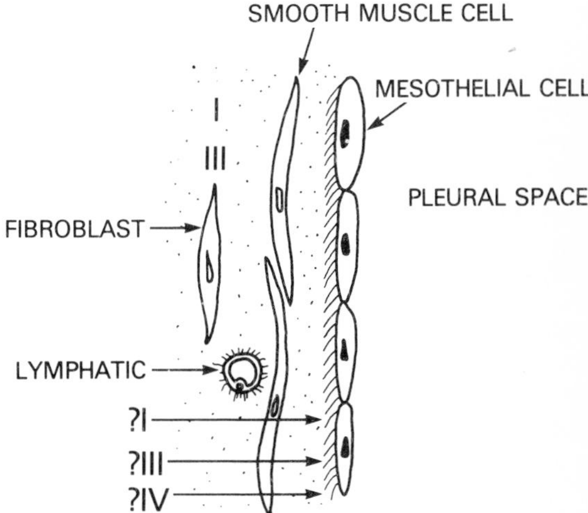

Fig. 24.4 Pleural collagen. The pleura has not been studied in detail and the collagens present are not well described. The visceral pleura forms the surface of the lung; it is lined by mesothelial cells which produce types I, III, and IV collagen. Smooth muscle cells and some fibroblasts are found beneath this layer and likely produce the collagens in the loose connective tissue.

collagen in lung have been made using hydroxyproline as a specific collagen marker (Hance & Crystal, 1975; Rennard et al, 1980). Other lung macromolecules do contain hydroxyproline (12 residues/1000 in elastin (Sandberg, 1976), 26/1000 in the C1q component of complement (Reid et al, 1972), and 8 to 12/1000 in two macromolecules of unknown aetiology found on the alveolar epithelial surface (Bhattacharyya et al, 1975)), but these noncollagen proteins are likely to contribute less than 5 per cent to the total lung hydroxyproline (Bradley et al, 1974). Thus, for most purposes, a measurement of hydroxyproline in lung tissue is 'specific' for collagen. Other methods, such as extraction by denaturation, have been used to quantitate lung collagen, but lack of specificity and the variable inefficiency has led to abandonment of these techniques.

In the adult, most lung collagen is insoluble. A variety of approaches have been used to extract intact collagen from lung, including techniques employing neutral salt, acetic acid, guanidine (Pierce, 1978; Bornstein & Traub, 1979), ultrasonic mechanical disruption (Richmond, 1980), and limited pepsin digestion (Pierce, 1968; Seyer, 1978; Madri & Furthmayr, 1979). For example, even with the relatively harsh method of pepsin digestion, only 15 to 30 per cent of total collagen can be extracted intact from the human lung (Madri & Furthmayer, 1979; Seyr, personal communication). Studies by Goldstein et all, 1978 suggest that this insolubility of lung collagen occurs soon after synthesis. For example, 1 day after [^{14}C]proline is administered intratracheally to hamsters, approximately 30 per cent of the newly synthesized collagen is soluble, but within 3 weeks less than 10 per cent of the collagen can be extracted (Goldstein et al, 1878).

It has been assumed that the relative insolubility of lung collagen results from the extracellular covalent interactions among collagen molecules (Juricova & Deyl, 1974; Szemenyei & Balint, 1973) and between collagen and other components of the extracellular matrix that form soon after the newly synthesized collagen molecule has been secreted from the cell (Hance & Crystal, 1975; Rennard et al, 1980; Bornstein & Traub, 1979). Lysyl oxidase, the enzyme responsible for collagen crosslinking, is present in lung (Brody et al, 1979), and the lysyl oxidase derived crosslinks, lysylnorleucine, hydroxylysylnorleucine, and dihydroxylysylnorleucine have been isolated from hydrolysates of lung collagen (Pickrell & Shafer, 1971). Moreover, dimeric and tremeric cross-linked collagen chains (termed β-chains and γ-chains, respectively) are routinely found in collagen preparations extracted from lung. Also, when animals are treated with cross-link inhibitors such as β-aminopropionitrile (Bradley et al, 1974) or penicillamine (Fedullo et al, 1979), a larger proportion of intact collagen can be extracted using conventional techniques. Thus, there is little doubt that lung collagen is processed after secretion and 'matures' into the insoluble fibres responsible for proper organ function.

TYPES OF COLLAGEN IN LUNG

The lung contains the entire spectrum of known collagen types (Figs. 24.1–24.4). As in other tissues, this heterogeneity has been evaluated using both chemical and immunofluorescent methodologies (Table 24.1). Most of the chemical information concerns the collagens of the alveolar structures, but using type-specific antibodies, the locations of most of the collagen types have been evaluated

Table 24.1 Collagen types in lung

Type	*Species*	*Method*	*Reference*
I*	Human	Immunofluorescence	Madri & Furthmayr, 1979, 1980
		Chemical	Alitalo (1980), Bradley et al (1974, 1975), Huang et al (1973), Hurst et al (1977), Last McLees et al (1977), Madri & Furthmayr (1979), Seyer (p.c.), Seyer et al (1976)
	Rabbit	Chemical	Crystal (1974), Bradley et al (1974)
	Porcine	Chemical	Seyer (personal comm.)
	Rat	Chemical	Reiser & Last (1980), Reiser et al (1979)
	Monkey	Chemical	Last (personal comm.)
	Baboon	Chemical	Collins et al
	Mouse	Chemical	Last (personal comm.)
	Sheep	Chemical	Last (personal comm.)
II	Human	Chemical	Hurst et al (1977)
		Immunofluorescence	Foidart et al (1979)
III	Human	Immunofluorescence	Madri & Furthmayer (1979, 1980), Wick & Crystal
		Chemical	Epstein & Munderloh (1975), Huang et al (1973), Hurst et al (1977), McLees et al (1977), Madri & Furthmayer (1979), Seyer (1978), Seyer et al (1976)
	Porcine	Chemical	Seyer (personal comm.)
	Rat	Chemical	Reiser & Last (1980), Reiser et al (1979)
	Monkey	Chemical	Last (personal comm.)
	Baboon	Chemical	Collins et al
	Mouse	Chemical	Last (personal comm.)
	Sheep	Chemical	Last (personal comm.)
IV	Human	Immunofluorescence	Madri & Furthmayer (1979, 1980), Seyer (1978), Wick & Crystal
	Porcine	Chemical	Seyer (personal comm.)
V	Human	Immunofluorescence	Madri & Furthmayer (1979, 1980), Seyer (1978)
		Chemical	Madri & Furthmayer (1979)
	Porcine	Chemical	Seyer (personal comm.)

*Type I trimer has not been identified in lung, although an epithelial cell strain derived from the cat lung in the late stage of fetal maturation (strain AK-D) produces type I trimer (as well as other collagen types).

in the pulmonary parenchyma, vasculature, airways, and pleura.

In the adult parenchyma, types I and III account for more than 90 per cent of the collagen. The best approximation of the relative amounts of these collagens comes from studies of human lung suggesting type I dominates type III in a ratio of 2 to 1 (Seyer, personal communication; Seyer et al, 1976, 1981). Type I is present throughout the interstitium of the alveolar structures and, like type I in other tissues, is thought to be the major collagen type comprising the banded fibres observed by electron miscroscopy (Huang et al, 1973). Immunofluorescent studies with type-specific antibodies have shown that type III collagen is found along with type I throughout the interstitium (Madri & Furthmayr, 1979, 1980; Wick & Crystal, unpublished). Collagen types I and III are also present in the connective tissue sheaths surrounding the tracheobronchial tree and the pulmonary arteries and veins as well as in the visceral pleura (Wick & Crystal, unpublished; Madri, personal communication).

Type II collagen in lung is confined to cartilage in the trachea and large bronchi (Bradley et al, 1974; Foidart et al, 1979). Type II collagen in tracheobronchial tree cartilage is thought to be in the form of thin, randomly dispersed fibres, but this has not been evaluated in detail (Rennard et al, 1980).

Type IV collagen has been localized to the epithelial and capillary basement membranes of the alveolar structures, where it represents about 5 per cent of parenchymal collagen (Rennard et al, 1980; Madri & Furthmayr, 1979, 1980; Wick & Crystal, unpublished). It is also found in the endothelial basement membranes of the pulmonary arteries and veins and the epithelial basement membranes of the tracheobronchial tree. The form of type IV collagen in these locations is unknown. It has also been recently observed that small amounts of type IV collagen are present as a very fine meshwork in the parenchymal interstitium (Wick & Crystal, unpublished).

Type V collagen is present in the alveolar structures but it is not clear whether it is limited to the endothelial and epithelial basement membranes or whether it is present in the interstitial matrix as well (Madri & Furthmayr, 1979, 1980; Wick & Crystal, unpublished). Like type IV collagen, type V is thought to represent approximately 5 per cent of parenchymal lung collagen (Rennard et al, 1980). Its anatomic form is unknown.

All available evidence suggests the collagen types present in lung are genetically identical to their counterparts in other organs. In this regard, most attention has been focused on collagen types I and III. When extracted from lung, the composite α-chains of collagen types have similar properties on carboxymethyl cellulose chromatograms and sodium-dodecyl sulphate acrylamide gels to comparable α-chains from other sources (Bradley et al, 1975; Bradley et al, 1974; McLees et al, 1977). In addition, CNBr peptides of α-chains from lung collagens I and III map on carboxymethyl cellulose and sodium-dodecyl sulphate acrylamide gels similarly to $\alpha 1(I)$, $\alpha 2$ and $\alpha 1(III)$ peptides from other tissues (Epstein & Munderloh, 1975; Reiser & Last, 1980). Although it has been shown that both type I (Bradley et al, 1975; Seyer et al, 1976; Epstein & Munderloh, 1975) and type III collagen from lung have a higher content of hydroxylysine than the collagens of the same type isolated from other organs, this likely results from differences in post-translational modifications to newly synthesized lung collagen rather than from differences in primary structure. The implications of these tissue specific modifications for the function of collagen in the lung are not known, but may be of significance since the hydroxylysine residues can be further modified by glycosylation and can be involved in collagen cross-linking (Hance & Crystal, 1975; Rennard, 1980; Bornstein & Traub, 1979).

PRODUCTION OF LUNG COLLAGEN

Collagen production by the lung has been demonstrated in vivo utilizing intravenous (Newman & Langer, 1975), intraperitoneal (Richmond & D'Auoust, 1976; Pierce et al, 1967; Metevier et al, 1978), or intratracheal (Goldstein et al, 1978) administration of radioactive tracers. In addition, a variety of in vitro methodologies have been used, including studies of isolated perfused and ventilated lung (Kerr et al, 1979), slices or minces of lung maintained in short-term culture (Bhatnager et al, 1978; Bradley et al, 1974; Collins et al, 1977; Greenberg et al, 1978; Hurst et al, 1977; Hussain et al, 1978; Last & Greenberg, 1979; Reiser et al, 1979), cultured lung cells (Alitalo, 1980; Clark et al, 1980; Hance et al, 1976; Kelley et al, 1979), and lung cell-free protein synthesizing components (Collins & Crystal, 1975; Tolstoshev et al, 1981). Most of these studies use the incorporation of labelled-proline into labelled hydroxyproline as evidence of collagen production, but sensitivity to Clostridial collagenase, solubility by hot trichloroacetic acid, and a variety of chromatographic and electrophoretic methods have also been used.

Quantitative estimates of collagen production by lung cells

It is difficult to state unequivocally how much collagen is produced by the whole lung (per cell per hr) because most studies utilize labelled tracer techniques but do not account for the specific activity of the intracellular tracer pool (Breul et al, 1980). For most species, the adult lung parenchymal cells devote an average of 2 to 5 per cent of their protein synthesizing machinery to collagen production. The best estimates of absolute amount of collagen produced suggest this represents approximately

2–4 × 10^4 collagen chains per cell per hr (averaged over all cells in the parenchyma) (Bradley et al, 1974, 1975; Collins & Jones, 1978). Once maturity is reached, the rate of collagen production by the lung parenchyma does not change (Collins & Jones, 1978; Newman & Langer, 1975). Studies of isolated pulmonary vasculature and airways have shown that these structures actively produce collagen, but their rate of collagen production has not been quantified (Bradley et al, 1974).

The alveolar structures of the normal adult lung contain six kinds of cells, including four parenchymal cells (fibroblasts, epithelial type I, epithelial type II, endothelial) (Fig. 24.1) and two inflammatory and immune effector cells (alveolar macrophages, lymphocytes). Of the parenchymal cells in normal lung, fibroblasts are the most abundant, comprising almost 40 per cent of all cells. Endothelial cells make up approximately one-third, and epithelial cells the remainder (Crapo et al, 1980). It is likely that all of these cells contribute to the collagen of the alveolar structures. Human lung fibroblasts in culture produce approximately 4.0–7.5 × 10^5 procollagen chains per cell per hr (Breul et al, 1980), close to what would be expected from the quantitative estimates of collagen production by the intact tissue. Although preliminary studies of type II epithelial cells isolated from adult rabbit lung suggested that this cell type did not produce collagen, a diploid feline lung parenchymal epithelial cell strain (AK–D) with characteristics of both type I and type II epithelial cells actively produced collagen in vitro (Fulmer et al, 1977; Elson et al, 1976). Interestingly, on the average, this cell produces more collagen (per cell per hr) than fibroblasts isolated from the lung of the same species, suggesting parenchymal epithelial cells may play a very important role in producing the collagenous extracellular matrix (Fulmer et al, 1977). Although lung endothelial cells have not been studied, endothelial cells from non-lung sources actively produce collagen (Howard et al, 1976; Jaffe et al, 1967; Barnes et al 1978), and thus it is likely that endothelial cells also contribute to parenchymal collagen production. Lung inflammatory and immune effector cells do not contribute directly to collagen production but they may have indirect effects by producing growth factors for lung parenchymal cells (Bitterman & Crystal, 1980; Bitterman et al, 1981), by producing fibronectin and thus modulating cellular and matrix organization and location (Villiger et al, 1980; Rennard et al, 1981), and perhaps by regulating the rate at which parenchymal cells produce collagen (Heppleston, 1979).

In contrast to cells of the lung parenchyma, quantitative collagen production has not been studied utilizing pure populations of cells isolated from the tracheobronchial tree or pulmonary vasculature. However, mesothelial cells from the rat pleura have been evaluated; these cells produce approximately 4 × 10^5 collagen chains per cell per hr (Rennard et al, 1981).

Types of collagen produced by lung cells

The adaptation of radioactive tracer technique to pieces of lung maintained in short-term culture has demonstrated, as expected, that the different lung structures synthesize the specific types of collagen found in each location (Figs. 24.1–24.4) (Hance & Crystal, 1975; Rennard et al, 1980). In a typical experiment of this genre, 1 to 2 mm^3 pieces of fresh lung are placed in culture medium with labelled proline for 4 to 6 hrs, the newly synthesized labelled collagens extracted, and the types identified by carboxymethyl cellulose chromatography, interrupted sodium dodecyl sulphate acrylamide gel electrophoresis, or CNBr mapping techniques. For example, pieces of lung parenchyma produce types I and III but not type II (Bradley et al, 1974, 1975; Crystal, 1974; Kelley et al, 1979; Tolstoshev, unpublished). Presumably these explants also produce small amounts of types IV (Last & Greenberg, 1979) and V, but this has not yet been evaluated fully.

In contrast, as expected from a cartilage-containing tissue, the major collagen produced by the tracheobronchial tree is type II (Bradley et al, 1974; Crystal, 1974). Although very little attention has been given to the large pulmonary blood vessels, it is known that they at least produce type I collagen (Crystal, 1974; Bradley et al, 1976).

To determine which cell types are responsible for production of each collagen type in the various lung structures, cell culture techniques have been utilized to evaluate pure populations of lung cells. This is a difficult technical problem, because the lung is a complex organ comprised of many cell types (Weibel et al, 1976). To date, the lung cells to be studied in this fashion are human (Alitalo, 1980; Clark et al, 1980; Hana et al, 1976; Kelley et al, 1979), rabbit (Hance et al, 1976), and feline parenchymal fibroblasts (Fulmer et al, 1977), feline parenchymal epithelial cells, and rat mesothelial cells (Rennard et al, 1981).

After the cell cultures have been established and the type and purity of the cells verified, these studies identify collagen production utilizing radioactive tracer techniques combined with column chromatography, interrupted sodium dodecyl sulphate gel electrophoresis, CNBr mapping, or enzyme-linked immunoassay method (ELISA). For example, such methods have shown that parenchymal fibroblasts produce type I and type III (Alitalo, 1980; Castor et al, 1979; Clark et al, 1980; Hance et al, 1976; Kelley et al, 1979; Kelman et al, 1977) and small amounts of type IV (Alitalo, 1980); most human lung fibroblasts produce I and III in a 6:1 to 10:1 ratio (Hance et al, 1976; Tolstoshev unpublished). A cell from fetal tissues which resembles both type I and type II epithelial cells produces (at least) types I and III and probably type I trimer (Bradley, unpublished; Fulmer et al, 1977). Recently, a strain of rat mesothelial cells has been shown to produce collagen types I, III and IV (Rennard et al, 1981).

It has been assumed that lung endothelial cells are similar to non-lung endothelial cells in terms of the types of collagen they produce, but endothelial cells cultured from lung have not been studied in this regard. Likewise, lung vascular and airway smooth muscle cells, and airway epithelial cells have not been evaluated in terms of collagen production.

Control of collagen production by lung cells

All available evidence suggests that the mechanisms utilized by lung cells to produce collagen are identical to those utilized by other cells in the body. The mRNA for type I collagen has been isolated from fetal sheep lung and translated efficiently in a heterologous cell-free system (Tolstoshev, unpublished), as have type I collagen polysomes from fetal rabbit lung (Collins & Crystal, 1975). On the average, cells from the lung parenchyma of a newborn sheep contain approximately 10^3 type I procollagen mRNA molecules per cell (Tolstoshev, unpublished). In contrast, confluent human fetal lung fibroblasts (strain HFL-1, American Type Culture Collection CCL153) contain 7×10^3 type I procollagen mRNA molecules per cell (Tolstoshev et al, 1981), consistent with the concept that the fibroblast, a cell comprising approximately 40 per cent of the parenchymal lung cells, is the major type I collagen producing cell in the alveolar structures.

There are some minor differences in the post-translational modifications of some lung collagens compared to collagen from other organs (see discussion in section on types of collagen). Nevertheless, although biochemical studies are limited, the lung enzymes relevant to the post-translation modification of collagen appear similar to those isolated from other tissues (Hance & Crystal, 1975). The polypeptide modifying enzymes prolyl hydroxylase (Halme et al, 1970; Ryhanen & Kivirikko, 1974), lysyl hydroxylase (Ryhanen & Kivirikko, 1974), and lysyl oxidase (Brody et al, 1979; Cronlund & Kagan, 1980), as well as glycosyl-transferases for the incorporation of glucose and galactose to the hydroxylysine residues of collagen have been measured in lung tissue obtained from several species (Spiro & Spiro, 1971). Although changes in the activity of some of these enzymes have been noted with growth, development (Brody et al, 1979; Ryhanen & Kivirikko, 1974), and in some models of disease (Cutroneo et al, 1975; Halme et al, 1970; Hussain et al, 1976; Kuttan et al, 1979; Ooshima et al, 1977; Orthoefer et al, 1976; Sneider et al, 1976; Thompson & Patrick, 1978; Valimaki et al, 1975), no clear relationship has been shown between the level of activity of an enzyme in lung tissue and either the amount or quality of the collagen produced.

Given the importance of collagen in influencing lung structure and function, it is not surprising that the amount of collagen produced by lung cells is well controlled. The internal mechanisms for this control seem to be complex and involve several steps along the entire pathway of biosynthesis from transcription of DNA into mRNA, translation of mRNA into protein, modification of the protein chains, and degradation before secretion of the final product (Bornstein & Traub, 1979; Hance & Crystal, 1975; Rennard et al, 1980). For example, human fetal lung fibroblasts produce the same amount of type I procollagen during both the log and confluent growth phases, even though confluent cells have two times the amount of type I procollagen mRNA than do log phase cells (Tolstoshev et al, 1981). In addition, the proportion of newly synthesized collagen undergoing intracellular degradation is known to be two- to threefold higher in log phase compared to confluent growth for these cells (Berg et al, 1980). Maintenance of a constant production rate of collagen by lung fibroblasts thus involves coordinated changes in (at least) transcription, translation and intracellular degradation. Moreover, these lung cells maintain a constant ratio of production of type I to type III collagen during growth (Hance & Crystal, 1977). Interestingly, different results have been obtained with skin fibroblasts (Abe et al, 1979), suggesting that the regulation of collagen production likely varies among tissues.

There has been a great deal of interest in the ability of exogenous factors (e.g., hormones, mediators from other cells) to modulate the amount of collagen produced by lung cells. For example, sex steroids (Morishige & Uetake, 1978; Takeda et al, 1975), glucocorticoids (Takeda et al, 1975), thyroxine (Hemberger & Shanker, 1978), α-adrenergic depletion (Ooshima et al, 1977), and hypophysectomy (Ooshima et al, 1977; Takeda et al, 1975) have been evaluated for their effect on lung collagen production. However, the results have been inconsistent and no definitive conclusions can be made concerning modulation of lung collagen production by these factors. There does, however, seem to be a role for mediators with β-agonist activity (e.g., epinephrine, norepinephrine) and prostaglandins of the E-series in suppressing collagen production by fibroblasts. In this context, acute exposure of lung fibroblasts to β-agonists or PGE_1 will decrease collagen production by 20 to 50 per cent (Baum et al, 1978). The mechanism for this suppression appears to be entirely at the post-translational level, and is mediated by a two–threefold increase in intracellular degradation. Since several types of lung cells can produce prostaglandins, this mechanism can provide a means for the coordinate behaviour of cells in lung tissue (Hyman et al, 1978).

In 1967, Heppleston & Styles (1967) suggested that macrophages that had ingested silica would, in turn, influence lung fibroblasts to produce more collagen (thus 'explaining' the lung fibrosis associated with inhalation of silica). Since that time, a number of experiments have been conducted to validate this observation and to examine the influence of mediators from inflammatory and immune effector cells on lung collagen production (Burrell & Anderson, 1973; Castor et al, 1979; Harrington et al, 1973; Heppleston, 1979; Nourse et al, 1975; Richards & Wusteman, 1974). Unfortunately, while the concept remains of interest, there has been no definitive demonstration of the ability of alveolar macrophages to influence collagen production by lung cells. Likewise, several investigators have suggested that activated mononuclear immune effector cells can influence lung fibroblasts to produce more collagen (Wahl et al, 1978), but definitive proof of this hypothesis is lacking. Most experiments designed to evaluate these questions have failed to take into account a variety of technical problems inherent in quantitating collagen production. These include variability of intracellular precursor pool sizes of the labelled tracer (Bruel et al, 1980), underhydroxylation of newly synthesized collagen, and failure to distinguish between newly synthesized collagen which is secreted intact and collagen that is degraded intracellularly and not secreted (Bienkowski et al, 1978). In addition, some of the studies designed to evaluate the influence of immune effector cell mediators on collagen production have failed to account for possible stimulatory effects on cell growth with resultant increases in the population of collagen producing fibroblasts. For example, it is now known that activated lung macrophages produce a growth factor that stimulates lung fibroblasts to replicate (Bitterman & Crystal, 1980; Bitterman et al, 1981). Thus, an increase in total collagen produced by a population of lung cells exposed to activated macrophages may result from an increase in the number of fibroblasts rather than an increase in the amount of collagen produced per cell. Lastly, many studies have failed to account for the heterogeneity of conventionally obtained lymphocyte and macrophage populations. Thus, although the interactions between immune effector cells and collagen producing cells undoubtedly have important implications for the composition of the extracellular matrix, the pathways and mechanisms involved remain largely unknown.

DESTRUCTION OF LUNG COLLAGEN

While it is known that the adult lung parenchyma actively produces collagen, it is also known that the total amount of collagen in the parenchyma does not change once maturity is reached (Bradley et al, 1974; Pierce, 1963). It is apparent, therefore, that to maintain this homeostasis, the normal lung must have processes to remove collagen at the same rate at which it is produced. Two distinct mechanisms are thought to account for this balance: (1) some of the cells normally present in the parenchyma produce collagenase; and (2) some parenchymal cells phagocytize extracellular collagen.

Collagenase

Two cells present in the normal alveolar structures, the alveolar macrophage (Harris & Cartwright, 1977; Horwitz & Crystal, 1976) and the fibroblast (Kelman et al, 1977), are capable of producing collagenases that can degrade at least some lung collagens (Table 24.2).

Table 24.2 Known collagenases in the lung in health and disease

Cell source	*Collagen type specificity* I	II	III	IV	V
A. Normal lung					
Alveolar macrophage*	Yes	Yes	Yes	?	?
Fibroblast**	Yes	Yes	Yes	?	?
B. Additional cell sources in lung disease					
Neutrophil†					
Collagenase	Yes	?	No	?	?
Elastase	Yes	?	Yes	Yes	Yes
Eosinophil (Davis et al, 1981)	Yes	?	Yes	?	?

*Demonstrated for the cells from the lungs of human (Kelman et al, 1977), rabbit (Horwitz & Crystal, 1976), dog (Senior et al, 1972), and guinea pig (Werb, 1978).

**Demonstrated for human lung fibroblasts (Kelman et al, 1977).

†Neutrophil enzymes are defined functionally: 'collagenase' cleaves the helical region of type I collagen only (Horwitz et al, 1977); 'elastase' cleaves a variety of substrates, including elastin and collagen (teleopeptides of I, the helical region of III close to the 'collagenase' site (Gadek et al, 1981), and probably several sites in IV) (Mainardi et al, 1980; Uitto et al, 1980).

Alveolar macrophages from a number of species produce a collagenase that attacks collagens I and III approximately at equal rates (Harris & Cartwright, 1977; Horwitz & Crystal, 1976). These macrophage enzymes have all the properties associated with 'classic' collagenases, i.e., they are metallo-enzymes active at neutral pH, and specifically cleave the collagen molecule at a single point 3/4 from the N-terminus of the molecule (Harris & Cartwright, 1977). In addition, the macrophage enzymes seem to be released from the cell in an inactive form, i.e., another neutral protease is required for activation. Nevertheless, it is not clear whether these macrophage collagenases are 'proenzymes' (as the skin fibroblast collagenase appears to be) or an active enzyme complexed with an inhibitor of some type. However, at least for the rabbit, it is known that the alveolar macrophage does secrete a neutral protease that is capable of activating the collagenase produced by the same cell population (Horwitz et al, 1976).

Like fibroblasts from other organs, human lung fibroblasts can produce a collagenase that degrades collagens I and III (Kelman et al, 1977). This collagenase is released in an inactive form, is a metallo-enzyme, and has a neutral pH optimum. Thus, the lung fibroblast is not only a major producer of collagens types I and III, but it also produces an enzyme capable of degrading these collagens.

The relative importance of the collagenases from alveolar macrophages and fibroblasts in maintaining lung collagen homeostasis is not known. It is thought that production of collagenase by the human alveolar macrophage appears to be constitutive, i.e., its production is not enhanced when the macrophage is 'activated' (Gadek et al, 1981). Thus, macrophage collagenase may play a role in the normal turnover of human lung collagen, but it is doubtful that it is important in disease states. In contrast, collagenase production by nonhuman alveolar macrophages can be modulated. For example, the process of phagocytosis stimulates guinea pig alveolar macrophages to release 3 to 10 times more collagenase (Werb, 1978).

It is important to realize that the lung has little, if any, defence against an active collagenase. The major antiprotease of the lower respiratory tract is α1-antityrypsin, a serum antiprotease of approximately 50 000 daltons that diffuses through the alveolar structures (Gadek et al, 1981). However, α1-antitrypsin does not inhibit the classic collagenases, and thus cannot modulate the action of macrophage or fibroblast collagenase. In addition, although the serum β1-globulin described by Woolley et al (1976) is an anticollagenase of the proper size to diffuse through the lung structures, it is present in such small amounts in serum that it does not play an important anticollagenase role in the lung. α2-macroglobulin is an effective anticollagenase (Eisen et al, 1970) but very little of this antiprotease is found in the lower respiratory tract, at least on the epithelial surface. For example, in normal humans there is about 500-fold more α1-antitrypsin present (on a mole for mole basis) in bronchoalveolar lavage fluid than α2-macroglobulin (Gadek, unpublished). Thus, even though α2-macroglobulin is a prominent serum anticollagenase, its size (725 000 daltons) apparently prohibits it from diffusing to the epithelial surface, although it may be present in the pulmonary interstitium (Mosher et al, 1977). In this regard, it is known that alveolar macrophages and lung fibroblasts can produce α2-macroglobulin in vitro. Nevertheless, the in vivo role of this macromolecule as an anticollagenase is unclear.

The role of other cells of the normal lung in producing collagenases is unknown. Likewise, there is currently no information explaining how collagen types II, IV and V are metabolized in the normal lung.

Phagocytosis

Although it is known that fibroblasts can ingest collagen fibrils (Tencate, 1972; Svoboda & Deporter, 1980), little attention has been given to the role of the lung cells in collagen phagocytosis. Recent studies by Sneider et al (1980) have shown that human lung fibroblast can phagocytize collagen, but the mechanisms by which this occurs and the importance of this phenomenon in normal collagen turnover are unknown. Macrophages have also been shown to phagocytize collagen (Svoboda & Deporter, 1980), including denatured collagen (Hormann & Jelinic, 1980). This process seems to require opsonization by fibronectin (Horman & Jelinic, 1980; Saba & Jaffe, 1980), a glycoprotein component of plasma (Yamada & Olden, 1978), lung tissue (Bray, 1978) and a prominent synthetic product of many lung cells including fibroblasts (Baum et al, 1977), smooth muscle (Burke & Ross, 1979) epithelial (Chen et al, 1977) and endothelial (Birdwell et al, 1978) cells and macrophages (Rennard et al, 1981; Villiger et al, 1980). The physiological role for such opsonization pathways in normal collagen metabolism is unknown.

LUNG COLLAGEN DURING ORGAN DEVELOPMENT

There is ample evidence for the role of collagen in influencing lung structure during early morphogenesis (Alescio, 1973; Loosli & Potter, 1951; Spooner & Faubian, 1980; Wessells & Cohen, 1968). Studies with lung buds have shown that collagen in the extracellular matrix modulates primordial lung structure and facilitates bronchial branching. For example, treatment of lung buds with collagenase alters existing morphology and, if collagen is not added, prevents the development of new buds in the rudimentary lung (Wessells & Cohen, 1968). Consistent with this observation, addition of the proline analogue azetidine to mouse embryonic lung decreases the number of lung buds formed (Alescio, 1973; Spooner & Faubian, 1980), even though epithelial growth is not affected, implying that collagen in the matrix plays a significant role in spatially organizing the epithelial tree. The mechanisms by which the amount and/or types of collagen provide a framework for early lung morphogenesis are unknown, but presumably are associated with the relationship of collagen to cell attachment proteins such as fibronectin and laminin.

As in other organs, changes in collagen content, extractability, types and production are associated with lung maturation. The most detailed studies concerning developmental changes in lung collagen content have been carried out in the rabbit (Bradley et al, 1974). There is a two–threefold increase in lung collagen content (collagen/dry weight) in the last trimester of fetal development and a twofold increase from birth to maturity. Collagen content remains constant after the lung stops growing (at approximately 3 months in the rabbit). This developmental accumulation of lung collagen is even more impressive when placed in the context of whole body growth. From 10 days before birth to 1 year after birth, rabbit lung collagen content increased fivefold, body weight increases 1000-fold, but lung weight increases only 100-fold (Crystal, 1974). Thus, while lung mass relative to body mass decreases, the amount of collagen per unit lung mass increases significantly. Interestingly, during the same period, total protein per unit lung mass does not change, further emphasizing the striking changes in lung collagen accumulation. These developmentally associated increases in collagen content are found in several different lung structures. For example, in the 1-week-old rabbit lung, blood vessels are 14 per cent collagen (amount collagen per dry weight of tissue) while bronchi are 15 per cent, and parenchyma 2.3 per cent. In contrast, in the 6-month-old rabbit lung, blood vessels are 19 per cent, bronchi 18 per cent and parenchyma 5.8 per cent, suggesting the largest developmental increase in collagen content occurs in the alveolar structures (Collins et al, unpublished). Studies in other species, while less extensive, confirm that lung collagen content increases with lung development. For example, in the 17th week of gestation, human fetal collagen content of the human lung parenchyma is 1.7 per cent (collagen/dry weight) while in the adult human it is approximately 20 per cent, a tenfold increase (Bradley et al, 1975).

Not only does lung collagen content increase with maturity, but its character changes as well. Several studies have shown that the extractability of lung collagen decreases with age, consistent with the concept that lung maturation is associated with increased interactions of collagen with itself and other extracellular matrix components (Bradley et al, 1974, 1975; Drodz et al, 1979; Hurst et al, 1977; Szemenyei & Balint, 1973). For example, almost twofold more collagen can be extracted with neutral salt and acetic acid from the human fetal lung compared to the adult human lung (Bradley et al, 1975). Age-related differences in lung collagen extractability have also been found in the rat; fivefold less collagen can be extracted from the lung of the 2-year-old rat compared to the 2-month-old rat (Szemenyei & Balint, 1973).

At least some species have age-related changes in the post-translational modification to collagen chains. For example, $\alpha 1(I)$ chains from the newborn rabbit lung parenchyma have a hydroxylysine to lysine ratio of 0.2, while $\alpha 1(I)$ chains from 4-month-old rabbit parenchyma have a ratio of 0.4 (Bradley et al, 1974). In contrast, the hydroxylysine to lysine ratios for $\alpha 1(I)$ chains are similar for human newborn and adult lungs (Hurst et al, 1977).

In addition to developmental changes in amounts of lung collagen, some species have marked developmental alterations in the rates of collagen production (Bradley et al, 1975; Garrett, 1978; Hurst et al, 1977; Newman & Langer, 1975; Tolstoshev, unpublished). For example, in the rabbit lung parenchyma, the rate of collagen production of the adult is fourfold less than that of the newborn (Bradley et al, 1974; Newman & Langer, 1975). Consistent with this developmental decrease in lung collagen production in the rabbit, the sheep lung also exhibits a decrease in collagen production from 60 days of fetal development compared to 140 days (Tolstoshev, unpublished). In both species, these decreases in lung collagen production seem to be controlled, at least in part, by the amount of collagen mRNA available for translation (Collins & Crystal, 1975; Tolstoshev, unpublished). In contrast, while the human fetal lung parenchyma produces more collagen per cell than adult human parenchyma, that difference is only about 30 per cent, much less than other species that have been evaluated (Bradley et al, 1975). Although there is no evidence that the post-translational enzymes that modify collagen are rate limiting, quantification of lysyl oxidase in the rabbit lung parenchyma has shown decreases in enzyme activity (per mg tissue protein) with increasing age (approximately three- to fourfold decrease from newborns compared to adults) (Brody et al, 1979). In contrast, there does not seem to be any changes in the proportion of collagen degraded intracellularly throughout rabbit lung maturation (Bienkowski et al, 1978).

While total collagen production significantly changes with fetal lung maturation, current evidence suggests the relative rates of production of collagen types I and III are constant. For example, in the developing sheep lung, production of type I collagen is three times that of type III in the 60-day lung, the 115-day lung, and the 145-day lung (Tolstoshev, unpublished).

It is not clear whether the changes in lung collagen production with development are due to changes in the level of collagen production by each collagen-producing cell or due to changes in the numbers or types of collagen-producing cells that are present. Although detailed studies of lung fibroblasts as a function of the age of the source tissue have not been carried out, preliminary studies of human lung fibroblasts obtained from adult lungs demonstrate somewhat lower rates of collagen production than fibroblasts derived from fetal lungs (Rennard & Crystal, unpublished). However, evaluation of fetal lung fibroblasts maintained in culture (Breul et al, 1980; Bradley et al, 1980) demonstrates that they produce similar amounts of collagen (per cell) over at least 25 population doublings, suggesting a stable phenotype for collagen production for these cells, at least during constant culture conditions.

One interesting approach to the study of collagen-related changes during lung development comes from study of the remaining lung after unilateral pneumonectomy. In a variety of species, including rabbit, cat, dog, or rat, if one lung is removed, the mass of the remaining lung increases over a short period to approximate that of both lungs. For example, when a left pneumonectomy is performed on a $2\frac{1}{2}$-month-old rabbit, total right lung mass increases within 1 month (Cowan & Crystal, 1975). This increase is accompanied by a doubling of the total amount of collagen in the right lung. Interestingly, this increase is preceded by a marked shift in the emphasis of the protein synthesizing machinery toward collagen. Prior to pneumonectomy, the lung devotes approximately 4 per cent of all protein synthesis to collagen; 2 weeks after pneumonectomy this has more than doubled (Crystal, 1974; Cowan & Crystal,

1975). Consistent with these observations, lung lysyl oxidase activity increases markedly following pneumonectomy (Brody et al, 1979). Interestingly, these marked shifts in collagen-related biochemical activity following pneumonectomy seem to be controlled by mechanical factors; obliteration of the pleural space remaining after resection of the left lung completely halts the increase in right lung growth and the concomitant shifts in collagen production and accumulation that normally occur after left pneumonectomy (Cowan & Crystal, 1975). Moreover, similar effects have been observed in normal lung after localized pulmonary irradiation (McBride et al, 1980). In humans, a similar phenomenon has been observed morphologically although biochemical studies have not been carried out (Snider & Karlinsky, 1977).

FUNCTION OF COLLAGEN IN THE NORMAL LUNG

The mechanical properties, abundance, and strategic location of collagen in lung all argue for a major role for collagen in modulating lung mechanical properties during respiration. However, the heterogeneity and complex interactions of the collagens, and the lack of specific 'probes' to modify only collagen, have made the study of this role of lung collagen difficult.

Although opinions vary among workers in the field, it is generally thought that a major role for collagen is to modulate lung volume-pressure relationships throughout the volume range, with the dominant influence being at large lung volumes where the high tensile strength of collagen limits lung expansion (Pierce, 1968; Snider & Karlinsky, 1977). Consistent with this concept are the observations that: (1) when animals are treated with crosslink inhibitors (Fedullo et al, 1979; Hoffman et al, 1971) or proline analogues (Riley et al, 1980), the lung becomes more compliant; (2) in patients with fibrotic lung disease, there is both a local accumulation of collagen and a shift toward relatively more type I collagen (Seyer et al, 1976); these individuals have smaller lungs that are less distensible than those of normals (Fulmer et al, 1979); (3) treatment of normal lung parenchyma with formaldehyde, an agent that induces artificial crosslinks among collagen (and other matrix components) causes the alveolar walls to be less compliant (Sugihara & Martin, 1975); (4) intratracheal instillation of collagenase permits greater lung expansion in saline-filled lungs where connective tissue forces predominate over surface tension (Karlinsky et al, 1976; Snider et al, 1977); and (5) in vitro exposure of lung parenchyma to Clostridial collagenase permits subsequent stretching with less force (Senior et al, 1975).

In addition to its role in defining lung mechanical properties, it is likely that collagen plays an important role in the topologic organization of lung cells. It is known that proteins that attach cells to collagen (Kleinman et al, 1981) (such as fibronectin and laminin) are present in lung (Bray, 1978; Foidart et al, 1980; Stenman & Vaheri, 1978). In this context, the localization, orientation, and form of the collagen in lung may determine parenchymal cell topography, not only during lung maturation, but also during normal cellular turnover and in response to injury (Vrako, 1972). In this context, derangement of the connective tissue matrix, as occurs in disease states, may severely limit the ability of the lung to heal normally.

LUNG COLLAGEN IN LUNG DISEASE

There are a variety of acquired and inherited disorders of man associated with abnormalities of lung collagen. Of these the fibrotic lung disorders have received the most attention.

Fibrotic lung disease

There are more than 130 different disorders of man that are grouped as the 'fibrotic lung diseases' or 'interstitial lung diseases' (Table 24.3). For a detailed description of these disorders, several reviews are available (Crystal et al, 1976, 1981; Fulmer & Crystal, 1976; Keogh & Crystal, 1981). In general, all interstitial lung disorders are characterized morphologically by fibrosis of the alveolar structures and functionally by decreased lung volumes and decreased lung compliance (i.e., 'stiff' lungs). There are also a variety of animal models of lung fibrosis (Hance & Crystal, 1975; Rennard et al, 1980) including those induced by bleomycin (Starcher et al, 1972; Fedullo et al, 1979; McCullough et al, 1978; Pozzi & Zanon, 1978; Sikic et al, 1978; Jones & Reeve, 1978; Marom et al, 1979; McCullough et al, 1978; Szapiel et al, 1979; Thrall et al, 1979; Snider et al, 1978; Jones, 1978; Aso et al, 1976; Snider et al, 1978; Goldstein et al, 1979; Kelley et al, 1980; Clark et al, 1980) (an antineoplastic agent used clinically in a variety of malignancies), paraquat (Reiser et al, 1979; Greenberg et al, 1978; Last & Greenberg, 1979; Thompson & Patrick, 1978; Kuttan et al, 1979; Greenberg et al, 1978; Khurana & Niden, 1979; Lam et al, 1979; Hussain & Bhatnagar, 1979; Hollinger et al, 1978; Hollinger & Chvapil, 1977; Popenoe & Loosti, 1978; Niden & Khurana, 1976) (a herbicide that is a powerful oxidant), radiation (Collins et al, 1977, 1978; Dubrawsky et al, 1978; Gerber et al, 1977; Jelenska et al, 1975; Jennings & Arden, 1961; Law et al, 1976; Metevier et al, 1978; Pickrell et al, 1975, 1976; Philips, 1966; Thyagarajen et al, 1976; Tombropoulos & Thomas 1970), N-nitroso-N-methylurethane (Barrett et al, 1979; Cantor et al, 1979; Ryan et al, 1978; Ryan, 1972), inhaled inorganic dusts (e.g., silica, asbestos), toxic gases (Autor & Stevens, 1978; Ayaz & Csallany, 1978; Bhatnagar et al, 1978; Chvapil & Peng, 1975; Drozdz et al, 1977; Frank et al, 1978; Haschek et al, 1979; Hesterberg & Last, 1981; Hugood, 1979; Hussain et al, 1976, 1978; Orthoefer

Table 24.3 Lung disorders in which lung collagen is relevant to the pathogenesis of the disease

Fibrotic lung disorders*
Known aetiology
Occupational and environmental inhalents
Drugs
Poisons
Radiation
Infectious agents
Other (chronic cardiac or renal disease, graft vs. host disease)
Unknown aetiology
Idiopathic pulmonary fibrosis
Chronic interstitial disease associated with the collagen-vascular disorders
Sarcoidosis
Histiocytosis-X
Goodpasture's syndrome
Idiopathic pulmonary hemosiderosis
Chronic eosinophilic pneumonia
Diffuse amyloidosis of lung
Lymphangioleiomyomatosis
Inherited disorders
Alveolar proteinosis
Liver disease associated with interstitial lung disease
Whipple's disease
Weber-Christian disease
Lymphocytic infiltrative disorders
Pulmonary vasculitis associated with interstitial lung disease
Proliferative vascular disease associated with interstitial lung disease
Pulmonary airway disease associated with interstitial lung disease
Destructive lung disorders**
Acquired emphysema
α1-antitrypsin deficiency
Disorders of the tracheobronchial tree
Relapsing polychondritis
Acquired tracheal stenosis
Wegener's granulomatosis
Hereditary disorders of connective tissue†
Marfan's syndrome
Ehlers-Danlos syndromes
Osteogenesis imperfecta

*Also termed 'interstitial lung disease'; the complete list of the fibrotic lung disorders has been reviewed.

**Mostly includes disorders associated with destruction of the lung parenchyma usually referred to as 'emphysema'. The major cause of 'acquired emphysema' is cigarette smoking.

†Disorders listed as those in which the defect is thought to involve collagen and in which lung abnormalities have been detected by X-ray or lung function tests.

et al, 1976; Richmond & D'Aoust, 1976) (high concentrations of oxygen, ozone, nitrogen dioxide), cigarette smoke (Hurst et al, 1977; Rosenkrantz et al, 1969), and a variety of immunological insults. While many of these models bear little relationship to the human fibrotic state, these models have enabled investigators to trace the development of pulmonary fibrosis in morphological, physiological, biochemical, and immunological terms.

Lung 'fibrosis' can be described as a disordering of the cellular architecture of the lung parenchyma associated with characteristic alterations of the interstitial connective tissue matrix. This includes localized accumulations of collagen (Greenberg et al, 1978), alterations in the types of collagen (Seyer et al, 1976) and derangement of the form of collagen (Basset et al, 1975).

While the disordering of the cellular architecture of the lung parenchyma is a central feature of pulmonary fibrosis, the mechanisms for this disordering are not well defined. From careful morphological studies it is known that the relative number of each parenchymal cell type changes and cellular topography is altered (Crapo et al, 1980). Since most parenchymal cell types produce collagen (see discussion above and Fig. 24.1), it is not hard to imagine how such changes in parenchymal cells could result in marked changes in parenchymal collagen. However, it is now known that matrix components such as collagen can significantly influence the movement (Gauss-Muller et al, 1980; Postlethwaite et al, 1978), location (Vrako, 1972), and perhaps the function of a variety of cells. Thus, it is not clear which comes first: changes in parenchymal cells which, in turn, produce an abnormal matrix; or an abnormal matrix which, in turn, modulates cellular disorganization. However, since there is convincing evidence that an accumulation of inflammatory and immune effector cells (i.e., 'alveolitis') precedes the 'fibrosis' in these disorders, it is likely that both cellular disorganization and matrix remodelling occur in parallel in the injured lung and represent mutually dependent processes (Rennard et al, 1980; Thompson & Patrick, 1978; Crystal et al, 1976; Fulmer & Crystal, 1979; Crystal et al, 1981; Keogh & Crystal, 1981; Crystal et al, 1981; Sikic et al, 1978; Jones & Reeve, 1978; Snider et al, 1978; Jones 1978; Aso et al, 1976; Greenberg et al, 1978; Popenoe & Loosti, 1978; Niden & Khurana, 1976; Jennings & Arden, 1961; Phillips, 1966; Pickerell et al, 1976; Barrett et al, 1979; Ryan et al, 1978; Ryan, 1972; Gross et al, 1977; Schoenberger et al, 1980; Chvapil & Peng, 1978; Hugood, 1979; Johnson & Ward, 1974; Richerson et al, 1971; Read, 1958; Brentjens et al, 1974; Van Toorn, 1970).

While the local accumulation of interstitial collagen seen morphologically in fibrotic lung disease is obvious to even the casual observer, it is very difficult to define and quantify biochemically. Data derived from a number of animal models have shown that total lung collagen can be elevated in pulmonary fibrosis (Crystal, 1974; Hance & Crystal, 1975; Rennard et al, 1980) (i.e., thus suggesting a net increase in collagen production or decrease in collagen destruction). However, in some animal models (Hance & Crystal, 1975; Rennard et al, 1980) and in all human biopsies evaluated to date, collagen content (amount/dry weight) in fibrotic disease has been found to be normal (Fulmer et al, 1980). There are several possible explanations for this: (1) total lung collagen has increased (i.e., a net accumulation of collagen takes place) but the mass of the lung is also increased (e.g., the lung is hypercellular); thus, the content (collagen/dry weight) will be unchanged if both total lung collagen and cell mass are increased proportionally; (2) the local accumulations of collagen seen morphologically are balanced by local decreases in parenchymal collagen in other regions; (3) what is seen morphologically as collagen is probably mostly type I (Hance & Crystal, 1975; Rennard et al, 1980) and thus shifts toward more type I collagen (see below) would be recognized morphologically as an accumulation of collagen even though total collagen (i.e., the sum of all types) may not have changed. Nevertheless, in spite of the failure of current biochemical technology to confirm the morphological observations, most investigators generally accept the morphological finding that there are local accumulations of collagen in the alveolar interstitium in these disorders.

The mechanism by which this collagen accumulates, however, is not clear. Although it is attractive to hypothesize that the fibrotic state is associated with a change in the differentiated state of parenchymal cells such that they produce more collagen (per cell), there is little convincing evidence that this occurs. Evaluation of biposies of human fibrotic lungs (i.e., for a disease such as idiopathic pulmonary fibrosis (IPF)), has demonstrated that rates of collagen production (averaged over all cells present) are normal (Fulmer et al, 1980). In contrast, studies of several animal models of pulmonary fibrosis have shown that rates of collagen production are elevated (Hollinger et al, 1978; Hussain & Bhatnager, 1979; Khurana & Niden, 1979; Kuttan et al, 1979; McCullough et al, 1978; Pickrell et al, 1976; Reiser et al, 1979). Even so, such observations can just as well be explained by the hypothesis that there has been a shift in the population of parenchymal cells such that there are more collagen-producing cells, Each cell could continue to produce the same amount of collagen but there would be an increase in the number of cells producing collagen. In this context, Crapo and colleagues have made morphometric counts of the cell populations in experimental oxygen toxicity demonstrating increased numbers of fibroblasts (Crapo et al, 1980). Consistent with this observation, Bitterman et al, have shown that alveolar macrophages recovered from the lungs of patients with fibrotic lung disease are actively releasing a growth factor that stimulates resting lung fibroblasts to replicate (Bitterman & Crystal, 1980).

One situation where increases in collagen production by individual fibroblasts may result in fibrosis is that caused by the β-blocking drugs. In rare patients, these drugs (propranolol, practolol, and metaproterenol) have resulted in fibrosis, including pulmonary fibrosis. Since β-agonists appear to reduce collagen production in normal lung fibroblasts (Baum et al, 1979), the 'resting β-adrenergic tone' of normal lung may partially suppress collagen production by these cells. In this context, loss of this tone in patients taking β-blocking agents may allow lung fibroblasts to produce more collagen, resulting in fibrosis.

The role of lung lymphocytes in the fibrotic lung disorders has not been fully clarified. In experimental models of bleomycin-induced fibrosis, there is conflicting evidence as to whether T-lymphocytes are necessary for the development of the fibrotic lesion (Szapiel et al, 1979). In idiopathic pulmonary fibrosis in humans, T-lymphocytes are normal (Hunninghake et al, 1981), but lung B-lymphocytes are producing elevated levels of immunoglobulins (Hunninghake et al, 1979), including IgG directed against type I collagen, a likely antigen for immune complex formation in this disease. Lung T-lymphocytes are increased and activated in pulmonary sarcoidosis (Hunninghake & Crystal, 1981; Hunninghake et al, 1980, 1981), but the relationship of this burden of activated T-lymphocytes to the interstitial fibrosis is unclear at this time.

In most fibrotic tissues, there seems to be a shift in the major collagens present such that there is more type I relative to type III. This seems to be true in lung as well, at least for idiopathic pulmonary fibrosis (Seyer et al, 1976). This observation is consistent with the observations that of all collagen types, type I collagen forms the least distensible collagen fibres in vivo and that patients with IPF have decreased lung compliance. In this context, the extent of fibrosis in the IPF lung observed morphologically correlates with the decrease in lung compliance quantified physiologically (Snider et al, 1977). However, recent studies of the lung in progressive systemic sclerosis have shown that the ratio of type I to type III in the parenchyma is similar to that in normals, suggesting that an increased I/III ratio may not be a universal part of the fibrosis of the interstitial lung disorders (Seyer et al, 1981). Interestingly, a study of one patient with scleroderma and a rapidly fatal course showed a decreased I/III ratio, although the methods used probably resulted in only partial extraction of lung collagen (Adam & Dostal, 1979).

Non-quantitative immunofluorescent studies of lung biopsies from patients with established fibrotic disease are consistent with the concept that there is increased amounts of type I collagen and decreased type III in the fibrotic parenchyma (Madri & Furthmayr, 1979, 1981; Wick & Crystal, unpublished). In addition, recent immunofluorescent studies (Wick & Crystal, unpublished) suggest that the relative proportions of types I and III are constantly changing as the disease progresses. Early in the disease, there appears to be an increase in type III, but with time, as the disease progresses, the type III fluorescence decreases and type I gradually increases. The result in established disease is a relative increase in the apparent I:III ratio compared to normal lung. Thus, the role of different collagen types in fibrotic lung disease will probably vary with both the category and stage of each disease.

The mechanisms by which the relative proportions of lung collagens change in fibrotic disease are unknown. It has been shown that the lung fibroblast is capable of producing both type I and III (Hance et al, 1976; Kelley et al, 1979), and the ratio of I/III produced by these cells is probably greater than that produced by other parenchymal lung cells (Hance & Crystal, 1975; Rennard et al, 1980), i.e. endothelial and epithelial cells. Since the relative proportion of fibroblasts increases in fibrotic diseases, the relative increase in type I may simply relate to an increase in the proportion of fibroblasts.

In addition to the accumulation and possible changes in type of lung collagen in fibrotic disease, morphological observations at the ultrastructural level demonstrate that interstitial collagen fibres (predominantly type I) to be twisted and frayed (Basset et al, 1975). One possible explanation for this observation is that inflammatory cells in the fibrotic lung release an active collagenase that destroys lung collagen. In this context, Gadek and colleagues have demonstrated that patients with IPF have active collagenase in their lower respiratory tract (Gadek et al, 1979). In addition, evaluation of this collagenase has shown that it is specific for type I collagen only, and thus is likely derived from the neutrophil (Table 24.2). Consistent with this observation, there is ample evidence that IPF is associated with the chronic accumulation of neutrophils in the alveolar structures (Hunninghake et al, 1981). It is also important to note that these several fibrotic lung disorders are associated with the accumulation of eosinophils in the lung parenchyma (Table 24.3) and that the eosinophil carries a collagenase capable of degrading collagens type I and III (Davis et al, 1981) (Table 24.2).

At the present time, therapy for the fibrotic lung disorders is not curative, at least for most patients. A variety of agents have been used to decrease collagen accumulation in experimental fibrotic lung disease (e.g., indomethacin (McCullough et al, 1978), corticosteroids (Halme et al, 1970; Hesterberg & Last, 1981; Reye & Bale, 1973; Rosenberg et al, 1980), colchicine (Dubrawsky et al, 1978), proline analogues (Kelley et al, 1980; Riley et al, 1980), cross-link inhibitors (Fedullo et al, 1979; Halme et al, 1970; Khurana & Niden, 1979)). However, in humans, most of the fibrotic lung disorders are chronic diseases in which local collagen accumulation, albeit progressive, occurs slowly. Lung collagen production, even if elevated on a local level, is probably less than normal collagen production in other organs. At some sites, such as bone, this normal collagen production probably exceeds that of the fibrotic lung. Thus, if agents that decrease production are to be effective in the fibrotic lung disorders, local specificity of action, achieved pharmacologically or by local administration of these agents, probably will be necessary.

The more rational therapeutic approach to these disorders is to attack the alveolitis stage of the disease where active inflammatory and immune effector cells are acting to alter cell populations and produce a variety of mediators that influence the collagenous matrix either directly or indirectly. For example, there is recent evidence that agents such as cyclophosphamide significantly reduce the accumulation of neutrophils in the lung parenchyma in IPF (Hunninghake et al, 1980), thus significantly decreasing a potential source of structural derangement in this disease.

Destructive lung disease

The destructive lung disorders, also called the emphysematous disorders, are chronic diseases in which there is actual loss, or dissolution, of the alveolar walls (Table 24.3). Most studies of lung connective tissue in emphysema have focused on lung elastin, and quantitative studies have shown no change in collagen content (Pierce, 1961, 1963; Wright et al, 1960; Keller & Mandi, 1972; Bruce et al, 1970; Mandle et al, 1977). Nevertheless, there is growing evidence that parenchymal collagen is abnormal in these disorders. Ultrastructural evaluation of emphysematous lung in man and rabbits demonstrates abnormal collagen fibres and focal accumulations of abnormal collagen (Yu et al, 1977; Belton et al, 1977; Martin & Boatman, 1965). It has been suggested that these changes in matrix lead to destruction by distorting the precise arrangement of the alveolar epithelium and capillaries (Huang, 1978). For example, this distortion of collagen fibres is accompanied by an apparent detachment of epithelial cells from their basement membrane (Yu et al, 1977; Huang, 1978). Thus the role of the collagenous matrix in defining tissue structure may be of paramount importance: qualitative changes in collagen and its associated cell attachment factors (McDonald et al, 1979) may lead to a loss of tissue integrity, ultimately resulting in emphysema.

The concept of destruction of collagen in pulmonary emphysema is supported by the presence of neutrophil collagenases in the lower respiratory tract of patients with α1-antitrypsin deficiency, a hereditary disorder associated with early onset emphysema (Gadek et al, 1981). Moreover, neutrophil elastase, often thought to be the major mediator of lung destruction in acquired emphysema, can attack the teleopeptides of type I (Gadek et al, 1981), the collagenase site of type III (Gadek et al, 1981), several sites in type IV (Mainardi et al, 1980; Uitto et al, 1980), and at least one site in type V.

Qualitative changes in lung collagen are also a prominent feature very early after inhalation of cadmium by rats (Dorvan & Hayes, 1981). This lesion subsequently 'matures' into a lesion closely resembling human centrilobular emphysema. Although a stimulation of collagen synthesis is a prominent early feature of this model, it appears to be accompanied by an increase in lung collagen turnover (Dorvan & Hayes, 1981).

Instillation of elastase or other proteases that cleave

elastin into the lungs of animals also results in emphysema (Karlinsky & Snider, 1978). Although similar lesions are not produced by collagenase, it is notable, however, that the elastase model shows a prominent stimulation of collagen synthesis (Kuhn et al, 1976; Yu & Keller, 1978; Collins et al, 1978) and is associated with an increase in lung collagen content (Kuhn et al, 1976; Collins et al, 1978). Thus, although the role of collagen metabolism in the development of emphysema is unclear, changes in collagen metabolism and structure appear to be present as early and prominent features.

Lastly, included with destructive lung disease are disorders that destroy the cartilage of large airways leading to obstruction to air flow. Immunological destruction due to anti-type II collagen antibodies with subsequent inflammation has been suggested in relapsing polychondritis (Foidart et al, 1979). In addition, a direct destruction of cartilage by inflammatory cells is a prominent feature of acquired tracheal stenosis (Feist et al, 1973) and Wegener's granulomatosis (Rosenberg et al, 1980). The relative importance of the destruction of collagen and the other connective tissue components in these disorders is unknown.

Hereditary disorders of connective tissue

Several of the heritable connective tissue diseases result in abnormal tissue collagen. Some patients with these diseases have been reported to have abnormal pulmonary function or structure (Reye & Bale, 1973; Dwyer & Troncale, 1965; Tueller et al, 1977; Chisolm et al, 1968; Fuleihan et al, 1963), although none of these cases has been characterized biochemically in lung. Furthermore, some patients have severe chest skeletal problems (e.g., osteogenesis imperfecta) and this further confounds interpretation of the collagen defect in their pulmonary parenchyma. Mice with lysyl oxidase deficiency develop emphysema (Rowe et al, 1977; Starcher et al, 1977), but since this same enzyme is required to cross-link elastin as well as collagen, it is not possible to interpret the role of collagen in the aetiology of this defect. Thus, at the present time little information is available concerning the role of collagen in the lung in these 'experiments of nature'.

Malignancy

It is becoming evident that tumour cells differ from their normal counterparts with regard to collagen synthesis as well as many other parameters. Moreover, the ability of tumour cells to degrade their matrix and to subsequently attach to collagen elsewhere may be of profound importance in the development of metastases (Liotta et al, 1980). To date, however, nothing is known about the metabolism of collagen and the development and metastasis of lung tumours. However, the ability of some cells to metastasize to the lung seems to correlate with both their ability to produce type IV collagenase (Liotta et al, 1980) (and thus penetrate the blood stream) and with their ability to adhere to type IV collagen (Murray et al, 1979) (and thus remain in the pulmonary capillary bed). Unfortunately, these studies depend on an in vitro measure of metastatic potential and whether the lung is affected specifically or merely because of the technique of the assay is unknown.

CONCLUSION

The involvement of collagen in normal lung function and alterations in its metabolism in disease is now beyond question. Less is known about the pathways involved in these changes in collagen metabolism. In addition to filling in the gaps in our knowledge of the amount, type, and metabolism of collagen in lung, perhaps the most important issues for the future include the interactions of collagen with the other components of the extracellular matrix and with the cellular constituents of the lung in both health and disease.

REFERENCES

Abe S, Steinman B U, Martin G R 1979 Density dependent modulation of types I and III collagen synthesis by fibroblasts in vitro. Nature 279: 442-44

Adam M, Dostal C 1979 Collagen heterogeneity in systemic scleroderma and other diseases. Journal of Clinical Chemistry and Clinical Biochemistry 17: 495-8

Alitalo K 1980 Production of interstitial and basement membrane procollagens by fibroblastic WI-38 cells from human embryonic lung. Biochemical and Biophysical Research Communications 93: 873-80

Alescio T 1973 Effect of a proline analogue, azetidine-2-carboxylic acid, on the morphogenesis in vitro of mouse embryonic lung. Journal of Embryology and Experimental Morphology 29: 439

Aso Y, Yoneda K, Kikkawa Y 1976 Morphological and biochemical study of pulmonary changes induced by bleomycin in mice. Laboratory Investigation 35: 558

Autor A P, Stevens J B 1978 Mechanism of oxygen detoxification in neonatal rat lung tissues. Photochemistry and Photobiology 28: 775

Ayaz K L, Csallany A S 1978 Long term NO_2 exposure of mice in the presence and absence of vitamin E. Effect of glutathione peroxidase. Archives of Environmental Health 33: 292

Barnes M J, Morton L F, Levene C I 1978 Synthesis of interstitial collagens by pig aortic endothelial cells in culture. Biochemical and Biophysical Research Communications 84: 646

Barrett C R, Bell A L L Jr, Ryan S F 1979 Alveolar epithelial injury causing respiratory distress in dogs. Chest 75: 705

Basset F, Soler P, Bernandin J F 1975 Contributions of electron microscopy to the study of interstitial pneumonias. Progress in Respiratory Research 8: 45

Baum B J, McDonald J A, Crystal R G 1977 Metabolic fate of major cell surface protein of normal human fibroblasts. Biochemical and Biophysical Research Communications 79: 8

Baum B J, Moss J, Breul S D, Crystal R G 1978 Association in normal human fibroblasts of elevated levels of adenosine 3':5'-monophosphate with a selective decrease in collagen production. Journal of Biological Chemistry 253: 3391

Belton J C, Crise N, McLaughlin R F, Tueller E E 1977 Ultrastructural alterations in collagen associated with microscopic foci of human emphysema. Human Pathology 8: 669

Berg R A, Schwartz M L, Crystal R G 1980 Regulation of the production of secretory proteins: intracellular degradation of newly synthesized 'defective' collagen. Proceedings of the National Academy of Sciences (USA) 72: 4746-50

Bhatnagar R S, Hussain M Z, Streifel J A, Tolentino M, Enriquez B 1978 Alteration of collagen synthesis in lung organ cultures by hyperoxic environments. Biochemical and Biophysical Research Communications 83: 392

Bhattacharyya S N, Passero M A, Di Augustine R P, Lynn W S 1975 Isolation and characterization of two hydroxyproline-containing glycoproteins from normal animal lung lavage and lamellar bodies. Journal of Clinical Investigation 55: 914

Bienkowski R, Baum B, Crystal R G 1978 Fibroblasts degrade newly synthesized collagen within the cell before secretion. Nature 276: 413-16

Bienkowski R, Cowan M J, McDonald J A, Crystal R G 1978 Degradation of newly synthesized collagen. Journal of Biological Chemistry 253: 4356-63

Birdwell C R, Gospodarowicz D, Nicholson G L 1978 Identification, localization and role of fibronectin in cultured bovine endothelial cells. Proceedings of the National Academy of Sciences (USA) 75: 3273

Bitterman P B, Crystal R G 1980 Pulmonary alveolar macrophages release a factor that stimulates human lung fibroblasts to replicate. American Review of Respiratory Disease 121: 58

Bitterman P B, Rennard S, Schoenberger C, Crystal R G 1981 Asbestos stimulates macrophages to release a factor causing human lung fibroblasts to replicate. Chest in press

Bornstein P, Traub W 1979 The chemistry and biology of collagen. In: Neurath H, Hiln R L (eds) The proteins, vol 4. Academic Press, New York

Bradley K H unpublished observations

Bradley K H, Breul S M, Crystal R G 1974 Lung collagen heterogeneity. Proceedings of the National Academy of Sciences (USA) 71: 2828

Bradley K H, Breul S, Crystal R G 1975 Collagen in the human lung: composition and quantitation of rates of synthesis. Journal of Clinical Investigation 55: 543

Bradley K H, McConnell S D, Crystal R G 1974 Lung collagen composition and synthesis: characterization and changes with age. Journal of Biological Chemistry 249: 2674

Bradley K H, Kawanami O, Ferrans V J, Crystal R G 1980 The fibroblast of human alveolar structures: a differentiated cell with a major role in lung structure and function. In: Harris C C, Trump B C, Stoner G S (eds) Methods in cell biology, vol 21. Academic Press, New York, p 37-6

Braley J F, Peterson L B, Dawson C A, Moore V L 1979 Effect of hypersensitivity on protein uptake across the air-blood barrier of isolated rabbit lungs. Journal of Clinical Investigation 63: 1103

Bray B A 1978 Cold insoluble globulin (fibronectin) in connective tissues of adult human lung and in trophoblast basement membrane. Journal of Clinical Investigation 62: 745

Brentjens J R, O'Connell D W, Pawlowski I B, Hsu K C, Andres G A 1974 Experimental immune complex disease of the lung. Journal of Experimental Medicine 140: 105

Breul S D, Bradley K H, Hance A J, Schafer M P, Berg R A, Crystal R G 1980 Control of collagen synthesis by human diploid lung fibroblasts. Journal of Biological Chemistry 255: 5250-60

Brody J S, Kagan H M, Manalo A B 1979 Lung lysyl oxidase activity in relation to lung growth. American Review of Respiratory Disease 120: 1289-96

Bruce R M, Adamson J S, Pierce J A 1970 Collagen and elastin content of the lung in anti-trypsin deficiency. Clinical Research 18: 89A

Burke J M, Ross R 1979 Synthesis of connective tissue macromolecules by smooth muscle. International Review of Connective Tissue Research 8: 119

Burrell R, Anderson M 1973 The induction of fibrogenesis by silica-treated alveolar macrophages. Environmental Research 6: 389-94

Burrell R, Flaherty D K, DeNee P B, Abraham J L, Gelderman A H 1974 The effect of lung antibody on normal lung structure and function. American Review of Respiratory Disease 109: 106

Cantor J O, Bray B, Ryan S, Mandl I, Turino G M 1979 Glycosaminoglycans and collagen synthesis in an animal model of pulmonary fibrosis. Federation Proceedings 38: 1373A

Castor C W, Heiss R R, Gray R H, Seidman J C 1979 Connective tissue formation by lung fibroblasts in vitro. American Review of Respiratory Disease 120: 107

Castor C W, Wilson S M, Heiss P R, Seidman J C 1979 Activation of lung connective tissue cells in vitro. American Review of Respiratory Disease 120: 101

Cate C C, Burrell R 1974 Lung antigen induced cell mediated immune injury in chronic respiratory diseases. American Review of Respiratory Diseaae 109: 114

Chen L B, Maitland N, Gallimore P H, McDougal J K 1977 Detection of the large external transformation sensitive protein on some epithelial cells. Experimental Cell Research 106: 39

Chisolm J S, Cherniak N S, Carton R W 1968 Results of pulmonary function testing in 5 persons with Marfan's syndrome. Journal of Laboratory and Clinical Medicine 71: 25

Chvapil M, Peng Y M 1975 Oxygen and lung fibrosis. Archives of Environmental Health 30: 528

Chvapil M, Bartos D, Bartos F 1973 Effect of long-term stress on collagen growth in the lung, heart and femur of young and adult rats. Gerentologica 19: 263

Clark J G, Overton J E, Marino B A, Uitto J, Starcher B C 1980 Collagen synthesis in bleomycin induced pulmonary fibrosis. Journal of Laboratory and Clinical Medicine 96: 943-53

Clark J G, Starcher B C, Uitto J 1980 Collagen in pulmonary fibrosis: bleomycin induced synthesis of type I procollagen by human lung and skin fibroblasts in cultures. Biochimica et Biophysica Acta 631: 359

Collins J F personal communication

Collins J F, Crystal R G 1975 Characterization of cell-free synthesis of collagen by lung polysomes in a heterologous system. Journal of Biological Chemistry 250: 7332

Collins J F, Durnin L S, Johanson W G Jr 1978 Papain-induced lung injury: alterations in connective tissue metabolism without emphysema. Experimental and Molecular Pathology 29: 29

Collins J, Fulmer J, Cowan M, Horwitz A, Crystal R unpublished observations

Collins J F, Jones M A 1978 Connective tissue proteins of the baboon lung: concentration, content and synthesis of collagen in the normal lung. Connective Tissue Research 5: 211

Collins J F, Jones M A, Durnin L S 1977 Collagen content and synthesis in the lungs of normal baboon and in baboon with experimental pulmonary fibrosis. Texas Journal of Science, Special Publication 3: 127

Collins J F, Johansen W G Jr, McCullough B, Jones B A, Waugh H J Jr 1978 Effects of compensatory lung growth in irradiation-induced regional pulmonary fibrosis in the baboon. American Review of Respiratory Disease 117: 1079-89

Collins J F, Strong G L, Johanson W G Jr, McCullough B 1978 Collagen and elastin metabolism in bleomycin-induced pulmonary fibrosis in the baboon. American Review of Respiratory Disease 117 (part 2): 323

Cowan M J, Crystal R G 1975 Lung growth after unilateral pneumonectomy: quantitation of collagen synthesis and content. American Review of Respiratory Disease 111: 267

Cronlund A L, Kagan H M 1980 Comparison of highly purified bovine lysyl and aortic lysyl oxidase. Federation Proceedings 39: 974A

Crapo J D, Barry B E, Fosone H A, Shelburne J 1980 Structural and biochemical changes in rat lung occurring during exposures to lethal and adaptive doses of oxygen. American Review of Respiratory Disease 112: 123-43

Crystal R G 1974 Lung collagen. Definition, diversity and development. Federation Proceedings 33: 2248

Crystal R G, Fulmer J D, Roberts W C, Moss J L, Line B R, Reynolds H Y 1976 Idiopathic pulmonary fibrosis: clinical, histologic, radiographic, physiologic, scintigraphic, cytologic and biochemical aspects. Annals of Internal Medicine 85: 769-88

Crystal R G, Gadek J E, Ferrans V J, Fulmer J D, Line B R, Hunninghake G W 1981 Interstitial lung disease: current concepts of pathogenesis, staging and therapy. American Journal of Medicine 70: 542-568

Crystal R G, Roberts W C, Hunninghake G W, Gadek J E, Fulmer J D, Line B R 1981 Pulmonary sarcoidosis: a disease characterized and perpetuated by activated lung T-lymphocytes. Annals of Internal Medicine 94: 73-94

Cutroneo K R, Guzman N A, Sharamy M M 1974 Evidence for a subcellular vesicular site for collagen prolyl hydroxylation. Journal of Biological Chemistry 249: 5989

Cutroneo K R, Stassen F L H, Cardinale G J 1975 Anti-inflammatory steroids and collagen metabolism: glucocorticoid mediated decrease of prolyl hydroxylase. Molecular Pharmacology 11: 44-51

Davis J M, Beckett S T, Bolton R E, Collings P, Middleton A P 1978 Mass and number of fibers in the pathogenesis of asbestos-related lung disease in rats. British Journal of Cancer 37: 673

Davis W B, Gadek J E, Fells G A, Crystal R G 1981 Role of eosinophils in connective tissue destruction. American Review of Respiratory Disease 123 (part 2): 55

Dorvan P A, Hayes J A 1981 Peribronchiolar scarring: New collagen formation in response to cadmium aerosol in press

Drodz M, Kucharz E, Olczyk K 1979 Age related changes in the content of fibrous proteins in the rat tissues. Acta Physiologia Polonicka 30: 3

Drozdz M, Kucharz E, Szyja J 1977 Effect of chronic exposure to nitrogen dioxide on collagen content in lung and skin of guinea pigs. Environmental Research 13: 369

Dubrawsky C, Dubrawsky N B, Withers H R 1978 The effect of colchicine on the accumulation of hydroxyproline and on lung compliance after irradiation. Radiation Research 73: 111

Dwyer E M, Troncale F 1965 Spontaneous pneumothorax and pulmonary disease in the Marfan syndrome. Annals of Internal Medicine 62: 1285

Eisen A Z, Bloch K J, Sakai T 1970 Inhibition of human skin collagenase by human serum. Journal of Laboratory of Clinical Medicine 75: 258

Elson N A, Karlinsky J B, Kelman J A, Rhoades R A, Crystal R G 1976 Differentiated properties of the type 2 alveolar cell: partial characterization of protein content, synthesis and secretion. Clinical Research 24: 464A

Epstein E H Jr, Munderloh N H 1975 Isolation and characterization of CNBr peptides of human $[\alpha 1(III)]_3$ collagen and tissue distribution of $[\alpha 1(I)]_2\alpha_2$ and $[\alpha 1(III)]_3$ collagens. Journal of Biological Chemistry 250: 9304-12

Fedullo A J, Karlinsky J B, Snider G L, Goldstein R H 1979 Biochemical and mechanical effects of penicillamine on normal and bleomycin fibrotic hamster lungs. American Review of Respiratory Disease 119 (part 2): 307

Feist J H, Johnson T H, Wilson R J 1973 Acquired tracheomalacia, etiology and differential diagnosis. Radiology 109: 577

Foidart J M, Abe S, Martin G R, Zizic T M, Barnett E V, Lawley T J, Katz S I 1979 Antibodies to type II collagen in relapsing polychondritis. New England Journal of Medicine 299: 1203-7

Foidart J M, Bere E W, Yaar M, Rennard S, Gullino M, Martin G R, Katz S I 1980 Distribution and immunoelectron microscopic localization of laminin, a noncollagenous basement membrane glycoprotein. Laboratory Investigation 42: 336-42

Frank L, Butcher J R, Roberts R J 1978 Oxygen toxicity in neonatal and adult animals of various species. Journal of Applied Physiology 45: 699

Fuleihan F J D, Suh S K, Shepard R H 1963 Some aspects of pulmonary function in the Marfan's syndrome. Bulletin of the Johns Hopkins Hospital 113: 320

Fulmer J D, Bienkowski R S, Cowan M J, Breul S D, Bradley K D, Ferrans V J, Roberts W C, Crystal R G 1980 Collagen concentration and rates of synthesis in idiopathic pulmonary fibrosis. American Review of Respiratory Disease 122: 289-301

Fulmer J D, Crystal R G 1979 Interstitial lung disease. In: Simmons D H (ed) Current polmonology II, vol 1. Houghton Mifflin, Boston Mass, p 1-65

Fulmer J, Elson N, Bradley K, Ferrans V, Crystal R G 1977 Comparison of type-specific collagens by lung epithelial and mesenchymal cells. Clinical Research 25: 503A

Fulmer J D, Von Gal E R, Roberts W C, Crystal R G 1979 Morphologic-physiologic correlates of the severity of fibrosis in idiopathic pulmonary fibrosis. Journal of Clinical Investigation 63: 665-76

Fung Y C B, Sobin S S, Lindal R G, Tremor H M, Bernick S, Wall R, Karspick M 1979 The connective tissue of the interalveolar wall. Federation Proceedings 38 (part 2): 1235

Gadek J E unpublished observations

Gadek J, Hunninghake G W, Fells G, Zimmerman R, Crystal R G 1981 Production of connective tissue-specific proteases by human alveolar macrophages is constitutive (nonregulatable). American Review of Respiratory Disease 123 (part 2): 55

Gadek J E, Hunninghake G W, Fells G A, Zimmerman R L, Keogh B A, Crystal R G 1981 Validation of the alpha-1-antitrypsin hypothesis: recovery of active connective tissue specific proteases from the lung of PiZ patients and reversal with alpha-1-antitrypsin replacement therapy. Clinical Research 49: 550A

Gadek J E, Kelman J A, Fells G A, Weinberger S E, Horwitz A L, Reynolds H Y, Fulmer J D, Crystal R G 1979 Collagenase in the lower respiratory tract of patients with idiopathic pulmonary fibrosis. New England Journal of Medicine 301: 737

Gadek J E, Zimmerman R L, Fells G A, Crystal R G 1981 Assessment of the protease-antiprotease theory of emphysema. Bulletin of European Physiopathology of Respiration in press

Garrett R J B 1978 Collagen and noncollagen protein synthesis in developing lung exposed to tobacco smoke. Environmental Research 17: 205-15

Gauss-Muller V, Kleinman H K, Martin G R, Schiffman E 1980 Role of attachment factors and attractants in fibroblast chemotaxis. Journal of Laboratory and Clinical Medicine 96: 1071-80

Goldstein R H, Faris B, Hu˙C L, Snider G L, Franzblau D 1978 The fate of newly synthesized lung collagen after endotracheal administration of ^{14}C-proline to hamsters. American Review of Respiratory Disease 117: 281

Goldstein R H, Lucey E C, Franzblau C, Snider G L 1979 Failure of mechanical properties to parallel changes in lung connective tissue composition in bleomycin-induced pulmonary fibrosis in hamsters. American Review of Respiratory Disease 120: 67

Gerber G B, Dancewicz A M, Bessemans B, Casale G 1977 Biochemistry of late effects in rat lung after hemithoracic irradiation. Acta Radiation Therapy and Physical Biology 16: 447

Greenberg D B, Lyons S A, Last J A 1978 Paraquat induced changes in the rate of collagen biosynthesis by rat lung explants. Journal of Laboratory of Clinical Medicine 92: 1033

Greenberg D B, Reiser K M, Last J A 1978 Correlation of biochemical and morphologic manifestations of acute pulmonary fibrosis in rats administered paraquat. Chest 74: 421

Gross P, Kociba R J, Sparschu G L, Norris J M 1977 The biologic response to titanium phosphate. Archives of Pathology and Laboratory Medicine 101: 550

Halme J, Uitto J, Kahanpaa K, Korhunen P, Lindy S 1970 Protocollagen proline hydroxylase activity in experimental pulmonary fibrosis of rats. Journal of Laboratory and Clinical Medicine 75: 355

Hance A J, Crystal R G 1975 The connective tissue of lung. American Review of Respiratory Disease 112: 657

Hance A J, Crystal R G 1977 Rigid control of the synthesis of collagen types I and III by cells in culture. Nature 268: 152-4

Harrington J S, Ritchie M, King P C, Miller K 1973 The in-vitro effects of silica-treated hamster macrophages on collagen production by hamster fibroblasts. Journal of Pathology 109: 21-37

Harris E D Jr, Cartwright E C 1977 Mammalian collagenases. In: Barrett A J (ed) Proteases in mammalian cells and tissues. North Holland Publishing Company, Amsterdam, p 249

Hance A J, Bradley K H, Crystal R G 1976 Lung collagen heterogeneity. Synthesis of type I and III collagen by rabbit and human lung cells in culture. Journal of Clinical Investigation 57: 102

Haschek W M, Meyer K R, Ullrich R L, Witschi H P 1979 Pulmonary fibrosis — a possible mechanism. Federation Proceedings 38 (part 2): 1155

Hemberger J A, Shanker L S 1978 Effect of thyroxine on permeability of the neonatal rat lung to drugs. Biology Neonatorum 34: 299

Heppleston A G 1979 Silica and asbestos: contrasts in tissue response. Annals of the New York Academy of Sciences 330: 725-40

Heppelston A G, Styles J A 1967 Activity of a macrophage factor in collagen formation by silica. Nature 214: 521

Hesterberg T W, Last J A 1981 Ozone induced acute pulmonary fibrosis in rats: prevention of increased rates of collagen synthesis by methylprednisolone. American Review of Respiratory Disease 123: 47-52

Hoffmann L, Blumenfeld O O, Mondshine R B, Park S S 1972 Effect of d-pencillamine on fibrous proteins of rats. Journal of Applied Physiology 33: 42

Hoffmann L, Mondshine R B, Park S S 1971 Effect of dl-penicillamine on elastic properties of rat lung. Journal of Applied Physiology 30: 508

Hollinger M A, Chvapil M 1977 Effect of paraquat on rat lung prolyl hydroxylase. Research Communications in Chemical Pathology and Pharmacology 16: 159

Hollinger M A, Zuckermann J E, Giri S N 1978 Effect of acute and chronic paraquat on rat lung collagen content. Research Communications in Chemical Pathology and Pharmacology 21: 295

Hormann H, Jelinic V 1980 Fibronectin VII. Binding of cold insoluble globulin and of denatured collagen by macrophages. Hoppe-Seyler's Zeitschrift fur Physiologie und Chemistrie 361: 379-87

Horwitz A, Crystal R G 1976 Collagenase from rabbit pulmonary alveolar macrophages. Biochemical and Biophysical Research Communications 69: 296

Horwitz A L, Hance A J, Crystal R G 1977 Granulocyte collagenase: selective digestion of type I over type III collagen. Proceedings of the National Academy of Sciences (USA) 74: 897

Horwitz A L, Kelman J A, Crystal R G 1976 Activation of alveolar macrophage collagenase by a neutral protease secreted by the same cell. Nature 264: 772

Howard B V, Macarak E J, Gunson D, Kefalides N A 1976 Characterization of the collagen synthesized by endothelial cells in culture. Proceedings of the National Academy of Sciences (USA) 73: 2361

Huang T W 1978 Composite epithelial and endothelial basal laminas in human lungs. American Journal of Pathology 93: 681

Huang T W, Carlson J R, Bray T M, Bradley B J 1977 3-methylindole-induced pulmonary injury in goats. American Journal of Pathology 87: 647

Hugood C 1979 Ultrastructural changes of rabbit lung after a 5 ppm nitric oxide exposure. Archives of Environmental Health 34: 12

Hurst D J, Kilburn K H, Baker W M 1977 Normal newborn and adult human lung collagen. Connective Tissue Research 5: 117

Hunninghake G W, Crystal R G 1981 Mechanisms of hypergammaglobulinemia in sarcoidosis: site of increased antibody production and role of T-lymphocytes. Journal of Clinical Investigation 67: 86–92

Hunninghake G W, Gadek J E, Young R C Jr, Kawanami O, Ferrans V J, Crystal R G 1980 Maintenance of granuloma formation in pulmonary sarcoidosis by T-lymphocytes within the lung. New England Journal of Medicine 302: 594-8

Hunninghake G W, Kawanami O, Ferrans V J, Young R C Jr, Roberts W C, Crystal R G 1981 Characterization of the inflammatory and immune effector cells in the lung parenchyma of patients with interstitial lung disease. American Review of Respiratory Disease 123: 407—412

Hunninghake G W, Keogh B A, Crystal R G 1980 Comparison of cyclophosphamide and corticosteroids on lung inflammatory immune responses in idiopathic pulmonary fibrosis. Clinical Research 28: 476A

Hunninghake G W, Schmit N, Rust M, Gadek J, Keogh B, Strumpf I, Crystal R G 1979 Lung immunoglobulin production in a chronic lung disease. Clinical Research 27: 493A

Hurst D S, Gilbert G L, McKenzie W N 1977 Effect of cigarette smoke on lung collagen synthesis. Clinical Research 25: 590A

Hussain M Z, Belton J C, Bhatnagar R S 1978 Macromolecular synthesis in organ cultures of neonatal rat lung. In vitro 14: 740

Hussain M Z, Bhatnagar R S 1979 Involvement of superoxide dismutase in the paraquat-induced enhancement of lung collagen synthesis in organ culture. Biochemical and Biophysical Research Communications 89: 71

Hussain M Z, Mustafa M G, Chow C K, Cross C E 1976 Ozone induced increase of lung proline hydroxylase and hydroxyproline content. Chest 69: 273

Hussain M Z, Streifel J A, Tolentino M, Enriquez B, Bhatnagar R S 1978 Macromolecular synthesis in lung organ cultures in high O_2 atmospheres. Federation Proceedings 37: 1529

Hyman A L, Spannhake E W, Kadowitz P J 1978 Prostaglandins and the lung. American Review of Respiratory Disease 117: 111-36

Jaffe E A, Minick R, Adelman B, Becker C G, Nachman R 1976 Synthesis of basement membrane collagen by cultured human endothelial cells. Journal of Experimental Medicine 144: 209

Jelenska M M, Dancewicz A M, Przygoda E 1975 Radiation-induced aldehydes in collagen. Acta Biochimica Polonica 22: 179

Jennings F L, Arden A 1961 Development of experimental radiation pneumonitis. Archives of Pathology 71: 437

Johnson K J, Ward P A 1974 Acute immunological pulmonary alveolitis. Journal of Clinical Investigation 54: 349

Jones A W 1978 Bleomycin lung damage: the pathology and nature of the lesion. British Journal of Diseases of the Chest 72: 321

Jones A W, Reeve N L 1978 Ultrastructure study of bleomycin-induced pulmonary changes in mice. Journal of Pathology 124: 227

Joubert J R, Ascah K, Moroz L A, Hogg J C 1976 Acute hypersensitivity pneumonitis in the rabbit. An animal model with horseradish peroxidase as antigen. American Review of Respiratory Disease 113: 503

Juricova M, Deyl Z 1974 Ageing processes in collagen from different tissues of rats. Advances in Experimental Medicine and Biology 53: 351

Karlinsky J B, Snider G L 1978 Animal models of emphysema. American Review of Respiratory Disease 117: 1109

Karlinsky J B, Snider G L, Franzblau C, Stone P J, Hoppin F G Jr 1976 In vitro effects of elastase and collagenase on mechanical properties of hamster lungs. American Review of Respiratory Disease 113: 769

Keller S, Mandl I 1972 Qualitative differences between normal and emphysematous human lung elastin. In: Mittman C (ed) Pulmonary emphysema and proteolysis. Academic Press, New York, p 251

Kelley J, Beaumont R T, Moehring J M 1979 Collagen phenotype in adult lung fibroblasts. American Review of Respiratory Disease 119: 323

Kelley J, Newman R A, Evans J N 1980 Bleomycin-induced pulmonary fibrosis in the rat. Prevention with an inhibition of collagen synthesis. Journal of Laboratory and Clinical Medicine 96: 954-65

Kelman J, Brin S, Horwitz A, Bradley K, Hance A, Breul S, Baum B, Crystal R G 1977 Collagen synthesis and collagenase production by human lung fibroblasts. American Review of Respiratory Disease 115 (part 2): 343

Keogh B A, Crystal R G 1981 Chronic interstitial lung disease. In: Current pulmonology II. Houghton Mifflin, Boston, Mass

Kerr S, Alper R, Kefalides N A, Fisher A B 1979 Relationship between alveolar pO_2 and collagen synthesis by perfused rat lung. American Review of Respiratory Disease 119 (part 2): 364

Khurana M, Niden A H 1979 The effect of penicillamine on pulmonary collagen synthesis in vivo. American Review of Respiratory Disease 119 (part 2): 324

Kleinman H K, Klebe R J, Martin G R Role of collagenous matrices in the adhesion and growth of cells 1981 Journal of Cell Biology 88: 473-485

Kuhn C, Yu S Y, Chraplyry M, Linder H E, Senior R 1976 The induction of emphysema with elastase. II. Changes in connective tissue. Laboratory Investigation 34: 372

Kuttan R, Meezan E, Brendel K, Lafranconi M, Sipes I G 1979 Effect of paraquat treatment on prolyl hydroxylase activity and collagen synthesis of rat lung and kidney. Research Communications in Chemical Pathology and Pharmacology 25: 257-68

Lam H F, Takezaum J, Van Stee E W 1979 The effect of paraquat and diquat on lung function measurement in rats. American Review of Respiratory Disease 119 (part 2): 327

Last J personal communication

Last J A, Greenberg D B 1979 Synthesis of type IV collagen by rat lungs in vitro. XIth International Congress of Biochemistry Abstracts: 696

Lavietes M H, Min B, Hagstrom J W C, Rochester D F 1977 Diffuse pulmonary granulomatous disease in the dog. American Review of Respiratory disease 116: 907

Law M P, Hornsey S, Field S B 1976 Collagen content of lungs of mice after X-irradiation. Radiation Research 65: 60

Liotta L A, Trygvasson K, Garbisa S, Hart I, Foltz C M, Shafis S 1980 Metastatic potential correlates with enzymatic degradation of basement membrane collagen. Nature 284: 67-8

Loosli C G, Potter E L 1951 The prenatal development of the human lung. Anatomic Record 109: 320A

Low F N 1978 Lung interstitium: development, morphology, fluid content. In: Staub N C (ed) Lung water and solute exchange. Marcel Dekker, Inc, New York

McBride J T, Wohl M E B, Streider D J, Jackson A L, Zwerdling R G, Grissom N T, Treves S, Williams A J, Schuster S 1980 Lung growth and airway function after lobectomy in infancy for congenital lobar emphysema. Journal of Clinical Investigation 66: 962-70

McCullough B, Collins J F, Johanson W G Jr, Grover F L 1978 Bleomycin-induced diffuse interstitial pulmonary fibrosis in baboons. Journal of Clinical Investigation 61: 79

McCullough B, Schneider S, Greene N D, Johanson W G 1978 Bleomycin induced lung injury to baboons: alteration of cells and immunoglobulins recoverable by bronchoalveolar lavage. Lung 155: 337

McDonald J, Baum B, Rosenberg D, Kelman J A, Brin S C, Crystal R G 1979 Destruction of a major extracellular adhesive glycoprotein (fibronectin) of human fibroblasts by neutral proteases from polymorphonuclear leukocyte granules. Laboratory Investigation 40: 350

McLees B D, Schleiter G, Pinnell S R 1977 Isolation of type III collagen from human adult parenchymal lung tissue. Biochemistry 16: 185

Mainardi C L, Dixit S N, Kang A H 1980 Degradation of type IV (basement membrane) collagen by a proteinase isolated from human polymorphonuclear leukocyte granules. Journal of Clinical Investigation 255: 5435-41

Madri J A, Furthmayr H 1979 Collagen polymorphism in the lung: an immunochemical study during the early and late stages of pulmonary fibrosis. Federation Proceedings 38 (part 2): 1407

Madri J A, Furthmayr H 1980 Collagen polymorphism in the lung: an immunochemical study of pulmonary fibrosis. Human Pathology 11: 353-66

Madri J A personal communication

Madri J A, Furthmayr H 1979 Isolation and tissue localization of type AB_2 collagen from normal lung parenchyma. American Journal of Pathology 94: 323

Mandl I, Darnule T V, Fierer J A, Keller S, Turino G M 1977 Elastin degradation in human and experimental emphysema. In: Sandberg L B, Gray W R, Franzblau C (eds) Elastin and elastic tissue. Plenum Press, New York, p 221

Marom Z, Weinberg K S, Fanburg B L 1979 Effect of bleomycin on collagenol ytic activity of the rat pulmonary macrophage. American Review of Respiratory Disease 119 (part 2): 334

Martin H B, Boatman E S 1965 Electron microscopy of human pulmonary emphysema. American Review of Respiratory Disease 91: 206

Metevier H, Legendre N, Darnule J, Masse R 1978 Renouvellment du collagene pulmonaire insoluble chez la rat adulte. C.R. Academy Sciences (Paris) 287: 1341

Metevier H, Masse R, Legendre N, Lafuma J 1978 Pulmonary connective tissue modifications induced by internal α irradiation. Radiation Research 75: 385

Moore V L, Hensley G T, Fink J N 1975 An animal model of hypersensitivity pneumonitis in the rabbit. Journal of Clinical Investigation 56: 937

Morishige W K, Uetake C A 1978 Receptors for androgen and estrogen in the lung. Endocrinology 102: 1827

Mosher D, Saksela O, Vaheri A 1977 Synthesis and secretion of alpha-2-macroglobulin by cultured adherent lung cells. Journal of Clinical Investigation 60: 1036

Murray J C, Liotta L, Rennard S I, Martin G R 1979 Adhesion characteristics of murine metastatic and non-metastatic cells in vitro. Cancer Research 40: 347-50

Newman R A, Langer R O 1975 Age related changes in the synthesis of connective tissues in the rabbit. Connective Tissue Research 3: 231

Niden A H, Khurana M 1976 An animal model for diffuse interstitial pulmonary fibrosis-chronic low dose paraquat ingestion. Federation Proceedings 35: 631

Nourse L D, Nourse P N, Botes H, Schwartz H M 1975 The effects of macrophages isolated from the lungs of guinea pigs dusted with silica on collagen biosynthesis by guinea pig fibroblasts in cell culture. Environmental Research 9: 115-27

Ooshima A, Fuller G C, Cardinale G J, Spector S, Udenfriend S 1977 Reduction of collagen biosynthesis in blood vessels and other tissues by reserpine and hypophysectomy. Proceedings of the National Academy of Sciences USA 74: 777

Orthoefer J G, Bhatnagar R S, Rahman A, Yang V Y, Lee S D, Stara J F 1976 Collagen and prolyl hydroxylase levels in lungs of beagles exposed to air pollutants. Environmental Research 12: 299

Phillips T L 1966 An ultrastructural study of the development of radiation injury in the lung. Radiology 87: 49

Pierce J A 1963 Age related changes in the fibrous proteins of the lungs. Archives of Environmental Health 6: 56

Pierce J A 1968 The elastic tissue of the lung. In: Liebow A A, Smith D E (eds) The lung. Williams & Wilkins Co, Baltimore Md, p 41

Pierce J A, Hocott J B, Ebert R V 1961 The collagen and elastin content of the lung in emphysema. Annals of Internal Medicine 55: 1210

Pierce J A, Resnick H, Henry P H 1967 Collagen and elastin metabolism in the lungs, skin, and bones of adult rats. Journal of Laboratory and Clinical Medicine 69: 485

Pickrell J A, Harris D V, Benjamin S A, Cuddihy R G, Pfleger R G, Manderly J L 1976 Pulmonary collagen metabolism after lung injury from inhaled $^{90}\gamma$ in fused clay particles. Experimental Molecular Pathology 25: 70

Pickrell J A, Harris D V, Hahn F F, Belasich J J, Jones R K 1975 Biological alterations resulting from chronic lung irradiation. III. Effect of partial ^{60}Co thoracic irradiation upon pulmonary collagen metabolism and fractionation in Syrian hamsters. Radiation Research 62: 133

Pickrell J A, Harris D V, Manderly J L, Hahn F F 1976 Altered collagen metabolism in radiation induced interstitial pulmonary fibrosis. Chest 69: 311

Pickrell J A, Schnizlein C T, Hahn F F, Snipes M G, Jones R K 1978 Radiation-induced pulmonary fibrosis: study of changes in collagen constituents in different lung regions of beagle dogs after inhalation of beta-emitting radionuclides. Radiation Research 74: 363

Pickrell J A, Harris D V, Pfleger R C, Benjamin S A, Belasich J J, Jones R K, McClellan R O 1975 Biological alterations resulting from chronic lung irradiation. Radiation Research 63: 299

Pickrell J A, Shafer J 1971 Lung connective tissue measurements. I. Amino acid analysis procedures for determination of canine connective tissue. Archives of Internal Medicine 127: 891

Popenoe D, Loosti C G 1978 The morphological effects of a single exposure of paraquat on the mouse lung. Proceedings of the Western Pharmalogical Society 21: 151

Postlethwaite A, Seyer J A, Kang A H 1978 Chemotactic attraction of human fibroblasts to types I, II and III collagens and collagen derived peptides. Proceedings of the National Academy of Sciences (USA) 75: 871

Pozzi E, Zanon P 1978 On the pathogenesis of bleomycin lung toxicity. International Journal of Pharamcology and Biopharmacology 16: 575

Read J 1958 The pathological changes produced by anti-lung serum. Journal of Pathology and Bacteriology 76: 403

Reid K B M, Lowe D M, Porter R R 1972 Isolation and characterization of C1q, a subcomponent of the first component of complement from human and rabbit sera. Biochemical Journal 130: 749

Reiser K M, Greenberg D B, Last J A 1979 Type I/III collagen ratios in lungs of rats with experimental pulmonary fibrosis, Federation Proceedings 38 (part2): 817

Reiser K M, Last J A 1980 Quantitation of specific collagen types from lungs of small mammals. Analytical Biochemistry 104: 87-98

Rennard S, Crystal R G unpublished observations

Rennard S, Bitterman P, Hunninghake G W, Gadek J, Crystal R G 1981 Alveolar macrophage fibronectin: a possible mediator of tissue remodelling in fibrotic lung disease. Clinical Research 49: 374A

Rennard S I, Ferrans V J, Bradley K H, Crystal R G 1980 Lung connective tissue. In: Witschi H (ed) Mechanisms of pulmonary toxicology. CRC Press Boca Raton, Fla pp 115-153

Rennard S, Jaurand M C, Bignon J, Salzman L, Kawanami O, Stier L, Davidson J, Ferrans V, Crystal R G 1981 Connective tissue production by pleural mesothelial cells. American Review of Respiratory Disease 123 (part 2): 144

Reye R D, Bale P M 1973 Elastic tissue in pulmonary emphysema in Marfan syndrome. Archives of Pathology 96: 427

Richerson H B, Cheny F H F, Bauserman S C 1971 Acute experimental hypersensitivity pneumonitis in rabbits. American Review of Respiratory Disease 104: 568

Richards R J, Jacoby F 1976 Light microscopic studies on the effects of chrysotile asbestos and fibre glass on the morphology and reticulum formation of cultured lung fibroblasts. Environmental Research 11: 112

Richards R J, Wusteman F S 1974 The effects of silica dust and alveolar macrophages on lung fibroblasts in vitro. Life Sciences 14: 355-64

Richmond V 1980 Increased lability of lung collagen crosslinks. Analytical Biochemistry 104: 277-83

Richmond V, D'Aoust B G 1976 Effect of intermittent hyperbaric oxygen on guinea pig lung elastin and collagen. Journal of Applied Physiology 41: 295

Riley D J, Berg R A, Edelman N H, Prockop D J 1980 Prevention of collagen deposition following pulmonary oxygen toxicity in the rat by cis-4-hydroxy-6-proline. Journal of Clinical Investigation 65: 642-51

Rosenberg D M, Weinberger S E, Fulmer J D, Flye M W, Fauci A S, Crystal R G 1980 Functional correlates of lung involvement in Wegener's granulomatosis: use of pulmonary function testing in staging and follow up. American Journal of Medicine 69: 387-94

Rosenkrantz H, Esber H J, Sprague R 1969 Lung hydroxyproline levels in mice exposed to cigarette smoke. Life Sciences 8: 571

Rowe D W, McGoodwin E B, Martin G R, Grahm D 1977 Decreased lysyl oxidase activity in the aneurysm-prone mottled mouse. Journal of Biological Chemistry 252: 939

Ryan S F, Barrett C R, Lavietes M H, Bell A L L, Rochester D F 1978 Volume-pressure and morphometric observations after acute alveolar injury in the dog from N-nitroso-N-methylurethane. American Review of Respiratory Disease 118: 735

Ryan S F 1972 Experimental fibrosing alveolitis. American Review of Respiratory Disease 105: 776

Ryhanen L, Kivirikko K I 1974 Developmental changes in protocollagen lysyl hydroxylase activity in the chick embryo. Biochimica et Biophysica Acta 343: 121

Saba T M, Jaffe E 1980 Plasma fibronectin (opsonic glycoprotein): its synthesis by vascular endothelial cells and role in cardiopulmonary integrity after trauma as related to reticulendothelial function. American Journal of Medicine 68: 577-94

Sandberg L B 1976 Elastin structure in health and disease. International Review of Connective Tissues 7: 159-210

Schoenberger C, Hunninghake G W, Gadek J, Crystal R G 1980 Role of alveolar macrophages in asbestosis: modulation of neutrophil migration to the lung following asbestos exposure. American Review of Respiratory Disease 121: 257

Seethanathan P, Radhakrishnamurthy B, Dalferes E R Jr, Berenson G S 1975 The composition of connective tissue macromolecules from bovine respiratory system. Respiratory Physiology 24: 347

Senior R, Bielefeld D R, Abensohn M K 1975 The effect of proteolytic enzymes on the tensile strength of human lung. American Review f Respiratory Disease 111: 184

Senior R M, Bielefeld D R, Jeffrey J J 1972 Collagenase activity in alveolar macrophages. Clinical Research 20: 88

Seyer J personal communication

Seyer J M 1978 Basement membrane associated collagens of human lungs. Federation Proceedings 37: 1527

Seyer J M, Hutcheson E T, Kang A H 1976 Collagen polymorphism in idiopathic chronic pulmonary fibrosis. Journal of Clinical Investigation 57: 1498

Seyer J M, Kang A H, Rodnan G 1981 Characterization of type I and type III collagens of the lung in progressive systemic sclerosis (scleroderma). Arthritis and Rheumatism 24: 625-631

Shannon B T, Love S H, Myrvik Q N 1979 Hyaluronic acid content of lungs of rabbits during a cell-mediated response in Bacillus Calmette Guerin (BCG). Federation Proceedings 38 (part 2): 1204

Sikic B I, Young D, Mimnaugh E G, Gram T E 1978 Quantification of bleomycin pulmonary toxicity in mice by changes in lung hydroxyproline content and morphometric histopathology. Cancer Research 38: 787

Singh J, Kaw J L, Pandey S D, Viswanathan P N, Zaidi S H 1977 Amino acid changes and pulmonary response of rats to silica dust. Environmental Research 14: 452

Sneider R E, Senior R M, Bielfeld D R 1976 Prolyl hydroxylase activity of human lung. Chest 69: 272-3

Snider G L, Celli B R, Goldstein R H, O'Brien J J, Lucey E G 1978 Chronic interstitial pulmonary fibrosis produced in hamsters by endotracheal bleomycin. American Review of Respiratory Disease 117: 289

Snider G L, Hayes J A, Korthy A L 1978 Chronic interstitial pulmonary fibrosis produced in hamsters by endotracheal bleomycin: pathology and stereology. American Review of Respiratory Disease 177: 1099

Snider G L, Karlinsky J B 1977 Relation between elastic behaviour and the connective tissues of the lung. In: Iaochim H L (ed) Pathobiology Annual 7: 115. Appleton-Century-Crofts, New York

Snider G L, Paz M A, Hall P, Gallop P M 1980 Phagocytosis of collagen fibres by human embryonic lung fibroblasts. American Review of Respiratory Disease 122 (part 2): 407

Snider G L, Sherter C B, Koo K W, Karlinsky J B, Hayes J A, Franzblau C 1977 Respiratory mechanics in hamsters following treatment with endotracheal elastase or collagenase. Journal of Applied Physiology 42: 206

Spiro R G, Spiro M J 1971 Studies on the biosynthesis of the hydroxylysine-linked disaccharide unit of basement membranes and collagens. III. Journal of Biological Chemistry 246: 4919

Spooner B S, Faubian J M 1980 Collagen involvement in the branching morphogenesis of embryonic lung and salivary gland. Developmental Biology 77: 84-102

Stacy B D, King E J 1954 Silica and collagen in the lungs of silicotic rats treated with cortisone. British Journal of Industrial Medicine 11: 192

Starcher B C, Kuhn C, Overton J E 1978 Increased elastin and collagen content in the lungs of hamsters receiving an intratracheal injection of bleomycin. American Review of Respiratory Disease 117: 299

Starcher B, Madoras J, Tepper A 1977 Lysyl oxidase deficiency in lung and fibroblasts from mice with hereditary emphysema. Biochemical and Biophysical Research Communications 78: 706

Stenman S, Vaheri A 1978 Distribution of a major connective tissue protein, fibronectin in normal human tissues. Journal of Experimental Medicine 147: 1054-64

Sugihara T, Martin C J 1975 Simulation of lung tissue properties in age and irreversible obstructive syndromes using an aldehyde. Journal of Clinical Investigation 56: 23

Svoboda E L, Deporter D A 1980 Phagocytosis of exogenous collagen by cultured murine fibroblasts and macrophages: a quantitative electron microscopic comparison. Journal of Ultrastructural Research 72: 169-72

Szapiel S V, Elson N A, Fulmer J D, Hunninghake G W, Crystal R G 1979 Bleomycin induced interstitial pulmonary disease in the nude, athymic mouse. American Review of Respiratory Disease 120: 893

Szemenyei C, Balint A 1973 Studies on the ageing process of the rat lung. Acta Morphologica and Academic Science of Hungary 21: 295

Takeda T, Suzuki Y, Yao C S 1975 Experimental studies on the effect of ageing and endocrine control on collagen formation in various organs. Acta Pathological Japan 25: 135

Tencate A R 1972 Morphological studies of fibroblasts in connective tissue undergoing rapid remodelling. Journal of Anatomy 112: 401

Thompson W D, Patrick R S 1978 Collagen prolyl hydroxylase levels in experimental paraquat poisoning. British Journal of Experimental Pathology 59: 288

Thrall R S, McCormick J R, Jack R M, McReynolds J A, Ward P A 1979 Bleomycin-induced pulmonary fibrosis in the rat: inhibition by indomethacin. American Journal of Pathology 95: 113

Thyagarajan P, Vakil V K, Sreenivasan A 1976 Effects of whole-body X-irradiation on some aspects of collagen metabolism in the rat. Radiation Research 66: 575

Tolstoshev P unpublished observations

Tolstoshev P, Berg R A, Rennard S I, Bradley K H, Trapnell B C, Crystal R G 1981 Procollagen production and procollagen messenger RNA level and activity in human lung fibroblasts during periods of rapid and stationary growth. Journal of Biological Chemistry 256: 3135-3140

Tombropoulos E G, Thomas G M 1970 Effect of 800 R thoracic X-irradiation on lung tissue biochemistry. Radiation Research 44: 76

Tueller E E, Criss N R, Belton J C, McLaughlin R F 1977 Idiopathic spontaneous pneumothorax. Chest 71: 419

Ueda E, Nishimura K, Nagasaka Y, Kokubu T, Yamamura Y 1975 Metabolism of vasoactive substances in the lung: change of metabolism and its significance in rabbits with experimental pneumonitis. Japanese Circulation Journal 39: 559

Uitto V J, Schwartz D, Veis A 1980 Degradation of basement membrane collagen by neutral proteases from human leukocytes. European Journal of Biochemistry 105: 409-17

Valimaki M, Jura K, Rantanen J, Ekfors T, Ninikowski J 1975 Collagen metabolism in rat lungs during chronic intermittent exposure to oxygen. Aviation, Space, and Environmental Medicine 46: 684

Van Toorn D W 1970 Experimental interstitial pulmonary fibrosis. Pathologica Europeana 5: 97

Villiger B, Kelley D G, Kuhn C, McDonald J A 1980 Human alveolar macrophage fibronectin: synthesis and ultrastructural localization. Clinical Research 28: 745A

Vrako R 1972 Significance of basal lamina for regeneration of injured lung. Virchows Archives of Pathology 355: 264

Wahl S M, Wahl L M, McCarthy J M 1978 Lymphocyte mediated activation of fibroblast proliferation and collagen production. Journal of Immunology 121: 942

Weibel E R, Gehr P, Haies D, Gil J, Bachofen M 1976 The cell population of the lung. In: Bouhuys A (ed) Lung cells in disease. North Holland Publishing Co, Amsterdam

Werb Z 1978 Biochemical actions of glucocorticoids on macrophages in culture. Specific inhibition of elastase, collagenase, and plasminogen activator secretion and effects on other metabolic functions. Journal of Experimental Medicine 147: 1695-712

Wessells N K, Cohen J H 1968 Effects of collagenase on developing epithelia in lung, ureteric bud, and pancreas. Developmental Biology 18: 294

Wick G, Crystal R G Unpublished observations

Woolley D E, Roberts D R, Evanson J M 1976 Small molecular $\beta 1$ serum protein which specifically inhibits human collagenases. Nature 261: 325

Wright G W, Kleinerman J, Zorn E M 1960 The elastin and collagen content of normal and emphysematous human lungs. American Review of Respiratory Disease 81: 938

Yamada K, Olden K 1978 Fibronectins — adhesive glycoproteins of cell surface and blood. Nature 275: 179

Yu S Y, Keller N R 1978 Synthesis of lung collagen in hamsters with elastase-induced emphysema. Experimental and Molecular Pathology 29: 37

Yu S Y, Sun C N, Still M F 1977 Ultrastructural changes of elastic tissue during elastase emphysema. Ibid: 39

25

Muscle

R. MAYNE

INTRODUCTION

Collagen is recognized as having several important functions as a structural component of all muscular tissues. It forms the linkages between the muscle and its associated connective tissues such as tendon or fascia, and also is the fibrillar component of the cell-to-cell connections which are present both between individual muscle cells and between the muscle cells and neighbouring capillaries plus other small blood vessels (Copenhaver et al, 1978). In this chapter, skeletal, cardiac and gastrointestinal muscle will be described. (For discussion of vascular smooth muscle see Ch. 20, and for uterine smooth muscle see Ch. 31. Muscle tendon junctions will also be described in Ch. 30.

NORMAL — MORPHOLOGY

Light microscopic observations

In skeletal muscle, each muscle fibre is surrounded by a thin sheath of connective tissue called the endomysium within which are located the endothelial cells of the capillary network, some pericytes and an occasional connective tissue cell or fibroblast. Several muscle fibres form a bundle or fascicle which is surrounded by the more dense connective tissue of the perimysium, and within which are located larger blood vessels, lymphatics and nerves. The fascicles collectively are surrounded by the outer dense connective tissue of the muscle or epimysium, which does not contain any blood vessels. In cardiac muscle, connective tissue surrounds the myocytes and an endomysium and perimysium can usually be recognized, the endomysium containing a very extensive capillary network. Within the endomysium, fibroblasts are sometimes encountered in addition to the endothelial cells and pericytes. Estimates by Enesco & Puddy (1964) for a variety of rat skeletal muscles showed that approximately 65 per cent of the nuclei which are observed in sections are located within the muscle fibres, whereas 25 per cent of the nonmuscle nuclei are located in the endomysium and 10 per cent in the perimysium. These results contrast with the results of Grove et al (1969) for rat cardiac muscle. These authors estimated that the muscle nuclei comprise only 26 per cent or less of the total nuclei present, the remainder being regarded as nuclei of connective tissue cells. However, the nuclei of endothelial cells must also have been included in this estimate.

Gastrointestinal smooth muscle does not contain an obvious endomysium or extensive capillary network, and many of the smooth muscle cells are in close contact to each other by both intermediate junctions and nexuses (gap junctions) (Gabella, 1979). However, the distribution of nexuses is quite variable both between different smooth muscles and also between species. For example, the circular smooth muscle of the guinea pig ileum has many nexuses, whereas these junctions cannot be found in the longitudinal smooth muscle (Gabella & Blundell, 1979). Recently, intramuscular septa of connective tissue have been described in guinea pig taenia coli, and to which groups or bundles of smooth muscle cells may attach to form a diffuse intramuscular tendon (Gabella, 1977).

Staining of all muscular tissues with an alkaline solution of a silver salt (an argyrophilic stain) reveals a fine network of 'reticular' fibrils which are in close proximity to the muscle cells and the neighbouring capillaries (Nagel, 1935; Bairati, 1937). It is now generally recognized that the reticular fibrils which stain with silver are collagenous, but it remains to be established for muscular tissues that these fibrils are composed of type III collagen as has been proposed for other tissues (see below and Nowack et al, 1976). Recently, Gabella (1976) has examined the distribution of the 'reticular' fibres in both stretched and contracted guinea pig taenia coli. During stretching the fibres were arranged almost in parallel to the muscle cells, whereas in contraction the fibres were transversely arranged. It is argued that during contraction the muscle cells in some way twist and form folds within which the fibres are contained.

The presence of elastin fibres can be demonstrated in all muscular tissues by staining with resorcein-fuchsin, and in some tissues (e.g. guinea pig taenia coli) the presence of these fibres has been confirmed by electron microscopy

(Gabella, 1977). The extracellular matrix between muscle cells will also stain with periodic acid-Schiff (PAS), this probably reflecting the glycoprotein or glycosaminoglycan content of the sarcolemma.* Electron microscopic observations suggest that all three layers of the sarcolemma are periodic acid-Schiff positive (Zacks et al, 1973a).

Electron microscopic observations

Transmission electron microscopy of thin sections

Examination of sections of frog skeletal muscle at high resolution in the electron microscope has shown that the sarcolemma consists of several different layers or structures (Mauro & Adams, 1961). The inner membrane or plasmalemma is of diameter 10 nm and is separated from the basal lamina by an electron translucent space, the lamina lucida, which is of unknown composition. The basal lamina itself is of width 30 to 50 nm and has the amorphous appearance typical of all basement membranes. Exterior to the basal lamina is a meshwork of collagen fibrils of approximate diameter 30 nm, each fibril appearing to be surrounded by a ruthenium red staining glycoprotein (Zacks et al, 1973a). In addition to the collagen fibrils, a meshwork of very fine fibrils ($\simeq$10 nm) can often be observed. These fibrils do not show any periodicity and are of unknown composition. Electron micrographs of preparations of skeletal muscle sarcolemma isolated by differential centrifugation show that the sarcolemma retains all of the above structures with the possible exception of the fine non-striated fibrils (Zacks et al, 1973b; Peter et al, 1974).

In cardiac muscle the organization of the extracellular matrix is very similar to skeletal muscle, except that the basal lamina is not so prominent (James & Sherf, 1978; Langer, 1978). Recently, Winegrad & Robinson (1978) have examined the ventricular muscle of frog and rat hearts after treatment with the Ca^{2+} chelator EGTA, and have observed a network of fine microthreads in addition to the collagen fibrils. The dimensions of each microthread were estimated to be 300 nm by 2 nm with a globular region at one end, and it was suggested that each microthread may be a collagen molecule which arose from the disruption of the collagen fibrils by the chelating action of EGTA. The type of collagen which makes up the microthreads is unknown, but the presence of a globular end suggests that it might by type III collagen, which is known to exist in tissues in part as a procollagen molecule from which the amino terminal extension peptide remains uncleaved (Timpl et al, 1975). The microthreads were also observed in heart muscle untreated with EGTA, and appeared to interact with both the collagen fibrils and also with the basal lamina. The authors proposed that the microthread network is involved both in the transmission of the force during contraction of the myocytes during systole, and also in restoring the relaxed state during diastole.

In gastrointestinal smooth muscle the cells are always surrounded by a basal lamina, which in grazing sections appears to have a microfibrillar structure (Gabella, 1979). The collagen fibrils appear to be attached to the basal lamina possibly through microfilament connections (Gabella, 1979). The collagen fibrils of the reticular lamina were found to be consistently of diameter 30 to 35 nm which is smaller than the 50 nm of the fibrils present in neighbouring connective tissues. In the smooth muscle of the guinea pig taenia coli numerous collagen fibrils were observed which in the moderately stretched muscle run roughly parallel to the muscle cells (Gabella, 1977; see (Fig. 25.1). The basal lamina is thin ($\simeq$ 20 nm in width) and, by analysis of serial sections, Gabella (1977) has described specialized end-to-end contacts between the smooth muscle cells where the basal lamina is markedly thickened and may be as much as 100 nm in width between the two cells. Undoubtedly, these apparently fused basal laminae are important for the transmission of force throughout the muscle and for coordinating the contraction of individual muscle cells. To what extent the collagen fibrils are directly or passively involved in contraction remains unclear, as does the extent and organization of the linkages between the collagen fibrils and the basal lamina.

Replica techniques

The organization of the collagen fibrils in the sarcolemma of striated muscle has occasionally been investigated in the electron microscope by the preparation of replicas of the muscle fibre surface using metal shadowing followed by digestion of the tissue with proteases and/or acid and alkali solutions. Reed & Rudall (1948) examined frog leg muscle fixed in a partially stretched state and observed that the collagen fibrils appeared to be arranged in part as spirals around the muscle fibres. Similar observations were made by Draper & Hodge (1949) with fragments of toad striated muscle prepared after homogenization. Whorls of collagen fibrils were observed which were arranged at roughly 45° to the fibre axis, this again suggesting a helical arrangement around the fibre. Schmalbruch (1974) has examined frog skeletal muscle fixed at different sarcomere lengths and has observed that with increasing stretch the collagen fibrils become more oriented with the fibre axis. This helical arrangement of the fibrils has been described by Mauro & Adams (1961) as a 'braid-like weave'.

Scanning electron microscopy

Recently, the technique of scanning electron microscopy has been used to examine the three dimensional organization of the larger collagen fibres which make up the connective tissue skeleton of both the heart (Caulfield &

* In this chapter the term sarcolemma will describe the external membrane of all muscle cells which is composed of the cell membrane, the lamina lucida, the basal lamina and any associated collagen fibrils of the reticular lamina.

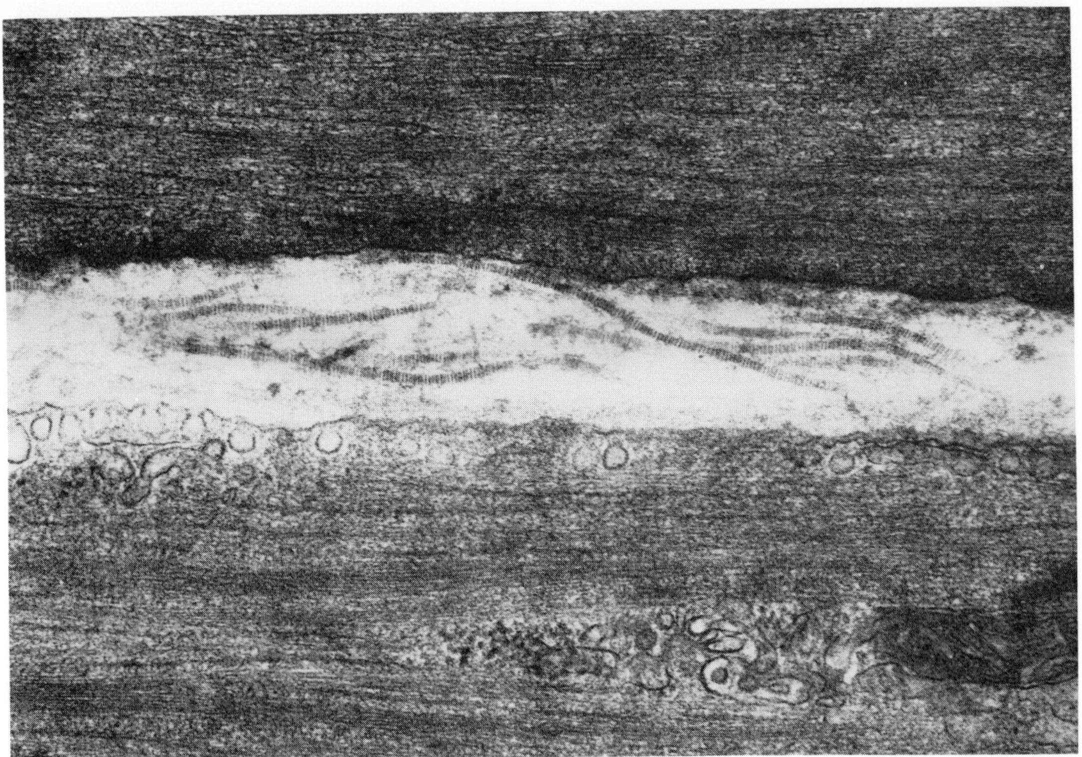

Fig. 25.1 Electron micrograph of a longitudinal section of guines pig taenia coli fixed in conditions of moderate stretch (×78 000). Note the numerous collagen fibrils which run roughly parallel to the smooth muscle cells, and the amorphous basement membrane which surrounds each cell. A collagen fibril can be observed in very close proximity to the plasmalemma, and may penetrate the basement membrane. (Micrograph kindly provided by Dr Giorgio Gabella, University College, London).

Borg, 1979) and skeletal muscle (Borg & Caulfield, 1980). In the heart, struts of collagen fibres of 120 to 150 nm in diameter were observed connecting each myocyte with a neighbouring myocyte (Fig. 25.2). These struts appear to spread out just before inserting directly into the basal lamina of the two cells. Insertion appears to occur close to the Z-bands and the presence of the struts may result in the alignment of the sarcomeres of neighbouring myocytes, and be in part responsible for co-ordinating the myocytes during diastole and systole without slippage occurring between the cells. An extensive network of fibres was also observed between the capillaries and the myocytes, and it was proposed that the arrangement of this network may be responsible for the maintenance of the patency of the capillaries during ventricular contraction. Similar myocyte to myocyte and myocyte to capillary connections were also observed in skeletal muscle (Borg & Caulfield, 1980).

NORMAL — BIOCHEMICAL AND IMMUNOFLUORESCENCE STUDIES

Comparison of collagen contents of muscular tissues

Recently, Gabella (1979) has estimated the collagen content of a variety of guinea pig tissues by determining hydroxyproline concentrations. Smooth muscles (taenia coli and myometrium) were found to have at least three times the collagen content when compared to the myocardium or sartorius muscle, and to have about one half of the concentration present in the aorta.

Skeletal muscle

Developmental studies

During the differentiation of chick skeletal muscle the accumulation of collagen closely parallels the accumulation of the muscle contractile proteins (Herrmann & Barry, 1955). Between days 13 and 17 of development, when muscle differentiation is most rapidly proceeding, the collagen concentration expressed as percentage wet weight of tissue increased seven times. To what extent the fibroblasts or connective tissue cells which are present in the developing muscle in small numbers, or the differentiating myoblasts and myotubes, are contributing to the increased collagen content is not known. Characterization of the collagen extracted by neutral salt from the muscle of 17 day lathyritic chick embryos has shown the presence of type I collagen (Ketley et al, 1976). Experiments have been performed in which clones of mononucleated cells derived from a single myoblast were

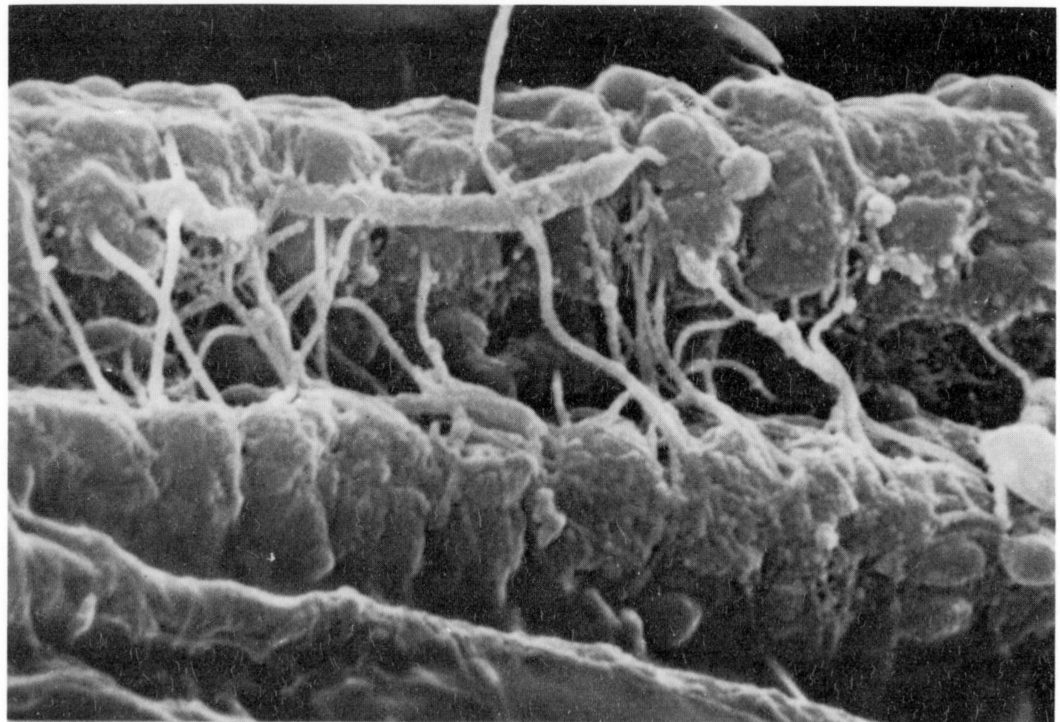

Fig. 25.2 Scanning electron micrograph of rabbit papillary heart muscle (×14 000). Two myocytes can be observed which are interconnected by numerous struts of collagen fibres. (Micrograph kindly provided by Dr T. K. Borg and Dr J. B. Caulfield, University of South Carolina, Columbia.)

grown in vitro and shown to synthesize collagen (Mayne et al, 1972; Abbott et al, 1974; Lipton, 1977). In one of these studies (Lipton, 1977) the incorporation of proline into hydroxyproline per DNA content was approximately 30 times less for clones derived from a myoblast when compared to clones of authentic fibroblasts, suggesting that myoblasts may not make a significant contribution to the total collagen content of muscle during in vivo development. Lipton (1977) also made the interesting observation with the electron microscope that only with mixed cultures of myoblasts and fibroblasts does a complete basal lamina and reticular lamina form in association with the developing myofibres. This result suggests that there may be an interaction between the fibroblast and the myofibre which promotes basal lamina and reticular fibre formation.

Recently, the biosynthesis of different collagen types was investigated in cultures of quail myoblasts both before and after fusion (Sasse et al, 1981). The advantage of using developing breast muscle from the quail is that myoblasts can be grown at clonal cell densities without the presence of contaminating fibroblasts (Konigsberg, 1971). Myoblasts before fusion were shown to synthesize types I, III and V collagen, the proportion of type III collagen increasing from 5 to 30 per cent as fusion proceeded. A small proportion of type V collagen was always synthesized during culture, most of this collagen being retained in the cell layer both before and after fusion. The results suggest that myoblasts in addition to authentic fibroblasts contribute to the collagen present in developing muscle.

It has been known for some time that a substratum of collagen will support myogenesis in vitro (Hauschka & Konigsberg, 1966), but the nature of the interaction between the collagen and the myoblast remains unclear. Native or denatured collagen are both equally effective, and some of the larger cyanogen bromide peptide fragments of type I collagen (α1(I)-CB7 and α1(I)-CB8) also have activity (Hauschka & White, 1971). However, another large cyanogen bromide peptide of type I collagen (α1(I)-CB6) did not possess activity, nor did various synthetic collagen-like polymers. Experiments in which substrata were made using different types of collagen (types I, II, III and IV) have shown that all are equally effective in supporting myogenesis (Ketley et al, 1976). Subtle differences may, however, arise with different collagen substrata. Recently, it was observed that myoblasts plated onto a substratum of type I collagen will align in parallel before fusion to form long myotubes. Myoblasts plated onto a substratum of type V collagen did not align, and formed only small myotubes (John & Lawson, 1980).

Myogenic cell lines

The myogenic lines of rat cells L6 and L8 originally developed by Yaffe and his colleagues (Yaffe, 1968; Richler

& Yaffe, 1970) have both been shown to synthesize collagen (Schubert et al, 1973; Garrels, 1979; Miranda et al, 1978). With the line L6, on reaching confluency, many of the cells will undergo fusion to form myotubes which will subsequently differentiate into myofibres. In the electron microscope an incomplete basal lamina was observed to form on the surface of the myotubes, and fibrillar collagen was present in the extracellular matrix (Schubert et al, 1973). Recently, it has been shown that the myotubes can be separated from the remaining mononucleated cells after fusion by sedimentation at 1 × gravity in a serum gradient (Garrels, 1979). Analysis of collagen biosynthesis by the myotubes alone showed that the rate of synthesis of collagen was less than one thousandth the rate of synthesis by the mononucleated cells, and from this result it was proposed that suppression of collagen biosynthesis probably occurs during myogenesis. Collagen biosynthesis has also been studied in the myogenic cell line L8, not before and after fusion of the myoblasts, but when fusion was prevented by the inclusion of dimethylsulfoxide in the culture medium (Miranda et al, 1978). Mononucleated cells grown in dimethylsulfoxide for several days continued to synthesize collagen, and measurements of hydroxyproline biosynthesis suggested that the rate of collagen biosynthesis had accelerated. Examination of the cultures in the electron microscope showed that large numbers of extracellular collagen fibrils were being assembled in the dimethylsulfoxide-treated cultures, and it was proposed that the cells had become similar to authentic fibroblasts. A similar proposal for a shift of myogenic cells towards a more fibroblastic behaviour has previously been made for the mononucleated cells which grew in vitro from clones of chick embryo myoblasts (Mayne et al, 1972; Abbott et al, 1974).

A detailed analysis of the collagen types synthesized by the myogenic cell lines L6 and L8 has not so far been reported. However, a human rhabdomyosarcoma cell line was recently analyzed for collagen types and shown to synthesize predominantly type III procollagen with smaller amounts of type IV and type V (AB) collagens (Krieg et al, 1979).

Collagen types present in skeletal muscle

Neutral salt- and acid-soluble collagen has been isolated from calf skeletal muscle, and the cyanogen bromide peptides derived from this collagen isolated and characterized (McClain, 1973). Cyanogen bromide peptides derived from type I collagen were the only peptides which could be identified. However, several recent analyses in which limited pepsin digestion was used to solubilize the collagen from adult bovine muscle (Duance et al, 1977) and 1-week-old chick limb muscle (Bailey et al, 1979) have shown the presence of type III and type V collagens in addition to type I collagen. Isolation of type IV collagen was not reported in these studies. Small amounts of fragments of type IV collagen can be isolated from chicken breast muscle after limited pepsin digestion followed by separation from the other collagen types by differential salt fractionation (Mayne & Zettergren, 1980).

In general, the results of the limited experiments so far performed characterizing the different collagen types present in skeletal muscle suggest that type I collagen is the predominant collagen which can be solubilized and that types III, IV and V collagen are all present.

Immunofluorescence studies with antibodies specific for different collagen types

Several studies have appeared attempting to localize the different collagen types in skeletal muscle using immunofluorescence staining techniques (Duance et al, 1977; Sasse et al, 1978; Krieg et al, 1979; Sanes & Hall, 1979; Duance et al, 1980). With antibodies prepared against types I, III and V (AB) collagen, Duance et al (1977), using frozen sections of bovine skeletal muscle, observed that staining for type I collagen was predominant in the epimysium and perimysium, whereas staining for type III collagen tended to localize in the perimysium, and for type V (AB) collagen in the endomysium. Similar findings have also been reported for chick skeletal muscle (Bailey et al, 1979), rat diaphragm (Sanes & Hall, 1979) and normal human muscle (Duance et al, 1980). The localization of type V collagen to the endomysium led Duance et al (1977) to propose that this collagen is located in the muscle basement membrane. Further evidence from haemagglutination titres of muscle cell medium (Bailey et al, 1979) suggests that the synthesis of type V collagen begins at the time of myotube formation, and would therefore indicate that type V collagen is a basement membrane collagen. However, other biochemical and immunofluorescence analyses of developing muscle have shown that type V collagen is synthesized by both myoblasts and myotubes, whereas types I and III collagen are only synthesized by myoblasts (Sasse et al, 1981). It is known from morphological observations that the basement membrane begins to form as the myotubes differentiate (Lipton, 1977). Other immunofluorescence studies have, however, shown that type IV collagen is located in the endomysium (Duance et al, 1980; Sanes & Hall, 1979), and immunofluorescence staining of mouse muscle showed localization of type III procollagen and type IV collagen, but not of type I procollagen, in the endomysium (Krieg et al, 1979). The latter result suggests that type III collagen may be a component of the reticular network between and around the muscle fibres, whereas type IV collagen is present in the basal lamina of the fibres.

Definition of the collagen types present in the sarcolemma of the muscle fibre is clearly of great importance in light of the known requirements for an intact sarcolemma both for successful muscle regeneration (Vracko & Benditt, 1972; Bischoff, 1975), and for the transmission of tension during muscle contraction (Street & Ramsey, 1965).

Cardiac muscle and heart valves

Developmental studies

Estimates of the collagen content of the embryonic chick heart by hydroxyproline analyses have shown that before hatching there is a continual net increase in collagen content per wet weight of heart tissue (Herrmann & Barry, 1955; Woessner et al, 1967), these results suggesting that collagen must have an increasingly important structural function during cardiac development. Similar increases in collagen concentration during development have also been reported for the rabbit heart, the stages of development which were analyzed ranging from the 28-day-old fetus to 6 months after birth (Caspari et al, 1976). In this latter study the concentration of collagen per wet weight of tissue present in the right ventricle was observed to increase with age, whereas the concentration in the left ventricle remained relatively constant, so that by 6 months of age the collagen concentration of the right ventricle was twice that of the left ventricle. Similar differences in collagen content have also been reported for the right and left ventricles of the adult cat heart (Buccino et al, 1969).

Ultrastructural studies of the developing chick heart have shown that the earliest cross-banded collagen fibrils which can be recognized are present in the cardiac jelly at about stage 10 of development (approximately 35 h, 9–10 somites), and these fibrils increase in number to stage 11 (approximately 43 h, 12–13 somites; Johnson et al, 1974). Analysis of the radioactively-labelled salt-extractable collagen obtained from the hearts of organ cultures of developing embryos has suggested that the collagen which is being synthesized at these early states is predominantly type I. The synthesis of type IV collagen was not detected in this study, although basal lamina-like material already appeared to be associated with both the endocardial and myocardial surfaces. Type IV collagen is normally not extracted by neutral salt solutions, and this may explain the inability to demonstrate type IV collagen biosynthesis in this study (Clark & Kefalides, 1974). In another study, the synthesis of different collagen types was investigated in organ cultures of chick ventricle between days 3 and 19 of development (Thompson et al, 1980). Radioactively-labelled collagen was isolated after limited pepsin digestion and analysis of collagen types was performed by polyacrylamide gel electrophoresis followed by fluorography of the gels. The results showed that type I collagen was synthesized throughout development, whereas the synthesis of type III collagen occurred only at later stages of development. Collagens tentatively identified as types IV and V were also synthesized by the cultures, type IV collagen being synthesized early in development and type V collagen at later stages.

Collagen types present in cardiac muscle

Type I and type III collagens have been isolated from bovine cardiac muscle after limited pepsin digestion followed by differential salt precipitation (Wiley & McClain, 1978). No evidence was found during these experiments for significant amounts of any additional collagen types, as had been suggested in an earlier publication (McClain, 1974). Analysis of the relative proportions of the cyanogen bromide peptides α1(I)-CB8 and α1(III)-CB8 after separation of CM-cellulose chromatography and subsequent agarose gel filtration suggested that approximately 25 per cent of the soluble collagen was type III, the remainder being type I. Similar results have also been reported by Epstein & Munderloh (1975), who showed the presence of both α1(I)-CB-8 and α1(III)-CB8 after cyanogen bromide cleavage of pepsin-solubilized human myocardium.

Collagen types present in heart valves

Collagen makes up approximately 50 per cent of the dry weight of heart valves (Bashey et al, 1967) and is highly cross-linked, the major cross-link having been identified as Δ^6-dehydro-5, 5' dihydroxylysinonorleucine (Collins et al, 1977), a cross-link which is typically found in hard tissues. Collagen of heart valves is insoluble in either neutral salt or acetic acid, and an initial attempt was made to characterize the collagen types by analysing the cyanogen bromide cleavage products derived from the insoluble collagen. The results suggested that in addition to type I collagen another collagen type might also be present (Morris & McClain, 1972). Subsequent experiments analyzing the collagen solubilized after limited pepsin digestion have demonstrated the presence of both type I and type III collagens in pig (Mannschott et al, 1976; Collins et al, 1977; Denning & Pinnell, 1979) and bovine heart valve (Bashey et al, 1978), with type I collagen being in excess. Jimenez & Bashey (1978) have recently shown that the solubilization of collagen from heart valves can be greatly facilitated by prior reduction of the tissue in the cold with dithiothreitol, this result suggesting that in vivo the collagen fibrils may be closely associated with disulphide-bonded proteins which prevent attack by pepsin. Preliminary evidence has also been presented that heart valves contain collagen chains similar or identical to the chains of type V (AB) collagen (Bashey et al, 1978; Denning & Pinnell, 1979).

Gastrointestinal smooth muscle

Collagen types present

At present, very little information is available concerning the different collagen types present in gastrointestinal smooth muscle. Analyses by Epstein & Munderloh (1975) of the relative proportions of α1(I)-CB8 and α1(III)-CB8 obtained after cyanogen bromide cleavage of human small intestine collagen have demonstrated that intestinal smooth muscle contains a high proportion of the type III collagen. Recently, the chicken gizzard (the lower part of the chicken stomach having mechanical but not digestive functions) has been introduced as a source of chicken collagens (Mayne & Zettergren, 1979; Mayne & Zettergren, 1980). In addition to type I collagen, significant amounts of types III, IV and V (AB) collagens have all been isolated from this tissue after limited pepsin digestion, and it appears likely that this tissue will serve as a useful source of these collagens. The finding of significant amounts of type IV collagen in this tissue was not surprising as the tissue consists predominantly of smooth muscle cells all of which are surrounded by a basement membrane.

ABNORMAL

Muscular dystrophy

During the progression of the Duchenne type of muscular dystrophy (x-linked recessive form) marked increases can be observed in the connective tissue of both the perimysium and endomysium, until finally the muscle is almost entirely replaced by connective tissue and fat (Engel, 1977; Dubowitz, 1978). It is generally assumed that the increased connective tissue arises as a consequence of replacement fibrosis, and may in part reflect a condensation of the endomysium and perimysium (Adams, 1976). Histologically, the deposition of connective tissue can often be observed during the preclinical stages of the disease (Pearson, 1963; Cazzato, 1968). This has led to the suggestion that the defect in muscular dystrophy may be directly associated with a defect either in the connective tissue itself (Bourne & Golarz, 1959; Duance et al, 1980), or, in the microcirculation causing ischaemia and associated connective tissue proliferation (Cazzato, 1968). Isolation of polysomes from muscle extracts of patients with Duchenne muscular dystrophy and investigation of protein synthesis has shown a greater than 5-fold increase in collagen biosynthesis when compared to normal controls (Ionasescu et al, 1971), the ribosomes from dystrophic muscle presumably being derived from the greatly increased fibroblast population. Duance et al (1980) have recently examined the immunofluorescence staining of dystrophic muscle with collagen type-specific antibodies. When compared to normal controls, increased immunofluorescence for type III and type IV collagens was observed, the type IV collagen being localized to basement membranes. Whether such changes can also be observed in preclinical muscular dystrophy has not been reported.

At present a major direction of research on the Duchenne form of muscular dystrophy is towards demonstrating that the defect lies in the plasmalemma of the muscle fibre (Somer et al, 1977; Rowland, 1980), and there is some electron microscopic evidence to support this contention (Mokri & Engel, 1975; Schmalbruch, 1975). The degradation of the muscle fibre as a consequence of a plamalemmal defect might result in the stimulation and proliferation of the satellite cells (Mauro, 1961) in an attempt to regenerate the fibre. Regeneration of fibres is known to occur during the progression of muscular dystrophy (Engel, 1977), and will probably occur within the previously existing basal lamina (Vracko & Benditt, 1972). Satellite cells are known to be present in considerable numbers in the early stages of Duchenne muscular dystrophy (Wakayama et al, 1979), but it is not known if metaplasia of these cells to connective tissue fibroblasts can occur. Several studies have shown that the mononucleated progeny of chick myoblasts grown in vitro can synthesize collagen (Mayne et al, 1972; Abbott et al, 1974; Lipton, 1977), as also can the myoblasts of the L8 established rat cell line (Miranda et al, 1978). It is therefore possible that 'fibroblastic' cells may, in fact, arise from satellite cells which are no longer competent to differentiate into muscle fibres. However, experiments with both quail and rat have shown that myoblasts which have been grown and labelled with tritiated thymidine in vitro will, when injected into a muscle, pass through the basal lamina and become incorporated into myofibres (Lipton & Schultz, 1979). The labelled cells do not appear to differentiate into the fibroblast population of the muscle.

Cardiac hypertrophy

Examination of histological sections of hypertrophied cardiac muscle has often suggested that the proportion of collagen is increased. However, several studies measuring the collagen content of human hearts by hydroxyproline determinations have shown that, either with increasing age or with hypertrophy of the diseased heart, the concentration of collagen per dry weight of tissue remains relatively unchanged (Oken & Boucek, 1957; Montfort & Pérez-Tamayo, 1962; Caspari et al, 1977). Examination of hypertrophied human hearts in the scanning electron microscope has suggested the presence of a much more extensive weave of collagen fibres with many of the struts appearing thicker (Caulfield & Borg, 1979).

Experimentally, cardiac hypertrophy can be induced in laboratory animals by constriction either of the aorta or the main pulmonary artery. In a series of experiments in which the ascending aortas of rats were constricted with silver bands, increases were observed in cardiac DNA synthesis, collagen content and collagen biosynthesis (Grove et al, 1969; Skosey et al, 1972). Autoradiography of sections of hearts from constricted rats after injection of tritiated thymidine showed that DNA synthesis was confined almost entirely to the connective tissue nuclei, although occasionally a labelled myocyte nucleus was also observed (Grove et al, 1969). Similar studies on the collagen content of hearts after experimentally-induced hypertrophy were reported by Bartosova et al (1969) who constricted the descending aorta of rats and obtained an increase in the total collagen content of the heart, but with little change in the collagen concentration. In this study rats were also exposed to hypoxia for 320 days to simulate high altitude. In this condition no change occurred in heart weight, but a significant increase in collagen content was obtained. In another study, a series of experiments were performed in which spontaneously hypertensive rats were compared to normotensive rats (Lund et al, 1979). The cardiac mass of the left ventricle of the hypertensive rats was increased but without any increase in the total collagen content. The collagen concentration of the left ventricle was therefore decreased. If, however, the hypertensive rats were placed in hypoxic conditions for 42 days the collagen concentration of the left ventricle was found to increase to a level similar to normotensive rats. Aortic constriction of normotensive rats resulted in cardiomegaly, but without change in collagen concentration, as had been found previously by other groups (Grove et al, 1969; Bartosova, 1969). All of the above results contrast with the results of Buccino et al (1969), who produced right ventricular hypertrophy in cats by constriction of the pulmonary artery and found increases in both the total collagen content and the collagen concentration not only in the hypertrophic right ventricle, but also in the unstressed left ventricle.

Myocardial infarction

Very little information is available concerning the nature and origin of the collagen present in myocardial scars which form as a result of myocardial infarctions. Analyses by Epstein & Munderloh (1975) of the cyanogen bromide peptides obtained from myocardial scar collagen have demonstrated the presence of both type I and type III collagen with type I collagen in excess. (For a more detailed discussion of scars see Ch. 27).

Diseased aortic valves

A single report has appeared of analyses made on the composition of the collagen present in the mitral valves of a patient suffering from prolapse and ruptured chordae tendinae (Hammer et al, 1979). Type I collagen was present in the valves in normal quantities whereas type III collagen and type V (AB) collagen appeared to be missing, and it was suggested that these deficiencies may have contributed to the malfunctioning valve.

Ehlers-Danlos type IV

A frequent cause of death in patients with this disorder is the rupture of an artery or the wall of the intestine, and it appears that the disorder is associated with a defect in the biosynthesis, secretion or correct formation of the fibrils of type III collagen (Byers et al, 1979; Pope et al, 1975). These results suggest that type III collagen is important in maintaining the integrity of the extracellular matrix and cell-to-cell connections of smooth muscle. A detailed description of this disorder together with the other Ehlers-Danlos syndromes is given in Chapter 16.

ABNORMAL

Scleroderma

During the progression of scleroderma, the oesophagus and to a lesser extent the small and large intestines are often affected (Hughes, 1977). In general, the smooth muscle of the muscularis layers becomes replaced by fibrous tissue, this often occurring focally and resulting in difficulties both in swallowing and in the absorption of digested food from the intestines. The stomach is very rarely affected. At present, little information exists concerning the nature of the collagen which is deposited in the gastrointestinal tract. One study suggested that the proportion of type III collagen to type I collagen was increased in the oesophagus and several other tissues of a patient affected by malignant systemic scleroderma (Adam et al, 1979). (For a more extensive discussion of scleroderma especially as the disease affects the skin, see Ch. 28).

CONCLUSIONS

Although several studies have now appeared attempting to characterize the different collagen types of muscular tissues by both biochemical and immunofluorescence staining techniques, many questions still remain unanswered with regard to the functional roles of the different collagens. It is still uncertain whether the basal lamina of muscle cells contains exclusively type IV collagen, or whether it also contains some type V (AB) collagen as some authors have suggested (Duance et al, 1977; Sasse et al, 1978). The function of type V collagen in all tissues remains obscure. In muscular tissues it has been isolated in significant amounts from chicken gizzard, heart and striated muscle, as have fragments of type IV collagen (Mayne & Zettergren, 1980). Another area of uncertainty is the potential relationship between type III collagen, the reticular fibres of classical histological staining techniques and the small fibrils of 35 nm diameter which appear to insert into the basal lamina. Although this relationship has often been suggested, it has not been satisfactorily demonstrated, and if these fibrils insert into the basal lamina how is this accomplished and what are the biochemical consequences during muscular contraction? The macro-organization of collagen fibres within heart muscle has recently been re-examined by scanning electron microscopy (Caulfield & Borg, 1979; Orenstein & Bloom, 1979) but many questions remain unanswered with regard to the several interactions of the collagen fibres which have now been described, and the possible functions of these interactions in muscular contraction.

REFERENCES

Abbott J, Schiltz J, Dientsman S, Holtzer H 1974 The phenotypic complexity of myogenic clones. Proceedings of the National Academy of Sciences USA 71: 1506

Adams R D 1976 Diseases of muscle: a study in pathology. Harper and Row, New York

Adam M, Dostal C, Deyl Z 1979 Collagen heterogeneity in systemic scleroderma and other diseases. The Journal of Clinical Chemistry and Clinical Biochemistry 17: 495

Bailey A J, Shellswell G B, Duance V C 1979 Identification and change of collagen types in differentiating myoblasts and developing chick muscle. Nature 278: 67

Bairati A 1937 Struttura e proprietà fisiche del sarcolemma della fibra muscolare striata. Zeitschrift für zellforschung und mikroskopische anatomie 27: 100

Bartosova D, Chvapil M, Korecky B, Poupa O, Rakusan K, Turek Z, Vizek M 1969 The growth of the muscular and collagenous parts of the rat heart in various forms of cardiomegaly. Journal of Physiology 200: 285

Bashey R I, Torii S, Angrist A 1967 Age-related collagen and elastin content of human heart valves. Journal of Gerontology 22: 203

Bashey R I, Bashey H M, Jimenez S A 1978 Characterization of pepsin-solubilized bovine heart-valve collagen. The Biochemical Journal 173: 885

Bischoff R 1975 Regeneration of single skeletal muscle fibres in vitro. The Anatomical Record 182: 215

Borg T K, Caulfield J B 1980 Morphology of connective tissue in skeletal muscle. Tissue and Cell 12: 197

Bourne G H, Golarz M N 1959 Human muscular dystrophy as an aberration of the connective tissue. Nature 183: 1741

Buccino R A, Harris E, Spann J F, Sonnenblick E H 1969 Response of myocardial connective tissue to development of experimental hypertrophy. American Journal of Physiology 216: 425

Byers P H, Holbrook K A, McGillvray B, MacLeod P M, Lowry R B 1979 Clinical and ultrastructural heterogeneity of type IV Ehlers-Danlos syndrome. Human Genetics 47: 141

Caspari P G, Gibson K, Harris P 1976 Changes in myocardial collagen in normal development and after β blockade. In: Harris P, Bing R J, Fleckenstein A (ed) Recent advances in studies on cardiac structure and metabolism, vol 7. University Park Press, Baltimore. p 99

Caspari P G, Newcomb M, Gibson K, Harris P 1977 Collagen in the normal and hypertrophied human ventricle. Cardiovascular Research 11: 554

Caulfield J B, Borg T K 1979 The collagen network of the heart. Laboratory Investigation 40: 364

Cazzato G 1968 Considerations about a possible role played by connective tissue proliferation and vascular disturbances in the pathogenesis of progressive muscular dystrophy. European Neurology 1: 158

Clark C C, Kefalides N A 1974 Type IV collagen: a universal component of basement membranes. Developmental Biology 40: f 1

Collins D, Lindberg K, McLees B, Pinnell S 1977 The collagen of heart valve. Biochimica et Biophysica Acta 495: 129

Copenhaver W M, Kelly D E, Wood R L 1978 Bailey's textbook of histology, 17th edn. Williams and Wilkins, Baltimore

Denning S, Pinnell S R 1979 Heart valve collagen — identification of two new species. Clinical Research 27: 162A

Draper M H, Hodge A J 1949 Studies on muscle with the electron microscope. 1. The ultrastructure of toad striated muscle. Australian Journal of Experimental Biology and Medicine 27: 465

Duance V C, Restall D J, Beard H, Bourne F J, Bailey A J 1977 The location of three collagen types in skeletal muscle. FEBS Letters 79: 248

Duance V C, Stephens H R, Dunn M, Bailey A J, Dubowitz V 1980 A role for collagen in the pathogenesis of muscular dystrophy. Nature 284: 470

Dubowitz V 1978 Muscle Disorders in Childhood. Saunders, London

Enesco M, Puddy D 1964 Increase in the number of nuclei and weight in skeletal muscle of rats of various ages. American Journal of Anatomy 114: 235

Engel W K 1977 Integrative histochemical approach to the defect of Duchenne muscular dystrophy. In: Rowland L P (ed) Pathogenesis of Human Muscular Dystrophies. Excerpta Medica, Amsterdam. p 277

Epstein E H, Munderloh N H 1975 Isolation and characterization of CNBr peptides of human $[\alpha 1(III)]_3$ collagen and tissue distribution of $[\alpha 1(I)]_2\alpha 2$ and $[\alpha 1(III)]_3$ collagens. The Journal of Biological Chemistry 250: 9304

Gabella G 1976 Structural changes in smooth muscle cells during isotonic contraction. Cell and Tissue Research 170: 187

Gabella G 1977 Arrangement of smooth muscle cells and intramuscular septa in the taenia coli. Cell and Tissue Research 184: 195

Gabella G 1979 Smooth muscle cell junctions and structural aspects of contraction. British Medical Bulletin 35: 213

Gabella G, Blundell D 1979 Nexuses between the smooth muscle cells of the guinea-pig ileum. Journal of Cell Biology 82: 239

Garrels J I 1979 Changes in protein synthesis during myogenesis in a clonal cell line. Developmental Biology 73: 134

Grove D, Zak R, Nair K G, Aschenbrenner V 1969 Biochemical correlates of cardiac hypertrophy IV observations on the cellular organization of growth during myocardial hypertrophy in the rat. Circulation Research 25: 473

Hammer D, Leier C U, Baba N, Vasko J S, Wooley C F, Pinnell S R 1979 Altered collagen composition in a prolapsing mitral valve with ruptured chordae tendinae. American Journal of Medicine 67: 863

Hauschka S D, Konigsberg I R 1966 The influence of collagen on the development of muscle colonies. Proceedings of the National Academy of Sciences USA 55: 119

Hauschka S D, White N K 1971 Studies of myogenesis in vitro. In: Banker B, Przybylski R, Van der Meulen J, Victor M (ed) Research concepts in muscle development and the muscle spindle. Excerpta Medica, Amsterdam. p 53

Herrman H, Barry S R 1955 Accumulation of collagen in skeletal muscle, heart and liver of the chick embryo. Archives of Biochemistry and Biophysics 55: 526

Hughes G R V 1977 Connective tissue diseases. Blackwell Scientific, Oxford

Ionasescu V, Zellweger H, Conway T W 1971 Ribosomal protein synthesis in Duchenne muscular dystrophy. Archives of Biochemistry and Biophysics 144: 51

James T N, Sherf L 1978 Ultrastructure of the myocardium. In: Hurst J W (ed) The heart, 4th edn. McGraw-Hill, New York. ch 6, p 57

Jimenez S A, Bashey R I 1978 Solubilization of bovine heart-valve collagen. Biochemical Journal 173: 337

John H A, Lawson H 1980 The effect of different collagen types used as substrata on myogenesis in tissue culture. Cell Biology International Reports 4: 841

Johnson R C, Manasek F J, Vinson W C, Seyer J M 1974 The biochemical and ultrastructural demonstration of collagen during early heart development. Developmental Biology 36: 252

Ketley J N, Orkin R W, Martin G R 1976 Collagen in developing chick muscle in vivo and in vitro. Experimental Cell Research 99: 261

Konigsberg I 1971 Diffusion-mediated control of myoblast fusion. Developmental Biology 26: 132

Krieg T, Timpl R, Alitalo K, Kurkinen M, Vaheri A 1979 Type III procollagen is the major collagenous component produced by a continuous rhabdomyosarcoma cell line. FEBS Letters 104: 405

Langer G A 1978 The structure and function of the myocardial cell surface. American Journal of Physiology 235: H461

Lipton B H 1977 Collagen synthesis by normal and bromodeoxyuridine-modulated cells in myogenic culture. Developmental Biology 61: 153

Lipton B H, Schultz E 1979 Developmental fate of skeletal muscle satellite cells. Science 205: 1292

Lund D D, Twietmeyer A, Schmid P G, Tomanek R J 1979 Independent changes in cardiac muscle fibres and connective tissue in rats with spontaneous hypertension, aortic constriction and hypoxia. Cardiovascular Research 13: 39

Mannschott P, Herbage D, Weiss M, Buffevant C 1976 Collagen heterogeneity in pig heart valves. Biochimica et Biophysica Acta 434: 177

Mauro A 1961 Satellite cell of skeletal muscle fibres. Journal of Biophysical and Biochemical Cytology 9: 493

Mauro A, Adams W R 1961 The structure of the sarcolemma of the frog skeletal muscle fibre. Journal of Biophysical and Biochemical Cytology 10: 177

Mayne R, Abbott J, Schiltz J 1972 Studies concerning the divergence of myoblast and fibroblast precursor cells during myogenesis in vitro. Journal of Cell Biology 55: 168a

Mayne R, Zettergren J G 1979 Basement membrane-like collagenous components isolated from adult chicken gizzard. Federation Proceedings 38: 818

Mayne R, Zettergren J G 1980 Type IV collagen from chicken muscular tissues. Isolation and characterization of the pepsin-resistant fragments. Biochemistry 19: 4065

McClain P E 1973 Isolation and characterization of the cyanogen bromide peptides from the $\alpha 1$ and $\alpha 2$ chains of soluble bovine striated muscle collagen. Biochimica et Biophysica Acta 310: 469

McClain P E 1974 Characterization of cardiac muscle collagen. The Journal of Biological Chemistry 249: 2303

Miranda A F, Nette E G, Khan S, Brockbank K, Schonberg M 1978 Alteration of myoblast phenotype by dimethyl sulfoxide. Proceedings of the National Academy of Sciences 75: 3826

Mokri B, Engel A G 1975 Duchenne dystrophy: electron microscopic findings pointing to a basic or early abnormality in the plasma membrane of the muscle fibre. Neurology 25: 1111

Montfort I, Pérez-Tamayo R 1962 The muscle-collagen ratio in normal and hypertrophied human hearts. Laboratory Investigation 11: 463

Morris S C, McClain P E 1972 Heterogeneity in the cyanogen bromide peptides from striated muscle and heart valve collagen. Biochemical and Biophysical Research Communications 47: 27

Nagel A 1935 Die mechanischen eigenschaften von perimysium internum und sarkolemm bei der quergestreiften muskelfaser. Zeitschrift für zellforschung und mikroskopische anatomie 22: 694

Nowack H, Gay S, Wick G, Becker U, Timpl R 1976 Preparation and use in immunohistology of antibodies specific for type I and type III collagen and procollagen. Journal of Immunological Methods 12: 117

Oken D E, Boucek R J 1957 Quantitation of collagen in human myocardium. Circulation Research 5: 357

Orenstein J M, Bloom S 1979 Longitudinally oriented fibrils on the surface of heart muscle cells. Journal of Cell Biology 83: 61a

Pearson C M 1963 Pathology of human muscular dystrophy. In: Bourne G H, Golarz M N (eds) Muscular dystrophy in man and animals. Karger, Basel/New York. p 1

Peter J B, Fiehn W, Nagatomo T, Andiman R, Stempel K, Bowman R 1974 Studies of sarcolemma from normal and diseased skeletal muscle. In: Milhorat A T (ed) Exploratory concepts in muscular dystrophy. Excerpta Medica, Amsterdam. p 479

Pope F M, Martin G R, Lichtenstein J R, Penttinen R, Gerson B, Rowe D W, McKusick V A 1975 Patients with Ehlers-Danlos syndrome type IV lack type III collagen. Proceedings of the National Academy of Sciences USA 72: 1314

Reed R, Rudall K M 1948 Electron microscope studies of muscle structure. Biochimica et Biophysica Acta 2: 19

Richler C, Yaffe D 1970 The in vitro cultivation and differentiation capacities of myogenic cell lines. Developmental Biology 23: 1

Rowland L P 1980 Biochemistry of muscle membranes in Duchenne muscular dystrophy. Muscle and Nerve 3: 3

Sanes J R, Hall Z W 1979 Antibodies that bind specifically to synaptic sites on muscle fiber basal lamina. Journal of Cell Biology 83: 357

Sasse J, von der Mark H, Kühl U, Dessau W, von der Mark K 1981 Origin of collagen types I, III and V in cultures of avian skeletal muscle. Developmental Biology 83: 79

Schmalbruch H 1974 The sarcolemma of skeletal muscle fibers as demonstrated by a replica technique. Cell and Tissue Research 150: 377

Schmalbruch H 1975 Segmental fiber breakdown and defects of the plasmalemma in diseased human muscles. Acta Neuropathologica 33: 129

Schubert D, Tarikas H, Humphreys S, Heinemann S, Patrick J 1973 Protein synthesis and secretion in a myogenic cell line. Developmental Biology 33: 18

Shellswell G B, Bailey A J, Duance V C, Restall D J 1980 Has collagen a role in muscle pattern formation in the developing chick wing? Journal of Embryology and Experimental Morphology 60: 245

Skosey J L, Zak R, Martin A F, Aschenbrenner V, Rabinowitz M 1972 Biochemical correlates of cardiac hypertrophy V labelling of collagen, myosin and nuclear DNA during experimental myocardial hypertrophy in the rat. Circulation Research 31: 145

Somer H, Willner J, Mawatari S, Rowland L P 1977 Surface membranes of skeletal muscle. In: Rowland L P (ed) Pathogenesis of Human Muscular Dystrophies. Excerpta Medica, Amsterdam. p 547

Street S F, Ramsey R W 1965 Sarcolemma: transmitter of active tension in frog skeletal muscle. Science 149: 1379

Thompson R P, Fitzharris T P, Denslow S, LeRoy E C 1979 Collagen synthesis in the developing chick heart. Texas Reports on Biology and Medicine 39: 305

Timpl R, Glanville R W, Nowack H, Wiedemann H, Fietzek P P, Kühn K 1975 Isolation, chemical and electron microscopical characterization of neutral-salt-soluble type III collagen and procollagen from fetal bovine skin. Hoppe-Seyler's Zeitschrift für Physiologishe Chemie 356: 1783

Vracko R, Benditt E P 1972 Basal lamina: the scaffold for orderly cell replacement. Journal of Cell Biology 55: 406

Wakayama Y, Schotland D L, Bonilla E, Orecchio E 1979 Quantitative ultrastructural study of muscle satellite cells in Duchenne dystrophy. Neurology 29: 401

Wiley E R, McClain P E 1978 Isolation and characterization of type III collagen from bovine cardiac muscle. International Journal of Biochemistry 9: 139

Winegrad S, Robinson T F 1978 Force generation among cells in the relaxing heart. European Journal of Cardiology 7 (Supplement): 63

Woessner J F, Bashey R I, Boucek R J 1967 Collagen development in heart and skin of the chick embryo. Biochimica et Biophysica Acta 140: 329

Yaffe D 1968 Retention of differentiation potentialities during prolonged cultivation of myogenic cells. Proceedings of the National Academy of Sciences USA 61: 477

Zacks S I, Sheff M F, Saito A 1973a Structure and staining characteristics of myofiber external lamina. Journal of Histochemistry and Cytochemistry 21: 703

Zacks S I, Vandenburgh H, Sheff M F 1973b Cytochemical and physical properties of myofiber external lamina. Journal of Histochemistry 21: 10

26

Placenta

R. BROWN

Until recently 'placenta' was not a word which would normally have appeared in association with collagen. This is not surprising since the placenta does not have an overt supportive function, other than maintaining its own shape. Three factors though, have made it an important tissue in contemporary collagen research. In the first place, it is relatively rich in the new collagen species, type V and in basement membrane collagen, type IV. Secondly, it is one of the few readily available human tissues. Thirdly, there has been a growing interest in recent years not only in these minor, or less common, collagen species but also in the non-structural function of collagen. That collagen has functions other than purely structural is implied by the diversity of collagen types present in very small amounts, and also by the collagen-like sequences of C1q and acetylcholinesterase (Ch. 2). The physiological role of $(Gly\text{–}X\text{–}Y)_n$ polymers is yet to be established but the placenta may be a good model to study, particularly in relation to basement membrane function (Ch. 17).

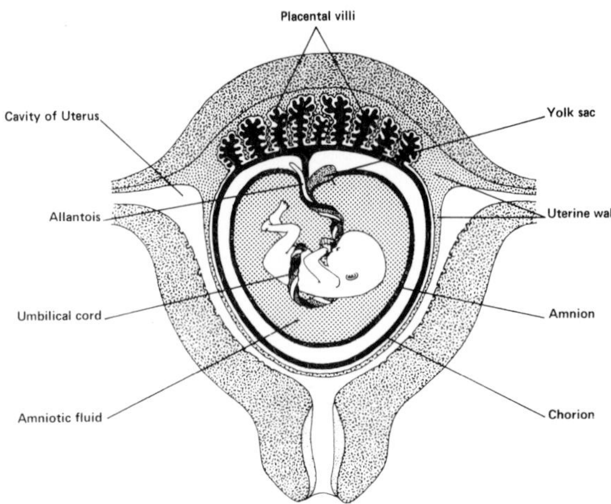

Fig. 26.1 Diagram of the human uterus and fetus showing the arrangement of the placental membranes.

PLACENTAL STRUCTURE AND COLLAGEN LOCATION

During its implantation in the uterine wall the embryo, surrounded by a chorionic membrane, becomes completely enveloped by uterine epithelium (the relationship of the fetal and uterine membranes is shown in Fig. 26.1). The chorion is thrown into folds or villi which proliferate and enlarge at one or more sites to leave the chorion and the wall of the uterus in intimate contact. The intimacy of this contact varies from species to species depending on how close the fetal tissues come to the maternal circulation. Capillaries from the allantoic sac vascularise these villi to form a functional placenta which then undergoes a gradual maturation until parturition (dealt with in detail by Jollie, 1964). There are a number of different types of placenta, classified on the basis of shape. Porcine and equine placentae are diffuse, covering the entire chorionic membrane (reviewed by Wynn, 1968, 1975a). The placenta in the ewe and cow consists of scattered tufts of villi which fit into thickened patches on the uterine wall, like fingers into a glove. In rodents, man and certain other primates the placenta is in the form of a single disc. A convenient form of classification is based on the maternal and fetal tissues which come into direct contact in the mature organ. Consequently, bovine, porcine, equine and ovine placentae are known as epitheliochorial since the chorionic membrane of the fetus comes into contact with the uterine epithelium (Wynn, 1975a; Perry et al, 1975; Steven, 1975). Rodents and primates, including man, produce the so-called haemochorial placenta where the outer cellular layer of the chorion (known as the trophoblast) is bathed by maternal blood.

Two types of placenta are considered here, the epitheliochorial and the haemochorial. The epitheliochorial form consists of villous capillaries (endothelial cells plus basement membrane) set in a connective tissue stroma and surrounded by the trophoblast. Juxtaposed to this, on the maternal side, is the uterine epithelium and stromal connective tissue which is fed by maternal capillaries. The evolution of the haemochorial placenta has eliminated all of the uterine layers from this arrangement. In this case, the fetal trophoblast is directly exposed to the maternal blood and, incidentally, the maternal immune system.

The human placenta

The structure of the human placenta has been reviewed by a number of authors (Wynn, 1975b; Fox, 1978; Wigglesworth, 1973; Thomsen & Hiersche, 1969) to whom it is worth referring for a detailed treatment of the subject.

The human placenta is a disc shaped organ reaching 15 to 20 cm in diameter at term. On the fetal side the major umbilical vessels feed into the centre and immediately branch out to the villi. The placental villi form a finely branched tree of folded chorionic membrane which invades the uterine wall at an early stage in placentation. At maturity they lie in large maternal sinuses, formed by the erosion of uterine blood vessels. The sinuses are packed with villi in such a way that the intervillous spaces are capillary-like in their dimensions (Bartels, 1970).

The trophoblast and its basement membrane

The trophoblastic layer in the mature human placenta consists of a single, continuous cell layer over the entire villous surface. Other mammals have further subdivisions of this cell layer, designated trophoblast I to III (Enders, 1965). In rats and mice the trophoblast takes the form of a continuous layer of trophoblastic giant cells. In contrast, the mature human trophoblast is a syncytium (know as the syncytiotrophoblast) formed by the breakdown of intercellular membranes. The trophoblast also contains a variable number of undifferentiated cells (Langhans cells or cytotrophoblasts Fig. 26.2) which are the precursors of the syncytiotrophoblast. During early placental development the trophoblastic layer consists entirely of cytotrophoblastic cells which later differentiate to form the syncytiotrophoblast. It is the cytotrophoblasts which are thought to produce the trophoblastic basement membrane, indeed, basement membrane thickening can accompany cytotrophoblastic hyperplasia (Fox, 1978).

In contrast to the cytotrophoblasts, the syncytium is synthetically very active (Wynn, 1975b) particularly in its thicker regions where the placental hormones are produced. Other areas of the trophoblast, known as vasculosyncytial membranes, are specialised for rapid gas exchange by having a thin layer of cytoplasm, lacking in microvilli and closely opposed to the underlying capillaries to facilitate diffusion (Fig. 26.2). Although the trophoblast is probably the most intensely studied region of the placenta its only direct relevance to placental collagen rests with the trophoblastic basement membrane. This structure supports both the syncytium and the cytotrophoblastic cells, isolating them from the underlying stroma. It is estimated to be about 100 to 300 nm thick in normal tissue (Verbeek et al, 1967) but dramatic thickening can accompany a number of diseases (Fox, 1968).

Basement membranes from other tissues such as kidney glomerulus and lens capsule are known to contain type IV collagen. This species is quite distinct from the interstitial collagen types (I, II and III) found in tendon, cartilage and skin (Miller, 1976). Glanville & Kuhn (1979) have found that antibodies to type IV collagen peptides from human placenta will bind to the basement membranes in skin and kidney glomeruli as well as placenta. It is also said that type V or AB collagen can be located by immunofluorescence in the basement membranes of a number of tissues, including the placenta (Bailey et al, 1979a; Glanville & Kuhn, 1979).

Collagen of the villous stroma

Within the villi themselves ultrastructural studies have shown the stroma to be rich in fibroblasts and the migratory Hofbauer cells. The placental fibroblast is not well investigated but comparison with other tissues would suggest that these cells are responsible for much of the turnover of interstitial stromal collagen (Kulonen & Pikkarainen, 1973). Hofbauer cells are most common in the immature placenta, normally decreasing in number after the 14th week. They are still present at maturity, particulary at the margins of lesions such as haemorrhagic infarcts and close to the trophoblastic basement membrane in diabetes (Jones & Fox, 1976b). Enders & King (1970) have suggested that these cells are in fact macrophages with large vacuolar inclusions and a high capacity for fluid uptake. If this is the case it would be tempting to speculate on their role in collagen turnover, since true macrophages can produce collagenase in culture (Wahl et al, 1975). At the ultrastructural level the stroma is rich in delicate striated fibrils of collagen. These are often matted and sometimes form a lattice (Thomsen & Hiersche, 1969). Since type IV collagen does not form striated fibrils these are presumably fibrils of types I and III collagen, both of which have been found in pepsin extracts of placenta. The only direct evidence for this, though, is the immunofluorescent studies of Faulk & Johnson (1977) and Johnson & Faulk (1978) on sections of human placenta. They found that the stroma of early (11 to 14 weeks) and mature placentae gave a strong reaction to a type I collagen antibody.

Collagen associated with the villous capillaries

The final component of the 'placental barrier' is the endothelial cell layer which will be considered as one unit with its basement membrane. The villous capillary is effectively an endothelial cell tube whose cells have tight overlapping junctions and rest on a basement membrane. Other cells such as pericytes are often associated with larger vessels, though their function is uncertain and structural modifications, such as fenestrae or pores in the endothelial cells have been reported (Jollie, 1964). Cultured endothelial cells and their capacity for collagen synthesis have recently become the subject of considerable interest (Ch. 20). However, it must be appreciated that endothelial cells are

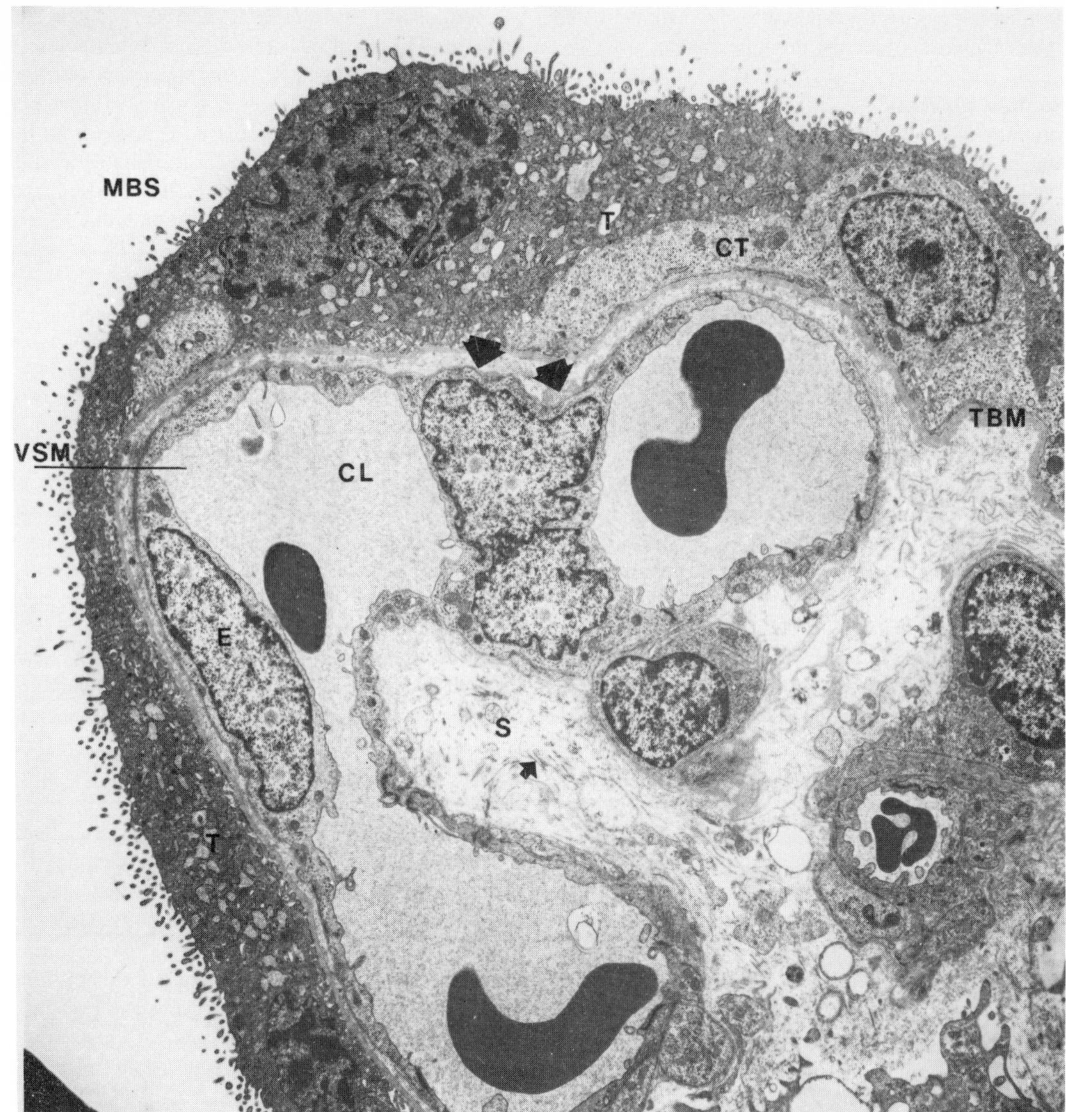

Fig. 26.2 Electron micrograph of a mature human placental villous (× 6250). Maternal blood system (MBS). Syncytiotrophoblast (T). Cytotrophoblast (CT). Trophoblastic basement membrane (TBM). Stroma (S). Capillary lumen (CL). Endothelial cell (E). Vasculo-syncytial membrane (VSM). Collagen fibrils (small arrow). Capillary basement membrane (large arrows). (Courtesy of Dr C.J.P. Jones, Hope Hospital, Salford, U.K.)

normally cultured from major blood vessels such as the aorta and umbilical vein. True capillary endothelial cells are not yet sufficiently well characterised to permit a comparison of their collagen synthesising capability with that of large vessel endothelial cells (Phillips et al, 1979). Sage et al (1979a) found that aortic endothelial cells secrete both fibronectin and type III procollagen into the culture medium. However only 3 per cent of the total protein in the medium was collagenous. The cell layer contained an even smaller amount, comprising 0.25 per cent of the total protein which was identified as types III, IV and V (or AB) collagen after pepsin digestion. Unfortunately, the site of accumulation in the placenta of this endothelial cell derived collagen is unknown. Other groups have reported the production of collagen by large vessel endothelial cells but not all have found the same species of collagen (Barnes et al, 1978; Howard et al, 1976; Mayne & Mayne, 1978) possibly due to variations in cell type or to their behaviour in vitro (McAuslan & Reilly, 1979; Sage et al, 1979a).

Damage to placental blood vessels could expose underlying structures to circulating platelets, possibly leading to aggregation and thrombus formation. The likelihood of this seems to depend on the collagen types exposed to the circulation. Type IV, in basement membrane, is said to have no platelet aggregating activity (Trelstad & Carvalho, 1979) but there is some disagreement over the effectiveness of type V collagen (Balleisen et al, 1979; Trelstad & Carvalho, 1979, see also Ch. 10). On the other hand, it is generally agreed that interstitial collagens are potent aggregating agents. It may be, then, that the basement membrane, rich in type IV collagen, forms the last barrier between circulating platelets and the interstitial stromal collagens. Breakdown of this barrier may contribute, for example, to fetal artery thrombosis in which the group of placental villi fed by the blocked vessel become avascular (Fox, 1978). Such a condition, however, rarely affects a large enough proportion of the villi to have any serious functional effect. It is thought that the vascular basement membrane is secreted once during the life of the endothelial cell and is subsequently maintained as a scaffolding for capillary support (Vracko & Benditt, 1970; Vracko, 1974). In certain conditions (e.g. diabetes) capillaries become surrounded by multiple layers of lamellae of basement membrane. It seems from experimental models, that these lamellae are formed by successive waves of endothelial cell replacement. Each wave lays down its own basement membrane, sometimes trapping cell debris between the lamellae. In some cases the endothelial cell layer is removed completely leaving an acellular tube of basement membrane which is eventually re-populated by new endothelial cells. This may give rise to the thickened basement membranes seen in some placentae and in diabetes mellitus as the new population of endothelial cells deposit a fresh layer of basement membrane. Structures known as vasculosyncytial membranes, found in the mature placental villi, are essential for the rapid gas exchange necessary as the fetus reaches term. In the human placenta at this stage dilated villous capillaries come to lie close to the trophoblastic basement membrane, effectively eliminating the stroma from the pathway for exchange. In addition, the syncytiotrophoblast becomes very thin in these regions leaving only a narrow band of syncytial cytoplasm, two basement membranes and the attenuated capillary endothelium separating the two circulations. On morphological grounds vasculosyncytial membranes probably contain an unusually high proportion of basement membrane in relation to cellular material and stroma (Fig. 26.2).

The parietal yolk sac as a model for placental basement membrane function

During the first 10 days of development, in rodents, the fetus is supplied with nutrients entirely by exchange across a yolk sac placenta. At maturity it consists of a layer of trophoblastic giant cells and an incomplete layer of yolk sac epithelium separated by an unusually thick basement membrane; Reichert's membrane. Reichert's membrane reaches a thickness of 7 μm after 10 to 12 days and so its formation clearly requires a considerable synthetic output. In culture, the rat parietal yolk sac Reichert's membrane is synthesised by the parietal endodern, the trophoblast making no apparent contribution (Pierce, 1970; Clark et al, 1975). About 10 per cent of the total protein secreted by these cells is collagen which becomes incorporated into the Reichert's membrane.

In mice the yolk sac epithelial cells do not form a continuous layer but move over the surface of the Reichert's membrane, laying down more basement membrane as they go. There may be a connection between this migration and the suggestion that type V collagen secretion accompanies epithelial cell migration (Stenn et al, 1979) since type V collagen is said to occur in some basement membranes (Bailey et al, 1979a). Working on parietal endoderm cells, Priest (1970) has pointed out that some clinical features of scurvy are consistent with a basement membrane lesion, particularly those associated with the vascular network. He found that these cells, in culture, produce less collagen and less total basement membrane in the absence of ascorbate. The mechanism seems to be related to the requirement of ascorbate by prolylhydroxylase (Prockop et al, 1976). In interstitial collagens a reduction in the level of prolyl hydroxylation results in an inhibition of their secretion. On the other hand, Maragoudakis et al (1978) have found that type IV collagen from parietal yolk sac endoderm cells is still secreted normally even with very low levels of hydroxylation. This underhydroxylated collagen does not get incorporated into the Reichert's membrane, though, probably because it is more susceptible to endogenous proteases than normally hydroxylated type IV collagen.

Placental basement membranes may be particularly at risk during vitamin C deficiency because of the heavy requirements for collagen synthesis imposed by the growing fetus. An analogous situation seems to exist in patients with rheumatoid arthritis. In this case rapid and prolonged connective tissue turnover can contribute to a subclinical ascorbate deficiency (Weiss, personal communication). Another possibility, suggested by Wideman et al (1964), is that ascorbate deficiency may contribute to the premature rupture of fetal membranes, probably by interfering with collagen synthesis. Indeed, ascorbate seems to be an important metabolite to the fetus as it is actively removed from the maternal circulation by the placenta (Hensliegh & Krantz, 1966).

Collagen produced by amniotic fluid cells

Two forms of cell are extracted with human amniotic fluid. They have different characteristics in culture and different patterns of collagen synthesis, resembling in one case fibroblasts and in the other endothelial or epithelial cells (Priest, 1977). Endothelial cells, cultured from amniotic fluid produce a type IV-like procollagen, rich in 3-hydroxyproline (Crouch & Bornstein, 1979; Crouch et al,

1980). The presence of this isomer of hydroxyproline is interesting since it is typical of type IV collagen from many sources but not, apparently, the placenta (Sage et al, 1979b). Apart from the value of a cell culture source of type IV collagen, Priest (1977) has suggested that amniotic fluid fibroblasts may prove useful in the early detection of inherited diseases of collagen such as Marfan syndrome.

THE PLACENTA AS A SOURCE OF COLLAGENS

Types I and III are the major constituents

It is worth pointing out that the bulk of the extractable placental collagen is interstitial, types I and III, despite the current use of placenta as a source of basement membrane-like collagens. Hong et al (1979) have reported that 58 per cent of the pepsin soluble collagen from bovine amnion precipitates at the same concentration of NaCl as type III collagen. This figure assumes that the species are adequately separated by differential salt precipitation but Ayad et al (in preparation) have found a similar amount (Table 26.1). They have also confirmed the identity of the precipitate by polyacrylamide gel electrophoresis. In the amnion and chorion membranes and in the placenta itself there is twice as much type III as type I. Hong et al (1979) found that 5 per cent of the amnion collagen was 'type VI' (this is a rarely used term for type V or AB collagen). Again, it is comparable with the value of 8 per cent obtained by Ayad et al. Indeed, the amnion seems to be the richest source of type V collagen yet described. These membranes do not seem to be particularly rich in type IV collagen relative to the other collagen types.

Most of the interstitial collagen is likely to come from the stroma in the case of the placenta and presumably plays an important role in the structural integrity of the organ. The reason for the large quantity of type III collagen is unknown. It may be that this is simply a function of all fetal tissues since the type III content of other fetal material is thought to be high in relation to that of the adult (Miller, 1976). On the other hand, the placenta is a grossly vascular organ and type III collagen has been associated with blood vessels. Both of these suggestions are rather vague and reflect the current inadequate understanding of the function of type III collagen. An important feature of most studies on placental collagen is that they start with a pepsin digestion of the tissue homogenate. However, the application of this technique needs a critical assessment. For example, it has been known for some time that animal collagens are far more susceptible than aged human collagens to proteolytic depolymerisation (Steven, 1966). The conditions of proteolysis (enzyme: substrate ratio; temperature; duration) can also affect the degree of type I collagen solubilisation (Weiss, 1976) and the fragmentation of pepsin sensitive type IV collagen (Glanville et al, 1979; Schuppan et al, 1980). Finally the use of certain extraction procedures such as extensive soaking of the homogenates in distilled water 1–2 days (Burgeson et al, 1976), neutral saline (Bailey et al 1979) and dilute acetic acid could allow endogenous proteases to modify the collagen peptides.

The pattern of reducible collagen cross-links found in the placenta is consistent with other tissues and similar to the uterus (Kao & Leslie, 1979). The number of cross-links rises steadily until the second trimester, presumably as new collagen is synthesised, and then decreases until term, as they mature. Substantial proportions of the two main forms of cross-link, dehydrodihydroxylysinonorleucine and dehydrohydroxlysinonorleucine, are present in the glycosylated form. In both cases they were found to contain the disaccharide glucosyl-galactose, supporting the view that basement membrane type IV collagen, rich in these residues, can participate in lysine derived cross-links (Tanzer & Kefalides, 1973).

Placental type IV: similarities to other basement membrane collagens

Human placental tissue was the first source, other than tissues consisting virtually entirely of basement membrane (lens capsule and glomerulus), from which type IV collagen was isolated. The type IV collagens described from the placenta have been identified largely on the basis of comparison with type IV from other sources (for a detailed

Table 26.1 The relative proportions of collagen species in pepsin extracts of foetal bovine membranes. 60% of the tissue hydroxyproline was solubilised after 48 hr pepsin digestion at 18°C. The collagen precipitates at various salt concentrations were checked by SDS polyacrylamide gel electrophoresis and quantitated (Woessner, 1961) by hydroxyproline estimation (Ayad, Abedin, Shuttleworth and Weiss in preparation).

Tissue	*% Type I*	*% Type III*	*% Type IV*	*% Type V*	*% 'cysteine-rich' aggregated fraction*
Amnion	27.8	59.6	2.6	7.9	2.1
Chorion	28.1	66.2	1.1	4.0	0.6
Placental villi	29.8	58.6	4.8	4.5	2.3

examination of basement membrane collagen in general the reader is referred to Chapter 17. For example, antobodies raised to placental type IV collagen bind to the basement membranes of cornea, lens capsule, glomerulus and skin (Glanville et al, 1979; Glanville & Kuhn, 1979) and show cross-reactivity with bovine lens capsule αI (IV) chain (Timpl et al 1979).

The limited sensitivity of type IV collagen to peptic cleavage is now well documented and is due to the presence of short discontinuities in the repeating sequence -gly–X–Y– of the triple helix. (Schuppa et al 1980; Schwartz & Veis 1978). Progressively longer pepsin digestion or treatment with higher enzyme: substrate ratios increases the yield of low molecular weight type IV peptides at the expense of the high molecular weight components. This effect is even more noticeable when disulphide bonds are broken in the digestion products by reduction and alkylation. These treatments frequently yield peptides well below 95K molecular weight, which is the αchain size of interstitial collagens corresponding to the pepsin resistant triple helix. Kresina & Miller (1979) have reported a similar phenomena using human placenta. They found that the peptides of about 50K were increased in proportion to the larger fragments after a second pepsin digestion. They conclude that the 50K peptides are a heterogeneous collection of degraded fragments from larger molecules or aggregates.

Four groups have recently reported the presence of a number of basement membrane-like collagen peptides from human placenta. (Glanville et al, 1979b; Bailey et al, 1979b; Kresina & Miller, 1979; Sage et al, 1979b).

The two predominant components in pepsin digests of type IV collagen from placenta both have a molecular weight of approximately 100K. Additional minor components are either derived from, or are precursors of, these two chains. Table 26.2 shows the relationship between the nomenclature and size of fragments derived from placental type IV collagen as quoted by various laboratories. The two types of chain are now designated 1(IV) and 2(IV) (Ch. 17) and can be separated on CM cellulose (Kresina & Miller, 1979).

In almost all reports, α_1(IV) chain components are more acidic and contain more hydroxylysine, serine, glutamic acid and valine but less arginine, threonine, alanine, isoleucine and phenylalanine than α_2(IV) chains. It is particularly interesting that placental type IV peptides do not seem to have the high proportion of 3-hydroxyproline found in collagen from other tissue sources. 3-hydroxyproline, then, may not be a good marker for placental basement membrane collagen. The α_1(IV) chain contains no $\frac{1}{2}$-cystine residues whereas the α_2(IV) chain contains one disulphide bond which on reduction gives rise to a 70K fragment as well as smaller fragments (15 to 25K).

Most of the reports of basement membrane-like placental collagens are in general agreement, though molecular weight estimates of the fragments are somewhat variable. The variability seems to be due to the anomalous behaviour of these highly hydroxylated and glycosylated peptides on gel filtration and electrophoresis. Variations in the conditions of pepsin digestion may also contribute by allowing cleavage at different positions within pepsin sensitive regions. This possibility is supported by the work of Glanville et al (1979) who found no $\frac{1}{2}$-cystine in their α_1(IV) and α_2(IV) chains, and an extra peptide (αI ^{11}(IV)) which was barely separable from their α_1(IV) chain. They used a sequential extraction involving

1. Pepsin digestion
2. Reduction and alkylation
3. Pepsin digestion

and may have exposed new sites to proteolysis after the cleavage of disulphide links.

A new basement membrane-like component has recently been described from pepsin extracts of human placenta. This appears to be a high molecular weight aggregate (HMW) which remains soluble under conditions which precipitate type IV collagen (Furoto & Miller, 1980), It has a molecular weight of over 300K when extracted but on reduction and alkylation it releases 3 major subunits of molecular weights 55K, 45K and 35K (Jander et al, 1981; Abedin et al, 1981). Furoto and Miller have isolated a number of basic and acidic peptides from the 40K fraction which are rich in cysteine. This high molecular weight

Table 26.2 Type IV collagen fragments from peptin digests of human placental villi

Parent chain	Bailey et al (1979b)	Glanville et al (1979b)	Kresina & Miller (1979)	Sage et al (1976b)
	170K			
			C^1	140K
α1(IV) (acidic)	100K	α(IV), α^{11}(IV)	C	100K 70K–I
			50K	
			D	
α2(IV) (basic)	70K	α^1(IV)	80K $50K_2$	70K–II

aggregate makes up the bulk of the 'cysteine rich' aggregate quoted in Table 26.1 for the amnion and chorion. However in the case of the placental villi, it is only approximately 50 per cent of this fraction, the remainder being another cysteine rich colalgen; 7S collagen which is thought to be a linkage protein for type IV procollagen molecule (Kuhn et al, 1981). Both these aggregates are collagenous in nature, although the HMW aggregate has less than one third glycine (see Ch. 1).

Type V collagen

The new collagen species, known as type V or AB collagen has been isolated from fetal membranes and placenta (the term AB collagen comes from the two chains: αA and αB). These two collagen chains are now known as α2(V) and α1(V) respectively (See Chap. 1). The fact that placenta was an early source of this collagen has lead to the fallacious impression that there is a special connection between type V collagen and the placenta. In fact, type V collagen is an ubiquitous species found in skin (Chung et al, 1978), lung (Madri et al, 1979) embryonic tendon (Jiminez et al, 1978) and synovial membrane (Brown et al, 1978). The strong association with the placenta has encouraged the belief that it is a form of basement membrane collagen but this now seems unlikely. The chain composition of type V collagen is also unresolved. A number of early reports using fetal membrane and placental type V estimated A and B chains to be in the ratio of 1:2 which lead to the widely quoted suggestion of an $(\alpha B)_2$ αA triple helix. Glanville et al (1978) presented evidence supporting this model, based on renaturation studies of the '$(\alpha B)_2$ αA' molecule. Rhodes & Millar (1978), however, suggested the homogenous chain content of $(\alpha A)_3$ and $(\alpha B)_3$ and supported their argument with evidence that these two molecules have different thermal denaturation points. They and other groups found much more variable A:B chain ratios, particularly in tissues other than placenta (Jiminez et al, 1978; Brown et al, 1978).

Recently, a related chain, αC(α3(V)), has been identified in synovial membrane, skin and placental villi (Brown et al 1978, Ayad et al, 1980; Sage & Bornstein, 1979), though not in the amnion and chorion. The relationship of αC to type V collagen is unknown. More recent studies have indicated that in fact the uterus is a richer source of α3(V) collagen chain than placental villi (Abedin et al, 1981). As in the case of type IV only small amounts of AB collagen are extractable from placenta. Sage & Bornstein (1979) found 6.5 per cent in pepsin extracts of human amnion and chorion but only 2 per cent in the placenta. Similarly, bovine amnion contains 5 to 8 per cent type V collagen though the placenta itself has much less (Hong et al, 1979; Ayad et al, 1980).

Placental type V collagen is made up of three separable chains αA, αB and αC. αA migrates on SDS polyacrylamide gel electrophoresis, slightly slower than α1(I) but can be distinguished from it since only αA gives a positive periodic acid Schiffs reaction indicating a high level of glycosylation (types I, II, III collagen chains do not give the periodic acid Schiffs reaction) αB, which is also PAS positive and contains twice as much hydroxylysine as αA, has a much lower electrophoretic mobility. In the case of bovine αB almost 75 per cent of the hydroxylysine residues carry the disaccharide, galactosyl-glucose (Hong et al, 1979). Indeed, it may be its characteristically high level of hydroxylation and glycosylation which make it easily separable from αA on SDS polyacrylamide gel electrophoresis. This separation is not a simple function of the relative molecular weights since cyanogen bromide peptide analysis of αB (Rhodes & Miller, 1979) suggests that it has a similar number of amino acids to interstitial α1 chains. Alternatively, it may be that the large hydrophobic amino acid residues, which are more common in the αB chain, contribute to its slower electrophoretic mobility. Neither chain contains any $\frac{1}{2}$-cystine, though the alanine content is consistently lower than interstitial collagens. The αC chain has a slightly higher electrophoretic mobility than αB and has been separated from the other two chains by ion-exchange chromatography (Sage & Bornstein, 1979). Its amino acid and carbohydrate compositions are similar to αB. The native type V molecule is not substantially degraded by mammalian collagenase (Sage & Bornstein, 1979; Hong et al, 1979). The location and function of this relatively minor component are largely a matter of speculation at present, though Stenn et al (1979) have suggested that it is produced by, and is necessary for, epithelial cell migration.

Placental pathology — does collagen have a significant role?
A general account of placental pathology is outside the scope of this chapter but has been covered in detail elsewhere (Robertson & Dixon, 1969; Fox, 1976; Fox, 1978). It is a difficult topic since morphological pathology is not easily related to functional impairment of the organ. The modern approach takes a broader view of fetomaternal blood flow and exchange and the factors affecting it. It is now thought that the large reserve of capacity for exchange which the placenta enjoys makes it rare for the fetus to suffer any real distress from this quarter (Fox, 1978).

Collagen is involved in placental abnormality in two ways; basement membrane thickening and fibrosis of the stroma.

Fibrosis of the villous stroma is a common abnormality. Collagen deposition in the villous stroma has been identified as early as the second month of gestation. After this it increases until midterm when it remains constant until parturition. Fibrosis of the stroma is easily identified histologically and occurs to some extent in all placentae. It is also found in association with a number of other conditions. Perivillous fibrin deposition, a common lesion with no apparent clinical significance, can result in extensive fibrosis. There is also an association with congenital syphilis, maternal diabetes and pre-eclampsia.

Fox (1978) has suggested that fibrosis results from a reduction in villous blood flow. Examples are seen following fetal death and fetal artery thrombosis. It is difficult to envisage a mechanism by which a reduced oxygen tension could account for this. On the contrary, limiting levels of oxygen can decrease the rate of collagen secretion by fibroblasts (Prockop et al, 1976). It is possible that a build up of steroid hormones resulting from a decreased perfusion, could stimulate collagen secretion (Fox, 1978) or suppress collagenolysis. Villous fibrosis, then, has the appearance of a secondary phenomena of debatable importance to the fetal well-being.

Thickening of the basement membrane. The trophoblastic basement membrane is first visible after six weeks gestation and increases in thickness until term. Some thickening is present in many functionally normal placentae (Fox, 1968) but unusually large affected areas are seen in some conditions. As in the case of fibrosis, increased thickening is associated with fetal hypoxia and intrauterine death. Consequently, it is possible to view this condition as a by-product of the repair process following hypoxic damage to the syncytium. By analogy with the model of Vracko (see p. 459) for basement membrane deposition, the proliferation of cytotrophoblastic cells in response to syncytial damage is likely to lead to thickening, each new cell secreting its own complement of basement membrane.

Basement membrane thickening is also associated with rhesus incompatibility, hypertension, pre-eclampsia and maternal diabetes though the mechanism is still uncertain. The focal thickening seen in diabetes is accompanied by granular inclusions and fine filaments (Jones & Fox, 1976a and b). There is however, no evidence for the deposition of immune complexes in this condition. Endothelial cell basement membrane is, in the main, unaffected.

Again it seems that this abnormality is best explained as a secondary effect. Although it does serve to increase the distance between the two circulations, this is of questionable significance compared with the initial insult which precipitated the thickening.

Future developments in the understanding of placental collagen will doubtless include a description of th structure and function of placental types IV and V collagen. In addition, the turnover of collagen in the placenta and fetal membranes may provoke some interest. For example, a potent inhibitor of mammalian collagenase and certain other metalloproteinases has been isolated from amniotic fluid (Murphy et al, 1981). On the other hand $\alpha2$ macroglobulin is absent from amniotic fluid and the total protease inhibitor activity (chiefly $\alpha1$ antitrypsin) is only 9 per cent of the maternal serum level (Bhat & Pattabiramen, 1980). There is still a great deal to explain in the interplay of collagenolytic enzymes, their inhibitors and hormones from the uterus and placenta during the development of the placenta. A number of the effects of hormones on collagenolytic enzymes have already been investigated in the uterus and cervix where there is good evidence for hormonal control of connective tissue turnover (Ch. 3 and Ellwood, 1980).

SUMMARY

With the single exception of type II, all of the known species of collagen can be extracted from human placenta. The most common types are III and I respectively, probably located in the villous stroma. Two basement membranes are found in the placental villi, one associated with the trophoblast the other with the villous capillaries. Both seem to contain type IV collagen similar to that found in other basement membranes in the body. The parietal yolk sac, a form of rodent placenta which can be grown in culture, has been used as a model for basement membrane function and secretion. Type V collagen is present in placenta but its function and location are uncertain. Connective tissue abnormalities include fibrosis and basement membrane thickening but these seem to have little functional significance.

ACKNOWLEDGEMENT

I am grateful to Drs Carolyn Jones, Shirley Ayad and Mohamed Abedin for their helpful criticism and to Dr Carolyn Jones for her electron micrographs.

REFERENCES

Abedin M Z, Ayad S, Weiss J B 1981 Type V collagen: The presence of appreciable amounts of $\alpha3$(V) chains in bovine uterus. Biochemical and Biophysical Research Communications 102: 1237

Ayad S, Abedin M Z, Weiss J B 1980 Non basement membrane collagen A, B and C α-chains: Type V and VI collagen? Biochemical Society Transactions 8: 324-5

Bailey A J, Duance V C, Sims T J, Beard H K 1979a Immunofluorescent localisation of basement membrane in skeletal muscle and placenta and preliminary characterisation of basement membrane in some other tissues. Frontiers in Matrix Biology 7: 49

Bailey A J, Sims T J, Duance V C, Light N D 1979b Partial characterisation of a second basement membrane collagen in human placenta. FEBS letters 99: 361

Balleisen L, Nowack H, Gay S, Timpl R 1979 Inhibition of collagen induced platelet aggregation by antibodies to distinct types of collagens. Biochemical Journal 184: 683

Barnes M J, Morton L F, Levene C I 1978 Synthesis of interstitial collagens by pig aortic endothelial cells in culture. Biochemical and Biophysical Research Communications 84: 646

Bartels H 1970 Prenatal respiration. Frontiers of biology 17. North Holland Research Monographs

Brentz M, Bachinger H P, Glanville R, Kuhn K 1978 Physical evidence for the assembly of A and B chains of human placental collagen in a single triple helix. European Journal of Biochemistry 92: 563

Bhat A R, Pattabiraman T N 1980 Comparative study of proteinase inhibitors in amniotic fluid and maternal serum. British Journal of Obstetrics and Gynaecology 87: 1109

Brown R A, Shuttleworth C A, Weiss J B 1978 Three new alpha chains of collagen from a non-basement membrane source. Biochemical and Biophysical Research Communications 80: 866

Burgeson R E, Adli F A, Kaitila I I, Hollister D W 1976 Fetal membrane collagens: identification of two new collagen alpha chains. Proceedings of the National Academy of Science U.S.A. 73: 2579

Chung E, Rhodes R K, Miller E J 1976 Isolation of three collagenous components of probable basement membrane origin from several tissues. Biochemical and Biophysical Research Communications 71: 1167

Clark C C, Tomichek E A, Koszalua T R, Minor R R, Kefalides N A 1975 The embryonic rat parietal yolk sac. Journal of Biological Chemistry 250: 5259

Crouch E, Bornstein P 1979 Characterisation of a type IV procollagen synthesised by human amniotic fluid cells in culture. Journal of Biological Chemistry 254: 4197

Crouch E, Sage H, Bornstein P 1980 Structural basis for apparent heterogeneity of collagens in human basement membranes: type IV procollagen contains two distinct chains. Proceedings of the National Academy of Science U.S.A. 77: 745

Dehm P, Kefalides N 1978 The collagenous component of lens basement membrane. Journal of Biological Chemistry 253: 6680

Dixit S N, Kang A H 1979 Anterior lens capsule collagens: Cyanogen bromide peptides of the C chain. Biochemistry 18: 5686

Ellwood D A 1980 The hormonal control of connective-tissue changes in the uterine cervix in pregnancy and at parturition. Biochemical Society Transactions 8: 662

Enders A C 1965 A comparative study of the fine structure of the trophoblast in several haemochorial placentae. American Journal of Anatomy 116: 29

Enders A C, King B F 1970 The cytology of Hofbauer cells. Anatomical Record 167: 231

Farquhar M G, Wissig S L, Palade G E 1961 Ferritin transfer across the normal glomerular capillary wall. Journal of Experimental Medicine 113: 47

Faulk W P, Johnson P M 1977 Immunological studies of human placentae: identification and distribution of proteins in mature villi. Clinical and Experimental Immunology 27: 365

Fox H 1968 Basement membrane changes in the villi of the human placenta. Journal of Obstetrics and Gynaecology of the British Commonwealth 75: 302

Fox H 1976 The histopathology of placental insufficiency. Journal of Clinical Pathology 29: supplement (Royal College of Pathologists) 10: 1

Fox H 1978 Pathology of the placenta. W B Saunders, London

Furoto D K, Miller E J 1980 Isolation of a unique collagenous fraction from limited pepsin digests of human placental tissue. Journal of Biological Chemistry 255: 290

Glanville R W, Kuhn K 1979a Preparation of two basement membranes from human placenta. Frontiers in Matrix Biology 7: 19

Glanville R W, Rauter A, Fietzek P P 1979b Isolation and characterisation of a native placental basement membrane collagen and its component alpha chains. European Journal of Biochemistry 95: 383

Heathcote J G, Sear C H J, Grant M E 1978 Studies on the assembly of the rat lens capsule. Biochemical Journal 176: 283

Hensleigh P A, Krantz K E 1966 Placental transfer of ascorbic acid. American Journal of Obstetrics and Gynaecology 96: 5

Hong B S, Davison P F, Cannon D J 1979 Isolation and characterisation of a distinct type of collagen from bovine foetal membranes and other tissues. Biochemistry 18: 4278

Howard B V, Macarak E J, Gunson D, Kefalides N 1976 Characterisation of the collagen synthesised by endothelial cells in culture. Proceedings of the National Academy of Science U.S.A. 73: 2361

Jander R, Rauterberg J, Voss B, Von Bassewitz D B 1981 A cysteine-rich collagenous protein from bovine placenta. Isolation of its constituent polypeptide chains and some properties of the non denatured protein. European Journal of Biochemistry 114: 17-25

Jiminez S A, Yankowski R, Bashey R I 1978 Identification of two new collagen alpha chains in extracts of lathyritic chick embryo tendons. Biochemical and Biophysical Research Communications 81: 1298

Johnson P M, Faulk W P 1978 Immunological studies of human placentae: Identification and distribution of proteins in immature chorionic villi. Immunology 34: 1027

Jollie W P 1964 Fine structural changes in placental labyrinth of the rat with increasing gestational age. Journal of Ultrastructural Research 10: 27

Jollie W P 1968 Fine structural changes of the rat parietal yolk sac with increasing age. American Journal of Anatomy 122: 513

Jones C J P, Fox H 1976a Placental changes in gestational diabetes. Obstetrics and Gynaecology 48: 274

Jones C J P, Fox H 1976b An ultra-structural and ultrahistochemical study of the placenta of the diabetic woman. Journal of Pathology 119: 91

Kao K T, Leslie J G 1979 Intermolecular cross-links in collagen of human placenta. Biochimica et Biophysica Acta 580: 366

Kefalides N A 1972 Isolation and characterisation of cyanogen bromide peptides from basement membrane collagen. Biochemical and Biophysical Research Communications 47: 1151

King B F 1972 The permiability of the guinea pig parietal yolk sac placenta to peroxidase and ferritin. American Journal of Anatomy 134: 365

Kresina T F, Miller E J 1979 Isolation and characterisation of basement membrane collagen from human placental tissue. Evidence for the presence of two genetically distinct collagen chains. Biochemistry 18: 3089

Kuhn K, Wiederman H, Timpl R, Ristelli J, Dieringer H, Voss T and Glanville R W 1981 Macromolecular structure of basement membrane collagens. Identification of 7S collagen as a cross-linking domain of 7S collagen. FEBS Letters 125: 123-8

Kulonen E, Pikkarainen J (eds) 1973 Biology of fibroblast. Academic Press, London

Madri J A, Furthmayer H 1979 Isolation and tissue localisation of type AB_2 collagen from normal lung parenchyma. American Journal of Pathology 94: 323

Maragoudakis M E, Kalinsky H J, Wasvary J 1978 Secretion without deposition of underhydroxylated basement membrane collagen by parietal yolk sacs. Biochimica et Biophysica Acta 538: 139

Mayne R, Mayne P M 1978 Characterisation of the collagenous components synthesised by cultured endothelial cells derived from pig thoracic aorta. Journal of Cell Biology 79: 147a

McAuslan B R, Reilly W 1979 A variant vascular endothelial cell line with altered growth characteristics. Journal of Cellular Physiology 101: 419

Miller E J 1976 Biochemical characteristics and biological significance of the genetically distinct collagens. Molecular and Cell Biochemistry 13: 165

Murphy G, Cawston T E, Reynolds J J 1981 An inhibitor of collagenase from human amniotic fluid. Biochemical Journal 195: 167

Perry J S, Heap R B, Ackland N 1975 The ultrastructure of the sheep placenta around the time of parturition. Journal of Anatomy 120: 561

Phillips P, Kumar P, Kumar S, Waghe M 1979 Isolation and characterisation of endothelial cells from rat and cow brain white matter. Journal of Anatomy 129: 261

Pierce G B 1970 Epithelial basement membrane: origin development and role in disease. In: Balazs E A (ed) Chemistry and molecular biology of the intercellular matrix, vol I. Academic Press, London, p 471

Priest R E 1970 Formation of epithelial basement membrane is restricted by scurvy in vitro and is stimulated by vitamin C. Nature 225: 744

Priest R E, Priest J H, Moinuddin J F, Keyser A J 1977 Differentiation in human amniotic fluid cell cultures I. Collagen Production. Journal of Medical Genetics 14: 157

Prockop D W, Berg R A, Kivirikko K I, Uitto J 1976 Intracellular steps in the biosynthesis of collagen In: Ramachandran G N, Reddi A H (eds) Biology of collagen. Plenum Press, New York, ch 5, p 163

Rhodes R K, Miller E J 1978 Physiochemical characterisation and molecular organisation of the collagen A and B chains. Biochemistry 17: 3442

Rhodes R K, Miller E J 1979 The isolation and characterisation of the cyanogen bromide peptides from the B chain of human collagen. Journal of Biological Chemistry 254: 12084

Robertson W B, Dixon H G 1969 Utero-placental pathology In: Klopper A, Diczfalusy E (eds) Fetus and placenta. Blackwell Scientific, Oxford, ch 2, p 33

Sage H, Bornstein P 1979a Characterisation of a novel collagen chain in human placenta and its relation to AB collagen. Biochemistry 18: 3815

Sage H, Crouch E, Bornstein P 1979a Collagen biosynthesis by bovine aotic endothelial cells in culture. Biochemistry 24: 5433

Sage H, Woodbury R G, Bornstein P 1979b Structural studies on human type IV collagen. The Journal of Biological Chemistry 254: 9893

Schuppan D, Timpl R, Glanville R W 1980 Discontinuities in the triple helical sequence gly–X–Y of basement membrane (Type IV) collagen. FEBS letters 115: 297-301

Schwartz D, Veis A 1978 Characterisation of basement membrane collagen of bovine anterior lens capsule via segment-long-spacing crystallites and the specific cleavage of the collagen by pepsin. FEBS letters 85: 326

Stenn K S, Madri J A, Roll F J 1979 Migrating epidermis produces AB_2 collagen and requires continual collagen synthesis for movement. Nature 277: 229

Steven D H 1975 Separation of the placenta in the ewe: An ultrastructural study. Quartery Journal of Experimental Physiology 60: 37

Steven F S 1966 The depolymerising action of pepsin on collagen. Molecular weights of the polypeptide chains. Biochimica et Biophysica Acta 130: 190

Tanzer M, Kefalides N A 1973 Collagen cross-links: Occurrence in basement membrane collagens. Biochemical Biophysical Research Communications 51: 775

Thomsen K, Hiersche H D 1969 The functional morphology of the placenta, the foetus, the membranes and the umbilical chord. In: Klopper A, Diczfalusy E (eds) Foetus and placenta. Blackwell Scientific, Oxford, ch 3, p 61

Timpl R, Glanville R W, Wick G, Martin G R 1979 Immunochemical studies on basement membrane (type IV) collagens. Immunology 38: 109

Trelstad R L, Carvalho A C A 1979 Type IV and type AB collagens do not elicit platelet aggregation or the serotonin release reaction. Journal of Laboratory and Clinical Medicine 93: 499

Verbeek J H, Robertson E M, Haust M D 1967 Basement membranes and adjacent tissue in term placenta. American Journal of Obstetrics and Gynaecology 99: 1136

Vracko R, Benditt E P 1970 Capillary basal lamina thickening. Journal of Cell Biology 47: 281

Vracko R 1975 Basal lamina scaffold — anatomy and significance for maintenance of orderly tissue structure. American Journal of Pathology 77: 314

Wahl L M, Wahl S M, Mergenhagen S E, Martin G R 1975 Collagenase production by lymphokine-activated macrophages. Science 187: 261

Wideman G L, Baird G H, Bolding O T 1964 Ascorbic acid deficiency and premature rupture of fetal membranes. American Journal of Obstetrics and Gynaecology 88: 592

Wigglesworth J S 1973 Development, anatomy and physiology of the placenta. In: Fox H, Langley F A (eds) Postgraduate obstetrical and gynaecological pathology. Pergamon Press, Oxford, ch 19, p 391

Woessner J F 1961 The determination of hydroxyproline in tissue and protein samples containing small proportions of this imino acid. Archives of Biochemistry and Biophysics 93: 440

Wynn R M 1968 Morphology of the placenta. In: Assali N S (ed) Biology of gestation I, the maternal organism. Academic Press, New York, ch 3. p 93

Weiss J B 1976 Enzymic degradation of collagen. International Review of Connective Tissue Research, vol 7, p 101-57

Wynn R M 1975a Principles of placentation and early human placental development. In: Gruenwald P (ed) The placenta. Medical and Technical Publications Ltd, Lancaster, ch 2, p 18

Wynn R M 1975b Fine structure of the placenta. In: Gruenwald P (ed) The placenta. Medical and Technical Publications Ltd, Lancaster, ch 4, p 56

27

Dermal scar

D. S. JACKSON

The ability to repair injured tissue is a biological adaptation essential to the survival of complex multicellular organisms. With the exception of those organs which have the capacity to regenerate completely, such as liver, the formation of fibrous tissue is the usual process of repair following most types of injury. The process is most obvious (and the most studied) in surface wounds involving loss of tissue or created by a surgical incision, the end product of which is a visible scar. Although the scar tissue contains several connective tissue components, the bulk of it is made up of collagen and it is this component which is the subject of this chapter.

MORPHOLOGY

Collagen fibres may be identified by the light microscope within the intercellular space 3 to 4 days after an incision and continue to increase in both number and size for several weeks (Ross, 1968). In the early stages the collagen is seen as thin silver-staining fibrils, but as they increase in number and thickness the fibres lose their silver staining capacity and take up the biological stains, such as Van Gieson, characteristic for mature collagen seen in tissues such as skin (Gilman, 1970).

Polarised light studies show that there is a generalised disorganisation of the wound collagen (Forrester, 1980). Normal collagen as seen for example in the dermis is birefringent but even after 100 days scar collagen is non-birefringent. This indicates a relatively disorganised structure at the molecular or small-fibril level.

This relative disorganisation is clearly seen when scar tissue is examined by scanning electron microscopy (SEM) and compared with adjacent normal dermis (Forrester, 1980). In unwounded dermis a regular pattern of fibre bundles is seen, with indications of a striated pattern in the individual fibrils (Fig. 27.1a). In contrast, in a 10-day-old wound the fibrils lie in a relatively haphazard fashion, with little evidence of collagen fibre substructure (Fig. 27.1b). With time the collagen fibrils appear to coalesce into large aggregates but normal network architecture, such as is seen in the dermis, is never restored (Forrester, 1980).

With the transmission electron microscope (TEM) collagen fibrils with the characteristic 67 nm repeating

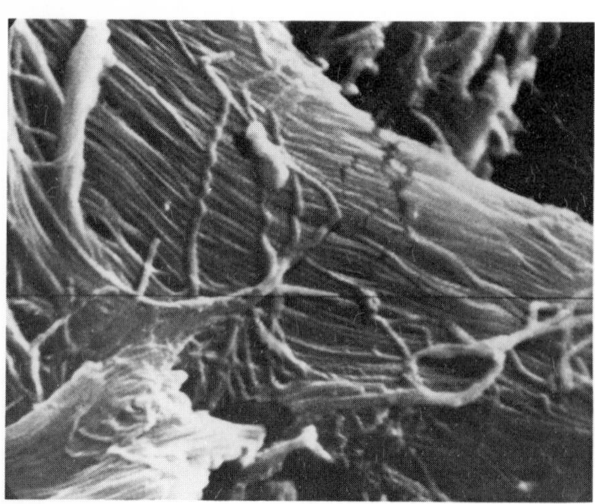
A

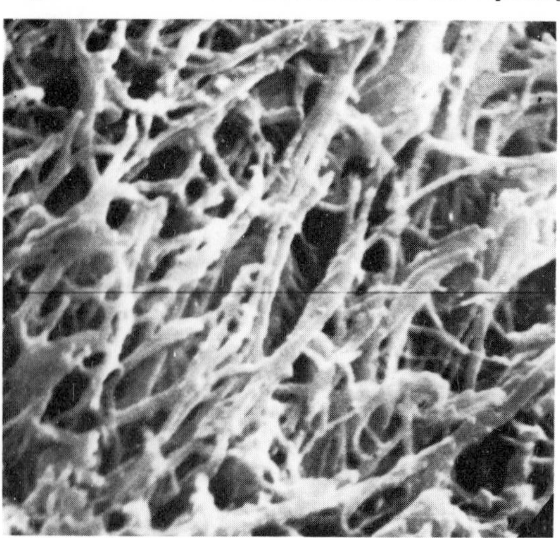
B

Fig. 27.1 SEM pictures of (A) normal dermis (B) 10-day-old normal wound. Magnification × 15,000. Kindly provided by Dr J. C. Forrester.

pattern can be identified by the third day. In punch biopsy wounds in the guinea pig Ross (1968) showed that as the wound gets older at least two separate populations of fibril size are present in the extracellular space. Both of these populations appeared to show an increase in fibril diameter with increasing age, with smaller fibrils closer to the cells (Ross, 1968).

In punch biopsy wounds in guinea pigs the fibrils in the larger population had a diameter of 40 nm at 5 days, increasing to 130 nm at 14 days. Those in the smaller population had a diameter of 20 nm at 5 days and 500 nm at 14 days. Various widths of collagen fibres from 65 to 150 nm were noted in 56-day-old linear wounds in the guinea pig dermis. In young surgical scars viewed both with the electron microscope and with light microscopy, the fibrils are initially narrower than those on the adjacent dermis, but increase in diameter as the scar ages (Ross, 1968).

However, when quantitative measurements are made on transverse sections through collagen fibrils in guinea pig wounds, a different pattern emerges (Forrest et al, 1972). At 1 week maturity the fibrils show a wide range of diameters ranging from 40 to 90 nm (Fig. 27.2 and 27.3) although there was some evidence of a biphasic distribution. However by the end of the second week the range of diameters had markedly narrowed to 40 to 60 nm and the median diameter had reduced from 80 nm to 50 nm.

BIOCHEMISTRY

Amino acid analysis

The amino acid analysis of insoluble scar collagen is very similar to that of collagen from the dermis in which the wound is made (Forrest & Jackson, 1971; Forrest et al, 1972; Barnes et al, 1975). However, there are significant differences between collagens sampled from early or late scars. In part, these may be related to the difficulties of purifying insoluble scar collagen since carbohydrate analyses suggest contamination with glycoprotein(s)

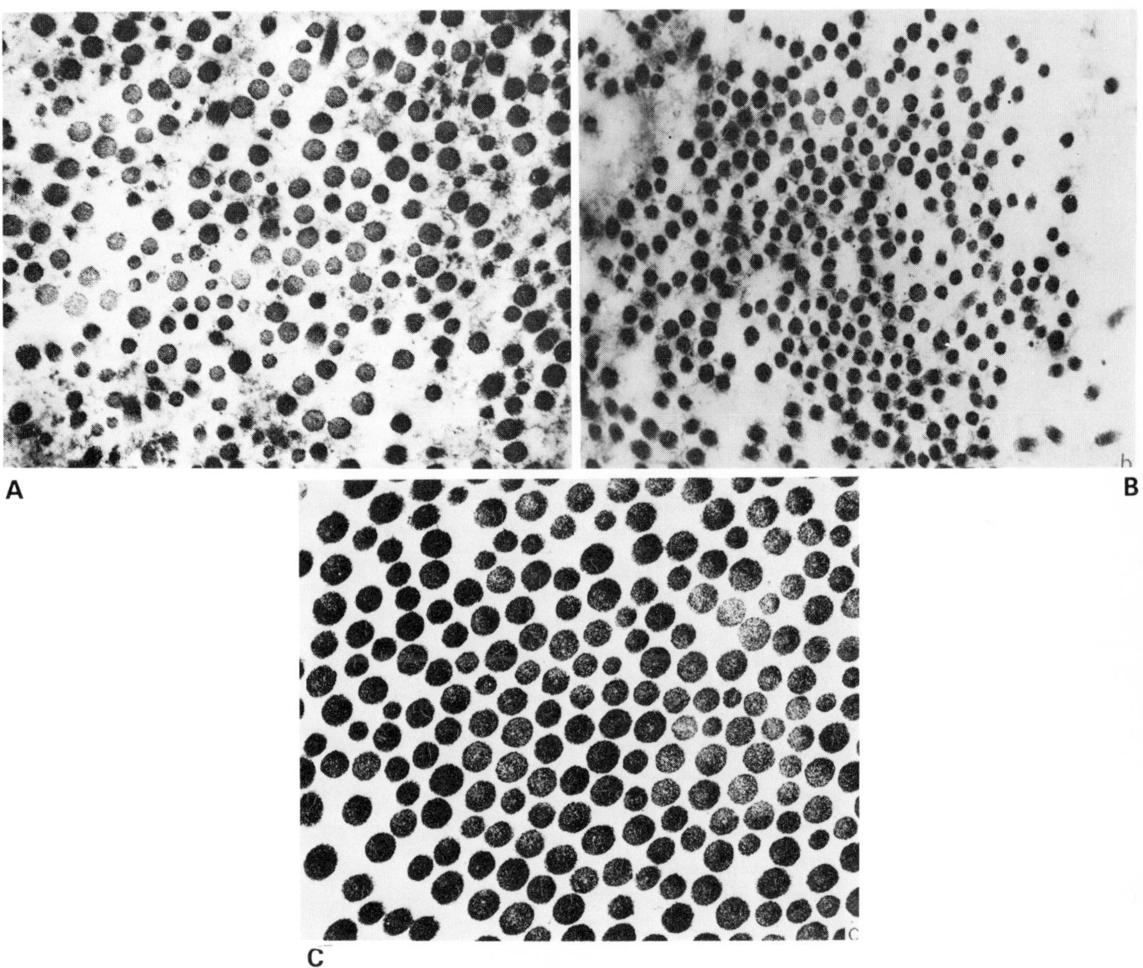

Fig. 27.2 TEM pictures of transverse section of collagen fibres of (A) 1 week scar, (B) 3 week scar, (C) normal dermis.

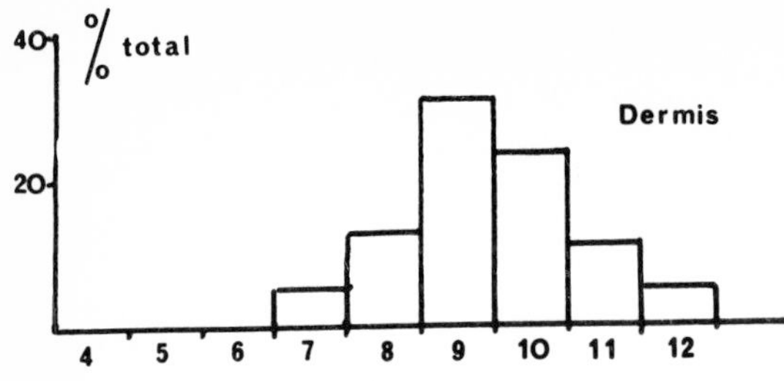

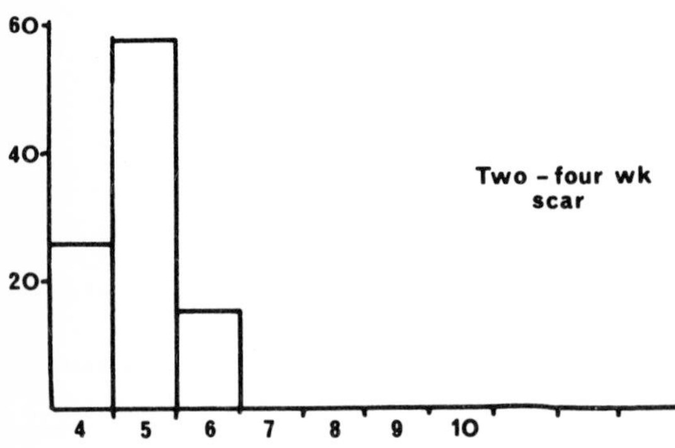

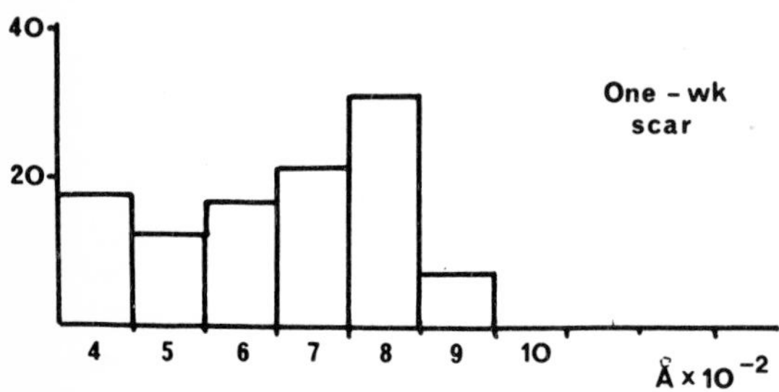

Fig. 27.3 Comparison of distribution of the diameters of collagen fibres from normal dermis and 1 and 2–4 week scar.

(Forrest et al, 1972a). Dermal collagen purified by extraction with EDTA contains virtually no hexoses except glucose and galactose attached to hydroxylysine. However scar collagen contains substantial amounts of fucose, mannose and hexosamine, in addition to glucose and galactose (Table 27.1).

However, quantitation of hydroxylysine and hydroxylysine glycosides also indicates other significant differences (Table 27.2).

Collagen from 1 to 2 week old guinea pig dermal scars contains 50 per cent more hydroxylysine (Forrest et al, 1972; Barnes et al, 1975, 1976) and there is a corresponding increase in glycosylation (Forrest et al, 1972a). In older wounds the hydroxylysine content is not significantly different from that of adjacent dermal collagen (Barnes et al, 1975). This change in the hydroxylation of lysine parallels that which occurs in dermis during growth and development. In embryonic skin collagen, hydroxylation of collagen lysine is relatively high (Barnes et al, 1971). After birth there is a rapid fall in hydroxylation of lysine (Barnes et al, 1971, 1974).

Cross-linking

The tensile strength of a scar increases rapidly over the first 15 days and more slowly thereafter, although it never reaches the strength of the original unwounded dermis (Dunphy & Jackson, 1962; Forrester, 1980). To some extent this may relate to the cross-links which form as the collagen is laid down. In guinea pig scar collagen there is a rapid decrease over the first 1 to 3 weeks on the degree of thermal solubilisation. When heated to 60 to 70°C in acetate buffer at pH 7, 40 per cent of the collagen is solubilised in a 1 week scar, but by the fourth week only 20 per cent is solubilised (Forrest et al, 1972a). The major cross-link in scar collagen is thermally stable (see below). This suggests that the thermally labile collagen represents

Table 27.1 Analyses of neutral sugars associated with EDTA-prepared collagens from dermis and dermal scar. The figures for total hexose expressed as residues of hexose/3000 amino acid residues are given as the mean ± the SD with the number of observations in parentheses.

Tissue	*Total hexose*	*Glu*	*Gal*	*Mann*	*Fuc*	*Gal + Glu*	*Gal/Glu*	*Hexosamine*
Dermis	9.1±0.1 (4)	3.3	5.2	0.6	—	8.5	1.6	4.5±0.2 (6)
Dermal scar (2-week wound)	36.7±4.2 (8)	17.3	13.4	4.0	2.0	30.7	0.8	24.0±1.7 (6)

Table 27.2 Quantitation of hydroxylysyl glycosides from dermis and dermal scar collagens. Results expressed as residues/3000 amino acid residues

Tissue	Total Hylys [a]	GluGalHyl [b]	GalHyl [b]	Gal + Glu	Gal/Glu
Dermis	19.2	3.1	2.0	8.2	1.6
Dermal scar (2 week wound)	25.2	5.2	1.3	11.7	1.2

[a] Determined from amino acid analysis of 6N HC1 hydrolysate of α amylase prepared collagen

[b] As determined from peak area ratios of Hyl: GluGalHyl: GalHyl from amino acid hydrolysate of EDTA prepared collagen

collagen not yet stabilised by covalent cross-links but that these cross-links form rapidly over the first 2 or 3 weeks. This is confirmed by similar studies on human scar collagen from 4 to 12 weeks maturity (Forrest & Jackson, 1971). Virtually all the collagen is thermally stable over the whole of this period.

The thermal stability is explained by the type of cross-links found in scar collagen. Several different types of collagen cross-links have been identified (see Ch. 9), but there are only two major cross-links found in scar collagen. These are derived either from one residue of allysine and one residue of hydroxylysine (hydroxylysinonorleucine) or from one residue of hydroxyallysine and one residue of hydroxylysine (dihydroxylysinonorleucine).

In guinea pig dermal scar collagen of 2 weeks duration, the major cross-link is dihydroxylysinonorleucine, with a small amount of hydroxylysinonorleucine (Forrest et al, 1972; Barnes et al, 1976). This is the reverse of the pattern found in unwounded dermis. The pattern remains unchanged for several weeks (Jackson & Mechanic, 1974), but thereafter changes with time and after a few months is very similar to that of dermis (Barnes et al, 1975). Similar results have been reported for human scar collagen (Bailey et al, 1975a).

This change in cross-link pattern is also seen during the growth and development of the dermis from embryonic to mature (Bailey & Robins, 1973). The underlying reason for the change in cross-link pattern in both these situations lies in the corresponding change in the degree of hydroxylation of lysine which was discussed above. The result is that the amino acid residue in the terminal peptide regions involved in the cross-linking process changes from hydroxyallysine to allysine, which interacting with an adjacent hydroxylysine residue giva rise to dihydroxynorleucine and hydroxynorleucine respectively.

The presence of dihydroxylysinonorleucine as the major cross-link explains the increased thermal stability of scar collagen discussed above. This cross-link in its unreduced form is a keto-imine which is heat stable in contrast to hydroxylysinonorleucine which is in the form of a Schiff's base which is thermally labile (Bailey et al, 1973). When scar collagens were heated in neutral buffer the stable cross-link was unaffected whereas the labile cross-link disappeared (Jackson et al, 1974).

Collagen types

The first investigations of the types of collagen occurring in scars were made on tissue derived from splinted wounds in the guinea pig. Only type I was found whereas both type I and III were found in unwounded dermis from the same animal (Shuttleworth & Forrest, 1974). Cells derived from the same tissue also produced only type I in culture (Harwood et al, 1974). These findings were confirmed by a comparison of the cyanogen bromide peptides of insoluble guinea pig skin and scar collagen (Shuttleworth et al, 1975).

However subsequent investigations on open unsplinted wounds in the guinea pig revealed the presence of both types I and III (Barnes et al, 1976). Initially it was felt that the difference between the two conflicting studies lay in the use of the splinted wound compared to the open wound (Jackson, 1978). However further investigations (Jackson & Cleary, unpublished work) showed that the difference lay in the ages of the guinea pigs used in the two studies. Shuttleworth & Forrest (1974) used 600 to 850 g animals whereas Barnes et al (1976) used young 250 g animals. When splinted wounds from 250 g animals were analysed the results were identical to those of Barnes et al (1976), i.e. the 10-day-old scar contained 9 per cent type III. With time the percentage of type III collagen falls so that by 21 days it has fallen to 7 per cent compared to 4 per cent in unwounded dermis (Barnes et al, 1976).

Similar studies have been reported in wound healing in rats (Clore et al, 1979) but the results, although showing a fall in the percentage of type III collagen, are somewhat different from those reported for guinea pig scar. These workers studied wounds from 10 hours up to 12 days after wounding. During this period the percentage type III collagen fell from 31 per cent to 15.5 per cent compared to 20 per cent for normal skin. However at 9 days the percentage type III (17.4) was lower than skin collagen, whereas in the guinea pig at 10 days the percentage type III in the scar is more than double that in the skin (Barnes et al, 1976). The finding of any collagen at all at 10 hours is surprising since fibroblasts capable of synthesising collagen are not seen in wounds until at least 72 hours (Ross, 1968). There have been no reports on collagen types in normal human scar, probably owing to the difficulty of obtaining such scar tissue free of adjacent dermis particularly in long standing scars. However, the finding of type III collagen in human hypertrophic scars suggests that the same phenomenon may occur in human wounds (Bailey et al, 1975b).

It has been suggested by Bailey and his coworkers (see for example Bailey et al, 1975) that the formation of collagen in a wound follows that which occurs in the development of the embryonic skin and the subsequent postnatal development. This proposal is based on the changes in lysine hydroxylation and the concomitant change in the cross-linking pattern which are features common to both normal dermis and scar tissue and on the changes in the proportions of the collagen types. However, although the parallel is clear in the case of hydroxylation and cross-linking, it is not so clear cut in the case of the collagen types. In the human infant dermis the ratio of type I to type III changed from 0.8 in the 15 week fetus to 3.6 at 3 months after birth (Epstein, 1974). In the guinea pig dermis the maximum rate of type III collagen synthesis is at 30 days of gestation and falls off rapidly thereafter. The rate of synthesis of type I is constant throughout. At 30 days the rate of synthesis of type III is over four times greater than that of type I, but less than one half at 70 days (Shuttleworth & Forrest, 1975). In contrast, although data is not available for very early wounds, even at 10 days post-wounding type I is by far the most preponderant collagen type. One further problem is that type III is the preponderant collagen in vascular tissue (Chung & Miller, 1974) and wound tissue is highly vascularised, particularly in the early stages of wound healing.

Biosynthesis

The source of the fibroblast appears to be perivascular mesenchymal cells which migrate into the wound, proliferating and differentiating into fibroblasts capable of synthesising collagen (Ross, 1968). Collagen synthesis begins about the third day after healing and collagen accumulates over the first 15 to 20 days (Forrester, 1980). This is paralleled by the appearance of the enzyme collagen prolyl hydroxylase which is detectable as early as the second day and the activity of which rises rapidly from the third to the sixth day, thereafter declining until it reaches the levels found in adjacent skin by the 18th day (Mussini et al, 1967). However collagen synthesis continues well beyond this period: in guinea pig dermal wounds the rate of synthesis is still higher than in the unwounded dermis 1 month after wounding, falling to the level of dermal collagen only after about four months (Barnes et al, 1976).

In human scar tissue, in spite of apparent clinical inactivity, collagen biosynthesis is demonstrable in vitro even after 20 years. Mature scars show lower rates of synthesis than normal skin although there is considerable variation between scars of similar duration (Craig et al, 1975a, b). This suggests that mature scar collagen has a low metabolic activity with biosynthesis in equilibrium with degradation.

PATHOLOGICAL SCARS

Hypertrophic and keloid

In the early stages of repair scars tend to have an excessive amount of tissue and only after a considerable length of time do they present the thin, white appearance characteristic of old scars (Peacock & Van Winkle, 1976). However, in some circumstances this late remodelling does not take place and scar tissue, including collagen, continues to increase and spread over a wider area than that of the original defect. These scars are referred to as hypertrophic or keloid. Although attempts have been made to distinguish between these types, conclusive tests have not been developed to separate them in clinical terms (Peacock & Van Winkle, 1976). However, changes in size and shape do appear to be different, with hypertrophic scars increasing in size over the first few months and then regressing or stabilising slowly, whereas keloid continue to increase in size and invade adjacent tissue and show little tendency to regress. Keloids may also have a hereditary component since the worst keloids are normally seen in certain black races.

Morphology

In general the fibrous structure shows an irregular pattern with a tendency to form sheets or nodules but there is some variation in the descriptions of different authors and between various hypertrophic and keloid scars described by the same author. With light microscopy, hypertrophic scars following burns show collagen fibres with a markedly irregular pattern. In some areas there are characteristic 'whorls' and in others the fibres tend to form into nodules (Larson et al, 1975). The same authors report that when examined by scanning electron microscopy the nodules appear to form by fusion of collagen fibrils into a homogeneous mat. Fibrils are rarely visible and when they are, they are randomly arranged. Other reports of hypertrophic scar (Brown & Gibson, 1975; Knapp et al, 1975) describe flatter collagen fibres in the form of sheets, or fibrils crossing over in all directions but in bundles loosely arranged in a wavy pattern. However, Brown & Gibson (1975) also report structure similar to those reported by Larson et al (1975). In another hypertrophic scar Brown & Gibson (1975) describe quite a different pattern of densely packed sheets with collagen fibres parallel to each other.

Knapp et al (1977) attempt to distinguish between hypertrophic and keloid scars and report that in keloid discrete fibre bundles were virtually absent. The fibres were in haphazardly connected sheets with random orientation but this is somewhat similar to the structures described by Brown & Gibson (1975) in what they classify as hypertrophic scars.

Using transmission electron microscopy Larson et al (1975) found that the diameter of the collagen fibrils in hypertrophic scars were much smaller than those of normal dermis with the fibrils packed very closely together. In a more detailed study Basom et al (1975) made very interesting observations concerning the subepithelial basement membrane. They claim that scar hypertrophy can be seen as early as 10 days after injury, when the basement membrane becomes convoluted and thickened. The thickening appears to be due to a reduplication resulting in the formation of multiple lamellae of basement membrane material. Since basement membrane collagen is thought to be type IV (see Ch. 17) one would expect that this collagen would be found in hypertrophic scars but thus far this has not been reported. After 1 month rapidly developing new collagen fibrils appear with random orientation and with age these fibrils appear to aggregate into bundles. There is also an increasing variability in the diameter of individual fibres, in contrast to normal scar where the range of fibril diameter narrows (Forrest et al, 1972). An interesting and unexplained change is reported to occur in the ability of fibres with diameters greater than 50 nm to take up stains such as uranyl acetate. They remain unstained even though fibrils with diameters less than 50 nm randomly distributed among them are adequately stained (Basom et al, 1975).

Biochemistry

The most striking feature of hypertrophic and keloid scars is the continuing build up of collagen over long periods of time compared to the remodelling and collagen loss in normal scars. In the normal scar collagen accumulates up to 21 days but does not increase thereafter, even though some collagen synthesis continues (Madden & Peacock, 1971). Collagen is therefore being removed as fast as it is formed. The continuing build up of collagen in hypertrophic and keloid scars may therefore be due to either collagen synthesis continuing at a higher rate, a failure of collagen removal, or a combination of both.

Continuing synthesis is indicated by several parameters which have been reported by a number of workers. The rate of synthesis of collagen in hypertrophic and keloid as measured in organ culture is three to four times higher than normal scar at 6 months post injury (Craig et al, 1975b). There is a steady fall in the rate of synthesis over a period of years with keloid reaching the level of mature normal scar after 2 to 3 years and hypertrophic scars after 4 to 5 years. Since collagen continues to accumulate during these periods it may be concluded that the defect may be a failure of collagen degradation. This conclusion is reinforced by the fact that even in adults the rate of synthesis of the abnormal scar collagen is less than in normal dermis after about one year (Craig et al, 1975a).

The continuing activity of hypertrophic and keloid scar is also indicated by the pattern of cross-links found in collagen from these tissues (Bailey et al, 1975a). As discussed above, in normal scar the pattern of cross-links changes from one in which dihydroxylysinonorleucine predominate to one in which hydroxylysinonorleucine is the predominant cross-link. Initially the ratio of these cross-links is about 3:1 in early wounds and plateaus to a ratio of 1:3, a ratio still found in a 10-year-old wound. This compares with the virtual absence of dihydroxylysinonorleucine in mature dermis and mature normal scar. Evidence for increased collagen biosynthesis may also be provided by the high solubility of collagen (Harris & Sjoedsma, 1966), and by high levels of proline hydroxylase (Cohen et al, 1975; Hayakawa et al, 1979) found in hypertrophic scars. The activity of lysyl oxidase, the enzyme whieh catalyses the first stage of cross-link formation is reported to be three times as high in hypertrophic and keloid scars as in normal dermis taken from the same patients (Knapp et al, 1977).

As in the early normal scar both type I and type III collagens are found in hypertrophic and keloid scars. Based on the weight of precipitates obtained by differential salt precipitation Bailey et al (1975b) reported a ratio of type I : type III of 2 : 1 for a 10-month-old hypertrophic scar, indicating a slightly higher amount of type III than is found in normal human dermis. In a more detailed report on the analysis of collagen from 35 samples of hypertrophic scars following burns Hayakawa et al (1979) also reported the presence of type III collagen. The age of the lesions varied from 22 days to 40 years and the ratio of type III to type I ranged from 0.72 at 22 days to 0.2 at 30 to 40 years compared to a mean value for normal dermis of 0.17. After 2 years the ratio gradually decreases to the range of normal dermis. The ratio of 0.72 at 22 days is very close to the 0.8 reported for embryonic skin (Epstein, 1974). These data provide very clear evidence in support of the idea first put forward by Barnes et al (1975a) that the pattern of change of collagen types and cross-links seen during the development of the skin also occurs during the formation of scar tissue. A similar pattern of high levels of type III is found in acute and chronic experimental granulation tissues (Bailey et al, 1975b) although these models are somewhat different from dermal scars.

Even a low rate of synthesis of collagen will, in the absence of a compensating degradation of collagen, lead over a long period to the accumulation of collagen which is seen in hypertrophic and keloid scars. Thus a defect in collagen degradation could be suspected as a cause of this accumulation of collagen. Collagen degradation in general is due to the activity of collagenase and other collagenolytic enzymes but the activity appears to be controlled by a complex system of inhibition and activation (see Woolley & Evanson, 1980 for reviews). Thus failure of collagen degradation could be due to the absence of collagenolytic enzymes, the presence of excess inhibitors or the absence of enzyme activators.

Collagenase activity in normal experimental wounds was first described by Grillo & Gross (1967) and has since been found in normal human scar (Milsom & Craig, 1973; Cohen et al, 1975). Milsom & Craig measured the collagenase activity of normal skin, mature scars, keloid and hypertrophic scars. Collagenase activity was found in all the tissues and there was a wide range of activities within each group. When compared with skin the majority of the specimens had similar activities but some specimens showed higher activities than the maximum seen for skin. Thus 3 specimens out of 12 of hypertrophic scar had greater than the maximum activity of skin, one very much higher. The majority of the keloid scars gave values within the limits of skin but two of the eight specimens examined gave activities appreciably higher than the skin maximum. Thus in general the collagenase activity of hypertrophic and keloid scars is no different than that of mature scar and normal and where values were different, the activities were higher rather than the expected lower values. The results of Cohen et al (1975) are similar although these workers detected no collagenase activity in normal skin. However, the in vivo situation may not be the same because of the presence of extracellular collagenase inhibitors which may not be present in vitro (Murphy & Sellers, 1980). Another possibility is that the enzyme is initially in the form of inactive zymogen which remains inactive in vivo in pathological scars, but which is activated by non-specific protease activity in vitro. Cohen et al (1975) have reported briefly that 'large amounts' of α_1-antitrypsin and α_2-macroglobulin can be detected by immunofluorescence in hypertrophic and keloid with 'detectable' amounts in normal scar and more in normal skin. However, α_1-antitrypsin is not a collagenase inhibitor and it is now known that there are a number of collagenase inhibitors besides α_2-macroglobulin. It must be concluded that the cause of the accumulation of excess fibrous tissue in hypertrophic and keloid scars is still unknown.

CONCLUSIONS

From the biochemical point of view the collagen of the mature dermal scar is identical to that of the original dermis. In the early stages of scar formation it is more akin to embryonic dermal collagen with a comparatively high ratio of type III: type I collagen, greater hydroxylation of lysine residues, greater glycosylation and with dihydroxylysinonorleucine as the major cross-link. By the time of maturity these parameters have changed towards those of mature dermis. However even to the naked eye the scar is different from normal dermis and bioengineering studies show that an apparently well healed wound is remarkably weak and brittle and remains less strong and more inextensible than the original dermis, even years after healing began.

Morphological studies make it clear that the reason for the relative weakness lies in the physical structure of the collagen fibres. Examined by light microscopy, birefringence, SEM and TEM, scar collagen has physical irregularities in fibre, shape and weave. In the early stages the fibres lie in a haphazard fashion compared to the regular array in the normal dermis. With time the collagen fibrils coalesce to form irregular masses with no evidence of collagen fibril substructure. Thus the microarchitecture of the wound is clearly abnormal.

In pathological scars the process of healing seems to be the same as in normal scars, but for reasons which are not clear, control of the process is lost. Biochemically the pathological scars remain 'immature' for long periods of time and morphologically the irregularity of fibre structure and microarchitecture are even more extreme than those of normal scars.

The mechanisms by which fibroblasts lay down the collagen in the precise array seen in the dermis and other connective tissues is unknown. Whatever these mechanisms are, they are clearly not operative in the formation of dermal scar collagen with the result that a wound heals by repair and not by regeneration of the original dermal structure.

REFERENCES

Bailey A J, Robins S P 1973 Development and maturation of the crosslinks in the collagen fibres of skin. In: Robert L (ed) Frontiers of matrix biology. ch 1, p 130

Bailey A J, Bazin S, Sims T J, Lelous M, Nicoletis C, Delauny A 1975a Characterisation of the collagen of human hypertrophic and normal scars. Biochimica et Biophysica Acta 405: 412

Bailey A J, Sims T J, Lelous M, Bazin S 1975b Collagen polymorphism in experimental granulation tissue. Biochemical and Biophysical Research Communications 66:

Barnes M J, Constable B J, Morton L F, Kodicek E 1971 Hydroxylysine in the N-terminal telopeptides from chick embryo and newborn rat. Biochemical Journal 125: 925

Barnes M J, Constable B J, Morton L F, Royce P M 1974 Age-related variations in hydroxylation of lysine and proline in collagen. Biochemical Journal 139: 461

Barnes M J, Morton L F, Bailey A J, Bennett R C 1975 Studies on collagen synthesis in the mature dermal scar in the guinea pig. Biochemical Society Transactions 3: 917

Barnes M J, Morton L F, Bennett R C, Bailey A J, Sims T J 1976 Presence of Type III collagen in guinea pig dermal scar. Biochemical Journal 157: 263

Basom C R, Townsend S F, Longacre J I, Berry H, Untertheiner R 1975 Ultrastructural changes during scar hypertrophy and following z-plasty. In: Gibson T, van der Meulen J C (eds) Wound healing. Foundation International Cooperation in Medical Sciences. p 165

Brown I A, Gibson T 1975 Pathological aspects of skin healing. In: Gibson T, van der Meulen J C (eds) Wound healing. Foundation International Cooperation in Medical Sciences. p 134

Chung E, Miller E J 1974 Collagen polymorphism: characterisation of molecules with the chain composition of $[\alpha 1\ III]_3$ in human tissues. Science 183: 1200

Clore J N, Cohen I K, Diegelmann R F 1979 Quantitation of collagen types I and III during wound healing in rat skin. Proceedings of the Society for Experimental Biology and Medicine 161: 337

Cohen I K, Diegelmann R F, Bryant C P, Keiser H R 1975 Collagen metabolism in keloid and hypertrophic scar. In: Gibson T, van der Meulen J C (eds) Wound healing. Foundation International Cooperation in Medical Sciences. p 69

Craig R D P, Schofield J D, Jackson D S 1975a Collagen biosynthesis in normal and hypertrophic scars and keloid as a function of the duration of the scar. British Journal of Surgery 62: 741

Craig R D P, Schofield J D, Jackson D S 1975b Collagen biosynthesis in normal human skin, normal hypertrophic scar and keloid. European Journal of Clinical Investigation 5: 69

Dunphy J E, Jackson D S 1962 Practical application of experimental studies in the care of the primarily closed wound. American Journal of Surgery 104: 273

Epstein E H 1974 [α1(III)]$_3$ human skin collagen. Release by pepsin digestion and preponderance in fetal life. Journal of Biological Chemistry 249: 3225

Forrest L, Jackson D S 1971 Intermolecular crosslinking of collagen in human and guinea pig scar tissue. Biochimica Biophysica Acta 229: 681

Forrest L, Dixon J, Jackson D S 1972a Comparative studies on insoluble collagen of guinea pig dermis and dermal scar tissue. Connective Tissue Research 1: 243

Forrest L, Shuttleworth C A, Jackson D S, Mechanic G 1972b A comparison between reducible intermolecular crosslinks of collagens from mature dermis and young dermal scar tissue of the guinea pig. Biochemical and Biophysical Research Communications 46: 1776

Forrester J C 1980 Collagen morphology in normal and wound tissue. In: Hunt T K (ed) Wound healing and wound infection. Theory and surgical practice' Appleton-Century-Crofts, New York. ch 10, p 118

Gillman T 1970 In: Campion R H, Gillman T, Rook S, Sims R T (eds) An introduction to the biology of the skin. Blackwell Scientific, Oxford. ch 6

Grillo H C, Gross J 1967 Collagenolytic activity during mammalian wound repair. Developmental Biology 15: 300

Harris E D, Sjoedsma A 1966 Solubility of collagen of hypertrophic scars. Lancet ii: 707

Harwood R, Grant M E, Jackson D S 1974 Influence of ascorbic acid on ribosomal patterns and collagen biosynthesis in the healing wound of scorbutic guinea pigs. Biochemical Journal 142: 641

Hayakawa T, Hashimoto Y, Myokei Y, Aoyama H, Izawa Y 1979 Changes in type of collagen during the development of human post-burn hypertrophic scars. Clinica Chimica Acta 93: 119

Jackson D S, Ayad S, Mechanic G 1974 Effect of heat on some collagen crosslinks. Biochimica et Biophysica Acta 336: 100

Jackson D S, Mechanic G 1974 Crosslink patterns of collagens synthesised by cultures of 3T6 and 3T3 fibroblasts and by fibroblasts of various granulation tissues. Biochimica et Biophysica Acta 336: 228

Jackson D S 1978 A possible effect of epithelialization on the type of collagen formed in scar tissue. In: Gasper H (ed) Collagen-platelet interaction. Schattauer Verlag, Stuttgart. p 389

Knapp T R, Daniels J R, Kaplan E N 1977 Pathological scar formation. Morphologic and biochemical correlates. American Journal of Pathology 86: 47

Larson D L, Linares H A, Baur P, Willis B, Abston S, Lewis S R 1975 Pathological aspects of skin healing in burns. In: Gibson T, van der Meulen J C (eds) Wound healing. Foundation International Cooperation in Medical Sciences. p 122

Madden J W, Peacock E E 1971 Studies on the biology of collagen during wound healing. III Dynamic metabolism of scar collagen and remodelling of dermal wounds. Annals of Surgery 174: 511

Milsom J P, Craig R D P 1973 Collagen degradation in cultured keloid and hypertrophic scar tissue. British Journal of Dermatology 89: 635

Murphy G, Sellers A 1980 The extracellular regulation of collagenase activity. In: Woolley D A, Evanson J M (eds) Collagenase in normal and pathological connective tissues' ch 4, p 65

Mussini E, Hutton J J, Udenfriend 1967 Collagen prolyl hydroxylase in wound healing, granuloma formation, scurvy and growth. Science 157: 927

Peacock E E, Van Winkle W 1976 Surgery and biology of wound repair, 2nd edn. W B Saunders & Company

Ross R 1968 The fibroblast and wound repair. Biological Reviews 43: 51

Shuttleworth C A, Forrest L 1974 Pepsin-solubilized collagens of guinea pig dermis and dermal scar. Biochimica et Biophysica Acta 365: 454

Shuttleworth C A, Forrest L 1975 Changes in guinea pig dermal collagen during development. European Journal of Biochemistry 55: 391

Shuttleworth C A, Forrest L, Jackson D S 1975 Comparison of the cyanogen bromide peptides of insoluble guinea pig skin and scar collagen. Biochimica et Biophysica Acta 379: 207

Wooley D E, Evanson J M (eds) 1980 Collagenase in normal and pathological connective tissues. Wiley & Son, Chichester UK

28

Skin

E. A. BAUER and J. UITTO

STRUCTURE AND FUNCTION

From a physiological standpoint, the skin serves one major function: it is the barrier between the body and the outside world. Additionally, however, this function must be performed in such a way as to permit maximum mobility and adaptability of the organism. Thus, the biological function of collagen, which represents over 70 per cent of the dry weight of skin, is to provide a structural framework underlying the epidermis and by interacting with other tissue macromolecules — such as proteoglycans and elastin — to provide the critical structural integrity necessary for the skin (Bauer & Uitto, 1979; Uitto & Eisen, 1979).

When viewed by conventional light microscopy and by electron microscopy, collagen comprises the major dermal component (Fig. 28.1). The predominant form of collagen found in the skin is type I collagen, comprising approximately 80 to 90 per cent of the total collagenous proteins (Epstein & Munderloh, 1978; Uitto, 1979). In addition, certain fibres, called reticulin fibres, and once thought to represent separate connective tissue elements because of their peculiar tinctorial properties (Seifter & Gallop, 1966), have been suggested to represent or to be derived from type III collagen (Gay & Miller, 1978; Uitto & Santa-Cruz, 1979).

The dermis, like other structures composed of connective tissue, contains fibroblasts which are the cellular source of most of the collagen found in the skin. Collagen, however, is a group of proteins with many specialized types and functions (Table 28.1) (Miller, 1976; Uitto & Lichtenstein, 1976; Bauer & Uitto, 1979). It is conceivable, therefore, that fibroblasts may not be the only source of collagen and that other cell types, such as smooth muscle cells and epidermal cells, may contribute to the synthesis of this family of macromolecules in the skin (Burke et al, 1977; Layman et al, 1977; Sage et al, 1979). In adult skin type I collagen constitutes 80 to 90 per cent of the dermal collagen. The remaining 10 to 15 per cent consists of type III collagen, while other forms, such as type I trimer, A-B (type V) and type IV collagens, represent less than 5 per cent of the total (Gay & Miller, 1978; Stenn et al, 1979; Uitto, 1979). In fetal skin, however, type III collagen is enriched in concentration (Chung & Miller, 1974; Epstein, 1974), suggesting developmental modulation of the

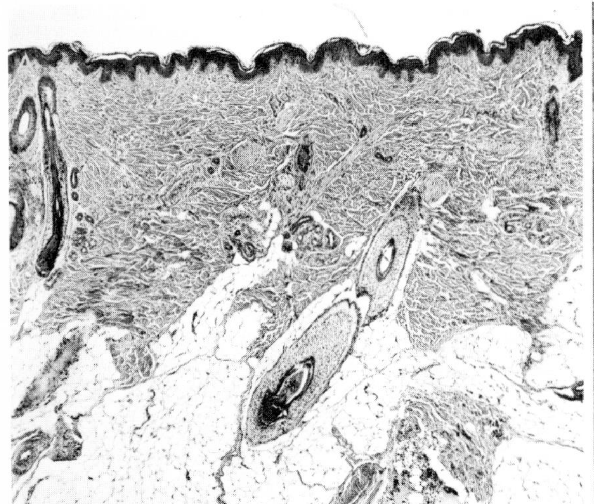

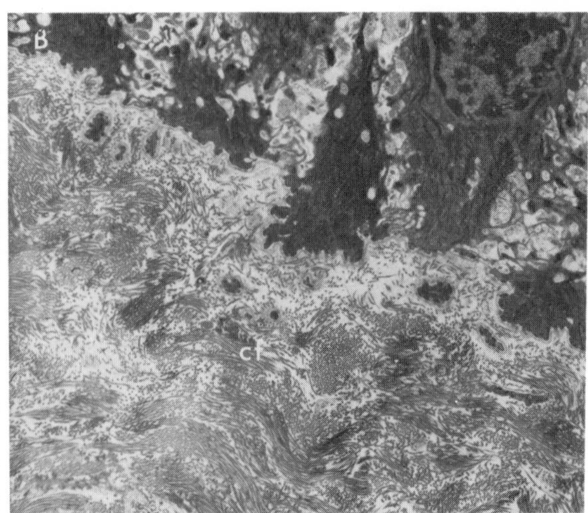

Fig. 28.1 Human skin. (A) Light micrograph. Hematoxylin and eosin. Original magnification, × 40. (B) Electron microscopy. Note the collagen fibrils (CF) in the dermis. Original magnification, × 8100.

Table 28.1 Genetically distinct collagens

Collagen type	*Chain composition*	*Chemical properties*	*Tissue distribution*
I	$[\alpha 1(I)]_2\alpha 2$	Hybrid molecule of two $\alpha 1$(I) chains plus one $\alpha 2$ chain. Low hydroxylysine	Dermis, bone, tendon; as well as most other connective tissue
I trimer	$[\alpha 1(I)]_3$	Similar to type I	Dermis, possibly other tissues
II	$[1(II)]_3$	Relatively high in hydroxylysine.	Hyaline cartilage
III	$[\alpha 1(III)]_3$	Interchain disulfide bonds. High in hydroxyproline and low in hydroxylysine. High glycine content.	Dermis, blood vessels, smooth muscle
IV	$[\alpha 1(IV)]_3$	High in hydroxylysine and glycosylated hydroxylysine. High hydroxyproline.	Epithelial and endothelial basement membranes
V	$\alpha A \alpha B$[a]	Similar to type IV	Basement membranes, placenta, possibly others

[a] The chain composition in each individual molecule is unknown.

synthesis and/or degradation of various genetic types of collagen. Similarly, the content of type III collagen is enhanced in blood vessels and other organs containing smooth muscle (Chung & Miller, 1974; Miller, 1976). Its critical role in these structures is emphasized by the propensity to cutaneous ecchymoses and to arterial and gastrointestinal rupture experienced by patients with the ecchymotic variety of Ehlers-Danlos syndrome (type IV) in which there is a deficiency of type III collagen (Pope et al, 1975; Byers et al, 1979; Uitto & Santa-Cruz, 1979; Jaffe et al 1981; Uitto et al, 1981).

The microanatomical distribution of the two major procollagen and collagen types in the skin has been studied using immunohistochemical techniques (Meigel et al, 1977). In these studies type I collagen can be found throughout the entire dermis, whereas type I procollagen appears to be localized to the uppermost, or papillary, dermis. Using specific antisera to type III procollagen and type III collagen, similar staining patterns are found with localization in the papillary dermis, the adventitia and the periadenexal structures. Thus, the type III immunological staining patterns also support the postulate that this collagen type plays a major role in vessel integrity.

Although the degree to which immunological staining patterns may be altered in certain diseases or in wound healing is still under investigation, it appears to be possible to extract type I and type III collagens from the skin without resorting to the use of proteolytic digestion (Lenaers & Lapiere, 1975). Thus, the combined use of biochemical and immunological techniques should provide considerable information on the modulation of these two dermal collagen components in disease' In this regard, it is of interest that in both naturally occurring human cutaneous scars (Weber et al, 1978) and in experimental wound healing in rat skin (Clore et al, 1979), there is an increase in the proportion of type III collagen. The approximate 2-fold increase in type III collagen observed early in the course of the wound healing process suggests that type III collagen may provide the basic lattice for subsequent healing events, such as guiding the influx of fibroblasts, establishing the vasculature, and leading to the deposition of type I collagen.

At least some, if not all, of the collagens associated with basement membrane are also found in the skin (Bornstein & Sage, 1980). The precise degree to which the various molecular species, such as $[\alpha 1(IV)]_3$ and $[\alpha 2(IV)]_3$ are present in skin is unknown, however, since the proteolytic digestion of tissue required for their isolation makes accurate quantitation difficult. The localization of basement membrane collagens in the skin in the subepithelial area as well as surrounding vascular structures suggests important biological functions for these types of collagen at the interface of various highly specialized tissues with other collagenous stroma. In the skin, the most obvious example of this is the interposition of the collagenous basement membrane between the epidermis and the interstitial collagens of the dermis. In addition, it is possible that these collagens may participate in the differentiation of cells (Gay & Miller, 1978).

As noted in Table 28.1, the principal collagens in the skin, types I and III, are composed of three polypeptide α-chains which exist in a unique triple-helical conformation. Type I collagen is a heteropolymer consisting of two identical $\alpha 1$(I) chains and one $\alpha 2$ chain which has a distinct primary structure (Piez et al, 1963). In contrast, type III collagen consists of three identical $\alpha 1$(III) chains joined by interchain disulphide bonds (see Ch. 00). The unique characteristics of these two skin collagens is demonstrated not only by their chemical properties (Table 28.1) but is further emphasized by their preferential cleavage by human skin collagenase. Welgus et al (1981), using essentially pure preparations both of human skin collagenase and of various collagen types, have shown that maximum rates of degradation vary with both the type and the species of origin of the collagen. Although the affinity of collagenase for all collagen types from all species is nearly identical to that for human type I collagen (apparent $K_m - 1 \times 10^{-6}$M), the maximum rates of degradation are greatest with types I and III collagens derived from the homologous dermal substrate; i.e., human skin collagenase preferentially cleaves human type I and type III collagens over type II collagen and fails to cleave types IV and V collagens et all. On the other hand, collagenase present in human polymorphonuclear leucocytes preferentially digests type I collagen over type III (Horwitz et al, 1977), yet the apparent K_m of leucocyte collagenase is of the same order of magnitude (—1μM) as that of human skin collagenase (Turto et al, 1977; Welgus et al, 1980). Finally, basement membrane collagen, type IV and A–B collagen (type V) appear to be resistant to cleavage by human skin collagenase. However, specific enzymes capable of degrading type IV collagen have been reported both in tissues and in polymorphonuclear leucocytes (Liotta et al, 1979; Uitto et al, 1980). Such findings suggest an intimate, and yet dynamic, structural-functional relationship for these proteins in the skin.

BIOSYNTHESIS OF COLLAGEN

Each of the genetically distinct types of collagen is initially synthesized as a precursor molecule, procollagen, which consists of three precursor polypeptides, pro-α chains (Table 28.2). The pro-α chains are larger than collagen α-chains, because they contain additional peptide sequences at both ends of the polypeptide (Tanzer et al, 1974; Byers et al, 1975; Fessler et al, 1975; Uitto et al, 1976; Fessler & Fessler, 1978; Prockop et al, 1979; Bornstein & Sage, 1980). The polypeptides undergo several modifications before the completed collagen molecules are deposited into extracellular fibres. These modifications include: (1) synthesis of hydroxyproline and hydroxylysine by hydroxylation of certain prolyl and lysyl residues; (2) glycosylation of the chains, particularly at hydroxylysyl residues; (3) chain association, disulphide bonding and triple helix formation; (4) proteolytic conversion of procollagen to collagen, and (5) fibre formation and intermolecular cross-link formation. In this scheme, steps 1 through 3 occur intracellularly, while conversion of procollagen to collagen and fibre formation (steps 4 and 5) occur extracellularly (Ch. 5).

Table 28.2 Post-translational modification reactions during the biosynthesis of collagen

Step	*Enzymes*	*Substrates and cofactors*
1. Prolyl and lysyl hydroxylation	Prolyl hydroxylase Lysyl hydroxylase	O_2 α-Ketoglutarate Ascorbate Fe^{2+} Peptidyl proline and lysine
2. Glycosylation	Glucosyl transferase Galactosyl transferase	UDP-Sugars Mn^{2+} Peptidyl hydroxylysine
3. Chain association, disulfide bonding and triple helix formation	—	—
4. Conversion of procollagen to collagen	Procollagen N-terminal protease Procollagen C-terminal protease	Procollagen Ca^{2+}
5. Fibre formation and inter-molecular cross-link formation	Lysyl oxidase	Lysine or hydroxylysine Cu^{2+} O_2

Synthesis of hydroxyproline and hydroxylysine

One of the characteristic features of collagen is the presence of relatively large amounts of hydroxyproline. Even though hydroxyproline accounts for about 10 per cent of the amino acids in collagen, there is no genetic code or transfer-RNA for this particular amino acid, and, therefore, free hydroxyproline is not incorporated into collagen polypeptides. Instead, hydroxyproline is synthesized by hydroxylation of certain prolyl residues which are already in peptide linkages (Cardinale & Udenfriend, 1974; Prockop et al, 1976)' The hydroxylation reaction is catalyzed by an enzyme, prolylhydoxylase, which has been purified and extensively characterized from various vertebrate tissues, including human skin (Cardinale & Udenfriend, 1974; Berg & Prockop, 1973; Kuutti et al, 1975; Tuderman et al, 1975). Prolylhydroxylase requires molecular oxygen, ferrous iron, α-ketoglutarate, and a reducing agent, such as ascorbic acid, as co-substrates or cofactors for the reaction. The enzyme recognizes prolyl residues only in the Y-position of the repeating triplet sequence X-Y-Gly of collagen (Ch. 5).

Hydroxylysine is the second amino acid characteristic of collagen, and during the intracellular biosynthesis of procollagen this amino acid serves as an attachment site for some of the sugar residues found in collagen (Prockop et al, 1976). The presence of hydroxylysine also plays a critical role in the formation of covalent cross-links which stabilize the extracellular matrix (see below).

Both prolylhydroxylase (Uitto et al, 1969; Uitto et al, 1970; Keiser et al, 1971; Fleckman et al, 1973; Tuderman & Kivirikko, 1977) and lysyl hydroxylase (Anttinen et al, 1973) have been measured in human skin. In each case, levels of the enzyme activities are highest in fetal skin, somewhat lower in infants and lowest in adults. Interestingly, when Tuderman & Kivirikko (1977) measured the amount of immunoreactive prolyl hydroxylase, about 13 to 19 per cent of the total enzyme protein was enzymatically active in fetal skin, while only to 2 to 4 per cent was active in adult skin. Although these enzymes in themselves do not appear to be rate-limiting in the collagen synthesis, they nevertheless appear to reflect the relative rates of synthesis, so that in most situations where collagen synthesis is increased, the activity of prolyl hydroxylase is increased (Prockop et al, 1976; Kivirikko & Risteli, 1976).

Glycosylation

Collagen is a glycoprotein containing galactosyl and glucosylgalactosyl residues attached to the molecule (Table

28.2). The sugar residues are attached to collagen polypeptides during intracellular biosynthesis in a sequential manner so that a galactosyl residue is added first to the molecule and then a glucose is attached to some of the galactosyl residues (Prockop et al, 1976; Kivirikko & Myllylä, 1979). These two glycosylation reactions are catalyzed by separate specific enzymes, collagen galactosyl transferase and collagen glucosyl transferase.

The function of the sugar residues in collagen or procollagen is not known. However, the degree of glycosylation of each molecule is affected not only by the primary structure but also by the rate of triple helix formation. First, since the hydroxylation of lysyl residues is inhibited by helix formation (Ryhänen & Kivirikko, 1974), a delay in helix formation is associated with an increase in the available hydroxylysine acceptor sites for sugar attachment. Secondly, the transferases catalyze glycosylations of the polypeptides only in a nonhelical conformation (Myllylä et al, 1975b; Oikarinen et al, 1976; Uitto et al, 1978). Thus, any delay in triple helix formation can increase the degree of glycosylation. Accordingly, type I procollagen, which requires the shortest time — approximately 10 minutes for triple-helix formation (Schofield et al, 1974) — manifests the least glycosylation. In contrast, type IV procollagen requires about 60 minutes for folding into the triple-helix and is high in glycosylated hydroxylysine residues (Grant et al, 1973). And finally, type II procollagen, which requires about 25 to 30 minutes for the formation of triple-helix, has intermediate levels of glycosylation (Uitto & Prockop, 1973).

Chain association, disulphide bonding and triple helix formation

One of the most critical steps in the intracellular synthesis of procollagen is the association of three pro-α chains and subsequent folding of the collagenous portions of the polypeptides into the triple-helical conformation (Fessler & Fessler, 1978; Prockop et al, 1976). This is fully discussed in chapter 5. During the process of chain association, the half-cystine residues on the extensions of the pro-α chains form interchain disulphide bonds linking three pro-α chains together (Uitto & Prockop, 1973; Harwood et al, 1977). The synthesis of interchain disulphide bonds closely parallels the rate at which the procollagen molecules fold into the triple-helical conformation (Schofield et al, 1974; Uitto & Prockop, 1974a). On this basis, it seems possible that the formation of interchain disulphide bonds may play a role in the helix formation during the biosynthesis of procollagen.

It should be emphasized that the primary structure of the collagenous portion of the molecule contains sufficient chemical information — and specificity — for formation of the triple helix to form under in vitro conditions. However, this spontaneous formation of helix proceeds extremely slowly, requiring approximately 24 h for one-half of the molecules to become helical. In contrast, biosynthetic studies indicate that chain association of the pro-α-chains into the triple helical conformation occurs in the cisternae of the rough endoplasmic reticulum, and the time course of the reaction (measured in minutes) suggests that the disulphide bonds on the carboxy-terminal extension peptides function to bring the three procollagen α-chains into register (Schofield et al, 1974; Uitto & Prockop, 1974a; Uitto & Prockop, 1973).

An equally critical, but as yet not fully explained, step is the requirement for correct recognition of procollagen α-chains. This is particularly the case when dealing with type I collagen, which requires the formation of the heteropolymer, $[\text{pro-}\alpha 1(\text{I})]_2\text{pro-}\alpha 2$. It has been suggested that the peptide extensions on the individual pro-α chains contain the specific information not only to place the chains in register for helix formation but also for proper association in a 2:1 ratio (Prockop et al, 1976). The necessity for such a putative recognition mechanism is further emphasized by the fact that in cultured fibroblasts there appears to be simultaneous synthesis of type I and type III procollagens in the same cell (Gay et al, 1976).

That all of these events are intimately tied to other post-translational events is emphasized by experiments dealing with the subcellular location of modification reactions. For example, the hydroxylations of prolyl and lysyl residues probably are initiated on the nascent chains in the cisternae of the rough endoplasmic reticulum, and these reactions are completed soon after the release of full-length polypeptide chains from the ribosomes (Miller & Udenfriend, 1970; Harwood et al, 1974; Uitto & Prockop, 1974b). Also, the glycosylation reactions are likely to start on the nascent chains soon after the synthesis of hydroxylysyl residues (Brownell & Veis, 1975). In addition, the enzymes catalyzing the hydroxylations or participating in the sugar attachment on the collagenous portion of the molecule do not function on substrates which are in a triple-helical conformation (Prockop et al, 1976; Kivirikko & Myllylä, 1979). It appears, therefore, that the post-translational modification reactions, such as the formation of hydroxylysine and attachment of the sugars, are regulated by the rate at which the collagen polypeptides fold into triple-helical conformation. Such a mechanism would also explain the considerable variability in the amount of hydroxylysine and in the degree of glycosylation of the hydroxylysyl residues encountered in various genetic types of collagen (see above).

Conversion of procollagen to collagen

After the initial synthesis of procollagen polypeptides in the rough endoplasmic reticulum, the polypeptides fold into the triple-helical conformation. The triple-helical procollagen molecules are then transported into the extracellular space by energy-requiring mechanisms (Kruse & Bornstein, 1975) involving Golgi vacuoles or vesicles of the smooth endoplasmic reticulum (Dehm & Prockop, 1972; Olsen & Prockop, 1974) and remain soluble until enzymatically converted to collagen. Once conversion occurs, the collagen molecules precipitate spontaneously under physiological temperature and ionic conditions. The conversion process is catalyzed by two specific enzymes which separately remove the amino-terminal and carboxy-terminal extensions from procollagen (Lapiere et al, 1971; Layman & Ross, 1973; Kohn et al, 1974; Goldberg et al, 1975; Tuderman et al, 1978; Leung et al, 1979). Both of the enzymes are relatively well-characterized and appear to require calcium for activity. Although enzymes capable of cleavaging the extension peptides have now been described from a number of sources, it is noteworthy that the initial demonstration of a defect in amino procollagen peptidase activity was in the hereditary skin disease of cattle, dermatosparaxis (Lapiere et al, 1971). In this disorder, defective processing of the procollagen molecule results in deficient intermolecular cross-linking, thus, causing the increased tissue friability characteristic of the disease (Bailey & Lapiere, 1973).

Fibre formation and intermolecular cross-link formation

After removal of extension peptides in the extracellular space, the collagen molecules spontaneously align to form fibres. These fibres, however, do not attain the necessary tensile strength until the molecules are linked together by specific, covalent cross-links (Bailey et al, 1974; Tanzer, 1976; Rucker & Murray, 1978). The most common cross-links in collagen are derived from lysine or hydroxylysine, and the formation of the cross-linked compounds involves enzymatic conversion of these two amino acids to corresponding aldehydes by the enzyme, lysyl oxidase (Pinnell & Martin, 1968; Siegel, 1974; Siegel & Fu, 1976). This first step, the enzymatic synthesis of an aldehyde derivative by removal of the ϵ-amino group of certain lysyl and hydroxylysyl residues, is followed by condensation of the aldehyde with an ϵ-amino group on an adjacent unmodified lysine or hydroxylysine to form a Schiff base type covalent cross-link.

The enzyme, lysyl oxidase, which catalyzes the first step of this reaction, functions in the extracellular space and has greater activity with fibrillar collagen than with denatured collagen or α-chains (Siegel et al, 1970). This enzyme requires copper as a cofactor, and its activity is readily inhibited by nitriles, such as β-aminopropionitrile, which are known to produce lathyrism in animals. Also, compounds such as D-penicillamine can prevent the cross-link formation by mechanisms which involve blocking of the reactive aldehydes formed from lysyl or hydroxylysyl residues (Desmukh & Nimni, 1969; Uitto & Lichenstein, 1976). Because the cross-links of collagen provide the tensile strength required in a functioning tissue, a defect in the formation of these covalent bonds can lead to a disturbance in connective tissue formation (Carnes, 1968).

Lysyl oxidase is synthesized and secreted into the extracellular space by cultured human skin fibroblasts (Layman et al, 1972) and these cells are also presumed to be the source of the enzyme in vivo. When measured in extracts of human skin, even though considerable variability has been observed in normal control subjects (Hayakawa et al, 1976), it appears that following a thermal burn, lysyl oxidase activity is low in granulation tissue but subsequently rises and is significantly elevated as wound healing evolves. Such studies clearly suggest that at a physiological level this enzyme functions to aid in the maintenance of appropriate tensile strength after tissue injury.

That the polymerization of collagen from skin is not a simple one-step phenomenon is emphasized by the in vitro studies of Trelstad et al (1976). Using electron microscopy, these investigators showed that several morphological stages of aggregation could be defined. Linear growth of collagen fibrils occurs by the tandem addition of collagen aggregates to each other and then to the ends of a subfibril. Lateral growth of the fibril occurs by the entwining of subfibrils. An extensive suprafibrillar order can also be observed with parallel, spiral and orthogonal sets of fibrils which may reflect the in vivo sequence of events. Recently Bruns et al (1978) have suggested that procollagen molecules associate intracellularly within vacuoles and are secreted as such into the extracellular compartment.

Irrespective of whether these in vitro observations are totally representative of initial in vivo events, it is clear that when collagen matures in the skin, it becomes progressively less soluble. Indeed, insoluble, collagen may represent as much as 98 per cent of the collagenous molecules in the skin. Extraction of skin collagen with neutral salt solutions or with acetic acid under nondenaturing conditions solubilized a portion of collagen which is significantly larger in fetuses and young children than in older individuals (Bakerman, 1962; Uitto et al, 1971; Uitto, 1972). The marked insolubility of the remaining polymeric collagen, which is attributable to intermolecular cross-links, make special extraction procedures, such as the use of enzyme digestion, chelating agents and cold alkali, essential (Steven, 1970; Francis & Macmillan, 1971). However, when careful extractions are carried out in normal subjects, it appears that a progressive, age-related stabilization of collagen occurs. In contrast, in certain diseases affecting connective tissues, such as homocystinuria, Werner's syndrome, osteogenesis imperfecta and others, the polymeric collagen is less stable than normal (Francis et al, 1973). Although the mechanism for increased age-related stability of the polymeric collagen is not totally known, it is noteworthy that an increase in intermolecular cross-links in collagen is associated with resistance to degradation by mammalian collagenase (Vater et al, 1979) suggesting that this type of collagen may not be subject to the same degradative forces which operate on more soluble forms of collagen.

Regulation of collagen biosynthesis by human skin fibroblasts in vitro

In order to understand fully the potential aberrations in the various collagen types in diseases affecting the skin, it is necessary first to examine those factors which modulate collagen synthesis in normal control cells. As noted above, in human skin, the two major interstitial collagens are type I and type III comprising about 80 and 15 per cent of the dermal collagen, respectively. Each of the genetically distinct types of collagen is synthesized as a precursor molecule, procollagen, and its biosynthesis involves unique reactions which are required for fibrillogenesis of collagen in normal connective tissues. A defect at any one of these reactions can lead to abnormal fibre formation and functionally defective collagen (Uitto & Prockop, 1974c). Biochemical studies during the past few years have demonstrated defects in the structure and metabolism of collagen in several connective tissue disorders and many of these studies employed cultured human skin fibroblasts (Bauer & Uitto, 1979; Minor, 1980; Freiberger & Pinnell, 1979). In many studies, however, culture conditions have not been rigorously controlled or optimized to yield unequivocal results from these cell culture systems.

Although immunohistochemical staining of cultured human skin fibroblasts has shown that the same cell in culture makes both type I and type III procollagens (Gay et al, 1976), factors which regulate or may alter their respective synthesis are poorly described. Thus, Uitto and associates (Booth et al, 1981; Uitto et al, 1980, Tan et al, 1981; Booth & Uitto, 1981) have examined the effects of cell density, pH, serum concentration and ascorbate content on the relative synthesis of types I and III procollagen. By dissecting each of these factors in cell culture, a reasonably clear picture of the appropriate conditions under which to examine collagen biosynthesis in human skin fibroblasts in vitro has emerged. Because such understanding of normal parameters required for reproducible data on collagen synthesis is critical to the appreciation of disease mechanisms, some of these experiments will be presented here in detail.

As shown in Figure 28.2, when normal human skin fibroblasts are incubated under various experimental conditions with radioactive proline and the formation of radioactive hydroxyproline in the non-dialyzable protein is used as an index of collagen formation, the cells rapidly incorporate [^{3}H] proline into nondialyzable protein and a significant amount of hydroxy[^{3}H]proline is detected after a 10 min labelling period. Examination of the medium hydroxy[^{3}H]proline separately from the cell fraction demonstrates that there is a considerable delay in the secretion of procollagen by the fibroblasts: over 60 min is required before any hydroxyproline can be detected in the medium. The secretion of the hydroxy[^{3}H]proline-containing macromolecules then proceeds linearly from 4 to 24 h of incubation.

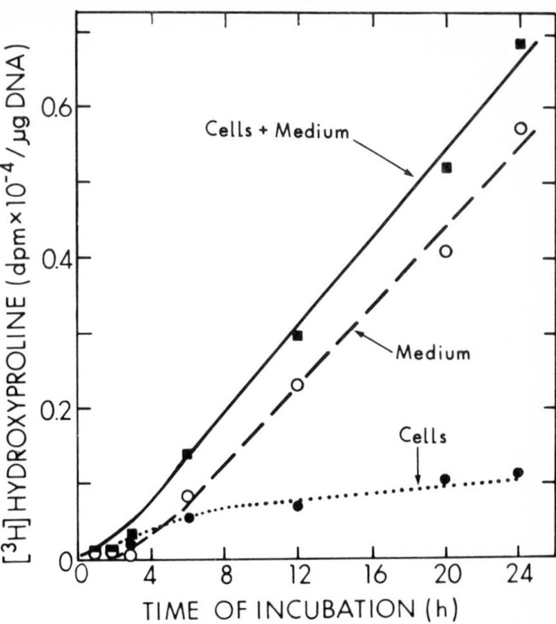

Fig. 28.2 Synthesis and secretion of procollagen by human skin fibroblasts. Cells in early confluent cultures were incubated in modified Dulbecco's modified Eagle's medium containing 20 per cent dialyzed fetal calf serum and 25 µg/ml ascorbic acid. After a 4 h preincubation, the cells were labelled with [^{3}H]proline. At the time points indicated the cell and medium fractions were removed and assayed for non-dialyzable hydroxy[^{3}H]proline and cellular DNA. •. . . . . .• cells; O------O, medium; ■——■, cells + medium. (Adapted from Booth et al, 1981).

In order to examine separately the synthesis of genetically distinct procollagens, the radioactive proteins recovered in the medium are chromatographed on DEAE-cellulose under conditions which separate human type I and type III procollagens (Smith et al, 1972; Lichtenstein et al, 1975; Uitto et al, 1976). In a typical chromatogram two major peaks of radioactivity can be observed (Fig 28.3). The first peak elutes as a symmetrical sharp peak and consists of a collagenous ^{3}H-labelled protein. Approximately 40 per cent of the [^{3}H]prolyl residues in the newly synthesized polypeptides are converted to hydroxyl[^{3}H]proline and about 90 per cent of the radioactivity in this peak can be digested with highly purified bacterial collagenase. On the basis of cyanogen bromide peptide mapping and α-chain composition, as estimated by carboxymethylcellulose chromatography and polyacrylamide gel electrophoresis in sodium dodecyl sulphate, the collagenous protein in the first peak, has been identified as type I [^{3}H]procollagen (Lichtenstein et al, 1975; Uitto et al, 1981). The second major area of radioactivity in most cases appears to represent a complex of ^{3}H-labelled proteins; it is usually relatively broad and it frequently displays several distinct peaks of radioactivity (Fig. 28.3). This complex, however, clearly contains collagenous proteins, since from 25 to 43 per cent of the [^{3}H]prolyl

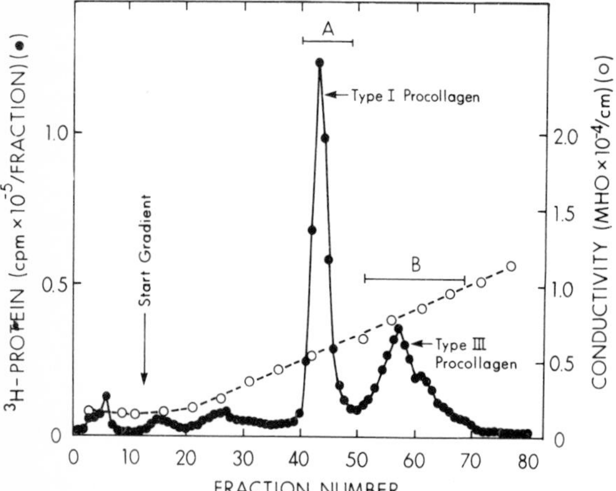

Fig. 28.3 DEAE-cellulose chromatography of partially purified medium ^{3}H-labelled proteins. Skin fibroblasts in early confluent cultures were labelled with [^{3}H]proline. After a 20 h labelling period, the medium ^{3}H-labelled protein was precipitated with 20 per cent $(NH_4)_2SO_4$ after addition of protease inhibitors. The precipitate was dissolved and chromatographed on DEAE-cellulose. The separated type I and type III procollagens were assayed, after pooling the fractions indicated by the horizontal bars by determining their hydroxy[^{3}H]proline content. (Adapted from Booth et al, 1981).

residues in the newly synthesized protein are converted to hydroxy[^{3}H]proline. Further purification of the hydroxy[^{3}H]proline-containing protein has allowed the identification of this macromolecule as type III. [^{3}H]Pro-collagen in the chromatograms is consistently separated from other [^{3}H]proline-labelled, noncollagenous proteins. The newly synthesized type I and type III procollagens, separated by DEAE-cellulose chromatography can be quantitated by assaying the radioactive hydroxyproline in the pooled areas, as indicated in Figure 28.3. Examination of the medium ^{3}H-labelled protein at 6, 12, and 20-h labelling points by DEAE-cellulose chromatography reveals essentially identical patterns. Thus, there is no apparent time-dependent alteration in the synthesis of the two procollagens.

As discussed above, a critical factor in regulating synthesis and secretion of procollagen is the concentration of ascorbic acid. When varying concentrations of ascorbic acid are added to the culture medium 4 h prior to and at the time of labelling, a marked stimulation of hydroxy[^{3}]proline synthesis occurs with as little as 1 μg/ml (5.6 μM) of ascorbic acid and maximal effects are seen with 5 to 50 μg/ml (Booth et al, 1981). It should be noted that the maximal stimulation by ascorbic acid varies with different cell lines, with the radioactive hydroxyproline in ascorbic acid-containing cultures being from 140 to 290 per cent of the controls. Such observations clearly illustrate how variable collagen synthesis can be even between normal cell strains and emphasize the caution required in dealing with diseased cells.

Since it has been suggested that serum concentration modulates the synthesis of procollagen by gingival fibroblasts (Narayanan & Page, 1977), it is important to evaluate this parameter in skin fibroblast cultures as well. When normal human skin fibroblasts are incubated in medium containing optimum concentrations of ascorbic acid (50 μg/ml) with variable concentrations of fetal calf serum, a dose-dependent effect on the synthesis of non-dialyzable hydroxy[^{3}H]proline occurs (Fig. 28.4). Both the cell protein and DNA content of the cultures increase as the serum concentration increases. At the same time, the hydroxy[^{3}H]proline synthesis per flask increases with increasing serum concentration up to 30 per cent. When the synthesis of hydroxy[^{3}H]proline is related to cellular protein or DNA, the range of 10 to 30 per cent serum concentration appears to produce a stimulation and on the whole, depending on the reference parameter used, the 20 per cent serum concentration appears to be optimal (Booth et al, 1981). Similar observations are made when heat-

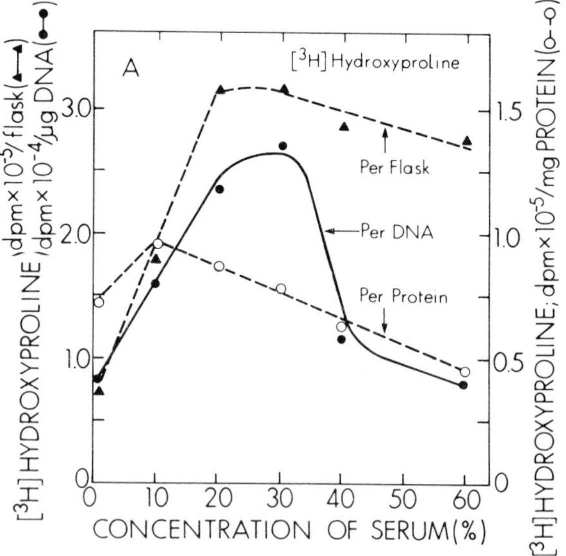

Fig. 28.4 Synthesis of [^{3}H]procollagen in the presence of varying concentrations of fetal calf serum. Cells in early confluency were first preincubated for 12 h in medium without serum and then for 4 h in medium containing 0–60 per cent dialyzed fetal calf serum and 50 μg/ml ascorbic acid. Cultures were labelled for 20 h with [^{3}H]proline and non-dialyzable hydroxy[^{3}H]proline in the cell and medium fractions, as well as cellular protein and DNA were determined. ▲------▲, synthesis of hydroxy[^{3}H]-proline, dpm (× 10^{-5})/flask; •——•, dpm (× 10^{-4})/μg DNA; O------O, dpm (× 10^{-5})/mg protein. (Adapted from Booth et al, 1981).

inactivated human serum is tested in the human skin fibroblast cultures (Tan et al, 1981).

Finally, maximum collagen synthesis in vitro is dependent upon an optimum culture density (Fig. 28.5). Examination of the synthesis of collagenous ^{3}H-labelled protein, measured as bacterial collagenase-released peptides, indicates that their formation is highest at the log phase of growth and decreases slightly thereafter. Examination of the hydroxy[^{3}H]proline in cell and medium fractions indicate, on the other hand, that procollagen synthesis, measured as formation of radioactive hydroxyproline, is highest about 1 day after the cells have reached visual confluency (Fig. 28.5).

Although some studies have suggested modulation of the synthesis of the various collagen types by some cells in vitro by serum or other factors (Narayanan & Page, 1977; Abe et al, 1979), no such change in the ratio of type I to type III collagen has been observed in adult human skin fibroblast cultures under rigidly controlled culture conditions (Booth et al, 1981). It should be emphasized that studies such as those discussed here, while forming a critical basis for examining regulatory mechanisms, do not in any way exclude any of the specific areas of control of synthesis which have been proposed. For example, studies have suggested a modulatory effect of corticosteroids on collagen synthesis (Ponec et al, 1977; Russell et al, 1978; Booth et al, 1981). Even more intriguing are the experiments suggesting that the binding of collagen (Goldberg, 1979) or

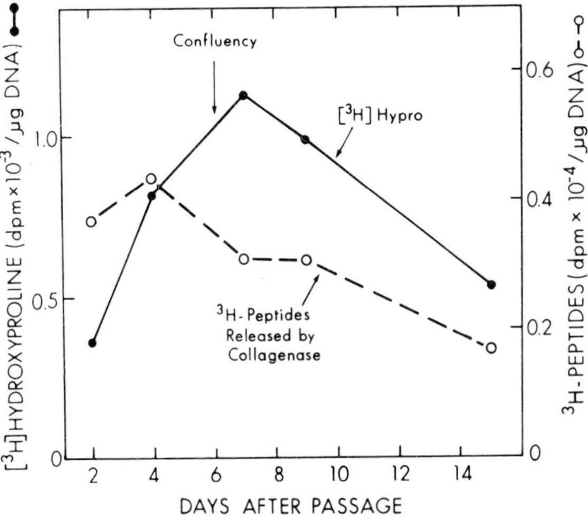

Fig. 28.5 Synthesis of [^{3}H]procollagen at different stages of cell growth. Cells were plated at low density and incubated in Dulbecco's modified Eagle's medium containing 20 per cent fetal calf serum. After varying time periods, the cells were labelled for 20 h with [^{3}H]proline in the presence of 50 μg/ml ascorbic acid. The cultures were assayed for collagenous proteins by measuring the non-dialyzable hydroxy[^{3}H]proline (hypro) or by assaying collagenase-released ^{3}H-labelled peptides. •——•, [^{3}H]hydroxyproline, dpm (× 10^{-3})/μg DNA; O------O, collagenase-released ^{3}H-labelled peptides, dpm (× 10^{-4})/μg DNA. (Adapted from Booth et al, 1981).

of the extension peptides of procollagen to the cell surface (Lichtenstein et al, 1973; Wiestner et al, 1979) may produce, in some as yet undefined manner, a feedback regulation of synthesis. These possibilities must now be explored in great detail both in control cell strains and in those derived from heritable and acquired diseases.

DEGRADATION OF SKIN COLLAGEN

In order to maintain the necessary tensile properties of the skin, specific mechanisms for controlled degradation of collagen must exist. Collagenases, enzymes capable of degrading native collagen, are now known to exist in a number of human and animal tissues and studies indicate that this group of enzymes occupy a crucial position in both the normal and pathological remodelling of collagen in vivo.

The most significant development in our understanding of normal connective tissue metabolism occurred when Gross & Lapiere (1962) demonstrated the first animal collagenase. Using an organ culture technique, these investigators showed that tissues taken from metamorphosing tadpoles could elaborate a collagenase which was capable of degrading native, reconstituted collagen under physiological conditions of temperature and pH. Since that time, specific collagenases have been isolated from a wide variety of animal and human sources (Gross, 1976) and systems have been developed which permit characterization of the normal parameters controlling collagenase biosynthesis and activity and, thus, of the degradation of collagen in general. In this section, we shall describe the properties and control of human skin collagenase.

The tissue and cell type responsible for the production of human skin collagenase in the skin have been defined using three different experimental conditions. Eisen (1969) initially cultured normal human skin explants on radioactive native reconstituted collagen gels. In these experiments, isolated epidermis and dermis were cultured separately, revealing the major site of collagenase production to be in the upper or papillary portion of the dermis (Eisen, 1969; Lazarus & Fullmer, 1969). It is of interest that under normal circumstances the epidermis contains essentially no collagenolytic activity, a finding which is in contrast to that in the anuran tadpole where the tailfin epidermis is the major source of collagenase (Eisen & Gross, 1965). These findings emphasize the difference which can be seen between species even when dealing with similar tissues of origin.

The development of a functionally specific antiserum to human skin collagenase (Bauer et al, 1970; Stricklin et al, 1978) permitted the precise localization of the enzyme by a second technique, immunofluoresence microscopy in tissue sections of human skin. With this technique, collagenase was found primarily in the papillary dermis (Reddick et al, 1974), i.e., in a location identical to that found by employing organ culture methods (Eisen, 1969). The collagen fibres showed pronounced staining for collagenase, suggesting that much of the enzyme present in the skin is extracellular and may be bound to its collagenous substrate. In certain circumstances cytoplasmic staining could also be seen in fibroblast-like cells scattered throughout the upper dermis.

In an extension of these studies, normal human skin fibroblasts grown in monolayer culture could be shown to stain for collagenase (Reddick et al, 1974). Furthermore, by radioimmunoassay (Bauer et al, 1972) the culture medium contained material immunologically identical to human skin collagenase, indicating that the fibroblast, indeed, is the major cell responsible for collagenase production in the human dermis. Despite the immunological evidence for the presence of collagenase in fibroblast cultures, enzymatic activity could not be found. This was initially attributed to inhibition of the enzyme by whole serum present in the culture medium. However, even when normal human skin fibroblasts were cultured in serum-free medium, it was still not possible to detect collagenase activity. The clarification of these findings occurred when it was demonstrated that normal human skin fibroblast cultures synthesized and secreted collagenase in an inactive, proenzyme form (Bauer et al, 1975; Stricklin et al, 1977), which required activation by another protease, such as trypsin, for detection.

More recently large scale cultures of human skin fibroblasts have been employed to purify and characterize human skin collagenase (Table 28.3). These studies have yielded quantitative amounts of the enzyme and indicate that human skin collagenase is synthesized and secreted as two proenzyme (zymogen) forms of approximately 60 000 and 55 000 daltons. It is noteworthy that recent studies on the biosynthesis of human skin collagenase in fibroblast cultures have revealed that the intracellular biosynthetic products at least in part are identical in molecular weight to the 60 000 and 55 000 dalton extracellular species (Valle & Bauer, 1979). These findings, thus, strongly support the concept that human skin collagenase is synthesized as a proenzyme. Each form can be converted to an active enzyme by trypsin, producing species of 50 000 and 45 000 daltons respectively. Alternatively, the proenzymes can undergo an autoactivation process without apparent change in molecular weight. In contrast to the cell culture system, where procollagenase is always seen, it is intriguing that in the serum-free organ culture system only active enzyme is found (Eisen et al, 1968; Stricklin et al, 1977) and that the procollagenase form can be found only when serum is added to the culture medium. This observation suggests that a serum-inhibitable proteolytic system is present in organ cultures which, like trypsin, is capable of converting the zymogen to active enzyme (Stricklin et al, 1977).

Table 28.3 Characteristics of human skin collagenase

Regulatory step	*Property*
Synthesis	In papillary dermis of the normal human skin
	By normal human skin fibroblasts in culture
	Two proenzyme forms of 60 000 and 55 000 daltons
	Controlled by steroid hormones and cyclic nucleotides
Activation	Proenzyme activation by a variety of proteases or by autoactivation
Substrate	Cleaves native collagen to produce two characteristic fragments, α^A and α^B
pH Optimum	Neutral, pH 7–8
Metal requirements	Intrinsic, Zn^{2+}
	Extrinsic, Ca^{2+}
Natural inhibitors	Whole serum
	α_2-macroglobulin
	β_1-anticollagenase
	Fibroblast-derived inhibitor

Detailed chemical comparisons reveal essentially no significant compositional differences between the two procollagenase forms or between the two tryptically activated enzymes (Stricklin et al, 1978). From the standpoint of control of collagen degradation, however, activation of the proenzymes represents a potential regulatory mechanism, since activation markedly alters the binding properties of the enzyme and results in tight binding to the substrate (Stricklin et al, 1978). Thus, the existence of a procollagenase produced by skin fibroblasts provides an important point for regulation of remodelling of collagen. Any imbalance in the system involving zymogen synthesis, secretion and subsequent activation could lead to abnormalities in collagen degradation in a variety of disease states.

Human skin collagenase, like a number of neutral proteases, has been shown to require calcium (Ca^{2+}) for optimum activity under physiologic conditions. Seltzer et al (1976) have shown that Ca^{2+} plays a dual role, acting both as an enzyme activator and, more critically, functioning as a thermal stabilizing cofactor to prevent the irreversible loss of enzyme activity by maintaining the tertiary structure of the enzyme. The precise definition of normal human skin collagenase as a Ca^{2+}-requiring enzyme has provided a valuable foundation for examining the properties of collagenase in the hereditary blistering disorder, recessive dystrophic epidermolysis bullosa, where an alteration in this property has been used to define the existence of a structurally altered collagenase (Bauer, 1977).

In addition to its requirement for extrisic Ca^{2+}, both replacement studies and atomic absorption analysis indicate that human skin collagenase has a second, intrinsic metal requirement, Zn^{2+} (Seltzer et al, 1977). Thus, the metal requirements of the enzyme make it clear that aberrant in vivo modulation of the tissue Ca^{2+} concentration or defective control of the insertion of Zn^{2+} as part of the biosynthetic process could have important implications in regulating collagenase activity.

Once collagenase is synthesized, secreted and activated, it may be subject to regulation by a variety of serum- and/or tissue-derived collagenase inhibitors. Initial studies (Eisen et al, 1970) showed that human serum, even in low concentrations, is a potent inhibitor of human skin collagenase. It is now clear that the major inhibitor in human serum is α_2-macroglobulin, which reacts with a molar equivalent of collagenase to form an irreversible enzyme-inhibitor complex (Abe & Nagai, 1972; Werb et al, 1974). It seems probable that the physiological importance of α_2-macroglobulin is to facilitate the clearing of enzyme-inhibitor complexes from the circulation to prevent the action of collagenase on collagen at sites distant from the collagenase synthesis (Ohlsson, 1971).

Woolley et al (1975, 1976) have described an apparently specific collagenase inhibitor, β_1-anticollagenase. This inhibitor has a molecular weight of approximately 40 000 daltons and is an effective inhibitor of all human collagenases examined but has no effect on a variety of serine, thiol, metallo- or carboxyl proteases. The possible relationship of this inhibitor to the collagenase inhibitor of approximately the same size isolated from human skin fibroblast cultures by Welgus et al (1979) remains to be determined.

Normal human skin fibroblast cultures which synthesize procollagenase also produce a specific inhibitor of the active form of human skin collagenase (Bauer et al, 1975). This inhibitor, which has been extensively purified from serum-free medium, is derived from the fibroblasts themselves as demonstrated by biosynthetic studies (Welgus et al, 1979). The inhibitor has an apparent molecular weight of 31 000 daltons, is remarkably heat stable and inhibits collagenase in a 1:1 molar ratio. The inhibitor derived from human skin fibroblasts is effective against all vertebrate collagenases but is not effective against noncollagenolytic proteases and collagenases of nonvertebrate origin. The existence of an apparently specific inhibitor of collagenase produced by fibroblasts offers another potential control mechanism for collagen degradation. Whether this inhibitor is present in vivo is, as yet, unknown.

It should be noted that a latent form of collagenase has been found in the culture medium of human fetal skin explants (Skinkai & Nagai, 1977). The inactive enzyme forms can be activated either with trypsin or, like the human skin fibroblast proenzyme, by incubation with chaotropic ions such as NaI. In contrast to the findings in the fibroblast system, however, these authors report the release of a small molecular weight inhibitor from the latent enzyme, which results in its activation. The relationship of these two experimental findings to each other is, as yet, unclear, but it may be that in the fetal explant system the association of enzyme and inhibitor occurs at a point subsequent to synthesis, secretion and activation of a proenzyme form.

Corticosteroids exert major effects on the metabolism of protein in mammals in a variety of systems. In view of the profound effects of these hormones in vivo, it was of interest to determine whether steroid hormones could effect the in vitro metabolism of collagen in human skin. Utilizing human skin in organ culture, it has been shown that either 10^{-7}M hydrocortisone or 10^{-8}M dexamethasone in the culture medium inhibits collagenase activity almost completely (Koob et al, 1974; Koob et al, 1980). It is of interest that concomitant with the inhibition of collagenase activity in the medium, there was complete cessation of endogeneous collagen degradation as measured by a marked reduction in the level of hydroxyproline-containing peptides in the culture medium. Furthermore, the decrease in collagenase activity in the medium is directly parallelled by a decrease in immunoreactive collagenase protein, suggesting that the steroid is inhibiting synthesis and/or secretion of the enzyme (Koob et al, 1980).

ACKNOWLEDGEMENTS

This work was supported by U.S.P.H.S. National Institutes of Health Grants AM 19537, AM 28450, GM 28833 and TO AM 07284 and by grants from the National Foundation-March of Dimes. Drs Bauer and Uitto are the recipients of Research Career Development Awards 5K04 AM 00077 and 7KO4 AM 00897 respectively. We wish to thank Dr Daniel J. Santa Cruz of the Department of Pathology, Washington University School of Medicine, for providing the photomicrographs of the skin.

REFERENCES

Abe S, Nagai Y 1972 Interaction between tadpole collagenase and human α_2-macroglobulin. Biochimica et Biophysica Acta 278: 125

Abe S, Steinmann B U, Wahl L M, Martin G R 1979 High cell density alters the ratio of type III to I collagen synthesis by fibroblasts. Nature 279: 442

Anttinen H, Orava S, Ryhanen L, Kivirikko K 1973 Assay of protocollagen lysyl hydroxylase activity in the skin of human subjects and changes in the activity with age. Clinica Chimica Acta 47: 289

Bailey A J, Lapiere CM 1973 Effect of an additional peptide extension of the N-terminus of collagen from dermatosparactic calves on the cross-linking of collagen. European Journal of Biochemistry 34: 91

Bailey A J, Robins S P, Balian G 1974 Biological significance of the intermolecular cross-links of collagen. Nature 251: 105

Bakerman S 1962 Quantitative extraction of acid-soluble human skin collagen with age. Nature 196: 375

Bauer E A 1977 Recessive dystrophic epidermolysis bullosa: evidence for an altered collagenase in fibroblast cultures. Proceedings of the National Academy of Sciences USA 74: 4646

Bauer E A, Eisen A Z, Jeffrey J J 1970 Immunologic relationship of a purified human skin collagenase to other human and animal collagenases. Biochimica et Biophysica Acta 206: 152

Bauer E A, Eisen A Z, Jeffrey J J 1972 Radioimmunoassay of human collagenase. Specificity of the assay and quantitative determination of in vivo and in vitro human skin collagenase. Journal of Biological Chemistry 247: 6679

Bauer E A, Stricklin G P, Jeffrey J J, Eisen A Z 1975 Collagenase production by human skin fibroblasts. Biochemical and Biophysical Research Communications 64: 232

Bauer E A, Uitto J 1979 Collagen in cutaneous diseases. International Journal of Dermatology 18: 251

Berg R A, Prockop D J 1973 Purification of [^{14}C]protocollagen and its hydroxylation by prolyl hydroxylase. Biochemistry 12: 3395

Booth B A, Polak K L, Uitto J 1970 Collagen biosynthesis by human skin fibroblasts. I. Optimization of the culture conditions for synthesis of type I and type III procollagens. Biochimica et Biophysica Acta 607: 145

Booth B A, Tan E M L, Oikarinen A, Uitto J 1981 Effects of glucocorticoids on collagen metabolism in cultured human skin fibroblasts: relevance to dermal atrophy. International Journal of Dermatology. In press

Booth B A, Uitto J 1981 Collagen biosynthesis by human skin fibroblasts. III. The effects of ascorbic acid on procollagen production and prolyl hydroxylase activity. Biochimica et Biophysica Acta 675: 117–122

Bornstein P, Sage H 1980 Structurally distinct collagen types. Annual Review of Biochemistry 49: 957

Brownell A G, Veis A 1975 The intracellular location of the glycosylation of hydroxylysine of collagen. Biochemical and Biophysical Research Communications 63: 371

Bruns R R, Hulmes D J S, Therrien S F, Gross J 1979 Procollagen segment-long-spacing crystallites: their role in collagen fibrillogenesis. Proceedings of the National Academy of Sciences USA 76: 313

Burke J M, Balian G, Ross R, Bornstein P 1977 Synthesis of types I and III procollagen and collagen by monkey aorta smooth muscle cells in vitro. Biochemistry 16: 3243

Byers P H, Click E M, Harper E, Bornstein P 1975 Interchain disulfide bonds in procollagen are located in a large nontriple-helical COOH-terminal domain. Proceedings of the National Academy of Sciences USA 72: 3009

Byers P H, Holbrook K A, McGillvray B, MacLeod P M, Lowry R B 1979 Clinical and ultrastructural heterogeneity of type IV Ehlers-Danlos syndrome. Human Genetics 47: 141

Cardinale G J, Udenfriend S 1974 Prolyl hydroxylase. Advances in Enzymology 41: 245

Carnes W H 1968 Copper and connective tissue metabolism. International Review of Connective Tissue Research 4: 197

Chung E, Miller E J 1974 Collagen polymorphism: characterization of molecules with chain composition $[\alpha 1(III)]_3$ in human tissues. Science 183: 1200

Clark C C, Kefalides N A 1976 Carbohydrate moieties of procollagen: incorporation of isotopically labeled mannose and glucosamine in propeptides of procollagen secreted by matrix-free chick embryo tendon cells. Proceedings of the National Academy of Sciences USA 73: 34

Clore J N, Cohen I K, Diegelmann R F 1979 Quantitation of collagen types I and III during wound healing in rat skin. Proceedings of the Society for Experimental Biology and Medicine 161: 337

Dehm P, Prockop D J 1972 Time lag in the secretion of collagen by matrix-free tendon cells and inhibition of the secretory process by colchicine and vinblastine. Biochimica et Biophysica Acta 264: 375

Desmukh K, Nimni M E 1969 A defect in the intramolecular and intermolecular cross-linking of collagen caused by penicillamine. II. Functional groups involved in the interaction process. Journal of Biological Chemistry 244: 1787

Eizen A Z 1969 Human skin collagenase: localization and distribution in normal human skin. Journal of Investigative Dermatology 52: 442

Eisen A Z, Bloch K J, Sakai T 1979 Inhibition of human skin collagenase by human serum. Journal of Laboratory and Clinical Medicine 75: 258

Eisen A Z, Gross J 1965 The role of epithelium and mesenchyme in the production of a collagenolytic enzyme and a hyaluronidase in the anuran tadpole. Developmental Biology 12: 408

Eisen A Z, Jeffrey J J, Gross J 1968 Human skin collagenase: isolation and mechanism of attack on the collagen molecule. Biochimica et Biophysica Acta 151: 637

Elsas L J, Miller R L, Pinnell S R 1978 Inherited human collagen lysyl hydroxylase deficiency: ascorbic acid response. Journal of Pediatrics 92: 378

Epstein E H 1974 $[\alpha 1(III)]$ Human skin collagen. Release by pepsin digestion and preponderance in fetal life. Journal of Biological Chemistry 249: 3225

Epstein E H, Munderloh N H 1978 Human skin collagen. Presence of type I and type III at all levels of dermis. Journal of Biological Chemistry 253: 1336

Fessler J H, Fessler L I 1978 Biosynthesis of procollagen. Annual Review of Biochemistry 47: 129

Fessler L I, Morris N P, Fessler J H 1975 Procollagen: biological scission of amino and carboxyl extension peptides. Proceedings of the National Academy of Sciences USA 72: 4905

Fleckman P H, Jeffrey J J, Eisen A Z 1973 A sensitive microassay for prolyl hydroxylase: activity in normal and psoriatic skin. Journal of Investigative Dermatology 60: 46

Francis M J O, Macmillan D C 1971 The extraction of polymeric collagen from biopsies of human skin. Biochimica et Biophysica Acta 251: 236

Francis M J O, Smith R, Macmillan D C 1973 Polymeric collagen of skin in normal subjects and in patients with inherited connective tissue disorders. Clinical Science 44: 429

Freiberger H F, Pinnell S R 1979 Heritable disorders of connective tissue. In: Moschella S L (ed) Dermatology update. Elsevier, New York. p 221

Gay S, Martin G R, Müller P K, Timpl R, Kühn K 1976 Simultaneous synthesis of types I and III collagen by fibroblasts in culture. Proceedings of the National Academy of Sciences USA 73: 4037

Gay S, Miller E J 1978 Collagen in the physiology and pathology of connective tissue. Gustav Fischer Verlag, Stuttgart

Goldberg B 1979 Binding of soluble type I collagen molecules to the fibroblast plasma membrane. Cell 16: 265

Goldberg B, Taubman M B, Radin B 1975 Procollagen peptidase: its mode of action on the native substrate. Cell 4: 45

Grant M E, Schofield J D, Kafalides N A, Prockop D J 1973 The biosynthesis of basement membrane collagen in embryonic chick lens. III. Intracellular formation of triple helix and the formation of aggregates through disulfide bonds. Journal of Biological Chemistry 248: 7432

Gross J 1976 Aspects of the animal collagenases. In: Ramachandran G N, Reddi A H (eds) Biochemistry of Collagen, Plenum, New York. p 275

Gross J, Lapiere C M 1962 Collagenolytic activity in amphibian tissues: a tissue culture assay. Proceedings of the National Academy of Sciences USA 48: 1014

Harwood R, Grant M E, Jackson D S 1974 Collagen biosynthesis. Characterization of subcellular fractions from embryonic chick fibroblasts and the intracellular localization of protocollagen prolyl and protocollagen lysyl hydroxylases. Biochemical Journal 144: 123

Harwood R, Merry A H, Wooley D E, Grant M E, Jackson D S 1977 The disulfide bonded nature of procollagen and the role of extension peptides in the assembly of the molecule. Biochemical Journal 161: 405

Hayakawa T, Hino M, Fuyamada H, Nagatsu T, Aoyama H, Izawa Y 1976 Lysyl oxidase activity in human normal skins and postburn scars. Clinica Chimica Acta 71: 245

Horwitz A L, Hance A J, Crystal R G 1977 Granulocyte collagenase: selective digestion of type I relative to type III collagen. Proceedings of the National Academy of Sciences USA 74: 897

Jaffe A S, Geltman E M, Rodey G E, Uitto J 1981 Mitral valve prolapse: a consistent manifestation of the type IV Ehlers-Danlos syndrome. The pathogenetic role of abnormal type III collagen synthesis. Circulation 64: 121-125

Jiminez S A, Harsch M, Murphy L, Rosenbloom J 1974 Effects of temperature on conformation, hydroxylation, and secretion of chick tendon procollagen. Journal of Biological Chemistry 249: 4480

Keiser H R, Stein H D, Sjoerdsma A 1971 Increased protocollagen proline hydroxylase activity in sclerodermatous skin. Archives of Dermatology 104: 57

Kivirikko K, Myllylä R 1979 Collagen glycosyltransferases. International Review of Connective Tissue Research 8: 23

Kivirikko K, Prockop D J 1972 Partial purification and characterization of protocollagen lysine hydroxylase from chick embryos. Biochimica et Biophysica Acta 258: 336

Kivirikko K, Risteli L 1976 Biosynthesis of collagen and its alteration in pathological states. Medical Biology 54: 159

Kohn L D, Isersky C, Zubnick J, Lenaers A, Lee G, Lapiere C M 1974 Calf tendon procollagen peptidase: its purification and endopeptidase mode of action. Proceedings of the National Academy of Sciences USA 71: 40

Koob T J, Jeffrey J J, Eisen A Z 1974 Regulation of human skin collagenase activity by hydrocortisone and dexamethasone in organ culture. Biochemical and Biophysical Research Communications 61: 1083

Koob T J, Jeffrey J J, Eisen A Z, Bauer E A 1980 Hormonal interactions in mammalian collagenase regulation. Comparative studies in human skin and rat uterus. Biochimica et Biophysica Acta 629: 13

Krane S M, Pinnell S R, Erbe R W 1972 Lysylprotocollagen hydroxylase deficiency in fibroblasts from siblings with hydroxylysine-deficient collagen. Proceedings of the National Academy of Sciences USA 69: 2899

Kruse N J, Bornstein P 1975 The metabolic requirements for transcellular movement and secretion of collagen. Journal of Biological Chemistry 250: 4841

Kuutti E R, Tuderman L, Kivirikko K 1975 Human prolyl hydroxylase. Purification partial characterization and preparation of antiserum to the enzyme. European Journal of Biochemistry 57: 18

Lapiere C M, Lenaers A, Kohn L D 1971 Procollagen peptidase: an enzyme excising the coordination peptides of procollagen. Proceedings of the National Academy of Sciences USA 68: 3054

Layman D L, Epstein E H, Dodson R F, Titus J L 1977 Biosynthesis of type I and III collagenas by cultured smooth muscle cells from human aorta. Proceedings of the National Academy of Sciences USA 74: 671

Layman D L, Narayanan A S, Martin G R 1972 The production of lysyl oxidase by human fibroblasts in culture. Archives of Biochemistry and Biophysics 149: 97

Layman D L, Ross R 1973 The production and secretion of procollagen peptidase by human fibroblasts in culture. Archives of Biochemistry and Biophysics 157: 451

Lazarus G S, Fullmer H M 1969 Collagenase production by human dermis in vitro. Journal of Investigative Dermatology 52: 545

Lenaers A, Lapiere C M 1975 Type III procollagen and collagen in skin. Biochimica et Biophysica Acta 400: 121

Leung M K K, Fessler L I, Greenberg D B, Fessler J H 1979 Separate amino and carboxyl procollagen peptidases in chick embryo tendon. Journal of Biological Chemistry 254: 224

Lichtenstein J R, Byers P H, Smith B O, Martin G R 1975 Identification of the collagenous proteins synthesized by cultured cells from human skin. Biochemistry 14: 1589

Lichtenstein J R, Martin G R, Kohn L D, Byers P H, McKusick V A 1973 Defect in conversion of procollagen to collagen in a form of Ehlers-Danlos syndrome. Science 182: 298

Liotta L A, Abe S, Gehron-Robey P, Martin G R 1979 Preferential digestion of basement membrane collagen by an enzyme derived from a metastatic murine tumor. Proceedings of the National Academy of Sciences USA 76: 2268

Meigel W N, Gay S, Weber L 1977 Dermal architecture and collagen type distribution. Archives of Dermatological Research 259: 1

Miller E J 1976 Biochemical characteristics and biological significance of the genetically-distinct collagens. Molecular and Cellular Biochemistry 13: 165

Miller R L, Udenfriend S 1970 Hydroxylation of proline residues in collagen nascent chains. Archives of Biochemistry and Biophysics 139: 104

Minor R R 1980 Collagen Metabolism. A comparison of diseases of collagen and diseases affecting collagen. American Journal of Pathology 98: 227

Myllyla R, Risteli L, Kivirikko K 1975a Assay of collagen galactosyltransferase and collagen glucosyltransferase activities and preliminary characterization of enzymic reactions with transferases from chick embryo cartilage. European Journal of Biochemistry 52: 401

Myllyla R, Risteli L, Kivirikko K 1975b Glucosylation of galactosylhydroxylysyl residues in collagen in vitro by collagen glucosyltransferase. Inhibition by triple-helical conformation of the substrate. European Journal of Biochemistry 58: 517

Narayanan A S, Page R C 1977 Serum modulates collagen types in human gingiva fibroblasts. Federation of European Biochemical Societies Letters 80: 221

Nist C, von der Mark K, May E D, Olsen B R, Bornstein P, Ross R, Dehm P 1975 Location of procollagen in chick corneal and tendon fibroblasts with ferritin-conjugated antibodies. Journal of Cell Biology 65: 75

Ohlsson K 1971 Interactions in vitro and in vivo between dog trypsin and dog plasma protease inhibitors. Scandinavian Journal of Clinical and Laboratory Investigation 28: 220

Oikarinen A, Anttinen H, Kivirikko K 1976 Hydroxylation of lysine and glycosylation of hydroxylysine during collagen biosynthesis in isolated chick embryo cartilage cells. Biochemical Journal 156: 545

Olsen B R, Guzman N A, Engel J, Condit C, Aase S 1977 Purification and characterization of a peptide from the carboxy-terminal region of chick tendon procollagen type I. Biochemistry 16: 3030

Olsen B R, Prockop D J 1974 Ferritin-conjugated antibodies used for labeling organelles involved in the cellular synthesis and transport of procollagen. Proceedings of the National Academy of Sciences USA 71: 2033

Piez K A, Eigner E A, Lewis M S 1963 The chromatographic separation and amino acid composition of the subunits of several collagens. Biochemistry 2: 58

Pinnell S R, Krane S M, Kenzora J E, Glimcher M J 1972 A heritable disorder of connective tissue. Hydroxylysine-deficient collagen disease. New England Journal of Medicine 286: 1013

Pinnell S R, Martin G R 1968 The cross-linking of collagen and elastin: enzymatic conversion of lysine in peptide linkage to an α-aminoadipic-w-simialdehyde (allysine) by an extract from bone. Proceedings of the National Academy of Sciences USA 61: 708

Ponec M, Hasper I, Vianden G D N E, Bachra B N 1977 Effects of glucocorticoids on primary human skin fibroblasts. II. Effects on total protein and collagen biosynthesis by confluent cell cultures. Archives of Dermatological Research 259: 125

Pope F M, Martin G R, Lichtenstein J R, Pentinen R P, Gerson B, Rowe D W, McKusick V A 1975 Patients with Ehlers-Danlos syndrome type IV lack type III collagen. Proceedings of the National Academy of Sciences USA 72: 1314

Prockop D J, Berg R A, Kivirikko K, Uitto J 1976 Intracellular steps in the biosynthesis of collagen. In: Ramachandran G N, Reddi A H (eds) Biochemistry of collagen. Plenum, New York. p 163

Prockop D J, Kivirikko K, Tuderman L, Guzman N A 1979 Biosynthesis of collagen and its disorders. New England Journal of Medicine 301: 13 and 77

Reddick M E, Bauer E A, Eisen A Z 1974 Immunocytochemical localization of collagenase in human skin and fibroblasts in monolayer culture. Journal of Investigative Dermatology 62: 361

Risteli L, Myllyla R, Kivirikko K 1976 Partial purification and characterization of collagen galactosyltransferase from chick embryos. Biochemical Journal 155: 145

Rucker R B, Murray J 1978 Cross-linking amino acids in collagen and elastin. American Journal of Clinical Nutrition 31: 1221

Russell J D, Russell S B, Trupin K M 1978 Differential effects of hydrocortisone on both growth and collagen metabolism of human fibroblasts from normal and keloid tissue. Journal of Cellular Physiology 97: 221

Ryhanen L 1976 Lysyl hydroxylase. Further purification and characterization of the enzyme from chick embryos and chick embryo cartilage. Biochimica et Biophysica Acta 438: 71

Ryhnaen L, Kivirikko K 1974 Hydroxylation of lysyl residues in native and denatured protocollagen by protocollagen lysyl hydroxylase in vitro. Biochimica et Biophysica Acta 343: 129

Sage H, Crouch E, Bornstein P 1979 Collagen synthesis by bovine aortic endothelial cells in culture. Biochemistry 18: 5433

Schofield J D, Uitto J, Prockop D J 1973 Formation of interchain disulfide bonds and helical structure during biosynthesis of procollagen by embryonic tendon cells. Biochemistry 13: 1801

Seifter S, Gallop P M 1966 The Structure Proteins. In: Neurath H (ed) The Proteins, Vol IV, 2nd edn. Academic Press, New York. ch 20, p 276

Seltzer J L, Jeffrey J J, Eisen A Z 1977 Evidence for mammalian collagenases as zinc ion metalloenzymes. Biochimica et Biophysica Acta 485: 179

Seltzer J L, Welgus H G, Jeffrey J J, Eisen A Z 1976 The function of Ca^{2+} in the action of mammalian collagenases. Archives of Biochemistry and Biophysics 173: 355

Shinkai H, Nagai Y 1977 A latent collagenase from embryonic human skin explants. Journal of Biochemistry 81: 1261

Siegel R C 1974 Biosynthesis of collagen cross-links: increased activity of purified lysyl oxidase with reconstituted collagen fibrils. Proceedings of the National Academy of Sciences USA 71: 4826

Siegel R C, Fu J C C 1976 Collagen cross-linking. Purification and specificity of lysyl oxidase. Journal of Biological Chemistry 251: 5779

Siegel R C, Pinnell S R, Martin G R Cross-linking of collagen and elastin. Properties of lysyl oxidase. Biochemistry 9: 4486

Smith B D, Byers P H, Martin G R 1972 Production of procollagen by human fibroblasts in culture. Proceedings of the National Academy of Sciences USA 69: 3260

Steinmann B, Gitzelmann R, Vogel A, Grant M E, Harwood R, Scar C H J 1975 Ehlers-Danlos syndrome in two siblings with deficient lysyl hydroxylase activity in cultured skin fibroblasts but only mild hydroxylysine deficit in skin. Helvetica Pediatrica Acta 30: 255

Stenn K S, Madri J A, Roll F J 1979 Migrating epidermis produces AB_2 collagen and requires continual collagen synthesis for movement. Nature 277: 229

Steven F S 1970 Polymeric collagen. In: Balazs E A (ed) Chemistry and molecular biology of the intercellular matrix. Academic Press, New York. p 43

Stricklin G P, Bauer E A, Jeffrey J J, Eisen A Z 1977 Human skin collagenase: isolation of precursor and active forms from both fibroblast and organ cultures. Biochemistry 16: 1607

Stricklin G P, Eisen A Z, Bauer E A, Jeffrey J J 1978 Human skin fibroblast collagenase: chemical properties of precursor and active forms. Biochemistry 17: 2331

Sussman M D, Lichtenstein J R, Nigra T, Martin G R, McKusick V A 1974 Hydroxylysine-deficient skin collagen in a patient with a form of Ehlers-Danlos syndrome. Journal of Bone and Joint Surgery 56A: 1228

Tan E M L, Uitto J, Bauer E A, Eisen A Z 1981 Human skin fibroblasts in culture: stimulation of procollagen synthesis by sera from normal human subjects and from patients with dermal fibroses. Journal of Investigative Dermatology 76: 462

Tanzer M L 1976 Cross-linking. In: Ramachandran G N, Reddi A H (eds) Biochemistry of collagen. Plenum, New York. p 137

Tanzer M L, Church R L, Yaeger J A, Wampler D E, Park E 1974 Procollagen: intermediate forms containing several types of peptide chains and noncollagen peptide extensions at NH_2 and COOH ends. Proceedings of the National Academy of Sciences USA 71: 3009

Trelstad R L, Hayaslir K, Gross J 1976 Collagen fibrillogenesis: intermediate aggregates and suprafibrillar order. Proceedings of the National Academy of Sciences USA 73: 4027

Tuderman L, Kivirikko K, Prockop D J 1978 Partial purification and characterization of a neutral protease which cleaves the N-terminal propeptides procollagen. Biochemistry 17: 2948

Tuderman L, Kuutti E-R, Kivirikko K 1975 Radioimmunoassay for human and chick prolyl hydroxylases. European Journal of Biochemistry 60: 399

Turto H, Lindy S, Uitto V-J, Wegelius O, Uitto J 1977 Human leukocyte collagenase. Characterization of enzyme kinetics by a new method. Analytical Biochemistry 83: 557

Uitto J 1972 Collagen biosynthesis in human skin. A review with emphasis on scleroderma. Annals of Clinical Research 3: 250

Uitto J 1979 Collagen polymorphism: isolation and partial characterization of α1(I)-trimer molecules in normal human skin. Archives of Biochemistry and Biophysics 192: 371

Uitto J, Booth B A, Polak J L 1981 Collagen biosynthesis by human skin fibroblasts. II. Isolation and further characterization of type I and type III procollagens synthesized in culture. Biochimica et Biophysica Acta, in press

Uitto J, Eisen A Z 1979 Collagen. In: Fitzpatrick T B, Eisen A Z, Wolff K, Freedberg I M, Austen K F (eds) Dermatology in general medicine. McGraw-Hill, New York. p 164

Uitto J, Halme J, Hannuksela M, Peltokallio P, Kivirikko K 1969 Protocollagen proline hydroxylase activity in the skin of normal human subjects and of patients with scleroderma. Scandinavian Journal of Clinical and Laboratory Investigation 23: 241

Uitto J, Hannuksela M, Rasmussen O 1970 Protocollagen proline hydroxylase activity in scleroderma and other connective tissue disorders. Annals of Clinical Research 2: 235

Uitto J, Tan E M L, Geltman E M, Rodey G E, Jaffe A S 1982 The Ehlers–Danlos syndrome type IV: clinical and biochemical studies in a family. In: Glimcher M, Bornstein P (eds) Workshop on inheritable disorders of connective tissue. C. V. Mosby, St. Louis

Uitto J, Lichtenstein J R 1976 Defects in the biochemistry of collagen in diseases of connective tissue. Journal of Investigative Dermatology 66: 59

Uitto J, Lichtenstein J R, Bauer E A 1976 Characterization of procollagen synthesized by matrix-free cells isolated from chick embryo tendons. Biochemistry 15: 4935

Uitto J, Ohlenschlaeger K, Lorenzen I 1971 Solubility of skin collagen in normal human subjects and patients with generalized scleroderma. Clinica Chimica Acta 31: 13

Uitto J, Prockop D J 1973 Rate of helix formation by intracellular procollagen and protocollagen. Evidence for a role for disulfide bonds. Biochemical and Biophysical Research Communications 55: 904

Uitto J, Prockop D J 1974a Biosynthesis of cartilage collagen. Influence of chain association and hydroxylation of prolyl residues on the folding of the polypeptides into the triple-helical conformation. Biochemistry 13: 4586

Uitto J, Prockop D J 1974b Hydroxylation of peptide-bound proline and lysine before and after chain completion of the polypeptide chains of procollagen. Archives of Biochemistry and Biophysics 164: 210

Uitto J, Prockop D J 1974c Molecular defects in collagen and the definition of 'collagen disease'. In: Good R A, Day S B, Yunis J J (eds) Molecular pathology. Thomas Springfield. p 670

Uitto J, Santa Cruz D J 1979 The Ehlers-Danlos syndrome (EDS) type IV: decreased synthesis of triple-helical type III procollagen by cultured skin fibroblasts. Journal of Investigative Dermatology 72: 274

Uitto V-J, Schwartz D, Veis A 1980 Degradation of basement membrane collagen by neutral proteases from human leukocytes. European Journal of Biochemistry 105: 409

Uitto V-J, Uitto J, Kao W W-Y, Prockop D J 1978 Procollagen polypeptides containing cis-4-hydroxy-L-proline are overglycosylated and secreted as non-helical pro-γ-chains. Archives of Biochemistry and Biophysics 185: 214

Valle K-J, Bauer E A 1979 Biosynthesis of collagenase by human skin fibroblasts in monolayer culture. Journal of Biological Chemistry 254: 10115

Vater C A, Harris E D, Siegel R C 1979 Native cross-links in collagen fibrils induce resistance to human synovial collagenase. Biochemical Journal 181: 639

Weber L, Meigel W N, Spier W 1978 Collagen polymorphism in pathologic human scars. Archives of Dermatological Research 261: 63

Welgus H G, Jeffrey J J, Eisen A Z 1981 The collagen substrate specificity of human skin fibroblast collagenase. Journal of Biological Chemistry 256: 9511

Welgus H G, Stricklin G P, Eisen A Z, Bauer E A, Cooney R V, Jeffrey J J 1979 A specific inhibitor of vertebrate collagenase produced by human skin fibroblasts. Journal of Biological Chemistry 254: 1938

Werb Z, Burleigh M C, Barrett A J, Starkey P M 1974 The interaction of α_2-macroglobulin with proteinases. Binding and inhibition of mammalian collagenases and other metal proteinases. Biochemical Journal 139: 359

Wiestner M, Kreig T, Horlein D, Glanville R W, Fietzek P, Müller P K 1979 Inhibiting effect of procollagen peptides on collagen biosynthesis in fibroblast cultures. Journal of Biological Chemistry 254: 7016

Woolley D E, Roberts D R, Evanson J M 1975 Inhibition of human collagenase activity by a small molecular weight serum protein. Biochemical and Biophysical Research Communications 66: 747

Woolley D E, Roberts D R, Evanson J M 1976 Small molecular weight β_1 serum protein which specifically inhibits collagenases. Nature 261: 235

29

Teeth

H. BIRKEDAL-HANSEN

INTRODUCTION

The tooth and its periodontium are composed of a number of distinct collagenous tissues. Each tissue serves one or more specialized functions required for the overall performance of the tooth as a delicate tool and a powerful weapon. Dental structure is closely related to function. To emphasize this point, details of the micromorphology of the individual tissues will be included in this chapter as needed. Each tooth is composed of a hollow core of dentin covered by enamel (crown) or cementum (root) (Fig. 29.1). The central part of the crown and root is made up of a loose connective tissue, the pulp. The dense connective tissue located between cementum and alveolar bone is the periodontal membrane. It is instrumental in securing anchorage of the tooth in the jaw by means of dense collagen fibre bundles (Sharpey's fibres) which insert in cementum on one side and in alveolar bone on the other. The periodontal membrane is continuous with the connective tissue of the gingiva, which connects the tooth with the oral mucosa.

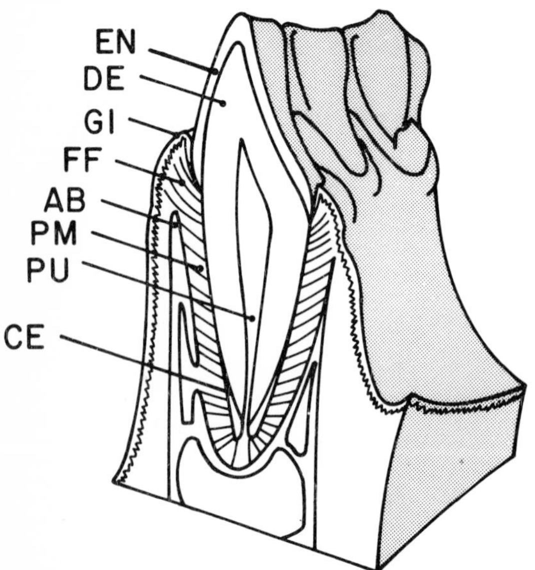

Fig. 29.1 Block diagram showing the relations between dental and supporting tissues. EN, enamel; DE, dentin; GI, gingiva; FF, free gingival fibres; AB, alveolar bone; PM, periodontal membrane, Sharpey's fibres; PU, pulp; CE, dental cementum.

ODONTOGENESIS

The formation of a tooth constitutes a wealth of complex and fascinating differentiation processes, epithelial-mesenchymal interactions, inductive effects and involutions which have often served as models in developmental biology. The cyto- and histodifferentiation in odontogenesis has been described in great detail at the light- and electron microscopic levels and recently the advent of monospecific antibodies to the different collagen types and their precursors has shed considerable light into extracellular matrix changes during odontogenesis.

Proliferation of the oral epithelium into the underlying menenchyme is the first histological evidence of odontogenesis. It leads to the formation of a continuous epithelial ridge, the dental lamina, which, in time, gives rise to all the teeth of the primary and permanent dentitions. From the dental lamina epithelial cells proliferate locally to form a small 'knot' which, together with underlying mesenchymal cells, constitute the early (bud stage) tooth germ (Fig. 29.2A). At this stage, epithelial and mesenchymal components are separated by a basement membrane which reacts strongly with antibodies to type IV collagen and fibronectin (Lesot et al, 1978; Thesleff et al, 1979). Gradually, the lower surface of the epithelial bud invaginates while the edges continue to proliferate deeper into the mesenchyme to give rise to a shell-shaped structure reminiscent of a tooth crown. At the same time the mesenchymal cells 'inside' the invagination proliferate to form a cell rich tissue, the dental papilla, which in time gives rise to both dentin and dental pulp (Fig. 29.2B). The shape and the size of the crown changes rapidly while the tooth germ passes through so-called 'cap' and 'bell' stages. The dental papilla, like the surrounding mesenchyme, initially produces both type I and III collagens. Along with its development into odontogenic mesenchyme, however, there is a marked decline in type III synthesis in the central

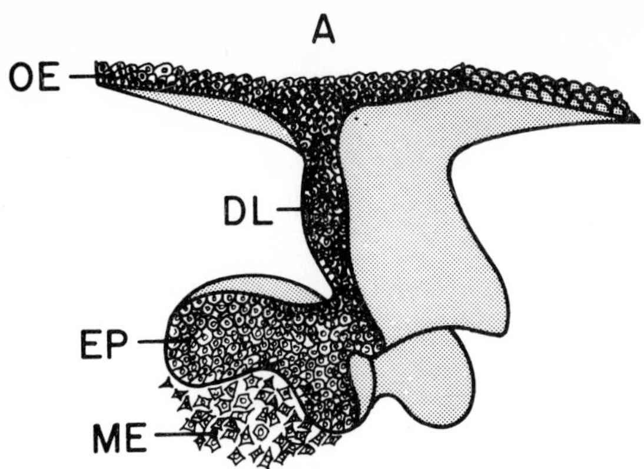

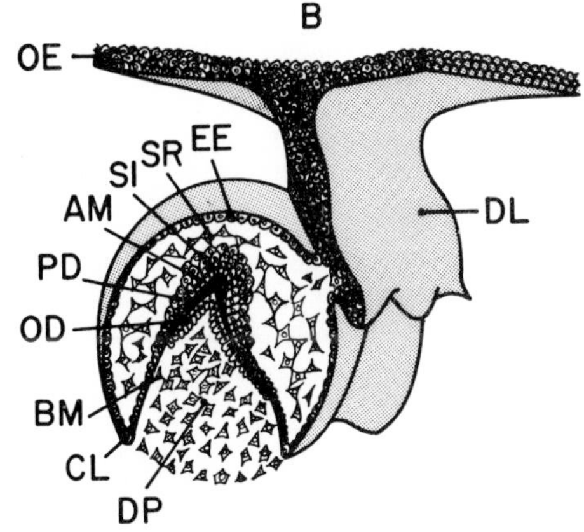

Fig. 29.2 Stages of development of a tooth crown. (A) *Bud stage.* The dental lamina (DL) which originates from the oral epithelium (OE) locally forms small proliferating epithelial 'buds' (EP). The lower surface has started to invaginate while the cells of the surrounding mesenchyme (ME) condense to form the early dental papilla. (B) *Bell stage.* The invagination has deepened and the epithelium has differentiated into several distinct epithelial structures, all of which participate in enamel formation. At the tip of the invagination the cells of the enamel epithelium (EE) have differentiated into ameloblasts (AM) which will soon start enamel matrix secretion. 'Outer' and 'inner' enamel epithelial cells (EE) remain separated from the mesenchyme by a basement membrane (BM). Stratum intermedium (SI) and the stellate reticulum (SR) occupy the space between the 'outer' and 'inner' enamel epithelium. On the mesenchymal side of the basement membrane odontoblasts (OD) have developed from the dental papilla (DP) and have started to secrete predentin (PD). Elongation of the crown is achieved by continued apical growth of the epithelial cells of the cervical loop (CL).

and incisal/cuspal part of the papilla, whereas type III synthesis continues around the proliferating edges (Thesleff et al, 1979). At the 'bottom' of the invagination (incisal/cuspal area), where the development is always most advanced, there is a complete stop of collagen type III synthesis.

During the cap and bell stages a number of distinct cell layers differentiate, each destined to play a unique role in the following formation of the tooth. On the inner side of the basement membrane, cells of the dental papilla differentiate into a seam of tall columnar odontoblasts, while epithelial cells on the other side of the basement membrane develop into ameloblasts. Initially, these two cell layers are in close contact, separated only by the basement membrane. At late bell stage, matrix synthesis starts with odontoblast secretion of predentin against the basement membrane (Fig. 29.2B). The matrix reacts strongly for collagen type I. Moreover, Thesleff et al (1979) noted staining with antisera against type III collagen in predentin but not in (mineralized) dentin. Cournil et al (1979) described a similar faint staining of predentin, but found that it disappeared after thorough absorption of the antibody preparation with type I collagen. Consequently, they interpreted the predentin type III collagen staining as an unspecific reaction. The presence, or not, of small amounts of type III collagen in normal predentin is of considerable interest since this type of collagen has recently been detected in mineralized dentin from patients suffering from osteogenesis and dentinogenesis imperfecta (Sauk et al, 1980) (see p. 495).

Ameloblasts start to secrete and mineralize the enamel matrix shortly after the odontoblasts have initiated predentin formation. Enamel does not contain collagen of any type. Mineralization of predentin starts when a zone of approximately 20 μm of unmineralized matrix has been laid down. Mineralization of dentin is an all or none process. Even with the resolution of the electron microscope, the transition between (mineralized) dentin and (unmineralized) predentin is quite abrupt. When dentin starts to mineralize, the basement membrane disappears (Eisenmann & Glick, 1972; Cournil et al, 1979).

The processes described above continue until the entire crown has been formed. When it has attained its final size, the cells of the odontogenic epithelium regroup to prepare for root formation. In the dental papilla, the development of odontoblasts and the secretion of dentin continues as before. The epithelium, which migrates in an apical direction, now consists of only a few cell layers without the intermediary layers characteristic of amelogenesis (stratum intermedium and stellate reticulum). This epithelium, which no longer engages in matrix secretion, is finally penetrated and disrupted by mesenchymal cells from the surroundings. These cells differentiate into *cementoblasts*, which form the cementum matrix, or into *fibroblasts*, which form the periodontal membrane. At some distance from the root surface, mesenchymal cells have already started to form the bone of the alveolar process and the jaw.

The role of collagenous matrices in the formation of a tooth is obvious. Evidence suggests that even at a very early stage the collagenous matrices play an important role in morphodifferentiation (Galbraith & Kollar, 1976). If collagen synthesis is impaired, for instance by addition in vitro of L-azetidine-2-carboxylic acid, a nonfunctional proline analogue, the subsequent morphodifferentiation is grossly affected. Addition to such cultures of exogenous procollagen partially reverses the effect. This was interpreted as evidence that the cells are able to process exogenous procollagen type I to support morphodifferentiation in tooth rudiments unable to synthesize procollagen themselves (Galbraith & Kollar, 1976). In similar experiments, addition of α, α-dipyridyl, a Fe^{2+}-chelator and hydroxylation inhibitor, to mouse molar rudiments rather surprisingly showed that the basal lamina (lamina densa) remained unaffected while the sub-basal fibrillar network disappeared within a day or two (Hetem et al, 1975). So, apparently the lamina densa collagen is turned over much slower than that of the sub-basal fibrillar network. Evidence of the role played by the basement membrane in odontoblast differentiation has been derived from in vitro experiments (Thesleff et al, 1978). After enzymatic dissociation of the embryonic tooth germ into its epithelial and mesenchymal components and intercalation of a controlled-pore-size filter, differentiation of odontoblasts on the mesenchymal side took place only if direct contact was established between the mesenchymal cells and the reformed (epithelial) basement membrane. The odontoblasts failed to differentiate if the basement membrane was not reformed.

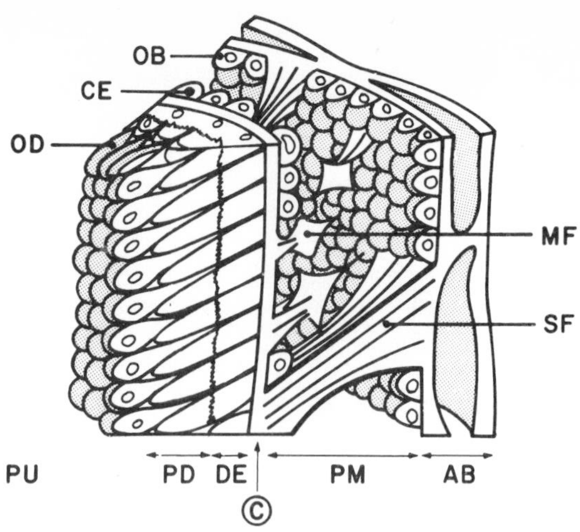

Fig. 29.3 Block diagram showing segment of tooth and supporting structures. Odontoblasts (OD) form dentin (DE) and predentin (PD) while gradually retreating into the pulp chamber (PU). A thin cytoplasmic process (Tomes' process) is left behind in the dentin and predentin matrices. The periodontal membrane connects the cementum (C) of the tooth with the alveolar bone of the jaw (AB) by means of dense Sharpey's fibre bundles (SF). Cementoblasts (CE) and osteoblasts (OB) secrete the respective tissue matrices. Sharpey's fibres are formed by fibroblasts (MF) which migrate from one hard tissue surface to the other while laying down a cable of collagen.

NORMAL DENTAL TISSUES

Dentin

Dentin is a highly mineralized tissue which forms the major part of the tooth. It is penetrated by numerous tubules ($\simeq$35 000 per mm^2) which extend through the entire width of the dentin (Fig. 29.3). The pulpal 1/3 of the length of each tubule is occupied by a cytoplasmic process extending from the corresponding odontoblast (Thomas, 1979). Each tubule represents the track of the movement of an odontoblast during dentinogenesis. The odontoblasts remain throughout life and continue to form dentin although at highly reduced rates with increasing age. Moreover, they serve as a dormant pool of cells which can be activated to resume rapid dentin formation in repair processes in connection with trauma or dental caries.

Demineralized dentin matrix is composed of tightly packed cross-banded collagen fibres without any distinctive pattern. Fibre diameters range from 200 to 700 A and increase throughout the predentin (Jessen, 1967; Johannesen & Bang, 1972). This has been interpreted as continued apposition of collagen molecules to the fibres during dentin formation.

In dentin as well as predentin, collagen is by far the major organic constituent. Noncollagenous proteins and proteoglycans account for only a few per cent of the matrix (Linde, 1973; Butler et al, 1979). However, this small noncollagenous fraction may be instrumental in the regulation of the precisely timed mineralization process (Weinstock & Leblond, 1973). Chemical and histochemical studies have indicated some differences in the composition of dentin and predentin, predominantly with regard to non-collagenous, acidic components such as phosphoproteins and proteoglycans (Weinstock & Leblond, 1973; Birkedal-Hansen, 1974; Carmichael et al, 1975).

Small amounts of collagen may be extracted from the predentin and odontoblast layers whereas the collagen of dentin itself is quite insoluble in neutral and acidic solvents and remains largely insoluble even under denaturing conditions (Carmichael et al, 1974; Munksgaard, 1979). Limited clevage with pepsin, known to release the major portion of skin and cartilage collagens, in dentin solubilizes only a minor fraction (Carmichael et al, 1977). Attempts to increase the soluble collagen fraction in animals by dietary supplements with the cross-link inhibitor β-aminopropionitrile have only been partly successful (Carmichael et al, 1974; Wolhllebe & Carmichael, 1979). It has, therefore, been suggested that the intermolecular cross-links of dentin collagen differ in some important ways from those of other tissues for instance by connecting the *helical* domains of two neighbouring molecules (Scott et al, 1976; Carmichael et al, 1973). Studies employing $NaB[^3H]_4$ reduction followed by characterization of the products released by acid hydrolysis have revealed several distinct reducible cross-links in dentin collagen. Dehydro-

$(OH)_2$-Lys-Norleu was the predominant type and one such cross-link is found per four collagen molecules (Mechanic et al, 1974; Carmichael et al, 1975; Scott et al, 1976; Kuboki et al, 1977 (See Ch. 9).

Studies aimed at identifying and characterizing dentin collagen have relied heavily on denatured chains extracted under dissociative conditions and on peptides generated from the insoluble residue by limited cleavage with CNBr (Volpin & Veis, 1973; Scott et al, 1976; Wohllebe & Carmichael, 1979). This peptide mapping technique has revealed that dentin matrix contains exclusively type I collagen with the chain composition $[\alpha\ 1\ (I)]_2\ \alpha_2\ (I)$ (Scott et al, 1976; Wohllebe & Carmichael, 1979). Amino acid analyses of insoluble dentin type I collagen and of the individual CNBr peptides have revealed a high degree of lysyl hydroxylation, as much as three times higher than in skin (Butler, 1973). Recent studies have not been able to substantiate early claims of presence of type III collagen in normal dentin (Volpin & Veis, 1973; Dodd & Carmichael, 1979). On the other hand, organ culture experiments have suggested that odontoblasts synthesize and secrete large amounts of a type I trimer with the chain composition $[\alpha 1\ (I)]_3$ (Munksgaard et al, 1978). Although the trimer has been extracted from rat and bovine predentin, this variant is a very minor component of dentin collagen in vivo (Wohllebe & Carmichael, 1978; Munksgaard, 1979).

Because of their polarity odontoblasts lend themselves well to the study of biosynthetic pathways in collagen secreting cells. The initial subcellular route of collagen synthesis is quite similar to that of other export proteins (Weinstock, 1972; Karim et al, 1979; Weinstock & Leblond, 1974). The packaging of the collagen in the odontoblasts prior to secretion, however, is quite unique. Saccules containing collagenous components can be identified at the endoplasmatic reticulum and the Golgi complex (Wesnstock, 1972; Karim et al, 1979). These saccules are gradually condensed and displaced to the peripheral parts of the cell while their contents become more and more reminiscent of SLS- or FLS-aggregates (See Ch. 1) before they are secreted to the dentin at the base of the odontoblast process (Weinstock & Leblond, 1974). It is of note that similar SLS-like structures have been identified in the extracellular predentin matrix in the vicinity of the odontoblast process (Warshawsky, 1972; Weinstock, 1977). Moreover, immunohistochemical studies have shown that predentin is endowed with type I procollagen, particularly the most newly synthesized matrix. The precise interpretation of these findings is unclear, but it has recently been suggested from another set of data that collagen fibrillogenesis may take place from intracellularly assembled procollagen FLS/SLS- aggregates (Bruns et al, 1979). It is conceivable then, that the SLS aggregates found in the predentin have been secreted as such but have yet failed to participate in fibril formation.

Not all matrix proteins follow the same schedule for extracellular processing. While collagen is laid down to form a new matrix at the predentin/odontoblast junction, phosphoproteins rapidly move through the predentin and are immobilized at the mineralization front (Weinstock & Leblond, 1973). The finding that phosphoproteins bind to collagen fibres right at the mineralization front has placed these proteins in a central role in the current concepts of regulation of dentin mineralization.

Once formed, the dentin matrix is quite stable and its collagen fibres are not turned over at a measurable rate (Borggreven et al, 1979). Only during shedding of the primary dentition is dentin again degraded. In that process, the entire root, cementum and dentin, matrices and minerals, are removed by multi-nucleated giant cells in a precisely timed and well regulated process.

Cementum

Cementum covers the root dentin and forms the dental side of the tooth suspension apparatus. In certain respects, cementum is closely related to bone but it deviates from bone in its lack of physiological remodelling and its relative acellularity. It is produced cooperatively by cementoblasts and fibroblasts, both derived from the periodontal membrane. The cementoblasts form a collagenous matrix with fibres parallel to the tooth surface (matrix fibres) while the fibroblasts form Sharpey's fibres perpendicular to the root surface and continuous with the dense fibre bundles of the periodontal membrane. The cementoblast may eventually become incorporated into the matrix, particularly in the apical region. In the cervical half of the root the cementum layer remains thin and acellular. The mineralization pattern is similar to that of bone. Crystals grow from discrete nuclei in the matrix and eventually form confluent mineralized foci. The core of the Sharpey's fibres, however, often remains unmineralized (Selvig, 1965). In certain species (rodents, herbivores) a thin layer of mineralized cementum-like tissue covers the enamel of the crown (Glimcher et al, 1964; Ainamo, 1970; Listgarten & Shapiro, 1974). A similar type of tissue may even be found in the fissures of human teeth (Silness et al, 1978). It is probably formed by mesenchymal cells which have penetrated the reduced enamel epithelium after enamel formation has been completed.

Early biochemical studies by Rodriguez & Wilderman (1972) confirmed the collagenous nature of cementum matrix. Cementum collagen is highly insoluble in acid and neutral solvents so the chain composition is best deduced from peptide mapping studies. CNBr peptide analyses have shown that demineralized bovine cementum is composed of type I collagen with a small admixture (less than 5 per cent) of type III (Birkedal-Hansen et al, 1977). These findings have recently gained support from immunofluorescent studies of the collagen type distribution in porcine periodontal tissues (Wang et al, 1980). It was shown that affinity purified, type specific anti-type III collagen stained Sharpey's fibre bundles which enter the cementum while other areas of the cementum matrix were unstained. In human teeth, however, Christner et al (1977) found no evidence of type III collagen. Cementum collagen has fewer reducible cross-links per molecule than dentin but, as in dentin, dehydro- $(OH)_2$- Lys-Norleu is the predominant reducible cross-link (Chovelon et al, 1975).

Gingiva and periodontal membrane

Collagen fibres are by far the major constituents of periodontal membrane and gingiva. The fibrils are assembled in bundles to form the *Sharpey's* fibres of the periodontal membrane and the *free gingival fibres* of the gingiva (Fig. 29.1). Autoradiographic data indicate that these fibre bundles are formed by fibroblasts which originate from the hard tissue surface and migrate across the periodontal space while leaving behind a heavy collagen cable (Garant & Cho 1979 a,b). Thus, each collagen fibre represents the track of a migrating fibroblast (Fig. 29.3). These findings are in keeping with newer concepts of collagen fibrillogenesis which suggest the fibril assembly takes place on the cell membrane and not in a random process in the surrounding tissue fluid (Trelstad & Hayashi, 1979). A mechanism such as this can more readily explain how genetically determined parameters such as fibre direction and fibre thickness remain under direct cellular control (Garant & Cho, 1979 a,b).

In humans and in certain animal species 10 to 30 per cent of the collagen of gingival and palatal mucosa can be solubilized in salt and dilute acid solutions (Schneir et al, 1975). Studies employing peptide mapping of the insoluble collagen fraction have provided evidence for the presence of both type I and type III collagen in gingiva and in periodontal membrane (Butler et al, 1975; Dabbous et al, 1979; Wang et al, 1980). Estimates of the proportion of type III relative to type I collagen have varied from 10 to 25 per cent. Similar figures were arrived at from another angle in studies of collagen biosynthesis in the rat periodontal membrane (Limeback & Sodek, 1979; Sodek & Limeback, 1979). These studies, moreover, suggested that type III collagen accumulates in the tissue in an intermediary proform. Both type I and type III are synthesized by periodontal membrane and gingival fibroblasts in culture at a ratio which can be modulated by the culture conditions (Narayan & Page, 1977; Limeback & Sodek, 1979; Engel et al, 1980) and therefore may not reflect the proportions secreted by the same cells in vivo. This is further reflected in the finding that gingival fibroblasts, like odontoblasts, secrete relatively high levels of type I trimer in vitro (Narayan & Page, 1976). The cross-links of the insoluble collagens of gingiva and periodontal membrane were investigated by Pearson et al (1975). As in other dental tissues the major cross-link identified after borohydride reduction was dehydro-$(OH)_2$-Lys-Norleu.

Collagen remodelling is faster in gingiva and periodontal membrane than at perhaps any other site (Kameyama, 1975; Rippin, 1976; Orlowski, 1976, 1978). In a comparative study, Sodek (1977) calculated a collagen turnover time of 2 days in rat periodontal membrane as opposed to 15 days in skin. Rapid periodontal remodelling is an expression of the continuous demand for break-down and reformation of collagen fibres in the adjustment of the teeth to one another and to the jaws. As an obvious example, the continuously erupting rat incisor moves at a rate of 0.5 mm per day relative to the jaw while maintaining its anchorage to the alveolar bone. Just how this is accomplished at the cellular level is not known in detail and it does represent a number of unresolved logistic problems. Two mechanisms seem possible: (1) fibroblasts in the periodontal membrane may sever existing fibres and reunite their fragments with others and with new fibres. It is an intriguing and almost inescapable possibility that periodontal fibroblasts can open and reunite periodontal collagen fibres which remain embedded with both ends in mineralized tissue; alternatively (2) periodontal fibroblasts may continually differentiate at the hard tissue surface, migrate across the periodontal membrane and insert new collagen fibres in the opposing hard tissue surface. Recent studies indicate that gingival and periodontal fibroblasts *are* polarized and that migration across the periodontal membrane *does* take place in the direction from the alveolar bone towards the cementum (Garant & Cho, 1979 a,b). These studies have, moreover, shown that the migrating cells on their way lay down a continuous collagen cable (see p. 490). However, insertion of new fibres in the hard tissue surface for all practical purposes is only possible on the bone side where remodelling is quite rapid. Reinsertion of new fibres in cementum would be entirely dependent on new cementum formation, a process which is extremely slow in the coronal part of the root.

The cellular events involved in the rapid removal of collagen in the periodontal membrane have not been satisfactorily accounted for either. Periodontal fibroblasts are often seen in the process of apparently engulfing whole collagen fibres (Listgarten, 1973; Yajima & Rose, 1977; Beertsen et al, 1978; Schellens et al, 1979). Although assembling collagen fibres in plasma membrane clefts give rise to very similar electron microscopic pictures (Trelstad & Hayashi, 1979), in vitro studies have strongly indicated that 'phagocytic' mechanisms may take part in the initial fragmentation of the fibres (Svoboda et al, 1979). On the other hand, there is little reason to doubt that the extracellular non-lysosomal protease collagenase, which is produced in large quantities by gingival and periodontal fibroblasts (Birkedal-Hansen et al, 1976 a,b) is involved in the collagen degradation process. A possible link between these apparently conflicting biochemical and ultrastructural data may exist, however, if collagenase proves to be a plasma membrane-associated enzyme. Although this idea has been expressed by several investigators, there is still very little data to support it (Horton et al, 1978).

Dental pulp

The dental pulp constitutes the remnant of the dental papilla which plays an important role in early odontogenesis. The pulp consists of a loose, highly vascularized connective tissue which serves throughout life to provide nutrients for the odontoblast layer. With continued dentin formation the pulp chamber gradually narrows over the years and the pulp becomes atrophic and fibrous. Studies of pulpal collagens employing biochemical and immunofluorescent techniques have revealed fibres of both type I and type III collagens (Lesot et al, 1978; Rao et al, 1979; Cournil et al, 1979; Shuttleworth et al, 1980). Staining with antibodies against type IV collagen, as expected, gave a marked reaction with the blood vessel walls of the dental papillae (Lesot et al, 1978; Thesleff et al, 1979).

Alveolar bone

The alveolar bone constitutes the 'jaw-side' of the suspension apparatus. The histological picture is dominated by the numerous Sharpey's fibres which enter from the periodontal membrane. Movement of the teeth during growth, development and ageing is accomplished entirely by remodelling of the walls of the bone socket. As a consequence, alveolar bone is constantly being rebuilt by intermittent formation and resorption. The biochemistry and pathology of bone collagen will be dealt with in detail elsewhere (see Ch. 19).

PATHOLOGICAL DENTAL TISSUES

Pathological formation or destruction of collagen are integral parts of a number of diseases of the oral cavity. Rather than surveying systematically the various dental diseases, most of which have virtually unknown pathogenic mechanisms, the following includes only the most interesting in the context of collagen metabolism. Collagen turnover rates of dental and periodontal tissues span the entire spectrum; it is extremely fast in gingiva and periodontal membrane while hardly measurable in cementum and dentin. These differences are clearly reflected in the types of diseases seen in each tissue. Most abnormalities which affect the slowly remodelling, or stationary, dental tissues such as dentin and cementum are acquired at the time when that particular part of the tooth is being formed. These tissues leave a permanent record of past insults and toxic influences. A number of local and systemic diseases experienced during early childhood may cause visible alterations of the dentin but only in a few of these are the specific mechanisms known (Pindborg, 1970).

Gingival hyperplasia

Certain hydantoin derivatives used in the treatment of epilepsy (5, 5-diphenylhydantoin) cause massive gingival hyperplasia in a large proportion of the patients. The mechanism of action of the drug in this regard, and the reason for its very tissue selective hyperplastic effect, are largely unknown. It has been suggested that the bacterial plaque which accumulates at the gingival margin serves as a local irritant necessary to promote the hyperplastic development. The hyperplastic gingiva consists of dense connective tissue dominated by type I collagen and with the same proportion of type III collagen as in normal gingiva (Ballard & Butler, 1974; Schneir et al, 1978). Fibroblasts isolated from the affected tissue produce collagen at a considerably faster rate than control cells (Hassel et al, 1976), but morphometric studies have shown a normal cell to fibre ratio in the affected tissue. Impairment of cellular growth control is therefore a more likely explanation of the gingival overgrowth than increased collagen formation by existing cells. Similarly, amino acid analyses of isolated collagen chains have *not* been able to substantiate that diphenylhydantoin inhibition of prolyl hydroxylation, as discovered in vitro (Liu & Bhatnagar, 1973, Blumenkrantz & Asboe-Hansen, 1974), plays a role in the pathogenesis (Schneir et al, 1978).

Periodontal disease

Periodontal disease is a chronic inflammatory condition which leads to gradual break-down of periodontal supporting structures and, finally, to loss of the teeth. It deserves detailed consideration because of its chronic, selectively destructive character. The break-down is a result of a gingival inflammation caused by bacteria accumulating in the vicinity of the gingival margin. At this location the micro-organisms are essentially out of reach of normal connective tissue defense mechanisms but close enough to influence adjoining epithelial and connective tissues by endotoxins, antigens and enzymes. The tissue response is a persisting chronic inflammation dominated by lymphocytes and plasma cells (Schroeder et al, 1973). Incident to this, the junctional epithelium separates from the enamel surface and a crevice is formed which permits further colonization by micro-organisms. During this process, gingival collagen is degraded and a recent study has indicated that type III collagen is broken down faster than type I (Hammouda et al, 1980). The lesion advances in apical direction with subsequent break-down of periodontal membrane and bone. The cementum, however, is not degraded. Loss of periodontal membrane and of alveolar bone is detrimental to the support and anchorage of the teeth in the jaw.

The persistence of a bacterial plaque which continues to

serve as an antigen is a key factor in the failure of the abortive healing efforts mounted by the tissue. Since the causative agent cannot be effectively removed a balance is established in which periodontal tissue is slowly sacrificed while host and parasite both remain 'alive'. Regeneration of Sharpey's fibres and of a functional periodontal membrane is possible under certain circumstances and does take place after trans- and replantation of exarticulated teeth. However, in periodontal disease two factors render healing much less favourable even if the plaque micro-organisms were removed: the destructed bone does not spontaneously grow back to its original level and the proliferating crevicular epithelium prevents reformation of continuous periodontal fibres.

Substantial interest has been devoted to the cellular mechanisms involved in collagen degradation both in normal and diseased periodontium. The permanent gingival cell population has a large potential for collagen breakdown as expected from the high normal turnover rate. As in skin, both collagen- and collagenase synthesis are much faster at the epithelial/connective tissue interface than deeper in the tissue, most likely because of the constant demand for remodelling at this particular area (Reddick et al, 1974; Birkedal-Hansen et al, 1976a; Pettigrew et al, 1978). Among the transient cells, PMN leucocytes and macrophages, which constitute 2 per cent each of the cells of inflamed gingiva, are capable of releasing collagenase to the surroundings (Lazarus et al, 1972; Horwitz & Crystal, 1976). Moreover, experimental evidence suggests that endotoxin and/or antigens released by plaque micro-organisms activate the macrophage population to secrete collagenase (Wahl et al, 1974, 1975).

The role of the crevicular epithelium in periodontal collagen break-down is an important, yet unresolved question. The main question to be answered is whether the epithelial cells migrate passively into the space opened to them during the inflammatory tissue destruction or make their way along the root surface by degrading the collagen fibres. Production of collagenase by gingival epithelial cells seems to occur only, or predominantly, in inflamed gingiva (Fullmer et al, 1969; Birkedal-Hansen et al, 1976a). A similar difference may exist between epithelial cells from normal and inflamed areas with respect to secretion of plasminogen activator (Lucas 1977). The plasminogen/plasmin system may be involved in collagen break-down and its regulation in a number of different ways. Plasmin serves as a potent activator of procollagenase (Eekhout & Vaes, 1977; Werb et al, 1978). It is well documented that it does not cleave type I collagen but its effect on other collagen types has not yet been sufficiently explored. It is conceivable that the gingival inflammation can induce secretion of collagenase and plasminogen activator in epithelial cells although direct evidence is still lacking and other roles for epithelial cells in modulating collagen metabolism are indeed possible. One such role has recently been indicated by the discovery of epithelial-mesenchymal cell interactions which result in increased collagenase secretion by fibroblasts in co-culture with epithelial cells (Johnson-Mueller & Gross, 1978).

The junctional epithelium allows passage of small amounts of interstitial body fluids from the connective tissue to the crevice. This 'crevicular fluid' can be collected by various means and its volume and composition can be determined and used as an inflammation parameter (Cimasoni, 1974). If the gingiva is inflamed, the crevicular fluid contains collagenase, elastase and complement cleavage products (Ohlsson et al, 1973; Golub et al, 1979; Kowashi et al, 1979; Patters et al, 1979). In the inflamed gingiva part, or maybe all, of this activity originated from the large number of PMN leucocytes which transmigrate the crevicular epithelium and pass to the oral cavity through the sulcus in an attempt to clear the pocket for micro-organisms. The identification of these compounds in the inflammatory exudate of the crevice underlines the potential significance of these enzymes and provides evidence that they are indeed operative in periodontal disease although their relative importance for the overall disease picture has not yet been established.

Vitamin C deficiency

Ascorbate, a co-factor for peptide hydroxylation, plays a key role in collagen formation. The effect of vitamin C deficiency on periodontal collagen metabolism has been known since the early, month-long sea voyages brought about the full complement of this avitaminosis. Loosening or loss of the teeth due to break-down of the periodontal structures were frequent symptoms. The aetiology most likely was a combination of an avitaminosis and a plaque induced periodontal disease resulting in a rampant net tissue break-down. In retrospect, it is clear that collagen metabolism was grossly affected in the terminal stages of the disease. Such severe cases are not seen any longer. In fact it has proven difficult to recreate the periodontal symptom complex in experimental vitamin C deficiency (Crandon et al, 1940; Burrill, 1946). Studies in guinea pigs have revealed that dentin formation may also be affected. Instead of normal dentin, an irregular, mineralized tissue is formed on the walls of the pulpal chamber (Pindborg, 1970).

Osteogenesis and dentinogenesis imperfecta

In the heritable disorder, dentinogenesis imperfecta, pathological changes are restricted to the teeth. The skeletal system remains unaffected. The enamel is poorly attached to the soft, underlying dentin. It readily fractures off and leaves the dentin core defenseless to abrasion. Characteristically, the pulp chamber is diminished or absent. Similar dental changes are seen in osteogenesis imperfecta along with the systemic abnormalities. Both are believed to affect matrix formation and mineralization although the pathogenic mechanism is unknown. Biosynthetic studies have suggested that fibroblasts derived from osteogenesis imperfecta patients have a deficient regulation of collagen synthesis resulting in an abnormally high proportion of type III collagen (Pentinen et al, 1975; Mueller et al, 1975; Fuji et al, 1977). Of considerable interest is the recent finding that dentin from both groups of patients stain positively for type III collagen with monospecific antibodies (Sauk et al, 1980). As previously mentioned, there is some uncertainty with respect to the presence of type III collagen in rodent predentin while it is generally accepted that it is absent in normal dentin irrespective of species. Its presence in dentin from osteogenesis imperfecta patients again raises the question whether collagen type III is in fact a transient component of predentin which is normally degraded before mineralization.

CONCLUSION

Apart from enamel hypoplasia, all dental diseases involve collagenous matrices one way or the other. Clearly, these diseases fall into two distinct categories set apart primarily by the rate of remodelling of the affected tissue. Dentin and cementum (and even enamel) are not remodelled and have essentially no repair mechanisms. As a consequence, defects acquired during their development remain throughout life. In contrast, diseases which affect the remodelling tissues, alveolar bone, gingiva and periodontal membrane are reversible and the damage can be amended. Examples include acute inflammatory conditions and traumatic injuries which heal very quickly and leave no cumulative, permanent record. That this is not the case in chronic periodontitis, the major disease of dental collagenous tissues, is largely due to the persistence of the causative micro-organisms.

REFERENCES

Ainamo J 1970 Morphogenetic and functional characteristics of coronal cementum in bovine molars. Scandinavian Journal of Dental Research 78: 378

Ballard J B, Butler W T 1974 Proteins of the Periodontium. Biochemical studies on the collagen and noncollagenous proteins of human gingivae. Journal of Oral Pathology 3: 176

Beertsen W, Brekelmans M, Everts V 1978 The site of collagen resorption in the periodontal ligament of the rodent molar. Anatomical Record 192: 305

Birkedal-Hansen H 1974 Distribution of carbohydrates in demineralized paraffin sections of the rat jaw. Scandinavian Journal of Dental Research 82: 113

Birkedal-Hansen H, Cobb C M, Taylor R E, Fullmer H M 1976a Fibroblastic origin of gingival collagenase. Archives of Oral Biology 21: 297

Birkedal-Hansen H, Cobb C M, Taylor R E, Fullmer H M 1976b Synthesis and release of procollagenase by cultured fibroblasts. Journal of Biological Chemistry 251: 3162

Birkedal-Hansen H, Butler W T, Taylor R E 1977 Proteins of the periodontium. Calcified Tissue Research 23: 39

Blumenkrantz N, Asboe-Hansen G 1974 Effect of diphenylhydantoin on connective tissue. Acta Neurologica Scandinavica 50: 302

Borggreven P M, Hoppenbrouwers P M M, Gorissen R 1979 Radiochemical determination of the metabolic activity of collagen in mature dentin. Journal of Dental Research 58: 2120

Bruns R R, Hulmes D J S, Therrien S F, Gross J 1979 Procollagen segment-long-spacing crystallites: their role in collagen fibrillogenesis. Proceedings of the National Academy of Sciences (USA) 76: 313

Burrill D Y 1946 Oral condition in experimental vitamin C and B deficiency. Journal of the American Dental Association 33: 594

Butler W T, Birkedal-Hansen H, Beegle W F, Taylor R E, Chung E 1975 Proteins of the periodontium. Identification of collagens with the $\alpha 1(I)_2\alpha 2$ and $\alpha 1(III)_3$ structures in bovine periodontal ligament. Journal of Biological Chemistry 250: 8907

Butler W T, Munksgaard E C, Richardson III W W 1979 Dentin proteins: chemistry, structure and biosynthesis. Journal of Dental Research 58(B): 817

Carmichael D J, Chovelon A, Pearson C H 1975 The composition of the insoluble collagenous matrix of bovine predentine. Calcified Tissue Research 17: 263

Carmichael D J, Dodd C M, Veis A 1977 The solubilization of bone and dentin collagens by pepsin. Effect of cross-linkages and noncollagen components. Biochimica et Biophysica Acta 491: 177

Carmichael D J, Dodd C M, Nawrot C F 1974 Studies on matrix proteins of normal and lathyritic rat bone and dentine. Calcified Tissue Research 14: 177

Chovelon A, Carmichael D J, Pearson C H 1975 The composition of the organic matrix of bovine cementum. Archives of Oral Biology 20: 537

Cimasoni G 1974 The crevicular fluid. In: Myers H M (ed) Monographs in Oral Science Vol 3. Karger, Basel

Christner P, Robinson P, Clark C C 1977 A preliminary characterization of human cementum collagen. Calcified Tissue Research 23: 147

Cournil I, Leblond C P, Pomponio J, Hand A R, Sederlof L, Martin G R 1979 Immunohistochemical localization of procollagens. Journal of Histochemistry and Cytochemistry 27: 1059

Crandon J H, Lund C C, Dill D B 1940 Experimental human scurvy. New England Journal of Medicine 22: 353

Dabbous M K, Seif M, Brinkley S B, Butler T, Braswell C W 1979 Gingival matrix proteins — the nature of insoluble bovine gingival collagen. Journal of Periodontal Research 14: 204

Dodd C M, Carmichael D J 1979 The collagenous matrix of bovine predentine. Biochimica et Biophysica Acta 577: 117

Eeckhout Y, Vaes G 1977 Further studies on the activation of procollagenase, the latent precursor of bone collagenase. Biochemical Journal 166: 21

Eisenmann D R, Glick P L 1972 Ultrastructure of initial crystal formation in dentin. Journal of Ultrastructure Research 41: 18

Engel D, Schroeder H E, Gay R, Clagett J 1980 Fine structure of cultured human gingival fibroblasts and demonstration of simultaneous synthesis of types I and III collagen. Archives of Oral Biology 25: 283

Fuji K, Kajiwara T, Kurosu H, Tanzer M L 1977 Osteogenesis imperfecta: altered content of type III collagen and proportion of the cross-links in skin. FEBS Letters 82: 251

Fullmer H M, Gibson W, Lazarus G S, Bladen H A, Whedon K A 1969 The origin of collagenase in periodontal tissues of man. Journal of Dental Research 48: 646

Galbraith D B, Kollar E J 1976 In vitro utilization of exogenous procollagen by embryonic tooth germs. Journal of Experimental Zoology 1976: 135

Garant P R, Cho M-I 1979a Cytoplasmic polarization of periodontal ligament fibroblasts. Journal of Periodontal Research 14: 95

Garant P R, Cho M-I 1979b Autoradiographic evidence of the coordination of the genesis of Sharpey's fibres with new bone formation in the periodontium of the mouse. Journal of Periodontal Research 14: 107

Glimcher M J, Friberg U A, Levine P T 1964 The identification and characterization of a calcified layer of coronal cementum in erupted bovine teeth. Journal of Ultrastructure Research 10: 76

Golub L M, Kaplan R, Mulvihill J E, Ramamurthy N S 1979 Collagenolytic activity of crevicular fluid and of adjacent gingival tissue. Journal of Dental Research 58: 2132

Hammouda O, Seif M, Sr., Brinkley B, Dabbous M K, Jurand J 1980 Gingival matrix collagen in chronic periodontitis. Journal of Dental Research 59: 17

Hassell T M, Page R C, Lindhe J 1978 Histologic evidence for impaired growth control in diphenylhydantoin gingival overgrowth in man. Archives of Oral Biology 23: 381

Hetem S, Kollar E J, Cutler L S, Yaeger J A 1975 Effect of α, α-dipyridyl on the basement membrane of tooth germs in vitro. Journal of Dental Research 54: 783

Horton J E, Wezeman F H, Kuettner K E 1978 Regulation of osteoclast-activating-factor (OAF)-stimulated bone resorption in vitro with an inhibitor of collagenase. In: Horton J E, Tarpley T M, Davis W F (eds) Mechanisms of localized bone loss. Special Supplement to Calcified Tissue Abstracts. p 127

Horwitz A L, Crystal R G 1976 Collagenase from rabbit pulmonary alveolar macrophages. Biochemical and Biophysical Research Communication 69: 296

Jessen H 1967 The ultrastructure of odontoblasts in perfusion fixed, demineralised incisors of adult rats. Acta Odontologica Scandinavica 25: 491

Johannessen J V, Bang G 1972 Transmission electron microscopy of sound demineralized guinea pig dentin. Scandinavian Journal of Dental Research 80: 213

Johnson-Muller B, Gross J 1978 Regulation of corneal collagenase production: epithelial-stromal cell interactions. Proceedings of the National Academy of Sciences (USA) 75: 4417

Kameyama Y 1975 Autoradiographic study of ^{3}H-proline incorporation by rat periodontal ligament, gingival connective tissue and dental pulp. Journal of Periodontal Research 10: 98

Karim A, Cournil I, Leblond C P 1979 Immunohistochemical localization of procollagens. Journal of Histochemistry and Cytoschemistry 27: 1070

Kowashi Y, Jaccard F, Cimasoni G 1979 Increase of free collagenase and natural protease activities in the gingival crevice during experimental gingivitis in man. Archives of Oral Biology 24: 645

Kuboki Y, Ohgushi K, Fusayama T 1977 Collagen biochemistry of the two layers of carious dentin. Journal of Dental Research 56: 1233

Lazarus G S, Daniels J R, Lian J, Burleigh M C 1972 Role of granulocyte collagenase in collagen degradation. American Journal of Pathology 68: 565

Lesot H, von der Mark K, Ruch J-V 1978 Localisation par immunofluoresence des types de collagene synthetises par l'ebauche dentaire chez l'embryon de Souris. Comptes Rendus de l'Academie des Sciences (Paris) 286: 765

Limeback H F, Sodek J 1979 Procollagen synthesis and processing in periodontal ligament in vivo and in vitro. European Journal of Biochemistry 100: 541

Linde A 1973 Glycosaminoglycans of the dental pulp. A biochemical study. Scandinavian Journal of Dental Research 81: 177

Listgarten M A 1973 Intracellular collagen fibrils in the periodontal ligament of the mouse, rat, hamster, guinea pig and rabbit. Journal of Periodontal Research 8: 335

Listgarten M A, Shapiro I M 1974 Fine structure and composition of coronal cementum in guinea-pig molars. Archives of Oral Biology 19: 679

Liu T Z, Bhatnagar R S 1973 Inhibition of protocollagen proline hydroxylase by dilantin. Proceedings of the Society of Experimental Biology and Medicine 142: 253

Lucas O N 1977 Increased fibrinolytic activity in the inflamed gingiva of beagle dogs. Journal of Dental Research 56: 1533

Mechanic G L, Kuboki Y, Shimokawa H, Nakamoto K, Sasaki S, Kawanishi Y 1974 Collagen crosslinks: direct quantitative determination of stable structural crosslinks in bone and dentin collagens. Biochemical and Biophysical Research Communications 60: 756

Müller P K, Lemmen C, Gay S, Meigel W N 1975 Disturbance in the regulation of the type of collagen synthesized in a form of osteogenesis imperfecta. European Journal of Biochemistry 59: 97

Munksgaard E C 1979 Collagen in Dentin. Journal de Biologie Buccale 7: 131

Munksgaard E C, Rhodes M, Mayne R, Butler W T 1978 Collagen synthesis and secretion by rat incisor odontoblasts in organ culture. European Journal of Biochemistry 82: 609

Narayanan A S, Page R C 1976 Biochemical characterization of collagens synthesized by fibroblasts derived from normal and diseased human gingiva. Journal of Biological Chemistry 251: 5464

Narayanan A S, Page R C 1977 Serum modulates collagen types in human gingiva fibroblasts. FEBS Letters 80: 221

Ohlsson K, Olsson I, Tynelius-Bratthall G 1973 Neutrophil leucocyte collagenase, elastase and serum protease inhibitors in human gingival crevices. Acta Odontologica Scandinavica 31: 51

Orlowski W A 1976 The incorporation of H^3-proline into the collagen of the periodontium of a rat. Journal of Periodontal Research 11: 96

Orlowski W A 1978 Metabolism of gingival collagen in the rat. Journal of Dental Research 57: 329

Patters M R, Schenkein H A, Weinstein A 1979 A method for detection of complement cleavage in gingival fluid. Journal of Dental Research 58: 1620

Pearson C H, Wohllebe M, Carmichael D J, Chovelon A 1975 Bovine periodontal ligament — an investigation of the collagen, glycosaminoglycan and insoluble glycoprotein components at different stages of tissue development. Connective Tissue Research 3: 195

Penttinen R P, Lichtenstein J R, Martin G R, McKusick V A 1975 Abnormal collagen metabolism in cultured cells in osteogenesis imperfecta. Proceedings of the National Academy of Sciences (USA) 76: 586

Pettigrew D W, Ho G H, Sodek D M, Brunette D M, Wang H-M 1978 Effect of oxygen tension and indomethacin on production of collagenase and neutral proteinase enzymes and their latent forms by porcine gingival explants in culture. Archives of Oral Biology 23: 767

Pindborg J J 1970 Pathology of the dental hard tissues. Munksgaard Copenhagen

Rao L G, Wang H M, Kalliecharan R, Heersche J N M, Sodek J 1979 Specific immunohistochemical localization of type I collagen in porcine periodontal tissues using the peroxidase-labelled antibody technique. Histochemical Journal 11: 73

Reddick M E, Bauer E A, Eisen A Z 1974 Immunocytochemical localization of collagenase in human skin and fibroblasts in monolayer culture. Journal of Investigative Dermatology 62: 361

Rippin J W 1976 Collagen turnover in the periodontal ligament under normal and altered functional forces. Journal of Periodontal Researoh 11: 101

Rodriguez M S, Wilderman M N 1972 Amino acid composition of the cementum matrix from human molar teeth. Journal of Periodontology 43: 438

Sauk J J, Gay R, Miller E J, Gay S 1980 Immunohistochemical localization of type III collagen in the dentin of patients with osteogenesis imperfecta and hereditary opalescent dentin. Journal of Oral Pathology In Press

Schellens J P M, Everts V, Beertsen W 1979 Resorption of connective tissue in the gingiva of the mouse incisor. Anatomical Record 195: 95

Schneir M, Ogata S, Fine A 1978 Confirmation that neither phenotype nor hydroxylation of collagen is altered in overgrown gingiva from diphenyl-hydantoin-treated patients. Journal of Dental Research 57: 506

Schneir M, Vogan I, Yu H, Yavelow J, Liu-Montcalm A, Furuto D 1975 Ability of salt and acetic acid to extract human and animal gingival collagen. Journal of Dental Research 54: 1095

Schroeder H E, Munzel-Pedrazzoli S, Page R 1973 Correlated morphometric and biochemical analysis of gingival tissue in early chronic gingivitis in man. Archives of Oral Biology 18: 899

Scott P G, Veis A, Mechanic G 1976 The identity of a cyanogen bromide fragment of bovine dentin collagen containing the site of an intermolecular cross-link. Biochemistry 15: 3191

Scott P G, Veis A 1976 The cyanogen bromide peptides of bovine soluble and insoluble collagens II. Tissue specific cross-linked peptides of insoluble skin and dentin collagen. Connective Tissue Research 4: 117

Selvig K A 1965 The fine structure of human cementum. Acta Odontologica Scandinavica 23: 423

Shuttleworth C A, Berry L, Wilson N 1980 Collagen synthesis in rabbit dental pulp fibroblast cultures. Archives of Oral Biology 25: 201

Silness J, Gustavsen F, Fejerskov O, Karring T, Loe H 1976 Cellular, afibrillar coronal cementum in human teeth. Journal of Periodontal Research 11: 331

Sodek J 1977 A comparison of the rates of synthesis and turnover of collagen and non-collagen proteins in adult rat periodontal tissues and skin using a microassay. Archives of Oral Biology 22: 655

Sodek J, Limeback H F 1979 Comparison of the rates of synthesis, conversion, and maturation of type I and type III collagens in rat periodontal tissues. Journal of Biological Chemistry 254: 20496

Svoboda E L A, Melcher A H, Brunette D M 1979 Stereological study of collagen phagocytosis by cultured periodontal ligament fibroblasts: time course and effect of deficient culture medium. Journal of Ultrastructure Research 68: 195

Thesleff I, Lehtonen E, Saxen L 1978 Basement membrane formation in transfilter tooth culture and its relation to odontoblast differentiation. Differentiation 10: 71

Thesleff I, Stenman S, Vaheri A, Timpl R 1979 Changes in the matrix proteins, fibronectin and collagen, during differentiation of mouse tooth germ. Developmental Biology 70: 116

Thomas H F 1979 The extent of the odontoblast process in human dentin. Journal of Dental Research 58: 2207

Trelstad R L, Hayashi K 1979 Tendon collagen fibrillogenesis: intracellular subassemblies and cell surface changes associated with fibril growth. Developmental Biology 71: 228

Volpin D, Veis A 1973 Cyanogen bromide peptides from insoluble skin and dentin bovine collagens. Biochemistry 12: 1452

Wahl L M, Wahl S M, Mergenhagen S E, Martin G R 1974 Collagenase production by endotoxin-activated macrophages. Proceedings of the National Academy of Sciences (USA) 71: 3598

Wahl L M, Wahl S M, Mergenhagen S E, Martin G R 1975 Collagenase production by lymphokine-activated macrophages. Science 187: 261

Wang H M, Nando V, Rao L G, Melcher A H, Heersche J N M, Sodek J 1980 Specific immunohistochemical localization of type III collagen in porcine periodontal tissues using the peroxidase-antiperoxidase method. Journal of Histochemistry and Cytochemistry 28: 1211

Warshawsky H 1972 The presence of atypical collagen fibrils in EDTA decalcified predentine and dentine of rat incisors. Archives of Oral Biology 17: 1745

Weinstock M 1972 Collagen formation — observations on its intracellular packaging and transport. Zeitschrift für Zellforschung 129: 455

Weinstock M 1977 Centrosymmetrical cross-banded structures in the matrix of rat incisor predentin and dentin. Journal of Ultrastructure Research 61: 218

Weinstock M, Leblond C P 1973 Radioautographic visualization of the deposition of a phosphoprotein at the mineralization front in the dentin of the rat incisor. Journal of Cell Biology 56: 838

Weinstock M, Leblond C P 1974 Synthesis, migration and release of precursor collagen by odontoblasts as visualized by radioautography after ^{3}H-proline administration. Journal of Cell Biology 60: 92

Werb Z, Mainardi C L, Vater C A, Harris E D 1977 Endogenous activation of latent collagenase by rheumatoid synovial cells. Evidence for a role of plasminogen activator. New England Journal of Medicine 296: 1017

Wohllebe M, Carmichael D J 1978 Type-I trimer and type I collagen in neutral-salt-soluble lathyritic-rat dentine. European Journal of Biochemistry 92: 183

Wohllebe M, Carmichael D J 1979 Biochemical characterization of guanidinium chloride-soluble dentine collagen from lathyritic-rat incisors. Biochemical Journal 181: 667

Yajima T, Rose G G 1977 Phagocytosis of collagen by human gingival fibroblasts in vitro. Journal of Dental Research 56: 1271

30

Tendon

P. F. DAVISON

A tendon is a band or cylinder of fibrous tissue through which the tension on a muscle is transmitted to an element of the skeleton or to another muscle. At either end of the tendon, the insertions, the structure must embody both its tensile function and the capacity to adhere to the adjoining tissue. The structural organization over the remaining length is Nature's design to serve only three functions, maintenance, the capacity for repair or growth, and the transmission of tensile stress. In adult tendons the tensile strength is derived from fascia of collagenous fibrils which outweigh the cells and other connective tissue components by a factor of four or more. In the adult this collagen is almost entirely type I. In view of the simplicity of the organization, composition and function it would seem that tendon should afford one of the easiest correlations between molecular structure and physiological function. However, there remain many unanswered questions ranging from the supramolecular organization to the disposition of the intermolecular cross-linking upon which the tensile strength of the tendon depends. Moreover, few experiments have been reported that define the turnover of tendon collagen, and although the fibrils within a tendon show a range of diameter which changes with age and disease, we know little about the molecular aspects of fibril growth or replacement following wounding. These points will be discussed at greater length in the succeeding sections.

This review emphasizes the molecular aspects of tendon structure; it updates and supplements a fine review by Elliott (1965).

ANATOMY

A tendon consists of bundles of fine filaments in which sparse cells are embedded, all within a sheath built of loose and dense connective tissue. The loose connective tissue is called the paratenon. A small tendon may comprise a single bundle, a larger one appears to be built from a tight packing of several bundles. These bundles are each wrapped in cylinders of a continuous, loose connective tissue, the endotenon, in which run fine vessels and nerves to the inner mass of the tendon. Columns of flattened cells, fibrocytes or fibroblasts, lie in the endotenon and in part ensheath the internal bundles of fibres (Fig. 30.1). Except in the embryo the tendon has a sparse capillary supply reflecting the large content of nonmetabolizing, extracellular tissue. Where it is necessary to minimize friction against adjacent surfaces the tendons often are enclosed in a collagenous tendon sheath. The inner part of the sheath closely wraps the tendon with usually narrow, circumferential collagen fibrils; the outer part may be fixed locally on adjacent bone; and between the two wrappings a thin lubricant solution which includes hyaluronic acid

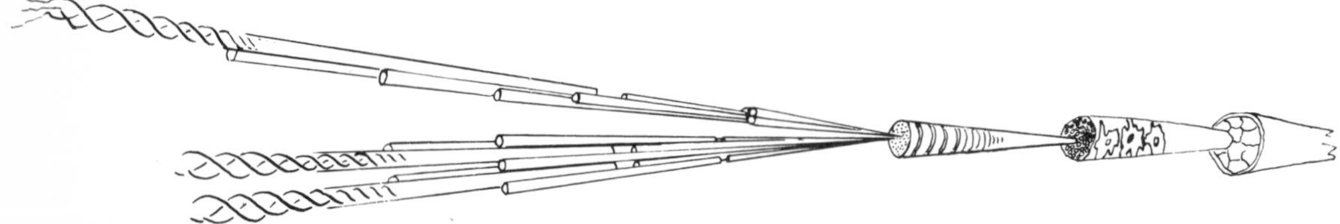

Fig. 30.1 Diagram of the hierarchical organization of the collagen molecules (left) in a tendon (right). The triple helix of coiled peptide chains is illustrated in three molecules, one of which shows the nonhelical telopeptides; the rest of the molecules are shown as simple cylinders. The width of the molecules is shown disproportionately large, the real length/width ratio is 200. Two postulated forms of molecular organization are shown: (top) the cylindrical 'Smith assembly' (also shown is a tetrad of such assemblies which may account for a filament of 8 nm diameter reported in tendons); and (below) a view of the quasi-hexagonal packing (Hulmes & Miller) selected to show the palisade of molecules in register in their longitudinal packing. Next (right) the banded fibril is seen; then the packed fibrils in the fibre bundle which is partly covered by a column of fibrocytes in the endotenon; and finally the ensheathed mass of fibre bundles that comprises the tendon.

reduces frictional resistance to the sliding of the tendon. In other areas where the tendon may slide over hardened surfaces (Gillard et al, 1977) or where it may form local attachments (e.g. along the vertebrae of the tail) the tendon may harden into fibrocartilage (see below).

If the surface of the tendon is cut the main bulk of the tendon can be easily teased apart to demonstrate a mass of colinear, apparently uninterrupted, fine filaments whose dimension cannot be determined by light microscopy but which can be shown by electron microscopy to range from 8 to 400 nm in various preparations. These filaments are usually referred to as collagen *fibrils*. In the bundle the fibrils are arranged to generate a coherent, wavy pattern so that the packed mass of them in the fibre under zero stress appears iridescent, with a sheen like watered silk. This crimping and the iridescence disappears reversibly with minor stretching of the fibril bundle (Kastelic et al, 1978).

In transverse section in the light microscope the packed fibrils of a tendon appears as an ensheathed, largely structureless mass in which cells are sparsely scattered. These fibrocytes appear star-like as they send long lamellipodia through the fascia of the fibrils (Fig. 30.2). In longitudinal sections these cells seem to be very elongated as they stretch along the columns of fibrils.

The binding of tendon to bone is accomplished through two transition zones, unmineralized fibrocartilage, mineralized fibrocartilage and then bone. In these regions the parallel collagen fibrils and the sparse elastin fibres course through a proteoglycan and polysaccharide-rich matrix characteristic of cartilage, and this matrix becomes progressively more mineralized as it nears the bone. The spicules of bone or mineralized cartilage which interdigitate with the collagen fibrils are called Sharpey's fibres; within the transition zones cells with the morphology of chondrocytes progressively replace the fibrocytes (Cooper & Misol, 1970). Since both the tendon and bone are built largely from a collagenous organic skeleton the transition would appear to be a simple one of progressive merging of the characteristics of both tissue but it is not clear if the fibrocartilage contains type II collagen, that characteristic of hyaline cartilage. If it does the transition zone may be structurally more complex than is presently appreciated.

The attachment of tendon to muscle, a largely acellular tissue to a largely cellular one, is more complex than the fibrocartilage insertion into bone. For years it was debated whether collagen fibrils attached to the fibrillar proteins of muscle, or to the sarcolemma. The latter is now affirmed and so the tension in the contracted myofilaments must be transmitted to the sarcolemma. The cells interdigitate between incoming collagen fibrils of the tendon and the fibrils appear to terminate in finger-like invaginations in the sarcolemma and on surface thickening on that membrane. Other fibrils of the tendon appear to penetrate and perhaps fuse with collagen of the perimysium and epimysium. How complete this contiguity is may be questioned, because it is reported that type III collagen forms a component of the epimysium, and most of the perimysium, and AB collagen is also present (Duance, et al, 1977). Thus, it must yet be determined whether fibrils of different collagen types fuse or interdigitate in this transition region around the muscle cells. For further structural details the reader is referred to Nakao (1976).

ULTRASTRUCTURE

At the electron microscope level the masses of packed, cylindrical fibrils are seen to be embedded in a lighter staining matrix. The diameters of the fibrils increase to maturity: they may show a large or small range of diameters in different tendons. The matrix is believed to be built from a proteoglycan and glycoprotein gel. It is readily penetrated by cellular processes which fill the interstices between the fibrils in most areas where the lamellipodia appear (Fig. 30.2).

When treated with electron stains, each fibril shows a banded staining pattern generated by the parallel, linearly organized collagen molecules. The staining shows a 64 to 67 nm period along the fibril length and the fine structure of the stained pattern is polarized consistently over as long a distance as can be followed in a micrograph, showing that the polarity of at least most of the molecules is maintained probably throughout the fibril; the polarity of adjacent fibrils is not consistent and roughly equal numbers are directed up or down along the tendon (Cooper & Misol, 1972). Many published micrographs of transverse sections show thin fibrils adjacent to, and apparently budding from the larger fibrils but this feature is not seen consistently and it may be a fixation or embedding artefact (Bouteille & Pease, 1971). However, it is possible that in older animals such budding-off may be an aspect of fibril breakdown (Parry et al, 1978).

In transverse section fibrils with positive staining give a punctate appearance that has been interpreted as evidence for a basic unit of organization, a 3 to 3.5 nm *filament* (as we shall refer to it) built from a polarized array of collagen molecules which themselves have a diameter of about 1.4 nm. Speculation has centred on the concept of a filament produced by the linear polymerization of 'Smith assemblies' (Smith, 1968) (See Ch. 3). Parry et al (1978) have postulated a similar subunit structure for the fibrils on the basis of their measurements of small fibril diameters — particularly in developing tissues — where the diameters appear to increase in increments of 80A. This dimension is plausibly equated with a tetrad of 'Smith cylinders' (see Fig. 30.1).

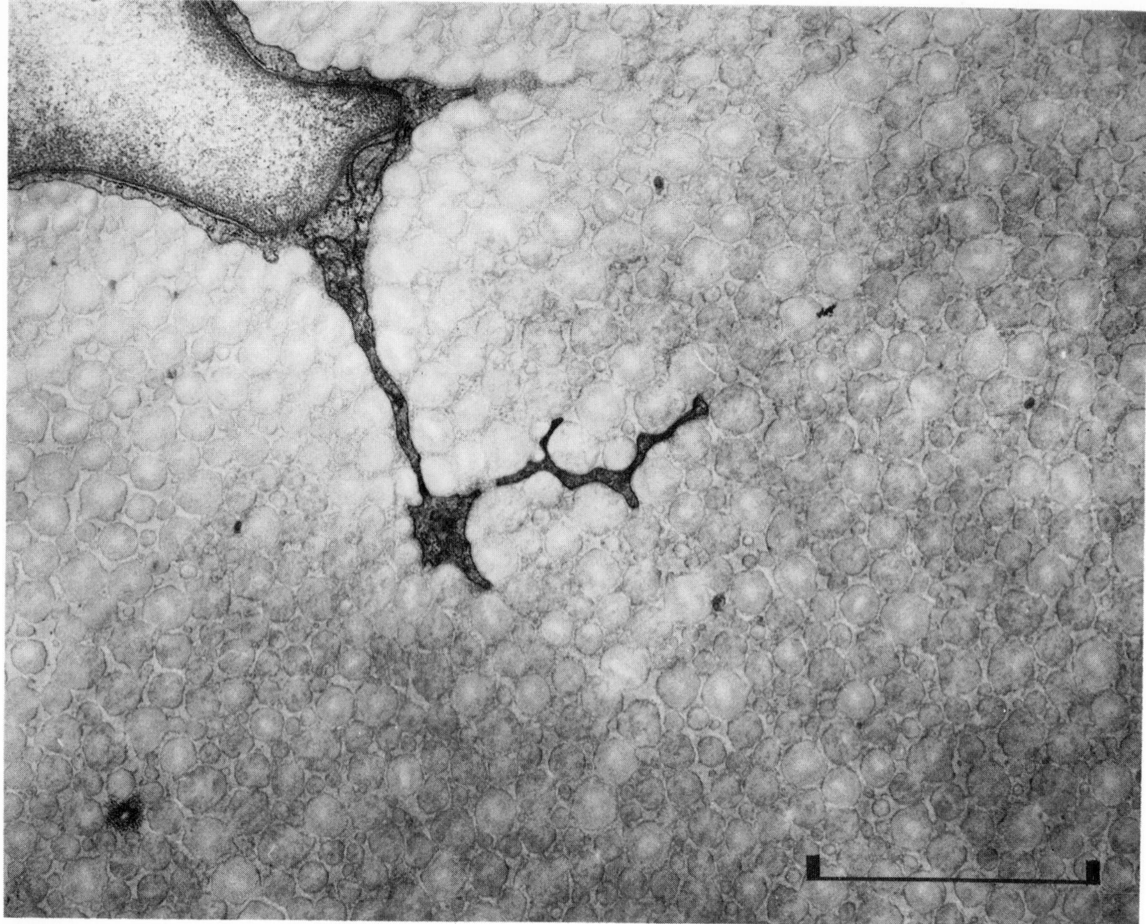

Fig. 30.2 Electron micrograph of transverse section of rat tail tendon showing a fibrocyte within the fibre bundle. The faintly stained fibrils appear as evenly spaced cylinders of various diameters. The pseudopodia of the cell penetrates the proteoglycan matrix between the fibrils. Stained with lead citrate. Bar indicates 5 μm. In a light micrograph the mass of fibrils appears structureless.

The 3.5 nm diameter attributed to the filaments is consistent with a prominent equatorial reflection seen in X-ray photographs of tendon. Fine filaments reconstituted from acid-soluble collagen have approximately the same diameter and the 67 nm period is detectable by X-rays in stretched masses of those fine filaments, implying the quarter-staggered assembly of collagen molecules can occur in such filaments (Veis et al, 1979). These observations are in accordance with Smith's model but there are difficulties in interpreting the disposition of intermolecular cross-links measured in these tissues with this model (see below). Whatever the internal organization of the filaments, they must be associated laterally in register to generate the band pattern seen across the stained fibril and the cross-linking within the filaments must be responsible for the tensile strength of the fibril and tendon. Some micrographs show the filaments in a fibril spiralling in a lazy helix (Bouteille & Pease, 1971). The crimp pattern of tendons must be generated either at the level of the twisting of the filaments or in the embedment of the fibrils in the matrix.

EMBRYONIC DEVELOPMENT

Tendons develop from local accretions of mesenchymal cells which in some locations subdivide to produce adjacent cellular assemblies from which will form the sheath as well as the tendon. Between the cells collagen fibrils appear progressively and their orientation becomes gradually established as the cellular fraction of the tissue mass is diluted by the steady synthesis of collagen and the matrix (Greenlee & Ross, 1967; Chaplin & Greenlee, 1975). As the arrangement of collagen fibrils begins to dominate the organization, the fibroblasts become arranged in columns or dispersed. The vascular supply becomes diluted by the progressive growth of the fibrillar mass of collagen until the mature tendon appears as a nearly avascular mass with a sparse cellular population. Around the digits the flexor tendon development is completed before the extensor tendon.

In the adult the collagen in the fibrils is entirely type I although other types have been reported in the endotenon.

In the embryo type I trimer collagen has been identified (Jiminez et al, 1977) as a significant component along with what is probably AB collagen as well as type I in chick tendons (Jiminez et al, 1978) and we have noted AB collagen in fetal bovine foot extensor tendons (Davison, unpublished). It may be significant that the ratio of type AB :type I parallels the diminishing cellular content of the developing tendon and some other tissues.

THE STRENGTH OF TENDONS: MATURATION AND AGEING

The ultimate tensile strength of tendons has probably never been accurately measured because clamping cannot be achieved that will exert the applied stress uniformly across the fibril bundles and clamping itself probably damages the structure; nevertheless it is apparent that tendons are strong enough to withstand several times the tension their attached muscles can impart. Over the working range the tensile elements, the *fibrils*, are essentially inextensible because X-ray analysis shows that the 67 nm spacing changes minimally. However, a tendon may be strained up to 5 per cent of its length before it is irreversibly damaged; as it is strained the crimp folding of the fibrils is lost and the imperfectly aligned fibrils become parallel to produce a more crystalline X-ray pattern.

The crimping of the fibres and the embedding of the fibrils in a hydrated matrix seems to be designed to give a structure resilient at low stress since the reversible loss of crimping occurs in the 'toe' of the stress-strain diagram (Viidik, 1972). The interaction with the matrix is presumably the explanation for the fact that type I fibrils can show a different periodicity, 64 nm in fibrocartilage and skin (e.g. Brodsky et al, 1980) and 670 nm in tendon, but this interaction appears to be only physical and no covalent linking of collagen to proteoglycan has been substantiated.

When a fetus or rapidly growing animal is injected with, or fed, an osteolathyrogen such as β-aminopropionitrile the collagenous tissues show a progressively diminished strength with continued dosage; bones are distorted, skin can be torn, and death often comes from aneurysms in major vessels. The lathyrogen inhibits the enzyme lysyl oxidase which effects cross-linking between newly synthesized collagen and elastin chains; cross-links are formed through the aldehydes the enzyme produces from lysyl and hydroxylysl residues in those chains. The tendons in lathyritic animals appear normal morphologically but have a diminished tensile strength. We can conclude that the ordered association of the collagen molecules into fibrils can be effected without cross-linking but that the lateral forces controlling this bonding generate little tensile strength. How little is not clear because the lathyrogen does not destroy cross-links already established so it would be difficult to test tissues containing no cross-linked collagen, but the obvious differences between the tensile strength of normal and severely lathyritic tissues shows that the greater part of the strength of a collagen fibril (and therefore a tendon) is dependent upon the formation of intermolecular cross-links.

Despite difficulties of measurement it appears that in a maturing animal the tensile strength of a tendon increases. This change probably results from two factors: a growth within each fibre of the fibrils at the expense of the matrix; and an increase in intermolecular cross-linking. The latter change is demonstrated by the diminished swelling of the tissue in denaturing solvents, the increasing resistance to proteolysis, and the increasing isometric tension which is produced on warming a tendon to 60° (thermal shrinkage) or the increased heat shrinkage that results from heating a dissected tendon under constant load.

Changes in heat shrinkage behaviour and enzymatic resistance continue beyond maturity and have been claimed to offer a measure of the age of the tissue (Hamlin et al, 1978; Viidik, 1979). However, the increasing heat shrinkage may result from a progressive conversion of thermally labile to stable bonds (see below) because there is no direct evidence of an increase in the number of intermolecular cross-links beyond maturity. The studies on isometric tension in heat shrinkage experiments on human and rat tendons showed a remarkable effect of oxygen in increasing maximal stress and presumably cross-linking (Mitchell & Rigby, 1975) but Robins & Bailey (1977) report that this oxygen effect does not relate to stabilization of labile cross-links but to another, unknown mechanism. Whether it has relevance to another population of reactive sites which in special circumstances can generate cross-links is not known.

There is no unchallenged evidence that tendons become stronger after maturation and the functionally necessary cross-links have been established. However, the progressive physical changes in skin and other connective tissues with ageing has provoked speculations that collagen cross-linking proceeds progressively and is the cause of the functional decrements and tissue changes of ageing (see Viidik, 1979). The search for increased cross-linking in tendon (see below) has not been successful and we conclude that the physical changes in ageing tissues must relate to decreased hydration, more dense packing and better order in collagen fibrils, and perhaps more physical or chemical interaction with the matrix components which themselves may be changed.

CROSS-LINKING

Soluble collagen can be extracted by acetic or other acids from tendons of young animals; less is extractable from older animal tendons. Flexor tendons yield less than extensor tendons in our experience. If the tendons are first reduced with sodium borohydride then virtually no acid-soluble collagen can be extracted from any except very young tendons. The acid solubility is due to the presence of acidlabile cross-links formed from aldehyde adducts (see Bailey et al, 1974). These cross-links are stabilized by reduction and the very small amount of collagen extractable after reduction probably indicates that most molecules are cross-linked very soon after fibril formation. The diminished yield of acid-soluble collagen from older animals results from a natural process of stabilization (that may include reduction) but the stabilized cross-links have not been unequivocally identified. The stabilization process appears to occur slowly through the animals' maturation and more slowly in the extensor than in the flexor tendon. However, some of the difference in the acid solubility of the flexor and tensor tendons may be a consequence of turnover, since newly synthesized collagen will presumably be cross-linked first with the labile cross-links.

Teleologically it seems strange that a significant fraction of collagen in young tendons that are designed, we presume, for tensile strength, should retain chemically labile cross-links whereas in other tissues (e.g., Houghton's jelly, cornea) where the demand for tensile strength is less obvious, the collagen is essentially insoluble in acid and the cross-links therefore have become stabilized. We may conclude that functionally the acid-labile cross-links are as suitable as the others and that their chemical vulnerability does not imply a diminished strength at neutral pH. Therefore the natural process that stabilizes the aldehyde adducts remains of uncertain biological significance. Another aspect of cross-link stabilization that presents a puzzle is why type I collagen that is selected for tissues of high tensile strength is the only collagen that shows significant acid solubility in young tissues.

To maximize the tensile strength of a collagen fibril there should be a covalent bond between each α-chain of one molecule and each chain in the next molecule in sequence. This continuity could be effected with one cross-link per α-chain if they were distributed optimally. However, some of the cross-links that have been identified bind 3 or 4 amino-acid residues and therefore are potentially polyvalent. Furthermore, in rapidly growing tissue or from young animals, free α-chain and β-components can be extracted with denaturants even if the labile cross-links are first stabilized by borohydride' Thus, cross-linking is not established in an orderly fashion from α-chain to α-chain but from molecule to molecule at first, so that some α-chains are freed if the triple-helix is disrupted by denaturation. However, from older tissues with the cross-links stabilized chemically or naturally very few α-chains can be extracted with denaturants so that linkage of every α-chain is ultimately achieved although some of these bonds may only join α-chains laterally, inter- or intramolecularly and may contribute little to tensile strength. This cross-linking appears to be achieved through perhaps no more than 2 cross-links per α-chain (see below).

The progressive decrease in solubility in the collagen of a tendon as the animal matures may correspond to the slow addition of cross-links to resident molecules in fibrils, or to the replacement of young fibrils as growth proceeds with later, more heavily cross-linked fibrils, or both.

The reducible cross-links in tendons of young and ageing animals have been analyzed and most have been identified (Tanzer, 1976). The populations of reducible, cross-linking adducts varies in different tendons and with age. The differences that involve the ratios of dehydro-hydroxylysinonorleucine (HLNL) and dehydrodihydroxy-lysineonorleucine (DHLNL) may be of little significance, reflecting only the different degrees of hydroxylation of certain lysyl residues in the α-chains. Variations in levels of hydroxylation occur in fetal compared to mature tissues (Barnes et al, 1971) and the variations may correspond to the rate of collagen biosynthesis, the more rapid the collagen secretion the less time to complete hydroxylation. As long as the adducts remain reducible, dehydro-HLNL is chemically more stable than dehydro-DHLNL but this difference may be irrelevant at neutral pH, and is ceratainly unimportant when the cross-link becomes stabilized and unreducible. We have yet to determine what controls the rate of stabilization of the cross-links, but the rate varies between different tendons, from tendons to other tissues and for different types of collagen.

The non-reducible cross-links have not been identified and hence cannot be summed with the reducible bonds (which can be enumerated) to give an estimate of total number of cross-links per α chain in mature collagen. There is a partial exception to this statement in the case of rat tissues. There the stabilization of cross-links is slow and an unusual amount of collagen can be extracted with reagents such as cysteamine which break the cross-linking aldimine adducts (Nimni, 1977). Measurements on solubilized rat collagen have indicated two to nine aldehyde residues per molecule; according to Deshmukh & Nimni (1971) some of these are in the helical lengths of the chains. This report has not been confirmed. Most analyses have shown that aldehydic residues are restricted to the amino- and carboxy-terminal telopeptides. The telopeptides that have been sequenced contain only one lysyl or hydroxylysyl residue so it seems that mature cross-linking may be accomplished with up to two cross-linking residues per α-chain.

The possibility of other types of cross-links besides aldehydes has prompted attempts to enumerate and localize the cross-links by identifying cross-linked peptides in collagen cleaved by cyanogen bromide (Davison, 1978; Light & Bailey, 1979). These experiments were directed to tendon (and later other tissues) where a single type of collagen is the predominant component so that other proteins would not confuse the interpretation of the peptide analyses. These authors concur in finding that from bovine tendons the yield and electrophoretic mobilities of many of the CNBr peptides do not differ between young and old animals. These peptides, α1 CB-4, -3,-8, α2CB-4, therefore are not significantly involved in cross-linking. Borohydride stabilization of labile cross-links resulted in significant changes in the peptides only for young bovine tendons, so by maturity the labile cross-links are either an insignificant fraction of the total or their function is duplicated (this mode of analysis can potentially enumerate the peptides that are cross-linked but not the number of cross-links that are involved). The novel information that these experiments provided was that the carboxyterminal peptide of the α1-chain, CB-6, is intermolecularly cross-linked to produce aggregates larger than β-components. Thus α1CB-6 without cross-links is virtually absent from the mature tendon, indicating an effective inter- and probably intra-molecular cross-linking. The carboxy-terminal peptide from the α2-chain (α2CB-3,5) also is somewhat depleted so it may be involved in the peptide polymer revealed by this analysis but α1CB-6 predominates and for brevity we will refer to this component as polyCB6.

The generation of aldehydes in the amino-terminal regions of the type I collagen chains has been well demonstrated and this is the only site where the intramolecular aldol cross-link has been found in acid-soluble collagen. One may specalate that the bonds involving poly-CB6 are those that render the molecule immediately acid-insoluble. Aldehydes have been reported in α1-CB6 but whether these are involved in producing poly-CB6 is not known.

The arrangement of collagen molecules in fibrils and the mode of assembly is not known. As mentioned previously speculations on organization have concentrated recently on the 'Smith' assembly (Smith, 1976), a cylinder of five collagen molecules each longitudinally displaced from its nearest neighbour by 67 nm. This displacement (234 amino acid residues) is greater than the length of α1CB-6 (186 residues) so unless the telopeptide can span that gap (and the lysyl residue that may be oxidized to allysine is only 17 residues (Fietzek & Kuhn, 1976) from the helix termination in calf collagen) lengthwise, polymerization of α1CB-6 through cross-linking is unlikely. Similarly the packing of cylinders of Smith assemblies presents a problem of arranging the 20 per cent of the molecules that are in register to build up poly-CB6 unless the telopeptides can worm around the diameter of these cylinders. A more recent proposal for collagen packing (Hulmes & Miller, 1979) appears to offer a simpler arrangement to permit planes of molecules to be found in register for extensive lateral cross-linking. Of course, such cross-linking contributes little to the longitudinal strength of the fibres only preserving the lateral order. Moreover, unless there is more than one cross-link per α1CB-6 telopeptide, aldol condensates cannot form the basis for the poly-CB6 cross-links because the cross-linking of two intramolecular chains would exhaust their potential. Nevertheless, the reports of laterally aligned assemblies of secreted molecules in fibroblast cultures synthesizing collagen (Bruns et al, 1979) raise the possibility that such assemblies are the biosynthetic precursors of fibrils in vivo; such assemblies may be the origin of poly-CB6.

The direct analysis of covalently linked collagen peptides labelled by ^{3}H-borohydride reduction of cross-links has provided a few positive identifications of cross-linking sites. Several findings had been made of a cross-link in tendons and other tissues between an aldehyde in α1CB-6 and the amino-terminal residue of α1CB-5 (e.g. Eyre & Glimcher, 1973; Hehkel et al, 1976). Cross-links from the amino-terminal aldehyde α1CB-1 to α1CB-6 have also been reported (see, Tanzer, 1976). Presuming that some adjacent molecules are staggered at multiples of 67 nm, the most economical way of building a tensile filament is through polymerization of subjacent collagen molecules with the minimal overlap of about 80 residues in the helical length of each α-chain; this is the overlap readily identified by electron microscopy of SLS aggregates derived from polymeric collagen and we are aware of no evidence for cross-linking at any other overlap. Thus the available data confirm that Nature builds tensile tissues like tendons from collagen polymerized through an 80 residue overlap and that across the width of the fibrils the molecules are staggered with a 67 nm periodicity but the mode of packing of adjacent molecules remains uncertain.

GROWTH, TURNOVER AND REPAIR

As a tendon matures it accumulates acid-resistant cross-links, the percentage of water drops, and the ratio collagen/proteoglycan increases. Under repeated stress a tendon will hypertrophy. As these changes occur there is a general increase in the diameters of the fibrils although in some tendons a bimodal or trimodal distribution of fibril diameters is developed (Parry et al, 1978). The increase in fibril diameter presumably indicates the accretion of collagen to each fibril by the progressive addition of individual molecules or filaments secreted by the fibrocytes ensheathing or penetrating the fibre bundle. In fetal development Trelstad & Hayashi (1978) have suggested that collagen fibrils are virtually spun from the secreting fibroblast like silk from a spider. To build upon a smooth cylinder by the accretion of secreted filaments would demand that these be small relative to the diameter of the fibril. Maybe this is the mode of fibril growth. Alternatively, the morphological changes with maturation could be explained by the catabolizing of the smaller fibrils and their replacement by wider ones. It is not yet clear if this process is compatible with the reports of limited turnover rates of tendon collagen in the mature animal. However, the turnover data derived from labelling studies may need reinvestigation if there is extensive reutilization of proline following catabolism so that isotope levels may not truly indicate fibril persistence (Jackson & Heininger, 1975).

Just as the mechanisms of fibril growth are not understood, so also do we lack a detailed understanding of repair. The tearing of tendons is a common injury although the natural site of rupture brought about by sudden stress is most usually at the bone insertion. Still, cut tendons also heal well if the damaged surfaces are sutured together. Healing follows the embryonic pattern with cell infiltration and the laying down first of fine, poorly oriented fibrils. Then the organization is progressively refined as the cut ends are penetrated and in part eroded by cell processes and invading cells. It is probable that these cells are not resident fibroblasts but activated or stem cells from the superficial connective tissue of the tendon; thus a tendon torn within a complete sheath does not heal (Peacock & Van Winkle, 1976). Through the area that they invade these cells secrete new, finer fibrils which later increase in diameter and become better oriented as the cell population drops and the restoration of the original structure becomes evident (Greenlee & Pike, 1971). This description does not tell us how the strength of the original tendon is re-established. At one time it was thought that fibrils fused. It now appears that fusion is rarely if ever seen so, if the tensile strength depends upon the continuity of the polymerized collagen, does continuity result from building a new insertion into old fibrils or by replacement of the old, interrupted fibrils with new? If the continuity of a fibril is established by the spinning of fibrils by fibroblasts, healing across gaps would demand a new mechanism for joining the ends; if molecules are simply secreted into the area of the wound, then the mechanisms that control the growth and ordering of the fibrils challenge further investigation.

DISEASES OF TENDONS

As a tissue tendons show a remarkable freedom from disease. The only clear evidence of failure of tendon function occurs in conditions where the formation or maintenance of cross-linking is interfered with or where the insertions into bone or muscle are not preserved. Thus, tendons are inadequate or weakened in experimental conditions such as osteolathyrism, induced by agents such as β-aminopropionitrile in growing animals; they are also weakened by treatment with penicillamine or cysteine which block aldehyde groups and prevent cross-linking, or chelate the copper ions required by the enzyme lysyl oxidase. A copper-deficient diet produces the same effect (Ganezar et al, 1977). These findings in tendons would probably also be found in homocysteinurics where the systemic collagenous disease implies a failure of the collagen fibrils to cross-link effectively (Kang & Trelstad, 1973).

In recent years a series of reports have described tendon ruptures in patients undergoing steroid therapy (see, Halpern et al, 1977). However, this occurrence is rare among such patients and the most frequent finding is rupture at the bone insertion. It seems probable that some aspect of bone replacement or fibrocartilage bonding is responsible for the failure, rather than the tendon structure itself.

The inherited diseases of connective tissue affect different tissues of the body to varying degrees. Thus each form of Ehlers-Danlos syndrome shows various levels of hyperextensibility of skin or joints, and the latter condition presumably is accompanied by lengthened tendons and ligaments; however, these seem adequate for function, and failure of these connectives is not common although tendon rupture has been reported in alkaptonuria. It appears that the safety margin built into the connectives is adequate for the inflicted stress despite incomplete fibre formation or cross-linking. The difference in the disease process in different tissues is exemplified in the dermatosparaxic condition described for cattle, sheep and cats (e.g. Hauset & Lapière, 1974; Patterson & Minor, 1977). These diseases are detected by the fragility of the skin, and microscopy reveals clear differences in fibre morphology (e.g. ribbons rather than cylinders) and/or fibre diameters and arrangement. Where the tendons have been examined, however, they seem not to be affected and the diseases are never presented on account of tendon rupture. We may deduce that a genetic defect so bad as to interfere with tendon morphogenesis or function would be lethal in other tissues.

Injuries or local infection may result in inflammation, tenosynovitis of the tendons and sheaths. Ideopathic, nodular inflammation commonly of the sheath, is termed villonodularsynovitis. The so-called giant cell tumours may arise as nodular growths in the tendon sheaths and they are common in the hands. These growths seem self-limited and are not malignant. The only notable malignancy of tendon or synovium is the synoviosarcoma (Ariel & Park, 1963).

Dupuytren's contracture is not primarily a disease of the tendon but it involves a fibrotic growth in the palmar fascia that develops into a length of connective tissue on the aponeurosis of the flexor tendons of the ring or little fingers (Luck, 1959). Subsequent contraction of that tissue results in the awkward flexion of those fingers. A similar contracture is seen in the foot. The frequent appearance of several such lesions on one hand suggest that this is not a simple tumour but results from a condition of the connective tissue. Bailey et al (1977) recently analyzed the collagens in the nodules and contractures and found significant amounts of type III collagen.

REFERENCES

Allain C, Le Lous M, Bazin S, Bailey A J, Delaumay A 1978 Isometric tension developed during heating of collagenous tissues. Biochimica et Biophysica Acta 533: 147–55

Ariel I M, Pack G T 1963 Synovial sarcoma. A review of 25 cases. New England Journal of Medicine 268: 1272-83

Bailey A J, Robins S P, Balian G 1974 Biological significance of the intermolecular cross-links in collagen. Nature 251: 105-9

Bailey A J, Sims T J, Gabbiani G, Bazin S, Le Lous M 1977 Collagen of Dupuytren's disease. Clinical science and molecular medicine 53: 499-502

Barres M J, Constable B J, Morton L F, Kodicek E 1971 Hydroxylysine in the N-terminal telopeptides of skin collagen from chick embryo and newborn rat. Biochemical Journal 125: 925-8

Bouteille M, Pease D C 1971 The tridimensional structure of native collagenous fibrils, their proteinaceous filaments. Journal of Ultrastructure Research 35: 314-38

Brodsky B, Eikenberry E F, Cassidy K 1980 An unusual collagen periodicity in skin. Biochimica et Biophysica Acta 621: 162-6

Bruns R R, Hulmes D J S, Therrien S F, Gross J 1979 Procollagen segment-long-spacing crystallites: their role in collagen fibrillogenesis. Proceedings of the National Academy of Sciences, US 76: 313-7

Chaplin D M, Greenlee T K 1975 The development of human digital tendons. Journal of Anatomy 120:253-64

Cooper R R, Misol S 1970 Tendon and ligament insertions. Journal of Bone and Joint Surgery 52A: 1-20

Davison P F 1978 Bovine tendons: ageing and collagen cross-linking. Journal of Biological Chemistry 253: 5635–41

Deshmukh K, Nimni M E 1971 Characterization of the aldehydes present on the cyanogen bromide peptides from mature rat skin collagen. Biochemistry 10: 1640-7

Duance V C, Restall D J, Beard H, Bourne F J, Bailey A J 1977 The location of three collagen types in muscle. FEBS Letters 79: 248–52

Elliott DH 1965 Structure and function of mammalian tendon. Biological Reviews 40: 392-421

Eyre D R, Glimcher M J 1973 Analysis of a cross-linked peptide from calf bone collagen: evidence that hydroxylysyl glycosides participates in the cross-link. Biochemical and Biophysical Research Communications 52: 663-70

Fietzek P P, Kühn K 1976 The primary structure of collagen. In: Hall D A, Jackson D S (eds) International review of connective tissue research vol 7. Academic Press, New York. p 1–60

Ganezer K S, Hart M L, Carnes W H 1977 Tensile properties of tendons in copper deficient swine. Proceedings of the Society for Experimental Biology and Medicine 153: 396–9

Gillard G C, Merrilees M J, Bell-Booth P G, Reilly M C, Flint M H 1977 The proteoglycan content and the axial periodicity of collagen in tendon. Biochemical Journal 163: 145–51

Greenlee T K, Pike D 1971 Studies on tendon healing in the rat. Journal of Plastic and Reconstructive Surgery 48: 260–70

Greenlee T K, Ross R 1967 The development of the rat flexor digital tendon, a fine structure study. Journal of Ultrastructure Research 18: 354–76

Halpern A A, Horowitz B G, Nagel D A 1977 Tendon ruptures associated with corticosteroid therapy. Western Journal of Medicine 127: 378–82

Hamlin C R, Luschin J M, Kohn R R 1978 Partial characterization of the age-related stabilizing factor of post-mature human collagen. Experimental Gerontology 13: 403–14

Hanset R, Lapière C M 1974 Inheritance of dermatopraxis in the calf. Journal of Heredity 65: 356-8

Henkel W, Rauterberg J, Stirtz T 1976 Isolation of a cross-linked cyanogen-bromide peptide from insoluble rabbit collagen. European Journal of Biochemistry 69: 223-31

Hulmes D J S, Miller A 1979 Quasihexagonal molecular packing in collagen fibrils. Nature 282: 878–80

Jackson S H, Heininger J A 1975 Proline recycling during collagen metabolism as determined by concurrent $^{18}O_2$and ^{3}H-labeling. Biochimica et Biophysica Acta 381: 359–67

Jimenez S A, Bashey R I, Benditt M, Yankowski R 1977 Identification of collagen α_1(I) trimer in embryonic chick tendons and calvaria. Biochemical and Biophysical Research Communications 78: 1354–60

Jimenez S A, Yankowski R, Bashey R I 1978 Identification of two collagen α-chains in extracts of lathyritic chick embryo tendons. Biochemical and Biophysical Research Communications 81: 1298–1306

Kang A H, Trelstad R L 1973 A collagen defect in homocystinuria. Journal of Clinical Investigation 52: 2571–8

Kastelic J, Galeski A, Baer E 1978 The multicomposite structure of tendon. Connective Tissue Research 6: 11–24

Light N D, Bailey A J 1979 Changes in cross-linking during ageing in bovine tendon collagen. FEBS Letters 97: 183–8

Luck J V 1959 Dupuytren's contracture. Journal of Bone and Joint Surgery 41: 635–44

Mitchell T W, Rigby B J 1975 In vivo and in vitro ageing of collagen examined using an isometric melting technique. Biochimica et Biophysica Acta 393: 531–41

Nakao T 1976 Some observations of the fine structure of the myotendinous junction in myotomal muscles in the tadpole tail. Cell and Tissue Research 161: 241–54

Nimni M E 1977 Mechanism of inhibition of collagen cross-linking by penicillamine. Proceedings of the Royal Society of Medicine, Supplement 3, 70: 65–72

Parry D A D, Craig A S, Barnes G R G 1978 Tendon and ligament from the horse: an ultrastructural study of collagen fibrils and elastic fibres as a function of age. Proceedings of the Royal Society of Medicine, Supplement B, 203: 293–321

Patterson D F, Minor R R 1977 Hereditary fragility and hypertensibility of the skin of cats. Laboratory Investigation 37: 170–9

Peacock E E, Van Winkle W 1976 Wound repair, 2nd edn. Saunders, Philadelphia

Robins S P, Bailey A J 1977 Some observations on the ageing in vitro of reprecipitated collagen fibres. Biochimica et Biophysica Acta 492: 408–14

Smith J W 1968 Molecular patterns in native collagen. Nature 219: 157–8

Tanzer M L 1976 Cross-linking. In: Ramachandran G N, Reddi A H (eds) Biochemistry of collagen. Plenum Press, New York, pp 137–62

Trelstad R L, Hayashi K 1979 Tendon collagen fibrillogenesis: Intracellular subassemblies and cell surface changes associated with fibril growth. Developmental Biology 71: 228–42

Veis A, Miller A, Leibovich S J, Traub W 1979 The limiting collagen microfibril. Biochimica et Biophysica Acta 576: 88–98

Viidik A 1972 Simultaneous mechanical and light microscopic studies of collagen fibres. Zeitschrift für Anatomie Entwicklungsgeschichte 136: 204–16

Viidik A 1979 Connective tissues — possible implications of the temporal changes for the ageing process. Mechanisms of Ageing and Development 9: 267–85

31

Uterus, cervix and ovary

J. F. WOESSNER

INTRODUCTION

Collagen in the uterus, cervix and ovaries performs a strictly mechanical function. In the uterus, great tensile strength is required to prevent this organ from rupturing during explusion of the baby. In the cervix, the collagen acts somewhat like drawstrings, holding the neck of the uterus firmly closed against the pressures of the growing fetus. In the ovary collagen supports the spherical structure of the growing Graafian follicle.

While these mechanical functions of collagen are certainly important, they are scarcely sufficient to warrant a separate chapter on these particular specialized tissues. Nor are there many pathological conditions of these tissues in which a central role can be ascribed to collagen. However, these tissues are of great interest because of the extremely dynamic state of their collagen. The uterine endometrium makes and destroys a collagenous framework every month of the adult reproductive life. The entire uterine framework grows about 6-fold in the last 3 months of pregnancy; then, all this scaffolding is dismantled within 2 to 3 weeks after parturition. The cervix must hold the uterus tightly closed until the end of pregnancy; then it must open to the widest possible extent in a very brief time. After this it, too, rapidly involutes to its normal resting size. In the follicle, collagen forms an impenetrable barrier to the escape of the ripe egg. Yet, in a few hours this barrier is destroyed and the egg leaves.

The major theme of this chapter, therefore, will be the dynamic state of collagen. What are the biochemical peculiarities of uterine and cervical collagen that might account for its rapid breakdown or that might arise during its rapid synthesis? What are the biological processes that account for the rapid degradation? Can the cervix and the follicle open without the destruction of collagen? While much is known, we still do not have satisfying answers to any of these questions.

It is timely to review this field now because 18 years have passed since the last major overview (Harkness, 1964). Where possible, the discussion will centre upon the human tissues. However, limited experimental work has been conducted on human subjects, so many of the topics will be illustrated by data drawn from studies on laboratory animals, especially the rat.

THE UTERUS

Most studies of uterine connective tissue have focused on the sexually mature organ. However, the collagenous structures of the human uterus in early development have been described by Herrera (1960). Cunha et al (1980) have provided an important review of the central role of the mesenchyme in controlling the differentiation of the accessory sexual structures including the uterus, vagina and cervix. Not only is this role highly significant in embryonic development, but it appears to continue into adult life and in disease processes such as cancer.

There is little information on the early growth of the human uterus in terms of its collagen content. Brown & Young (1970) and Partridge & Brown (1972) have studied collagen development in the prepubertal sow uterus. The size of the uterus depends on caloric intake; with low calorie diets the uterus is smaller and contains less collagen/organ. The proportion of collagen, however, remains fairly constant.

Collagen chemistry of the mature human uterus

The mature human uterus weighs about 50 to 70 g, excluding the cervix; of this weight, about 80 per cent is water. One gram of wet tissue contains 172 mg of protein of which two-thirds is stromal protein (Schwalm & Cretius, 1958). However, stromal protein includes all protein that is not soluble or contractile. Collagen, based on hydroxyproline content, amounts to about 22 mg per gram of wet tissue (Cretius, 1959).

Early studies of the amino acid composition of uterine collagen (Kao et al, 1967) showed a fairly typical composition; however, cysteic acid was also found. We now know from the subsequent work of Chung & Miller (1974) that the human uterus contains type III collagen as well as type I, and that this type III contains cysteine. Typing depends on first solubilizing the different forms of collagen by digesting the tissue residue with pepsin. Kao & Leslie

(1977) have shown a ratio of type I: type III of 80:20. Only 50 per cent of the uterine collagen could be solubilized, so the composition of the remaining 50 per cent is not known. However, indirect evidence such as trypsin digestibility suggests that these proportions may be correct for the entire uterine collagen. In addition to types I and III, the uterus contains small amounts of type V collagen (Chung et al, 1976).

Direct analysis of the cross-linking pattern of human uterine collagen, following reduction by sodium borohydride, shows the presence of typical reduced cross-links. The main types, each accounting for 20 to 24 per cent of the total, are dihydroxylysinonorleucine, hydroxylysinonorleucine and histidinohydroxymerodesmosine (Kao et al, 1976). In addition, small amounts of dihydroxynorleucine and various glycosylated links are present. Uterine leiomyomas show the same pattern of cross-links in their collagen. This is of interest because Henkel et al (1979) have recently shown the location of two cross-links in type III collagen of leiomyoma. One link is hydroxylysinonorleucine and the other is a novel trifunctional link. Both links originate in the N-terminal nonhelical region of the molecule and join to the helical regions of adjacent chains.

We have no data on the absolute numbers of reducible (or especially of nonreducible) cross-links in uterine collagen. Cretius (1965) and Kao et al (1967) have both commented on the small proportion of collagen that can be extracted from homogenized uterus with neutral salt and citrate buffer solutions (typically 1 to 2 per cent each). These results point to extensive cross-linking. However, that this cross-linking is less extensive in uterine collagens than it is in the collagens of other tissues is borne out by studies of thermal shrinkage. Uterine collagen has a shrinkage temperature of 55°C compared to 61°C for collagen from fascia and tendon (Brown et al, 1958). Further evidence discussed later supports the conclusion that the cross-linking is adequate to give strength to the collagen fibres, but it may not be as extensive as in other tissues. Uterine collagen may remain like a young collagen during the reproductive life.

The metabolic turnover of uterine collagen has been studied in the rat. The content of collagen in the rat uterus is similar to that in the human: about 20 to 30 mg/g wet tissue (Kao & McGavack, 1959). Kao et al (1961a) labelled young rats with U-^{14}C-lysine and then followed the loss of labelled collagen for 90 days. The half-life was found to be 12 days. Studies by the same workers (1961b) with old rats gave similar results although the half-life lengthened to about 40 days. This is still the fastest collagen turnover that they observed and exceeded that in aorta, skin and tendon. The rat uterus is a suitable tissue for the in vitro synthesis of collagen by tissue slices (Kao et al, 1964a). Enzymes involved in collagen synthesis, including prolyl hydroxylase (Salvador & Tsai, 1973b) and glycosyltransferases (Spiro & Spiro, 1971), can be readily demonstrated.

Anatomical distribution of uterine collagen

The myometrial wall

Reference is made to Figure 31.1, which depicts the human uterus. The cervix is that portion of the uterus below the internal os. The remaining portion is the uterus proper or the corpus. This is a muscular organ, the myometrium, with an inner lining or mucosa called the endometrium.

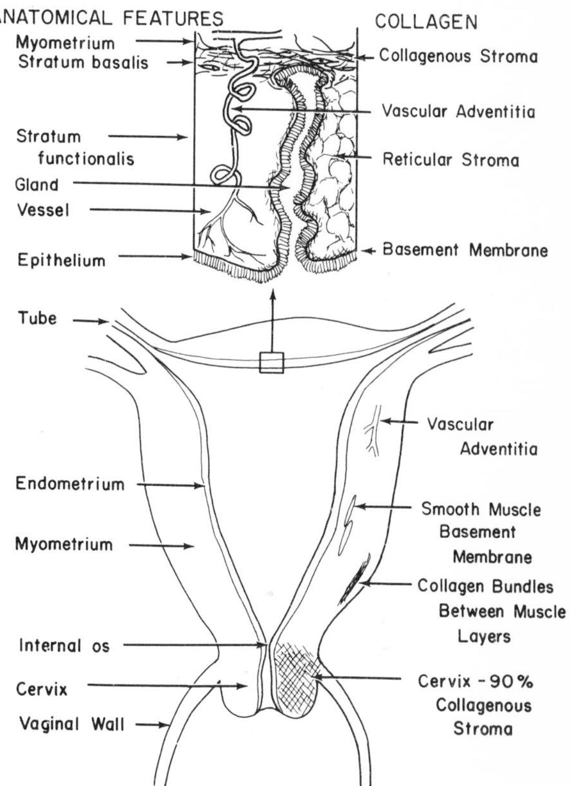

Fig. 31.1 Schematic diagram of the human uterus showing anatomical features and the location of collagenous structures. The endometrium is enlarged above; cells are greatly enlarged in proportion to the depth of the endometrial layer.

The classical description of the histology of the human uterine wall was published by Stieve (1929). He concentrated largely on the muscle fibres, but he noted fibrocytes between the muscle bundles, which produce fibres of collagen. Jaeger (1965) observed that the connective tissue becomes denser as one moves from the upper uterus to the cervix. Histologically, there is little collagen between muscle cells, but large collagenous septa occur between muscle bundles. Schwalm & Dubrauszky (1966) have provided a more quantitative picture by means of histometric measurements on 40 uteri. They distinguish an outer, middle and inner wall of the corpus. At the upper end of the corpus these layers contain 25 to 30, 35 and 40 per cent, respectively, of muscle fibre volume. In the isthmus these values fall to 18, 21 and 25 per cent, and in the cervix all drop to approximately 5 per cent. The remaining volume is occupied by connective tissue plus vasculature. Overall, the corpus consists of about 28 per cent muscle, and connective tissue comprises much of the remainder. Strauss (1969) places the connective tissue fibre volume at 34 per cent and the ground substance at 22 per cent. Strauss also determined the collagen content chemically (25 mg/g wet weight) and showed clearly that the histochemical fibre volume does not correlate well with the biochemical fibre content due to large variations in intrafibre ground substance and degree of hydration in various physiological states. The paper of Dubrauszky et al (1971) should be referred to for excellent micrographs showing the appearance of the wavy bundles of collagen fibres and their relationship to the muscle bundles.

The electron microscope shows that most of the smooth muscle cells are surrounded by a typical basal membrane (Koenig, 1971). Wherever muscle cells do not touch, the intervening space is filled with fibroblasts, collagen fibres and ground substance. Some of the wall collagen is finely fibrillar and argentophilic, the so-called reticulin fibres (Cretius, 1965). Wu et al (1978) have shown that cultured endometrium grows out 90 per cent smooth muscle cells, and that 26 per cent of the collagen they produce is type III collagen. Whether type III collagen in vivo is produced by the myometrial smooth muscle cells, or whether it is chiefly associated with the extensive vasculature remains to be determined. Ross & Klebanoff (1971) present presumptive evidence that in the mouse uterus, the myometrial smooth muscle cells are a major source of collagen synthesis.

The endometrium and the menstrual cycle

The endometrial collagen, in contrast to the myometrial collagen, undergoes considerable alteration with the menstrual cycle, so it is necessary to consider the various stages separately. The endometrium or mucosa may be divided into 3 zones: the stratum basalis, the stratum functionalis and the epithelium (compare Fig. 31.1). In the proliferative phase (days 5 to 14 of the menstrual cycle), silver staining (Dubrauszky & Schmitt, 1958) reveals a network of moderately thick fibres in the basal layer, especially around vessels and glands. Fibres also connect the endometrium to the myometrium. In the functionalis, this network of reticulin is much finer, although it increases gradually during the proliferative phase. In the secretory phase (days 15 to 27) the basal layer changes little, but the functionalis shows a very marked increase in fine argentophilic fibres. The enlarged stromal cells become enclosed in 'baskets' of reticulin fibres and the glands and vessels are densely covered.

The final phase of desquamation (days 28, 1, 2) involves extensive destruction of the reticulin network (Staemmler, 1953). The lower part of the endometrial stroma becomes oedematous and the fibres lose their silver-staining tendency and seem to dissolve until the network is gone, except around vessels and glands. Staemmler attributes this to lytic enzymes and considers it a critical step necessary for normal menstruation. A basement membrane underlies the epithelial cells which line the lumen and the glands. When the reticulin network disintegrates, the basement membranes of the glandular cells remain intact (Craig & Danziger, 1963).

Electron microscope studies reveal in slightly more detail what was found by light microscopy (Wetzstein & Wagner, 1960; Hoffmeister & Schulz, 1961). The fibres of reticulin, recognized as collagen by their characteristic cross-striations, build up in concentration during the cycle. Fibrils have a diameter of about 25 to 28 nm.

Various observations made from the middle to the end of the cycle suggest an intracellular localization of part of the collagen. Hoffmeister & Schulz (1961) see cytoplasmic collagen fibres in fibroblasts of the endometrium during rapid synthesis. They postulate that when the cells are synthesizing and secreting large quantities of collagen, the cell membrane may become momentarily disrupted in certain regions. Nemetschek-Gansler et al (1977) observe curious banded associations of collagen with a spacing about 90 nm. These forms are interpreted, by comparison to other tissues, as a stage in the degradation of type III collagen (although this is not firmly established). Some of these forms can be seen inside phagocytic cells. Dubrauszky & Schmitt (1960) note that by the middle of the cycle, 2 to 5 per cent of the ripe fibre bundles are taken into the cytoplasm of fibroblastic cells. They think the fibres are taken in, not formed internally, Wienke et al (1968) localize intracellular collagen at days 15 to 20 to lysosomal vacuoles. In the involutionary phase, by day 25, Sengel & Stoebner (1970) visualize some of the predecidual cells developing macrophage-like activity and containing vacuoles filled with striated fragments of collagen. These are believed to represent heterophagosomes engaged in collagen digestion. It may be that both points of view are correct. Earlier in the cycle when synthesis predominates, part of the collagen may be in the cell in the process of leaving. Later, it may be phagocytized as destruction commences.

Due to difficulties in sampling and timing, there have not been any quantitative studies of collagen changes during the human cycle. However, the rat has been studied by a number of workers. In this case the cycle is about 5 days long. Harkness et al (1957) failed to see differences in uterine collagen on the various days of the cycle. Smith & Kaltreider (1963) and Morgan (1963a) claimed to find cyclic differences, but their results did not agree very closely. Yochim & Blahna (1976) appear to have resolved the issue by first separating the endometrium from the myometrium. The myometrium contains about 90 per cent of the uterine mass and 98 per cent of its collagen. The remaining 2 per cent of collagen in the endometrium shows cyclic changes as great as 4-fold (Fig. 31.2). The greatest amount of collagen is found at proestrus.

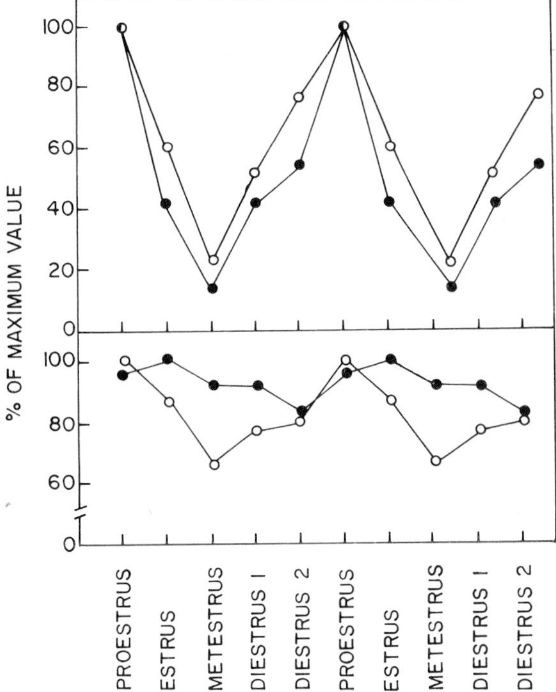

Fig. 31.2 Collagen (●) and wet weight (O) changes in the endometrium (upper panel) and myometrium (lower panel) of the cycling rat. 100% is 0.5 mg collagen and 43.3 mg wet weight in the upper panel (endometrium) and 472 mg wet weight and 25 mg collagen in the bottom panel (myometrium). (Data are taken from Yochim & Blahna, 1976.)

At this same time point, Kao et al (1964a) find the most active synthesis of collagen by uterine slices, and Amma et al (1978) find high levels of prolyl hydroxylase. Collagen then falls to a low at metestrus. At this time endometrial stromal cells contain phagocytized collagen which is membrane-bounded and seems to be undergoing degradation (Dyer & Peppler, 1977). In particular, figures showing circular coils of collagen are unlikely to represent fibres extending beyond the cell membrane. The cells involved are largely in the upper region near the endothelium and are difficult to classify between macrophages and fibroblasts.

Some interesting collagen forms underlie the basement lamina of mouse epithelial cells (Rowlatt, 1969). These are banded fibrils of 400 nm length with a symmetrical band pattern. They seem to be dimeric aggregates of tropocollagen having both ends attached to the basement membrane.

The uterus in pregnancy

Endometrial changes

Microscopic study of the pregnant uterus has focused on the endometrium, whereas quantitative chemistry has been applied to the entire organ, which is largely myometrium. An early consequence of pregnancy is the transformation of endometrial stromal cells to decidual cells (Liebig & Stegner, 1977). This process begins in the late secretory phase of the menstrual cycle, when reticular cells reach a predecidual stage. If pregnancy ensues, these cells continue their development and, by the sixth week, they become partly-developed decidual cells. The upper region of the endometrium at this stage forms a decidua compacta covered by a surface epithelium with a broad multilamellar basement membrane. Under the compacta lie large polygonal decidual cells embedded in thick collagen envelopes; this is the middle, or spongiosa, zone. Each decidual cell becomes enveloped by a 'basket' of fine reticulin fibrils (Craig & Danziger, 1963; Dubrauszky & Schmitt, 1958). The maximum formation of decidual cells is at 14 to 16 weeks; this is also the end of the period of reticulin increase and the time at which the fibre tinctorial properties become altered (Chernysheva, 1957). By 18 weeks, decidual cells begin to undergo regressive changes (Liebig & Stegner, 1977). Many cells show collagen inclusions in invaginations of the cell; this may help to anchor the cells (Wessel, 1959). Reticulin and collagen also build up a framework around the many enlarging vessels of the endometrium (Craig & Danziger, 1963).

A special event at one point in the endometrium is the implantation or nidation of the blastocyst. This topic falls under the heading of the placenta (see Ch. 26). However, it should be noted that the connective tissue of the endometrium offers a barrier to implantation. After the blastocyst attaches to the epithelial cells, the developing trophoblast must penetrate several collagenous structures: the basement membrane of the epithelial cell layer, the collagenous fibres of the stroma and adventitia around the blood vessel to which connection must be made, and finally the basement membrane of the vessel endothelial layer. Wislocki & Dempsey (1948) have pointed out the fact of trophoblastic attack on collagen, but there have not yet been any studies of collagenases that might function to break through these various types of collagen.

Myometrial changes

In the pregnant uterus, there is a considerable development in fibrocytes in the myometrial wall, with extensive deposition of collagen between the muscle layers (Stieve, 1929). This increase in collagen does not keep pace with muscle development, however, so there is a gradual decline in the proportion of collagen (Dubrauszky et al, 1971). Histometric measurements indicate that collagen drops from 25 per cent of the myometrial volume in the first trimester of pregnancy to 18 per cent in the last trimester. Strauss (1969) performed an elegant study combining morphometry with biochemistry. During the growth of the uterus from the nongravid state to term, the percentage of area occupied by connective tissue fibres remains constant at 35 per cent, whereas the collagen content declines from 25 to 14.5 mg/gram wet weight. This discrepancy is due to an increase in ground substance within the fibre structure as pregnancy advances. Muscle fibres increase from 25 per cent of uterine volume in early pregnancy to 50 per cent at term (Schwalm & Dubrauszky, 1966).

The uterus at term

The growth of the human uterus in pregnancy is truly amazing. Zimmer (1965) estimates that the volume increased 150-fold, including the conceptus, and the surface area 30-fold. The growth of weight and collagen have been tabulated by Woessner & Brewer (1963), Montfort & Pérez-Tamayo (1961), and Morrione & Seifter (1962). The wet weight increases 10- to 16-fold (depending on previous pregnancies) to about 1 kg. The collagen content increases 7- to 8-fold to about 35 g total. Most of this growth occurs in the last trimester.

In spite of this very extensive and rapid growth of collagen, the finished product seems to have full mechanical strength to resist the large forces generated during expulsion of the baby. Histologically, the collagen fibres appear normal at term. There is some softening and depolymerization of the ground substance (Narik, 1960). There is a dissociation of reticular fibres to finer fibrils and a further fragmentation of these occasioned by labour (Chernysheva, 1957). Biochemically, too, the collagen appears to be normal in terms of solubility and shrinkage temperature (Cretius, 1965; Cretius et al, 1966). However, an experiment by Woessner (1963) suggests this newly-formed collagen may be less highly cross-linked than mature collagen. The rate of digestion of this collagen by bacterial collagenase from *Clostridium histolyticum* was 2-fold faster than the rate for nongravid uterine collagen and 4-fold faster than that for postmenopausal uterine collagen.

Mechanical factors in the uterine growth of pregnancy

The question is often raised as to the relative contributions to uterine growth of hormonal status and the pressure exerted by the growing fetuses. The best answers to this question have come from studies on bicornuate uteri, since there is always a contralateral control available. Harkness & Harkness (1956) postulated that mechanical factors were of major importance in uterine growth, since both horns of the rat uterus showed minimal growth in 12 days of pregnancy; then from 12 to 21 days, the pregnant horn grew tremendously, while the nonpregnant horn showed little further growth. Thus, only 75 per cent of a total increase of 600 per cent could be attributed to hormonal influences. Moreover, the size and collagen content of a horn at term were directly related to the number of fetuses in that horn.

Cullen & Harkness (1968) ovariectomized mature rats, then instituted a regimen of oestradiol, progesterone and relaxin that would mimic the conditions on day 17 of pregnancy. They injected 200 mg of paraffin wax daily through the vagina into one uterine horn. This produced a 5-fold increase in uterine weight and a 3-fold increase in collagen content in comparison to the control horn (Fig. 31.3). These increases are equivalent to those found in pregnancy.

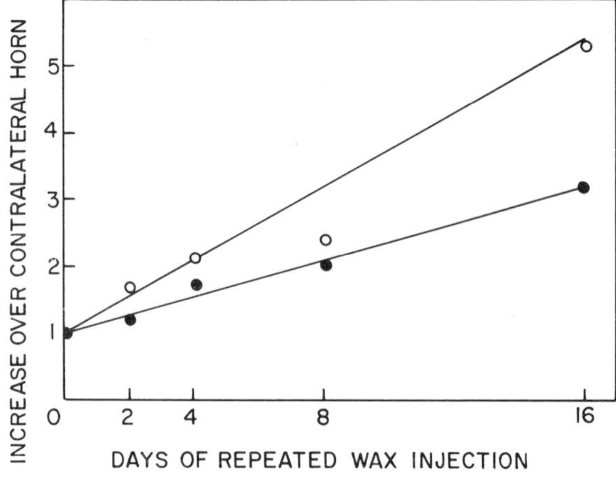

Fig. 31.3 Effect of mechanical stretching on uterine collagen (●) and wet weight (O). Paraffin wax 0.2 g was injected into the uterus each day of the experiment. The starting value of 1 = 120 mg wet weight and 3.3 mg of collagen. Changes in the contralateral horn which received no mechanical stimulus were subtracted as a control. (Data from Cullen & Harkness, 1968.)

Takács & Verzár (1968) used untreated rats, gave a single injection of 2 g of paraffin and achieved a 4-fold increase in weight; however, collagen increased only 50 per cent. It may be concluded that hormones alone produce minimal collagen growth, but they do govern the response produced by distension.

The removal of the fetuses is essential to involution. Wray (1979) removed fetuses on day 18 of pregnancy and replaced them with Silgel dummies. By 7 days post partum this region of the horn showed no involution; indeed, it had increased collagen, while the contralateral horn had completely involuted.

Deciduoma formation

The uterine endometrium can be artificially induced to decidualize and form a maternal placenta (deciduoma) if it is subjected to certain stimuli, such as scratching, when it is in the progestational state. Again, the human uterus has not been studied extensively for obvious reasons. Most frequently, rats are used. First, stimulation of the cervix with a rod at oestrus induces pseudopregnancy. On the fourth day, the endometrial lining is scratched along the length of one horn, and by the eighth day, a large deciduoma is fully developed. Microscopy reveals two families of cells: large and small decidual cells (Wolfe & Wright, 1942). There is considerable formation of reticulin and collagen, particularly around the small cells. Most of the endometrium is involved in this process. There is also a considerable stretching of the myometrium, with separation of muscle bundles and deposition of intervening connective tissue (Lobel et al, 1965a).

Beyond the ninth day, the deciduoma regresses,and by the 20–21st day, it is gone. The deciduoma begins to cleave away from the uterine wall and undergoes degeneration involving autophagy and heterophagy by macrophages (Lobel et al, 1965b). The reticulin and collagen fibres are among the last components to be degraded.

Jeffrey et al (1975) quantitated these changes. In their experiments the deciduomata grew for 8 days (12th day of pseudopregnancy), achieving a mass of about 3 g and a collagen content of about 25 mg (Fig. 31.4). These represent 10-fold and 5-fold increases over control horns. Resorption began on day 12, but collagen breakdown did not begin until about day 15. At this time collagenase production by cultured deciduoma tissue began to rise and reached a peak when the tissue was cultured on day 17. The production of collagenase was blocked by progesterone in the culture medium.

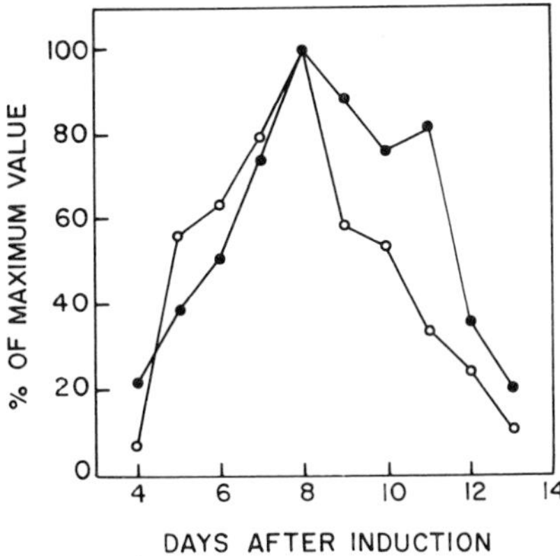

Fig. 31.4 Changes in wet weight (O) and collagen (●) in deciduomata induced in the uterine horns of rats on the fourth day of pseudopregnancy. The maximum values were 3.2 g wet weight and 25.4 mg collagen. (Data are taken from Jeffrey et al, 1975.)

Uterine involution

The human uterus

The tremendous growth of the uterus and its extensive collagen framework serve no useful function after delivery, so both are rapidly undone and the uterus is restored to an approximation of its original nongravid state, ready for another reproductive cycle. It has proved quite difficult to study this process in the human because there is rarely occasion to remove the uterus 1 to 2 weeks after parturition. However, an outline of the involutionary process may be sketched (Fig. 31.5) based on a few reports. What strikes one's attention is that in comparison to the rate of uterine growth and collagen formation in pregnancy, the resorption of the uterus and the breakdown

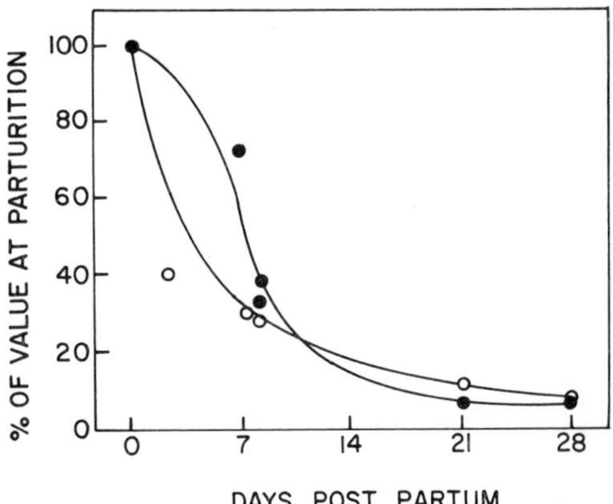

Fig. 31.5 Post partum involution of the human uterus. The initial values are 100 = 1000 g wet weight (O) and 35 g collagen (●). The curve is drawn with considerable freedom, based on the results for rats (Fig. 31.8) and giving particular weight to the 7–9 day period where there are 4–5 measurements. (Data are taken from Montfort & Pérez-Tamayo, 1961; Morrione & Seifter, 1962 and Woessner & Brewer, 1963.)

of collagen in involution occur at a truly phenomenal rate — the uterus is back to its normal size within 3 weeks post partum. In lactating women involution continues beyond this point and produces a hyperinvolution at 4 to 8 weeks (Morrione & Seifter, 1962; Woessner & Brewer, 1963). These authors also note that collagen is degraded in vitro by uterine enzymes at acid pH (3 to 4), but not at neutral pH. There is little accumulation of collagen degradation products in the uterus: only a few per cent of the collagen is soluble, and there is an increase in free hydroxyproline to about 1 per cent of the total tissue content of hydroxyproline (Weossner & Brewer, 1963). Trypsin digests 12 to 21 per cent of the collagen (Hertel & Schmitt, 1968). This was once thought to indicate the presence of partially degraded collagen, but is now known merely to reflect the presence of type III collagen (Miller et al, 1976).

Histologically, the involuting uterus contains increased numbers of macrophages, lymphocytes, mast cells and eosinophils in the myometrial layers. Fibres become disorganized and lose their argyrophilia (Morrione & Seifter, 1962). Stieve (1929) attributes most of the breakdown to the destruction of fibrocytes and fibres and the carrying off of debris by monocytes and macrophages. A small part of the collagen, in the endometrial layer, may be lost by sloughing into the lumen, especially at the placental site (Anderson & Davis, 1968).

The rat uterus

Interest in the mechanisms that produce the tremendous rates of collagen breakdown in involution coupled with the difficulty of working with human tissue, has led a number of workers to study involution in the rat uterus. The process is even more rapid here, being about 90 per cent complete within 96 hours post partum.

The pioneering work on this problem was done by the Harnkesses in the early 1950's. In their first paper (Harkness & Harkness, 1954) they showed the rapid growth of uterine weight and collagen during the last week of pregnancy: both parameters increase 5- to 6-fold. Then, immediately following parturition, there is a rapid loss of weight and collagen that is well advanced by 3 days post partum and essentially complete by 6 days. At term, the uterus contains about 60 mg of collagen, and during involution, 90 per cent of this collagen is degraded. The finer details of this collagen breakdown were reported in 1956 (Harkness & Moralee). There is a delay of 12 to 24 hours in the initiation of collagen breakdown; then an extreme rate of degradation (half-life of 24 hours) is attained. The breakdown process must be due to catabolism within the tissue, since hydroxyproline does not leave through the lumen. These results have been amply verified by Montfort & Pérez-Tamayo (1961) and Woessner (1962). Figure 31.6 shows results I have obtained with 300 rats. In a search for metabolic breakdown products, I showed (1962) that the soluble forms of collagen increase slightly

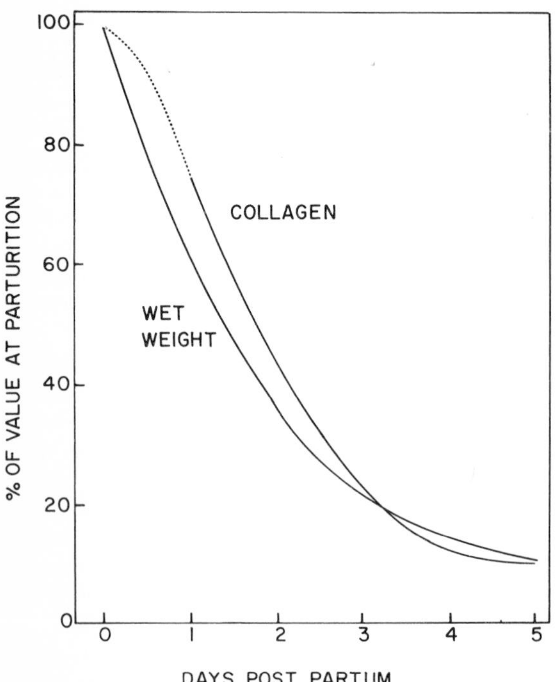

Fig. 31.6 Post partum involution of the rat uterus. The initial values are 100 = 2.65 g wet weight (O) and 64.5 mg collagen (●). These curves are based on data from 300 rats studied over a 20 year period. (From Woolley D W, Evanson J M 1980 Collagenase in normal and pathological connective tissue, Wiley, London, with permission.)

during involution, peptide products are barely detectable and free hydroxyproline rises about 5-fold to 100 μg/g wet tissue by 70 hours post partum. This indicates that collagen molecules, once entering on the breakdown pathway, pass rapidly through intervening stages to the level of free amino acids. Less than 15 per cent of the hydroxyproline is excreted in the urine; the remainder is probably oxidized in tissues such as the lung.

The collagen which is laid down in pregnancy is cross-linked and insoluble, but it is not as firmly linked as collagen from nongravid uteri. Heating the collagen to 65°C for 10 minutes releases 11 per cent of the collagen, whereas at the end of involution only 6 per cent is labile. In the human uterus, the collagen at term is digested twice as rapidly as normal by bacterial collagenase (Woessner, 1963). While these changes would aid a more rapid breakdown of collagen during involution, they cannot begin to account for the extremely rapid rates observed.

Mechanisms of collagen breakdown in involution: collagenase. While this topic is covered by Werb (Ch. 7), and by Pérez-Tamayo (Ch. 8), it is worth discussing briefly here because the uterus displays such rapid breakdown and also illustrates several pathways in one tissue. A great deal of enzymatic and morphological information is available on the rat uterus.

The rise in soluble collagen and free hydroxyproline during collagen breakdown clearly points to a proteolytic mechanism of degradation. It now appears that such proteolyis may involve both intracellular and extracellular enzymes. The beginnings of both pathways were traced out in 1962. Gross & Lapière (1962) cultured slices of rat uterus on collagen gels and demonstrated the production of extracellular collagenase. Woessner (1962) homogenized rat uteri and showed the presence of an intracellular cathepsin that digested collagen at pH 3.5.

Uterine collagenase was first obtained in quantity by tissue culture methods (Jeffrey & Gross, 1970). The enzyme was partially purified and shown to be a typical collagenase: metal-dependent and capable of cutting the collagen helix. Tissue cultured from nongravid uterus produces no enzyme; there is only a brief period between 12 and 72 hours post partum when the tissue will produce enzyme. This is just the time of most rapid breakdown of collagen (Jeffrey et al, 1971a). Ryan & Woessner (1971) were able to demonstrate collagenase directly in homogenates of the involuting uterus. The enzyme cannot be extracted readily from tissue homogenates; but the insoluble portion of such homogenates contains both collagen and collagenase, possibly in intimate association. Incubation of uterine 'pellets' releases hydroxyproline-containing peptides in proportion to the enzyme activity present. Weeks et al (1976) then developed a procedure for extracting the enzyme by heating in 0.1M $CaCl_2$ at 60°C for 4 minutes. Direct tissue assay of the enzyme, taking into account both latent and active forms of the enzyme

(Weossner, 1979a) has shown that collagenase is barely detectable during pregnancy and at the moment of parturition. It then rises to a maximum at 24 hours post partum and declines to low values by 5 days post partum. The uterus is one of the first physiological systems of collagen resorption in which it has been possible to trace the course of enzyme activity by direct tissue assay. The close agreement of enzyme activity with collagen breakdown rate is good circumstantial evidence that collagenase is involved in this breakdown.

Uterine collagenase is under the control of the ovarian hormones, oestradiol and progesterone. Uterine fragments in culture do not produce collagenase if progesterone is added to the medium (Jeffrey et al, 1971b). Oestradiol has no effect in this system. In the living animal, on the other hand, oestradiol inhibits the post-partum resorption of collagen (Woessner, 1969). Progesterone will also produce inhibition but only when administered in sublethal doses (Halme & Woessner, 1975). The treatments with oestradiol and progesterone appear to act by reducing the tissue levels of collagenase (Woessner, 1979a). The reduction of oestradiol is exactly proportional to the reduction of collagen breakdown, lending further support to the hypothesis that uterine collagen is degraded by collagenase. It is not yet clear why cultured uterine tissue is sensitive to progesterone and not oestradiol, while in vivo, the situation is reversed. The culture work must be re-examined in the light of more recent information on the existence of latent forms of collagenase produced in vitro.

Uterine collagenase is under further controls besides the hormonal ones. The enzyme is found in the tissue in a latent form, probably as an enzyme-inhibitor complex. Even at the peak of involution, only 35 per cent of the enzyme is recovered in a free form (Woessner, 1979a). The uterus also contains a serine proteinase which is able to activate the latent collagenase (Woessner, 1977). However, even latent enzyme appears to be absent until after parturition. Either a cell type in the uterus, such as the fibroblast, is not activated to produce collagenase until a signal arrives in the form of low oestrogen and progesterone levels; or else a new cell type arrives after parturition, e.g., the macrophage.

Collagenase only initiates collagen breakdown, it cannot complete it. Further digestion may take place intracellularly (next section) or may continue by means of a battery of enzymes including specialized peptidases (Woessner, 1979b; Ryan & Woessner, 1972).

Mechanisms of collagen breakdown in involution: lysosomal digestion. In contrast to the biochemical data which point to a central role for collagenase in involution, the morphological data point to an important role for the phagocytosis and lysosomal digestion of collagen. Luse & Hutton (1964) were the first to describe intracellular collagen fragments in fibroblasts of the involuting rat uterus. Electron microscopy established the banded nature of the collagen. Schwarz & Güldner (1967) saw many phagocytized collagen fibres in cells they identified as histiocytes. These fibres are seen maximally at 2 to 3 days post partum and are confined to the myometrium. The collagen fragments are clearly enclosed in membranes and can be seen in various stages of degradation. Parakkal (1969) obtained striking electron micrographs of the mouse uterus showing macrophages packed with collagen-containing vacuoles. Acid phosphatase is in these same vacuoles. Later, he repeated this work with rats. The macrophages are present in the uterus near the end of pregnancy, but do not stain for acid phosphatase (Parakkal, 1972). Within 4 hours after parturition, enzyme staining becomes apparent in macrophages below the endometrium lining. These cells soon spread through the endometrium and then into the myometrium. By 3 days they are throughout the uterus ingesting and digesting collagen. The same events are seen in nongravid contralateral horns, indicating hormonal rather than mechanical control of the process. Brandes & Anton (1969) include fibroblasts and smooth muscle cells as participants in collagen phagocytosis. Collagen phagocytosis by fibroblasts has also been observed in the involuting human uterus (Okamura et al, 1976).

Tansey & Padykula (1978) examined the endometrial layer of the rat uterus after treatment with 100 μg oestradiol or 40 mg progesterone (doses previously shown to inhibit involution). Oestradiol treatment reduces the numbers of eosinophils, heterophils and macrophages. The macrophages are reduced by a blocking of the conversion of tissue monocytes to macrophages. At the same time there is less breakdown of collagen in the deeper layers of the endometrium. Unfortunately, the myometrium, containing the bulk of collagen, was not studied.

If ingestion of collagen and digestion within the lysosomal system of one or more cell types represents a major pathway of collagen degradation, it may be asked 'what are the responsible enzymes?' Woessner (1962) showed that uterine homogenates digested collagen at pH 3.5 to 4.0; this would be consistent with intralysosomal protease action. Lysosomal enzymes increase in concentration some 3- to 5-fold during post partum involution, a finding consistent with a role of lysosomal cathepsins in this process (Woessner, 1965). Schaub (1964) found that acid collagenolytic activity increases in pregnancy and still more post partum. It is inhibited by p-chloromercuribenzoate; this suggests that a thiol cathepsin is responsible. Etherington (1973) described the enzyme activity as collagenolytic cathepsin and showed that activity rose to a peak 2 days after parturition. Burleigh (1977) has reviewed the digestion of collagen by acid cathepsins and concluded that cathepsin B and collagenolytic cathepsin are two distinct lysosomal thiol proteinases which can degrade collagen at 37°C. Woessner (1978) has found that the uterus contains both cathepsin B and collagenolytic cathepsin and that the latter may be quantitatively more important in collagen breakdown.

It has not yet been resolved whether collagen digestion within cells requires prior action of collagenase. It might be postulated that damage by collagenase is a signal for phagocytosis to commence. Agents such as oestradiol inhibit involution to the same extent that they reduce collagenase activity. This would be consistent with collagenases being involved in initiating the breakdown of all collagen. However, it has been possible to find some agents such as triamcinolone which retard breakdown without reducing collagenase (Woessner, unpublished results). Therefore, the possibility must be left open that the uterus contains two independent pathways of collagen degradation.

Effects of hormones on uterine collagen

The menstrual/oestrus cycle provides one example of how changing hormonal levels affect the deposition and removal of collagen. However, the effects of oestradiol in this case are limited largely to the endometrium, which comprises only a few per cent of the total uterine collagen. Striking effects can be demonstrated on myometrial collagen by two methods: administering oestradiol to immature animals produces a gain in collagen, and ovariectomizing mature animals causes a loss. Most of the data illustrating the effects of these treatments have come from studies on rats, since humans are generally not amenable to study. However, the atrophy of the postmenopausal human uterus is a direct analogue to ovariectomy effects. The losses and gains of collagen are probably not due to direct effects on collagen synthetic and degradative pathways but to effects on uterine size. The collagen framework subsequently adjusts itself to the changing mechanical requirements.

Burack et al (1942) administered oestradiol to immature rats. In short-term experiments, there is increasing deposition of collagen and transformation of reticulin to collagen. In long-term experiments (up to 300 days) myometrial collagen becomes denser as the uterine wall thickens. In quantitative studies, Salvador & Tsai (1973a) injected 5 μg oestradiol per day into 19-day old rats. The results are illustrated in Figure 31.7. Both wet weight and collagen increase in comparison to control values; however, the collagen increase lags behind the weight increase and does not increase in the same proportion. The rise in collagen is accompanied by a striking increase in prolyl hydroxylase. Kao & Hitt (1974) have shown that oestradiol also stimulates the formation of reducible cross-links in rat uterine collagen.

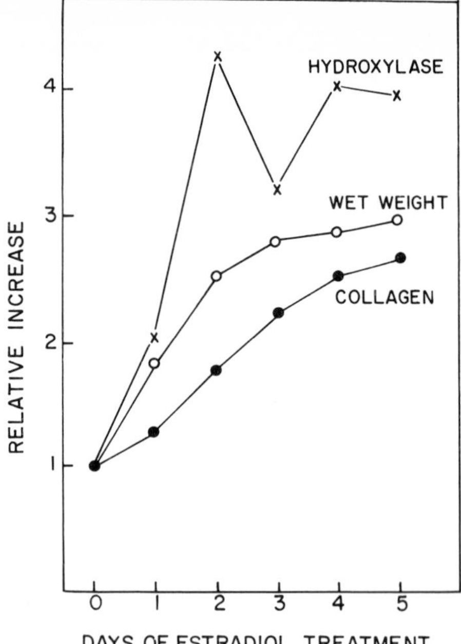

Fig. 31.7 Relative increases in collagen (●), wet weight (O) and prolyl hydroxylase activity (x) when immature 20-day old rats were given daily injections of 5 μg oestradiol. The starting point is 1 = 18 mg wet weight and 1.8 mg collagen. Subsequent values are corrected for the growth observed in untreated controls. (Data are taken from Salvador & Tsai, 1973a, b.)

Ovariectomy effects on rat uterine collagen

Harkness et al (1956) ovariectomized mature female rats (180 g) and found a slow involution of the uterus out to 6 weeks. Uterine wet weight fell from 330 mg to 78 mg. Collagen changes are illustrated in Figure 31.8. Other workers have observed more striking decreases in collagen (Kao et al, 1964b; Morgan, 1963b). Those of Smith & Kaltreider (1963) are also illustrated in Figure 31.8. The loss of collagen is relatively slow in this situation, and again is never quite as extensive as the loss in weight. Ovariectomy leads to decreased synthesis of collagen by

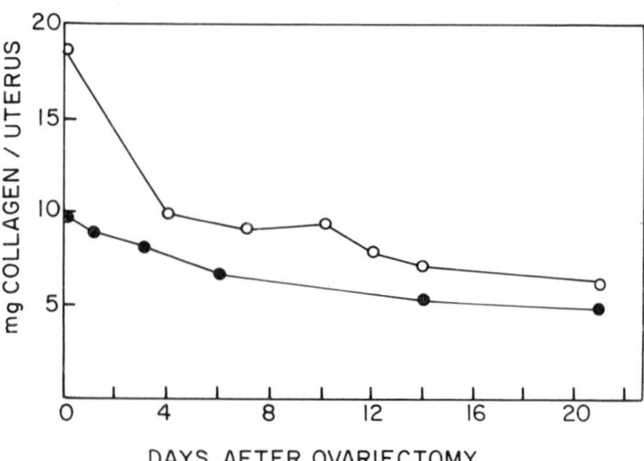

Fig. 31.8 Loss of collagen from the uteri of mature female rats after ovariectomy. (Data are taken from Harkness et al, 1956, ● and from Smith & Kaltreider, 1963, O.)

uterine slices in vitro (Kao et al, 1964b). A limiting factor may be prolyl hydroxylase activity which decreases by 85 per cent (whole organ basis) within 3 weeks (Salvador & Tsai, 1973b). There is no information on what happens to the rate of collagen breakdown.

Treatment with oestradiol tends to reverse the effects of ovariectomy. If rats are ovariectomized and held until involution of the uterus is complete, uterine growth can be stimulated with oestradiol. Two- to 4-fold increases in collagen were produced (Cullen & Harkness, 1960, 1964; Morgan, 1963b). Relaxin and progesterone do not augment the effects of oestradiol. It is also possible to administer appropriate doses of oestradiol which will completely block involution following ovariectomy (Smith & Kaltreider, 1963).

Slices of uterus from ovariectomized rats synthesize only 7 per cent as much collagen in vitro as do normal uterine slices (Kao et al, 1964b). Synthetic activity can be restored to normal if the rats are treated with 1 μg oestradiol for 3 days. Oestradiol is more effective than oestrone or oestriol, and progesterone has no effect. Prolyl hydroxylase may be a limiting factor in collagen synthesis. The depressed levels of this enzyme in the uteri of ovariectomized rats are rapidly restored to normal by oestradiol treatment (Kao et al, 1969; Salvador & Tsai, 1973b).

Hormonal effects on collagen breakdown during involution

In the rat, pregnancy comes to an end when progesterone levels drop. Oestradiol also drops at the time of parturition. The absence of one or both of these hormones may be essential for the rapid breakdown of collagen in the post partum period. If rats are ovariectomized at parturition, involution proceeds at the normal rapid pace for 2 days. However, it then continues on without abating to 12 days, resulting in a tremendous hyperinvolution (Morrione & Ru, 1964). The uterus shrinks to one-tenth its normal size; it weighs 32 mg and contains only 0.4 mg of collagen. This suggests that the slowly rising oestradiol and progesterone of the post partum ovary may limit the extent of involution in the normal case. Lactation also suppresses the return of ovarian function, possibly through prolactin action. The uteri of nonlactating rats do not show a hyperinvolution; their weight and collagen losses stop when normal values are reached (Grant, 1965; Woessner, 1962). Maintenance of high levels of hormones immediately post partum will also retard collagen breakdown. Oestradiol (Woessner, 1969) and progesterone (Halme & Woessner, 1975) are both effective. Oestradiol acts to inhibit collagen breakdown in this situation, as opposed to the cases mentioned above where it stimulates collagen synthesis. This has been shown in three ways: by the failure of prelabelled collagen to break down at the normal rate, by the failure of free hydroxyproline to rise in the tissue and by the lack of stimulation of radioactive labelling of collagen (Ryan & Woessner, 1972). The effect of oestradiol appears to be due to its action in reducing collagenase activity (p. 513).

Finally, oestradiol is important in the restoration of mature collagen fibres in the endometrial stroma following parturition. Suckling prevents the deposition of dense collagen fibres until after weaning (22 to 30 days; Fainstat, 1965). If the pups are removed to block lactation, an oestrus cycle ensues, and at the second oestrus (about 7 days post partum), collagen appears (Fainstat, 1963). If the rat is ovariectomized at parturition, no collagen is seen by 17 days, but if 1 μg oestradiol is given daily, mature fibres appear in the endometrium by 2 to 3 days and in the myometrium by 5 to 6 days. Progesterone has no effect (Fainstat, 1962).

Uterine ageing

The postmenopausal human uterus undergoes a gradual process of atrophy related to a diminished production of sex hormones by the ovary. In the endometrium, the superficial layers tend to be lost, but the basalis persists. Cell loss leads to an increased concentration of reticulin, (see Ch. 1), which is arranged in bands parallel to the surface (Craig & Danziger, 1963). In the myometrium, muscle mass diminishes and the intervening reticulin coalesces to form prominent collagen bands. The uterine artery and related vessels also diminish in size (Lapina, 1947). This histological picture is borne out by quantitative studies (Cretius, 1959; Strauss, 1969) showing a 25 to 100 per cent increase in collagen/g wet weight of tissue. The higher value appears more reliable.

The involution of old age, as well as post partum involution, offers a paradigmatic illustration of the difficulty of evaluating collagen metabolism on the basis of histology or concentration studies. Thus, during pregnancy, collagen concentration declines to a low point and then rises to a maximum during involution. Likewise, in atrophy due to age, the concentration of collagen doubles. These results give a totally false impression of the metabolic processes, the true nature of which can only be fully appreciated when the total collagen content of the organ is taken into consideration. Thus, in pregnancy, the collagen is increasing by 700 to 800 per cent in a tremendous burst of synthesis, which, however, is exceeded by a still more rapid synthesis of other components which dilute the collagen and reduce its concentration. In the involution following parturition. collagen breakdown approaches the highest rates found in any tissue. Yet, since this process lags behind the loss of other components of the uterus, there is a rising concentration of collagen and the fibres are more closely packed in histological section. So it is, too, with the involution of old age. The gain of collagen is only an apparent gain; when the entire organ is measured (Woessner, 1963), about 50 per cent of the collagen is found to be lost. This is a slow process, commencing at the menopause. In order to see the effect of age clearly, it is necessary to cancel out the effects of parity (number of births). Even though post partum involution reduces the size and collagen content of the uterus to about half the normal value, this phase is rapidly passed and the uterus returns to a final resting state larger than it was before pregnancy. With repeated pregnancies, the collagen level increases until, after eight or more births, it is double the content in virgin uteri.

There are also changes in the properties of uterine collagen with age. The shrinkage temperature, which is similar to that of fetal collagen in adult uterus rises from 55°C to 58°C, but does not reach the value of 61°C found in old fascia (Brown et al, 1958). Reducible cross-links remain fairly high, even in 82-year old collagen (Kao et al, 1976). However, fluorescence of collagen, which is lacking in most mature uteri, becomes uniformly bright in postmenopausal uteri (Brown et al, 1958). This may correspond to the development of a novel reduced cross-link of the pyridinoline type discovered by Fujimoto (1980). If so, it would help to explain the higher shrinkage temperature and the two-fold increase in resistance to digestion by clostridial collagenase (Woessner, 1963). Postmenopausal collagen still has an amino acid composition resembling reticulin (Harding, 1963) which points to the continuing existence of type III collagen in old age.

The rat uterus does not offer a very close analogy to the human uterus since it continues to increase in its total weight and collagen content throughout life (Árvay et al, 1971; Kao & Hitt, 1974). However, there is a lower rate of synthesis and turnover of collagen in old age (2 years; Kao et al, 1961b). The cross-linking pattern shifts from a 10:1 ratio of dihydroxylysinonorleucine: hydroxylysinonorleucine to a 4:1 ratio. As the collagen increases with age, so do the reducible cross-links, but at a slower rate. Thus, at 25 months, there is about 35 per cent less reducible cross-link/mg collagen that at 6 weeks of age. This is not a very pronounced decrease. Multiple parity does not increase the collagen content of the rat's uterus (Rundgren, 1974).

Uterine disease

Fibroids, or leiomyomas, are relatively common in the human. Any mature uterus that makes its way to the biochemistry laboratory after surgery usually contains a number of fibroids of varying sizes. The collagen in these tissues does not seem to differ very much from that of normal uterine tissue. The collagen content is a little higher: 5.2 mg/g wet tissue compared to 3.7 mg for normal tissue (Purkayastha & Roy, 1956). Korchagin & Pashkova (1974) state that the collagen content of these leiomyomas is correlated with the age of the woman. There appears to be about 20 per cent type III collagen in this tissue (Chung & Miller, 1974). No change can be detected in the cross-linking pattern (Kao et al, 1976). A novel cross-link has been isolated from leiomyoma by Henkel et al (1979), but this may be unique to type III collagen rather than unique to the myoma.

Another problem of clinical interest is that of irregular shedding of the uterine lining in the menses. Dallenbach-Hellweg & Bornebusch (1970) have observed that in such cases there is a failure of the disintegration of the endometrial reticulin fibres. They postulate that the cyclic drop in progesterone triggers the release of relaxin from endometrial cells and this, in turn, induces disintegration of the reticulin fibres. The progestin contraceptives tend to override this process. At the appropriate time, oestrogen levels drop, water is lost from the tissue, the endometrium shrinks, and arteries and veins collapse, producing ischaemia. But without the drop in progesterone, the reticulin fibres hold the endometrium firmly anchored and shedding is delayed, patchy and irregular.

Sedlis & Kim (1971) report on a series of patients whose endometrium shows a thick collagen band immediately beneath the epithelial cell layer. This is restricted to cases of anovulation and Stein-Levinthal syndrome. Agrawal & Fox (1972) dispute this causal relationship. In any event, the finding is of limited diagnostic value since only 17 per cent of anovulatory patients showed the band.

THE CERVIX

The human cervix and its dilatation

The uterine cervix is considered separately from the corpus uterus because of its distinctive structure and function. Danforth (1947) was one of the first proponents of the concept that the cervix is a passive connective tissue structure, whereas the uterus is an active muscular organ. While small amounts of smooth muscle tissue are found in the cervix, typically on the order of 10 per cent (Dubrauszky, 1965; Schwalm & Dubrauszky, 1966), this tissue does not seem to play an important role in governing the opening and closing of the cervix. There is a sharp transition from uterus to cervix at the level of the internal os (Fig. 31.1). The cervix consists of a heavy mass of stromal tissue and is lined with an endometrial or mucosal layer, which has an underlying basement membrane. This membrane has been studied by electron microscopy (Younes et al, 1965; Garska, 1966) and is a typical collagenous structure. However, as in the corpus, there is not much contribution from the basement membrane and mucosa to the total collagen content of the cervix.

The cervix is of particular interest because of its ability to open to a 10 cm aperture at term to permit the passage of the baby from the womb. Descriptions of the changes that take place in the cervix as parturition approaches are based largely on light microscopy. Biochemical changes have been measured largely in biopsies, not in the entire cervix, so there is little solid information on net changes, only on concentration changes.

The muscle and collagen content of the cervix both increase during pregnancy, but in relatively small proportion to the growth of the uterus (Danforth, 1947). As term approaches the collagen fibres become more widely separated by increased ground substance and oedematous change (Stieve, 1929). Instead of smooth, parallel wavy bundles or sheets of collagen, there is more disarray, fragmentation and splitting up of bundles while reticulin becomes more luxuriant and thicker (Voutsa et al, 1963; Runge & Riehm, 1952; Danforth et al, 1960). How this contributes to increased distensibility is not clear. Ferenczy (1980) believes there is an actual loss of collagen; he supports this by an electron microscopic demonstration of collagen phagocytosis and intralysosomal digestion by histiocytes in the early post partum period. However, there is little biochemical data to support these views.

The cervix at the time of labour contains 82.6 per cent water, compared to 78 per cent in nongravid cervix. Collagen is only 24.4 mg/g wet tissue compared to 35.5 mg in controls (Cretius, 1959). Similar figures have been presented by Danforth et al (1960) and Strauss (1969); in their studies collagen concentration dropped 50 per cent. However, it is not clear if this is an absolute decrease or only a dilution by water and other components. Indeed, if the cervix grows, there may be more collagen in toto by term. Anderson & Turnbull (1969) summed up the results of hydroxyproline measurements by concluding that the concentration of collagen is not correlated with changes in the physical state of the cervix and the onset of labour.

It has been postulated by Berwind (1954) that the cementing substances between fibres are broken down, loosening the ties between fibrils. Buckingham et al (1962) could find no striking changes in hexosamine concentration near term. On the other hand, Kondo (1972), Karube et al (1975) and Breen et al (1975) all find an increase in glycosaminoglycans and/or glycoprotein in the cervix at term. Von Maillot et al (1979) have performed detailed analyses of the various types of glycosaminoglycans. At the time of early labour, hyaluronate is 29 per cent of the total and chondroitin 7 per cent. Chondroitin sulphates have dropped from 55 per cent to 31 per cent which should lower tissue rigidity, and keratan sulphate has risen from 17 to 33 per cent which may limit the diameter of collagen fibrils. However, the total glyosaminoglycans/g dry weight show no change over nongravid controls.

Quantitation of collagen and ground substance carbohydrates has not given a clear answer as to the mechanism of cervical dilatation. Therefore, attention has been turned to the physical properties of the collagen, with a view to demonstrating reduced fibre stability or strength. Danforth & Buckingham (1964) extracted cervical tissue with 0.15M NaCl, 0.5M NaCl, and citrate buffer. They solubilized a total of 25 per cent of the dilated cervix in this way, compared to 15 per cent soluble in controls. But this preliminary data has not been fully substantiated. Cretius (1965) extracted only 3 to 4 per cent of the collagen by such means, and this value was only slightly higher at term than in controls. Von Maillot & Zimmermann (1976) extracted 11 per cent at full dilatation compared to 3 per cent in early pregnancy and 6 per cent in early labour. These changes do not involve a very large fraction of the collagen, but they at least occur at the proper time and indicate either a partial degradation of collagen or an increased accessibility of solvents to the fibres. Kleissl et al (1978) lean to the view that collagen is being degraded. The soluble collagen, upon electrophoresis, does not give typical α- and β-bands. They suggest it is degraded to smaller pieces, but this has not been proven.

Collagen typing indicates that the cervix, like the uterus, contains type III as well as type I collagen. Type III is about 20 per cent of the total (Kleissl et al, 1978). This value does not change from nongravid to term; however, type I collagen can be readily extracted by pepsin digestion from the cervix at term, whereas 50 per cent of type I is unextracted from the nonpregnant cervix (Ito et al, 1979). This suggests a reduced extent of cross-linking of type I collagen in the cervix at term. It would also fit nicely with the thesis of Veis (1980) that digestion of non-helical extension peptides of collagen by nonspecific neutral proteases might weaken the interconnections between fibrils sufficiently to allow slippage. The cross-links after reduction are typically dihydroxylysinonorleucine, plus hydroxylysinonorleucine and histidinohydroxymerodesmosine (Kleissl et al, 1978).

Collagenase can be detected directly in cervical tissue (Kitamura et al, 1979), but it increases only slightly from the nongravid to the term cervix (1.7 to 2.2 units). Cultured cervical tissue releases collagenase into the medium. If patients close to term are treated with dehydroepiandrosterone, their tissue in culture forms collagenase sooner and to a higher level than that of untreated women. However, the collagenase changes are not large compared to those seen in uterine involution and the hormonal control would have to be quite different from that in the uterus. The cervix also contains a neutral protease of the serine class (Ito et al, 1980). It is not known if this rises near term nor if it could solubilize collagen.

It must be concluded that we have a very poor understanding of the reasons why the human cervix is able to undergo its sudden extreme change in extensibility.

Dilatation of the rat cervix

The rat again offers the advantage that the entire tissue may be excised at any time of pregnancy or parturition. This has enabled many groups to obtain data on the collagen changes in the entire tissue, not just on concentration changes. Figure 31.9 summarizes the results obtained by a number of researchers. There is definitely a decrease of collagen concentration in the cervix at term; but, as in the case of the uterus, this decrease is due to a growth of

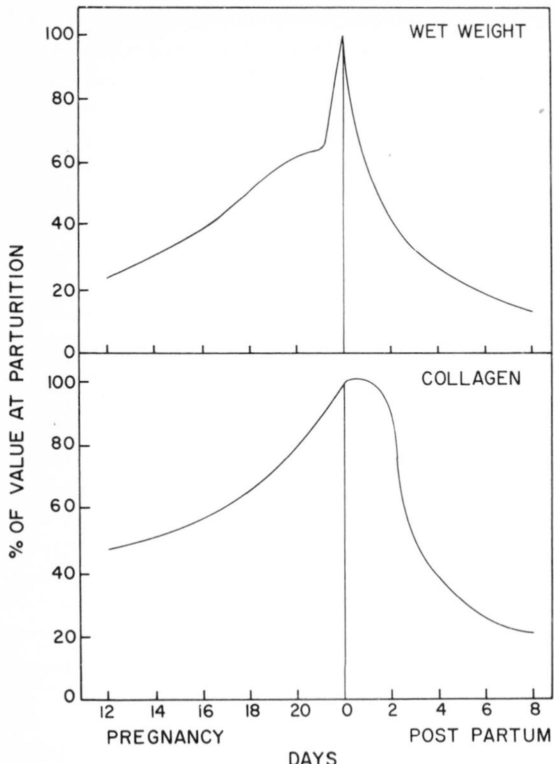

Fig. 31.9 Changes in the wet weight and collagen of the rat cervix during pregnancy and post partum. The maximum values are 100 = 235 g wet weight and 8.5 mg collagen. (The data are taken from Harkness & Moralee, 1956; Harkness & Harkness, 1961; Harkness & Nightingale, 1962; Bryant et al, 1968 and Zarrow & Yochim, 1961.)

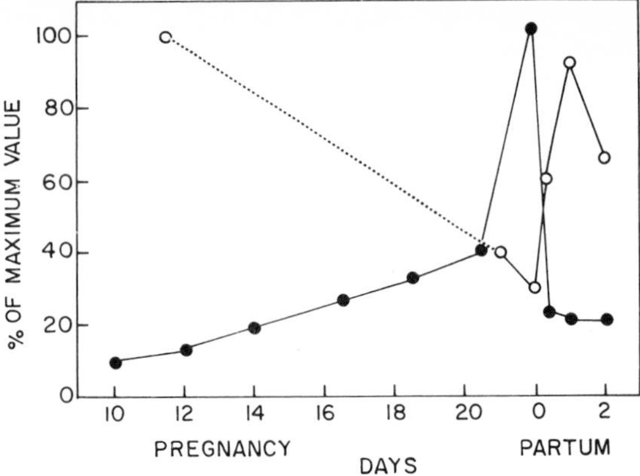

Fig. 31.10 Mechanical properties of the rat cervix during pregnancy, parturition and immediate post partum period. The internal circumference of the cervix (●) achieved a maximum value of 100 = 5.1 mm. A ring of cervical tissue had two rods placed through it and weights were suspended from one rod to determine the weight (O) needed to rupture the tissue ring. The maximum weight (100%), at 12 days of pregnancy, was 975 g. The dotted line indicates uncertainty as to the path of the curve in this region. (Data are taken from Harkness & Harkness, 1959b; 1961.)

collagen (2-fold) which fails to keep pace with a growth in wet weight (5-fold). The result is that, while there may be a dilution of collagen at term, there is certainly much more collagen in the total cervix than there is in the nongravid state. Glycosaminoglycans, as total hexosamine, show a sharp 3-fold rise within 24 hours of parturition, and this is accompanied by a 3-fold increase in water (Bryant et al, 1968).

The rat cervix has also offered a very useful system for the study of mechanical properties of the cervix. Harkness & Harkness (1959a) adopted the simple expedient of placing two rods through a loop cut from the cervix, hanging on weights and determining the extent of stretching and the load required to break the loop. The properties of the cervix show little change up to 12 days of pregnancy; the inner circumference then rises linearly to about 15 mm at term (Fig. 31.10). The circumference just before the loop ruptures under load increases to 34.5 mm. Along with this extensibility increase, the resistance to breaking declines. A 975 g load is required to rupture a control loop, but only 300 g at term. Even allowing for the lower concentration of collagen, the strength is halved. However, the most revealing experiment is one in which a 50 g weight is hung on the loop. At 12 days of pregnancy, there is some initial stretching and then little further lengthening with time. At term, the stretching just continues indefinitely until finally the loop ruptures. The uterus in early pregnancy behaves as if made up of elastic elements; the term uterus, of viscous elements. That is, it seems that the fibres must be slipping past one another in a viscous medium until the tissue breaks.

With respect to the idea of collagen degradation by collagenase, it is found that there is indeed a very extensive breakdown of cervical collagen, but this does not begin until about 48 hours post partum and requires a week to complete (Fig. 31.10). Therefore, breakdown does not seem to be involved in dilatation. Moreover, the breaking strength of the cervix recovers within 24 hours of parturition, and the inner circumference decreases within this same period. These changes seem much too rapid to be due to changes in collagen structure or cross-linking.

In the rat, dilatation of the cervix appears to require the action of the hormone relaxin. This is shown by ovariectomizing rats at day 12 to 16 of pregnancy, then treating with progesterone and oestrogen. Extensibility is significant only when relaxin is included in the regimen (Zarrow & Yochim, 1961; Hollingsworth et al, 1979).

A proposed mechanism of dilatation

After all of these human and animal studies extending over 30 years, there is still not a clear explanation of dilatation. I lean to the hypothesis that the connective tissue state is altered so that there is some slippage of the fibres of collagen past one another. In the last third of pregnancy, collagen increases at least two-fold (in the rat). If this collagen were laid down in fibrils that were sufficiently separated by glycosaminoglycan matrix, there would be little cross-linking between fibrils. However, cross-linking within fibrils may be normal, producing normal tensile strength.

While the fibres are not firmly cross-linked, they are held together by the glycosaminoglycan cement substances. Near term, the proportions of glycosaminoglycans shift and the total amount increases. Within a short time, a good deal of water comes in, making the tissue oedematous and producing still greater separation of the fibres. It is possible at this time that the cement substances are also broken down by the action of neutral proteinases. At this point fibres could be pulled past one another to a tremendous extent by a small but continuous force. If the force is too large, the tissue will break without tremendous extension (Harkness & Harkness, 1959a). The same sort of viscous extensibility can be produced by trypsin treatment (Harkness & Harkness, 1959b), which these authors indicate would not attack collagen. Within 24 hours of parturition, degraded glycosaminoglycans would wash out of the tissue, and new glycosaminoglycans would be synthesized. The collagen fibres would be much closer together with a firmer ground substance, and the mechanical properties would be almost back to normal. Then involution would restore the cervix to its normal size.

This hypothesis is quite similar to that of Veis (1980) except that it is proposed that a neutral proteinase, such as that reported by Ito et al (1980), would attack the cement substances to permit movement of the fibres through a viscous medium, whereas Veis proposes that the proteinase would cut off terminal extension peptides of collagen, disrupting cross-linking and permitting fibre slippage. These two hypotheses are not mutually exclusive, and neither invokes the action of collagenase.

THE OVARY

The connective tissue framework of the mature human ovary

The embryological development of the human ovary and its connective tissue elements has been reviewed by Gillman (1948) and will not be covered here. The surface of the mature ovary is covered with a single-celled layer of germinal epithelium resting on a thin basement membrane. Directly beneath this is a dense fibrous layer known as the tunica albuginea. The ovary may be divided into the cortex and medulla. The cortex contains the primordial and developing follicles. The medullary region is more fibrous, with strands of collagen and interspersed interstitial cells. The ovary is richly vascularized and much of the collagen content of the ovary is associated with the vessel walls, especially in the medullary region. Petry (1950) has presented beautiful illustrations of the collagen fibres in the human ovary; this has been supplemented by additional studies of Ferner & Dietel (1953). There are coarser collagen fibres in the medullary region, supporting the vessels; in the cortex the fibres are more of the reticulin type, forming fine but dense networks and baskets around the follicles. Many of these fibres appear to continue vertically towards the ovarian surface, passing through the albuginea and then spreading out parallel to the ovarian surface.

Petkov (1978a, b) has made detailed electron microscopic studies of ovarian collagen resulting in three interesting observations: (1) The fibroblasts in the ovary, when actively laying down fibres, often show disturbances in their cell membranes. The membranes disappear or 'dissolve' in certain areas so that the cytoplasm is in direct contact with the extracellular space. Collagen fibres then seem to be growing directly out of the cytoplasm and from extracellular vesicles. (2) Stromal fibrils have diameters of 30 to 120 nm with some sort of regular bridges between fibrils. Under treatments that produce partial separation of the fibrils, the alignment and banding pattern is still maintained. (3) The ovarian collagen fibrils are made up of filaments. The filaments in turn comprise three to five subfilaments of 3.0 to 4.5 nm diameter. The illustrations remind one of the pictures of the microfibrillar structure of collagen proposed on the basis of X-ray diffraction studies (Miller & Parry, 1973). The filaments pass in a spiral manner around the fibril with a pitch of 1.04–1.12 μm and an angle of inclination of 75–86°.

Follicular maturation

Follicles begin to form by the 56th day of human embryonic development, and most of the promordial follicles have developed by the time of birth (Peters, 1978). At age 15 there are 400 000 primordial follicles, and by age 35 about 60 000 remain (Bjersing, 1978). These primordial follicles consist of an oocyte accompanied by one or more granulosa cells, and the whole is enclosed in a basement membrane.

Maturation occurs in three stages (Bjersing, 1978): (1) In the primary follicle, the simple squamous epithelium is replaced by a single row of columnar epithelium. Already the follicle is anchored to the tunica albuginea by connective tissue fibres (Petry, 1949). (2) The secondary follicle develops two to six layers of cells in the stratum granulosum. (3) The tertiary follicle (Fig. 31.11 A, B) is distinguished by a fluid-filled central chamber, the antrum, containing an enlarged oocyte. The basement membrane around the antrum and membrana granulosa has expanded considerably but is still intact. At the early tertiary stage (2.5 to 3.5 mm) several coats or thecae can be distinguished. The theca interna consists of three regions (Schaar, 1976): an inner layer of spindle-shaped cells lying on the outer surface of the basement membrane; a central zone of large

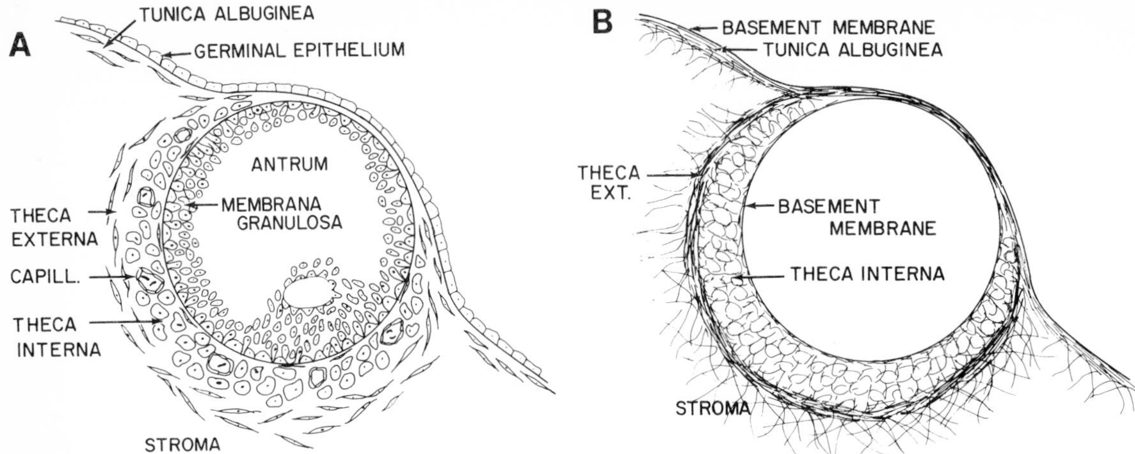

Fig. 31.11 Schematic diagram of the Graafian follicle. A, cellular structures. B, collagenous structures. The microscopic features of cells and collagen have been exaggerated in scale for clarity.

round vacuolar cells richly supplied by capillaries; and an outer region of more spindle-shaped cells. Each cell in the theca interna is surrounded by a dense basketwork of fine reticulin fibres. As this zone grows, the collagen increases in parallel.

The outermost layer of the follicle is the theca externa. This consists almost entirely of connective tissue with thicker collagen fibres than in the interna. This layer blends into the surrounding stroma but is denser and more concentric (Petry, 1950).

The tertiary or Graafian follicle undergoes further growth to a diameter of about 15 mm before ovulation occurs. Since the diameter of the primordial follicle is only 49 μm, this is a tremendous growth. This growth is opposed by the tunica albuginea of the follicle so that most of the growth is at the expense of the underlying ovary which is compressed and displaced. Petry (1949) illustrates how the adjacent stroma is compacted and the fibre network becomes denser around the ovary. At the same time there is a considerable amount of new collagen deposited in the thecae. During the final surge of growth, the albuginea thins out and the follicle protrudes above the surface of the ovary (Fig. 31.11a). The theca externa is also compacted in this apical region. A dense network of collagen fibres covers the apex of the follicle (Petry, 1950).

Follicular rupture (ovulation)

The dense meshwork of collagen fibres at the apex of the follicle led Petry (1950) to conclude that the egg could never make its way out unless these fibres were broken or destroyed. Espey (1978) has enumerated the collagenous layers separating the egg from freedom: the basement membrane under the germinal epithelium, the tunica albuginea, the theca externa, the theca interna and the basement membrane beneath the granulosa cells. These layers thin out considerably during the final stage of follicle growth, but they still remain intact. Of course, the egg must also penetrate the membrane granulosa, an extensive capillary network, and the outermost epithelial layer, but it is the collagen layers which seemingly offer the greatest impediment to escape. Considerable attention has been given to this problem, and various 'ovulatory' enzymes have been invoked to soften or destroy the intervening connective tissues.

A small circumscribed area within the region bulging from the surface of the ovary becomes further elevated and forms a stigma. Prior to rupture of the follicle, this area becomes weakened and thinned. The connective tissue fibres become swollen and fail to support the small vessels which collapse and cause the stigma to blanch (Petry, 1950). The fibres thin out and do not take the silver stain very well. Since the fibres are weakened, the stigma protrudes further.

It is very difficult to obtain a human ovary at the moment of ovulation, so much of the experimental work on ovulation has been carried out on the rabbit. Administration of human chorionic gonadotropin to a virgin rabbit leads to maturation and rupture of a number of follicles within 10 to 11 hours. The earliest signs of breakdown in the apical region were noted by Bjersing & Cajander (1974b). The first change is in the basement membrane underlying the germinal epithelium which covers the ovary. Oedema, cell necrosis, and collagen fragmentation become visible in this area. The theca externa also shows signs of degeneration by 8 hours. By 9.5 hours, portions of the theca externa on other sides of the follicle show collagen degeneration. At this time the tunica albuginea is also disintegrating. Another change that is noted at about 8 hours is the poking of granulosa cells through the basal lamina into the theca interna. The basement membrane beneath the granulosa begins to disintegrate several hours prior to ovulation. This would permit the entry of materials from the exterior capillaries into the antrum (Bjersing & Cajander, 1974a).

Quantitative measurements show that the apical wall of the rabbit follicle thins to 20 per cent of its initial thickness just prior to ovulation, and collagen fibres per square micron fall from 53 to 15 (Espey, 1967). The follicle is easily separated from the ovary at this time.

An ovulatory protease?

Lipner (1973) has reviewed results bearing on this question up to 1972. Proteolytic enzymes were first invoked by Schochet (1916) to explain egg release. He showed that follicular fluid digested fibrin and other proteins. Various proteinases have been reported in the intervening years, but only three will be considered here: lysosomal cathepsins, plasmin and collagenase.

Cajander & Bjersing (1976) attribute lytic activity to the germinal epithelial cells. In the rabbit, these cells become filled with dark lysosomal granules which appear to be discharged in the direction of the tunica albuginea. Rawson & Espey (1977) deny a role to these cells and their enzymes, because it is possible to scrape off the epithelium without preventing follicle rupture. However, this does not eliminate the lysosomal hypothesis since other cells in the follicle could well produce the necessary cathepsins. Homogenates of sow ovary can digest collagen at pH 4 (Lee & Malvin, 1970). This activity is possible due to thiol proteinases such as cathepsin B (Burleigh, 1977). In rabbit follicles, cathepsin B activity rises to a peak just prior to rupture (Motohashi et al, 1977).

Strickland & Beers (1976) believe that the granulosa cells hold the key to ovulation. These cells, in the rat ovary, produce plasminogen activator, which rises in those follicles destined to ovulate. Plasminogen activator is also produced by granulosa cells in culture when stimulated with luteinizing hormone or follicle-stimulating hormone. Plasminogen activator would activate plasmin that enters the follicular fluid from the circulation near the time of ovulation. Plasmin can attack the basement membrane and can weaken the follicular wall. This hypothesis receives further support from studies on the bovine follicle (Takayama, 1979). Plasmin activity increases as the follicle grows, but remains low in follicles that fail to rupture.

Espey & Rawson (1979) find certain attractive features in the hypothesis of Strickland & Beers (1976), and they add the thought that plasmin could also activate latent collagenase. However, they also offer serious objections and point out that plasmin alone cannot digest collagen. Espey (1971) assigns a central role to the fibroblasts of the theca and particularly to multivasicular bodies extruded from fibroblastic extensions. These bodies increase 9-fold in the rabbit follicle within 8 hours after administration of gonadotropin. These bodies might be a source of collagenase (compare Schwarz & Güldner, 1967). Rabbit follicles contain an enzymatic activity that hydrolyses the synthetic peptide carbobenzyl-oxy-Pro-Leu-Gly-Pro-Leu, a substrate for clostridial collagenase (Espey & Rondell, 1967). At the time this activity was thought to be collagenase, but subsequent work (Morales & Woessner, 1977) has shown that activity is more likely due to a peptidase and not to a collagenase. More recently, Espey & Coons (1976) have cultured follicles on collagen gels and shown that collagenase is released. However, the enzyme activity was present at all stages and did not seem to be correlated temporally with ovulation. Somewhat similar results have been obtained in my laboratory (Morales et al, 1978a). A micromethod was developed for the direct estimation of collagenase activity in rat follicular tissue. When this method was applied to the study of ovulation (Morales et al, 1978b), it was found that collagenase activity increases with growth of the follicle but does not show further increases at the time of ovulation.

Most recently, Espey (1980) has offered a theoretical paper stressing the parallelism between uterine involution and ovulation. In both cases there must be a drop in oestradiol and progesterone as a signal to turn on collagenase production. Prostaglandin E can act as an inflammatory stimulus to activate fibroblasts to produce latent collagenase and plasminogen activator or other serine proteinases. Macrophages and leucocyte responses are noted in both tissues. However, the last and most important step remains the degradation of collagen!

Follicular atresia

As the follicles mature, they may go completely through the ripening process to the point of rupture and still fail to yield an egg. At any point along the way, for reasons not readily perceived, a follicle may stop maturing and undergo a process of regression or atresia. In the human, 99.9 per cent of all follicles undergo atresia before reaching the point of ovulation (Byskov, 1978). This process of atresia requires a few days to 1 month depending on the follicle's size. In tertiary follicles, granulosa cells die and are phagocytized. The antrum collapses and is invaded by connective tissue. The basement membrane and the connective tissue elements persist as a scar in the centre of the ovary. While connective tissue proliferation is seen in the early phases of tertiary atresia, the general impression is that there is, by the end of the process, a considerable diminution of collagen fibres (Petry, 1949).

Similar observations have been made on obliterative atresia in the cow ovary (as opposed to cystic atresia undergone by full-sized follicles). Connective tissue from the theca grows into the antrum until it is obliterated by fibroblastic cells. The collagen fibres of the theca interna coalesce with the basement membrane, and the whole becomes hyalinized to form a 'glass membrane' (Priedkalns et al, 1968).

Corpus luteum formation

The human corpus luteum reaches its full secretory 'bloom' by 8 to 10 days after ovulation. It is heavily vascularized by 7 days; this process contributes to the connective tissue content of the wall of the corpus luteum (Harrison, 1962). Also, the cavity of the corpus luteum becomes lined with connective tissue by day 8. Judging from studies in other species, the hypothesis that ovulation is essentially an inflammatory reaction is at least partly justified. The formation of the corpus luteum has some of the aspects of connective tissue repair processes that follow inflammation. Connective tissue cells migrate in from the adjacent stroma and cover over the ruptured stigma and apex region (Van Blerkom & Motta, 1978). In the sheep, shortly after ovulation, discontinuities can be seen in the basement membrane (Van Lennep & Madden, 1965). It is through these gaps that capillary endothelium reaches the granulosa cells. Presumably, fibroblasts also enter here to line the cavity. In the sow, the remnants of folded basement membrane form the foundation for thick supporting collagenous septae, which give the corpus a lobulate appearance (Corner, 1919). Delicate reticulin fibres form a dense basketwork supporting the individual luteal cells.

Luteolysis

If pregnancy does not ensue in the human, the corpus luteum is referred to as the corpus luteum of menstruation. By day 10 to 11 after ovulation, it begins to undergo regression (or retrogression). The luteal cells begin to shrink and more connective tissue fibres are laid down between these cells, together with ground substance, to form a fibrohyaline material. The early matrix has fine filaments of 3 to 5 nm, and later, collagen fibres are seen. The collagen fibres between cells remain unoriented and do not form bundles. The fibrohyaline mass persists, while the cells are destroyed by autophagy and heterophagy, and is finally reduced to a collagenous scar — the corpus albicans (Van Lennep & Madden, 1965).

If pregnancy does occur, then these changes of luteolysis are delayed until near the end of pregnancy. It is not clear if luteolysis involves a final net destruction of collagen, but this seems likely. Macrophages are abundant during luteal regression and are involved in ingesting senescent luteal cells and debris (Paavola, 1979, guinea pig). Perhaps these cells are also involved in collagen resorption? Much clearer evidence for collagen disappearance, especially in the theca externa, has been obtained in the rabbit (Koering & Thor, 1978).

CONCLUSION

The uterus, cervix and ovary are all found to have a collagen framework which is essential to maintain the mechanical function of the organ or tissue. Yet, in each tissue, there arises a critical juncture when this framework is an obstacle to normal function, and it must be rapidly dismantled. I have made some rough calculations in Table 31.1 of the rate at which collagen can be synthesized and degraded. These rates are necessarily approximate, since they involve determining slopes of curves whose shapes are only vaguely discernible. Yet it is clear that collagen can be doubled or halved in 1 to 2 days in several of these tissues. These are truly phenomenal rates. A still cruder calculation is made of the amounts of collagen that 1 g of tissue can synthesize or degrade in 24 hours. The record synthesis appears to be in the very young rat uterus stimulated with oestrogen, and the record breakdown may be in the cervix (where the concentration of collagen is the highest).

These various tissues of the reproductive tract have provided a number of important insights into collagen metabolism, and they promise to yield still more information in the immediate future.

Table 31.1 Magnitude of collagen changes in the reproductive tract

A. Synthesis	*Doubling time (Days)*	*Collagen synthesis (mg/g wet wt in 24 h)*
Endometrium in cycle — rat	1	12
Growing pregnant uterus — human	100	0.5
Growing pregnant uterus — rat	3	6
Uterus with wax insert — rat	8	4
Deciduoma formation — rat	2	2
Estrogen-stimulated uterus — rat	2.5	25
Cervix in pregnancy — rat	8	12
Maturing follicle — rat	2	3
B. Degradation	*Half-life (Days)*	*Collagen degradation (mg/g wet wt in 24 h)*
Endometrium in cycle — human	3	—
Endometrium in cycle — rat	1	5
Deciduoma regression — rat	1	1
Post-partum uterus — human	3	6
Post-partum uterus — rat	1	12
Uterus after ovariectomy — rat	21	2
Post-partum cervix — rat	1.5	34

REFERENCES

Agrawal K, Fox H 1972 Subepithelial endometrial collagen. American Journal of Obstetrics and Gynecology 114: 172-5

Amma M K P, Singh J, Sareen K 1978 Changes in rat plasma hydroxyproline during estrus and estrogen treatment. Indian Journal of Experimental Biology 16: 806-8

Anderson A B, Turnbull A C 1969 Relationship between length of gestation and cervical dilatation, uterine contractility and other factors during pregnancy. American Journal of Obstetrics and Gynecology 105: 1207-14

Anderson W R, Davis J 1968 Placental site involution. American Journal of Obstetrics and Gynecology 102: 23-33

Árvay A, Takács I, Ladányi P, Balogh Á, Benkö K 1971 The effect of intensive nervous stimulation on certain physico-chemical properties of rat tail tendon and uterus collagen. Gerontologia 17: 157-69

Berwind T 1954 Elektronenmikroskopische Untersuchungen am Fasersystem der Cervix uteri der Frau. Archiv für Gynäkologie 184: 459-68

Bjersing L 1978 Maturation, morphology and endocrine function of the follicular wall in mammals. In. Jones R E (ed) The Vertebrate Ovary. Plenum, New York. 181-214

Bjersing L, Cajander S 1974a Ovulation and the mechanism of follicle rupture. IV. Ultrastructure of membrane granulosa of rabbit Graafian follicles prior to induced ovulation. Cell and Tissue Research 153: 1-14

Bjersing L, Cajander S 1974b Ovulation and the mechanism of follicle rupture. V. Ultrastructure of tunica albuginea and theca externa of rabbit Graafian follicles prior to induced ovulation. Cell and Tissue Research 153: 15-30

Brandes C, Anton E 1969 Lysosomes in uterine involution: intracytoplasmic degradation of myofilaments and collagen. Journal of Gerontology 24: 55-69

Breen M, Sittig R A, Blacik L J, Borcherding M, Weinstein H G 1975 Collagen and glycosaminoglycan content in the parturient cervix. Federation Proceedings 34: 636

Brown P C, Consden R, Glynn L E 1958 Observation on the shrink temperature of collagen and its variation with age and disease. Annals of Rheumatic Diseases 17: 196-208

Brown R G, Young L G 1970 Connective tissue metabolism in swine. I. Growth 34: 369-77

Bryant W M, Greenwell J E, Weeks P M 1968 Alterations in collagen organization during dilatation of the cervix uteri. Surgery Gynecology and Obstetrics 126: 27-39

Buckingham J C, Selden R, Danforth D N 1962 Connective tissue changes in the cervix during pregnancy and labor. Annals of the New York Academy of Science 97: 733-42

Burack E, Wolfe J M, Wright A W 1942 Effects of administration of estrogen on connective tissues of the genital tract of the rat. Endocrinology 30: 335-43

Burleigh M C 1977 Degradation of collagen by non-specific proteinases. In: Barrett A J (ed) Proteinases in Mammalian Cells and Tissues. North Holland, New York. pp 286-309

Byskov A G 1978 Follicular atresia. In: Jones R E (ed) The Vertebrate Ovary. Plenum, New York. pp 533-62

Cajander S, Bjersing L 1976 Further studies of the surface epithelium covering preovulatory rabbit follicles with special reference to lysosomal alteration. Cell and Tissue Research 169: 129-41

Chernysheva L I 1957 [Reticulo-fibrous structure of the human uterus during pregnancy and the puerperium]. Leningrad. Pervyi Leningradskii Meditsinskii Institut. Kafeda Akusherstva i Ginekologii. Sbornik Nauchnykh Trudov 1: 116-26

Chung E, Miller E J 1974 Collagen polymorphism: characterization of molecules with the chain composition $[\alpha 1(III)]_3$ in human tissues. Science 183: 1200-1

Chung E, Rhodes R K, Miller E G 1976 Isolation of three collagenous components of probable basement membrane origin from several tissues. Biochemical and Biophysical Research Communications 71: 1167-74

Corner G W 1919 On the origin of the corpus luteum of the sow from both granulosa and theca interna. American Journal of Anatomy 26: 117-83

Craig J M, Danziger S 1963 Reticulum and collagen in the human endometrium. American Journal of Obstetrics and Gynecology 86: 421-9

Cretius K 1959 Der Kollagengehalt menschlicher Uterusmuskulatur. Bibliotheca Gynaecologica Suppl. Gynaecologia No. 20: 68-89

Cretius K 1965 Zur molekularen Struktur des Bindegewebes im menschlichen Uterus. Archiv für Gynäkologie 202: 43-6

Cretius K, Hannig K, Beier G 1966 Untersuchungen zur Löslichkeit und zum Verhalten des Kollagens im nichtschwangeren und im schwangeren menschlichen Uterus. Archiv für Gynäkologie 203: 329-53

Cullen B M, Harkness R D 1960 The effect of hormones on the physical properties and collagen content of the rat's uterine cervix. Journal of Physiology (London) 152: 419-36

Cullen B M, Harkness R D 1964 Effects of ovariectomy and of hormones on collagenous framework of the uterus. American Journal of Physiology 206: 621-7

Cullen B M, Harkness R D 1968 Collagen formation and changes in cell population in the rat's uterus after distension with wax. Quarterly Journal of Experimental Physiology 53: 33-42

Cunha G R, Chung L W K, Shannon J M, Reese B A 1980 Stromalepithelial interactions in sex differentiation. Biology of Reproduction 22: 19-42

Dallenbach-Hellweg G, Bornebusch C G 1970 Histologische Untersuchungen über die Reaktion des Endometrium bei der verzögerten Abstossung. Archiv für Gynäkologie 208: 235-46

Danforth D N 1947 The fibrous nature of the human cervix and its relation to the isthmic segment in gravid and nongravid uteri. American Journal of Obstetrics and Gynecology 53: 541-57

Danforth D N, Buckingham J C 1964 Connective tissue mechanisms and their relation to pregnancy. Obstetrical and Gynecological Survey 19: 715-32

Danforth D N, Buckingham J C, Roddick J W Jr 1960 Connective tissue changes incident to cervical effacement. American Journal of Obstetrics and Gynecology 80: 939-45

Dubrauszky V 1965 Weitere Beobachtungen zum Aufbauder Uteruswand in der Schwangerschaft. Archiv für Gynäkologie 202: 41-3

Dubrauszky V, Schmitt H 1958 Mikroskopische und elektronenmikroskopische Untersuchungen am Gitterfasersystem der Corpusmucosa während des Cyclus und der Gestation. Archiv für Gynäkologie 191: 212-23

Dubrauszky V, Schmitt H 1960 Die Entstehung der Bindegewebsfibrillen im Korpusendometrium. Gynaecologia 150: 103-12

Dubrauszky V, Schwalm H, Fleischer M 1971 Das Bindegewebsfasersystem des Myometrium während der Geschlechtsreife, der Menopause und der Gravidität. Archiv für Gynäkologie 210: 276-93

Dyer R F, Peppler R D 1977 Intracellular collagen in the nonpregnant and IUD-containing rat uterus. Anatomical Record 187: 241-8

Espey L L 1967 Ultrastructure of the apex of the rabbit Graafian follicle during the ovulatory process. Endocrinology 81: 267-76

Espey L L 1971 Decomposition of connective tissue in rabbit ovarian follicles by multivesicular structures of thecal fibroblasts. Endocrinology 88: 437-44

Espey L L 1978 Ovulation. In: Jones R E (ed) The vertebrate ovary. Plenum, New York. pp 503-32

Espey L L 1980 Ovulation as an inflammatory reaction — a hypothesis. Biology of Reproduction 22: 73-106

Espey L L, Coons P J 1976 Factors which influence ovulatory degradation of rabbit ovarian follicles. Biological Reproduction 14: 233-45

Espey L L, Rawson J M R 1979 Regarding the role of plasminogen activator in ovulation. In: Midgley A R, Sadler W A (eds) Ovarian follicular development and function. Raven Press, New York. pp 155-8

Espey L L, Rondell P 1967 Estimation of mammalian collagenolytic activity with a synthetic substrate. Journal of Applied Physiology 23: 757-61

Etherington D J 1973 Collagenolytic-cathepsin and acid-proteinase activities in the rat uterus during post partum involution. European Journal of Biochemistry 32: 126-9

Fainstat T 1962 Hormonal basis for collagen bundle generation in uterine stroma. Extracellular studies of uterus. Endocrinology 71: 878-87

Fainstat T 1963 Extracellular studies of uterus. II. Regeneration of collagen bundles in uterine stroma after parturition. American Journal of Anatomy 112: 371-88

Fainstat T 1965 Endocrine effects of suckling mirrored by collagen changes in endometrium. V. Extracellular studies of uterus. American Journal of Obstetrics and Gynecology 91: 504-17

Ferenczy A 1980 The ultrastructure of the human cervix. In: Naftolin F, Stubblefield P G (eds) Dilatation of the uterine cervix. Raven Press, New York. pp 27-44

Ferner H, Dietel H 1953 Über das menschliche Ovarialstroma und den Einbau der Primärfollikel. Zeitschrift für Zellforschung und mikroskopische Anatomie 38: 139-47

Fujimoto D 1980 Evidence for natural existence of pyridinoline cross-link in collagen. Biochemical and Biophysical Research Communications 93: 948-53

Garska W 1966 Morphology of the basement membrane in inflammatory conditions and erosions of the cervix uteri. Acta Medica Polona 7: 383-99

Gillman J 1948 The development of the gonads in man, with a consideration of the role of fetal endocrines and the histogenesis of ovarian tumors. Contributions to Embryology, Carnegie Institution of Washington Contribution 32: 83-131

Grant R A 1965 Chemical changes in the uterus of the rat during late pregnancy and post partum involution. The effects of lactation and hormone treatment. Journal of Reproduction and Fertility 9: 285-99

Gross J, Lapière C M 1962 Collagenolytic activity in amphibian tissues: a tissue culture assay. Proceedings of the National Academy of Science, USA 48: 1014-22

Halme J, Woessner J F Jr 1975 Effect of progesterone on collagen breakdown and tissue collagenolytic activity in the involuting rat uterus. Journal of Endocrinology 66: 357-62

Harding J J 1963 Amino acid composition of human collagens from adult dura mater and postmenopausal uterus. Biochemical Journal 86: 574-6

Harkness R D 1964 Physiology of the connective tissues of the reproductive tract. In: Hall D E (ed) International review of connective tissue research, vol 2. Academic Press, New York. pp 155-211

Harkness M L R, Harkness R D 1954 The collagen content of the reproductive tract of the rat during pregnancy and lactation. Journal of Physiology (London) 123: 492-500

Harkness M L R, Harkness R D 1956 The distribution of the growth of collagen in the uterus of the pregnant rat, Journal of Physiology (London) 132: 492-501

Harkness M L R, Harkness R D 1959a Changes in the physical properties of the uterine cervix of the rat during pregnancy. Journal of Physiology (London) 148: 524-7

Harkness M L R, Harkness R D 1959b Effect of enzymes on mechanical properties of tissues. Nature 183: 1821-2

Harkness M L R, Harkness R D 1961 The mechanical properties of the uterine cervix of the rat during involution after parturition. Journal of Physiology (London) 156: 112-20

Harkness R D, Moralee B E 1956 The time course and route of loss of collagen from the rat's uterus during post partum involution. Journal of Physiology (London) 132: 502-8

Harkness R D, Nightingale M A 1962 The extensibility of the cervix uteri of the rat at different times of pregnancy. Journal of Physiology (London) 160: 214-20

Harkness M L R, Harkness R D, Moralee B E 1956 Loss of collagen from the uterus of the rat after ovariectomy and from the nonpregnant horn after parturition. Quarterly Journal of Experimental Phsyiology 41: 254-62

Harkness M L R, Harkness R D, Moralee B E 1957 Effect of the oestrous cycle and of hormones on the collagen content of the uterus of the rat. Journal of Physiology (London) 135: 270-80

Harrison R J 1962 The structure of the ovary. C. Mammals. In: Zuckerman S (ed) The Ovary. Academic Press, New York. 143-87

Henkel W, Rauterberg J, Glanville R W 1979 Isolation of cross-linked peptides from insoluble human leiomyoma. The involvement of the N-terminal, non-helical region of type III collagen in intermolecular cross-linking. European Journal of Biochemistry 96: 249-56

Herrera V E 1960 Collagen structure of the uterus during fetal development. Anales Dessarolo 8: 67-77

Hertel H, Schmitt W 1968 Spontane Uterusperforation bei Endomyometritis puerpalis durch erhölten Kollagenabbau. Archiv für Gynäkologie 206: 456-64

Hoffmeister H, Schulz H 1961 Light optical and electronoptical findings in the endometrium of the sexually mature woman during the proliferation and secretion phase with special reference to fiber structures. Beitraege zur Pathologischen Anatomie und zur Allgemeinen Pathologie 124: 415-46

Hollingsworth M, Isherwood C N M, Foster R W 1979 Effects of oestradiol benzoate, progesterone, relaxin and ovariectomy on cervical extensibility. Journal of Reproduction and Fertility 56: 471-7

Ito A, Ihara H, Mori Y 1980 Partial purification and characterization of a novel neutral proteinase from human uterine cervix. Biochemical Journal 185: 443-50

Ito A, Kitamura K, Mori Y, Hirakawa S 1979 The change in solubility of type I collagen in human uterine cervix in pregnancy at term. Biochemical Medicine 21: 262-70

Jaeger J 1965 Zur Ultrastruktur des bindegewebigen Anteils der Uterusmuskulatur. Archiv für Gynäkologie 202: 59-62

Jeffrey J J, Gross J 1970 Collagenase from rat uterus. Isolation and partial characterization. Biochemistry 9: 268-73

Jeffrey J J, Coffey R J, Eisen A Z 1971a Studies on uterine collagenase in tissue culture. I. Relationship of enzyme production to collagen metabolism. Biochimica Biophysica Acta 252: 136-42

Jeffrey J J, Coffey R J, Eisen A Z 1971b Studies on uterine collagenase in tissue culture. II. Effect of steroid hormones on enzyme production. Biochimica Biophysica Acta 252: 143-50

Jeffrey J J, Koob T J, Eisen A Z 1975 Hormonal regulation of mammalian collagenases. In: Burleigh P M C, Poole A R (eds) Dynamics of connective tissue macromolecules. North Holland, Amsterdam. pp 147-56

Kao K Y T, Hitt W E 1974 The intermolecular cross-links in rat uterine collagen. Biochimica Biophysica Acta 371: 501-10

Kao K Y T, Leslie J G 1977 Polymorphism in human uterine collagen. Connective Tissue Research 5: 127-9

Kao K Y T, McGavack T H 1959 Connective tissue: I. Age and sex influence on protein composition of rat tissues. Proceedings of the Society for Experimental Biology and Medicine 101: 153-7

Kao K Y T, Hilker D M, McGavack T H 1961a Connective tissue IV. Synthesis and turnover of proteins in tissues of rats. Proceedings of the Society for Experimental Biology and Medicine 106: 121-4

Kao K Y T, Hilker D M, McGavack T H 1961b Connective tissues V. Comparison of synthesis and turnover of collagen and elastin in tissues of rat at several ages. Proceedings of the Society for Experimental Biology and Medicine 106: 335-8

Kao K Y T, Hitt W E, Bush A T, McGavack T H 1964a Connective tissue XI. Factors affecting collagen synthesis by rat uterine slices. Proceedings of the Society for Experimental Biology and Medicine 115: 422-4

Kao K Y T, Hitt W E, Bush A T, McGavack T H 1964b Connective tissue. XII Stimulating effects of oestrogens on collagen synthesis in rat uterine slices. Proceedings of the Society for Experimental Biology and Medicine 117: 86-97

Kao K Y T, Hitt W E, Dawson R L, McGavack T H 1967 Connective tissue. XIV. Preparation and amino acid composition of soluble collagen from human uterus. Archives of Biochemistry and Biophysics 120: S18-24

Kao K Y T, Arnett W M, McGavack T H 1969 Effect of endometrial phase, ovariectomy, oestradiol and progesterone on uterine protocollagen hydroxylase. Endocrinology 85: 1057-61

Kao K Y T, Hitt W E, Leslie J G 1976 The intermolecular cross-links in uterine collagens of guinea pig, pig, cow and human beings. Proceedings of the Society for Experimental Biology and Medicine 151: 385-99

Karube H, Kanke Y, Mori Y 1975 Increase of structural glycoprotein during dilatation of human cervix in pregnancy at term. Endocrinologia Japonica 22: 445-8

Kitamura K, Ito A, Mori Y, Hirakawa S 1979 Changes in the human uterine cervical collagenase with special reference to cervical ripening. Biochemical Medicine 22: 332-8

Kleissl H P, Van der Rest M, Naftolin F, Glorieux F H, De Leon A 1978 Collagen changes in the human uterine cervix at parturition. American Journal of Obstetrics and Gynecology 130: 748-53

Koenig B Jr 1971 Das Verhalten zwishchen glatten Muskelzellen und Bindegewebe menschlicher Uteri. Anatomischer Anzeiger 129: 541-50

Koering M J, Thor M J 1978 Structural changes in the regressing corpus luteum of the rabbit. Biology of Reproduction 17: 719-33

Kondo T 1972 Histochemical studies on the human cervix uteri. 2. Acid mucopolysaccharides of the human cervix uteri during pregnancy. Nagoya Medical Journal 17: 111-21

Korchagin G M, Pashkova V S 1974 [Relationship between the amount of stroma in uterine myomas and the patient's age]. Akusherstvo i Ginekologiia 1974 (10): 61

Lapina Z V 1947 [Arteries and veins of the human uterus in relation to its growth]. Akusherstvo i Ginekologiia 33(1): 18-22

Lee C Y, Malvin R 1970 Acid proteolytic activity of the sow ovarian follicle. Federation Proceedings 29: 643

Liebig W, Stegner H-E 1977 Die Dezidualisation der endometrialen Stromazelle. Elektronenmikroskopische Untersuchungen. Archiv für Gynäkologie 223: 19-31

Lipner H 1973 Mechanism of mammalian ovulation. In: Greep R O (ed) Handbook of Physiology, Section 7. Endocrinology 2, Part 1. American Physiological Society, Washington. 409-37

Lobel B L, Tic L, Shelesnyak M C 1965a Studies on the mechanism of nidation. XVII. Part 3. Formation of deciduomata. Acta Endocrinology 50: 517-36

Lobel B L, Tic L, Shelesnyak M C 1965b Studies on the mechanism of nidation XVII. Part 4. Regression of deciduomata. Acta Endocrinology 50: 537-59

Luse S, Hutton R 1964 An electronmicroscopic study of the fate of collagen in the post-partum rat uterus. Anatomical Record 148: 308

Miller A, Parry D A D 1973 Structure and packing of microfibrils in collagen. Journal of Molecular Biology 75: 441-7

Miller E J, Finch J E Jr, Chung E, Butler W T, Robertson P B 1976 Specific cleavage of the native type III collagen molecule with trypsin. Archives of Biochemistry and Biophysics 173: 631-7

Montfort I, Pérez-Tamayo R 1961 Studies on uterine collagen during pregnancy and puerperium. Laboratory Investigation 10: 1240-58

Morales T I, Woessner J F Jr 1977 PZ-peptidase from chick embryos. Purification, properties, and action on collagen peptides. Journal of Biological Chemistry 252: 4855-60

Morales T I, Woessner J F Jr, Howell D S, Marsh J M, LeMaire W J 1978a A microassay for the direct demonstration of collagenolytic activity in Graafian follicles of the rat. Biochimica Biophysica Acta 524: 428-34

Morales T I, Woessner J F, Marsh J M, LeMaire W J 1978b Collagenase in Graafian follicles. Abstracts of 60th Meeting of the Endocrine Society. 501

Morgan C F 1963a Temporal variations in the collagen, non-collagen protein and hexosamine of the uterus and vagina. Proceedings of the Society for Experimental Biology and Medicine 112: 690-4

Morgan C F 1963b A study of oestrogenic action on the collagen, hexoasmine, and nitrogen content of skin, uterus and vagina. Endocrinology 73: 11-19

Morrione T G, Ru M Z 1964 Injury influence on resorption of uterine collagen. Archives of Pathology 78: 591-600

Morrione T G, Seifter S 1962 Alteration in the collagen content of the human uterus during pregnancy and post partum involution. Journal of Experimental Medicine 115: 357-65

Motohashi T, Okamura H, Okazaki T, Morikawa H, Nishimura T 1977 A study on ovarian lysosomal enzyme activities during ovulation in rodents. Proceedings II Asian Congress of Obstetrics and Gynecology, Bankok. 860-72

Narik G 1960 Histochemische Darstellung der Schwangerschaftsveränderungen im Bindegewebe des Myometrium. Zeitschrift für Geburtschilfe und Gynäkologie 155: 329-35

Nemetschek-Gansler H, Meinel A, Nemetschek T 1977 Ueber Vorkommen und Bedeutung extra- und intracellulärer periodisch gebänderter filamentärer Assoziate. Virchow's Archiv A. Pathologie Anatomie Histologie 375: 185-96

Okamura H, Koshiba H, Yoshida Y, Nishimura T 1976 An ultrastructural study of collagen degradation in human involuting uterus. Acta Obstetrica et Gynaecologica Japonica 23: 179-84

Paavola L G 1979 Cellular mechanisms involved in luteolysis. In: Channing C P, Marsh J M, Sadler W A (eds) Ovarian follicular and corpus luteum function. Plenum Press, New York. pp 527-33

Parakkal P F 1969 Involvement of macrophages in collagen resorption. Journal of Cell Biology 41: 345-54

Parakkal P F 1972 Macrophages: time course and sequence of their distribution in the post partum uterus. Journal of Ultrastructure Research 40: 284-91

Partridge I G, Brown R G 1972 The influence of dietary energy upon the uterus of the prepuberal gilt. II. Growth 36: 113-23

Peters H 1978 Folliculogenesis in mammals. In: Jones R E (ed) The vertebrate ovary. Plenum Press, New York. pp 121-44

Petkov R 1978a Ultrastructure of collagen fibril. 1. Some features of structure of collagen fibril. Anatomischer Anzeiger 144: 301-18

Petkov R 1978b Ultrastructure of collagen fibril. 2. Evidence of spiral organization of fibril. Anatomischer Anzeiger 144: 485-501

Petry G 1949 Die Ursachen der Ovulation. Zeitschrift für Geburtshilfe und Gynäkologie 130: 236-40

Petry G 1950 Die Konstruktion des Eierstockbindegewebes und dessen Bedeutung für den ovariellen Zyklus. Zeitschrift für Zellforschung und mikroskopische Anatomie 35: 1-32

Priedkalns J, Weber A F, Zemjanis R 1968 Qualitative and quantitative morphological studies of the cells of the membrane granulosa, theca interna and corpus luteum of the bovine ovary. Zeitschrift für Zellforschung und mikroskopische Anatomie 85: 501-20

Purkayastha R, Roy S C 1956 Amino acids in human uterine tissue — normal, fibroid or malignant. Annals of Biochemistry and Experimental Medicine 16: 97-100

Rawson J R, Espey L L 1977 Concentration of electron dense granules in the rabbit ovarian surface epithelium during ovulation. Biology of Reproduction 17: 561-6

Ross R, Klebanoff S J 1971 The smooth muscle cell. I. In vivo synthesis of connective tissue proteins. Journal of Cell Biology 50: 159-72

Rowlatt C 1969 Subepithelial fibrils associated with the basal lamina under simple epithelia in mouse uterus: possible tropocollagen aggregates. Journal of Ultrastructural Research 26: 44-51

Rundgren A 1974 Physical properties of connective tissue as influenced by single and repeated pregnancies in the rat. Acta Physiologica Scandinavica, Suppl. 417: 1-138

Runge H, Riehm H 1952 Über die Beteiligung des Kollagenfasersystems an der Dehnung der Cervix uteri sub partu. Archiv für Gynäkologie 181: 400-16

Ryan J N, Woessner J F Jr 1971 Mammalian collagenase. Direct demonstration in homogenates of involuting rat uterus. Biochemical and Biophysical Research Communications 44: 144-9

Ryan J N, Woessner J F Jr 1972 Oestradiol inhibits collagen breakdown in the involuting rat uterus. Biochemical Journal 127: 705-15

Salvador R A, Tsai I 1973a Accumulation of collagen in the uterus of the immature rat administered oestradiol–17β. Biochemical Pharmacology 22: 37-46

Salvador R A, Tsai I 1973b Collagen proline hydroxylase activity in the uterus of the rat during rapid collagen synthesis in vivo. Archives of Biochemistry and Biophysics 154: 583-92

Schaar H 1976 Funktionelle Morphologie der Theca interna im Bläschenfollikel des menschlichen Ovars. Acta Anatomica 94: 283-98

Schaub M C 1964 Distribution and variation of a collagen-degrading enzyme in the uterus of pregnant rats. Experientia 20: 675-6

Schochet S S 1916 A suggestion as to the process of ovulation and ovarian cyst formation. Anatomical Record 10: 447-57

Schwalm H, Cretius K 1958 Über den Gehalt der menschlichen Uterusmuskulatur an contractilen Proteinen, an wasserlöslichen Proteinen und an Stromaeiweiss. Archiv für Gynäkologie 191: 271-82

Schwalm H, Dubrauszky V 1966 The structure of the musculature of the human uterus — muscles and connective tissue. American Journal of Obstetrics and Gynecology 94: 391-404

Schwarz W, Güldner F-H 1967 Elektronenmikroskopische Untersuchungen des Kollagenabbaus im Uterus der Ratte nach der Schwangerschaft. Zeitschrift für Zellforschung und mikroskopische Anatomie 83: 416-26

Sedlis A, Kim N G 1971 Significance of the endometrial subepithelial collagen band. Obstetrics and Gynecology 38: 264-9

Sengel A, Stoebner P 1970 Ultrastructure de l'endomètre humain normal. I. Le chorion cytogène. Zeitschrift für Zellforschung und mikroskopische Anatomie 109245-59

Smith O W, Kaltreider N B 1963 Collagen content of the nonpregnant rat uterus as related to the functional responses to oestrogen and progesterone. Endocrinology 73: 619-28

Spiro R G, Spiro M J 1971 Studies on the biosynthesis of the hydroxylysine-linked disaccharide unit of basement membranes and collagens. III. Journal of Biological Chemistry 246: 4919-25

Staemmler M 1953 Untersuchung über die Bedeutung der Gitterfasern im Stroma der Uterusschleimhaut. I. Archiv für Gynäkologie 182: 445-60

Stieve H 1929 Muskulatur and Bindegewebe in der Wand der menschlichen Gebärmutter ausserhalb und während der Schwangerschaft, während der Geburt and des Wochenbettes. Zeitschrift für mikroskopische-anatomische Forschung 17: 371-518

Strauss G 1969 Funktionsbedingte Unterschiede der Feinstruktur des kollagenen Bindegewebes menschlicher Uteri. Archiv für Gynäkologie 208: 147-77

Strickland S, Beers W H 1976 Studies on the role of plasminogen activator in ovulation. Journal of Biological Chemistry 251: 5694-702

Takács I, Verzár F 1968 Macromolecular ageing of collagen. III. Stimulation of collagen production in the skin and uterus. Gerontologia 14: 126-32

Takayama S 1979 [The role of protease in the ovarian follicle wall at ovulation]. Nippon Naibumpi Gakkai Zasshi 55: 761-75

Tansey T R, Padykula H A 1978 Cellular responses to experimental inhibition of resorption in the post partum rat uterus. Anatomical Record 191: 287-309

Van Blerkom J, Motta P 1978 A scanning electron microscopic study of the luteo-follicular complex. III. Repair of ovulated follicle and formation of the corpus luteum. Cell and Tissue Research 189: 131-53

Van Lennep E W, Madden L M 1965 Electron microscopic observations on the involution of the human corpus luteum of menstruation. Zeitschrift für Zellforschung 66: 365-80

Veis A 1980 Cervical dilatation: a proteolytic mechanism for loosening the collagen fibre network. In: Naftolin F, Stubblefield P G (eds) Dilatation of the uterine cervix. Raven Press, New York. pp 195-202

Von Maillot K, Zimmermann B K 1976 Solubility of collagen of uterine cervix during pregnancy and labour. Archiv für Gynäkologie 220: 275-80

Von Maillot K, Stuhlsatz H W, Mohanaradhakrishnan V, Greiling H 1979 Changes in the glyosaminoglycans distribution pattern in the human uterine cervix during pregnancy and labor. Ameracan Journal of Obstetrics and Gynecology 135: 503-6

Voutsa N, Beveridge G C, Foraker A G 1963 The uterine cervix at term: glycogen, mast cells and connective tissue elements. Obstetrics and Gynecology 22: 108-14

Weeks J G, Halme J, Woessner J F Jr 1976 Extraction of collagenase from the involuting rat uterus. Biochimica Biophysica Acta 445: 205-14

Wessel W, 1959 Die menschlichen Deciduazellen und ihre 'Kollageneinschlüsse' in Elektronenmikroskop. Virchow's Archiv für pathologische Anatomie 332: 224-35

Wetzstein R, Wagner H 1960 Elektronenmikroskopische Untersuchungen am menschlichen Endometrium. Anatomischer Anzeiger 108: 362-75

Wienke E C Jr, Cavazos F, Hall D V, Lucas F V 1968 Ultrastructure of the human endometrial stroma cell during the menstrual cycle. American Journal of Obstetrics and Gynecology 102: 65-77

Wislocki G B, Dempsey E W 1948 The chemical histology of the human placenta and decidua with reference to mucopolysaccharides, glycogen, lipids and acid phosphatase. American Journal of Anatomy 83: 1-42

Woessner J F Jr 1962 Catabolism of collagen and non-collagen protein in the rat uterus during post partum involution. Biochemical Journal 83: 304-14

Woessner J F Jr 1963 Age-related changes of the human uterus and its connective tissue framework. Journal of Gerontology 18: 220-26

Woessner J F Jr 1965 Acid hydrolases of the rat uterus in relation to pregnancy, post partum involution and collagen breakdown. Biochemical Journal 97: 855-66

Woessner J F Jr 1969 Inhibition by oestrogen of collagen breakdown in the involuting rat uterus. Biochemical Journal 112: 637-46

Woessner J F Jr 1977 A latent form of collagenase in the involuting rat uterus and its activation by a serine proteinase. Biochemical Journal 161: 535-42

Woessner J F Jr 1978 Collagenolytic cathepsin of the involuting rat uterus. Federation Proceedings 37: 1530

Woessner J F Jr 1979a Total, latent and active collagenase during the course of post partum involution of the rat uterus. Effect of oestradiol. Biochemical Journal 180: 95-102

Woessner J F Jr 1979b Separation of collagenase and a metal-dependent endopeptidase of rat uterus that hydrolyzes a heptapeptide related to collagen. Biochimica Biophysica Acta 571: 313-20

Woessner J F Jr, Brewer T H 1963 Formation and breakdown of collagen and elastin in the human uterus during pregnancy and post partum involution. Biochemical Journal 89: 75-82

Wolfe J M, Wright A W 1942 Fibrous connective tissue of artificially induced material placenta in rat with particular reference to the relationship between reticulum and collagen. American Journal of Pathology 18: 431-61

Wray S 1979 Localized inhibition of uterine resorption in rats containing dummy fetuses after parturition. Journal of Physiology (London) 287: 2-1

Wu C H, Rojkind M, Rifas L, Seifter S 1978 Biosynthesis of type I and type III collagens by cultured uterine smooth muscle cells. Archives of Biochemistry and Biophysics 188: 294-300

Yochim J M, Blahna D G 1976 Effects of estrone and progesterone on collagen and ascorbic acid content in the endometrium and myometrium of the rat. Journal of Reproduction and Fertility 47: 79-82

Younes M S, Steele H D, Robertson E M, Bencosme S A 1965 Correlative light and electron microscope study of the basement membrane of the human ectocervix. American Journal of Obstetrics and Gynecology 92: 163-71

Zarrow M X, Yochim J 1961 Dilatation of the uterine cervix of the rat and accompanying changes during the oestrous cycle, pregnancy and following treatment with oestradiol, progesterone and relaxin. Endocrinology 69: 292-304

Zimmer F 1965 Die Uterus vergrössering in der Schwangerschaft. Archiv für Gynaekologie 202: 31-40

Appendix

The primary structure

DIANE GALLOWAY

INTRODUCTION

Two methods have been used for determining the primary structure of collagen α-chains. The original method is peptide sequencing, in which the chain is first digested by cyanogen bromide, which breaks the peptide bond after methionine residues, giving rise to small peptides (CB peptides). These are further digested to produce shorter peptides in which the sequence of individual amino acids can be identified. The numbering of the CB peptides refers to their elution order in ion exchange chromatography. Their positions in the molecule must then be determined by one of two methods. Their individual SLS patterns may be compared with the overall SLS pattern of the whole collagen molecule. Alternatively, a different set of peptides may be produced from the α-chain by enzymatic degradation, and regions of overlap can then be identified between the peptides obtained by these two types of digestion. This method has revealed large parts of the sequences of collagen types I, II and III, but work on types IV and V has still to be done.

The more recent method involves analysis of the sequence of bases in the procollagen gene; from this the amino acid sequence of procollagen can be predicted. This does not of course allow identification of the amino acids hydroxyproline and hydroxylysine, which result from post-translational modifications. However it does provide information about the N- and C-terminal procollagen peptides which are removed enzymatically at the cell surface. (They are not normally available for study by traditional peptide sequencing, unless a deficiency of the relevant gene prevents their removal; this is true of the amino-terminal extension in dermatosporaxis.) The procollagen genes, in common with all vertebrate genes so far studied, except that for interferon, contain non-coding sequences (introns) which interrupt their coding sequences (exons). In the following tables the positions of the introns will not be indicated. However, according to American workers (J. Wozney, D. Hanahan, V. Tate, H. Boedtker and P. Doty 1981 Nature 294: 129–35) the proα2(I) collagen gene is the most highly interrupted gene so far examined. Information already obtained from gene sequencing refers only to type I collagen. It is anticipated that details of the other collagen types will be available soon.

In the following tables, the results obtained by the two methods are presented side by side for comparison.

Key to symbols used in the tables

Ala	Alanine
Arg	Arginine
Asn	Asparagine
Asp	Aspartic acid
Asx	Asparagine or Aspartic acid
Cys	Cysteine
Gln	Glutamine
Glu	Glutamic acid
pGlu	Pyroglutamic acid
Glx	Glutamine or Glutamic acid
Gly	Glycine
His	Histidine
Hyl	Hydroxylysine
Hyp	Hydroxyproline
Ile	Isoleucine
Leu	Leucine
Lys	Lysine
Met	Methionine
Phe	Phenylalanine
Pro	Proline
Ser	Serine
Thr	Threonine
Trp	Tryptophan
Tyr	Tyrosine
Val	Valine

Table 1. The N-terminal procollagen peptides

Residue no.	**a. Revealed by protein sequencing**							
	α1(I) chain			α2(I) chain			α1(II) chain	α1(III) chain
	Bovine	*Rat*	*Chick*	*Bovine*	*Rat*	*Chick*	*Bovine*	*Bovine*
1*	pGlu**							
2	Glu							
3	Glu							
4	Gly							
5	Gln							
6	Glu							
7	Glu							
8	Gly		pGly					
9	Gln		Gly					
10	Glu		Glu					pGlu
11	Glu		Glu					Gln
12	Asp		Asp					Glu
13	Ile		Ile					Ala
14	Pro		Gln					Val
15	Pro		Thr					Asp
16	Val		Gly					Gly
17	Thr		Ser					Gly
18	Cys		Cys					Cys
19	Val		Val					Ser
20	Gln		Gln					His
21	Asp		Asp					Leu
22	Gly		Gly					Gly
23	Leu		Leu					Gln
24	Arg							Ser
25	Tyr		Tyr					Tyr
26	His		Asn					Ala
27	Asp		Asp					Asp
28	Arg							Arg
29	Asp		Asp					Asp
30	Val		Val					Val
31	Trp		Trp					Trp
32	Lys							Lys
33	Pro		Pro					Pro
34	Val		Glu					Glu
35	Pro		Pro					Pro
36	Cys		Cys					Cys
37	Gln							Gln
38	Ile							Ile
39	Cys							Cys
40	Val							Val
41	Cys							Cys
42	Asp							Asp
43	Asn							Ser
44	Gly							Gly
45	Asn							Ser
46	Val							Val
47	Leu							Leu
48	Cys							Cys
49	Asp							Asp
50	Asp							Asp
51	Val							Ile
52	Ile							Ile
53	Cys							Cys
54	Asp							Asp
55	Gln							Asp
56	Leu							Gln

*Numbering of residues refers to the bovine α1(I) sequence, both for the N-terminal procollagen peptides and for the N-terminal region of the collagen molecules.

**The ring structure of pyroglutamic acid is formed from glutamine when the N-terminal group is exposed.

Table 1. The N-terminal procollagen peptides—*(contd)*

Residue no.	**a. Revealed by protein sequencing**							
	$\alpha 1$(I) chain			$\alpha 2$(I) chain			$\alpha 1$(II) chain	$\alpha 1$(III) chain
	Bovine	*Rat*	*Chick*	*Bovine*	*Rat*	*Chick*	*Bovine*	*Bovine*
57	Lys							Glu
58	Asp							Leu
59	Cys							Asp
60	Pro							Cys
61	Asn							Pro
62	Ala							Asn
63	Lys							Pro
64	Val							Glu
65	Pro							Ile
66	Thr							Pro
67	Asp							Phe
68	Glu							Gly
69	Cys							Glu
70	Cys							Cys
71	Pro							Cys
72	Val							Ala
73	Cys							Val
74	Pro							Cys
75	Glu							Pro
76	Gly							Gln
77	Gln							Pro
78	Glu							Pro
79	Ser							Thr
80	Pro							Ala
81	Thr							Pro
82	Asp							Thr
83	Gln							Arg
84	Glu							Pro
85	Thr							Pro
86	Thr							Asp
87	Gly							Gly
88	Val							Gln
89	Glu							*Gly**
90	Gly							*Pro*
91	Pro							*Gln*
92	Lys							*Gly*
93	Gly							*Pro*
94	Asp							*Lys*
95	Thr							Gly
96	Gly							Asp
97	Pro							Hyp
98	Arg							Gly
99	Gly							Pro
100	Pro							Hyp
101	Arg							Gly
102	Gly							Ile
103	Pro							Hyp
104	Ala							Gly
105	Gly							Arg
106	Pro							Asn
107	Hyp							Gly
108	Gly							Asp
109	Arg							Hyp
110	Asp		Asp					Gly
111	Gly		Gly					Pro
112	Ile		Ile					Hyp
113	Hyp		Hyp					Gly
114	Gly		Gly					Ser

*Symbols in italics indicate that the sequence has not been confirmed

Table 1. The N-terminal procollagen peptides—*(contd)*

Residue no.	a. Revealed by protein sequencing							
	α1(I) chain			α2(I) chain			α1(II) chain	α1(III) chain
	Bovine	*Rat*	*Chick*	*Bovine*	*Rat*	*Chick*	*Bovine*	*Bovine*
115	Gln		Gln					Hyp
116	Pro		Hyp					Gly
117	Gly		Gly					Ser
118	Leu		Leu					Hyp
119	Hyp		Hyp					Gly
120	Gly		Gly					Ser
121	Pro		Pro					Hyp
122	Hyp		Hyp					Gly
123	Gly		Gly					Pro
124	Pro		Pro					Hyp
125	Hyp		Hyp					Gly
126	Gly							Ile
127	Pro							Cys
128	Hyp							Glu
129	Gly							Ser
130	Pro							Cys
131	Hyp							Pro
132	Gly							Thr
133	Leu							Gly
134	Gly							Gly
135	Gly							Gln
136	Asn							Asn
137	Phe							Tyr
138	Ala							Ser
139	Pro							Pro

Table 2. The N-terminal non-helical region of the collagen molecule

Residue no.	a. Revealed by protein sequencing								b. Revealed by nucleotide sequencing		
	α1(I) chain			α2(I) chain			α1(II) chain	α1(III)	α1(I) chain	α2(I) chain	
	Bovine	*Rat*	*Chick*	*Bovine*	*Rat*	*Chick*	*Bovine*	*Bovine*	*Chick*	*Bovine*	*Chick*
								pGlu			
								Tyr			
								Glu			
								Ala			
1	pGlu	pGlu	pGlu					Tyr			Asn
2	Leu	Met	Met					Asp			Phe
3	Ser	Ser	Ser					Val			Ala
4	Tyr	Tyr	Tyr					Lys			Ala
5	Gly	Gly	Gly			pGlu		Ser			Gln
6	Tyr	Tyr	Tyr		pGlu	Tyr		Gly			Tyr
7	Asp	Asp	Asp		Tyr	Asp		Val			Asp
8	Glu	Glu	Glu	pGlu	Ser	Pro		Ala			Pro
9	Lys	Lys	Lys	Phe	Asp	Ser		Gly			Ser
10	Ser	Ser	Ser	Asp	Lys	Lys		Gly			Lys
11	Thr	Ala	Ala	Ala	Gly	Ala		Gly			Ala
12	Gly	Gly	Gly	Lys	Val	Ala		Ile			Ala
13	Ile	Val	Val	Gly	Ser	Asp		Ala			Asp
14	Ser	Ser	Ala	Gly	Ala	Phe		Gly			Phe
15	Val	Val	Val	Gly	Gly	Gly		Tyr			Gly
16	Pro	Pro	Pro	Pro	Pro	Pro		Hyp			Pro

Table 3. The helical region of the collagen molecule

Residue no.	**a. Revealed by protein sequencing**								**b. Revealed by nucleotide sequencing**		
	α1(I) chain			α2(I) chain			α1(II) chain	α1(III) chain	α1(I) chain	α2(I) chain	
	Bovine	*Rat*	*Chick*	*Bovine*	*Rat*	*Chick*	*Bovine*	*Bovine*	*Chick*	*Bovine*	*Chick*
1	Gly	Gly	Gly	Gly	Gly	Gly	Gly	Gly		Gly	Gly
2	Pro	Pro	Pro	Pro	Pro	Pro	Val	Pro		Pro	Pro
3	Met	Met	Met	Met	Met	Met	Met	Ala		Met	Met
4	Gly	Gly	Gly	Gly	Gly		Gly	Gly		Gly	Gly
5	Pro	Pro	Pro	Leu	Leu		Pro	Pro		Leu	Leu
6	Ser	Ser	Ala	Met	Met		Met	Hyp		Met	Met
7	Gly	Gly	Gly	Gly	Gly		Gly	Gly		Gly	Gly
8	Pro	Pro	Pro	Pro	Pro		Pro	Pro		Pro	Pro
9	Arg	Arg	Arg	Arg	Arg		Arg	Hyp		Arg	Arg
10	Gly	Gly	Gly	Gly	Gly		Gly	Gly		Gly	Gly
11	Leu	Leu	Leu	Pro	Pro		Pro	Pro		Pro	Pro
12	Hyp	Hyp	Hyp	Hyp	Hyp		Hyp	Hyp		Pro	Pro
13	Gly	Gly	Gly	Gly	Gly		Gly	Gly		Gly	Gly
14	Pro	Pro	Pro	Ala	Ala		Pro	Thr		Ala	Ala
15	Hyp	Hyp	Hyp	Ser	Val		Ala	Ser		Ser	Ser
16	Gly	Gly	Gly	Gly	Gly		Gly	Gly		Gly	Gly
17	Ala	Ala	Ala	Ala	Ala		Ala	His		Ala	Pro
18	Hyp	Hyp	Hyp	Hyp	Hyp		Hyp	Hyp		Pro	Pro
19	Gly	Gly	Gly	Gly	Gly		Gly	Gly		Gly	Gly
20	Pro	Pro	Pro	Pro	Pro		Pro	Ala		Pro	Pro
21	Gln	Gln	Gln	Gln	Gln		Gln	Hyp		Gln	Pro
22	Gly	Gly	Gly	Gly	Gly		Gly	Gly		Gly	Gly
23	Phe	Phe	Phe	Phe	Phe		Phe	Ala		Phe	Phe
24	Gln	Gln	Gln	Gln	Gln		Gln	Hyp		Gln	Gln
25	Gly	Gly	Gly	Gly	Gly		Gly	Gly		Gly	Gly
26	Pro	Pro	Pro	Pro	Pro		Asn	Tyr		Pro	Val
27	Hyp	Hyp	Hyp	Hyp	Ala		Pro	Gln		Pro	Pro
28	Gly	Gly	Gly	Gly	Gly		Gly	Gly		Gly	Gly
29	Glu	Glu	Glu	Glu	Glu		Glu	Pro		Glu	Glu
30	Hyp	Hyp	Hyp	Hyp	Hyp		Hyp	Hyp		Pro	Pro
31	Gly	Gly	Gly	Gly	Gly		Gly	Gly		Gly	Gly
32	Glu	Glu	Glu	Glu	Glu		Glu	Glu		Glu	Glu
33	Hyp	Hyp	Hyp	Hyp	Hyp		Hyp	Hyp		Pro	Pro
34	Gly	Gly	Gly	Gly	Gly		Gly	Gly		Gly	Gly
35	Ala	Ala	Ala	Gln	Gln		Val	Gln		Gln	Gln
36	Ser	Ser	Ser	Hyp	Hyp		Ser	Ala		Thr	Thr
37	Gly	Gly	Gly	Gly	Gly		Gly	Gly		Gly	Gly
38	Pro	Pro	Pro	Pro	Pro		Pro	Pro		Pro	Pro
39	Met	Met	Met	Ala	Ala		Met	Ala		Ala	Gln
40	Gly	Gly	Gly	Gly	Gly		Gly	Gly		Gly	Gly
41	Pro	Pro	Pro	Ala	Pro		Pro	Pro		Ala	Pro
42	Arg	Arg	Arg	Arg	Arg		Arg	Hyp		Arg	Arg
43	Gly	Gly	Gly	Gly	Gly		Gly	Gly		Gly	Gly
44	Pro	Pro	Pro	Pro	Pro		Pro	Pro		Pro	Pro
45	Hyp	Hyp	Ala	Ala	Hyp		Hyp	Hyp		Pro	Pro
46	Gly	Gly	Gly	Gly	Gly		Gly	Gly		Gly	Gly
47	Pro	Pro	Pro	Pro	Pro		Pro	Ala		Pro	Pro
48	Hyp	Hyp	Hyp	Hyp	Hyp		Hyp	Ile		Pro	Pro
49	Gly	Gly	Gly	Gly			Gly	Gly		Gly	Gly
50	Lys	Lys	Lys	Lys			Lys	Pro		Lys	Lys
51	Asn	Asn	Asn	Ala			Hyp	Ser		Ala	Ala
52	Gly	Gly	Gly	Gly			Gly	Gly		Gly	Gly
53	Asp	Asp	Asp	Glu			Asp	Lys		Glu	Glu
54	Asp	Asp	Asp	Asp			Asp	Asp		Asp	Asp
55	Gly	Gly	Gly	Gly			Gly	Gly		Gly	Gly
56	Glu	Glu	Glu	His			Glu	Glu		His	His
57	Ala	Ala	Ala	Hyp			Ala	Ser		Pro	Pro
58	Gly	Gly	Gly	Gly			Gly	Gly		Gly	Gly
59	Lys	Lys	Lys	Lys			Lys	Arg		Lys	Lys
60	Pro	Pro	Pro	Pro			Hyp	Hyp		Pro	Pro

Table 3. The helical region of the collagen molecule—*(contd)*

Residue no.	a. Revealed by protein sequencing								b. Revealed by nucleotide sequencing		
	α1(I) chain			α2(I) chain			α1(II) chain	α1(III) chain	α1(I) chain	α2(I) chain	
	Bovine	*Rat*	*Chick*	*Bovine*	*Rat*	*Chick*	*Bovine*	*Bovine*	*Chick*	*Bovine*	*Chick*
61	Gly	Gly	Gly	Gly			Gly	Gly		Gly	Gly
62	Arg	Arg	Arg	Arg			Lys	Arg		Arg	Arg
63	Hyp	Hyp	Hyp	Hyp			Ser	Hyp		Pro	Pro
64	Gly	Gly	Gly	Gly			Gly	Gly		Gly	Gly
65	Glu	Gln	Gln	Glu			Glu	Pro		Glu	Glu
66	Arg	Arg	Arg	Arg			Arg	Arg		Arg	Arg
67	Gly	Gly	Gly	Gly			Gly	Gly		Gly	Gly
68	Pro	Pro	Pro	Val			Pro	Phe		Val	Val
69	Hyp	Hyp	Hyp	Pro			Hyp	Hyp		Pro	Ala
70	Gly	Gly	Gly	Gly			Gly	Gly		Gly	Gly
71	Pro	Pro	Pro	Pro			Pro	Pro		Pro	Pro
72	Gln	Gln	Gln	Gln			Gln	Hyp		Gln	Gln
73	Gly	Gly	Gly	Gly			Gly	Gly			
74	Ala	Ala	Ala	Ala			Ala	Met			
75	Arg	Arg	Arg	Arg			Arg	Hyl			
76	Gly	Gly	Gly	Gly			Gly	Gly			
77	Leu	Leu	Leu	Phe			Phe	Pro			
78	Hyp	Hyp	Hyp	Hyp			Hyp	Ala			
79	Gly	Gly	Gly	Gly			Gly	Gly			
80	Thr	Thr	Thr	Thr			Thr	Met			
81	Ala	Ala	Ala	Hyp			Hyp	Hyp			
82	Gly	Gly	Gly	Gly			Gly	Gly			
83	Leu	Leu	Leu	Leu			Leu	Phe			
84	Hyp	Hyp	Hyp	Hyp			Hyp	Hyp			
85	Gly	Gly	Gly	Gly			Gly	Gly			
86	Met	Met	Met	Phe			Val	Met			
87	Hyl	Hyl	Hyl	Hyl			Hyl	Hyl			
88	Gly	Gly	Gly	Gly			Gly	Gly			
89	His	His	His	Ile			His	His			
90	Arg	Arg	Arg	Arg			Arg	Arg			
91	Gly	Gly	Gly	Gly			Gly	Gly			
92	Phe	Phe	Phe	His			Tyr	Phe			
93	Ser	Ser	Ser	Asn			Hyp	Asp			
94	Gly	Gly	Gly	Gly			Gly	Gly			
95	Leu	Leu	Leu	Leu			Leu	Arg			
96	Asp	Asp	Asp	Asp			Asp	Asn			
97	Gly	Gly	Gly	Gly			Gly	Gly			
98	Ala	Ala	Ala	Leu			Ala	Glu			
99	Lys	Lys	Lys	Thr			Hyl	Hyl			
100	Gly	Gly	Gly	Gly			Gly	Gly			
101	Asp	Asn	Gln	Gln			Glu	Glu			
102	Ala	Thr	Hyp	Hyp			Ala	Hyp			
103	Gly	Gly	Gly	Gly			Gly	Gly			
104	Pro	Pro	Pro	Ala			Ala	Ala			
105	Ala	Ala	Ala	Hyp			Hyp	Hyp			
106	Gly	Gly	Gly	Gly			Gly	Gly			
107	Pro	Pro	Pro	Val			Val	Leu			
108	Lys	Lys	Lys	Hyl			Hyl	Lys			
109	Gly	Gly	Gly	Gly			Gly	Gly			
110	Glu	Glu	Glu	Glu			Glu	Glu			
111	Hyp	Hyp	Hyp	Hyp			Ser	Asn			
112	Gly	Gly	Gly	Gly			Gly	Gly			
113	Ser	Ser	Ser	Ala			Ser	Val			
114	Hyp	Hyp	Hyp	Hyp			Hyp	Hyp			
115	Gly	Gly	Gly	Gly			Gly	Gly			
116	Glu	Glx	Glu	Glu			*Glx*	Glu			
117	Asn	Asx	Asn	Asn			*Asx*	Asp			
118	Gly	Gly	Gly	Gly			*Gly*	Gly			
119	Ala	Ala	Ala	Thr			*Ser*	Ala			
120	Hyp	Hyp	Hyp	Hyp			*Hyp*	Hyp			

Table 3. The helical region of the collagen molecule—*(contd)*

Residue no.	a. Revealed by protein sequencing								b. Revealed by nucleotide sequencing		
	α1(I) chain			α2(I) chain			α1(II) chain	α1(III) chain	α1(I) chain	α2(I) chain	
	Bovine	*Rat*	*Chick*	*Bovine*	*Rat*	*Chick*	*Bovine*	*Bovine*	*Chick*	*Bovine*	*Chick*
121	Gly	Gly	Gly	Gly			Gly	Gly			
122	Gln	Gln	Gln	Gln			Pro	Pro			
123	Met	Met	Met	Hyl			Met	Met			
124	Gly	Gly		Gly			Gly	Gly			
125	Pro	Pro		Ala			Pro	Pro			
126	Arg	Arg		Arg			Arg	Arg			
127	Gly	Gly		Gly			Gly	Gly			
128	Leu	Leu		Leu			Leu	Ala			
129	Hyp	Hyp		Hyp			Hyp	Hyp			
130	Gly	Gly		Gly			Gly	Gly			
131	Glu	Glu		Glu			Glu	Glu			
132	Arg	Arg		Arg			Arg	Arg			
133	Gly	Gly		Gly			Gly	Gly			
134	Arg	Arg		Arg			Arg	Arg			
135	Hyp	Hyp		Val			Thr	Hyp			
136	Gly	Gly		Gly			Gly	Gly			
137	Ala	Pro		Ala			Pro	Leu			
138	Hyp	Hyp		Hyp			Ala	Hyp			
139	Gly	Gly		Gly			Gly	Gly			
140	Pro	Ser		Pro			Ala	Ala			
141	Ala	Ala		Ala			Ala	Ala			
142	Gly	Gly		Gly			Gly	Gly			
143	Ala	Ala		Ala			Ala	Ala			
144	Arg	Arg		Arg			Arg	Arg			
145	Gly	Gly		Gly			Gly	Gly			
146	Asn	Asp		Ser			Asn	Asn			
147	Asp	Asp		Asp			Asp	Asp			
148	Gly	Gly		Gly			Gly	Gly			
149	Ala	Ala		Ser			Gln	Ala			
150	Thr	Val		Val			Hyp	Arg			
151	Gly	Gly		Gly			Gly	Gly			
152	Ala	Ala		Pro			Pro	Ser			
153	Ala	Ala		Val			Ala	Asp			
154	Gly	Gly		Gly			Gly	Gly			
155	Pro	Pro		Pro			Pro	Gln			
156	Hyp	Hyp		Ala			Hyp	Hyp			
157	Gly	Gly		Gly			Gly	Gly			
158	Pro	Pro		Pro			Pro	Pro			
159	Thr	Thr		Ile			Val	Hyp			
160	Gly	Gly		Gly			Gly	Gly			
161	Pro	Pro		Ser			Pro	Pro			
162	Ala	Thr		Ala			Ala	Hyp			
163	Gly	Gly		Gly			Gly	Gly			
164	Pro	Pro		Pro			Gln	Thr			
165	Hyp	Hyp		Hyp			Hyp	Ala			
166	Gly	Gly		Gly			Gly	Gly			
167	Phe	Phe		Phe			Phe	Phe			
168	Hyp	Hyp		Hyp			Hyp	Hyp			
169	Gly	Gly		Gly			Gly	Gly			
170	Ala	Ala		Ala			Ala	Ser			
171	Val	Ala		Hyp			Hyp	Hyp			
172	Gly	Gly		Gly			Gly	Gly			
173	Ala	Ala		Pro			Ala	Ala			
174	Lys	Lys		Hyl			Hyl	Lys			
175	Gly	Gly		Gly			Gly	Gly		Gly	Gly
176	Glu	Glu		Glu			Glu	Glu		Glu	Glu
177	Gly	Ala		Leu			Ala	Val		Leu	Ile
178	Gly	Gly		Gly			Gly	Gly		Gly	Gly
179	Pro	Pro		Pro			Pro	Pro		Pro	Pro
180	Gln	Gln		Val				Ala		Val	Ala

Table 3. The helical region of the collagen molecule—*(contd)*

Residue no.	a. Revealed by protein sequencing								b. Revealed by nucleotide sequencing		
	α1(I) chain			α2(I) chain			α1(II) chain	α1(III) chain	α1(I) chain	α2(I) chain	
	Bovine	*Rat*	*Chick*	*Bovine*	*Rat*	*Chick*	*Bovine*	*Bovine*	*Chick*	*Bovine*	*Chick*
181	Gly	Gly		Gly			Gly	Gly		Gly	Gly
182	Pro	Ala		Asn			Ala	Ser		Asn	Asn
183	Arg	Arg		Hyp			Arg	Hyp		Pro	Glu
184	Gly	Gly		Gly				Gly		Gly	Gly
185	Ser	Ser		Pro				Ser		Pro	Pro
186	Glu	Glu		Ala				Ser		Ala	Thr
187	Gly	Gly		Gly				Gly		Gly	Gly
188	Pro	Pro		Pro				Ala		Pro	Pro
189	Gln	Gln		Ala				Hyp		Ala	Ala
190	Gly	Gly		Gly				Gly		Gly	Gly
191	Val	Val		Pro				Gln		Pro	Pro
192	Arg	Arg		Arg				Arg		Arg	Arg
193	Gly	Gly		Gly			Gly	Gly		Gly	Gly
194	Glu	Glu		Glu			Glu	Glu		Glu	Glu
195	Hyp	Hyp		Val			Hyp	Hyp		Val	Ile
196	Gly	Gly		Gly			Gly	Gly		Gly	Gly
197	Pro	Pro		Leu			Thr	Pro		Leu	Leu
198	Hyp	Hyp		Hyp			Hyp	Gln		Pro	Pro
199	Gly	Gly		Gly			Gly	Gly		Gly	Gly
200	Pro	Pro		Leu			Ser	His		Leu	Ser
201	Ala	Ala		Ser			Hyp	Ala		Ser	Ser
202	Gly	Gly		Gly			Gly	Gly		Gly	Gly
203	Ala	Ala		Pro			Pro	Ala		Pro	Pro
204	Ala	Ala		Val			Ala	Hyp		Val	Val
205	Gly	Gly		Gly			Gly	Gly		Gly	Gly
206	Pro	Pro		Pro			Ala	Pro		Pro	Pro
207	Ala	Ala		Hyp			Ala	Hyp		Pro	Pro
208	Gly	Gly		Gly			Gly	Gly		Gly	Gly
209	Asn	Asn		Asn			Asn	Pro		Asn	Asn
210	Hyp	Hyp		Ala			Hyp	Hyp		Ala	Pro
211	Gly	Gly		Gly			Gly	Gly		Gly	Gly
212	Ala	Ala		Pro			Thr	Ser		Pro	Ala
213	Asp	Asp		Asn			Asp	Asp		Asn	Asn
214	Gly	Gly		Gly			Gly	Gly		Gly	Gly
215	Glu	Gln		Leu			Ile	Ser		Leu	Leu
216	Hyp	Hyp		Hyp			Hyp	Hyp		Pro	Pro
217	Gly	Gly		Gly			Gly	Gly		Gly	Gly
218	Ala	Ala		Ala			Ala	Gly		Ala	Ala
219	Lys	Lys		Hyl			Hyl	Lys		Lys	Lys
220	Gly	Gly		Gly			Gly	Gly		Gly	Gly
221	Ala	Ala		Ala			Ser	Glu		Ala	Ala
222	Asn	Asn		Ala			Ala	Met		Ala	Ala
223	Gly	Gly		Gly			Gly	Gly		Gly	Gly
224	Ala	Ala		Leu			Ala	Pro		Leu	Leu
225	Hyp	Hyp		Hyp			Hyp	Ala		Pro	Pro
226	Gly	Gly		Gly			Gly	Gly		Gly	Gly
227	Ile	Ile		Val			Ile	Ile		Val	Val
228	Ala	Ala		Ala			Ala	Hyp		Ala	Ala
229	Gly	Gly		Gly			Gly	Gly		Gly	Gly
230	Ala	Ala		Ala			Pro	Ala		Ala	Ala
231	Hyp	Hyp		Hyp			Hyp	Hyp		Pro	Pro
232	Gly	Gly		Gly			Gly	Gly		Gly	Gly
233	Phe	Phe		Leu			Phe	Leu		Leu	Leu
234	Hyp	Hyp		Hyp			Hyp	Ile		Pro	Pro
235	Gly	Gly		Gly			Gly	Gly		Gly	Gly
236	Ala	Ala		Pro			Ala	Ala		Pro	Pro
237	Arg	Arg		Arg			Arg	Arg		Arg	Arg
238	Gly	Gly		Gly			Gly	Gly		Gly	Gly
239	Pro	Pro		Ile			Pro	Pro		Ile	Ile
240	Ser	Ser		Hyp			Hyp	Hyp		Pro	Pro

Table 3. The helical region of the collagen molecule—*(contd)*

Residue no.	a. Revealed by protein sequencing								b. Revealed by nucleotide sequencing		
	α1(I) chain			α2(I) chain			α1(II) chain	α1(III) chain	α1(I) chain	α2(I) chain	
	Bovine	*Rat*	*Chick*	*Bovine*	*Rat*	*Chick*	*Bovine*	*Bovine*	*Chick*	*Bovine*	*Chick*
241	Gly	Gly		Gly			Gly	Gly		Gly	Gly
242	Pro	Pro		Pro			Pro	Pro		Pro	Pro
243	Gln	Gln		Val			Gln	Hyp		Val	Pro
244	Gly	Gly		Gly			Gly	Gly		Gly	Gly
245	Pro	Pro		Ala			Ala	Thr		Ala	Pro
246	Ser	Ser		Ala			Thr	Asn		Ala	Ala
247	Gly	Gly		Gly			Gly	Gly		Gly	Gly
248	Pro	Ala		Ala			Pro	Val		Ala	Pro
249	Hyp	Hyp		Thr			Leu	Hyp		Thr	Ser
250	Gly	Gly		Gly			Gly	Gly		Gly	Gly
251	Pro	Pro		Ala			Pro	Gln		Ala	Ala
252	Lys	Lys		Arg			Hyl	Arg		Arg	Arg
253	Gly	Gly		Gly			Gly	Gly		Gly	Gly
254	Asn	Asn		Leu			Gln	Ala		Leu	Leu
255	Ser	Ser		Val				Ala		Val	Val
256	Gly	Gly		Gly				Gly		Gly	Gly
257	Glu	Glu		Glu				Glu		Glu	Glu
258	Hyp	Hyp		Hyp				Hyp		Pro	Pro
259	Gly	Gly		Gly				Gly		Gly	Gly
260	Ala	Ala		Pro				Lys		Pro	Pro
261	Hyp	Hyp		Ala				Asn		Ala	Ala
262	Gly	Gly		Gly				Gly		Gly	Gly
263	Asn	Asn		Ser				Ala		Ser	Ala
264	Lys	Lys		Hyl				Lys		Lys	Lys
265	Gly	Gly		Gly				Gly		Gly	Gly
266	Asp	Asp		Glu				Asp		Glu	Glu
267	Thr	Thr		Ser				Hyp		Ser	Ser
268	Gly	Gly		Gly				Gly		Gly	Gly
269	Ala	Ala		Asn				Pro		Asn	Asn
270	Lys	Lys		Lys				Arg		Lys	Lys
271	Gly	Gly		Gly				Gly		Gly	Gly
272	Glu	Glu		Glu				Glu		Glu	Glu
273	Hyp	Hyp		Hyp				Arg		Pro	Pro
274	Gly	Gly		Gly				Gly		Gly	Gly
275	Pro	Pro		Ala				Glu		Ala	Ala
276	Thr	Ala		Val				Ala		Val	Ala
277	Gly	Gly		Gly				Gly		Gly	Gly
278	Ile	Val		Gln				Ser		Gln	Pro
279	Gln	Gln		Hyp				Hyp		Pro	Pro
280	Gly	Gly		Gly				Gly		Gly	Gly
281	Pro	Pro		Pro				Ile		Pro	Pro
282	Hyp	Hyp		Hyp				Ala		Pro	Pro
283	Gly	Gly		Gly				Gly		Gly	Gly
284	Pro	Pro		Pro				Pro		Pro	Pro
285	Ala	Ala		Ser				Lys		Ser	Ser
286	Gly	Gly		Gly				Gly		Gly	Gly
287	Glu	Glu		Glu				Glu		Glu	Glu
288	Glu	Glu		Glu				Asp		Glu	Glu
289	Gly	Gly		Gly				Gly		Gly	Gly
290	Lys	Lys		Lys				Lys		Lys	Lys
291	Arg	Arg		Arg				Asp		Arg	Arg
292	Gly	Gly		Gly				Gly		Gly	Gly
293	Ala	Ala		Ser				Ser		Ser	Ser
294	Arg	Arg		Thr				Hyp		Thr	Asn
295	Gly	Gly		Gly				Gly		Gly	Gly
296	Glu	Glu		Glu				Glu		Glu	Glu
297	Hyp	Hyp		Ile				Hyp		Ile	Pro
298	Gly	Gly		Gly				Gly		Gly	Gly
299	Pro	Pro		Pro				Ala		Pro	Ser
300	Ala	Ser		Ala				Asn		Ala	Ala

Table 3. The helical region of the collagen molecule—*(contd)*

Residue no.	a. Revealed by protein sequencing								b. Revealed by nucleotide sequencing		
	α1(I) chain			α2(I) chain			α1(II) chain	α1(III) chain	α1(I) chain	α2(I) chain	
	Bovine	*Rat*	*Chick*	*Bovine*	*Rat*	*Chick*	*Bovine*	*Bovine*	*Chick*	*Bovine*	*Chick*
301	Gly	Gly		Gly				Gly		Gly	Gly
302	Leu	Leu		Pro				Leu		Pro	Pro
303	Hyp	Hyp		Hyp				Hyp		Pro	Pro
304	Gly	Gly		Gly				Gly		Gly	Gly
305	Pro	Pro		Pro				Ala		Pro	Pro
306	Hyp	Hyp		Hyp				Ala		Pro	Ala
307	Gly	Gly		Gly				Gly		Gly	Gly
308	Glu	Glu		Leu				Glu		Leu	Leu
309	Arg	Arg		Arg				Arg		Arg	Arg
310	Gly	Gly		Gly				Gly		Gly	Gly
311	Gly	Gly		Asn				Val		Asn	Glu
312	Hyp	Hyp		Hyp				Hyp		Pro	Pro
313	Gly	Gly		Gly				Gly		Gly	Gly
314	Ser	Ser		Ser				Phe		Ser	Ser
315	Arg	Arg		Arg				Arg		Arg	Arg
316	Gly	Gly		Gly				Gly		Gly	Gly
317	Phe	Phe		Leu				Pro		Leu	Leu
318	Hyp	Hyp		Hyp				Ala		Pro	Pro
319	Gly	Gly		Gly				Gly		Gly	Gly
320	Ala	Ala		Ala				Ala		Ala	Ala
321	Asp	Asp		Asp				Asn		Asp	Asp
322	Gly	Gly		Gly				Gly		Gly	Gly
323	Val	Val		Arg				Leu		Arg	Arg
324	Ala	Ala		Ala				Hyp		Ala	Ala
325	Gly	Gly		Gly				Gly		Gly	Gly
326	Pro	Pro		Val				Glu		Val	Val
327	Lys	Lys		Met				Lys		Met	Met
328	Gly	Gly		Gly	Gly	Gly		Gly			Gly
329	Pro	Pro		Pro	Pro	Pro		Pro			Pro
330	Ala	Ala		Ala	Hyp	Ala		Hyp			Ala
331	Gly	Gly		Gly	Gly	Gly		Gly			Gly
332	Glu	Glu		Ser	Asn	Asn		Asp			Asn
333	Arg	Arg		Arg	Arg	Arg		Arg			Arg
334	Gly	Gly		Gly	Gly	Gly		Gly			Gly
335	Ala	Ser		Thr	Thr	Ala		Gly			Ala
336	Hyp	Hyp		Ala	Ser	Ser		Hyp			Ser
337	Gly	Gly		Gly	Gly	Gly		Gly			Gly
338	Pro	Pro		Pro	Pro	Pro		Pro			Pro
339	Ala	Ala		Ala	Ala	Ala		Ala			Val
340	Gly	Gly		Gly	Gly	Gly		Gly			Gly
341	Pro	Pro		Val	Val	Val		Pro			Ala
342	Lys	Lys		Arg	Arg	Lys		Arg			Lys
343	Gly	Gly		Gly	*Gly*	Gly		Gly			Gly
344	Ser	Ser		Pro	*Pro*	Pro		Val			Pro
345	Hyp	Hyp		Asn	*Asx*	Asn		Ala			Asn
346	Gly	Gly		Gly	*Gly*	Gly		Gly			Gly
347	Glu	Glu		Asp	*Asx*	Asp		Glu			Asp
348	Ala	Ala		Ser	*Ala*	Ala		Hyp			Ala
349	Gly	Gly		Gly	*Gly*	Gly		Gly			Gly
350	Arg	Arg		Arg	*Arg*	Arg		Arg			Arg
351	Hyp	Hyp		Hyp	*Hyp*	Hyp		Asn			Pro
352	Gly	Gly		Gly	*Gly*	Gly		Gly			Gly
353	Glu	Glu		Glu	*Glx*	Glu		Leu			Glu
354	Ala	Ala		Hyp	*Hyp*	Hyp		Hyp			Pro
355	Gly	Gly		Gly	*Gly*	Gly		Gly			Gly
356	Leu	Leu		Leu	*Leu*	Leu		Gly			Leu
357	Hyp	Hyp		Met	Met	Met		Hyp			Met
358	Gly	Gly		Gly	Gly	Gly		Gly			Gly
359	Ala	Ala		Pro	Pro	Pro		Leu			Pro
360	Lys	Lys		Arg	Arg	Arg		Arg			Arg

Table 3. The helical region of the collagen molecule—*(contd)*

Residue no.	a. Revealed by protein sequencing								b. Revealed by nucleotide sequencing		
	α1(I) chain			α2(I) chain			α1(II) chain	α1(III) chain	α1(I) chain	α2(I) chain	
	Bovine	*Rat*	*Chick*	*Bovine*	*Rat*	*Chick*	*Bovine*	*Bovine*	*Chick*	*Bovine*	*Chick*
361	Gly	Gly		Gly	Gly	Gly		Gly			
362	Leu	Leu		Phe	Leu	Leu		Ile			
363	Thr	Thr		Hyp	Hyp	Hyp		Hyp			
364	Gly	Gly		Gly	Gly	Gly		Gly			
365	Ser	Ser		Ser	Ser	Gln		Ser			
366	Hyp	Hyp		Hyp	Hyp	Hyp		Hyp			
367	Gly	Gly		Gly	Gly	Gly		Gly			
368	Ser	Ser		Asn	Asn	Ser		Gly			
369	Hyp	Hyp		Ile	Val	Hyp		Hyp			
370	Gly	Gly		Gly	Gly	Gly		Gly			
371	Pro	Pro		Pro	Pro	Pro		Ser			
372	Asp	Asp		Ala	Ala	Ala		Asn			
373	Gly	Gly		Gly	Gly	Gly		Gly			
374	Lys	Lys		Lys	Lys	Lys		Lys			
375	Thr	Thr		Glu	Glu	Glu		Hyp			
376	Gly	Gly		Gly	Gly	Gly		Gly			
377	Pro	Pro		Pro	Pro	Pro		Pro			
378	Hyp	Hyp		Val	Val	Val		Hyp			
379	Gly	Gly		Gly	Gly	Gly		Gly			Gly
380	Pro	Pro		Leu	Leu	Phe		Ser			Phe
381	Ala	Ala		Hyp	Hyp	Hyp		Gln			Pro
382	Gly	Gly		Gly	Gly	Gly		Gly			Gly
383	Gln	Glx		Ile	Ile	Ala		Glu			Ala
384	Asn	Asx		Asp	Asp	Asp		Thr			Asp
385	Gly	Gly		Gly	Gly	Gly		Gly			Gly
386	Arg	Arg		Arg	Arg	Arg		Arg			Arg
387	Hyp	Hyp		Hyp	Hyp	Val		Hyp			Val
388	Gly	Gly		Gly	Gly	Gly		Gly			Gly
389	Pro	Pro		Pro	Pro	Pro		Pro			Pro
390	Hyp	Ala		Ile	Ile	Ile		Hyp			Ile
391	Gly	Gly		Gly	Gly	Gly		Gly			Gly
392	Pro	Pro		Pro	Pro	Pro		Ser			Pro
393	Hyp	Hyp		Ala	Ala	Ala		Hyp			Ala
394	Gly	Gly		Gly	Gly	Gly		Gly			Gly
395	Ala	Ala		Pro	Pro	Asn		Pro			Asn
396	Arg	Arg		Arg	Arg	Arg		Arg			Arg
397	Gly	Gly		Gly	Gly	Gly		Gly			Gly
398	Gln	Gln		Glu	Glx	Glu		Gln			Glu
399	Ala	Ala		Ala	Ala	Hyp		Hyp			Pro
400	Gly	Gly			Gly	Gly		Gly			Gly
401	Val	Val			Ala	Asn		Val			Asn
402	Met	Met			Ile	Ile		Met			Phe
403	Gly	Gly	Gly		Gly	Gly	Gly	Gly			Gly
404	Phe	Phe	Phe		Phe	Phe	Phe	Phe			Phe
405	Hyp	Hyp	Hyp		Hyp	Hyp	Hyp	Hyp			Pro
406	Gly	Gly	Gly			Gly	Gly	Gly			Gly
407	Pro	Pro	Pro			Pro	Pro	Pro			Pro
408	Lys	Lys	Lys			Lys	Hyl	Lys			Lys
409	Gly	Gly	Gly			Gly	Gly	Gly			Gly
410	Ala	Thr	Ala			Pro	Ala	Asn			Pro
411	Ala	Ala	Ala			Thr	Asn	Asp			Thr
412	Gly	Gly	Gly			Gly	Gly	Gly			Gly
413	Glu	Glu	Glu			Glu	Glu	Ala			Glu
414	Hyp	Hyp	Hyp			Hyp	Hyp	Hyp			Pro
415	Gly	Gly	Gly			Gly	Gly	Gly			Gly
416	Lys	Lys	Lys			Lys	Lys	Lys			Lys
417	Ala	Ala	Hyp			Hyp	Ala	Asn			Pro
418	Gly	Gly	Gly			Gly	Gly	Gly			Gly
419	Glu	Glu	Glu			Glu	Glu	Glu			Glu
420	Arg	Arg	Arg			Lys	Hyl	Arg			Lys

Table 3. The helical region of the collagen molecule—*(contd)*

Residue no.	a. Revealed by protein sequencing								b. Revealed by nucleotide sequencing		
	α1(I) chain			α2(I) chain			α1(II) chain	α1(III) chain	α1(I) chain	α2(I) chain	
	Bovine	*Rat*	*Chick*	*Bovine*	*Rat*	*Chick*	*Bovine*	*Bovine*	*Chick*	*Bovine*	*Chick*
421	Gly	Gly	Gly			Gly	Gly	Gly			Gly
422	Val	Val	Ala			Asn	Leu	Gly			Asn
423	Hyp	Hyp	Hyp			Val	Hyp	Hyp			Val
424	Gly	Gly	Gly			Gly	Gly	Gly			Gly
425	Pro	Pro	Pro			Leu	Ala	Gly			Leu
426	Hyp	Hyp	Hyp	Ala		Ala	Hyp	Hyp			Ala
427	Gly	Gly	Gly	Gly		Gly	Gly	Gly			Gly
428	Ala	Ala	Ala	Ala		Pro	Leu	Pro			Pro
429	Val	Val	Val	Arg		Arg	Arg	Gln			Arg
430	Gly	Gly	Gly	Gly		Gly	Gly	Gly			
431	Pro	Pro	Ala	Ala		Ala	Leu	Pro			
432	Ala	Ala	Ala	Hyp		Hyp	Hyp	Ala			
433	Gly	Gly	Gly	Gly		Gly	Gly	Gly			
434	Lys	Lys	Lys	Pro		Pro	Lys	Lys			
435	Asp	Asp	Asp	Asp		Glu	Asp	Asn			
436	Gly	Gly	Gly	Gly		Gly	Gly	Gly			
437	Glu	Glu	Glu	Asn		Asn	Glu	Glu			
438	Ala	Ala	Ala	Asn		Asn	Thr	Thr			
439	Gly	Gly	Gly	Gly		Gly	Gly	Gly			
440	Ala	Ala	Ala	Ala		Ala	Ala	Pro			
441	Gln	Gln	Gln	Gln		Gln	Ala	Gln			
442	Gly	Gly	Gly	Gly		Gly	Gly	Gly			
443	Pro	Ala	Pro	Pro		Pro	Pro	Pro			
444	Hyp	Hyp	Pro	Hyp		Hyp	Hyp	Hyp			
445	Gly	Gly	Gly	Gly		Gly	Gly	Gly			
446	Pro	Pro	Pro	Leu		Val	Pro	Pro			
447	Ala	Ala	Thr	Gln		Thr	Ala	Thr			
448	Gly	Gly	Gly	Gly		Gly	Gly	Gly			
449	Pro	Pro	Pro	Val		Asn	Pro	Pro			
450	Ala	Ala	Ala	Gln		Gln	Ala	Ser			
451	Gly	Gly	Gly	Gly		Gly	Gly	Gly			
452	Glu	Glu	Glu	Glu		Ala	Glu	Asp			
453	Arg	Arg	Arg	Lys		Lys	Arg	Lys			
454	Gly	Gly	Gly	Gly		Gly	Gly	Gly			
455	Glu	Glu	Glu	Glu		Glu	Glu	Asp			
456	Gln	Gln	Gln	Gln		Thr	Gln	Thr			
457	Gly	Gly	Gly	Gly		Gly	Gly	Gly			
458	Pro	Pro	Pro	Pro		Pro	Ala	Pro			
459	Ala	Ala	Ala	Ala		Ala	Hyp	Hyp			
460	Gly	Gly	Gly	Gly		Gly	Gly	Gly			
461	Ser	Ser	Ala	Pro		Pro	Pro	Pro			
462	Hyp	Hyp	Hyp	Hyp		Hyp	Ser	Gln			
463	Gly	Gly	Gly	Gly		Gly	Gly	Gly			
464	Phe	Phe	Phe	Phe		Phe	Phe	Leu			
465	Gln	Gln	Gln	Gln		Gln	Gln	Gln			
466	Gly	Gly	Gly	Gly		Gly	Gly	Gly			
467	Leu	Leu	Leu	Leu		Leu	Leu	Leu			
468	Hyp	Hyp	Hyp	Hyp		Hyp	Hyp	Hyp			
469	Gly	Gly	Gly	Gly		Gly	Gly	Gly			
470	Pro	Pro	Pro	Pro		Pro	Pro	Thr			
471	Ala	Ala	Ala	Ala		Ser	Hyp	Ser			
472	Gly	Gly	Gly	Gly		Gly	Gly	Gly			
473	Pro	Pro	Pro			Pro	Pro	Pro			
474	Hyp	Hyp	Hyp	Ala		Ala	Hyp	Hyp			
475	Gly	Gly	Gly	Gly		Gly	Gly	Gly			
476	Glu	Glu	Glu	Glu		Glu	Glu	Glu			
477	Ala	Ala	Ala	Ala		Ala	Hyp	Asn			
478	Gly	Gly	Gly	Gly		Gly	Gly	Gly			
479	Lys	Lys	Lys	Lys		Lys	Lys	Lys			
480	Hyp	Hyp	Hyp			Hyp	Hyp	Hyp			

Table 3. The helical region of the collagen molecule—*(contd)*

Residue no.	**a. Revealed by protein sequencing**								**b. Revealed by nucleotide sequencing**		
	α1(I) chain			α2(I) chain			α1(II) chain	α1(III) chain	α1(I) chain	α2(I) chain	
	Bovine	*Rat*	*Chick*	*Bovine*	*Rat*	*Chick*	*Bovine*	*Bovine*	*Chick*	*Bovine*	*Chick*
481	Gly	Gly	Gly			Gly	Gly	Gly			
482	Glu	Glx	Glu			Glu	Asp	Glu			
483	Gln	Glx	Gln			Arg	Gln	Hyp			
484	Gly	Gly	Gly			Gly	Gly	Gly			
485	Val	Val	Val			Leu	Val	Pro			
486	Hyp	Hyp	Hyp			His	Pro	Lys			
487	Gly	Gly	Gly			Gly	Gly	Gly			
488	Asp	Asp	Asn			Glu	Glu	Glu			
489	Leu	Leu	Ala			Phe	Ala	Ala			
490	Gly	Gly	Gly	Gly		Gly	Gly	Gly			
491	Ala	Ala	Ala	Leu		Val	Ala	Ala			
492	Hyp	Hyp	Hyp	Hyp		Hyp	Hyp	Hyp			
493	Gly	Gly	Gly	Gly		Gly	Gly	Gly			
494	Pro	Pro	Pro	Pro		Pro	Leu	Ile			
495	Ser	Ser	Ala	Ala		Ala	Val	Hyp			
496	Gly	Gly	Gly	Gly		Gly	Gly	Gly			
497	Ala	Ala	Ala	Ala		Pro	Pro	Gly			
498	Arg	Arg	Arg	Arg		Arg	Arg	Lys			
499	Gly	Gly	Gly	Gly		Gly	Gly	Gly			
500	Glu	Glu	Glu	Glu		Glu	Glu	Asp			
501	Arg	Arg	Arg	Arg		Arg	Arg	Ser			
502	Gly	Gly	Gly	Gly		Gly	Gly	Gly			
503	Phe	Phe	Phe	Pro		Leu	Phe	Ala			
504	Hyp	Hyp	Hyp	Hyp		Hyp	Hyp	Hyp			
505	Gly	Gly	Gly	Gly		Gly	Gly	Gly			
506	Glu	Glu	Glu	Glu		Glu	Glu	Glu			
507	Arg	Arg	Arg	Arg		Ser	Arg	Arg			
508	Gly	Gly	Gly	Gly		Gly	Gly	Gly			
509	Val	Val	Val	Ala		Ala	Ser	Pro			
510	Glu	Gln	Gln	Ala		Val	Hyp	Hyp			
511	Gly	Gly	Gly	Gly		Gly	Gly	Gly			
512	Pro	Pro	Pro	Pro		Pro	Ser	Ala			
513	Hyp	Hyp	Hyp	Thr		Ala	Gln	Gly			
514	Gly	Gly	Gly	Gly		Gly	Gly	Gly			
515	Pro	Pro	Pro	Pro		Pro	Leu	Pro			
516	Ala	Ala	Gln	Ile		Ile	Gln	Hyp			
517	Gly	Gly	Gly	Gly		Gly	Gly	Gly			
518	Pro	Pro	Pro	Ser		Ser	Ala	Pro			
519	Arg	Arg	Arg	Arg		Arg	Arg	Arg			
520	Gly	Gly	Gly	Gly		Gly	Gly	Gly			
521	Ala	Asn	Ala	Pro		Pro	Leu	Gly			
522	Asn	Asn	Asn	Ser		Ser	Hyp	Ala			
523	Gly	Gly	Gly	Gly		Gly	Gly	Gly			
524	Ala	Ala	Ala	Pro		Pro	Thr	Pro			
525	Hyp	Hyp	Hyp	Hyp		Hyp	Hyp	Hyp			
526	Gly	Gly	Gly	Gly		Gly	Gly	Gly			
527	Asn	Asx	Asn	Pro		Pro	Thr	Pro			
528	Asp	Asx	Asp	Asp		Asp	Asp	Glu			
529	Gly	Gly	Gly	Gly		Gly	Gly	Gly			
530	Ala	Ala	Ala	Asn		Asn	Pro	Gly			
531	Lys	Lys	Lys	Lys		Lys	Hyl	Lys			
532	Gly	Gly	Gly	Gly		Gly	Gly	Gly			
533	Asp	Asp	Asp	Gln		Glu	Ala	Ala			
534	Ala	Thr	Ala	Ala		Hyp	Ala	Ala			
535	Gly	Gly	Gly	Gly		Gly	Gly	Gly			
536	Ala	Ala	Ala	Ala		Asn	Pro	Pro			
537	Hyp	Hyp	Hyp	Val		Val	Ala	Hyp			
538	Gly	Gly	Gly			Gly	Gly	Gly			
539	Ala	Ala	Ala			Pro	Pro	Pro			
540	Hyp	Hyp	Hyp			Ala	Hyp	Hyp			

Table 3. The helical region of the collagen molecule—*(contd)*

Residue no.	a. Revealed by protein sequencing								b. Revealed by nucleotide sequencing		
	α1(I) chain			α2(I) chain			α1(II) chain	α1(III) chain	α1(I) chain	α2(I) chain	
	Bovine	*Rat*	*Chick*	*Bovine*	*Rat*	*Chick*	*Bovine*	*Bovine*	*Chick*	*Bovine*	*Chick*
541	Gly	Gly	Gly			Gly	Gly	Gly			
542	Ser	Ser	Asn			Ala	Ala	Ser			
543	Gln	Gln	Glu			Hyp	Gln	Ala			
544	Gly	Gly	Gly			Gly	Gly	Gly			
545	Ala	Ala	Pro			Pro	Pro	Thr			
546	Hyp	Hyp	Hyp			Ala	Hyp	Hyp			
547	Gly	Gly	Gly			Gly	Gly	Gly			
548	Leu	Leu	Leu			Pro	Leu	Leu			
549	Gln	Glx	Glu			Hyp	Gln	Gln			
550	Gly	Gly	Gly			Gly	Gly	Gly			
551	Met	Met	Met			Ile	Met	Met			
552	Hyp		Hyp			Hyp	Hyp	Hyp			
553	Gly		Gly			Gly	Gly	Gly			
554	Glu		Glu			Glu	Glu	Glu			
555	Arg		Arg			Arg	Arg	Arg			
556	Gly		Gly			Gly	Gly	Gly			
557	Ala		Ala			Val	Ala	Gly			
558	Ala		Ala			Ala	Ala	Hyp			
559	Gly		Gly			Gly	Gly	Gly			
560	Leu		Leu			Val	Ile	Gly			
561	Hyp		Hyp			Hyp	Ala	Hyp			
562	Gly		Gly			Gly	Gly	Gly			
563	Pro		Ala			Gly	Pro	Pro			
564	Lys		Lys			Lys	Hyl	Lys			
565	Gly		Gly			Gly	Gly	Gly			
566	Asp		Asp			Glu	Asp	Asp			
567	Arg		Arg			Lys	Arg	Lys			
568	Gly		Gly			Gly	Gly	Gly			
569	Asp		Asp			Ala	Asp	Glu			
570	Ala		Hyp			Hyp	Val	Hyp			
571	Gly		Gly			Gly	Gly	Gly			
572	Pro		Pro			Leu	Glu	Ser			
573	Lys		Lys			Arg	Lys	Ser			
574	Gly		Gly			Gly	Gly	Gly			
575	Ala		Ala			Asp	Pro	Val			
576	Asp		Asp			Thr	Glu	Asp			
577	Gly		Gly			Gly	Gly	Gly			
578	Ala		Ala			Ala	Ala	Ala			
579	Pro		Pro			Thr	Hyp	Pro			
580	Gly		Gly			Gly	Gly	Gly			
581	Lys		Lys			Arg	Lys	Lys			
582	Asp		Asp			Asp	Asp	Asp			
583	Gly		Gly			Gly	Gly	Gly			
584	Val		Leu			Ala	Gly	Pro			
585	Arg		Arg			Arg	Arg	Arg			
586	Gly		Gly			Gly	Gly	Gly			
587	Leu		Leu			Leu	Leu	Pro			
588	Thr		Thr			Hyp	Thr	Thr			
589	Gly		Gly			Gly	Gly	Gly			
590	Pro		Pro			Ala	Pro	Pro			
591	Ile		Ile			Ile	Ile	Ile			
592	Gly		Gly			Gly	Gly	Gly			
593	Pro		Pro			Ala	Pro	Pro			
594	Hyp		Hyp			Hyp	Hyp	Hyp			
595	Gly		Gly			Gly	Gly	Gly			
596	Pro		Pro			Pro	Pro	Pro			
597	Ala		Ala			Ala	Ala	Ala			
598	Gly		Gly			Gly	Gly	Gly			
599	Ala		Ala			Gly	Ala	Gln			
600	Hyp		Hyp			Ala	Asn	Hyp			

Table 3. The helical region of the collagen molecule—*(contd)*

Residue no.	a. Revealed by protein sequencing								b. Revealed by nucleotide sequencing		
	α1(I) chain			α2(I) chain			α1(II) chain	α1(III) chain	α1(I) chain	α2(I) chain	
	Bovine	*Rat*	*Chick*	*Bovine*	*Rat*	*Chick*	*Bovine*	*Bovine*	*Chick*	*Bovine*	*Chick*
601	Gly		Gly			Gly	Gly	Gly			
602	Asp		Asp			Asp	Glu	Asp			
603	Lys		Lys			Arg	Hyl	Lys			
604	Gly		Gly			Gly	Gly	Gly			
605	Glu		Glu			Glu	Glu	Glu			
606	Ala		Ala			Gly	Val	Ser			
607	Gly		Gly			Gly	Gly	Gly			
608	Pro		Pro			Pro	Pro	Ala			
609	Ser		Hyp			Ala	Hyp	Hyp			
610	Gly		Gly			Gly	Gly	Gly			
611	Pro		Pro			Pro	Pro	Val			
612	Ala		Ala			Ala	Ala	Hyp			
613	Gly		Gly			Gly	Gly	Gly			
614	Pro		Pro			Pro	Thr	Ile			
615	Thr		Thr			Ala	Ala	Ala			
616	Gly		Gly			Gly	Gly	Gly			
617	Ala		Ala			Ala	Ala	Pro			
618	Arg		Arg			Arg	Arg	Arg			
619	Gly		Gly			Gly	Gly	Gly			
620	Ala		Ala			Ile	Ala	Gly			
621	Hyp		Hyp			Hyp	Hyp	Hyp			
622	Gly		Gly			Gly	Gly	Gly			
623	Asp		Asp			Glu	Glu	Glu			
624	Arg		Arg			Arg	Arg	Arg			
625	Gly		Gly			Gly	Gly	Gly			
626	Glu		Glu			Glu	Glu	Glu			
627	Hyp		Hyp			Hyp	Thr	Gln			
628	Gly		Gly			Gly	Gly	Gly			
629	Pro		Pro			Pro	Pro	Pro			
630	Hyp		Hyp			Val	Hyp	Hyp			
631	Gly		Gly			Gly	Gly	Gly			
632	Pro		Pro			Pro	Pro	Pro			
633	Ala		Ala			Ser	Ala	Ala			
634	Gly		Gly			Gly	Gly	Gly			
635	Phe		Phe			Phe	Phe	Phe			
636	Ala		Ala	Ala		Ala	Ala	Hyp			
637	Gly		Gly	Gly		Gly	Gly	Gly			
638	Pro		Pro	Pro		Pro	Pro	Arg			
639	Hyp		Hyp	Ala		Hyp	Hyp	Hyp			
640	Gly		Gly	Gly		Gly	Gly	Gly			
641	Ala		Ala	Ala		Ala	Ala	Gln			
642	Asp		Asp	Ala		Ala	Asp	Asn			
643	Gly		Gly	Gly		Gly	Gly	Gly			
644	Gln		Gln	Gln		Glu	Gln	Glu			
645	Hyp		Hyp	Hyp		Hyp	Pro	Hyp			
646	Gly		Gly	Gly		Gly	Gly	Gly			
647	Ala		Ala	Ala		Ala	Ala	Ala			
648	Lys		Lys	Hyl		Lys	*Hyl*	Lys			
649	Gly		Gly	Gly		Gly	Gly	Gly			
650	Glu		Glu	Glu		Glu	Glu	Glu			
651	Hyp		Thr	Arg		Arg	Gln	Arg			
652	Gly		Gly	Gly		Gly	Gly	Gly			
653	Asp		Asp	Thr		Pro	Glu	Ala			
654	Ala		Ala	Lys		Lys	Ala	Hyp			
655	Gly		Gly	Gly		Gly	Gly	Gly			
656	Ala		Ala	Pro		Pro	Gln	Glu			
657	Lys		Lys	Val		Lys	*Hyl*	Lys			
658	Gly		Gly	Gly		Gly	Gly	Gly			
659	Asp		Asp	Glu		Glu	Asp	Glu			
660	Ala		Ala	Gln		Thr	Ala	Gly			

Table 3. The helical region of the collagen molecule—*(contd)*

Residue no.	a. Revealed by protein sequencing								b. Revealed by nucleotide sequencing		
	α1(I) chain			α2(I) chain			α1(II) chain	α1(III) chain	α1(I) chain	α2(I) chain	
	Bovine	*Rat*	*Chick*	*Bovine*	*Rat*	*Chick*	*Bovine*	*Bovine*	*Chick*	*Bovine*	*Chick*
661	Gly		Gly	Gly		Gly	Gly	Gly			
662	Pro		Pro	Pro		Pro	Ala	Pro			
663	Hyp		Hyp	Val		Thr		Hyp			
664	Gly		Gly	Gly		Gly		Gly			
665	Pro		Pro	Pro		Ala		Ala			
666	Ala		Ala	Gln		Ile		Ala			
667	Gly		Gly	Gly		Gly		Gly			
668	Pro		Pro	Pro		Pro		Pro			
669	Ala		Thr	Val		Ile		Ala			
670	Gly		Gly	Gly		Gly		Gly			
671	Pro		Ala	Ala		Ala		Gly			
672	Hyp		Hyp	Ala		Ser		Ser			
673	Gly		Gly	Gly		Gly		Gly			
674	Pro		Pro	Pro		Pro		Pro			
675	Ile		Ala	Hyp		Hyp		Ala			
676	Gly		Gly			Gly		Gly			
677	Asn		Glx			Pro		Pro			
678	Val		Val			Val		Hyp			
679	Gly		Gly			Gly		Gly			
680	Ala		Ala			Ala		Pro			
681	Hyp		Hyp			Ala		Gln			
682	Gly		Gly			Gly		Gly			
683	Pro		Pro			Pro		Val			
684	Hyl		Hyl			Ala		Lys			
685	Gly		Gly			Gly		Gly			
686	Ala		Ala			Pro		Glu			
687	Arg		Arg			Arg		Arg			
688	Gly		Gly			Gly		Gly			
689	Ser		Ser			Asp		Ser			
690	Ala		Ala			Ala		Hyp			
691	Gly		Gly			Gly		Gly			
692	Pro		Pro			Pro		Gly			
693	Hyp		Hyp			Hyp		Hyp			
694	Gly		Gly			Gly		Gly			
695	Ala		Ala			Met		Ala			
696	Thr		Thr		Thr	Thr		Ala			
697	Gly		Gly		Gly	Gly		Gly			
698	Phe		Phe		Phe	Phe		Phe			
699	Hyp		Hyp		Hyp	Hyp		Hyp			
700	Gly		Gly		Gly	Gly		Gly			
701	Ala		Ala		Ala	Ala		Gly			
702	Ala		Ala		Ala	Ala		Arg			
703	Gly		Gly		Gly	Gly		Gly			
704	Arg		Arg		Arg	Arg		Pro			
705	Val		Val		Thr	Val		Hyp			
706	Gly		Gly		Gly	Gly		Gly			
707	Pro		Pro		Pro	Thr		Pro			
708	Hyp		Hyp		Hyp	Hyp		Hyp			
709	Gly		Gly		Gly	Gly		Gly			
710	Pro		Pro		Pro	Pro		Ser			
711	Ser		Ser		Ser	Ala		Asn			
712	Gly		Gly		Gly	Gly		Gly			
713	Asn		Asn		Ile	Ile		Asn			
714	Ala		Ile		Thr	Thr		Hyp			
715	Gly		Gly		Gly	Gly		Gly			
716	Pro		Leu		Pro	Pro		Pro			
717	Hyp		Hyp		Hyp	Hyp		Hyp			
718	Gly		Gly		Gly	Gly		Gly			
719	Pro		Pro		Pro	Pro		Ser			
720	Hyp		Hyp		Hyp	Hyp		Ser			

Table 3. The helical region of the collagen molecule—*(contd)*

Residue no.	a. Revealed by protein sequencing								b. Revealed by nucleotide sequencing		
	α1(I) chain			α2(I) chain			α1(II) chain	α1(III) chain	α1(I) chain	α2(I) chain	
	Bovine	*Rat*	*Chick*	*Bovine*	*Rat*	*Chick*	*Bovine*	*Bovine*	*Chick*	*Bovine*	*Chick*
721	Gly		Gly		Gly	Gly		Gly			
722	Pro		Pro		Ala	Pro		Ala			
723	Ala		Ala		Ala	Ala		Hyp			
724	Gly		Gly		Gly	Gly		Gly			
725	Lys		Lys		Lys	Lys		Lys			
726	Glu		Glx		Glu	Asp		Asp			
727	Gly		Gly		Gly	Gly		Gly			
728	Ser		Ser		Ile	Pro		Pro			
729	Lys		Lys	Arg	Lys	Arg		Hyp			
730	Gly		Gly	Gly	Gly	Gly		Gly			
731	Pro		Pro	Pro	Pro	Leu		Pro			
732	Arg		Arg	Arg	Arg	Arg		Hyp			
733	Gly		Gly	Gly	Gly	Gly		Gly			
734	Glu		Glu	Asp	Asp	Asp		Ser			
735	Thr		Thr	Gln	Gln	Val		Asn			
736	Gly		Gly	Gly	Gly	Gly		Gly			
737	Pro		Pro	Pro	Pro	Pro		Ala			
738	Ala		Ala	Val	Val	Val		Hyp			
739	Gly		Gly	Gly	Gly	Gly		Gly			
740	Arg		Arg	Arg	Arg	Arg		Ser			
741	Hyp		Hyp	Ser		Thr		Hyp			
742	Gly		Gly	Gly		Gly		Gly			
743	Glu		Glu	Glu		Glu		Ile			
744	Val		Hyp	Thr		Gln		Ser			
745	Gly		Gly	Gly		Gly		Gly			
746	Pro		Pro	Ala		Ile		Pro			
747	Hyp		Ala	SerThr		Ala		Lys			
748	Gly		Gly	Gly		Gly		Gly			
749	Pro		Pro	Pro		Pro		Asp			
750	Hyp		Hyp	SerThr		Hyp		Ser			
751	Gly		Gly	Gly		Gly		Gly			
752	Pro		Pro	Phe		Phe		Pro			
753	Ala		Hyp	Val		Ala		Hyp			
754	Gly		Gly	Gly		Gly		Gly			
755	Glu		Glu	Glu		Glu		Glu			
756	Lys		Lys	Lys		Lys		Arg			
757	Gly		Gly	Gly		Gly		Gly			
758	Ala		Ser	Pro		Pro		Ala			
759	Hyp		Hyp	SerThr		Ser		Hyp			
760	Gly		Gly	Gly		Gly		Gly			
761	Ala		Ala	Glu		Glu		Pro			
762	Asp		Asp	Hyp		Ala		Gln			
763	Gly		Gly	Gly		Gly		Gly			
764	Pro		Pro	ThrSer		Ala		Pro			
765	Ala		Ile	Ala		Ala		Hyp			
766	Gly		Gly	Gly		Gly		Gly			
767	Ala		Ala	Pro		Pro		Ala			
768	Hyp		Hyp	Hyp		Hyp		Hyp			
769	Gly		Gly	Gly		Gly		Gly			
770	Thr		Thr	Pro		Thr		Pro			
771	Pro		Pro	Hyp		Hyp		Leu			
772	Gly		Gly	Gly		Gly		Gly			
773	Pro		Pro	Pro		Pro		Ile			
774	Gln		Gln	Gln		Gln		Ala			
775	Gly		Gly	Gly		Gly		Gly			
776	Ile		Ile	Leu		Ile		Leu			
777	Ala		Ala	Leu		Leu		Thr			
778	Gly		Gly	Gly		Gly		Gly			
779	Gln		Gln	Ala		Ala		Ala			
780	Arg		Arg	Hyp		Hyp		Arg			

Table 3. The helical region of the collagen molecule—*(contd)*

Residue no.	a. Revealed by protein sequencing								b. Revealed by nucleotide sequencing		
	α1(I) chain			α2(I) chain			α1(II) chain	α1(III) chain	α1(I) chain	α2(I) chain	
	Bovine	*Rat*	*Chick*	*Bovine*	*Rat*	*Chick*	*Bovine*	*Bovine*	*Chick*	*Bovine*	*Chick*
781	Gly		Gly	Gly		Gly		Gly			
782	Val		Val	Phe		Ile		Leu			
783	Val		Val	Leu		Leu		Ala			
784	Gly		Gly	Gly		Gly		Gly			
785	Leu		Leu	Leu		Leu		Pro			
786	Hyp		Hyp	Hyp		Hyp		Hyp			
787	Gly		Gly	Gly		Gly		Gly			
788	Gln		Gln	Ser		Ser		Met			
789	Arg		Arg	Arg		Arg		Hyp			
790	Gly		Gly	Gly		Gly		Gly			
791	Glu		Glu	Glu		Glu		Ala			
792	Arg		Arg	Arg		Arg		Arg			
793	Gly		Gly	Gly		Gly		Gly			
794	Phe		Phe	Leu		Leu		Ser			
795	Hyp		Hyp	Hyp		Hyp		Hyp			
796	Gly		Gly	Gly		Gly		Gly			
797	Leu		Leu	Val		Ile		Pro			
798	Hyp		Hyp	Ala		Ala		Gln			
799	Gly		Gly	Gly		Gly		Gly			
800	Pro		Pro	Ser		Ala		Ile			
801	Ser		Ser	Val		Thr		Lys			
802	Gly		Gly	Gly		Gly		Gly			
803	Glu		Glu	Glu		Glu		Glu			
804	Hyp		Hyp	Hyp		Hyp		Asn			
805	Gly		Gly	Gly		Gly		Gly			
806	Lys		Lys	Pro		Pro		Lys			
807	Gln		Gln	Leu		Leu		Hyp			
808	Gly		Gly	Gly				Gly			
809	Pro		Pro	Ile				Pro			
810	Ser		Ser	Ala				Ser			
811	Gly		Gly	Gly				Gly			
812	Ala		Ala	Pro				Gln			
813	Ser		Ser	Hyp				Asn			
814	Gly		Gly	Gly				Gly	Gly		
815	Glu		Glu	Ala				Glu	Glu		
816	Arg		Arg	Arg				Arg	Arg		
817	Gly		Gly	Gly				Gly	Gly		
818	Pro		Pro	Pro				Pro	Pro		
819	Hyp		Hyp	Hyp				Hyp	Pro		
820	Gly		Gly	Gly				Gly	Gly		
821	Pro		Pro	Asn				Pro	Pro		
822	Met		Met	Val				Gln	Met		
823	Gly		Gly	Gly				Gly	Gly		
824	Pro		Pro	Asn				Leu	Pro		
825	Hyp		Hyp	Hyp				Hyp	Pro		
826	Gly		Gly	Gly				Gly	Gly		
827	Leu		Leu	Val				Leu	Leu		
828	Ala		Ala	Asn				Ala	Ala		
829	Gly		Gly	Gly				Gly	Gly		
830	Pro		Pro	Ala				Thr	Pro		
831	Hyp		Hyp	Hyp				Ala	Pro		
832	Gly		Gly	Gly				Gly	Gly		
833	Glu		Glu	Glu				Glu	Glu		
834	Ser		Ala	Ala				Hyp	Ala		
835	Gly		Gly	Gly				Gly	Gly		
836	Arg		Arg	Arg				Arg	Arg		
837	Glu		Glu	Asp				Asp	Glu		
838	Gly		Gly	Gly				Gly	Gly		Gly
839	Ala		Ala	Asn				Asn	Ala		Asn
840	Hyp		Hyp	Hyp				Hyp	Pro		Pro

Table 3. The helical region of the collagen molecule—*(contd)*

Residue no.	a. Revealed by protein sequencing								b. Revealed by nucleotide sequencing		
	α1(I) chain			α2(I) chain			α1(II) chain	α1(III) chain	α1(I) chain	α2(I) chain	
	Bovine	*Rat*	*Chick*	*Bovine*	*Rat*	*Chick*	*Bovine*	*Bovine*	*Chick*	*Bovine*	*Chick*
841	Gly		Gly	Gly				Gly	Gly		Gly
842	Ala		Ala	Asn				Ser	Ala		Asn
843	Glu		Glu	Asp				Asp	Glu		Asp
844	Gly		Gly	Gly				Gly	Gly		Gly
845	Ser		Ala	Pro				Leu	Ala		Pro
846	Hyp		Hyp	Hyp				Hyp	Pro		Pro
847	Gly		Gly	Gly				Gly	Gly		Gly
848	Arg		Arg	Arg				Arg	Arg		Arg
849	Asp		Asp	Asp				Asp	Asp		Asp
850	Gly		Gly	Gly				Gly	Gly		Gly
851	Ser		Ala	Gln				Ala	Ala		Ala
852	Hyp		Ala	Hyp				Hyp	Ala		Pro
853	Gly		Gly	Gly				Gly	Gly		Gly
854	Ala		Pro	His				Ala	Pro		Phe
855	Lys		Lys	Lys				Lys	Lys		Lys
856	Gly		Gly	Gly				Gly	Gly		Gly
857	Asp		Asp	Glu				Asp	Asp		Glu
858	Arg		Arg	Arg				Arg	Arg		Arg
859	Gly		Gly	Gly				Gly	Gly		Gly
860	Glu		Glu	Thr				Glu	Glu		Ala
861	Thr		Thr	Hyp				Asn	Thr		Pro
862	Gly		Gly	Gly				Gly	Gly		Gly
863	Pro		Pro	Asn				Ser	Pro		Asn
864	Ala		Ala	Ala				Hyp	Ala		Pro
865	Gly		Gly	Gly				Gly	Gly		Gly
866	Pro		Pro	*Pro*				Ala	Pro		Pro
867	Hyp		Hyp	*Hyp*				Hyp	Pro		
868	Gly		Gly	*Gly*				Gly	Gly		
869	Ala		Ala	*Ala*				Ala	Ala		
870	Hyp		Hyp	*Hyp*				Hyp	Pro		
871	Gly		Gly	*Gly*				Gly	Gly		
872	Ala		Ala	*Ala*				His	Ala		
873	Hyp		Hyp	*Val*				Hyp	Pro		
874	Gly		Gly	*Gly*				Gly	Gly		
875	Ala		Ala	*Pro*				Pro	Ala		
876	Hyp		Pro	*Val*				Hyp	Pro		
877	Gly		Gly	*Gly*				Gly	Gly		
878	Pro		Pro	*Pro*				Pro	Pro		
879	Val		Val	*Val*				Val	Val		
880	Gly		Gly	*Gly*				Gly	Gly		Gly
881	Pro		Pro	*Glu*				Pro	Pro		Pro
882	Ala		Ala	*Pro*				Ala	Ala		Ser
883	Gly		Gly	*Gly*				Gly	Gly		Gly
884	Lys		Lys	Lys				Lys	Lys		Lys
885	Ser		Asn	Leu				Ser	Asn		Pro
886	Gly		Gly	Gly				Gly	Gly		Gly
887	Asp		Asp	Asn				Asp	Asp		Asn
888	Arg		Arg	Arg				Arg	Arg		Arg
889	Gly		Gly	Gly				Gly	Gly		Gly
890	Glu		Glu	Glu				Glu	Glu		Asn
891	Thr		Thr	Hyp				Thr	Thr		Pro
892	Gly		Gly	Gly				Gly	Gly		Gly
893	Pro		Pro	Pro				Pro	Pro		Pro
894	Ala		Ala	Ala				Ala	Ala		Val
895	Gly		Gly	Gly				Gly	Gly		Gly
896	Pro		Pro	Ala				Pro	Pro		Pro
897	Ile		Ala	Val				Ser	Ala		Val
898	Gly		Gly	Gly				Gly	Gly		Gly
899	Pro		Pro	Pro				Ala	Pro		Pro
900	Val		Hyp	Ala				Hyp	Pro		Ala

Table 3. The helical region of the collagen molecule—*(contd)*

Residue no.	a. Revealed by protein sequencing								b. Revealed by nucleotide sequencing		
	α1(I) chain			α2(I) chain			α1(II) chain	α1(III) chain	α1(I) chain	α2(I) chain	
	Bovine	*Rat*	*Chick*	*Bovine*	*Rat*	*Chick*	*Bovine*	*Bovine*	*Chick*	*Bovine*	*Chick*
901	Gly		Gly	Gly				Gly	Gly		Gly
902	Pro		Pro	Ala				Pro	Pro		Ala
903	Ala		Ala	Val				Ala	Ala		Phe
904	Gly		Gly	Gly				Gly	Gly		Gly
905	Ala		Ala	Pro				Ser	Ala		Pro
906	Arg		Arg	Arg				Arg	Arg		Arg
907	Gly		Gly	Gly				Gly	Gly		Gly
908	Pro		Pro	Pro				Pro	Pro		Leu
909	Ala		Ala	Ser				Hyp	Ala		Ala
910	Gly		Gly	Gly				Gly	Gly		Gly
911	Pro		Pro	Pro				Pro	Pro		Pro
912	Gln		Gln	Gln				Gln	Gln		Gln
913	Gly		Gly	Gly				Gly	Gly		Gly
914	Pro		Pro	Ile				Pro	Pro		Pro
915	Arg		Arg	Arg				Arg	Arg		Arg
916	Gly		Gly	Gly				Gly	Gly		Gly
917	Asx		Asp	Asp				Asp	Asp		Glu
918	Hyl		Hyl	Asp				Hyl	Lys		Lys
919	Gly		Gly	Gly				Gly	Gly		Gly
920	Glx		Glu	Glu				Glu	Glu		Glu
921	Thr		Thr	Hyp				Thr	Thr		His
922	Gly		Gly	Gly				Gly	Gly		Gly
923	Glx		Glu	Asp				Glu	Glu		Asp
924	Glx		Gln	Lys				Arg	Gln		Lys
925	Gly		Gly	*Gly*				Gly	Gly		Gly
926	Asp		Asp	*Asp*				Ala	Asp		His
927	Arg		Arg	*Val*				Met	Arg		Arg
928	Gly		Gly	*Gly*				Gly	Gly		Gly
929	Ile		Met	*Leu*				Ile	Met		Leu
930	Hyl		Hyl	*Hyl*				Hyl	Lys		Pro
931	Gly		Gly	Gly				Gly	Gly		Gly
932	His		His	Asp				His	His		Leu
933	Arg		Arg	Arg				Arg	Arg		Lys
934	Gly		Gly	Gly				Gly	Gly		Gly
935	Phe		Phe	His				Phe	Phe		His
936	Ser		Ser	Asn				Hyp	Ser		Asn
937	Gly		Gly	Gly				Gly	Gly		Gly
938	Leu		Leu	Leu				Asn	Leu		Leu
939	Gln		Gln	Gln				Hyp	Gln		Gln
940	Gly		Gly	Gly				Gly	Gly		Gly
941	Pro		Pro	Leu				Ala	Pro		Leu
942	Hyp		Hyp	Hyp				Hyp	Pro		Pro
943	Gly		Gly	Gly				Gly	Gly		Gly
944	Pro		Pro	Leu				Ser	Pro		Leu
945	Hyp		Hyp	Ala				Hyp	Pro		Ala
946	Gly		Gly	Gly				Gly	Gly		Gly
947	Ser		Ala	His				Pro	Ala		Gln
948	Hyp		Hyp	His				Ala	Pro		His
949	Gly		Gly	Gly				Gly	Gly		Gly
950	Glu		Glu	Asp				His	Glu		Asp
951	Gln		Gln	Gln				Gln	Gln		Gln
952	Gly		Gly	Gly				Gly	Gly		Gly
953	Pro		Pro	Ala				Ala	Pro		Pro
954	Ser		Ser	Hyp				Val	Ser		Pro
955	Gly		Gly	Gly				Gly	Gly		Gly
956	Ala		Ala	Ala				Ser	Ala		Asn
957	Ser		Ser	Val				Hyp	Ser		Asn
958	Gly		Gly	Gly				Gly	Gly		Gly
959	Pro		Pro	Pro				Pro	Pro		Pro
960	Ala		Ala	Ala				Ala	Ala		Ala

Table 3. The helical region of the collagen molecule—*(contd)*

Residue no.	**a. Revealed by protein sequencing**								**b. Revealed by nucleotide sequencing**		
	α1(I) chain			α2(I) chain			α1(II) chain	α1(III) chain	α1(I) chain	α2(I) chain	
	Bovine	*Rat*	*Chick*	*Bovine*	*Rat*	*Chick*	*Bovine*	*Bovine*	*Chick*	*Bovine*	*Chick*
961	Gly		Gly	Gly				Gly	Gly		Gly
962	Pro		Pro	Pro				Pro	Pro		Pro
963	Arg		Arg	Arg				Arg	Arg		Arg
964	Gly		Gly	Gly				Gly	Gly		Gly
965	Pro		Pro	Pro				Pro	Pro		Pro
966	Hyp		Hyp	Ala				Val	Pro		His
967	Gly		Gly	Gly				Gly	Gly		Gly
968	Ser		Ser	Pro				Pro	Ser		Pro
969	Ala		Ala	Ser				Ser	Ala		Ser
970	Gly		Gly	Gly				Gly	Gly		Gly
971	Ser		Ala	Pro				Pro	Ala		Pro
972	Hyp		Ala	Ala				Pro	Ala		His
973	Gly		Gly	Gly				Gly	Gly		Gly
974	Lys		Lys	Lys				Lys	Lys		Lys
975	Asp		Asp	Ile				Asp	Asp		Asp
976	Gly		Gly	Gly				Gly	Gly		Gly
977	Leu		Leu	Glu				Ala	Leu		Arg
978	Asn		Asn	Hyp				Ser	Asn		Asn
979	Gly		Gly	Gly				Gly	Gly		Gly
980	Leu		Leu	Ala				His	Leu		Leu
981	Hyp		Hyp	Val				Hyp	Pro		Pro
982	Gly		Gly	Gly				Gly	Gly		Gly
983	Pro		Pro	Pro				Pro	Pro		Pro
984	Ile		Ile	Ala				Ile	Ile		Ile
985	Gly		Gly	Gly				Gly	Gly		Gly
986	Hyp		Hyp	*Ala*				Pro	Pro		Pro
987	Hyp		Hyp	*Hyp*				Hyp	Pro		Ala
988	Gly		Gly	*Gly*				Gly	Gly		Gly
989	Pro		Pro	*Ile*				Pro	Pro		Val
990	Arg		Arg	Asp				Arg	Arg		Arg
991	Gly		Gly	Gly				Gly	Gly		Gly
992	Arg		Arg	Ser				Asn	Arg		Ser
993	Thr		Thr	Gln				Arg	Thr		His
994	Gly		Gly	Gly				Gly	Gly		Gly
995	Asp		Glu	Ser				Glu	Glu		Ser
996	Ala		Val	Gln				Arg	Val		Gln
997	Gly		Gly	Gly				Gly	Gly		Gly
998	Pro		Pro	Pro				Ser	Pro		Pro
999	Ala		Val	Ala				Glu	Val		Ala
1000	Gly		Gly	Gly				Gly	Gly		Gly
1001	Pro		Pro	Pro				Ser	Pro		Pro
1002	Hyp		Hyp	Hyp				Hyp	Pro		Pro
1003	Gly		Gly	Gly				Gly	Gly		Gly
1004	Pro		Pro	Pro				His	Pro		Pro
1005	Hyp		Hyp	Hyp				Hyp	Pro		Pro
1006	Gly		Gly	Gly				Gly	Gly		Gly
1007	Pro		Pro	Pro				Gln	Pro		Pro
1008	Hyp		Hyp	Hyp				Hyp	Pro		Pro
1009	Gly		Gly	Gly				Gly	Gly		Gly
1010	Pro		Pro	Pro				Pro	Pro		Pro
1011	Hyp		Hyp	Hyp				Hyp	Pro		Pro
1012	Gly		Gly	Gly				Gly	Gly		Gly
1013	Pro		Pro	Pro				Pro	Pro		Pro
1014	Pro		Pro	Pro				Hyp	Pro		Asn
1015								Gly			
1016								Ala			
1017								Hyp			
1018								Gly			
1019								Pro			
1020								Cys			

Table 4. The C-terminal non-helical region of the collagen molecule

Residue no.	a. Revealed by protein sequencing								b. Revealed by nucleotide sequencing		
	$\alpha 1$(I) chain			$\alpha 2$(I) chain			$\alpha 1$(II) chain	$\alpha 1$(III) chain	$\alpha 1$(I) chain	$\alpha 2$(I) chain	
	Bovine	*Rat*	*Chick*	*Bovine*	*Rat*	*Chick*	*Bovine*	*Bovine*	*Chick*	*Bovine*	*Chick*
1	Ser		Ser	Ser				Cys	Ser		Gly
2	Gly		Gly	Gly				Gly	Gly		Gly
3	Gly		Gly	Gly				Ala	Gly		Gly
4	Tyr		Phe	Tyr				Gly	Phe		Tyr
5	Asp		Asp	Glu				Gly	Asp		Glu
6	Leu		Leu	Phe				Val	Phe		Val
7	Ser			*				Ala	Ser		Gly
8	Phe							Ala	Phe		Phe
9	Leu							Ile	Leu		Asp
10	Pro							Ala	Pro		Ala
11	Gln							Gly	Gln		Glu
12	Pro							Val	Pro		Tyr
13	Pro							Gly	Pro		Tyr
14	Gln							Ala	Gln		Arg
15	Gln							Glu	Glu		Ala
16	Glx								Lys		
17	Lys								Ala		
18	Ala								His		
19	His								Asp		
20	Asp							Lys	Gly		
21	Gly							Gly	Gly		
22	Gly							Asp	Arg		
23	Arg							Gly	Tyr		
24	Tyr							Phe	Tyr		
25	Tyr							Ala	Arg		
26								Pro	Ala		
27								Tyr			
28								Arg			
								*			

* This region has not yet been sequenced, so the length of the chain is still unknown.

Table 5. The C-terminal procollagen peptides

Residue no.	b. Revealed by nucleotide sequencing		
	$\alpha 1$(I) chain	$\alpha 2$(I) chain	
	Chick	*Bovine*	*Chick*
1	Asp		Asp
2	Asp		Gln
3	Ala		Pro
4	Asn		Ser
5	Val		Leu
6	Met		Arg
7	Arg		Pro
8	Asp		Lys
9	Arg		Asp
10	Asp		Tyr
11	Leu		Glu
12	Glu		Val
13	Val		Asp
14	Asp		Ala
15	Thr		Thr
16	Thr		Leu
17	Leu		Lys
18	Lys		Thr
19	Ser		Leu
20	Leu		Asn
21	Ser		Asn

Table 5. The C-terminal procollagen peptides—*(contd)*

Residue no.	**b. Revealed by nucleotide sequencing**		
	α1(I) chain	α2(I) chain	
	Chick	*Bovine*	*Chick*
22	Gln		Gln
23	Gln		Ile
24	Ile		Glu
25	Glu		Thr
26	Asn		Leu
27	Ile		Leu
28	Arg		Thr
29	Ser		Pro
30	Pro		Glu
31	Glu		Gly
32	Gly		Ser
33	Thr		Lys
34	Arg		Lys
35	Lys		Asn
36	Asn		Pro
37	Pro		Ala
38	Ala		Arg
39	Arg		Thr
40	Thr		Cys
41	Cys		Arg
42	Arg		Asp
43	Asp		Leu
44	Leu		Arg
45	Lys		Leu
46	Met		Ser
47	Cys		His
48	His		Pro
49	Gly		Glu
50	Asp		Trp
51	Trp		Ser
52	Lys		Ser
53	Ser		Gly
54	Gly		Phe
55	Glu		Ser
56	Tyr		Trp
57	Trp		Ile
58	Ile		Ala
59	Asp		Pro
60	Pro		Asn
61	Asn		His
62	Gln		Gly
63	Gly		Cys
64	Cys		Thr
65	Asn		Ala
66	Leu		Asp
67	Asp		Ala
68	Ala		Ile
69	Ile		Arg
70	Lys		Ala
71	Val		Tyr
72	Tyr		Cys
73	Cys		Asp
74	Asn		Phe
75	Met		Ala
76	Glu		Thr
77	Thr		Gly
78	Gly		Glu
79	Glu		Thr
80	Thr		Cys
81	Cys		Ile

Table 5. The C-terminal procollagen peptides—*(contd)*

Residue no.	b. Revealed by nucleotide sequencing		
	α1(I) chain	α2(I) chain	
	Chick	*Bovine*	*Chick*
82	Val		His
83	Tyr		Ala
84	Pro		Ser
85	Thr		Leu
86	Gln		Glu
87	Ala		Asp
88	Thr		Ile
89	Ile		Pro
90	Ala		Thr
91	Gln		Lys
92	Lys		Thr
93	Asn		Trp
94	Trp		Tyr
95	Tyr		Val
96	Leu		Asp
97	Ser		Lys
98	Lys		Asn
99	Asn		Pro
100	Pro		Lys
101	Lys		Asp
102	Glu		Lys
103	Lys		Lys
104	Lys		His
105	His		Ile
106	Val		Trp
107	Trp		Phe
108	Phe		Gly
109	Gly		Glu
110	Glu		Thr
111	Thr		Ile
112	Met		Asn
113	Ser		Gly
114	Asp		Gly
115	Gly		Thr
116	Phe		Gln
117	Gln		Phe
118	Phe		Glu
119	Val		Tyr
120	Tyr		Asn
121	Gly		Gly
122	Gly		Glu
123	Glu		Gly
124	Gly		Val
125	Cys		Thr
126	Asn		Thr
127	Pro		Lys
128	Val		Asp
129	Val		Met
130	Val		Ala
131	Ala		Thr
132	Ile		Gln
133	Gln		Leu
134	Leu		Ala
135	Thr		Phe
136	Phe		Met
137	Leu		Arg
138	Arg		Leu
139	Leu		Leu
140	Met		Ala
141	Ser		Asn

Table 5. The C-terminal procollagen peptides—*(contd)*

Residue no.	b. Revealed by nucleotide sequencing		
	α1(I) chain	α2(I) chain	
	Chick	*Bovine*	*Chick*
142	Thr		His
143	Glu		Ala
144	Ala		Ser
145	Thr		Gln
146	Gln		Asn
147	Asn		Ile
148	Val		Thr
149	Thr		Thr
150	Tyr		His
151	His		Cys
152	Cys		Lys
153	Lys		Asn
154	Asn		Ser
155	Ser		Ile
156	Val		Ala
157	Ala		Tyr
158	Tyr		Met
159	Met		Asp
160	Asp		Glu
161	His		Glu
162	Asp		Thr
163	Thr		Gly
164	Gly		Asn
165	Asn		Leu
166	Leu		Lys
167	Lys		Lys
168	Lys		Ala
169	Ala		Val
170	Leu		Ile
171	Leu		Leu
172	Leu		Gln
173	Gln		Gly
174	Gly		Ser
175	Ala		Asn
176	Asn		Asp
177	Glu		Val
178	Ile		Glu
179	Glu		Leu
180	Ile		Arg
181	Arg		Ala
182	Ala		Glu
183	Glu		Gly
184	Gly		Asn
185	Asn		Ser
186	Ser		Arg
187	Arg		Phe
188	Phe		Thr
189	Thr		Phe
190	Tyr		Ser
191	Gly		Val
192	Val		Leu
193	Thr		Val
194	Glu		Asp
195	Asp		Gly
196	Gly		Cys
197	Cys		Ser
198	Thr		Lys
199	Ser		Lys
200	His		Asn
201	Thr		Asn

Table 5. The C-terminal procollagen peptides—*(contd)*

Residue no.	**b. Revealed by nucleotide sequencing**		
	α1(I) chain	α2(I) chain	
	Chick	*Bovine*	*Chick*
202	Gly		Lys
203	Ala		Thr
204	Trp		Gly
205	Gly		Lys
206	Lys		Thr
207	Thr		Ile
208	Val		Ile
209	Ile		Glu
210	Glu		Tyr
211	Tyr		Arg
212	Lys		Thr
213	Thr		Asn
214	Thr		Lys
215	Lys		Pro
216	Thr		Ser
217	Ser		Arg
218	Arg		Leu
219	Leu		Pro
220	Pro		Ile
221	Ile		Leu
222	Ile		Asp
223	Asp		Ile
224	Leu		Ala
225	Ala		Pro
226	Pro		Leu
227	Met		Asp
228	Asp		Ile
229	Val		Gly
230	Gly		Gly
231	Ala		Ala
232	Pro		Asp
233	Asp		Gln
234	His		Glu
235	Glu		Phe
236	Phe		Gly
237	Gly		Leu
238	Ile		His
239	Asp		Ile
240	Ile		Gly
241	Gly		Pro
242	Pro		Val
243	Val		Cys
244	Cys		Phe
245	Phe		Lys
246	Leu		

REFERENCES FOR PEPTIDE SEQUENCING

In the following references, all residue numbers with prefix pN or pC refer to N-terminal and C-terminal procollagen peptides. Numbers with superscript ^{N} or ^{C} refer to the non-helical regions at each end of the collagen molecule. Other numbers refer to the helical region of the collagen molecule. Thus 1^N–3 means all residues from number 1 of the N-terminal non-helical region to number 3 of the helical region inclusive. For the helical region only, the peptides are identified in the first column in the standard way eg α1–CB2,4,5 means the cyanogen bromide peptides numbered 2, 4 and 5 of the α1 chain. α1–CB6A means the first part of peptide number 6.

Peptides	*Residues*	*References*
α1(I) Chain, Bovine		
	pN1–pN139	Hörlein D, Fietzek P P, Wachter E, Lapière C M, Kühn K 1979 Eur. J. Biochem. 99: 31-8
α1–CB0,1	1^N–3	Rauterberg J, Timpl R, Furthmayr H 1972 Eur. J. Biochem. 27: 231-7
α1–CB2,4,5	4–123	Fietzek P P, Kühn K 1975 Eur. J. Biochem. 52: 77-82
α1–CB8	124–402	Glanville R W, Breitkreutz D, Meitinger M, Fietzek P P (in preparation)
α1–CB3	403–551	Fietzek P P, Wendt P, Kell I, Kühn K 1972 FEBS Letters 26: 74-6
α1–CB7	613–618*	Kleinman H K, McGoodwin E B, Martin G R, Klebe R J, Fietzek P P, Woolley D E 1978 J. Biol. Chem. 253: 5642-6
	552–822	Fietzek P P, Rexrodt F W, Hopper K E, Kühn K 1973 Eur. J. Biochem. 38: 396-400
α1–CB6A	823–935	Wendt P, von der Mark K, Rexrodt F W, Kühn K 1972 Eur. J. Biochem. 30: 169-83
α1–CB6B	936–1014, 1^C–4^C	Fietzek P P, Rexrodt F W, Wendt P, Stark M, Kühn K 1972 Eur. J. Biochem. 30: 163-8
	5^C–25^C	Rauterberg J, Fietzek P P, Rexrodt F W, Becker U, Stark M, Kühn K 1972 FEBS Letters 21: 75-9

* As a result of three additional amino acids being found in this region, the numbering of all subsequent amino acids in the chain has been altered.

Peptides	*Residues*	*References*
α1(I) Chain, Rat		
α1–CB0	1^N–4^N	Reported in Piez K A 1976 In: Ramachandran G N, Reddie A H (eds) Biochemistry of Collagen. Plenum Press
α1–CB1	5^N–3	Kang A H, Bornstein P, Piez K A 1967 Biochemistry 6: 788-95
α1–CB2	4–39	Bornstein P 1967 Biochemistry 6: 3082-93
α1–CB4	40–86	Butler W T, Ponds S L 1971 Biochemistry 10: 2076-81
α1–CB5	87–123	Butler W T 1970 Biochemistry 9: 44-50
α1–CB8A	124–222	Balian G, Click E M, Bornstein P 1971 Biochemistry 10: 4470-8
α1–CB8B	223–402	Balian G, Click E M, Hermodson M A, Bornstein P 1972 Biochemistry 11: 3798-806
α1–CB3	403–551	Butler W T, Underwood S P, Finch J E Jr 1974 Biochemistry 13: 2946-53
α1–CB7	552–822	Sequence not available
α1–CB6	823–1014	Sequence not available

Peptides	*Residues*	*References*
α1(I) Chain, Chick		
	pN (incomplete)	Pesciotta D M, Silkowitz M H, Fietzek P P, Graves P N, Berg R A, Olsen B R 1980 Biochemistry 19: 2447-54
α1–CB0,1,2	1^N–39	Kang A H, Gross J 1970 Biochemistry 9: 796-804
α1–CB4,5	40–123	Kang A H, Dixit S N, Corbett C, Gross J 1975 J. Biol. Chem. 250: 7428-34
α1–CB8	124–402	Sequence not available
α1–CB3	403–551	Dixit S N, Kang A H, Gross J 1975 Biochemistry 14: 1929-33
α1–CB7	607–617*	Highberger J H, Corbett C, Kang A H, Gross J 1978 Biochem. Biophys. Res. Commun. 83: 43-9
	552–822	Highberger J H, Corbett C, Kang A H, Gross J 1975 Biochemistry 14: 2872-81
α1–CB6A	823–929	Dixit S N, Seyer J M, Oronsky A O, Corbett C, Kang A H, Gross J 1975 Biochemistry 14: 1933-8
α1–CB6B	930–6^C	Dixit S N, Seyer J M, Kang A H, Gross J 1978 Biochemistry 17: 5719–22

* See note under α1(I) Chain, Bovine.

References for peptide sequencing—*(contd)*

Peptides	*Residues*	*References*
α2(I) Chain, Bovine		
α2–CB1,0	1^N–6	Fietzek P P, Breitkreutz D, Kühn K 1974 Biochem. Biophys. Acta. 365: 305-10
α2–CB4A	7–48	Fietzek P P, Kell I, Kühn K 1972 FEBS Letters 26: 66-8
α2–CB4B	49–327	Fietzek P P, Rexrodt F W 1975 Eur. J. Biochem. 59: 113-8
α2–CB2	328–357	Fietzek P P, Furthmayr H, Kühn K 1974 Eur. J. Biochem. 47: 257–61
α2–CB3A	358–393	Fietzek P P, Kühn K 1974 Hoppe-Seyler's Z. Physiol. Chem. 355: 647–50
α2–CB3B,5	394–1014 (incomplete)	Reported in Bornstein P, Traub W 1979 In: Neurath H, Hill R L (eds) The Proteins 4: 411-631 Academic Press, New York
	1^C–6^C	Fietzek P P, Kühn K 1976 Int. Rev. Connect. Tissue Res. 7: 1-60
α2(I) Chain, Rat		
α2–CB1	1^N–3	Kang A H, Bornstein P, Piez K A 1967 Biochemistry 6: 788-95
α2–CB0	4–6	Reported in Bornstein P, Traub W 1979 In: Neurath H, Hill R L (eds) The Proteins 4: 411-631. Academic Press, New York
α2–CB4A	7–48	Fietzek P P, Kell I, Kühn K 1972 FEBS Letters 26: 66-8
α2–CB4B	49–327	Sequence not available
α2–CB2	328–357	Highberger J H, Kang A H, Gross J 1971 Biochemistry 10: 610-6
α2–CB3A	358–405	Fietzek P P, Kühn K 1974 Hoppe-Seyler's Z. Physiol. Chem. 355: 647-50
α2–CB3B	406–695	Sequence not available
α2–CB5A	696–740	Fietzek P P, Kühn K 1973 FEBS Letters 36: 289-91
α2–CB5B	741–1014	Sequence not available
α2(I) Chain, Chick		
α2–CB1	1^N–3	Kang A H, Gross J 1970 Biochemistry 9: 796-804
α2–CB0	4–6	Sequence not available
α2–CB4	7–327	Sequence not available
α2–CB2	328–357	Highberger J H, Kang A H, Gross J 1971 Biochemistry 10: 610-6
α2–CB3A	358–489	Dixit S N, Seyer J M, Kang A H 1977 Eur. J. Biochem. 73: 213-21
α2–CB3B	490–695	Dixit S N, Seyer J M, Kang A H 1977 Eur. J. Biochem. 81: 599-607
α2–CB5A	696–807	Dixit S N, Mainardi C L, Seyer J M, Kang A H 1979 Biochemistry 18: 5416-22
α2–CB5B	808–1014	Sequence not available
α1(II) Chain, Bovine		
α1(II)–CB2,3, 6,12,11A	1–162	Butler W T, Miller E J, Finch J E Jr 1976 Biochemistry 15: 3000–6
	163–179 181–183 193–254	Reported in Bornstein P, Traub W 1979 In: Neurath H, Hill R L (eds) The Proteins 4: 411-631. Academic Press, New York
	255–402	Sequence not available
α1(II)–CB8A	403–477	Butler W T, Miller E J, Finch J E Jr, Inagami T 1974 Biochem. Biophys. Res. Commun. 57: 190-5
	478–551	Reported in Bornstein P, Traub W 1979 In: Neurath H, Hill R L (eds) The Proteins 4: 411-631. Academic Press, New York
α1(II)–CB10A	552–662	Francis G, Butler W T, Finch J E Jr 1978 Biochem. J. 175: 921-30
	663–end	Sequence not available
α1(III) Chain, Bovine		
	pN1–pN130	Brandt A, Hörlein D, Bruckner P, Timpl R, Fietzek P P, Glanville R W (preliminary data)
	1^N–20^N	Glanville R W, Fietzek P P 1976 FEBS Letters 71: 99-102
α1(III)–CB3, 7,6	1–222	Fietzek P P, Allmann H, Rauterberg J, Henkel W, Wachter E, Kühn K 1979 Hoppe-Seyler's Z. Physiol. Chem. 360: 809-20

References for peptide seqencing—*(contd)*

Peptides	*Residues*	*References*
α1(III)-CB1, 8,10,2	223–402	Dewes H, Fietzek P P, Kühn K 1979 Hoppe-Seyler's Z. Physiol. Chem. 360: 821-32
α1(III)-CB4	403–551	Bentz H, Fietzek P P, Kühn K 1979 Hoppe-Seyler's Z. Physiol. Chem. 360: 833-40
α1(III)-CB5	552–788	Lang H, Glanville R W, Fietzek P P, Kühn K 1979 Hoppe-Seyler's Z. Physiol. Chem. 360: 841-50
α1(III)-CB9A	789–927	Dewes H, Fietzek P P, Kühn K 1979 Hoppe-Seyler's Z. Physiol. Chem. 360: 851-60
α1(III)-CB9B	928–1020	Allmann H, Fietzek P P, Glanville R W, Kühn K 1979 Hoppe-Seyler's Z. Physiol. Chem. 360: 861-8
	1^C–28^C	Glanville R W, Allmann H, Fietzek P P 1976 Hoppe-Seyler's Z. Physiol. Chem. 357: 1663-5 Fietzek P P, Allmann H, Bentz H, Dewes H, Glanville R W, Henkel W, Lang H, Rauterberg J, Wachter E, Kühn K (unpublished data)

REFERENCES FOR NUCLEOTIDE SEQUENCING

Residues	*References*
α1(I) Chain, Chick	
814–1014 1^C–26^C pC1–pC103	Fuller F, Boedtker H 1981 Biochemistry 20: 999-1006
pC104–pC246	Showalter A M, Pesciotta D M, Eikenberry E F, Yamamoto T, Pastan I, de Crombrugghe B, Fietzek P P, Olsen B R 1980 FEBS Letters 111: 61-5
α2(I) Chain, Bovine	
1–72 175–327	Wozney J, Boedtker H (in preparation) Wozney J, Hanahan D, Tate V, Boedtker, Doty P 1981 Nature 294: 129-35
α2(I) Chain, Chick	
1^N–16^N 1–36 175–360	Wozney J, Boedtker H (in preparation) Wozney J, Hanahan D, Tate V, Boedtker H, Doty P 1981 Nature 294: 129-35
37–72 379–429 838–866 880–909	Yamada, Y, Avvedimento V E, Mudryj M, Ohkubo H, Vogeli G, Irani M, Pastan I, de Crombrugghe B 1980 Cell. 22: 887-92
910–1014 1^C–15^C pC1–pC245	Dickson L A, Ninomiya Y, Bernard M P. Pesciotta D M, Parsons J, Green G, Eikenberry E F, de Crombrugghe B, Vogeli G, Pastan I, Fietzek P P, Olsen B R 1981 J. Biol. Chem. 256: 8407-15

NOTE ON HUMAN α1(III) COLLAGEN, ADDED IN PROOF
(Seyer J M, Kang A H 1981 Biochemistry 20: 2621-7)

This differs from α1(III) bovine collagen as follows*:

20	Ser	213	Asn	311	Ala	393	Ser	542	Ala	665	Val	752	Gln	921	Hyp
23	Ser	234	Met	320	Pro	432	Hyp	558	Leu	669	Hyp	756	Lys	927	Ala
39	Ser	243	Ala	323	Ile	450	Gly	560	Ser	701	Ala	758	Ser	950	Gln
65	Glu	245	Ala	330	Ala	471	Gly	572	Gly	704	Leu	761	Ala	954	Ile
68	Leu	248	Ala	332	Glu	488	Asp	573	Hyp	719	Pro	776	Ile	978	Thr
74	Ile	251	Leu	335	Ala	494	Ala	575	Ala	720	Ala	791	Pro	980	Ser
80	Ile	254	Gly	344	Ala	500	Asn	578	Val	722	Ser	800	Val		
102	Ala	266	Glu	353	Val	501	Ala	606	Gly	732	Ala	804	Ala		
113	Leu	278	Thr	362	Met	512	Leu	611	Leu	734	Asn	851	Ser		
119	Ser	281	Val	372	Asp	513	Ala	620	Ser	735	Thr	854	Gly		
204	Gln	282	Hyp	384	Ser	515	Ala	627	Thr	743	Val	891	Ser		
212	Ile	284	Ala	392	Pro	518	Leu	647	Gly	750	Ala	908	Ala		

*Columns read downwards

ACKNOWLEDGEMENTS

I am grateful to the following for providing data before its publication: R. W. Glanville, D. Breitkreutz, M. Meitinger, P. P. Fietzek, A. Brandt, D. Hörlein, P. Bruckner, R. Timpl, H. Allmann, H. Bentz, H. Dewes, W. Henkel, H. Lang, J. Rauterberg, E. Wachter, K. Kühn, J. Wozney, H. Boedtker, D. Hanahan, V. Tate, P. Doty.

Index

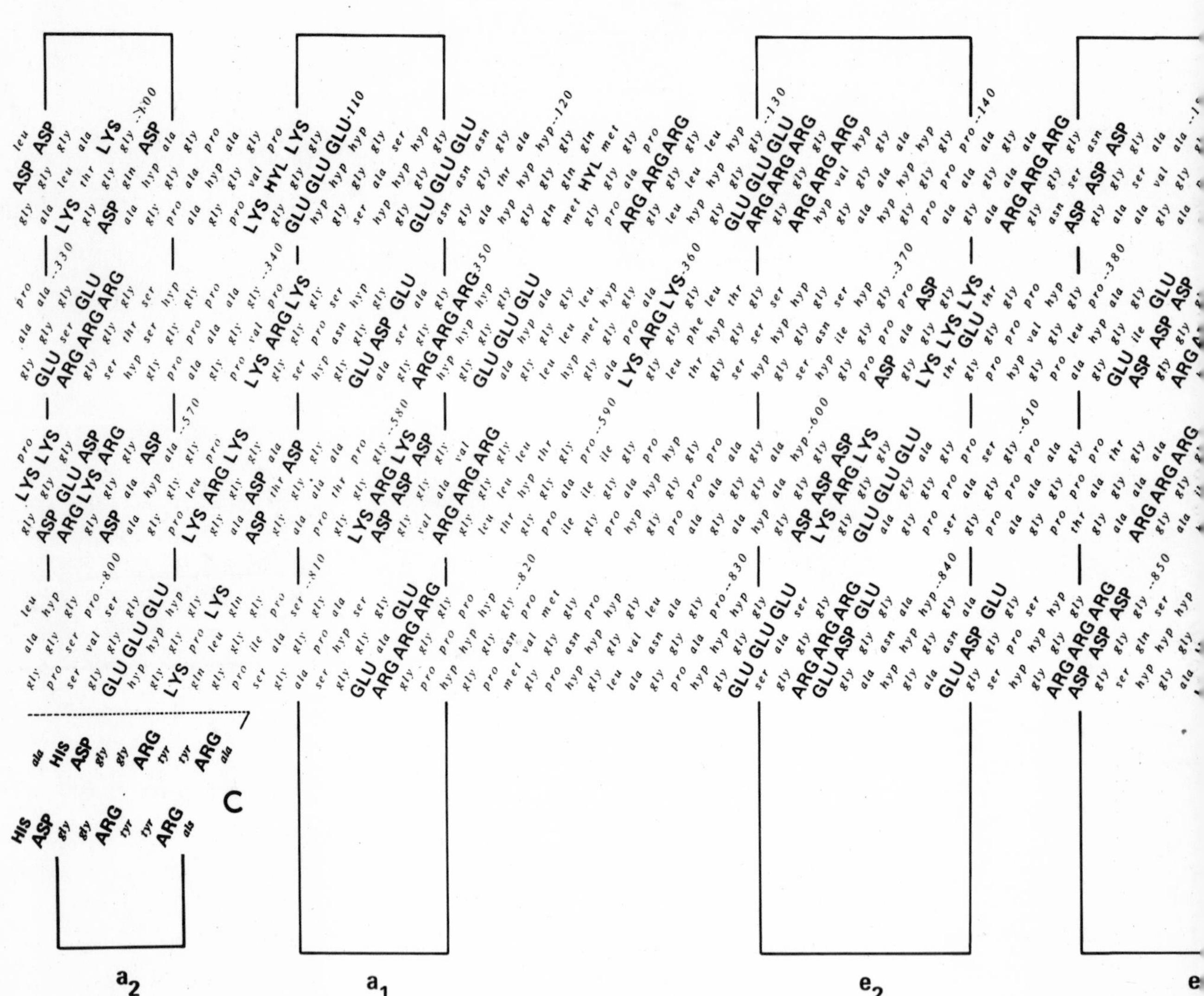

C
a_2
a_1
e_2